Signs & Symptoms

A 2-in-1 Reference for Nurses

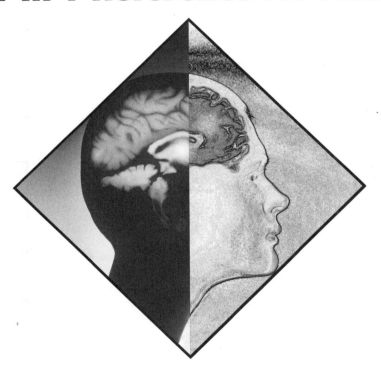

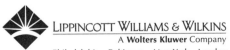

LIPPINCOTT WILLIAMS & WILKINS
A **Wolters Kluwer** Company

Philadelphia · Baltimore · New York · London
Buenos Aires · Hong Kong · Sydney · Tokyo

STAFF

Executive Publisher
Judith A. Schilling McCann, RN, MSN

Editorial Director
David Moreau

Clinical Director
Joan M. Robinson, RN, MSN

Senior Art Director
Arlene Putterman

Editorial Project Manager
Jaime Stockslager Buss

Clinical Project Manager
Marcy Caplin, RN, MSN

Editors
Julie Munden, Liz Schaeffer

Copy Editors
Kimberly Bilotta (supervisor),
Scotti Cohn, Heather Ditch,
Shana Harrington, Dorothy P. Terry,
Pamela Wingrod

Designer
Debra Moloshok (project manager)

Digital Composition Services
Diane Paluba (manager), Joyce Rossi Biletz,
Richard Eng, Donna S. Morris

Manufacturing
Patricia K. Dorshaw (director),
Beth Janae Orr

Editorial Assistants
Megan L. Aldinger, Tara L. Carter-Bell,
Linda K. Ruhf

Librarian
Wani Z. Larsen

Indexer
Barbara Hodgson

SS2IN1—D N O S A J J M A
06 05 04   10 9 8 7 6 5 4 3 2 1

Library of Congress
Cataloging-in Publication Data

Signs & symptoms : a 2-in-1 reference for nurses.
    p. ; cm.
Includes bibliographical references and index.
  1. Nursing assessment—Handbooks, manuals,
etc. 2. Symptoms—Handbooks, manuals, etc. I.
Title: Signs and symptoms. II. Lippincott
Williams & Wilkins.
  [DNLM: 1. Nursing Assessment—methods—
Handbooks. 2. Signs and
Symptoms—Handbooks. WY 49 S578 2004]
RT48.S553 2004
616.07'5—dc22
ISBN 1-58255-318-1 (alk. paper)   2003023645

Contents

Contributors

Peggy D. Baikie, RNC, MS, NNP, PNP
Senior Instructor
University of Colorado Health Sciences
    Center
School of Nursing
Denver

Barbara Broome, RN, PhD, CNS
*Assistant Dean and Chair —
    Community/Mental Health*
University of South Alabama College of
    Nursing
Mobile

David J. Clugston, MSN, CRNP
Director of Resident Care
Rydal (Pa.) Park

Sue M. Enns, MHS, PA-C
Assistant Professor
Wichita (Kans.) State University

Kenneth R. Harbert, PhD, CHES, PA-C
*Professor and Chair, Department of PA
    Studies*
Philadelphia College of Osteopathic
    Medicine

Janice D. Hausauer, RN, MS, FNP
Adjunct Assistant Professor
Montana State University College of
    Nursing
Bozeman

Bobbie L. Hunter, RN, MSN, CFNP
Nursing Instructor
Columbus (Ga.) Technical College

Nathan C. Kindig, PA-C
Department Head
Branch Medical Annex Wahiawa
Naval Medical Clinic
Pearl Harbor, Hawaii

Manuel D. Leal, PA-C, MPAS
Department Head
Naval Medical Clinic
Pearl Harbor, Hawaii

Eric G. Neilson, MD
*Hugh Jackson Morgan Professor of
    Medicine; Chairman, Department of
    Medicine; Physician-in-Chief*
Vanderbilt University School of
    Medicine
Nashville, Tenn.

Glenn H. Nordehn, DO
Assistant Professor
University of Minnesota School of
    Medicine
Duluth

Marlene L. Roman, RN, MSN, ARNP
*Medical-Surgical Clinical Nurse
    Specialist*
North Broward Medical Center
Pompano Beach, Fla.

Barbara L. Sauls, EdD, PA-C
*Clinical Director Physician Assistant
    Program*
King's College
Wilkes Barre, Pa.

Alexander John Siomko, RN, MSN,
    BC, CRNP
Staff Nursing — Telemetry
Methodist Hospital Division of Thomas
    Jefferson University Hospital
Philadelphia

Dominique A. Thuriere, MD
*Chief of Mental Health and Behavioral
    Sciences*
Bay Pines (Fla.) VA Medical Center

David Toub, MD
Medical Director for Clinical Informatics
Doctor Quality
Conshohocken, Pa.

Foreword

There's no doubt that nurses have many important responsibilities. They serve as the primary channel for assessing patients, implementing care, and providing patient teaching. In the past, these responsibilities were facilitated by extended hospital stays and office visits. Nurses had more time to provide such care.

Today, however, nurses work in a much different environment. The demands are greater. Patients live longer and therefore have greater health care needs. In addition, the age of technology has increased the acuity of patients. Patients are more likely to demand the most up-to-date information and expect to have such information available to them immediately.

Unfortunately, both the novice and the experienced clinician are constrained by the amount of time allotted to provide care. Nurses need to have immediate and easy access to the most up-to-date information possible when assessing patients or care may be misdirected.

Signs & Symptoms: A 2-in-1 Reference for Nurses responds to this need for quick and easy access to information. The book features a unique two-column format to cover 215 common signs and symptoms. The inner column provides a comprehensive explanation for each sign or symptom, covering all key nursing tasks from obtaining a history to providing patient counseling. Each entry includes an overview of the main disorders associated with a particular sign or symptom. Within the entry, *Emergency actions* icons help identify critical situations and their appropriate interventions. *Cultural cues* offer tips and insights regarding how a patient's cultural background may impact the assessment process or the presentation of a sign or symptom.

Complementing the inner column text are easily scannable tables and illustrations that help to clarify concepts. *Assessment tips* focus on building assessment skills. *Associated disorder* sidebars offer an in-depth look at the most common causes of certain signs or symptoms.

The outer bulleted columns contain summaries of the most important aspects of the inner column text. The nurse can rapidly review key concepts, such as the primary causes of a specific sign or symptom, questions to ask when obtaining a history, and the special considerations associated with a sign or symptom.

In today's complex work environments, nurses have less time, less backup, and fewer resources on hand to provide quality patient care. It's essential for them to have the proper tools to assist them during the assessment process and the selection of appropriate patient treatment. It's equally essential for nurses to have a resource on hand that can enhance their knowledge base and validate their decisions, for as we all know, evidence-based practice is essential to providing the highest quality of professional patient care. So, whether you are an experienced clinician who needs to quickly identify the common causes of abdominal pain or you are a novice nurse who wants more detailed information about tracheal deviation, *Signs & Symptoms: A 2-in-1 Reference for Nurses* is the all-in-one resource for you.

Elizabeth K. Hall, RN, MSN, CFNP, CGNP
Assistant Professor of Clinical Nursing
Columbia University School of Nursing
Director, Family Nurse Practitioner Program
Nagle Avenue Family Practice
New York

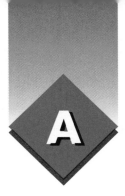

ABDOMINAL DISTENTION

Abdominal distention refers to increased abdominal girth—the result of increased intra-abdominal pressure forcing the abdominal wall outward. Distention may be mild or severe, depending on the amount of pressure. It may be localized or diffuse and may occur gradually or suddenly. Acute abdominal distention may signal life-threatening peritonitis or acute bowel obstruction.

Fluid and gas are normally present in the GI tract but not in the peritoneal cavity. However, if fluid and gas can't pass freely through the GI tract, abdominal distention occurs. In the peritoneal cavity, distention may reflect acute bleeding, accumulation of ascitic fluid, or air from perforation of an abdominal organ.

Abdominal distention doesn't always signal disease. For example, in anxious patients or those with digestive distress, localized distention in the left upper quadrant can result from aerophagia—the unconscious swallowing of air. Generalized distention can result from the ingestion of fruits or vegetables with large quantities of unabsorbable carbohydrates, such as legumes, or from abnormal food fermentation by microbes. Don't forget to rule out pregnancy in all females with abdominal distention.

 EMERGENCY ACTIONS If the patient displays abdominal distention, quickly check for signs of hypovolemia, such as pallor; diaphoresis; hypotension; rapid, thready pulse; rapid, shallow breathing; decreased urine output; poor capillary refill; and altered mentation. Ask the patient if he's experiencing severe abdominal pain or difficulty breathing. Find out about any recent accidents, and observe the patient for signs of trauma and peritoneal bleeding, such as Cullen's sign or Turner's sign. Then auscultate all abdominal quadrants, noting rapid and high-pitched, diminished, or absent bowel sounds. (If you don't hear bowel sounds immediately, listen for at least 5 minutes.) Gently palpate the abdomen for rigidity. Remember that deep or extensive palpation may increase pain.

If you detect abdominal distention and rigidity along with abnormal bowel sounds and the patient complains of pain, begin emergency interventions. Place the patient in the supine position, administer oxygen, and insert an I.V. line for fluid replacement. Prepare to insert a nasogastric tube to relieve acute intraluminal distention. Reassure the patient, and prepare him for surgery.

HISTORY

If the patient's abdominal distention isn't acute, ask about its onset and duration and associated signs. A patient with localized distention may report a sensation of

Key facts about abdominal distention

✦ Increased abdominal girth
✦ Occurs when increased fluid and gas can't pass freely through the GI tract
✦ Can be mild or severe
✦ May reflect acute bleeding, accumulation of ascitic fluid, or air from perforation of an abdominal organ

In an emergency

If you detect abdominal rigidity and abnormal bowel sounds and the patient complains of pain:
✦ Place the patient in the supine position.
✦ Administer oxygen.
✦ Insert an I.V. line for fluid replacement.
✦ Prepare to insert an NG tube to relieve acute intraluminal distention.
✦ Prepare the patient for surgery.

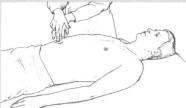

ASSESSMENT TIP

Detecting ascites

To differentiate ascites from other causes of distention, check for shifting dullness and fluid wave as described here.

SHIFTING DULLNESS
Step 1. With the patient in a supine position, percuss from the umbilicus outward to the flank, as shown at right. Draw a line on the patient's skin to mark the change from tympany to dullness.

Step 2. Turn the patient onto his side. (Note that this positioning causes ascitic fluid to shift.) Percuss again, as shown at right, and mark the change from tympany to dullness. Any difference between these lines can indicate ascites.

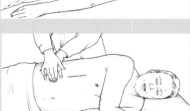

FLUID WAVE
Have another person press deeply into the patient's midline to prevent vibration from traveling along the abdominal wall. Place one of your palms on one of the patient's flanks, as shown at right. Strike the opposite flank with your other hand. If you feel the blow in the opposite palm, ascitic fluid is present.

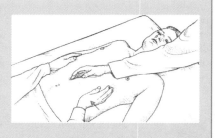

Key history points
◆ Onset and duration of distention
◆ Associated signs, including abdominal pain, fever, nausea, vomiting, anorexia, altered bowel habits, and weight gain or loss
◆ Medical history, including GI or biliary disorders, chronic constipation, abdominal surgery, and recent accidents

Critical assessment steps
◆ Perform a complete physical examination.
◆ Observe the recumbent patient for abdominal asymmetry.
◆ Assess abdominal contour.
◆ Observe the umbilicus.
◆ Inspect the abdomen for signs of inguinal or femoral hernia and for incisions.
◆ Auscultate for bowel sounds, abdominal friction rubs, and bruits.
◆ Percuss and palpate the abdomen.
◆ Prepare the patient for pelvic examination or genital examination as appropriate.
◆ Measure abdominal girth for a baseline value.

pressure, fullness, or tenderness in the affected area. A patient with generalized distention may report a bloated feeling, a pounding heart, and difficulty breathing when lying flat or breathing deeply. The patient may also feel unable to bend at his waist. Be sure to ask about abdominal pain, fever, nausea, vomiting, anorexia, altered bowel habits, and weight gain or loss.

Obtain a medical history, noting GI or biliary disorders that may cause peritonitis or ascites, such as cirrhosis, hepatitis, and inflammatory bowel disease. (See *Detecting ascites*.) Also note chronic constipation. Has the patient recently had abdominal surgery, which can lead to abdominal distention? Ask about recent accidents, even minor ones, like falling off a stepladder.

PHYSICAL ASSESSMENT

Perform a complete physical examination. Don't restrict the examination to the patient's abdomen because you could miss important clues to the cause of his abdominal distention. Stand at the foot of the bed and observe the recumbent patient for abdominal asymmetry to determine if distention is localized or generalized. Then assess abdominal contour by stooping at his side. Inspect for tense, glistening skin and bulging flanks, which may indicate ascites. Observe the umbilicus. An everted umbilicus may indicate ascites or umbilical hernia. An inverted umbilicus may indicate distention from gas; it's also common in obesity. Inspect the abdomen for signs of inguinal or femoral hernia and for incisions that may point to adhesions. Both may lead to intestinal obstruction. Then auscultate for bowel sounds, abdominal friction rubs (indicating peritoneal inflammation), and bruits (indicating an aneurysm). Listen for succussion splash — a splashing sound normally heard in the stomach when the patient moves or when palpation disturbs the viscera. However, an abnormally loud splash indicates fluid accumulation, suggesting gastric dilation or obstruction.

Next, percuss and palpate the abdomen to determine if distention results from air, fluid, or both. A tympanic note in the left lower quadrant suggests an air-filled descending or sigmoid colon. A tympanic note throughout a generally distended abdomen suggests an air-filled peritoneal cavity. A dull percussion note throughout a generally distended abdomen suggests a fluid-filled peritoneal cavity. Shifting of dullness laterally with the patient in the decubitus position also indicates a fluid-filled abdominal cavity. A pelvic or intra-abdominal mass causes local dullness upon percussion and should be palpable. Obesity causes a large abdomen without shifting dullness, prominent tympany, or palpable bowel or other masses, and with generalized, rather then localized, dullness.

Palpate the abdomen for tenderness, noting whether it's localized or generalized. Watch for peritoneal signs and symptoms, such as rebound tenderness, guarding, rigidity, McBurney's point, obturator sign, and psoas sign. Female patients should undergo a pelvic examination; males, a genital examination. All patients who report abdominal pain should undergo a digital rectal examination with fecal occult blood testing. Finally, measure abdominal girth for a baseline value. Mark the flanks with a felt-tipped pen as a reference for subsequent measurements.

MEDICAL CAUSES

Abdominal cancer

Generalized abdominal distention may occur when the cancer — most commonly ovarian, hepatic, or pancreatic — produces ascites (usually in a patient with a known tumor). It's an indication of advanced disease. Shifting dullness and a fluid wave accompany distention. Associated signs and symptoms may include severe abdominal pain, an abdominal mass, anorexia, jaundice, GI hemorrhage (hematemesis or melena), dyspepsia, and weight loss that progresses to muscle weakness and atrophy.

Abdominal trauma

When brisk internal bleeding accompanies trauma, abdominal distention may be acute and dramatic. Associated signs and symptoms of this life-threatening disorder include abdominal rigidity with guarding, decreased or absent bowel sounds, vomiting, tenderness, and abdominal bruising. Pain may occur over the trauma site or over the scapula if abdominal bleeding irritates the phrenic nerve. Signs of hypovolemic shock (such as hypotension and rapid, thready pulse) appear with significant blood loss.

Bladder distention

Various disorders cause bladder distention which, in turn, causes lower abdominal distention. Slight dullness on percussion above the symphysis pubis indicates mild bladder distention. A palpable, smooth, rounded, fluctuant suprapubic mass suggests severe bladder distention; a fluctuant mass extending to the umbilicus indi-

Medical causes

Abdominal cancer

✦ Generalized distention may result from cancer-produced ascites.
✦ Associated signs and symptoms may include severe abdominal pain, an abdominal mass, anorexia, jaundice, GI hemorrhage (hematemesis or melena), dyspepsia, weight loss, and muscle weakness and atrophy.

Abdominal trauma

✦ Acute and dramatic distention may occur with brisk internal bleeding.
✦ Associated signs and symptoms include abdominal rigidity with guarding, decreased or absent bowel sounds, vomiting, tenderness, abdominal bruising, pain over the trauma site or scapula, and signs of hypovolemic shock (if blood loss is significant).

Bladder distention

✦ Lower abdominal distention results from bladder distention.
✦ Additional signs and symptoms depend on the severity of distention.

Cirrhosis
- Ascites causes generalized distention.
- The patient may report a feeling of fullness or weight gain.

Gastric dilation (acute)
- Left-upper-quadrant distention is characteristic, but presentation varies.

Heart failure
- Ascites causes generalized distention.
- Hallmark signs and symptoms include peripheral edema, jugular vein distention, dyspnea, and tachycardia.

Irritable bowel syndrome
- Periodic intestinal spasms may cause intermittent, localized distention.
- Lower abdominal pain or cramping typically accompanies intestinal spasms.

Large-bowel obstruction
- Constipation precedes dramatic distention.
- Loops of the large bowel may become visible on the abdomen.

Mesenteric artery occlusion (acute)
- Abdominal distention usually occurs several hours after the sudden onset of severe, colicky periumbilical pain and rapid or forceful bowel evacuation.

cates extremely severe bladder distention. Urinary dribbling, frequency, or urgency may occur with urinary obstruction. Suprapubic discomfort is also common.

Cirrhosis
With cirrhosis, ascites causes generalized distention and is confirmed by a fluid wave and shifting dullness. Umbilical eversion and caput medusae (dilated veins around the umbilicus) are common. The patient may report a feeling of fullness or weight gain. Associated findings include vague abdominal pain, fever, anorexia, nausea, vomiting, constipation or diarrhea, bleeding tendencies, severe pruritus, palmar erythema, spider angiomas, leg edema and, possibly, splenomegaly. Hematemesis, encephalopathy, gynecomastia, or testicular atrophy may also be seen. Jaundice is usually a late sign. Hepatomegaly occurs initially; however, the liver may not be palpable if the patient has advanced disease.

Gastric dilation (acute)
Left-upper-quadrant distention is characteristic of acute gastric dilation, but the presentation varies. The patient usually complains of epigastric fullness or pain and nausea (with or without vomiting). Physical examination reveals tympany, gastric tenderness, and a succussion splash. Initially, visible peristalsis may occur. Later, hypoactive or absent bowel sounds confirm ileus. The patient may be pale and diaphoretic and may exhibit tachycardia or bradycardia.

Heart failure
Generalized abdominal distention due to ascites typically accompanies severe cardiovascular impairment and is confirmed by shifting dullness and a fluid wave. Signs and symptoms of heart failure are numerous and depend on the disease stage and degree of cardiovascular impairment. Hallmarks include peripheral edema, jugular vein distention, dyspnea, and tachycardia. Common associated signs and symptoms include hepatomegaly (which may cause right-upper-quadrant pain), nausea, vomiting, productive cough, crackles, cool extremities, cyanotic nail beds, nocturia, exercise intolerance, nocturnal wheezing, diastolic hypertension, and cardiomegaly.

Irritable bowel syndrome
Irritable bowel syndrome may produce intermittent, localized distention—the result of periodic intestinal spasms. Lower abdominal pain or cramping typically accompanies these spasms. The pain is usually relieved by defecation or by passage of intestinal gas and is aggravated by stress. Other possible signs and symptoms include diarrhea that may alternate with constipation or normal bowel function; nausea; dyspepsia; straining and urgency at defecation; feeling of incomplete evacuation; and small, mucus-streaked stools.

Large-bowel obstruction
Dramatic abdominal distention is characteristic of large-bowel obstruction, a life-threatening disorder; in fact, loops of the large bowel may become visible on the abdomen. Constipation precedes distention and may be the only symptom for days. Associated findings include tympany, high-pitched bowel sounds, and the sudden onset of colicky lower abdominal pain that becomes persistent. Fecal vomiting and diminished peristaltic waves and bowel sounds are late signs.

Mesenteric artery occlusion (acute)
In acute mesenteric artery occlusion, a life-threatening disorder, abdominal distention usually occurs several hours after the sudden onset of severe, colicky periumbilical pain accompanied by rapid (even forceful) bowel evacuation. The pain later becomes constant and diffuse. Related signs and symptoms include severe abdomi-

nal tenderness with guarding and rigidity, absent bowel sounds and, occasionally, a bruit in the right iliac fossa. The patient may also experience vomiting, anorexia, diarrhea, or constipation. Late signs include fever, tachycardia, tachypnea, hypotension, and cool, clammy skin. Abdominal distention or GI bleeding may be the only clue if pain is absent.

Nephrotic syndrome

Nephrotic syndrome may produce massive edema, causing generalized abdominal distention with a fluid wave and shifting dullness. It may also produce elevated blood pressure, hematuria or oliguria, fatigue, anorexia, depression, pallor, periorbital edema, scrotal swelling, and skin striae.

Ovarian cysts

Typically, large ovarian cysts produce lower abdominal distention accompanied by umbilical eversion. Because they're thin walled and fluid filled, these cysts produce a fluid wave and shifting dullness — signs that mimic ascites. Lower abdominal pain and a palpable mass may be present.

Paralytic ileus

Paralytic ileus, which produces generalized distention with a tympanic percussion note, is accompanied by absent or hypoactive bowel sounds and, occasionally, extreme distress and vomiting. The patient may be severely constipated or may pass flatus and small, liquid stools.

Peritonitis

In peritonitis, a life-threatening disorder, abdominal distention may be localized or generalized, depending on the extent of peritonitis. Fluid accumulates first within the peritoneal cavity and then within the bowel lumen, causing a fluid wave and shifting dullness. Typically, distention is accompanied by sudden and severe abdominal pain that worsens with movement. Rebound tenderness and abdominal rigidity may be present.

Associated signs and symptoms usually include hypoactive or absent bowel sounds, fever, chills, hyperalgesia, nausea, and vomiting. Also, the skin over the patient's abdomen may appear taut. Signs of shock, such as tachycardia and hypotension, appear with significant fluid loss into the abdomen.

Small-bowel obstruction

Abdominal distention, which is characteristic of small-bowel obstruction, is most pronounced during late obstruction, especially in the distal small bowel. Auscultation reveals hypoactive or hyperactive bowel sounds, whereas percussion produces a tympanic note. Accompanying signs and symptoms of this life-threatening disorder include colicky periumbilical pain, constipation, nausea, and vomiting; the higher the obstruction, the earlier and more severe the vomiting. Rebound tenderness reflects intestinal strangulation with ischemia. Associated signs and symptoms include drowsiness, malaise, and signs of dehydration. Signs of hypovolemic shock appear with progressive dehydration and plasma loss.

Toxic megacolon (acute)

Acute toxic megacolon is a life-threatening complication of infectious or ulcerative colitis. It produces dramatic abdominal distention that usually develops gradually and is accompanied by a tympanic percussion note, diminished or absent bowel sounds, and mild rebound tenderness. The patient also presents with abdominal pain and tenderness, fever, tachycardia, and dehydration.

Medical causes
(continued)

Nephrotic syndrome
✦ Massive edema causes generalized distention with a fluid wave and shifting dullness.

Ovarian cysts
✦ Lower abdominal distention is accompanied by umbilical eversion.
✦ Lower abdominal pain and a palpable mass may be present.

Paralytic illeus
✦ Generalized distention occurs with a tympanic percussion note.

Peritonitis
✦ Abdominal distention may be localized or generalized, depending on the extent of peritonitis.
✦ Typically, distention is accompanied by sudden and severe abdominal pain that worsens with movement.
✦ Rebound tenderness and abdominal rigidity may be present.

Small-bowel obstruction
✦ Abdominal distention is most pronounced during late obstruction, especially in the distal small bowel.

Toxic megacolon (acute)
✦ Dramatic abdominal distention usually develops gradually.
✦ Distention is accompanied by a tympanic percussion note, diminished or absent bowel sounds, and mild rebound tenderness.

Special considerations

+ Position the patient comfortably, using pillows for support.
+ Place the patient on his left side to help flatus escape.
+ If the patient has ascites, elevate the head of the bed to ease his breathing.
+ Administer drugs to relieve pain.
+ Offer emotional support.

Peds points

+ Distention may be difficult to observe in pediatric patients; it may be found on palpation.
+ In neonates, abdominal distention caused by ascites usually results from GI or urinary perforation; in older children, from heart failure, cirrhosis, or nephrosis.
+ Other causes in pediatric patients include congenital malformations of the GI tract, hernia that produces intestinal obstruction, overeating, and constipation.

Geri points

+ Don't confuse distention with a potbelly, a common effect of aging.

Teaching points

+ Slow-breathing techniques
+ Food and fluid restrictions
+ Oral hygiene

Key facts about abdominal mass

+ Manifests as localized swelling in one abdominal quadrant
+ May signify an enlarged organ, a neoplasm, an abscess, a vascular defect, or a fecal mass

SPECIAL CONSIDERATIONS

Position the patient comfortably, using pillows for support. Place him on his left side to help flatus escape. Or, if he has ascites, elevate the head of the bed to ease his breathing. Administer drugs to relieve pain, and offer emotional support.

Prepare the patient for diagnostic tests, such as abdominal X-rays, endoscopy, laparoscopy, ultrasonography, computed tomography scan or, possibly, paracentesis.

PEDIATRIC POINTERS

Because a young child's abdomen is normally rounded, distention may be difficult to observe. Fortunately though, a child's abdominal wall is less developed than an adult's, making palpation easier. When percussing the abdomen, remember that children normally swallow air when eating and crying, resulting in louder-than-normal tympany. Minimal tympany with abdominal distention may result from fluid accumulation or solid masses. To check for abdominal fluid, test for shifting dullness instead of for a fluid wave. (In a child, air swallowing and incomplete abdominal muscle development make the fluid wave difficult to interpret.)

Some children won't cooperate with a physical examination. Try to gain the child's confidence, and consider allowing him to remain in the parent's or caregiver's lap. You can gather clues by observing the child while he's coughing, walking, or even climbing on office furniture. Also, perform a gentle rectal examination.

In neonates, abdominal distention caused by ascites usually results from GI or urinary perforation; in older children, from heart failure, cirrhosis, or nephrosis. Besides ascites, congenital malformations of the GI tract (such as intussusception and volvulus) may cause abdominal distention. A hernia may cause distention if it produces an intestinal obstruction. In addition, overeating and constipation can cause distention.

GERIATRIC POINTERS

As people age, fat tends to accumulate in the lower abdomen and near the hips, even when body weight is stable. This accumulation, together with weakening abdominal muscles, commonly produces a potbelly, which some elderly patients interpret as fluid collection or evidence of disease.

PATIENT COUNSELING

If the patient's anxiety triggers air swallowing or deep breathing that causes discomfort, advise him to take slow breaths. If the patient has an obstruction or ascites, explain food and fluid restrictions. Stress good oral hygiene to prevent dry mouth.

ABDOMINAL MASS

Commonly detected on routine physical examination, an abdominal mass is a localized swelling in one abdominal quadrant. Typically, this sign develops insidiously and may represent an enlarged organ, a neoplasm, an abscess, a vascular defect, or a fecal mass.

Distinguishing an abdominal mass from a normal structure requires skillful palpation. At times, palpation must be repeated with the patient in a different position. A palpable abdominal mass is an important clinical sign and usually represents a serious—and perhaps life-threatening—disorder.

ASSESSMENT TIP

Performing an abdominal assessment

When performing an abdominal assessment, use this sequence:
1. Inspection
2. Auscultation
3. Percussion
4. Palpation.

Palpating or percussing the abdomen before you auscultate can change the character of the patient's bowel sounds, resulting in an inaccurate assessment.

EMERGENCY ACTIONS If the patient has a pulsating midabdominal mass and severe abdominal or back pain, suspect an aortic aneurysm. Quickly take his vital signs. Because the patient may require emergency surgery, withhold food and fluids until the patient is examined. Prepare to administer oxygen and to start an I.V. infusion for fluid and blood replacement. Obtain routine preoperative tests, and prepare the patient for angiography. Frequently monitor blood pressure, pulse, respirations, and urine output. Be alert for signs of shock, such as tachycardia, hypotension, and cool, clammy skin, which may indicate significant blood loss.

HISTORY

If the patient's abdominal mass doesn't suggest an aortic aneurysm, continue with a detailed history. Ask the patient if the mass is painful. If so, ask if the pain is constant or if it occurs only on palpation. Is it localized or generalized? Determine if the patient was aware of the mass. If he was, find out if he noticed any change in the size or location of the mass.

Next, review the patient's medical history, paying special attention to GI disorders. Ask the patient about GI symptoms, such as constipation, diarrhea, rectal bleeding, abnormally colored stools, and vomiting. Has the patient noticed a change in appetite? If the patient is female, ask whether her menstrual cycles are regular and when the first day of her last menses was.

CULTURAL CUE *When taking a health history, consider your patient's ethnic background. For example, Japanese patients are at higher risk for gastric cancer than non-Japanese patients and cirrhosis tends to be more common in Native American patients than in patients of other ethnic backgrounds.*

PHYSICAL ASSESSMENT

A complete physical assessment should be performed. Be sure to auscultate for bowel sounds in each quadrant. Listen for bruits or friction rubs, and check for enlarged veins. Lightly palpate and then deeply palpate the abdomen, assessing any painful or suspicious areas last. Note the patient's position when you locate the mass. Some masses can be detected only with the patient in a supine position; others require a side-lying position. (See *Performing an abdominal assessment.*)

Estimate the size of the mass in centimeters. Determine its shape. Is it round or sausage shaped? Describe its contour as smooth, rough, sharply defined, nodular, or irregular. Determine the consistency of the mass. Is it doughy, soft, solid, or hard? Also, percuss the mass. A dull sound indicates a fluid-filled mass; a tympanic sound, an air-filled mass.

Sequence for abdominal assessment
1. Inspection
2. Auscultation
3. Percussion
4. Palpation

In an emergency
If the patient has a pulsating midabdominal mass and severe abdominal or back pain:
✦ Quickly take vital signs.
✦ Withhold food and fluids until the patient is examined.
✦ Prepare to administer oxygen and to start an I.V. infusion for fluid and blood replacement.
✦ Be alert for signs of shock.

Key history points
✦ Extent of pain
✦ Changes in size or location of mass
✦ History of GI disorders
✦ Associated GI symptoms
✦ Description of menstrual cycles

Critical assessment steps
✦ Lightly palpate and then deeply palpate the abdomen, assessing painful or suspicious areas last.
✦ Estimate the size of the mass in centimeters and determine its shape and consistency.
✦ Determine if the mass moves with your hand or in response to respiration.

Next, determine if the mass moves with your hand or in response to respiration. Is the mass free-floating or attached to intra-abdominal structures? To determine whether the mass is located in the abdominal wall or the abdominal cavity, ask the patient to lift his head and shoulders off the examination table, thereby contracting his abdominal muscles. While these muscles are contracted, try to palpate the mass. If you can, the mass is in the abdominal wall; if you can't, the mass is within the abdominal cavity. (See *Abdominal masses: Locations and causes.*)

After the abdominal examination is complete, perform pelvic, genital, and rectal examinations.

MEDICAL CAUSES

Medical causes

Abdominal aortic aneurysm

An abdominal aortic aneurysm may persist for years, producing only a pulsating periumbilical mass with a systolic bruit over the aorta. However, it may become life-threatening if the aneurysm expands and its walls weaken. In such cases, the patient initially reports constant upper abdominal pain or, less often, low back or dull abdominal pain. If the aneurysm ruptures, he'll report severe abdominal and back pain. After rupture, the aneurysm no longer pulsates.

Associated signs and symptoms of rupture include mottled skin below the waist, absent femoral and pedal pulses, lower blood pressure in the legs than in the arms, mild to moderate tenderness with guarding, and abdominal rigidity. Signs of shock — such as tachycardia and cool, clammy skin — appear with significant blood loss.

Bladder distention

A smooth, rounded, fluctuant suprapubic mass is characteristic of bladder distention. With extreme distention, the mass may extend to the umbilicus. Severe suprapubic pain and urinary frequency and urgency may also occur.

Cholecystitis

With cholecystitis, deep palpation below the liver border may reveal a smooth, firm, sausage-shaped mass. However, with acute inflammation, the gallbladder is usually too tender to be palpated. Cholecystitis can cause severe right-upper-quadrant pain that may radiate to the right shoulder, chest, or back; abdominal rigidity and tenderness; fever; pallor; diaphoresis; anorexia; nausea; and vomiting. Recurrent attacks usually occur 1 to 6 hours after meals. Murphy's sign (inspiratory arrest elicited when the examiner palpates the right upper quadrant as the patient takes a deep breath) is common.

Cholelithiasis

With cholelithiasis, a stone-filled gallbladder usually produces a painless right-upper-quadrant mass that's smooth and sausage-shaped. However, passage of a stone through the bile or cystic duct may cause severe right-upper-quadrant pain that radiates to the epigastrium, back, or shoulder blades. Accompanying signs and symptoms include anorexia, nausea, vomiting, chills, diaphoresis, restlessness, and low-grade fever. Jaundice may occur with obstruction of the common bile duct. The patient may also experience intolerance to fatty foods and frequent indigestion.

Colon cancer

A right-lower-quadrant mass may occur with cancer of the right colon, which may also cause occult bleeding with anemia and abdominal aching, pressure, or dull cramps. Associated findings include weakness, fatigue, exertional dyspnea, vertigo,

---

Medical causes

Abdominal aortic aneurysm

✦ A pulsating periumbilical mass develops.
✦ The mass occurs with a systolic bruit over the aorta.

Bladder distention

✦ A smooth, rounded, fluctuant suprapubic mass develops.
✦ With extreme distention, the mass may extend to the umbilicus.

Cholecystitis

✦ Deep palpation below the liver border may reveal a smooth, firm, sausage-shaped mass.

Cholelithiasis

✦ A painless, smooth, and sausage-shaped mass develops in the right upper quadrant.

Colon cancer

✦ With cancer of the right colon, a right-lower-quadrant mass may occur.
✦ With cancer of the left colon, a palpable mass produces rectal bleeding and pressure and intermittent abdominal fullness or cramping.

Abdominal masses: Locations and causes

The location of an abdominal mass provides an important clue to the causative disorder. Here are the disorders responsible for abdominal masses in each of the four abdominal quadrants.

RIGHT UPPER QUADRANT
- ✦ Aortic aneurysm (epigastric area)
- ✦ Cholecystitis or cholelithiasis
- ✦ Gallbladder, gastric, or hepatic cancer
- ✦ Hepatomegaly
- ✦ Hydronephrosis
- ✦ Pancreatic abscess or pseudocysts
- ✦ Renal cell cancer

LEFT UPPER QUADRANT
- ✦ Aortic aneurysm (epigastric area)
- ✦ Gastric cancer (epigastric area)
- ✦ Hydronephrosis
- ✦ Pancreatic abscess (epigastric area)
- ✦ Pancreatic pseudocysts (epigastric area)
- ✦ Renal cell cancer
- ✦ Splenomegaly

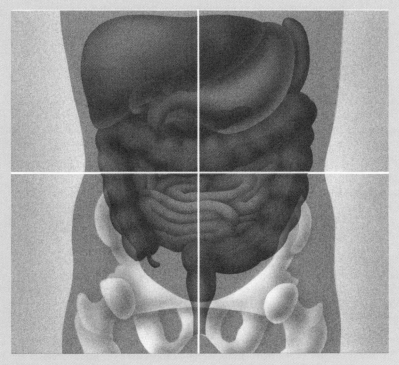

RIGHT LOWER QUADRANT
- ✦ Bladder distention (suprapubic area)
- ✦ Colon cancer
- ✦ Crohn's disease
- ✦ Ovarian cyst (suprapubic area)
- ✦ Uterine leiomyomas (suprapubic area)

LEFT LOWER QUADRANT
- ✦ Bladder distention (suprapubic area)
- ✦ Colon cancer
- ✦ Diverticulitis
- ✦ Ovarian cyst (suprapubic area)
- ✦ Uterine leiomyomas (suprapubic area)
- ✦ Volvulus

Medical causes
(continued)

Crohn's disease
+ Tender, sausage-shaped masses are usually palpable in the right lower quadrant and, at times, in the left lower quadrant.
+ Colicky right-lower-quadrant pain and diarrhea are common.

Diverticulitis
+ A left-lower-quadrant mass that's usually tender, firm, and fixed may develop.

Gallbladder cancer
+ A moderately tender, irregular mass may develop in the right upper quadrant.

Gastric cancer
+ An epigastric mass may develop.

Hepatic cancer
+ A tender, nodular mass in the right upper quadrant or right epigastric area develops.
+ Pain is aggravated by jolting.

Hepatomegaly
+ A firm, blunt, irregular mass in the epigastric region or below the right costal margin develops.

Hydronephrosis
+ A smooth, boggy mass develops in one or both flanks.

and signs and symptoms of intestinal obstruction, such as obstipation and vomiting.

Occasionally, cancer of the left colon also causes a palpable mass. Usually though, it produces rectal bleeding, intermittent abdominal fullness or cramping, and rectal pressure. The patient may also report fremitus and pelvic discomfort. Later, he develops obstipation, diarrhea, or pencil-shaped, grossly bloody, or mucus-streaked stools. Typically, defecation relieves pain.

Crohn's disease
With Crohn's disease, tender, sausage-shaped masses are usually palpable in the right lower quadrant and, at times, in the left lower quadrant. Attacks of colicky right-lower-quadrant pain and diarrhea are common. Associated signs and symptoms include fever, anorexia, weight loss, hyperactive bowel sounds, nausea, abdominal tenderness with guarding, and perirectal, skin, or vaginal fistulas.

Diverticulitis
Most common in the sigmoid colon, diverticulitis may produce a left-lower-quadrant mass that's usually tender, firm, and fixed. It also produces intermittent abdominal pain that's relieved by defecation or passage of flatus. Other findings may include alternating constipation and diarrhea, nausea, low-grade fever, and a distended and tympanic abdomen.

Gallbladder cancer
Gallbladder cancer may produce a moderately tender, irregular mass in the right upper quadrant. Accompanying it is chronic, progressively severe epigastric or right-upper-quadrant pain that may radiate to the right shoulder. Associated signs and symptoms include nausea, vomiting, anorexia, weight loss, jaundice and, at times, hepatosplenomegaly.

Gastric cancer
Advanced gastric cancer may produce an epigastric mass. Early findings include chronic dyspepsia and epigastric discomfort, whereas late findings include weight loss, a feeling of fullness, fatigue and, occasionally, coffee-ground vomitus or melena.

Hepatic cancer
Hepatic cancer produces a tender, nodular mass in the right upper quadrant or right epigastric area accompanied by severe pain that's aggravated by jolting. Other effects include weight loss, weakness, anorexia, nausea, fever, dependent edema and, occasionally, jaundice and ascites. A large tumor can also cause a bruit or hum.

Hepatomegaly
Hepatomegaly produces a firm, blunt, irregular mass in the epigastric region or below the right costal margin. Associated signs and symptoms vary with the causative disorder but commonly include ascites, right-upper-quadrant pain and tenderness, anorexia, nausea, vomiting, leg edema, jaundice, palmar erythema, spider angiomas, gynecomastia, testicular atrophy and, possibly, splenomegaly.

Hydronephrosis
Enlarging one or both kidneys, hydronephrosis produces a smooth, boggy mass in one or both flanks. Other findings vary with the degree of hydronephrosis. The patient may have severe colicky renal pain or dull flank pain that radiates to the groin, vulva, or testes. Hematuria, pyuria, dysuria, alternating oliguria and polyuria, nocturia, accelerated hypertension, nausea, and vomiting may also occur.

Ovarian cyst

A large ovarian cyst may produce a smooth, rounded, fluctuant mass, resembling a distended bladder, in the suprapubic region. Large or multiple cysts may also cause mild pelvic discomfort, low back pain, menstrual irregularities, and hirsutism. A twisted or ruptured cyst may cause abdominal tenderness, distention, and rigidity.

Pancreatic abscess

Occasionally, pancreatic abscess may produce a palpable epigastric mass accompanied by epigastric pain and tenderness. The patient's temperature usually rises abruptly but may climb steadily. Nausea, vomiting, diarrhea, tachycardia, and hypotension may also occur.

Renal cell cancer

Usually occurring in only one kidney, renal cell carcinoma produces a smooth, firm, nontender mass near the affected kidney. Accompanying it are dull, constant abdominal or flank pain and hematuria. Other signs and symptoms include elevated blood pressure, fever, and urine retention. Weight loss, nausea, vomiting, and leg edema occur in late stages.

Splenomegaly

The lymphomas, leukemias, hemolytic anemias, and inflammatory diseases are among the many disorders that may cause splenomegaly. Typically, the smooth edge of the enlarged spleen is palpable in the left upper quadrant. Associated signs and symptoms vary with the causative disorder but commonly include a feeling of abdominal fullness, left-upper-quadrant abdominal pain and tenderness, splenic friction rub, splenic bruits, and low-grade fever.

Uterine leiomyomas (fibroids)

If large enough, a uterine leiomyoma (common, benign uterine tumor) can produce a round, multinodular mass in the suprapubic region. The patient's chief complaint is usually menorrhagia; she may also experience a feeling of heaviness in the abdomen, and pressure on surrounding organs may cause back pain, constipation, and urinary frequency or urgency. Edema and varicosities of the lower extremities may develop. Rapid fibroid growth in perimenopausal or postmenopausal women needs further evaluation.

SPECIAL CONSIDERATIONS

Discovery of an abdominal mass commonly causes anxiety. Offer emotional support to the patient and his family as they await the diagnosis. Position the patient comfortably, and administer drugs for pain or anxiety as needed.

If an abdominal mass causes bowel obstruction, watch for indications of peritonitis — abdominal pain and rebound tenderness — and for signs of shock, such as tachycardia and hypotension.

PEDIATRIC POINTERS

Detecting an abdominal mass in an infant can be quite a challenge. However, these tips will make palpation easier for you:
✦ Allow an infant to suck on his bottle or pacifier to prevent crying, which causes abdominal rigidity and interferes with palpation. Avoid tickling him because laughter also causes abdominal rigidity.
✦ Reduce the infant's apprehension by distracting him with cheerful conversation.
✦ Rest your hand on the infant's abdomen for a few moments before palpation. If he remains sensitive, place his hand under yours as you palpate.

Medical causes
(continued)

Ovarian cyst
✦ A smooth, rounded, fluctuant mass may develop in the suprapubic region.

Pancreatic abscess
✦ Occasionally, a palpable epigastric mass may develop.
✦ Epigastric pain and tenderness occur.

Renal cell cancer
✦ A smooth, firm, nontender mass develops near the affected kidney.

Splenomegaly
✦ The spleen is palpable in the left upper quadrant.

Uterine leiomyomas (fibroids)
✦ A round, multinodular mass may develop in the suprapubic region.
✦ Menorrhagia, feeling of heaviness in the abdomen, back pain, constipation, and urinary frequency and urgency may occur.

Special considerations
✦ Offer emotional support to the patient and his family.
✦ Position the patient comfortably.
✦ Administer drugs for pain or anxiety as needed.
✦ If bowel obstruction occurs, watch for indications of peritonitis and shock.

Peds points

✦ In neonates, most abdominal masses result from renal disorders.

✦ In older infants and children, abdominal masses are usually caused by enlarged organs.

Geri points

✦ Ultrasonography is used to evaluate a prominent midepigastric mass in thin, elderly patients.

Teaching points

✦ Explanation of diagnostic tests

Key facts about abdominal pain

✦ Arises from the abdominopelvic viscera, the parietal peritoneum, or the capsules of the liver, kidney, or spleen

✦ May be acute or chronic, diffuse or localized

✦ Is produced by stretching or tension of the gut wall, traction on the peritoneum or mesentery, vigorous intestinal contraction, inflammation, ischemia, and sensory nerve irritation

In an emergency

✦ Quickly take the patient's vital signs.

✦ Palpate pulses below the waist.

✦ Be alert for signs of hypovolemic shock.

✦ Obtain I.V. access.

✦ Prepare the patient for emergency surgery as needed.

✦ Consider allowing the child to remain on the parent's or caregiver's lap.
✦ Perform a gentle rectal examination.

In neonates, most abdominal masses result from renal disorders, such as polycystic kidney disease or congenital hydronephrosis. In older infants and children, enlarged organs, such as the liver and spleen, usually cause abdominal masses.

Other common causes include Wilms' tumor, neuroblastoma, intussusception, volvulus, Hirschsprung's disease (congenital megacolon), pyloric stenosis, and abdominal abscess.

GERIATRIC POINTERS

Ultrasonography should be used to evaluate a prominent midepigastric mass in thin, elderly patients.

PATIENT COUNSELING

Carefully explain diagnostic tests, which may include blood and urine studies, abdominal X-rays, barium enema, computed tomography scans, ultrasonography, radioisotope scans, and gastroscopy or sigmoidoscopy. A pelvic or rectal examination is usually indicated.

ABDOMINAL PAIN

Abdominal pain usually results from a GI disorder, but it can be caused by a reproductive, genitourinary (GU), musculoskeletal, or vascular disorder; drug use; or ingestion of toxins. At times, such pain signals life-threatening complications.

Abdominal pain arises from the abdominopelvic viscera, the parietal peritoneum, or the capsules of the liver, kidney, or spleen. It may be acute or chronic, diffuse or localized. Visceral pain develops slowly into a deep, dull, aching pain that's poorly localized in the epigastric, periumbilical, or lower midabdominal (hypogastric) region. In contrast, somatic (parietal, peritoneal) pain produces a sharp, more intense, and well-localized discomfort that rapidly follows the insult. Movement or coughing aggravates this pain. (See *Abdominal pain: Types and locations.*)

Pain may also be referred to the abdomen from another site with the same or similar nerve supply. This sharp, well-localized, referred pain is felt in skin or deeper tissues and may coexist with skin hyperesthesia and muscle hyperalgesia.

Mechanisms that produce abdominal pain include stretching or tension of the gut wall, traction on the peritoneum or mesentery, vigorous intestinal contraction, inflammation, ischemia, and sensory nerve irritation.

 EMERGENCY ACTIONS If the patient is experiencing sudden and severe abdominal pain, quickly take his vital signs and palpate pulses below the waist. Be alert for signs of hypovolemic shock, such as tachycardia and hypotension. Obtain I.V. access. Emergency surgery may be required if the patient also has mottled skin below the waist and a pulsating epigastric mass or rebound tenderness and rigidity.

HISTORY

If the patient has no life-threatening signs or symptoms, take his history. Ask him if he has had this type of pain before. Have him describe the pain — for example dull, sharp, stabbing, or burning. Ask if anything relieves the pain or makes it worse. Ask the patient if the pain is constant or intermittent and when the pain began. Constant, steady abdominal pain suggests organ perforation, ischemia, or inflammation

Abdominal pain: Types and locations

AFFECTED ORGAN	VISCERAL PAIN	PARIETAL PAIN	REFERRED PAIN
Stomach	Middle epigastrium	Middle epigastrium and left upper quadrant	Shoulders
Small intestine	Periumbilical area	Over affected site	Midback (rare)
Appendix	Periumbilical area	Right lower quadrant	Right lower quadrant
Proximal colon	Periumbilical area and right flank for ascending colon	Over affected site	Right lower quadrant and back (rare)
Distal colon	Hypogastrium and left flank for descending colon	Over affected site	Left lower quadrant and back (rare)
Gallbladder	Middle epigastrium	Right upper quadrant	Right subscapular area
Ureters	Costovertebral angle	Over affected site	Groin; scrotum in men, labia in women (rare)
Pancreas	Middle epigastrium and left upper quadrant	Middle epigastrium and left upper quadrant	Back and left shoulder
Ovaries, fallopian tubes, and uterus	Hypogastrium and groin	Over affected site	Inner thighs

or blood in the peritoneal cavity. Intermittent, cramping abdominal pain suggests the patient may have obstruction of a hollow organ.

If the pain is intermittent, find out the duration of a typical episode. In addition, ask the patient where the pain is located and if it radiates to other areas.

Find out if movement, coughing, exertion, vomiting, eating, elimination, or walking worsens or relieves the pain. The patient may report abdominal pain as indigestion or gas pain, so have him describe it in detail.

Ask the patient about substance abuse and any history of vascular, GI, GU, or reproductive disorders. Ask the female patient about the date of her last menses, changes in her menstrual pattern, or dyspareunia.

Ask the patient about appetite changes. Ask about the onset and frequency of nausea or vomiting. Find out about increased flatulence, constipation, diarrhea, and changes in stool consistency. When was his last bowel movement? Ask about urinary frequency, urgency, or pain. Is his urine cloudy or pink?

PHYSICAL ASSESSMENT

Perform a physical assessment. Take the patient's vital signs, and assess skin turgor and mucous membranes. Inspect his abdomen for distention or visible peristaltic waves and, if indicated, measure his abdominal girth.

Key history points
+ Previous abdominal pain
+ Description of pain
+ Factors that worsen or relieve pain
+ History of substance abuse
+ History of vascular, GI, GU, or reproductive disorders
+ Menstrual history, as appropriate
+ Appetite
+ GI changes such as increased flatulence, constipation, diarrhea, stool consistency, bowel movements, urinary frequency and urgency, or pain

Critical assessment steps
+ Take the patient's vital signs.
+ Assess skin turgor and mucous membranes.
+ Inspect the patient's abdomen for distention or visible peristaltic waves and, if indicated, measure his abdominal girth.
+ Auscultate for bowel sounds and characterize their motility.
+ Percuss all quadrants, noting the percussion sounds.
+ Palpate the entire abdomen for masses, rigidity, and tenderness.
+ Check for CVA tenderness, abdominal tenderness with guarding, and rebound tenderness.

Assessing abdominal vascular sounds

Use the bell of your stethoscope to auscultate for vascular sounds at the sites shown in the illustration.

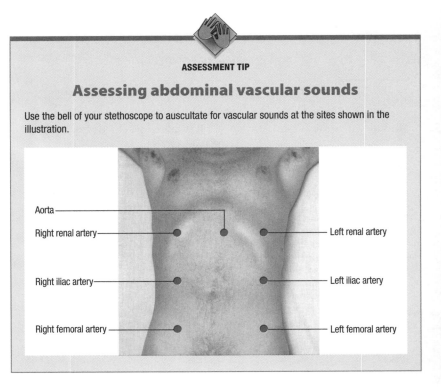

Medical causes

Abdominal aortic aneurysm (dissecting)

- Initially, dull lower abdominal, lower back, or severe chest pain may appear.
- Pain becomes constant in the upper abdomen.

Abdominal trauma

- Generalized or localized abdominal pain occurs with ecchymoses on the abdomen, abdominal tenderness, and vomiting.
- Abdominal rigidity occurs with hemorrhage into the peritoneal cavity.
- Bowel sounds are decreased or absent.

Adrenal crisis

- Severe abdominal pain appears early.
- Other signs and symptoms include nausea, vomiting, dehydration, profound weakness, anorexia, and fever.

Auscultate for bowel sounds and characterize their motility. Percuss all quadrants, noting the percussion sounds. Palpate the entire abdomen for masses, rigidity, and tenderness. Check for costovertebral angle (CVA) tenderness, abdominal tenderness with guarding, and rebound tenderness. (See *Assessing abdominal vascular sounds.*)

MEDICAL CAUSES

Abdominal aortic aneurysm (dissecting)

Dissecting abdominal aortic aneurysm, a life-threatening disorder, may initially produce dull lower abdominal, lower back, or severe chest pain. Typically, it produces constant upper abdominal pain, which may worsen when the patient lies down and may abate when he leans forward or sits up. Palpation may reveal an epigastric mass that pulsates before rupture but not after it.

Other findings may include mottled skin below the waist, absent femoral and pedal pulses, lower blood pressure in the legs than in the arms, mild to moderate abdominal tenderness with guarding, and abdominal rigidity. Signs of shock, such as tachycardia and tachypnea, may appear.

Abdominal trauma

With abdominal trauma, generalized or localized abdominal pain occurs with ecchymoses on the abdomen, abdominal tenderness, vomiting and, with hemorrhage into the peritoneal cavity, abdominal rigidity. Bowel sounds are decreased or absent. The patient may have signs of hypovolemic shock, such as hypotension and a rapid, thready pulse.

Adrenal crisis

With adrenal crisis, severe abdominal pain appears early, along with nausea, vomiting, dehydration, profound weakness, anorexia, and fever. Later signs are progressive loss of consciousness; hypotension; tachycardia; oliguria; cool, clammy skin; and increased motor activity, which may progress to delirium or seizures.

Anthrax, GI

GI anthrax is an acute infectious disease that's caused by eating meat contaminated with the gram-positive, spore-forming bacterium *Bacillus anthracis.* Initial signs and symptoms include loss of appetite, nausea, vomiting, and fever. Late signs and symptoms include abdominal pain, severe bloody diarrhea, and hematemesis.

Appendicitis

With appendicitis, a life-threatening disorder, pain initially occurs in the epigastric or umbilical region. Anorexia, nausea, or vomiting may occur after the onset of pain. Pain localizes at McBurney's point in the right lower quadrant and is accompanied by abdominal rigidity, increased tenderness (especially over McBurney's point), rebound tenderness, and retractive respirations. Later signs and symptoms include malaise, constipation (or diarrhea), low-grade fever, and tachycardia.

Cholecystitis

In cholecystitis, severe pain in the right upper quadrant may arise suddenly or increase gradually over several hours, usually after meals. It may radiate to the right shoulder, chest, or back. Accompanying the pain are anorexia, nausea, vomiting, fever, abdominal rigidity, tenderness, pallor, and diaphoresis. Murphy's sign (inspiratory arrest elicited when the examiner palpates the right upper quadrant as the patient takes a deep breath) is common.

Cholelithiasis

A patient with cholelithiasis may suffer sudden, severe, and paroxysmal pain in the right upper quadrant lasting several minutes to several hours. The pain may radiate to the epigastrium, back, or shoulder blades. The pain is accompanied by anorexia, nausea, vomiting (sometimes bilious), diaphoresis, restlessness, and abdominal tenderness with guarding over the gallbladder or biliary duct. The patient may also experience fatty food intolerance and frequent indigestion.

Cirrhosis

With cirrhosis, dull abdominal aching occurs early and is usually accompanied by anorexia, indigestion, nausea, vomiting, constipation, or diarrhea. Subsequent right-upper-quadrant pain worsens when the patient sits up or leans forward. Associated signs include fever, ascites, leg edema, weight gain, hepatomegaly, jaundice, severe pruritus, bleeding tendencies, palmar erythema, and spider angiomas. Gynecomastia and testicular atrophy may also be present.

Crohn's disease

An acute attack of Crohn's disease causes severe cramping pain in the lower abdomen, typically preceded by weeks or months of milder cramping pain. Crohn's disease may also cause diarrhea, hyperactive bowel sounds, dehydration, weight loss, fever, abdominal tenderness with guarding and, possibly, a palpable mass in a lower quadrant. Abdominal pain is usually relieved by defecation. Milder chronic signs and symptoms include right-lower-quadrant pain with diarrhea, steatorrhea, and weight loss. Complications include perirectal or vaginal fistulas.

Cystitis

With cystitis, abdominal pain and tenderness are usually suprapubic. Associated signs and symptoms include malaise, flank pain, low back pain, nausea, vomiting, urinary frequency and urgency, nocturia, dysuria, fever, and chills.

Medical causes
(continued)

Anthrax, GI
- Initial signs and symptoms include loss of appetite, nausea, vomiting, and fever.
- Abdominal pain, severe bloody diarrhea, and hematemesis are late signs and symptoms.

Appendicitis
- After initially occurring in the epigastric or umbilical region, pain localizes at McBurney's point in the right lower quadrant.

Cholecystitis
- Severe pain in the right upper quadrant may arise suddenly or increase gradually over several hours, usually after meals.

Cholelithiasis
- Sudden, severe, and paroxysmal pain in the right upper quadrant may occur.

Cirrhosis
- Dull abdominal aching occurs early.
- Pain in the right upper quadrant worsens when the patient sits up or leans forward.

Crohn's disease
- Acute attacks result in severe cramping pain in lower abdomen.
- Weeks or months of milder cramping pain typically precede an attack.
- Chronic signs and symptoms include right-lower-quadrant pain with diarrhea, steatorrhea, and weight loss.

Cystitis
- Abdominal pain and tenderness are usually suprapubic.

Medical causes
(continued)

Diverticulitis
+ Intermittent, diffuse left-lower-quadrant pain usually occurs in mild cases.
+ Rupture causes severe left-lower-quadrant pain.

Duodenal ulcer
+ Pain is localized and steady, gnawing, burning, aching, or hungerlike.
+ Pain typically occurs 2 to 4 hours after a meal.

Ectopic pregnancy
+ Pain occurs in lower abdomen and may be sharp, dull, or cramping, and constant or intermittent.
+ Rupture of the fallopian tube produces sharp lower abdominal pain, which may radiate to the shoulders and neck.

Endometriosis
+ Constant, severe pain in the lower abdomen usually begins 5 to 7 days before the start of menses.

E. coli O157:H7
+ Abdominal cramps, watery or bloody diarrhea, nausea, vomiting, and fever occur after eating contaminated foods.

Gastric ulcer
+ Diffuse, gnawing, burning pain in the left upper quadrant or epigastric area occurs 1 to 2 hours after meals.
+ Pain may be relieved by ingesting food or antacids.

Diverticulitis
Mild cases of diverticulitis usually produce intermittent, diffuse left-lower-quadrant pain, which is sometimes relieved by defecation or passage of flatus and worsened by eating. Other signs and symptoms include nausea, constipation or diarrhea, low-grade fever and, in many cases, a palpable abdominal mass that's usually tender, firm, and fixed. Rupture causes severe left-lower-quadrant pain, abdominal rigidity and, possibly, signs and symptoms of sepsis and shock (high fever, chills, and hypotension).

Duodenal ulcer
With a duodenal ulcer, localized abdominal pain—described as steady, gnawing, burning, aching, or hungerlike—may occur high in the midepigastrium, slightly off-center, usually on the right. The pain usually doesn't radiate unless pancreatic penetration occurs. It typically begins 2 to 4 hours after a meal and may cause nocturnal awakening. Ingestion of food or antacids brings relief until the cycle starts again, but it also may produce weight gain. Other symptoms include changes in bowel habits and heartburn or retrosternal burning.

Ectopic pregnancy
Lower abdominal pain may be sharp, dull, or cramping, and constant or intermittent in ectopic pregnancy, a potentially life-threatening disorder. Vaginal bleeding, nausea, and vomiting may occur, along with urinary frequency, a tender adnexal mass, and a 1- to 2-month history of amenorrhea. Rupture of the fallopian tube produces sharp lower abdominal pain, which may radiate to the shoulders and neck and become extreme with cervical or adnexal palpation. Signs of shock (such as pallor, tachycardia, and hypotension) may also appear.

Endometriosis
With endometriosis, constant, severe pain in the lower abdomen usually begins 5 to 7 days before the start of menses and may be aggravated by defecation. Depending on the location of the ectopic tissue, the pain may be accompanied by constipation, abdominal tenderness, dysmenorrhea, dyspareunia, and deep sacral pain.

Escherichia coli O157:H7
Escherichia coli O157:H7 is an aerobic, gram-negative bacillus that causes foodborne illness. Most strains of *E. coli* are harmless and are part of the normal intestinal flora of healthy humans and animals. *E. coli* O157:H7, one of hundreds of strains of the bacterium, can produce a powerful toxin and cause severe illness. Eating undercooked beef or other foods contaminated with the bacteria causes the disease. Signs and symptoms include watery or bloody diarrhea, nausea, vomiting, fever, and abdominal cramps. In children younger than age 5 and elderly adults, hemolytic uremic syndrome may develop and may ultimately lead to acute renal failure.

Gastric ulcer
In a patient with a gastric ulcer, diffuse, gnawing, burning pain in the left upper quadrant or epigastric area commonly occurs 1 to 2 hours after meals and may be relieved by ingestion of food or antacids. Vague bloating and nausea after eating are common. Indigestion, weight change, anorexia, and episodes of GI bleeding also occur.

Gastritis
With acute gastritis, the patient experiences rapid onset of abdominal pain that can range from mild epigastric discomfort to burning pain in the left upper quadrant. Other typical features include belching, fever, malaise, anorexia, nausea, bloody or

coffee-ground vomitus, and melena. However, significant bleeding is unusual, unless the patient has hemorrhagic gastritis.

Gastroenteritis

With gastroenteritis, cramping or colicky abdominal pain, which can be diffuse, originates in the left upper quadrant and radiates or migrates to the other quadrants, usually in a peristaltic manner. It's accompanied by diarrhea, hyperactive bowel sounds, headache, myalgia, nausea, and vomiting.

Heart failure

Right-upper-quadrant pain commonly accompanies these hallmarks of heart failure: jugular vein distention, dyspnea, tachycardia, and peripheral edema. Other findings include nausea, vomiting, ascites, productive cough, crackles, cool extremities, and cyanotic nail beds. Clinical signs are numerous and vary according to the stage of the disease and amount of cardiovascular impairment.

Hepatitis

Liver enlargement from any type of hepatitis causes discomfort or dull pain and tenderness in the right upper quadrant. Associated signs and symptoms may include dark urine, clay-colored stools, nausea, vomiting, anorexia, jaundice, malaise, and pruritus.

Herpes zoster

Herpes zoster of the thoracic, lumbar, or sacral nerves can cause localized abdominal and chest pain in the areas served by these nerves. Pain, tenderness, and fever can precede or accompany erythematous papules, which rapidly evolve into grouped vesicles.

Intestinal obstruction

Short episodes of intense, colicky, cramping pain alternate with pain-free intervals in intestinal obstruction. Accompanying signs and symptoms of this life-threatening disorder may include abdominal distention, tenderness, and guarding; visible peristaltic waves; high-pitched, tinkling, or hyperactive sounds proximal to the obstruction and hypoactive or absent sounds distally; obstipation; and pain-induced agitation. In jejunal and duodenal obstruction, nausea and bilious vomiting occur early. In distal small- or large-bowel obstruction, nausea and vomiting are commonly feculent. Complete obstruction produces absent bowel sounds. Late-stage obstruction produces signs of hypovolemic shock, such as hypotension and tachycardia.

Irritable bowel syndrome

With irritable bowel syndrome, lower abdominal cramping or pain is aggravated by ingestion of coarse or raw foods and may be alleviated by defecation or passage of flatus. Related findings include abdominal tenderness, diurnal diarrhea alternating with constipation or normal bowel function, and small stools with visible mucus. Dyspepsia, nausea, and abdominal distention with a feeling of incomplete evacuation may also occur. Stress, anxiety, and emotional lability intensify the symptoms.

Listeriosis

Listeriosis is a serious infection that's caused by eating food contaminated with the bacterium *Listeria monocytogenes*. This food-borne illness primarily affects pregnant women, neonates, and those with weakened immune systems. Signs and symptoms include fever, myalgia, abdominal pain, nausea, vomiting, and diarrhea. If the infection spreads to the nervous system, meningitis may develop; signs and

---

Medical causes
(*continued*)

Gastritis
+ Onset of pain is rapid.
+ Pain ranges from mild epigastric discomfort to burning in the left upper quadrant.

Gastroenteritis
+ Cramping or colicky pain originates in the left upper quadrant and then radiates or migrates to the other quadrants.

Heart failure
+ Right-upper-quadrant pain is common.

Hepatitis
+ Liver enlargement causes discomfort or dull pain and tenderness in the right upper quadrant.

Herpes zoster
+ Abdominal and chest pain may occur in the areas served by the nerves affected by the infection.

Intestinal obstruction
+ Short episodes of intense, colicky, cramping pain alternate with pain-free intervals.

Irritable bowel syndrome
+ Lower abdominal cramping or pain is aggravated by ingestion of coarse or raw foods.
+ Pain may be alleviated by defecation or passage of flatus.

Listeriosis
+ Abdominal pain, fever, myalgia, nausea, vomiting, and diarrhea occur after eating contaminated food.

Medical causes
(continued)

Mesenteric artery ischemia
+ Sudden, severe abdominal pain develops after 2 to 3 days of colicky periumbilical pain and diarrhea.
+ Condition tends to occur in patients older than age 50 with chronic heart failure, cardiac arrhythmia, cardiovascular infarct, or hypotension.

Ovarian cyst
+ Torsion or hemorrhage related to an ovarian cyst causes pain and tenderness in the right or left lower quadrant.

Pancreatitis
+ In acute pancreatitis, fulminating, continuous upper abdominal pain may radiate to both flanks and to the back.
+ In chronic pancreatitis, severe left-upper-quadrant or epigastric pain radiates to the back.

Pelvic inflammatory disease
+ Pain occurs in the right or left lower quadrant.
+ Extent of pain ranges from vague discomfort to deep, severe, and progressive pain.

Perforated ulcer
+ Sudden, severe, and prostrating epigastric pain may radiate through the abdomen to the back or right shoulder.

symptoms include fever, headache, nuchal rigidity, and change in level of consciousness (LOC).

Mesenteric artery ischemia

Always suspect mesenteric artery ischemia in patients older than age 50 with chronic heart failure, cardiac arrhythmia, cardiovascular infarct, or hypotension who develop sudden, severe abdominal pain after 2 to 3 days of colicky periumbilical pain and diarrhea. Initially, the abdomen is soft and tender with decreased bowel sounds. Associated findings include vomiting, anorexia, alternating periods of diarrhea and constipation and, in late stages, extreme abdominal tenderness with rigidity, tachycardia, tachypnea, absent bowel sounds, and cool, clammy skin.

Ovarian cyst

Torsion or hemorrhage related to an ovarian cyst causes pain and tenderness in the right or left lower quadrant. Sharp and severe if the patient suddenly stands or stoops, the pain becomes brief and intermittent if the torsion self-corrects or dull and diffuse after several hours if it doesn't. Pain is accompanied by slight fever, mild nausea and vomiting, abdominal tenderness, a palpable abdominal mass and, possibly, amenorrhea. Abdominal distention may occur if the patient has a large cyst. Peritoneal irritation, or rupture and ensuing peritonitis, causes high fever and severe nausea and vomiting.

Pancreatitis

Life-threatening acute pancreatitis produces fulminating, continuous upper abdominal pain that may radiate to both flanks and to the back. To relieve this pain, the patient may bend forward, draw his knees to his chest, or move restlessly about. Early findings include abdominal tenderness, nausea, vomiting, fever, pallor, tachycardia and, in some patients, abdominal rigidity, rebound tenderness, and hypoactive bowel sounds. Turner's sign (ecchymosis of the abdomen or flank) or Cullen's sign (a bluish tinge around the umbilicus) signals hemorrhagic pancreatitis. Jaundice may occur as inflammation subsides.

Chronic pancreatitis produces severe left-upper-quadrant or epigastric pain that radiates to the back. Abdominal tenderness, a midepigastric mass, jaundice, fever, and splenomegaly may occur. Steatorrhea, weight loss, maldigestion, and diabetes mellitus are common.

Pelvic inflammatory disease

Pelvic inflammatory disease causes pain in the right or left lower quadrant that ranges from vague discomfort that's worsened by movement, to deep, severe, and progressive pain. Sometimes, metrorrhagia precedes or accompanies the onset of pain. Extreme pain accompanies cervical or adnexal palpation. Associated findings include abdominal tenderness, a palpable abdominal or pelvic mass, fever, occasional chills, nausea, vomiting, urinary discomfort, and abnormal vaginal bleeding or purulent vaginal discharge.

Perforated ulcer

With perforated ulcer, a life-threatening disorder, sudden, severe, and prostrating epigastric pain may radiate through the abdomen to the back or right shoulder. Other signs and symptoms include boardlike abdominal rigidity, tenderness with guarding, generalized rebound tenderness, absent bowel sounds, grunting and shallow respirations and, in many cases, fever, tachycardia, hypotension, and syncope.

Peritonitis

With peritonitis, a life-threatening disorder, sudden and severe pain can be diffuse or localized in the area of the underlying disorder; movement worsens the pain.

The degree of abdominal tenderness usually varies according to the extent of disease. Typical findings include fever; chills; nausea; vomiting; hypoactive or absent bowel sounds; abdominal tenderness, distention, and rigidity; rebound tenderness and guarding; hyperalgesia; tachycardia; hypotension; tachypnea; and positive psoas and obturator signs.

Pleurisy
Pleurisy may produce upper abdominal or costal margin pain referred from the chest. Characteristic sharp, stabbing chest pain increases with inspiration and movement. Many patients have a pleural friction rub and rapid, shallow breathing; some have a low-grade fever.

Pneumonia
Lower-lobe pneumonia can cause pleuritic chest pain and referred, severe upper abdominal pain, tenderness, and rigidity that diminish with inspiration. It can also cause fever, shaking chills, achiness, headache, blood-tinged or rusty sputum, dyspnea, and a dry, hacking cough. Accompanying signs include crackles, egophony, decreased breath sounds, and dullness on percussion.

Pneumothorax
Pneumothorax is a potentially life-threatening disorder that can cause pain across the upper abdomen and costal margin that's referred from the chest. Characteristic chest pain arises suddenly and worsens with deep inspiration or movement. Accompanying signs and symptoms include anxiety, dyspnea, cyanosis, decreased or absent breath sounds over the affected area, tachypnea, and tachycardia. Watch for asymmetrical chest movements on inspiration.

Prostatitis
With prostatitis, vague abdominal pain or discomfort in the lower abdomen, groin, perineum, or rectum may develop. Other findings include dysuria, urinary frequency and urgency, fever, chills, low back pain, myalgia, arthralgia, and nocturia. Scrotal pain, penile pain, and pain on ejaculation may occur in chronic cases.

Pyelonephritis (acute)
Progressive lower quadrant pain in one or both sides, flank pain, and CVA tenderness characterize acute pyelonephritis. Pain may radiate to the lower midabdomen or to the groin. Additional signs and symptoms include abdominal and back tenderness, high fever, shaking chills, nausea, vomiting, and urinary frequency and urgency.

Renal calculi
Depending on the location of renal calculi, severe abdominal or back pain may occur. However, the classic symptom is severe, colicky pain that travels from the CVA to the flank, suprapubic region, and external genitalia. The pain may be excruciating or dull and constant. Pain-induced agitation, nausea, vomiting, abdominal distention, fever, chills, hypertension, and urinary urgency with hematuria and dysuria may occur.

Sickle cell crisis
Sudden, severe abdominal pain may accompany chest, back, hand, or foot pain in sickle cell crisis. Associated signs and symptoms include weakness, aching joints, dyspnea, and scleral jaundice. Sickle cell crisis is the hallmark of sickle cell disease and tends to appear periodically after age 5.

Medical causes
(continued)

Peritonitis
+ Sudden and severe pain can be diffuse or localized in the area of the underlying disorder.
+ Movement worsens the pain.

Pleurisy
+ Upper abdominal or costal margin pain is referred from the chest.
+ Sharp chest pain increases with inspiration and movement.

Pneumonia
+ Pleuritic chest pain occurs with referred, severe upper abdominal pain, tenderness, and rigidity that diminish with inspiration.

Pneumothorax
+ Pain refers from the chest across the upper abdomen and costal margin.

Prostatitis
+ Vague abdominal pain or discomfort in the lower abdomen, groin, perineum, or rectum may develop.

Pyelonephritis (acute)
+ Progressive lower quadrant pain occurs in one or both sides.
+ Pain may radiate to the lower midabdomen or the groin.

Renal calculi
+ Depending on the location of calculi, severe abdominal or back pain may occur.

Sickle cell crisis
+ Sudden, severe abdominal pain may accompany chest, back, hand, or foot pain.

Medical causes
(continued)
Smallpox (variola major)
+ Abdominal pain, high fever, malaise, prostration, severe headache, and backache appear initially.

Splenic infarction
+ Sudden, severe pain in the left upper quadrant occurs along with chest pain.
+ Pain commonly radiates to the left shoulder.

Ulcerative colitis
+ Initially, vague abdominal discomfort leads to cramping lower abdominal pain.
+ Pain may become steady and diffuse, increasing with movement and coughing.

Uremia
+ Generalized or periumbilical pain that shifts and varies in intensity occurs.

Other causes
+ Salicylates
+ NSAIDs

Special considerations
+ Have the patient lie in a supine position with his head flat on the table, arms at his sides, and knees slightly flexed.
+ Monitor for complications.
+ Withhold analgesics.
+ Withhold food and fluids.
+ Prepare for I.V. infusion and insertion of an NG or other intestinal tube.
+ Peritoneal lavage or abdominal paracentesis may be required.

Smallpox (variola major)
Initial signs and symptoms of smallpox include high fever, malaise, prostration, severe headache, backache, and abdominal pain. A maculopapular rash develops on the mucosa of the mouth, pharynx, face, and forearms and then spreads to the trunk and legs. Within 2 days, the rash becomes vesicular and later pustular. The lesions develop at the same time, appear identical, and are more prominent on the face and extremities. The pustules are round, firm, and embedded in the skin. After 8 to 9 days, the pustules form a crust, and later the scab separates from the skin leaving a pitted scar. In fatal cases, death results from encephalitis, extensive bleeding, or secondary infection.

Splenic infarction
Sudden, severe pain in the left upper quadrant occurs along with chest pain that may worsen on inspiration in splenic infarction. Pain commonly radiates to the left shoulder with splinting of the left diaphragm, abdominal guarding and, occasionally, a splenic friction rub.

Ulcerative colitis
Ulcerative colitis may begin with vague abdominal discomfort that leads to cramping lower abdominal pain. As the disorder progresses, pain may become steady and diffuse, increasing with movement and coughing. The most common symptom — recurrent and possibly severe diarrhea with blood, pus, and mucus — may relieve the pain. The abdomen may feel soft, squashy, and extremely tender. High-pitched, infrequent bowel sounds may accompany nausea, vomiting, anorexia, weight loss, and mild, intermittent fever.

Uremia
Characterized by generalized or periumbilical pain that shifts and varies in intensity, uremia causes diverse GI signs and symptoms, such as nausea, anorexia, vomiting, and diarrhea. Abdominal tenderness that changes in location and intensity may occur, along with vision disturbances, bleeding, headache, decreased LOC, vertigo, and oliguria or anuria. Chest pain may occur secondary to pericardial effusion. Localized or diffuse pruritus is common.

OTHER CAUSES
Drugs
Salicylates and nonsteroidal anti-inflammatories commonly cause burning, gnawing pain in the left upper quadrant or epigastric area, along with nausea and vomiting.

SPECIAL CONSIDERATIONS
Help the patient find a comfortable position to ease his distress. The patient should lie in a supine position with his head flat on the table, arms at his sides, and knees slightly flexed to relax the abdominal muscles. Monitor him closely because abdominal pain can signal a life-threatening disorder. Especially important indications include tachycardia, hypotension, clammy skin, abdominal rigidity, rebound tenderness, a change in the pain's location or intensity, or sudden relief from the pain.

Withhold analgesics from the patient because they may mask symptoms. Also withhold food and fluids because surgery may be needed. Prepare for I.V. infusion and insertion of a nasogastric or other intestinal tube. Peritoneal lavage or abdominal paracentesis may be required.

You may have to prepare the patient for a diagnostic procedure, which may include a pelvic and rectal examination; blood, urine, and stool tests; X-rays; barium studies; ultrasonography; endoscopy; and biopsy.

PEDIATRIC POINTERS

Because a child typically has difficulty describing abdominal pain, you should pay close attention to nonverbal cues, such as wincing, lethargy, or unusual positioning (such as a side-lying position with knees flexed to the abdomen). Observing the child while he coughs, walks, or climbs may offer some diagnostic clues. Also, remember that a parent's description of the child's complaints is a subjective interpretation of what the parent believes is wrong.

In children, abdominal pain can signal a disorder with greater severity or different associated signs than in adults. Appendicitis, for example, has higher rupture and mortality rates in children, and vomiting may be the only other sign. Acute pyelonephritis may cause abdominal pain, vomiting, and diarrhea, but not the classic urologic signs found in adults. Peptic ulcer, which is becoming increasingly common in teenagers, causes nocturnal pain and colic that, unlike peptic ulcer in adults, may not be relieved by food.

Abdominal pain in children can also result from lactose intolerance, allergic-tension-fatigue syndrome, volvulus, Meckel's diverticulum, intussusception, mesenteric adenitis, diabetes mellitus, juvenile rheumatoid arthritis, and many uncommon disorders such as heavy metal poisoning. Remember, too, that a child's complaint of abdominal pain may reflect an emotional need, such as a wish to avoid school or to gain adult attention.

GERIATRIC POINTERS

Advanced age may decrease the manifestations of acute abdominal disease. Pain may be less severe, fever less pronounced, and signs of peritoneal inflammation diminished or absent.

PATIENT COUNSELING

Prepare the patient for diagnostic testing by explaining what to expect before, during, and after the procedure. Explain any food and fluid restrictions. Discuss the importance of reporting changes in bowel habits and monitoring stools for blood. Discuss proper positioning to alleviate symptoms.

ABDOMINAL RIGIDITY

Detected by palpation, abdominal rigidity refers to abnormal muscle tension or inflexibility of the abdomen. Also known as *abdominal muscle spasm* or *involuntary guarding,* rigidity may be voluntary or involuntary. Voluntary rigidity reflects the patient's fear or nervousness upon palpation; involuntary rigidity reflects potentially life-threatening peritoneal irritation or inflammation. (See *Recognizing voluntary rigidity,* page 22.)

Involuntary rigidity most commonly results from GI disorders but may also result from pulmonary and vascular disorders and from the effects of insect toxins. Usually, it's accompanied by fever, nausea, vomiting, and abdominal tenderness, distention, and pain.

In an emergency

+ Quickly take the patient's vital signs.
+ Prepare to administer oxygen and to insert an I.V. line for fluid and blood replacement.
+ Anticipate the need for drugs to support blood pressure.
+ Prepare the patient for catheterization.
+ Monitor intake and output.
+ Be aware that an NG tube may have to be inserted to relieve abdominal distention.
+ Prepare the patient for laboratory tests and X-rays.

Key history points

+ Onset of abdominal rigidity
+ Associated abdominal pain
+ Location of rigidity
+ Aggravating and alleviating factors
+ Other signs and symptoms

Critical assessment steps

+ Inspect the abdomen for peristaltic waves.
+ Check for a visibly distended bowel loop.
+ Auscultate bowel sounds.
+ Perform light palpation to locate the rigidity and to determine its severity.
+ Check for poor skin turgor and dry mucous membranes.

ASSESSMENT TIP

Recognizing voluntary rigidity

Distinguishing voluntary from involuntary abdominal rigidity is a must for accurate assessment. Review this comparison so that you can quickly tell the two apart.

Voluntary rigidity is:
+ usually symmetrical
+ more rigid on inspiration (expiration causes muscle relaxation)
+ eased by relaxation techniques, such as positioning the patient comfortably and talking to him in a calm, soothing manner
+ painless when the patient sits up using his abdominal muscles alone.

Involuntary rigidity is:
+ usually asymmetrical
+ equally rigid on inspiration and expiration
+ unaffected by relaxation techniques
+ painful when the patient sits up using his abdominal muscles alone.

EMERGENCY ACTIONS After palpating abdominal rigidity, quickly take the patient's vital signs. Even though the patient may not appear gravely ill or have markedly abnormal vital signs, abdominal rigidity calls for emergency actions. Prepare to administer oxygen and to insert an I.V. line for fluid and blood replacement. The patient may require drugs to support blood pressure. Also prepare him for catheterization, and monitor intake and output. A nasogastric tube may have to be inserted to relieve abdominal distention. Because emergency surgery may be necessary, the patient should be prepared for laboratory tests and X-rays.

HISTORY

If the patient's condition allows further assessment, take a brief history. Find out when the abdominal rigidity began. Is it associated with abdominal pain? If so, did the pain begin at the same time? Determine whether the abdominal rigidity is localized or generalized. Is it always present? Has its site changed or remained constant? Next, ask about aggravating or alleviating factors, such as position changes, coughing, vomiting, elimination, and walking. Then explore other signs and symptoms.

PHYSICAL ASSESSMENT

Inspect the abdomen for peristaltic waves, which may be visible in very thin patients. Also check for a visibly distended bowel loop. Next, auscultate bowel sounds. Perform light palpation to locate the rigidity and to determine its severity. Avoid deep palpation, which may exacerbate abdominal pain. Finally, check for poor skin turgor and dry mucous membranes, which indicate dehydration.

MEDICAL CAUSES

Abdominal aortic aneurysm (dissecting)

Mild to moderate abdominal rigidity occurs with dissecting abdominal aortic aneurysm, a life-threatening disorder. Typically, it's accompanied by constant upper abdominal pain that may radiate to the lower back. The pain may worsen when the patient lies down and may be relieved when he leans forward or sits up. Before rupture, the aneurysm may produce a pulsating mass in the epigastrium, accompanied by a systolic bruit over the aorta. However, the mass stops pulsating after rupture. Associated signs and symptoms include mottled skin below the waist, absent femoral and pedal pulses, lower blood pressure in the legs than in the arms, and mild to moderate tenderness with guarding. Significant blood loss causes signs of shock, such as tachycardia, tachypnea, and cool, clammy skin.

Insect toxins

Insect stings and bites, especially black widow spider bites, release toxins that can produce generalized, cramping abdominal pain, usually accompanied by rigidity. These toxins may also cause low-grade fever, nausea, vomiting, tremors, and burning sensations in the hands and feet. Some patients develop increased salivation, hypertension, paresis, and hyperactive reflexes. Children commonly are restless, have an expiratory grunt, and keep their legs flexed.

Mesenteric artery ischemia

Mesenteric artery ischemia is a life-threatening disorder that's characterized by 2 to 3 days of persistent, low-grade abdominal pain and diarrhea leading to sudden, severe abdominal pain and rigidity. Rigidity occurs in the central or periumbilical region and is accompanied by severe abdominal tenderness, fever, and signs of shock, such as tachycardia and hypotension. Other findings may include vomiting, anorexia, diarrhea, and constipation. Always suspect mesenteric artery ischemia in patients older than age 50 with a history of heart failure, arrhythmia, cardiovascular infarct, or hypotension.

Peritonitis

Depending on the cause of peritonitis, abdominal rigidity may be localized or generalized. For example, if an inflamed appendix causes local peritonitis, rigidity may be localized in the right lower quadrant. If a perforated ulcer causes widespread peritonitis, rigidity may be generalized and, in severe cases, boardlike.

Peritonitis also causes sudden and severe abdominal pain that can be localized or generalized. In addition, it can produce abdominal tenderness and distention, rebound tenderness, guarding, hyperalgesia, hypoactive or absent bowel sounds, nausea, and vomiting. Usually, the patient also displays fever, chills, tachycardia, tachypnea, and hypotension.

SPECIAL CONSIDERATIONS

Continue to monitor the patient closely for signs of shock. Position him as comfortably as possible. The patient should lie in a supine position with his head flat on the table, arms at his sides, and knees slightly flexed to relax the abdominal muscles. Withhold analgesics until a tentative diagnosis has been made because they may mask other symptoms. Also withhold food and fluids and administer an I.V. antibiotic because emergency surgery may be required. Prepare the patient for diagnostic tests, which may include blood, urine, and stool studies; chest and abdominal X-rays; a computed tomography scan; magnetic resonance imaging; peritoneal lavage; and gastroscopy or colonoscopy. A pelvic or rectal examination may also be done.

PEDIATRIC POINTERS

Voluntary rigidity may be difficult to distinguish from involuntary rigidity if associated pain makes children restless, tense, or apprehensive. However, in any child with suspected involuntary rigidity, your priority is early detection of dehydration and shock, which can rapidly become life-threatening.

Medical causes

Abdominal aortic aneurysm (dissecting)
✦ Mild to moderate abdominal rigidity occurs.

Insect toxins
✦ Rigidity usually accompanies generalized, cramping abdominal pain.

Mesenteric artery ischemia
✦ Sudden, severe abdominal pain and rigidity occur in the central or periumbilical region after 2 to 3 days of persistent, low-grade abdominal pain and diarrhea.

Peritonitis
✦ Rigidity is localized or generalized depending on the cause of peritonitis.

Special considerations
✦ Monitor the patient closely for signs of shock.
✦ Position the patient in a supine position with his head flat on the table, arms at his sides, and knees slightly flexed.
✦ Withhold analgesics until a tentative diagnosis has been made.
✦ Withhold food and fluids.
✦ Administer an I.V. antibiotic because emergency surgery may be required.

Peds points
✦ Abdominal rigidity in children can stem from gastric perforation, hypertrophic pyloric stenosis, duodenal obstruction, meconium ileus, intussusception, cystic fibrosis, celiac disease, and appendicitis.

Geri points

◆ Advanced age and impaired cognition decrease pain perception and intensity.
◆ Weakening of abdominal muscles may decrease muscle spasms and rigidity.

Teaching points

◆ Explanation of diagnostic tests and surgery

Key facts about accessory muscle use

◆ Stabilizes the thorax during respiration when breathing requires extra effort
◆ May indicate acute respiratory distress, diaphragmatic weakness, fatigue, or chronic respiratory disease

In an emergency

◆ Look for signs of acute respiratory distress.
◆ Quickly auscultate for abnormal, diminished, or absent breath sounds.
◆ Check for airway obstruction and, if detected, attempt to restore airway patency.
◆ Begin suctioning and manual or mechanical ventilation.
◆ Assess oxygen saturation using pulse oximetry, if available.
◆ Administer oxygen.

Key history points

◆ Onset, duration, and severity of signs and symptoms
◆ Medical and family history, including respiratory and cardiac disorders
◆ Past trauma, testing, or therapy
◆ Smoking and occupational hazards

Abdominal rigidity in children can stem from gastric perforation, hypertrophic pyloric stenosis, duodenal obstruction, meconium ileus, intussusception, cystic fibrosis, celiac disease, and appendicitis.

GERIATRIC POINTERS

Advanced age and impaired cognition decrease pain perception and intensity. Weakening of abdominal muscles may decrease muscle spasms and rigidity.

PATIENT COUNSELING

Explain and prepare the patient for diagnostic testing and surgery. Because the patient may be gravely ill, keep your explanations short and simple and take measures to reduce his anxiety.

ACCESSORY MUSCLE USE

When breathing requires extra effort, the accessory muscles—the sternocleidomastoid, scalene, pectoralis major, trapezius, internal intercostal, and abdominal muscles—stabilize the thorax during respiration. Some accessory muscle use normally takes place during such activities as singing, talking, coughing, defecating, and exercising. (See *Accessory muscles: Locations and functions.*) However, more pronounced use of these muscles might signal acute respiratory distress, diaphragmatic weakness, or fatigue. It may also result from chronic respiratory disease. Typically, the extent of accessory muscle use reflects the severity of the underlying cause.

 EMERGENCY ACTIONS If the patient displays increased accessory muscle use, immediately look for signs of acute respiratory distress, including decreased level of consciousness, shortness of breath when speaking, tachypnea, intercostal and sternal retractions, cyanosis, external breath sounds (such as wheezing or stridor), diaphoresis, nasal flaring, and extreme apprehension or agitation. Quickly auscultate for abnormal, diminished, or absent breath sounds. Check for airway obstruction and, if detected, attempt to restore airway patency. Insert an airway or intubate the patient. Then begin suctioning and manual or mechanical ventilation. Assess oxygen saturation using pulse oximetry if available. Then administer oxygen. You may need to use a high flow rate initially, but be attentive to the patient's respiratory drive (too much oxygen may decrease respiratory drive). If the patient has chronic obstructive pulmonary disease (COPD), use only a low flow rate for mild COPD exacerbations. An I.V. line also may be required.

HISTORY

If the patient's condition allows, question him thoroughly. Ask him about the onset, duration, and severity of associated signs and symptoms, such as dyspnea, chest pain, cough, or fever.

Explore his medical history, focusing on respiratory disorders, such as infection or COPD. Ask about cardiac disorders such as heart failure, which may lead to pulmonary edema; also inquire about neuromuscular disorders such as amyotrophic lateral sclerosis, which may affect respiratory muscle function. Note a history of allergies or asthma. Because collagen vascular diseases can cause diffuse infiltrative lung disease, ask about such conditions as rheumatoid arthritis and lupus erythematosus.

Accessory muscles: Locations and functions

Physical exertion and pulmonary disease usually increase the work of breathing, taxing the diaphragm and external intercostal muscles. When this happens, accessory muscles provide the extra effort needed to maintain respirations. The upper accessory muscles assist with inspiration, whereas the upper chest, sternum, internal intercostal, and abdominal muscles assist with expiration.

With inspiration, the scalene muscles elevate, fix, and expand the upper chest. The sternocleidomastoid muscles raise the sternum, expanding the chest's anteroposterior and longitudinal dimensions. The pectoralis major elevates the chest, increasing its anteroposterior size, and the trapezius raises the thoracic cage.

With expiration, the internal intercostals depress the ribs, decreasing the chest size. The abdominal muscles pull the lower chest down, depress the lower ribs, and compress the abdominal contents, which exerts pressure on the chest.

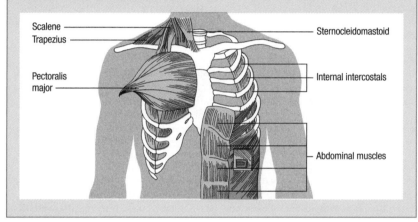

Ask about recent trauma, especially to the spine or chest. Find out if the patient has recently undergone pulmonary function testing or received respiratory therapy. Ask about smoking and occupational exposure to chemical fumes or mineral dusts such as asbestos. Explore the patient's family history for such disorders as cystic fibrosis and neurofibromatosis, which can cause diffuse infiltrative lung disease.

PHYSICAL ASSESSMENT

Perform a detailed chest assessment, noting abnormal respiratory rate, pattern, or depth. Assess the color, temperature, and turgor of the patient's skin, and check for clubbing.

MEDICAL CAUSES

Acute respiratory distress syndrome

In acute respiratory distress syndrome (ARDS), accessory muscle use increases in response to hypoxia. It's accompanied by intercostal, supracostal, and sternal retractions on inspiration and by grunting on expiration. Other characteristics of this life-threatening disorder include tachypnea, dyspnea, diaphoresis, diffuse crackles, and a cough with pink, frothy sputum. Worsening hypoxia produces anxiety, tachycardia, and mental sluggishness.

Critical assessment steps

◆ Perform a detailed chest assessment, noting abnormal respiratory rate, pattern, or depth.
◆ Assess the color, temperature, and turgor of the patient's skin.
◆ Check for clubbing.

Medical causes

ARDS

◆ Accessory muscle use increases in response to hypoxia.
◆ Intercostal, supracostal, and sternal retractions occur on inspiration.
◆ Grunting occurs on expiration.

Medical causes
(continued)

Airway obstruction
✦ Accessory muscle use increases.
✦ Inspiratory stridor, dyspnea, tachypnea, gasping, wheezing, coughing, drooling, intercostal retractions, cyanosis, and tachycardia occur.

ALS
✦ Accessory muscle use increases because the diaphragm is affected by the disorder.
✦ Other signs and symptoms include muscle atrophy and weakness and incoordination.

Asthma
✦ Accessory muscle use increases during acute attacks.
✦ Severe dyspnea, tachypnea, wheezing, productive cough, nasal flaring, and cyanosis occur.

Chronic bronchitis
✦ Productive cough and exertional dyspnea precede accessory muscle use that may be chronic.

Emphysema
✦ Increased accessory muscle use occurs with progressive exertional dyspnea and a minimally productive cough.

Pneumonia
✦ Increased accessory muscle use is accompanied by a sudden high fever with chills.

Pulmonary edema
✦ Increased accessory muscle use is accompanied by dyspnea, tachypnea, orthopnea, crepitant crackles, wheezing, and a cough with pink, frothy sputum.

Airway obstruction
Acute upper airway obstruction can be life-threatening—fortunately, most obstructions are subacute or chronic. Typically, this disorder increases accessory muscle use. Its most telling sign, however, is inspiratory stridor. Associated signs and symptoms include dyspnea, tachypnea, gasping, wheezing, coughing, drooling, intercostal retractions, cyanosis, and tachycardia.

Amyotrophic lateral sclerosis
Typically, amyotrophic lateral sclerosis (ALS) affects the diaphragm more than the accessory muscles. As a result, increased accessory muscle use is characteristic. Other signs and symptoms of this progressive motor neuron disorder include fasciculations, muscle atrophy and weakness, spasticity, bilateral Babinski's reflex, and hyperactive deep tendon reflexes. Incoordination makes carrying out routine activities difficult for the patient. Associated signs and symptoms include impaired speech; difficulty chewing or swallowing and breathing; urinary frequency and urgency; and, occasionally, choking and excessive drooling. (*Note:* Other neuromuscular disorders may produce similar signs and symptoms.) Although the patient's mental status remains intact, his poor prognosis may cause periodic depression.

Asthma
During acute asthma attacks, the patient usually displays increased accessory muscle use. Accompanying it are severe dyspnea, tachypnea, wheezing, productive cough, nasal flaring, and cyanosis. Auscultation reveals faint or possibly absent breath sounds, musical crackles, and rhonchi. Other signs and symptoms include tachycardia, diaphoresis, and apprehension caused by air hunger. Chronic asthma may also cause barrel chest.

Chronic bronchitis
With chronic bronchitis, a form of COPD, increased accessory muscle use may be chronic and is preceded by a productive cough and exertional dyspnea. Chronic bronchitis is accompanied by wheezing, basal crackles, tachypnea, jugular vein distention, prolonged expiration, barrel chest, and clubbing. Cyanosis and weight gain from edema account for the characteristic label of "blue bloater." Low-grade fever may occur with secondary infection.

Emphysema
With emphysema, a form of COPD, increased accessory muscle use occurs with progressive exertional dyspnea and a minimally productive cough. Sometimes called a "pink puffer," the patient will display pursed-lip breathing and tachypnea. Associated signs and symptoms include peripheral cyanosis, anorexia, weight loss, malaise, barrel chest, and clubbing. Auscultation reveals distant heart sounds; percussion detects hyperresonance.

Pneumonia
Bacterial pneumonia usually produces increased accessory muscle use. Initially, this infection produces sudden high fever with chills. Its associated signs and symptoms include chest pain, productive cough, dyspnea, tachypnea, tachycardia, expiratory grunting, cyanosis, diaphoresis, and fine crackles.

Pulmonary edema
With acute pulmonary edema, increased accessory muscle use is accompanied by dyspnea, tachypnea, orthopnea, crepitant crackles, wheezing, and a cough with pink, frothy sputum. Other findings include restlessness, tachycardia, ventricular gallop, and cool, clammy, cyanotic skin.

Pulmonary embolism

Although signs and symptoms vary with the size, number, and location of the emboli, this life-threatening disorder may cause increased accessory muscle use. Commonly, it produces dyspnea and tachypnea that may be accompanied by pleuritic or substernal chest pain. Other signs and symptoms include restlessness, anxiety, tachycardia, productive cough, low-grade fever and, with a large embolus, hemoptysis, cyanosis, syncope, jugular vein distention, scattered crackles, and focal wheezing.

Spinal cord injury

Depending on the location and severity of a spinal cord injury, increased accessory muscle use may occur. An injury below Ll typically doesn't affect the diaphragm or accessory muscles, whereas an injury between C3 and C5 affects the upper respiratory muscles and diaphragm, causing increased accessory muscle use.

Associated signs and symptoms of spinal cord injury include unilateral or bilateral Babinski's reflex; hyperactive deep tendon reflexes; spasticity; and variable or total loss of pain and temperature sensation, proprioception, and motor function. Horner's syndrome (unilateral ptosis, pupillary constriction, facial anhidrosis) may occur with lower cervical cord injury.

Thoracic injury

With thoracic injury, increased accessory muscle use may occur, depending on the type and extent of injury. Associated signs and symptoms of this potentially life-threatening injury include an obvious chest wound or bruising, chest pain, dyspnea, cyanosis, and agitation. Signs of shock, such as tachycardia and hypotension, occur with significant blood loss.

SPECIAL CONSIDERATIONS

If the patient is alert, elevate the head of the bed to make his breathing as easy as possible. Encourage him to get plenty of rest and to drink plenty of fluids to liquefy secretions. Administer oxygen. Prepare him for such tests as pulmonary function studies, chest X-rays, lung scans, arterial blood gas analysis, complete blood count, and sputum culture.

PEDIATRIC POINTERS

Because an infant's or a child's accessory muscles tire sooner than an adult's muscles, these patients are more likely to encounter respiratory distress that can rapidly precipitate respiratory failure. Upper airway obstruction — caused by edema, bronchospasm, or a foreign object — usually produces respiratory distress and increased accessory muscle use. Disorders associated with airway obstruction include acute epiglottitis, croup, pertussis, cystic fibrosis, and asthma. Supraventricular, intercostal, or abdominal retractions indicate accessory muscle use.

GERIATRIC POINTERS

Because of age-related loss of elasticity in the rib cage, accessory muscle use may be part of an older person's normal breathing pattern.

PATIENT COUNSELING

Because labored breathing can make the patient apprehensive, provide a calm environment and encourage him to perform relaxation techniques while you provide interventions to reduce the work of breathing.

Medical causes
(continued)

Pulmonary embolism
+ Accessory muscle use may increase.

Spinal cord injury
+ Injury between C3 and C5 affects the upper respiratory muscles and diaphragm, causing increased accessory muscle use.

Thoracic injury
+ Increased accessory muscle use may occur depending on the type and extent of injury.

Special considerations
+ If the patient is alert, elevate the head of the bed to make his breathing as easy as possible.
+ Encourage the patient to get plenty of rest and to drink plenty of fluids to liquefy secretions.
+ Administer oxygen.

Peds points
+ Upper airway obstruction usually produces respiratory distress and increased accessory muscle use.
+ Disorders associated with airway obstruction include acute epiglottitis, croup, pertussis, cystic fibrosis, and asthma.
+ Supraventricular, intercostal, or abdominal retractions indicate accessory muscle use.

Geri points
+ Because of age-related loss of elasticity in the rib cage, accessory muscle use may be part of an older person's normal breathing pattern.

Teaching points

+ Relaxation techniques
+ Resources to stop smoking
+ Measures to prevent infection
+ Explanation of prescribed drugs
+ Pursed-lip, diaphragmatic breathing
+ Coughing and deep-breathing exercises

Key facts about agitation

+ Refers to a state of hyperarousal, increased tension, and irritability
+ Can lead to confusion, hyperactivity, and overt hostility
+ Can arise gradually or suddenly
+ Can last for minutes or months

Key history points

+ Severity of agitation
+ Diet and known allergies
+ Past or present illnesses, trauma, stress, and sleep patterns
+ Drug and alcohol use

Critical assessment steps

+ Check for signs of drug abuse.
+ Obtain baseline vital signs and neurologic status.

Medical causes

Affective disturbance

+ Agitation may occur in depressed and manic phases and in personality disorders.
+ Psychomotor agitation may involve an inability to sit still, hand-wringing, pacing, and irritability.

Alcohol withdrawal syndrome

+ Mild to severe agitation occurs along with hyperactivity, tremors, and anxiety.

If appropriate, stress how smoking endangers the patient's health, and refer him to an organized program to stop smoking. Also, teach him how to prevent infection. Explain the purpose of prescribed drugs, such as bronchodilators and mucolytics, and make sure he knows their dosage and schedule.

Show the patient with a chronic lung disorder how to perform pursed-lip, diaphragmatic breathing and coughing and deep-breathing exercises.

AGITATION

Agitation refers to a state of hyperarousal, increased tension, and irritability that can lead to confusion, hyperactivity, and overt hostility. Agitation can result from a toxic (poisons), metabolic, or infectious cause; brain injury; or a psychiatric disorder. It can also result from pain, fever, anxiety, drug use and withdrawal, hypersensitivity reactions, and various disorders. It can arise gradually or suddenly and last for minutes or months. Whether it's mild or severe, agitation worsens with increased fever, pain, stress, or external stimuli.

Agitation alone merely signals a change in the patient's condition. However, it's a useful indicator of a developing disorder.

HISTORY

Determine the severity of the patient's agitation by examining the number and quality of agitation-induced behaviors, such as emotional lability, confusion, memory loss, hyperactivity, and hostility. Obtain a history from the patient or a family member, including diet and known allergies.

Ask if the patient is being treated for any illnesses. Has he had any recent infections, trauma, stress, or changes in sleep patterns? Ask the patient about prescribed or over-the-counter drug use, including supplements and herbal medicines. Ask about alcohol intake.

PHYSICAL ASSESSMENT

Perform a complete physical examination. Check for signs of drug abuse, such as needle tracks and dilated pupils. Obtain baseline vital signs and neurologic status for future comparison.

MEDICAL CAUSES

Affective disturbance

Agitation may occur in depressed and manic phases of affective disturbance and in personality disorders, such as borderline and antisocial personality disorders. In its depressive form, chronic anxiety occurs with varying severity. The hallmark is depressed mood upon awakening, which eases during the day. Psychomotor agitation may be characterized by an inability to sit still, hand-wringing, pacing, and irritability. Other findings in manic states may include decreased sleep, pressured speech, and grandiosity.

Alcohol withdrawal syndrome

With alcohol withdrawal syndrome, mild to severe agitation occurs. It may be accompanied by hyperactivity, tremors, and anxiety. With delirium tremens, the potentially life-threatening stage of alcohol withdrawal, severe agitation accompanies hallucinations, insomnia, diaphoresis, and depressed mood. Pulse rate and temperature rise as withdrawal progresses; status epilepticus, cardiac exhaustion, and shock can occur.

Anxiety

Anxiety produces varying degrees of agitation. The patient may be unaware of his anxiety or may complain of it without knowing its cause. Other findings include nausea, vomiting, diarrhea, cool and clammy skin, frontal headache, back pain, insomnia, and tremors.

Chronic renal failure

Moderate to severe agitation occurs with chronic renal failure, marked especially by confusion and memory loss. The agitation is accompanied by diverse signs and symptoms, such as nausea, vomiting, anorexia, mouth ulcers, ammonia breath odor, GI bleeding, pallor, edema, dry skin, and uremic frost.

Dementia

Mild to severe agitation related to dementia can result from many common syndromes, such as Alzheimer's and Huntington's diseases. The patient may display a decrease in memory, attention span, problem-solving ability, and alertness. Hypoactivity, wandering behavior, hallucinations, aphasia, and insomnia may also occur.

Drug withdrawal syndrome

In drug withdrawal syndrome, mild to severe agitation occurs. Related findings vary with the drug but include anxiety, abdominal cramps, diaphoresis, and anorexia. With narcotic or barbiturate withdrawal, a decreased level of consciousness (LOC), seizures, and elevated blood pressure, heart rate, and respiratory rate can also occur.

Hepatic encephalopathy

Agitation occurs with fulminating hepatic encephalopathy. Other findings include drowsiness, stupor, fetor hepaticus (musty, sweet breath odor), asterixis, and hyperreflexia. Lethargy, aberrant behavior, and apraxia may also occur.

Hypersensitivity reaction

Moderate to severe agitation may be the first sign of a hypersensitivity reaction. Depending on the severity of the reaction, agitation may be accompanied by urticaria, pruritus, and facial and dependent edema.

With anaphylactic shock, a potentially life-threatening reaction, agitation occurs rapidly along with apprehension, urticaria or diffuse erythema, skin that's warm and moist, paresthesia, pruritus, edema, dyspnea, wheezing, stridor, hypotension, and tachycardia. Abdominal cramps, vomiting, and diarrhea can also occur.

Hypoxemia

Beginning as restlessness, agitation rapidly worsens with hypoxemia. The patient may be confused and have impaired judgment and motor coordination. He may also have tachycardia, tachypnea, dyspnea, and cyanosis.

Increased intracranial pressure

With increased intracranial pressure (ICP), agitation usually precedes other early signs and symptoms, such as headache, nausea, and vomiting. ICP produces respiratory changes, such as Cheyne-Stokes, cluster, ataxic, or apneustic breathing; sluggish, nonreactive, or unequal pupils; widening pulse pressure; tachycardia; decreased LOC; seizures; and motor changes, such as decerebrate or decorticate posture.

Medical causes
(continued)

Anxiety
+ Varying degrees of agitation result.

Chronic renal failure
+ Moderate to severe agitation occurs, marked especially by confusion and memory loss.

Dementia
+ Mild to severe agitation can result from many common syndromes, such as Alzheimer's and Huntington's diseases.

Drug withdrawal syndrome
+ Mild to severe agitation occurs.
+ Related findings vary with the drug but include anxiety, abdominal cramps, diaphoresis, and anorexia.

Hepatic encephalopathy
+ Patients may experience agitation, drowsiness, stupor, fetor hepaticus, asterixis, and hyperreflexia.

Hypersensitivity reaction
+ Moderate to severe agitation may be the first sign.
+ Urticaria, pruritus, and facial and dependent edema may occur.

Hypoxemia
+ Agitation starts as restlessness, then rapidly worsens.

Increased ICP
+ Agitation precedes other early signs and symptoms, such as headache, nausea, and vomiting.

Medical causes
(continued)

Organic brain syndrome
✦ Agitation manifests as hyperactivity, emotional lability, confusion, and memory loss.

Post–head trauma syndrome
✦ Agitation is characterized by disorientation, loss of concentration, angry outbursts, and emotional lability.

Vitamin B$_6$ deficiency
✦ Agitation ranges from mild to severe.
✦ Other effects include seizures, peripheral paresthesia, and dermatitis.

Other causes
✦ CNS stimulants
✦ Radiographic contrast media

Special considerations
✦ Monitor the patient's vital signs and neurologic status.
✦ Eliminate stressors.
✦ Provide adequate lighting.
✦ Maintain a calm environment.
✦ Allow the patient time to sleep.
✦ Ensure a balanced diet, and provide vitamin supplements and hydration.
✦ Remain calm, nonjudgmental, and nonargumentative.

Peds points
✦ In children, agitation accompanies the expected childhood diseases as well as more severe disorders that can lead to brain damage.
✦ In neonates, agitation can stem from alcohol or drug withdrawal.

Organic brain syndrome

With organic brain syndrome, agitation is manifested as hyperactivity, emotional lability, confusion, and memory loss. Slurred or incoherent speech and paranoid behavior may also occur.

Post–head trauma syndrome

Shortly after — or even years after — head trauma, mild to severe agitation develops, characterized by disorientation, loss of concentration, angry outbursts, and emotional lability. Other findings include fatigue, wandering behavior, and poor judgment.

Vitamin B$_6$ deficiency

With vitamin B$_6$ deficiency, agitation can range from mild to severe. Other effects include seizures, peripheral paresthesia, and dermatitis. Oculogyric crisis may also occur.

OTHER CAUSES

Drugs

Mild to moderate agitation, which is commonly dose related, develops as an adverse reaction to central nervous system stimulants — especially appetite suppressants, such as amphetamines and amphetamine-like drugs; sympathomimetics such as ephedrine; caffeine; and theophylline.

Radiographic contrast media

Reaction to the contrast medium injected during various diagnostic tests produces moderate to severe agitation along with other signs of hypersensitivity.

SPECIAL CONSIDERATIONS

Because agitation can be an early sign of many different disorders, continue to monitor the patient's vital signs and neurologic status while the cause is being determined. Eliminate stressors, which can increase agitation. Provide adequate lighting, maintain a calm environment, and allow the patient ample time to sleep. Ensure a balanced diet, and provide vitamin supplements and hydration.

Remain calm, nonjudgmental, and nonargumentative. Use restraints sparingly because they tend to increase agitation. If appropriate, prepare the patient for diagnostic tests, such as computed tomography scanning, skull X-rays, magnetic resonance imaging, and blood studies.

PEDIATRIC POINTERS

A common sign in children, agitation accompanies the expected childhood diseases as well as more severe disorders that can lead to brain damage: hyperbilirubinemia, phenylketonuria, vitamin A deficiency, hepatitis, frontal lobe syndrome, increased ICP, and lead poisoning. In neonates, agitation can stem from alcohol or drug withdrawal if the mother abused these substances.

When evaluating an agitated child, remember to use words that he can understand and to look for nonverbal clues. For instance, if you suspect that pain is causing agitation, ask him to tell you where it hurts, but be sure to watch for other indicators, such as wincing, crying, or moving away.

GERIATRIC POINTERS

Any deviation from an older person's usual activities or rituals may provoke anxiety or agitation. Any environmental change, such as a transfer to a nursing home or a visit from a stranger in the patient's home, may trigger a need for treatment.

PATIENT COUNSELING

Orient the patient with agitation to the unit and its procedures and routines. Provide reassurance and emotional support. Explain the need to reduce stressors and maintain a quiet environment.

Geri points

✦ Deviation from usual activities or an environmental change may provoke agitation.

Teaching points

✦ Orientation to the unit and its procedures and routines
✦ Stress-reduction measures

ALOPECIA

Alopecia (hair loss) usually develops gradually and affects the scalp; it may be diffuse or patchy. It can be classified as scarring or nonscarring. Scarring alopecia (permanent hair loss) results from hair follicle destruction, which smoothes the skin surface, erasing follicular openings. Nonscarring alopecia (temporary hair loss) results from hair follicle damage that spares follicular openings, allowing future hair growth.

One of the most common causes of alopecia is the use of certain chemotherapeutic drugs. Alopecia may also result from the use of other drugs; radiation therapy; a skin, connective tissue, endocrine, nutritional, or psychological disorder; a neoplasm; an infection; a burn; or exposure to toxins. Anxiety, high fever, and even certain hairstyles or grooming methods may also cause alopecia. (See *Recognizing patterns of alopecia,* page 32.)

Aging, genetic predisposition, and hormonal changes may contribute to gradual hair thinning and hairline recession. This type of alopecia occurs in about 40% of adult men and may also occur in postmenopausal women.

 CULTURAL CUE People who have fine and relatively scanty hair, such as natives of tropical areas, may not recognize their alopecia right away.

HISTORY

If the patient isn't receiving a chemotherapeutic drug or radiation therapy, begin by asking when he first noticed the hair loss or thinning. Does it affect the scalp alone, or does it occur elsewhere on the body? Is it accompanied by itching or rashes? Then carefully explore other signs and symptoms to help distinguish between normal and pathologic hair loss. Ask about recent weight change, anorexia, nausea, vomiting, excessive stress, and altered bowel habits. Also ask about urinary tract changes, such as hematuria or oliguria. Has the patient been especially tired or irritable? Does he have a cough or difficulty breathing? Ask about joint pain or stiffness and about heat or cold intolerance. Inquire about exposure to insecticides. If the patient is female, find out if she has had menstrual irregularities and note her pregnancy history. If the patient is male, ask about sexual dysfunction, such as decreased libido or impotence.

Next, ask about hair care. Does the patient frequently use a hot blow-dryer or electric curlers? Does he periodically dye, bleach, or perm his hair? If the patient is black, ask if he uses a hot comb to straighten his hair or a long-toothed comb to achieve an Afro look. Does he ever braid the hair in cornrows? Check for a family history of alopecia, and ask what age relatives were when they started experiencing hair loss. Also ask about nervous habits, such as pulling the hair or twirling it around a finger.

Key facts about alopecia

✦ Loss of hair
✦ Can be scarring (permanent; follicles are destroyed) or nonscarring (temporary; follicles are damaged)

Key history points

✦ Onset of hair loss or thinning
✦ Affected areas
✦ Associated signs and symptoms, such as itching and rashes
✦ Menstrual irregularities (in females)
✦ Sexual dysfunction (in males)
✦ Hair care and habits
✦ Family history

Critical assessment steps

- ✦ Assess the extent and pattern of scalp hair loss.
- ✦ Inspect the underlying skin for follicular openings, erythema, loss of pigment, scaling, induration, broken hair shafts, and hair regrowth.
- ✦ Examine the rest of the skin for jaundice, edema, hyperpigmentation, pallor, or duskiness. Note the size, color, texture, and location of any lesions.
- ✦ Examine nails for vertical or horizontal pitting, thickening, brittleness, or whitening.
- ✦ Palpate for lymphadenopathy, enlarged thyroid or salivary glands, and masses in the abdomen or chest.

Medical causes

Alopecia areata
- ✦ Well-circumscribed patches of nonscarring scalp alopecia develop.
- ✦ Patches of alopecia are bordered by loose hairs with rough, brushlike tips on narrow, less-pigmented shafts.

Recognizing patterns of alopecia

Distinctive patterns of alopecia result from different causes. The illustrations below show four of the most common patterns.

Tinea capitis, a fungal infection, produces irregular bald patches with scaly, red lesions.

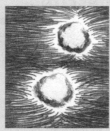

Trauma from habitual hair pulling or injudicious grooming habits may cause permanent peripheral alopecia.

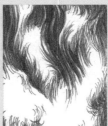

Alopecia areata causes expanding patches of nonscarring hair loss bordered by "exclamation point" hairs.

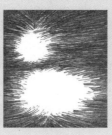

Chemotherapeutic drugs produce diffuse, yet temporary, hair loss.

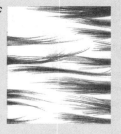

PHYSICAL ASSESSMENT

Begin the physical assessment by taking the patient's vital signs and then assessing the extent and pattern of scalp hair loss. Is it patchy or symmetrical? Is the hair surrounding a bald area brittle or lusterless? Is it a different color from other scalp hair? Does it fall out easily? Inspect the underlying skin for follicular openings, erythema, loss of pigment, scaling, induration, broken hair shafts, and hair regrowth.

Then examine the rest of the skin. Note the size, color, texture, and location of any lesions. Check for jaundice, edema, hyperpigmentation, pallor, or duskiness. Examine nails for vertical or horizontal pitting, thickening, brittleness, or whitening. As you do so, watch for fine tremors in the hands. Observe the patient for muscle weakness and ptosis. Palpate for lymphadenopathy, enlarged thyroid or salivary glands, and masses in the abdomen or chest.

 CULTURAL CUE *Be aware that hair distribution may vary depending on the patient's ethnic background. For example, Chinese males tend to lack facial hair and Koreans tend to have less body hair.*

MEDICAL CAUSES

Alopecia areata
Alopecia areata is usually marked by well-circumscribed patches of nonscarring scalp alopecia without skin changes. Occasionally, the patches also appear on the beard, axillae, pubic area, arms, legs, or the entire body (alopecia universalis). "Exclamation point" hairs—loose hairs with rough, brushlike tips on narrow, less-pigmented shafts—typically border expanding patches of alopecia. Although this disorder is recurrent, hair growth usually returns after several months. In about 20% of patients, alopecia areata also causes horizontal or vertical nail pitting.

Arterial insufficiency

Patchy alopecia occurs with arterial insufficiency, typically on the lower extremities, and is accompanied by thin, shiny, atrophic skin and thickened nails. The skin turns pale when the patient's legs are elevated and dusky when they're dependent. Associated signs include weak or absent peripheral pulses, cool extremities, paresthesia, leg ulcers, and intermittent claudication.

Burns

Full-thickness or third-degree burns completely destroy the dermis and epidermis, leaving translucent, charred, or ulcerated skin. Scarring or keloid formation associated with these burns causes permanent alopecia.

Cutaneous T-cell lymphoma

More common in older patients, cutaneous T-cell lymphoma may be associated with alopecia mucinosa in its first, or premycotic, stage. Scattered papules or plaques may occur on clothed areas, such as breasts and buttocks, or a zebralike pattern of scaly erythema may form on the trunk. Alopecia may persist through the plaque and tumor stages.

Exfoliative dermatitis

With exfoliative dermatitis, a transient disorder, loss of scalp and body hair is preceded by several weeks of generalized scaling and erythema. Nail loss commonly occurs, along with pruritus, malaise, fever, weight loss, lymphadenopathy, and gynecomastia.

Fungal infections

Tinea capitis (scalp ringworm), the most common fungal infection, produces irregular balding areas, scaling, and erythematous lesions. As these lesions enlarge, their centers heal, causing the classic ring-shaped appearance. Surrounding the balding areas are broken scalp hairs. When they break off at the scalp surface, hairs resemble black dots. Other findings include pruritus and thick, whitish nails.

Hodgkin's disease

With Hodgkin's disease, permanent alopecia may occur if the lymphoma infiltrates the scalp. It's accompanied by edema, pruritus, and hyperpigmentation. Associated signs vary with the degree and location of lymphadenopathy.

Hypopituitarism

In adults, hypopituitarism varies greatly, depending on its severity and the number of deficient hormones. Gonadotropin deficiency in the female causes sparse or absent pubic and axillary hair accompanied by infertility, amenorrhea, and breast atrophy. A similar deficiency in the male decreases facial and body hair and causes infertility, decreased libido, impotence, poor muscle development, and undersized testes, penis, and prostate gland. A human growth hormone deficiency at an early age may cause short stature. Deficiency of thyroid-stimulating hormone produces signs of hypothyroidism; deficiency of corticotropin produces signs of adrenocortical insufficiency.

Hypothyroidism

In hypothyroidism, the hair on the face, scalp, and genitals thins and becomes dull, coarse, and brittle. Most characteristic, though, is loss of the outer third of the eyebrows. Typically, it's preceded by fatigue, constipation, cold intolerance, and weight gain. Other signs and symptoms include dry, flaky, inelastic skin; puffy face, hands, and feet; hoarseness; thick, brittle nails; slow mental function; bradycardia; menorrhagia; and myalgia.

Medical causes
(continued)

Arterial insufficiency
+ Patchy alopecia occurs, typically on the lower extremities.

Burns
+ Scarring or keloid formation from full-thickness or third-degree burns causes permanent alopecia.

Cutaneous T-cell lymphoma
+ Alopecia mucinosa may occur in the premycotic stage and may persist through the plaque and tumor stages.

Exfoliative dermatitis
+ Loss of scalp and body hair is preceded by several weeks of generalized scaling and erythema.

Fungal infections
+ Tinea capitis produces irregular balding areas, scaling, and erythematous lesions.

Hodgkin's disease
+ Permanent alopecia may occur if lymphoma infiltrates the scalp.

Hypopituitarism
+ In females, sparse or absent pubic and axillary hair, infertility, and breast atrophy occur.
+ In males, decreased facial and body hair, infertility, decreased libido, impotence, and poor muscle development occur.

Hypothyroidism
+ Hair on the face, scalp, and genitals thins and becomes dull, coarse, and brittle.
+ Hair loss in the outer one-third of the eyebrows occurs.

Medical causes
(continued)
Lupus erythematosus
+ Hair becomes brittle and falls out in patches.
+ Broken hairs commonly appear above the forehead.

Myotonic dystrophy
+ Premature baldness occurs in the adult form.

Protein deficiency
+ Hair becomes brittle, fine, dry, and thin.

Sarcoidosis
+ Scarring alopecia occurs if sarcoidosis infiltrates the scalp.

Seborrheic dermatitis
+ Hair loss on the scalp may occur, beginning at the vertex and frontal areas.

Skin metastasis
+ Scarring alopecia may develop slowly along with scalp induration and atrophy.

Thyrotoxicosis
+ Diffuse hair loss occurs.
+ Hair loss may be accentuated at the temples.

Other causes
+ Allopurinol
+ Antithyroid drugs
+ Beta-adrenergic blockers
+ Carbamazepine
+ Chemotherapeutic agents
+ Colchicine
+ Excessive doses of vitamin A
+ Gentamicin

Lupus erythematosus
Hair loss is a chief complaint of patients with either discoid or systemic lupus. Hair tends to become brittle and may fall out in patches; short, broken hairs (known as *lupus hairs*) commonly appear above the forehead. Both types of lupus are characterized by raised, red, scaling plaques with follicular plugging, telangiectasia, and central atrophy. Facial plaques typically assume a distinctive butterfly pattern.

With systemic lupus, however, the rash may vary in severity from malar erythema to discoid lesions. Unlike discoid lupus, systemic lupus affects multiple body systems. It may produce photosensitivity, weight loss, fatigue, lymphadenopathy, arthritis, emotional lability, and other signs and symptoms.

Myotonic dystrophy
Premature baldness characterizes the adult form of myotonic dystrophy, a muscular dystrophy. However, myotonia — the inability to normally relax a muscle after its contraction — is its primary sign. Associated signs include muscle wasting and cataracts.

Protein deficiency
Protein deficiency produces brittle, fine, dry, and thinning hair and, occasionally, changes in its pigment. Characteristic muscle wasting may be accompanied by edema, hepatomegaly, apathy, irritability, anorexia, diarrhea, and dry, flaky skin.

Sarcoidosis
Sarcoidosis may produce scarring alopecia if it infiltrates the scalp. Accompanied by various lesions on the face and the oral and nasal mucosa, it may also produce fever, weight loss, fatigue, lymphadenopathy, substernal pain, cough, shortness of breath, visual muscle weakness, arthralgia, myalgia, and cranial nerve palsies.

Seborrheic dermatitis
Erupting in areas with many sebaceous glands and in skin folds, seborrheic dermatitis may produce hair loss on the scalp. Alopecia begins at the vertex and frontal areas and may spread to other scalp areas. The patient's skin is reddened and dry with branlike scales that flake off easily. Pruritus is common.

Skin metastasis
Occasionally, cancer from an internal site such as the lung metastasizes to the skin, causing scarring alopecia that may develop slowly along with scalp induration and atrophy. Related findings include weight loss, fever, altered bowel habits, abdominal pain, and lymphadenopathy.

Thyrotoxicosis
Diffuse hair loss, possibly accentuated at the temples, occurs with thyrotoxicosis. Hair becomes fine, soft, and friable. The skin becomes uniformly flushed and thickened, marked by red, raised, pruritic patches. Characteristically, this disorder produces fine tremors, nervousness, an enlarged thyroid, sweating, heat intolerance, amenorrhea, palpitations, weight loss despite increased appetite, diarrhea and, possibly, exophthalmos.

OTHER CAUSES

Drugs
Chemotherapeutic agents — such as bleomycin, cyclophosphamide, dactinomycin, daunorubicin, doxorubicin, fluorouracil, and methotrexate — may cause patchy, reversible alopecia a few weeks after administration. Hair loss is usually limited to the scalp but, with long-term chemotherapy, it may also affect the axillae, arms, legs,

face, and pubic area. New hair, which may differ in thickness, texture, and color from the patient's original hair, may begin to grow after the drug is discontinued or between successive treatments.

Other common drugs may cause diffuse hair loss on the scalp a few weeks after administration. These include allopurinol, antithyroid drugs, beta-adrenergic blockers, carbamazepine, colchicine, gentamicin, heparin, hormonal contraceptives, indomethacin, lithium, methysergide, trimethadione, valproic acid, excessive doses of vitamin A, and warfarin. Hair growth usually returns when these drugs are discontinued.

Radiation therapy

As do certain drugs, radiation therapy produces temporary reversible hair loss a few weeks after exposure. Because X-rays damage hair follicles at the site of therapy, head or scalp X-rays cause the most obvious hair loss.

SPECIAL CONSIDERATIONS

Alopecia can have a devastating impact on the patient's self-image, especially if it's extensive and occurs suddenly, as with chemotherapeutic drugs. Make sure you explain to the patient that this hair loss is reversible. Occasionally, scalp hypothermia methods — such as a cryogen, an ice-filled cap, or a scalp tourniquet — may be used before, during, and after drug administration to cause scalp vasoconstriction, thus decreasing drug delivery to the hair follicles and minimizing hair loss. However, these methods are contraindicated in patients with circulating malignant cancer cells (for example, patients with lymphoma) or scalp metastasis.

A skin biopsy may be performed to determine the cause of the alopecia, especially if skin changes are evident. Microscopic examination of a plucked hair may also aid diagnosis.

For patients with partial baldness or alopecia areata, topical application of minoxidil (a common antihypertensive that also produces hair growth) for several months stimulates localized hair growth. However, hair loss may recur if the drug is discontinued.

PEDIATRIC POINTERS

Alopecia normally occurs during the first 6 months of life, as either a sudden, diffuse hair loss or a gradual thinning that's hardly noticeable. Reassure the infant's parents that this hair loss is normal and temporary. If bald areas result because the infant is left in one position for too long, advise the parents to change his position regularly.

Common causes of alopecia in children include use of chemotherapy or radiation therapy, seborrheic dermatitis (known as *cradle cap*), alopecia mucinosa, tinea capitis, and hypopituitarism. Tinea capitis may produce a kerion lesion — a boggy, raised, tender, and hairless lesion. Trichotillomania, a psychological disorder more common in children than adults, may produce patchy baldness with stubby hair growth due to habitual hair pulling. Other causes include progeria and congenital hair shaft defects such as trichorrhexis nodosa.

PATIENT COUNSELING

Encourage gentle hair care to avoid further hair loss. Also, suggest a wig, cap, or scarf, if appropriate. Remind the patient to cover his head in cold weather to prevent loss of body heat. Encourage patients who are frequently exposed to the sun to use sunblock to decrease the risk of skin cancer.

Other causes
(continued)
+ Heparin
+ Hormonal contraceptives
+ Indomethacin
+ Lithium
+ Methysergide
+ Radiation therapy
+ Trimethadione
+ Valproic acid
+ Warfarin
+ Radiation therapy

Special considerations
+ Explain to the patient that hair loss resulting from chemotherapy is reversible.
+ A skin biopsy may be performed.
+ Microscopic examination of a plucked hair may aid diagnosis.
+ For patients with partial baldness or alopecia areata, topical application of minoxidil for several months stimulates localized hair growth.

Peds points
+ Alopecia normally occurs during the first 6 months of life.
+ Common causes of alopecia in children include use of chemotherapy or radiation therapy, seborrheic dermatitis, alopecia mucinosa, tinea capitis, hypopituitarism, trichotillomania, progeria, and congenital hair shaft defects.

Teaching points
+ Hair care
+ Head wear and hairpieces, if appropriate
+ Head protection (sunblock, hat)

AMENORRHEA

The absence of menstrual flow, amenorrhea can be classified as primary or secondary. With primary amenorrhea, menstruation fails to begin before age 16. With secondary amenorrhea, it begins at an appropriate age but later ceases for 3 or more months in the absence of normal physiologic causes, such as pregnancy, lactation, or menopause.

Pathologic amenorrhea results from anovulation or physical obstruction to menstrual outflow, such as from an imperforate hymen, cervical stenosis, or intrauterine adhesions. Anovulation itself may result from hormonal imbalance, debilitating disease, stress or emotional disturbances, strenuous exercise, malnutrition, obesity, or anatomic abnormalities, such as congenital absence of the ovaries or uterus. Amenorrhea may also result from drug or hormonal treatments. (See *How amenorrhea develops,* pages 38 and 39.)

HISTORY

Begin by determining whether the amenorrhea is primary or secondary. If it's primary, ask the patient at what age her mother first menstruated because age of menarche is fairly consistent in families. Form an overall impression of the patient's physical, mental, and emotional development because these factors as well as heredity and climate may delay menarche until after age 16.

If menstruation began at an appropriate age but has since ceased, determine the frequency and duration of the patient's previous menses. Ask her about the onset and nature of any changes in her normal menstrual pattern, and determine the date of her last menses. Find out if she has noticed any related signs, such as breast swelling or weight changes.

Determine when the patient last had a physical examination. Review her health history, noting especially any long-term illnesses such as anemia or use of hormonal contraceptives. Ask about exercise habits, especially running, and whether she experiences stress on the job or at home. Probe the patient's eating habits, including the number and size of daily meals and snacks, and ask if she has gained weight recently.

PHYSICAL ASSESSMENT

Observe her appearance for secondary sex characteristics or signs of virilization. If you're responsible for performing a pelvic examination, check for anatomic aberrations of the outflow tract, such as cervical adhesions, fibroids, or an imperforate hymen.

MEDICAL CAUSES

Adrenal tumor

In a patient with an adrenal tumor, amenorrhea may be accompanied by acne, thinning scalp hair, hirsutism, increased blood pressure, truncal obesity, and psychotic changes. Asymmetrical ovarian enlargement in conjunction with rapid onset of virilizing signs is usually indicative.

Adrenocortical hyperplasia

In a patient with adrenocortical hyperplasia, amenorrhea precedes characteristic cushingoid signs, such as truncal obesity, moon face, buffalo hump, bruises, purple striae, hypertension, renal calculi, psychiatric disturbances, and widened pulse pressure. Acne, thinning scalp hair, and hirsutism typically appear.

Adrenocortical hypofunction

Besides amenorrhea, adrenocortical hypofunction may cause fatigue, irritability, weight loss, increased pigmentation (including bluish black discoloration of the areolas and mucous membranes of the lips, mouth, rectum, and vagina), nausea, vomiting, and orthostatic hypotension.

Anorexia nervosa

Anorexia nervosa, a psychological disorder, can cause either primary or secondary amenorrhea. Related findings include significant weight loss, a thin or emaciated appearance, compulsive behavior patterns, blotchy or sallow complexion, constipation, reduced libido, decreased pleasure in once-enjoyable activities, dry skin, loss of scalp hair, lanugo on the face and arms, skeletal muscle atrophy, and sleep disturbances.

Congenital absence of the ovaries and uterus

Congenital absence of the ovaries and uterus results in primary amenorrhea and absence of secondary sex characteristics. Primary amenorrhea occurs with congenital absence of the uterus. The patient may not develop breasts.

Corpus luteum cysts

Corpus luteum cysts may cause sudden amenorrhea as well as acute abdominal pain and breast swelling. Examination may reveal a tender adnexal mass and vaginal and cervical hyperemia.

Hypothyroidism

Deficient thyroid hormone levels can cause primary or secondary amenorrhea. Typically vague, early findings include fatigue, forgetfulness, cold intolerance, unexplained weight gain, and constipation. Subsequent signs include bradycardia; decreased mental acuity; dry, flaky, inelastic skin; puffy face, hands, and feet; hoarseness; periorbital edema; ptosis; dry, sparse hair; and thick, brittle nails. Other common findings include anorexia, abdominal distention, decreased libido, ataxia, intention tremor, nystagmus, and delayed reflex relaxation time, especially in the Achilles tendon.

Pituitary infarction

Pituitary infarction usually causes postpartum failure to lactate and failure to resume menses. Although associated signs and symptoms depend on the infarction's severity, they include headaches, visual field defects, oculomotor palsies, and an altered level of consciousness. The patient may also lose pubic and axillary hair.

Pituitary tumor

Amenorrhea may be the first sign of a pituitary tumor. Associated findings include headache, vision disturbances such as bitemporal hemianopia, and acromegaly. Cushingoid signs include moon face, buffalo hump, hirsutism, hypertension, truncal obesity, bruises, purple striae, widened pulse pressure, and psychiatric disturbances.

Polycystic ovary syndrome

In polycystic ovary syndrome, menarche typically occurs at a normal age and is followed by irregular menstrual cycles, oligomenorrhea, and secondary amenorrhea or periods of profuse bleeding may alternate with periods of amenorrhea. Obesity, hirsutism, slight deepening of the voice, and enlarged, "oysterlike" ovaries may also accompany this disorder.

Medical causes
(continued)

Adrenocortical hypofunction
- ✦ Amenorrhea, fatigue, irritability, weight loss, increased pigmentation, nausea, vomiting, and orthostatic hypotension may result.

Anorexia nervosa
- ✦ Primary or secondary amenorrhea may occur.
- ✦ Characteristic related findings include weight loss, emaciated appearance, and dry skin.

Congenital absence of ovaries and uterus
- ✦ Primary amenorrhea and absence of secondary sex characteristics occur.

Corpus luteum cysts
- ✦ Amenorrhea may be sudden.
- ✦ Abdominal pain and breast swelling may develop.

Hypothyroidism
- ✦ Amenorrhea may be primary or secondary.

Pituitary infarction
- ✦ The postpartum patient fails to lactate and resume menses.

Pituitary tumor
- ✦ Amenorrhea may be the first sign.
- ✦ Associated findings include headache, vision disturbances, and acromegaly.

Polycystic ovary syndrome
- ✦ Irregular menstrual cycles, oligomenorrhea, and secondary amenorrhea or periods of profuse bleeding may alternate with periods of amenorrhea.

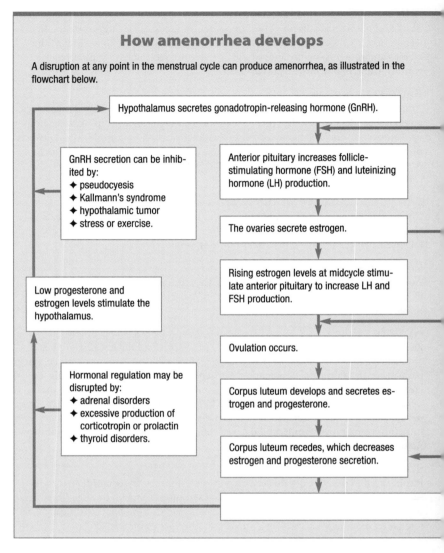

How amenorrhea develops

A disruption at any point in the menstrual cycle can produce amenorrhea, as illustrated in the flowchart below.

Hypothalamus secretes gonadotropin-releasing hormone (GnRH).

GnRH secretion can be inhibited by:
◆ pseudocyesis
◆ Kallmann's syndrome
◆ hypothalamic tumor
◆ stress or exercise.

Anterior pituitary increases follicle-stimulating hormone (FSH) and luteinizing hormone (LH) production.

The ovaries secrete estrogen.

Rising estrogen levels at midcycle stimulate anterior pituitary to increase LH and FSH production.

Low progesterone and estrogen levels stimulate the hypothalamus.

Ovulation occurs.

Hormonal regulation may be disrupted by:
◆ adrenal disorders
◆ excessive production of corticotropin or prolactin
◆ thyroid disorders.

Corpus luteum develops and secretes estrogen and progesterone.

Corpus luteum recedes, which decreases estrogen and progesterone secretion.

Medical causes
(continued)

Pseudoamenorrhea
◆ An anatomic anomaly obstructs menstrual flow, causing primary amenorrhea.

Testicular feminization
◆ Primary amenorrhea may indicate this form of male pseudohermaphroditism.

Thyrotoxicosis
◆ Thyroid hormone overproduction may result in amenorrhea.

Turner's syndrome
◆ Primary amenorrhea and failure to develop secondary sex characteristics may signal this syndrome.

Pseudoamenorrhea
With pseudoamenorrhea, an anatomic anomaly such as imperforate hymen obstructs menstrual flow, causing primary amenorrhea and, possibly, cyclic episodes of abdominal pain. Examination may reveal a pink or blue bulging hymen.

Testicular feminization
Primary amenorrhea may signal testicular feminization, a form of male pseudohermaphroditism. The patient, outwardly female but genetically male, shows breast and external genital development but scant or absent pubic hair.

Thyrotoxicosis
Thyroid hormone overproduction may result in amenorrhea. Classic signs and symptoms include an enlarged thyroid (goiter), nervousness, heat intolerance, diaphoresis, tremors, palpitations, tachycardia, dyspnea, weakness, and weight loss despite increased appetite.

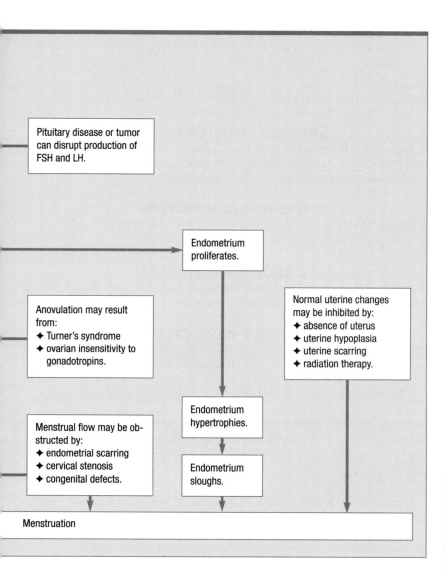

Pituitary disease or tumor can disrupt production of FSH and LH.

Endometrium proliferates.

Anovulation may result from:
◆ Turner's syndrome
◆ ovarian insensitivity to gonadotropins.

Normal uterine changes may be inhibited by:
◆ absence of uterus
◆ uterine hypoplasia
◆ uterine scarring
◆ radiation therapy.

Endometrium hypertrophies.

Menstrual flow may be obstructed by:
◆ endometrial scarring
◆ cervical stenosis
◆ congenital defects.

Endometrium sloughs.

Menstruation

Turner's syndrome

Primary amenorrhea and failure to develop secondary sex characteristics may signal Turner's syndrome, a syndrome of genetic ovarian dysgenesis. Typical features include short stature, webbing of the neck, low nuchal hairline, a broad chest with widely spaced nipples and poor breast development, underdeveloped genitalia, and edema of the legs and feet.

OTHER CAUSES

Drugs

Busulfan, chlorambucil, injectable or implanted contraceptives, cyclophosphamide, and phenothiazines may cause amenorrhea. Hormonal contraceptives may cause anovulation and amenorrhea after they're discontinued.

Other causes
◆ Busulfan
◆ Chlorambucil
◆ Cyclophosphamide
◆ Hormonal contraceptives (when discontinued)
◆ Injectable or implanted contraceptives
◆ Irradiation of the abdomen
◆ Phenothiazines
◆ Surgical removal of both ovaries

Special considerations

+ In patients with secondary amenorrhea, rule out pregnancy before starting diagnostic testing.

Peds points

+ Adolescent girls are prone to amenorrhea caused by emotional upsets stemming from school, social, or family problems.

Geri points

+ In women older than age 50, amenorrhea usually represents the onset of menopause.

Teaching points

+ Explanation of treatment and expected outcomes
+ Discussion of fears
+ Referral to psychological counseling if necessary

Key facts about anhidrosis

+ An abnormal deficiency of sweat
+ Classified as generalized (complete) or localized (partial)
+ Results from neurologic and skin disorders; congenital, atrophic, or traumatic changes to sweat glands; and the use of certain drugs

In an emergency

If anhidrotic asthenia is suspected:
+ Start rapid cooling measures.
+ Frequently check vital signs and neurologic status until the patient's temperature drops below 102° F (38.9° C).
+ Place the patient in an air-conditioned room.

Radiation therapy

Irradiation of the abdomen may destroy the endometrium or ovaries, causing amenorrhea.

Surgery

Surgical removal of both ovaries or the uterus produces amenorrhea.

SPECIAL CONSIDERATIONS

In patients with secondary amenorrhea, physical and pelvic examinations must rule out pregnancy before diagnostic testing begins. Typical tests include progestin withdrawal, serum hormone and thyroid function studies, and endometrial biopsy.

PEDIATRIC POINTERS

Adolescent girls are especially prone to amenorrhea caused by emotional upsets, typically stemming from school, social, or family problems.

GERIATRIC POINTERS

In women older than age 50, amenorrhea usually represents the onset of menopause.

PATIENT COUNSELING

After diagnosis, answer the patient's questions about the type of treatment that will be provided and its expected outcome. Because amenorrhea can cause severe emotional distress, provide emotional support. Be sure to encourage the patient to discuss her fears and, if necessary, refer her for psychological counseling.

ANHIDROSIS

Anhidrosis, an abnormal deficiency of sweat, can be classified as generalized (complete) or localized (partial). Generalized anhidrosis can lead to life-threatening impairment of thermoregulation. Localized anhidrosis rarely interferes with thermoregulation because it affects only a small percentage of the body's eccrine (sweat) glands.

Anhidrosis results from neurologic and skin disorders; congenital, atrophic, or traumatic changes to sweat glands; and the use of certain drugs. Neurologic disorders disturb central or peripheral nervous pathways that normally activate sweating, causing retention of excess body heat and perspiration. The absence, obstruction, atrophy, or degeneration of sweat glands can produce anhidrosis at the skin surface, even if neurologic stimulation is normal.

Anhidrosis may go unrecognized until significant heat or exertion fails to raise sweat. However, localized anhidrosis commonly provokes compensatory hyperhidrosis in the remaining functional sweat glands — which, in many cases, is the patient's chief complaint.

EMERGENCY ACTIONS If you detect anhidrosis in a patient whose skin feels hot and flushed, ask if it's accompanied by nausea, dizziness, palpitations, and substernal tightness. If it is, quickly take a rectal temperature and other vital signs and assess level of consciousness (LOC). If the patient's rectal temperature is higher than 102.2° F (39° C) and is accompanied by tachycardia, tachypnea, altered blood pressure, and decreased LOC, suspect life-threatening anhidrotic asthenia (heatstroke). Start rapid cooling measures, such as immersing the patient in ice or very cold water and giving I.V. fluid replacements. Continue these measures, and frequently check vital signs and neurologic status, until the patient's temperature drops below 102° F (38.9° C). Then place him in an air-conditioned room.

HISTORY

If anhidrosis is localized or the patient reports local hyperhidrosis or unexplained fever, take a brief history. Ask the patient to characterize his sweating during heat spells or strenuous activity. Does he usually sweat slightly or profusely? Ask about recent prolonged or extreme exposure to heat and about the onset of anhidrosis or hyperhidrosis. Obtain a complete medical history, focusing on neurologic disorders, skin disorders such as psoriasis, autoimmune disorders such as scleroderma, systemic diseases that can cause peripheral neuropathies such as diabetes mellitus, and drug use.

PHYSICAL ASSESSMENT

Perform a neurologic assessment to detect a disorder of the central or peripheral nervous system as a cause of anhidrosis. Inspect skin color, texture, and turgor. If you detect any skin lesions, document their location, size, color, texture, and pattern.

MEDICAL CAUSES

Anhidrotic asthenia

Also known as *heatstroke,* anhidrotic asthenia is a life-threatening disorder that causes acute, generalized anhidrosis. In early stages, sweating may still occur and the patient may be rational, but his rectal temperature may already exceed 102.2° F (39° C). Associated signs and symptoms include severe headache and muscle cramps, which later disappear; fatigue; nausea and vomiting; dizziness; palpitations; substernal tightness; and elevated blood pressure followed by hypotension. Within minutes, anhidrosis and hot, flushed skin develop, accompanied by tachycardia, tachypnea, and confusion progressing to seizure or loss of consciousness.

Burns

Depending on their severity, burns may destroy eccrine glands, causing permanent anhidrosis in affected areas. Blistering, edema, and increased pain or loss of sensation may also occur.

Miliaria crystallina

Miliaria crystallina is an usually innocuous form of miliaria that causes anhidrosis and tiny, clear, fragile blisters, usually under the arms and breasts. This form of miliaria typically occurs in the neonate and can be widespread.

Miliaria profunda

If severe and extensive, miliaria profunda can progress to life-threatening anhidrotic asthenia. Typically, it produces localized anhidrosis with compensatory facial hyperhidrosis. Whitish papules appear mostly on the trunk but also on the extremities. Associated signs and symptoms include inguinal and axillary lymphadenopathy, weakness, shortness of breath, palpitations, and fever.

Miliaria rubra

Also known as *prickly heat*, miliaria rubra, which typically produces localized anhidrosis, can progress to life-threatening anhidrotic asthenia if it becomes severe and extensive (although this is a rare occurrence). Small, erythematous papules

Medical causes
(continued)

Nervous system disorders

+ Cerebral cortex and brain stem lesions may cause anhidrotic palms and soles.
+ Peripheral neuropathy causes anhidrosis over the legs.

Spinal cord lesions

+ Anhidrosis may occur symmetrically below the level of the lesion.
+ Compensatory hyperhidrosis occurs in adjacent areas.

Other causes

+ Anticholinergics

Special considerations

To evaluate anhidrosis:
+ Wrap the patient in an electric blanket or place him in a heated box to observe sweat patterns.
+ Apply a topical agent to detect sweat on the skin.
+ Administer a systemic cholinergic drug to stimulate sweating.

Peds points

+ Common causes of anhidrosis in infants include miliaria rubra and congenital skin disorders.
+ Infants are anhidrotic for several weeks after birth.

Teaching points

+ Ways to stay cool, such as maintaining a cool environment, moving slowly during warm weather, and avoiding strenuous exercise and hot foods
+ Anhidrotic effects of drugs

with centrally placed blisters appear on the trunk and neck and, rarely, on the face, palms, or soles. Pustules may also appear in extensive and chronic miliaria. Related symptoms include paroxysmal itching and paresthesia.

Nervous system disorders

Cerebral cortex and brain stem lesions may cause anhidrotic palms and soles, along with various motor and sensory disturbances specific to the site of the lesions.

Anhidrosis over the legs, caused by peripheral neuropathy, commonly appears with compensatory hyperhidrosis over the head and neck. Associated findings mainly involve extremities and include glossy red skin; paresthesia, hyperesthesia, or anesthesia in hands and feet; diminished or absent deep tendon reflexes; flaccid paralysis and muscle wasting; footdrop; and burning pain.

Spinal cord lesions

Anhidrosis may occur symmetrically below the level of a spinal cord lesion, with compensatory hyperhidrosis in adjacent areas. Other findings depend on the site and extent of the lesion but may include partial or total loss of motor and sensory function below the lesion as well as impaired cardiovascular and respiratory function.

OTHER CAUSES

Drugs

Anticholinergics, such as atropine and scopolamine, can cause generalized anhidrosis.

SPECIAL CONSIDERATIONS

Because even a careful evaluation can be inconclusive, you may need to administer specific tests to evaluate anhidrosis. These include wrapping the patient in an electric blanket or placing him in a heated box to observe the skin for sweat patterns, applying a topical agent to detect sweat on the skin, and administering a systemic cholinergic drug to stimulate sweating.

PEDIATRIC POINTERS

In infants and children, miliaria rubra and congenital skin disorders, such as ichthyosis and anhidrotic ectodermal dysplasia, are the most common causes of anhidrosis.

Because delayed development of the thermoregulatory center renders the infant — especially a premature one — anhidrotic for several weeks after birth, caution parents against overdressing their infant.

PATIENT COUNSELING

Advise the patient with anhidrosis to remain in cool environments, to move slowly during warm weather, and to avoid strenuous exercise and hot foods. Warn him about the anhidrotic effects of any drugs he's receiving.

ANOREXIA

Anorexia, a lack of appetite in the presence of a physiologic need for food, is a common symptom of GI and endocrine disorders and is characteristic of certain severe psychological disturbances such as anorexia nervosa. It can also result from such factors as anxiety, chronic pain, poor oral hygiene, increased blood temperature due to hot weather or fever, and changes in taste or smell that normally accompany aging. Anorexia also can result from drug therapy or abuse. Short-term anorexia rarely jeopardizes health, but chronic anorexia can lead to life-threatening malnutrition.

HISTORY

Find out previous minimum and maximum weights. Ask about involuntary weight loss greater than 10 lb (4.5 kg) in the last month. Explore dietary habits, such as when and what the patient eats. Ask what foods he likes and dislikes and why. The patient may identify tastes and smells that nauseate him and cause loss of appetite. Ask about dental problems that interfere with chewing, including poor-fitting dentures. Ask if he has difficulty or pain when swallowing or if he vomits or has diarrhea after meals. Ask the patient how frequently and intensely he exercises.

Check for a history of stomach or bowel disorders, which can interfere with the ability to digest, absorb, or metabolize nutrients. Find out about changes in bowel habits. Ask about alcohol use and drug use and dosage.

If the medical history doesn't reveal an organic basis for anorexia, consider psychological factors. Ask the patient if he knows what's causing his decreased appetite. Situational factors — such as a death in the family or problems at school or at work — can lead to depression and subsequent loss of appetite. Be alert for signs of malnutrition, consistent refusal of food, and a 7% to 10% loss of body weight in the preceding month.

PHYSICAL ASSESSMENT

Perform a complete physical examination. Take the patient's vital signs and weight. (See *Is your patient malnourished?* page 44.)

MEDICAL CAUSES

Acquired immunodeficiency syndrome

With acquired immunodeficiency syndrome (AIDS), an infection or Kaposi's sarcoma affecting the GI or respiratory tract may lead to anorexia. Other findings include fatigue, afternoon fevers, night sweats, diarrhea, cough, bleeding, lymphadenopathy, oral thrush, gingivitis, and skin disorders, including persistent herpes zoster and recurrent herpes simplex, herpes labialis, or herpes genitalis.

Adrenocortical hypofunction

With adrenocortical hypofunction, anorexia may begin slowly and subtly, causing gradual weight loss. Other common signs and symptoms include nausea and vomiting, abdominal pain, diarrhea, weakness, fatigue, malaise, vitiligo, bronze-colored skin, and purple striae on the breasts, abdomen, shoulders, and hips.

Alcoholism

Chronic anorexia commonly accompanies alcoholism, eventually leading to malnutrition. Other findings include signs of liver damage (jaundice, spider angiomas, ascites, edema), paresthesia, tremors, increased blood pressure, bruising, GI bleeding, and abdominal pain.

Anorexia nervosa

With anorexia nervosa, chronic anorexia begins insidiously and eventually leads to life-threatening malnutrition, as evidenced by skeletal muscle atrophy, loss of fatty tissue, constipation, amenorrhea, dry and blotchy or sallow skin, alopecia, sleep disturbances, distorted self-image, anhedonia, and decreased libido. Paradoxically,

---

Is your patient malnourished?

When assessing a patient with anorexia, be sure to check for these common signs of malnutrition.

HAIR
- Dull, dry, thin, fine, straight, and easily plucked
- Areas of light or dark spots and hair loss

FACE
- Generalized swelling
- Dark areas on cheeks and under eyes
- Lumpy or flaky skin around the nose and mouth
- Enlarged parotid glands

EYES
- Dull appearance
- Dry and either pale or red membranes
- Triangular, shiny gray spots on conjunctivae
- Red, fissured eyelid corners
- Bloodshot ring around cornea

LIPS
- Red and swollen, especially at corners

TONGUE
- Swollen, purple, and raw-looking, with sores or abnormal papillae

TEETH
- Missing, or emerging abnormally
- Visible cavities or dark spots
- Spongy, bleeding gums

NECK
- Swollen thyroid gland

SKIN
- Dry, flaky, swollen, and dark, with lighter or darker spots, some resembling bruises
- Tight and drawn, with poor skin turgor

NAILS
- Spoon-shaped, brittle, and ridged

MUSCULOSKELETAL SYSTEM
- Muscle wasting
- Knock-knee or bowlegs
- Bumps on ribs
- Swollen joints
- Musculoskeletal hemorrhages

CARDIOVASCULAR SYSTEM
- Heart rate above 100 beats/minute
- Arrhythmias
- Elevated blood pressure

ABDOMEN
- Enlarged liver and spleen

REPRODUCTIVE SYSTEM
- Decreased libido
- Amenorrhea

NERVOUS SYSTEM
- Irritability
- Confusion
- Paresthesia in hands and feet
- Loss of proprioception
- Decreased ankle and knee reflexes

Medical causes
(continued)

Appendicitis
- Anorexia follows the abrupt onset of generalized or localized epigastric pain, nausea, and vomiting.
- Anorexia can continue as pain localizes in the right lower quadrant (McBurney's point) and other signs and symptoms appear.

Cancer
- Chronic anorexia occurs along with possible weight loss, weakness, apathy, and cachexia.

the patient commonly exhibits extreme restlessness and vigor and may exercise avidly. Many patients also have complicated food preparation and eating rituals.

Appendicitis
With appendicitis, anorexia closely follows the abrupt onset of generalized or localized epigastric pain, nausea, and vomiting. It can continue as pain localizes in the right lower quadrant (McBurney's point) and other signs and symptoms appear: abdominal rigidity, rebound tenderness, constipation (or diarrhea), slight fever, and tachycardia.

Cancer
With cancer, chronic anorexia occurs along with possible weight loss, weakness, apathy, and cachexia. Other findings may include nausea, vomiting, oral lesions, and changes in bowel habits.

Chronic renal failure

Chronic anorexia is common and insidious in chronic renal failure. It's accompanied by changes in all body systems, such as nausea, vomiting, mouth ulcers, ammonia breath odor, metallic taste in the mouth, GI bleeding, constipation or diarrhea, drowsiness, confusion, tremors, pallor, dry and scaly skin, pruritus, alopecia, purpuric lesions, and edema.

Cirrhosis

With cirrhosis, anorexia occurs early and may be accompanied by weakness, nausea, vomiting, constipation or diarrhea, and dull abdominal pain. It continues after these early signs and symptoms subside and is accompanied by lethargy, slurred speech, bleeding tendencies, ascites, severe pruritus, dry skin, poor skin turgor, hepatomegaly, fetor hepaticus, jaundice, edema of the legs, gynecomastia, and right-upper-quadrant pain.

Crohn's disease

With Crohn's disease, chronic anorexia causes marked weight loss. Associated signs vary according to the site and extent of the lesion but may include diarrhea, abdominal pain, fever, abdominal mass, weakness, perianal or vaginal fistulas and, rarely, clubbing of the fingers. Acute inflammatory signs and symptoms — right-lower-quadrant pain, cramping, tenderness, flatulence, fever, nausea, diarrhea (including nocturnal), and bloody stools — mimic those of appendicitis.

Depressive syndrome

Anorexia reflects anhedonia in depressive syndrome. Accompanying signs and symptoms include poor concentration, indecisiveness, delusions, menstrual irregularities, decreased libido, insomnia or hypersomnia, fatigue, mood swings, poor self-image, and gradual social withdrawal.

Gastritis

With acute gastritis, the onset of anorexia may be sudden. The patient may experience postprandial epigastric distress, accompanied by nausea, vomiting (commonly hematemesis), fever, belching, hiccups, and malaise.

Hepatitis

With viral hepatitis (hepatitis A, B, C, or D), anorexia begins in the preicteric phase, accompanied by fatigue, malaise, headache, arthralgia, myalgia, photophobia, nausea and vomiting, mild fever, hepatomegaly, and lymphadenopathy. It may continue through the icteric phase, along with mild weight loss, dark urine, clay-colored stools, jaundice, right-upper-quadrant pain and, possibly, irritability and severe pruritus.

Signs and symptoms of nonviral hepatitis usually resemble those of viral hepatitis but may vary, depending on the cause and extent of liver damage.

Hypopituitarism

Anorexia usually develops slowly in hypopituitarism, which usually begins with hypergonadism. Accompanying signs and symptoms vary with the disorder's severity and the number and type of deficient hormones. Such signs and symptoms include amenorrhea; decreased libido; lethargy; cold intolerance; pale, thin, and dry skin; dry, brittle hair; and decreased temperature, blood pressure, and pulse rate.

Hypothyroidism

Anorexia is common and usually insidious in patients with hypothyroidism (thyroid hormone deficiency). Typically, vague early findings include fatigue, forgetfulness, cold intolerance, unexplained weight gain, and constipation. Subsequent find-

Medical causes
(continued)

Chronic renal failure
- Chronic anorexia is common and insidious.

Cirrhosis
- Anorexia occurs early and continues after other early signs and symptoms subside.
- Weakness, nausea, vomiting, constipation or diarrhea, and dull abdominal pain also occur.

Crohn's disease
- Anorexia causes marked weight loss.
- Associated signs may include diarrhea, abdominal pain, fever, abdominal mass, weakness, perianal or vaginal fistulas and, rarely, clubbing of the fingers.

Depressive syndrome
- Anorexia reflects anhedonia in depressive syndrome.

Gastritis
- Onset of anorexia may be sudden.
- Patient may experience postprandial epigastric distress, accompanied by nausea, vomiting (commonly hematemesis), fever, belching, hiccups, and malaise.

Hepatitis
- In viral hepatitis, anorexia begins in preicteric phase and may continue through icteric phase.

Hypopituitarism
- Anorexia usually develops slowly.
- Accompanying signs and symptoms, such as amenorrhea, decreased libido, and lethargy, vary with the disorder's severity and the number and type of deficient hormones.

Medical causes
(continued)

Hypothyroidism
+ Anorexia is usually insidious.
+ Vague early findings include fatigue, forgetfulness, cold intolerance, unexplained weight gain, and constipation.

Pernicious anemia
+ Insidious anorexia may cause considerable weight loss.

Other causes
+ Amphetamines
+ Chemotherapeutic agents
+ Digoxin toxicity
+ Radiation therapy
+ Some antibiotics
+ Sympathomimetics
+ Total parenteral nutrition

Special considerations
+ Promote protein and calorie intake by providing high-calorie snacks or frequent, small meals.
+ Take a 24-hour diet history daily.
+ Maintain strict calorie and nutrient counts for meals.
+ In severe malnutrition, provide supplemental nutrition.

Peds points
+ Anorexia occurs in many illnesses but usually resolves promptly.
+ In preadolescent or adolescent girls, be alert for subtle signs of anorexia nervosa.

Teaching points
+ Explanation of condition
+ Good nutrition
+ Oral hygiene
+ Target weight, daily weight, and weight log

ings include decreased mental stability; dry, flaky, and inelastic skin; edema of the face, hands, and feet; ptosis; hoarseness; thick, brittle nails; coarse, broken hair; and signs of decreased cardiac output such as bradycardia. Other common findings include abdominal distention, menstrual irregularities, decreased libido, ataxia, intention tremor, nystagmus, dull facial expression, and slow reflex relaxation time.

Pernicious anemia
With pernicious anemia, insidious anorexia may cause considerable weight loss. Related findings include the classic triad of burning tongue, general weakness, and numbness and tingling in the extremities; alternating constipation and diarrhea; abdominal pain; nausea and vomiting; bleeding gums; ataxia; positive Babinski's and Romberg's signs; diplopia and blurred vision; irritability, headache, malaise, and fatigue.

OTHER CAUSES

Drugs
Anorexia results from the use of amphetamines, chemotherapeutic agents, sympathomimetics such as ephedrine, and some antibiotics. It also signals digoxin toxicity.

Radiation therapy
Radiation treatments can cause anorexia, possibly as the result of metabolic disturbances.

Total parenteral nutrition
Maintenance of blood glucose levels by I.V. therapy may cause anorexia.

SPECIAL CONSIDERATIONS
Because the causes of anorexia are diverse, diagnostic procedures may include thyroid function studies, endoscopy, upper GI series, gallbladder series, barium enema, liver and kidney function tests, hormone assays, computed tomography scans, ultrasonography, and blood studies to assess nutritional status.

Promote protein and calorie intake by providing high-calorie snacks or frequent, small meals. You should encourage the patient's family to supply his favorite foods to help stimulate his appetite. Take a 24-hour diet history daily. The patient may consistently exaggerate his food intake (common in patients with anorexia nervosa), so you'll need to maintain strict calorie and nutrient counts for the patient's meals. In severe malnutrition, provide supplemental nutrition, such as total parenteral nutrition or oral nutritional supplements.

Because anorexia and poor nutrition increase susceptibility to infection, monitor the patient's vital signs and white blood cell count and closely observe any wounds.

PEDIATRIC POINTERS
In children, anorexia commonly accompanies many illnesses but usually resolves promptly. However, if the patient is a preadolescent or adolescent girl, be alert for subtle signs of anorexia nervosa.

PATIENT COUNSELING
Teach the patient about his specific condition. Also teach him the importance of good nutrition. Encourage him to perform oral hygiene before meals. Review the patient's target weight and instruct him to weigh himself and keep a weight log.

ANOSMIA

Although usually an insignificant consequence of nasal congestion or obstruction, anosmia—absence of the sense of smell—occasionally heralds a serious defect. Temporary anosmia can result from any condition that irritates and causes swelling of the nasal mucosa and obstructs the olfactory area in the nose, such as heavy smoking, rhinitis, or sinusitis. Permanent anosmia usually results when the olfactory neuroepithelium or any part of the olfactory nerve is destroyed. Permanent or temporary anosmia can also result from inhaling irritants, such as cocaine or acid fumes, that paralyze nasal cilia. Anosmia may also be reported—without an identifiable organic cause—by patients suffering from hysteria, depression, or schizophrenia.

Because combined stimulation of taste buds and olfactory cells produces the sense of taste, anosmia is usually accompanied by ageusia, loss of the sense of taste.

HISTORY

Begin the patient history by asking about the onset and duration of anosmia and related signs and symptoms—stuffy nose, nasal discharge or bleeding, postnasal drip, sneezing, dry or sore mouth and throat, loss of sense of taste or appetite, excessive tearing, and facial or eye pain. Pinpoint any history of nasal disease, allergies, or head trauma. Ask about heavy smoking and the use of prescribed or over-the-counter nose drops or nasal sprays. Be sure to rule out cocaine use.

PHYSICAL ASSESSMENT

Inspect and palpate nasal structures for obvious injury, inflammation, deformities, and septal deviation or perforation. Observe the contour and color of the nasal mucosa and the size and color of the turbinates. Check for polyps, which appear as translucent, white masses around the middle meatus. Note the source and character of any nasal discharge. Palpate the sinus areas for tenderness and contour.

Assess the patient for nasal obstruction by occluding one nostril at a time with your thumb as the patient breathes quietly; listen for breath sounds and for sounds of moisture or mucus. Test olfactory nerve (cranial nerve I) function by having the patient identify common odors.

MEDICAL CAUSES

Anterior cerebral artery occlusion
Permanent anosmia may follow vascular damage involving the olfactory nerve in anterior cerebral artery occlusion. Associated signs and symptoms include contralateral weakness and numbness (especially in the leg), confusion, and impaired motor and sensory functions.

Degenerative brain disease
Anosmia may accompany Alzheimer's disease, Parkinson's disease, and other degenerative central nervous system disorders. Associated findings include dementia, tremor, rigidity, and gait disturbance.

Head trauma
Permanent anosmia may follow head trauma that results in damage to the olfactory nerve. Associated findings depend on the type and severity of the trauma but may include epistaxis, headache, nausea and vomiting, altered level of consciousness, blurred or double vision, raccoon eyes, Battle's sign, and otorrhea.

Medical causes
(continued)

Lead poisoning
- Anosmia may be permanent or temporary, depending on the extent of damage to the nasal mucosa.

Neoplasm (brain, nasal, or sinus)
- Anosmia may be permanent if a neoplasm destroys or displaces the olfactory nerve.

Pernicious anemia
- Anosmia may be temporary or permanent.
- Symptom is accompanied by the classic triad of weakness; sore, pale tongue; and numbness and tingling in the extremities.

Polyps
- Temporary anosmia occurs when multiple polyps obstruct nasal cavities.

Rhinitis
- Temporary anosmia occurs.

Septal fracture
- Anosmia is usually temporary, caused by airflow obstruction.
- Septal repositioning alleviates the symptom.

Septal hematoma
- Anosmia is temporary, resolving with repair of the nasal mucosa or absorption of the hematoma.

Sinusitis
- Anosmia is temporary.

Lead poisoning
Anosmia related to lead poisoning may be permanent or temporary, depending on the extent of damage to the nasal mucosa. Associated findings include abdominal pain, weakness, headache, nausea, vomiting, constipation, wristdrop or footdrop, lead line on the gums, metallic taste, seizures, delirium and, possibly, coma.

Neoplasm (brain, nasal, or sinus)
Anosmia may be permanent if a neoplasm destroys or displaces the olfactory nerve. Associated signs and symptoms include unilateral or bilateral epistaxis, swelling and tenderness in the affected area, vision disturbances, decreased tearing, and elevated intracranial pressure.

Pernicious anemia
With pernicious anemia, anosmia may be temporary or permanent and is accompanied by the classic triad of weakness; sore, pale tongue; and numbness and tingling in the extremities. Related findings include distortion of taste, pallor, headache, irritability, dizziness, nausea, vomiting, diarrhea, and shortness of breath.

Polyps
Temporary anosmia occurs when multiple polyps obstruct nasal cavities. Nasal obstruction may also be accompanied by a sensation of fullness in the face, nasal discharge, headache, and shortness of breath. Associated clinical features are usually the same as those of allergic rhinitis. Examination reveals the smooth, pale, grape-like polyp clusters.

Rhinitis
With common acute *viral rhinitis*, temporary anosmia occurs with nasal congestion; sneezing; watery or purulent nasal discharge; red, swollen nasal mucosa; dryness or a tickling sensation in the nasopharynx; headache; low-grade fever; and chills.

With *allergic rhinitis*, temporary anosmia accompanies nasal congestion; itching mucosa; pale, edematous turbinates; thin nasal discharge; sneezing; tearing; and headache.

With *atrophic rhinitis*, anosmia resolves with successful treatment of the disorder. Purulent, yellow-green, foul-smelling crusts on sclerotic mucous membranes are characteristic, with paradoxical nasal congestion in an airway that's more open than normal. Turbinates are thin and atrophic. The nasopharynx and pharynx appear smooth, dry, and shiny, rather than pink and moist.

With *vasomotor rhinitis*, temporary anosmia is accompanied by chronic nasal congestion, watery nasal discharge, postnasal drip, sneezing, and pale nasal mucosa.

Septal fracture
Anosmia resulting from septal fracture is usually temporary, caused by airflow obstruction, and returns with septal repositioning. Examination reveals septal deviation, swelling, epistaxis, hematoma, nasal congestion, and ecchymoses.

Septal hematoma
Anosmia resulting from septal hematoma is temporary, resolving with repair of the nasal mucosa or absorption of the hematoma. Associated signs and symptoms include epistaxis; dusky red, inflamed nasal mucosa; headache; and mouth breathing.

Sinusitis
With sinusitis, temporary anosmia may be associated with nasal congestion; sinus pain, tenderness, and swelling; severe headache; watery or purulent nasal discharge;

postnasal drip; inflamed throat and nasal mucosa; enlarged, purulent turbinates; malaise; low-grade fever; and chills.

OTHER CAUSES

Drugs
Anosmia can result from prolonged use of nasal decongestants, which produces rebound nasal congestion. Occasionally, it results from naphazoline, a local decongestant that may paralyze nasal cilia. It can also result from reserpine and, less commonly, amphetamines, phenothiazines, and estrogen, which cause nasal congestion.

Radiation therapy
Permanent anosmia may follow radiation damage to the nasal mucosa or olfactory nerve.

Surgery
Temporary anosmia may result from damage to the olfactory nerve or nasal mucosa during nasal or sinus surgery. Permanent anosmia accompanies a permanent tracheostomy, which disrupts nasal breathing.

SPECIAL CONSIDERATIONS

If anosmia results from nasal congestion, administer a local decongestant or antihistamine and provide a vaporizer or humidifier to prevent mucosal drying and to help thin purulent nasal discharge. Advise the patient to avoid excessive use of local decongestants, which can lead to rebound nasal congestion.

If anosmia doesn't result from simple nasal congestion, prepare the patient for diagnostic tests, such as sinus transillumination, skull X-ray, or computed tomography scan.

Although permanent anosmia usually doesn't respond to treatment, vitamin A given orally or by injection occasionally provides improvement.

PEDIATRIC POINTERS

Anosmia in children usually results from nasal obstruction by a foreign body or enlarged adenoids.

PATIENT COUNSELING

Advise the patient not to overuse nose drops and sprays. If the patient breathes through his mouth because of nasal obstruction or congestion, encourage oral hygiene.

ANURIA

Clinically defined as urine output of less than 100 ml in 24 hours, anuria indicates either urinary tract obstruction or acute renal failure due to various mechanisms. (See *Major causes of acute renal failure,* page 50.) Fortunately, anuria is rare; even in renal failure the kidneys usually produce at least 75 ml of urine daily.

Because urine output is easily measured, anuria rarely goes undetected. However, without immediate treatment, it can rapidly cause uremia and other complications of urine retention.

Other causes
+ Amphetamines
+ Estrogen
+ Nasal or sinus surgery
+ Phenothiazines
+ Prolonged use of decongestants
+ Radiation therapy
+ Reserpine

Special considerations
For anosmia from nasal congestion:
+ Give a local decongestant or antihistamine.
+ Provide a vaporizer or humidifier.
+ Advise against excessive use of local decongestants.

Peds points
+ Anosmia in children usually results from nasal obstruction by a foreign body or enlarged adenoids.

Teaching points
+ Proper use of nose drops and sprays
+ Oral hygiene

Key facts about anuria
+ Clinically defined as urine output of less than 100 ml in 24 hours
+ Indicates either urinary tract obstruction or acute renal failure

In an emergency

◆ Determine if urine formation is occurring and intervene appropriately.
◆ Prepare to catheterize.
◆ If you collect more than 75 ml of urine, suspect lower urinary tract obstruction.
◆ If you collect less than 75 ml, suspect renal dysfunction or obstruction higher in the urinary tract.

Key history points

◆ Changes in voiding pattern
◆ Amount of fluid normally ingested and amount ingested in last 24 to 48 hours
◆ Time and amount of last urination
◆ Previous renal or urinary tract disease
◆ Drug use
◆ Previous abdominal, renal, or urinary tract surgery

Critical assessment steps

◆ Inspect and palpate the abdomen for asymmetry, distention, or bulging.
◆ Inspect the flank area for edema or erythema; percuss and palpate the bladder.
◆ Palpate the kidneys anteriorly and posteriorly, and percuss them at the costovertebral angle.

Medical causes

Acute tubular necrosis
◆ Anuria occurs occasionally; oliguria is more common.

Glomerulonephritis (acute)
◆ Anuria or oliguria occurs.

Major causes of acute renal failure

PRERENAL CAUSES
◆ Decreased cardiac output
◆ Hypovolemia
◆ Peripheral vasodilation
◆ Renovascular obstruction
◆ Severe vasoconstriction

INTRARENAL CAUSES
◆ Acute tubular necrosis
◆ Glomerulonephritis
◆ Renovascular occlusion
◆ Vasculitis

POSTRENAL CAUSES
◆ Bladder obstruction
◆ Ureteral obstruction
◆ Urethral obstruction

EMERGENCY ACTIONS After detecting anuria, your priorities are to determine if urine formation is occurring and to intervene appropriately. Prepare to catheterize the patient to relieve any lower urinary tract obstruction and to check for residual urine. You may find that an obstruction hinders catheter insertion and that urine return is cloudy and foul smelling. If you collect more than 75 ml of urine, suspect lower urinary tract obstruction; if you collect less than 75 ml, suspect renal dysfunction or obstruction higher in the urinary tract.

HISTORY

Begin by obtaining a complete history. First ask about any changes in the patient's voiding pattern. Determine the amount of fluid he normally ingests each day, the amount of fluid he ingested in the last 24 to 48 hours, and the time and amount of his last urination. Review his medical history, noting especially previous kidney disease, urinary tract obstruction or infection, prostate enlargement, renal calculi, neurogenic bladder, or congenital abnormalities. Ask about drug use and about any abdominal, renal, or urinary tract surgery.

PHYSICAL ASSESSMENT

Take the patient's vital signs. Inspect and palpate the abdomen for asymmetry, distention, or bulging. Inspect the flank area for edema or erythema, and percuss and palpate the bladder. Palpate the kidneys both anteriorly and posteriorly, and percuss them at the costovertebral angle. Auscultate over the renal arteries, listening for bruits.

MEDICAL CAUSES

Acute tubular necrosis
Oliguria (occasionally anuria) is a common finding in acute tubular necrosis. It precedes the onset of diuresis, which is heralded by polyuria. Associated findings reflect the underlying cause and may include signs and symptoms of hyperkalemia (muscle weakness, cardiac arrhythmias), uremia (anorexia, nausea, vomiting, confusion, lethargy, twitching, seizures, pruritus, uremic frost, and Kussmaul's respirations), and heart failure (edema, jugular vein distention, crackles, and dyspnea).

Glomerulonephritis (acute)
Acute glomerulonephritis produces anuria or oliguria. Related effects include mild fever, malaise, flank pain, gross hematuria, facial and generalized edema, elevated blood pressure, headache, nausea, vomiting, abdominal pain, and signs and symptoms of pulmonary congestion (crackles, dyspnea).

Hemolytic-uremic syndrome

Anuria commonly occurs in the initial stages of hemolytic-uremic syndrome and may last from 1 to 10 days. The patient may experience vomiting, diarrhea, abdominal pain, hematemesis, melena, purpura, fever, elevated blood pressure, hepatomegaly, ecchymoses, edema, hematuria, and pallor. He may also show signs of upper respiratory tract infection.

Renal artery occlusion (bilateral)

Bilateral renal artery occlusion produces anuria or severe oliguria, commonly accompanied by severe, continuous upper abdominal and flank pain; nausea and vomiting; decreased bowel sounds; fever up to 102° F (38.9° C); and diastolic hypertension.

Renal vein occlusion (bilateral)

Bilateral renal vein occlusion occasionally causes anuria; more typical signs and symptoms include acute low back pain, fever, flank tenderness, and hematuria. Development of pulmonary emboli—a common complication—produces sudden dyspnea, pleuritic pain, tachypnea, tachycardia, crackles, pleural friction rub and, possibly, hemoptysis.

Urinary tract obstruction

Severe urinary tract obstruction can produce acute and sometimes total anuria, alternating with or preceded by burning and pain on urination, overflow incontinence or dribbling, increased urinary frequency and nocturia, voiding of small amounts, or altered urine stream. Associated findings include bladder distention, pain and a sensation of fullness in the lower abdomen and groin, upper abdominal and flank pain, nausea and vomiting, and signs of secondary infection, such as fever, chills, malaise, and cloudy, foul-smelling urine.

OTHER CAUSES

Diagnostic tests

Contrast media used in radiographic studies can cause nephrotoxicity, producing oliguria and, rarely, anuria.

Drugs

Many classes of drugs can cause anuria or, more commonly, oliguria through their nephrotoxic effects. Antibiotics, especially the aminoglycosides, are the most commonly seen nephrotoxins. Anesthetics, heavy metals, ethyl alcohol, and organic solvents can also be nephrotoxic. Adrenergics and anticholinergics can cause anuria by affecting the nerves and muscles of micturition to produce urine retention.

SPECIAL CONSIDERATIONS

If catheterization fails to initiate urine flow, prepare the patient for diagnostic studies—such as ultrasonography, cystoscopy, retrograde pyelography, and renal scan—to detect any obstruction higher in the urinary tract. If these tests reveal an obstruction, prepare him for immediate surgery to remove the obstruction, and insert a nephrostomy or ureterostomy tube to drain the urine. If these tests fail to reveal an obstruction, prepare the patient for further kidney function studies.

Carefully monitor the patient's vital signs and intake and output, initially saving any urine for inspection. Restrict daily fluid allowance to 600 ml more than the previous day's total urine output. Restrict foods and juices high in potassium and sodium, and make sure the patient maintains a balanced diet with controlled pro-

Hemolytic-uremic syndrome
+ Anuria occurs in the initial stages and lasts 1 to 10 days.

Renal artery occlusion (bilateral)
+ Anuria or severe oliguria occurs.

Renal vein occlusion (bilateral)
+ Anuria sometimes develops with low back pain, fever, flank tenderness, and hematuria.

Urinary tract obstruction
+ Acute or total anuria may alternate with or precede other signs and symptoms.

Other causes
+ Adrenergics, anesthetics, antibiotics, and anticholinergics
+ Contrast media
+ Ethyl alcohol, heavy metals, and organic solvents

Special considerations
+ If there's obstruction, prepare patient for surgery; insert a nephrostomy or ureterostomy tube to drain the urine.
+ Monitor vital signs and intake and output, initially saving urine for inspection.
+ Restrict daily fluid allowance to 600 ml more than the previous day's total urine output.
+ Restrict foods and juices high in potassium and sodium.
+ Have the patient maintain a balanced diet and control protein.
+ Record fluid intake and output, and weigh the patient daily.

Peds points

+ In neonates, anuria is the absence of urine output for 24 hours.
+ Anuria in children commonly results from loss of renal function.

Geri points

+ Hospitalized or bedridden patients may be unable to generate pressure to void if they remain in a supine position.

Teaching tips

+ Fluid and dietary restrictions
+ Nephrostomy or ureterostomy tube care

Key facts about anxiety

+ Produces a nonspecific feeling of uneasiness or dread
+ Causes physical or psychological discomfort (mild) or an incapacitating or life-threatening reaction (severe)

Key history points

+ Chief complaint
+ Duration of anxiety
+ Precipitating or exacerbating factors
+ Medical history, including drug use

tein levels. Provide low-sodium hard candy to help decrease thirst. Record fluid intake and output, and weigh the patient daily.

PEDIATRIC POINTERS

In neonates, anuria is defined as the absence of urine output for 24 hours. It can be classified as primary or secondary. Primary anuria results from bilateral renal agenesis, aplasia, or multicystic dysplasia. Secondary anuria, associated with edema or dehydration, results from renal ischemia, renal vein thrombosis, or congenital anomalies of the genitourinary tract. Anuria in children commonly results from loss of renal function.

GERIATRIC POINTERS

In elderly patients, anuria is a gradually occurring sign of underlying disease. Hospitalized or bedridden elderly patients may be unable to generate the necessary pressure to void if they remain in a supine position.

PATIENT COUNSELING

Teach the patient about maintaining fluid restrictions and about dietary modifications, such as restricting potassium and sodium, as needed. If the patient had a nephrostomy or ureterostomy, show him how to care for the tube.

ANXIETY

A subjective reaction to a real or imagined threat, anxiety is a nonspecific feeling of uneasiness or dread. It may be mild, moderate, or severe. Mild anxiety may cause slight physical or psychological discomfort. Severe anxiety may be incapacitating or even life-threatening.

Everyone experiences anxiety from time to time — it's a normal response to actual danger, prompting the body (through stimulation of the sympathetic and parasympathetic nervous systems) to purposeful action. It's also a normal response to physical and emotional stress, which can be produced by virtually any illness. In addition, anxiety can be precipitated or exacerbated by many nonpathologic factors, including lack of sleep, poor diet, and excessive intake of caffeine or other stimulants. However, excessive, unwarranted anxiety may indicate an underlying psychological problem.

HISTORY

If the patient displays acute, severe anxiety, quickly take his vital signs and determine his chief complaint; this will serve as a guide for how to proceed. For example, if the patient's anxiety occurs with chest pain and shortness of breath, you might suspect myocardial infarction and act accordingly. While examining the patient, try to keep him calm. Suggest relaxation techniques, and talk to him in a reassuring, soothing voice. Uncontrolled anxiety can alter vital signs and exacerbate the causative disorder.

If the patient displays mild or moderate anxiety, ask about its duration. Is the anxiety constant or sporadic? Did he notice any precipitating factors? Find out if the anxiety is exacerbated by stress, lack of sleep, or excessive caffeine intake and alleviated by rest, tranquilizers, or exercise. Obtain a complete medical history, especially noting drug use.

PHYSICAL ASSESSMENT

Perform a physical examination, focusing on any complaints that may trigger or be aggravated by anxiety.

If the patient's anxiety isn't accompanied by significant physical signs, suspect a psychological basis. Determine the patient's level of consciousness (LOC) and observe his behavior. If appropriate, refer the patient for psychiatric evaluation.

MEDICAL CAUSES

Acute respiratory distress syndrome
With acute respiratory distress syndrome (ARDS), acute anxiety occurs along with tachycardia, mental sluggishness and, in severe cases, hypotension. Other respiratory signs and symptoms include dyspnea, tachypnea, intercostal and suprasternal retractions, crackles, and rhonchi.

Anaphylactic shock
Acute anxiety usually signals the onset of anaphylactic shock. It's accompanied by urticaria, angioedema, pruritus, and shortness of breath. Soon, other signs and symptoms develop: light-headedness, hypotension, tachycardia, nasal congestion, sneezing, wheezing, dyspnea, barking cough, abdominal cramps, vomiting, diarrhea, and urinary urgency and incontinence.

Angina pectoris
Acute anxiety may either precede or follow an attack of angina pectoris. An attack produces sharp and crushing substernal or anterior chest pain that may radiate to the back, neck, arms, or jaw. The pain may be relieved by nitroglycerin or rest, which eases anxiety.

Asthma
During allergic asthma attacks, acute anxiety occurs with dyspnea, wheezing, productive cough, accessory muscle use, hyperresonant lung fields, diminished breath sounds, coarse crackles, cyanosis, tachycardia, and diaphoresis.

Autonomic hyperreflexia
The earliest signs of autonomic hyperreflexia may be acute anxiety accompanied by severe headache and dramatic hypertension. Pallor and motor and sensory deficits occur below the level of the lesion; flushing occurs above it.

Cardiogenic shock
With cardiogenic shock, acute anxiety is accompanied by cool, pale, clammy skin; tachycardia; weak, thready pulse; tachypnea; ventricular gallop; crackles; jugular vein distention; decreased urine output; hypotension; narrowing pulse pressure; and peripheral edema.

Chronic obstructive pulmonary disease
Acute anxiety, exertional dyspnea, cough, wheezing, crackles, hyperresonant lung fields, tachypnea, and accessory muscle use characterize chronic obstructive pulmonary disease (COPD). Other signs and symptoms include barrel chest, pursed-lip breathing, and finger clubbing (late in the disease).

Heart failure
Acute anxiety is commonly the first symptom of inadequate oxygenation in a patient with heart failure. Associated findings include restlessness, shortness of breath, tachypnea, decreased LOC, edema, crackles, ventricular gallop, hypotension, diaphoresis, and cyanosis.

Critical assessment steps
+ Focus physical examination on complaints that trigger or are aggravated by anxiety.
+ Assess LOC and observe behavior.

Medical causes

ARDS
+ Acute anxiety occurs along with tachycardia and mental sluggishness.

Anaphylactic shock
+ Acute anxiety signals the onset of anaphylactic shock.

Angina pectoris
+ Acute anxiety may precede or follow an attack.

Asthma
+ Acute anxiety occurs with dyspnea, wheezing, and other signs and symptoms of asthma.

Autonomic hyperreflexia
+ Anxiety, severe headache, and hypertension may be early signs.

Cardiogenic shock
+ Acute anxiety is accompanied by such signs and symptoms as cool, pale, clammy skin; tachycardia; and weak, thready pulse.

COPD
+ Acute anxiety occurs with exertional dyspnea, cough, wheezing, crackles, hyperresonant lung fields, tachypnea, and accessory muscle use.

Heart failure
+ Acute anxiety is a symptom of inadequate oxygenation.

Medical causes
(continued)

Hyperthyroidism
+ Acute anxiety may be an early sign.

Hyperventilation syndrome
+ Anxiety, pallor, circumoral and peripheral paresthesia occur.

Hypochondriasis
+ Patient has mild to moderate chronic anxiety.

Hypoglycemia
+ Anxiety is mild to moderate.

Mitral valve prolapse
+ Patient may feel panic.

Mood disorder
+ Anxiety may be the chief complaint.
+ In depressive form, chronic anxiety occurs with varying severity.

Myocardial infarction
+ Acute anxiety occurs with persistent, crushing substernal pain that may radiate.

Obsessive-compulsive disorder
+ Chronic anxiety occurs along with thoughts or impulses to perform ritualistic acts.
+ Anxiety builds if the patient can't perform rituals.

Pheochromocytoma
+ Acute, severe anxiety accompanies persistent or paroxysmal hypertension.

Phobias
+ Chronic anxiety occurs along with persistent fear of an object, activity, or situation.

Hyperthyroidism

Acute anxiety may be an early sign of hyperthyroidism. Classic signs and symptoms include heat intolerance, weight loss despite increased appetite, nervousness, tremor, palpitations, sweating, an enlarged thyroid, and diarrhea. Exophthalmos may occur.

Hyperventilation syndrome

Hyperventilation syndrome produces acute anxiety, pallor, circumoral and peripheral paresthesia and, occasionally, carpopedal spasms. Other signs and symptoms include chest pain, tachycardia, belching, flatus, and dizziness.

Hypochondriasis

Mild to moderate chronic anxiety occurs with hypochondriasis. The patient focuses more on the belief that he has a specific serious disease than on the actual symptoms. Difficulty swallowing, back pain, light-headedness, and upset stomach are common complaints. The patient tends to "physician hop" and isn't reassured by favorable physical examinations and laboratory test results.

Hypoglycemia

Anxiety resulting from hypoglycemia is usually mild to moderate and associated with hunger, mild headache, palpitations, blurred vision, weakness, and diaphoresis. Other signs and symptoms include nervousness, dizziness, and tingling and numbness around the mouth.

Mitral valve prolapse

Panic may occur in patients with mitral valve prolapse, referred to as the click-murmur syndrome. The disorder also may cause paroxysmal palpitations accompanied by sharp, stabbing, or aching precordial pain. Its hallmark is a midsystolic click, followed by an apical systolic murmur.

Mood disorder

Anxiety may be the patient's chief complaint in the depressive or manic form of mood disorder. With the depressive form, chronic anxiety occurs with varying severity. Associated findings include dysphoria; anger; insomnia or hypersomnia; decreased libido, energy, and concentration; appetite disturbance; multiple somatic complaints; and suicidal thoughts. With the manic form, the patient's chief complaint may be a reduced need for sleep, hyperactivity, increased energy, rapid or pressured speech and, in severe cases, paranoid ideas and other psychotic symptoms.

Myocardial infarction

With myocardial infarction, a life-threatening disorder, acute anxiety commonly occurs with persistent, crushing substernal pain that may radiate to the left arm, jaw, neck, or shoulder blades. It can be accompanied by shortness of breath, nausea, vomiting, diaphoresis, and cool, pale skin.

Obsessive-compulsive disorder

Chronic anxiety occurs with obsessive-compulsive disorder, along with recurrent, unshakable thoughts or impulses to perform ritualistic acts. The patient recognizes these acts as irrational but can't control them. Anxiety builds if he can't perform these acts and diminishes after he does.

Pheochromocytoma

Acute, severe anxiety accompanies the cardinal sign of pheochromocytoma: persistent or paroxysmal hypertension. Common associated signs and symptoms include tachycardia, diaphoresis, orthostatic hypotension, tachypnea, flushing, severe headache, palpitations, nausea, vomiting, epigastric pain, and paresthesia.

Phobias

With phobias, chronic anxiety occurs along with persistent fear of an object, activity, or situation that results in a compelling desire to avoid it. The patient recognizes the fear as irrational but can't suppress it.

Postconcussion syndrome

Postconcussion syndrome may produce chronic anxiety or periodic attacks of acute anxiety. Associated signs and symptoms include irritability, insomnia, dizziness, and mild headache. The anxiety is usually most pronounced in situations demanding attention, judgment, or comprehension.

Posttraumatic stress disorder

Posttraumatic stress disorder occurs in patients who have experienced an extreme traumatic event. It produces chronic anxiety of varying severity and is accompanied by intrusive, vivid memories and thoughts of the traumatic event. The patient also relives the event in dreams and nightmares. Insomnia, depression, and feelings of numbness and detachment are common.

Pulmonary edema

With pulmonary edema, acute anxiety occurs with dyspnea, orthopnea, cough with frothy sputum, tachycardia, tachypnea, crackles, ventricular gallop, hypotension, and thready pulse. The patient's skin may be cool, clammy, and cyanotic.

Pulmonary embolism

Hypoxia resulting from a pulmonary embolus may lead to acute anxiety and restlessness. The patient may also experience dyspnea, tachypnea, chest pain, tachycardia, blood-tinged sputum, and low-grade fever.

Somatoform disorder

Somatoform disorder, which usually begins in young adulthood, is characterized by anxiety and multiple somatic complaints that can't be explained physiologically. The symptoms aren't produced intentionally but are severe enough to significantly impair functioning. Pain disorder, conversion disorder, and hypochondriasis are examples of a somatoform disorder.

OTHER CAUSES

Drugs

Many drugs cause anxiety, especially sympathomimetics and central nervous system stimulants. In addition, many antidepressants may cause paradoxical anxiety.

SPECIAL CONSIDERATIONS

Supportive care can help relieve anxiety. Provide a calm, quiet atmosphere and make the patient comfortable. Encourage him to express his feelings and concerns freely. If it helps, take a short walk with him while you're talking. Or, try anxiety-reducing measures, such as distraction, relaxation techniques, or biofeedback.

PEDIATRIC POINTERS

Anxiety in children usually results from painful physical illness or inadequate oxygenation. Its autonomic signs tend to be more common and dramatic than in adults.

Medical causes
(continued)

Postconcussion syndrome
✦ Chronic anxiety or periodic attacks of acute anxiety may occur, especially in situations demanding attention, judgment, or comprehension.

Posttraumatic stress disorder
✦ Chronic anxiety occurs with thoughts of the traumatic event.

Pulmonary edema
✦ Acute anxiety occurs along with dyspnea, orthopnea, cough with frothy sputum, tachycardia, tachypnea, crackles, ventricular gallop, hypotension, and thready pulse.

Pulmonary embolism
✦ Hypoxia may result in acute anxiety and restlessness.

Somatoform disorder
✦ Anxiety and multiple somatic complaints that can't be explained are severe enough to impair functioning.

Other causes
✦ Antidepressants
✦ CNS stimulants
✦ Sympathomimetics

Special considerations
✦ Provide a calm, quiet atmosphere.
✦ Encourage the patient to express his feelings and concerns freely.

Peds points
✦ Anxiety's autonomic signs tend to be more common and dramatic in children than in adults.

Geri points

+ Distractions from ritualistic activity may provoke anxiety or agitation.

Teaching tips

+ Relaxation techniques
+ Verbalization of anxiety
+ Identification of stressors
+ Coping mechanisms

Key facts about aphasia (dysphasia)

+ Impaired expression or comprehension of written or spoken language
+ Reflects disease or injury of the brain's language centers

In an emergency

+ Look for signs and symptoms of increased ICP.
+ If you detect increased ICP, administer mannitol I.V. to decrease cerebral edema.

Key history points

+ History of headaches, hypertension, seizure disorders, or drug use
+ Preaphasia ability to communicate and perform routine tasks

Critical assessment steps

+ Check for obvious signs of neurologic deficit.
+ Take the patient's vital signs and assess his LOC.
+ Assess the patient's pupillary response, eye movements, and motor function.

GERIATRIC POINTERS

In elderly patients, distractions from the patient's ritualistic activity may provoke anxiety or agitation.

PATIENT COUNSELING

Teach the patient relaxation techniques and practice them with him. Encourage the patient to verbalize his anxiety and listen to him attentively. Help the patient identify and explore coping mechanisms that he used in the past. Work with the patient to identify stressors and guide him in effective coping skills.

APHASIA

Aphasia (also called *dysphasia*), impaired expression or comprehension of written or spoken language, reflects disease or injury of the brain's language centers. (See *Where language originates.*) Depending on severity, aphasia may slightly impede communication or may make it impossible. It can be classified as Broca's, Wernicke's, anomic, or global. Anomic aphasia eventually resolves in more than 50% of patients, but global aphasia is usually irreversible. (See *Identifying types of aphasia,* page 58.)

 EMERGENCY ACTIONS Quickly look for signs and symptoms of increased intracranial pressure (ICP), such as pupillary changes, decreased level of consciousness (LOC), vomiting, seizures, bradycardia, widening pulse pressure, and irregular respirations. If you detect increased ICP, administer mannitol I.V. to decrease cerebral edema. Also, make sure that emergency resuscitation equipment is readily available to support respiratory and cardiac function, if necessary. You may have to prepare the patient for emergency surgery.

HISTORY

If the patient doesn't display signs of increased ICP, or if his aphasia has developed gradually, perform a thorough neurologic examination, starting with the patient's history. You'll probably need to obtain this history from the patient's family or companion because of the patient's impairment. Ask if the patient has a history of headaches, hypertension, seizure disorders, or drug use. Also ask about the patient's ability to communicate and to perform routine activities before aphasia began.

PHYSICAL ASSESSMENT

Check for obvious signs of neurologic deficit, such as ptosis or fluid leakage from the nose and ears. Take the patient's vital signs and assess his LOC. Be aware, though, that assessing LOC is typically difficult because the patient's verbal responses may be unreliable. Also, recognize that dysarthria (impaired articulation due to weakness or paralysis of the muscles necessary for speech) or speech apraxia (inability to voluntarily control the muscles of speech) may accompany aphasia; so speak slowly and distinctly, and allow the patient ample time to respond. Assess the patient's pupillary response, eye movements, and motor function, especially his mouth and tongue movement, swallowing ability, and spontaneous movements and gestures. To best assess motor function, first demonstrate the motions and then have the patient imitate them.

Where language originates

Aphasia reflects damage to one or more of the brain's primary language centers, which, in most persons, are located in the left hemisphere. Broca's area lies next to the region of the motor cortex that controls the muscles necessary for speech. Wernicke's area is the center of auditory, visual, and language comprehension. It lies between Heschl's gyrus, the primary receiver of auditory stimuli, and the angular gyrus, a "way station" between the brain's auditory and visual regions. Connecting Wernicke's and Broca's areas is a large nerve bundle, the arcuate fasciculus, which enables repetition of speech.

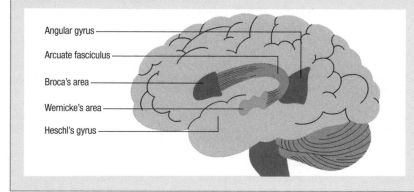

Angular gyrus
Arcuate fasciculus
Broca's area
Wernicke's area
Heschl's gyrus

MEDICAL CAUSES

Alzheimer's disease

With Alzheimer's disease, a degenerative disease, anomic aphasia may begin insidiously and then progress to severe global aphasia. Associated signs and symptoms include behavioral changes, loss of memory, poor judgment, restlessness, myoclonus, and muscle rigidity. Incontinence is usually a late sign.

Brain abscess

Any type of aphasia may occur with brain abscess. Usually, aphasia develops insidiously and may be accompanied by hemiparesis, ataxia, facial weakness, and signs of increased ICP.

Brain tumor

A brain tumor may cause any type of aphasia. As the tumor enlarges, other aphasias may occur along with behavioral changes, memory loss, motor weakness, seizures, auditory hallucinations, visual field deficits, and increased ICP.

Creutzfeldt-Jakob disease

Creutzfeldt-Jakob disease is a rapidly progressive dementia accompanied by neurologic signs and symptoms, such as myoclonic jerking, ataxia, aphasia, vision disturbances, and paralysis. It generally affects adults ages 40 to 65.

Encephalitis

Encephalitis usually produces transient aphasia. Its early signs and symptoms include fever, headache, and vomiting. Seizures, confusion, stupor or coma, hemiparesis, asymmetrical deep tendon reflexes, positive Babinski's reflex, ataxia, myoclonus, nystagmus, ocular palsies, and facial weakness may accompany aphasia.

Medical causes

Alzheimer's disease
+ Anomic aphasia may begin insidiously and then progress to severe global aphasia.

Brain abscess
+ Any type of aphasia may occur.
+ Aphasia may be accompanied by hemiparesis, ataxia, facial weakness, and signs of increased ICP.

Brain tumor
+ Any type of aphasia may occur.
+ Other signs and symptoms appear as tumor enlarges.

Creutzfeldt-Jakob disease
+ Aphasia is accompanied by dementia.

Encephalitis
+ Transient aphasia occurs.
+ Early signs and symptoms include fever, headache, and vomiting.

Identifying types of aphasia

The location of the lesion as well as its signs and symptoms help to differentiate between types of aphasia.

TYPE	LOCATION OF LESION	SIGNS AND SYMPTOMS
Anomic aphasia	Temporal-parietal area; may extend to angular gyrus, but sometimes poorly localized	Patient's understanding of written and spoken language is relatively unimpaired. His speech, although fluent, lacks meaningful content. Word-finding difficulty and circumlocution are characteristic. Rarely, the patient also displays paraphasias.
Broca's aphasia (expressive aphasia)	Broca's area; usually in third frontal convolution of left hemisphere	Patient's understanding of written and spoken language is relatively spared, but speech is nonfluent, evidencing word-finding difficulty, jargon, paraphasias, limited vocabulary, and simple sentence construction. He can't repeat words and phrases. If Wernicke's area is intact, he recognizes speech errors and shows frustration. He's commonly hemiparetic.
Global aphasia	Broca's and Wernicke's area	Patient has profoundly impaired receptive and expressive ability. He can't repeat words or phrases and can't follow directions. His occasional speech is marked by paraphasias or jargon.
Wernicke's aphasia (receptive aphasia)	Wernicke's area; usually in posterior or superior temporal lobe	Patient has difficulty understanding written and spoken language. He can't repeat words or phrases and can't follow directions. His speech is fluent but may be rapid and rambling, with paraphasias. He has difficulty naming objects (anomia) and is unaware of speech errors.

Medical causes
(continued)

Head trauma
+ Aphasia occurs suddenly.
+ Condition may be transient or permanent, depending on the extent of brain damage.

Seizures
+ Transient aphasia may occur if the seizures involve the language centers.

Stroke
+ Stroke is the most common cause of aphasia.

Head trauma
Any type of aphasia may accompany severe head trauma; typically, aphasia occurs suddenly and may be transient or permanent, depending on the extent of brain damage. Associated signs and symptoms include blurred or double vision, headache, pallor, diaphoresis, numbness and paresis, cerebrospinal otorrhea or rhinorrhea, altered respirations, tachycardia, behavioral changes, and increased ICP.

Seizures
Seizures and the postictal state may cause a transient aphasia if the seizures involve the language centers.

Stroke
The most common cause of aphasia, stroke may also produce Wernicke's, Broca's, or global aphasia. Associated findings include decreased LOC, right-sided hemiparesis, homonymous hemianopia, paresthesia, and loss of sensation. These signs and symptoms may appear on the left side if the right hemisphere contains the language centers. (See *Associated disorder: Stroke.*)

ASSOCIATED DISORDER

Stroke

Stroke, also known as *cerebrovascular accident* or *brain attack,* is a sudden impairment of cerebral circulation in one or more blood vessels. A stroke interrupts or diminishes oxygen supply and commonly causes serious damage to or necrosis of brain tissue. The sooner the circulation returns to normal after a stroke, the better the chances are for a full recovery. However, about 50% of the patients who survive a stroke remain permanently disabled and experience a recurrence within weeks, months, or years. It's the leading cause of admission to long-term care.

Stroke is the third most common cause of death in the United States and the most common cause of neurologic disability. It strikes over 500,000 people per year and is fatal in approximately 50% of these cases.

CAUSES

Stroke typically results from one of three causes:
+ thrombosis of the cerebral arteries supplying the brain or of the intracranial vessels, occluding blood flow
+ embolism from thrombus outside the brain, such as in the heart, aorta, or common carotid artery
+ hemorrhage from an intracranial artery or vein, such as from hypertension, ruptured aneurysm, arteriovenous malformation, trauma, hemorrhagic disorder, or septic embolism.

Predisposing factors for stroke include:
+ hypertension
+ history of transient ischemic attacks
+ cardiac disease, including arrhythmias, coronary artery disease, acute myocardial infarction, dilated cardiomyopathy, and valvular disease
+ diabetes
+ familial hyperlipidemia
+ cigarette smoking
+ increased alcohol intake
+ obesity
+ sedentary lifestyle
+ use of hormonal contraceptives.

DIAGNOSIS

The diagnosis of stroke is based on observation of clinical features, a history of risk factors, and the results of diagnostic tests:
+ Computed tomography scan shows evidence of hemorrhagic stroke immediately but may not show evidence of thrombotic infarction for 48 to 72 hours.
+ Magnetic resonance imaging may identify ischemic or infarcted areas and cerebral swelling.
+ Positron emission tomography scanning provides data on cerebral metabolism and cerebral blood flow changes, especially in ischemic stroke.
+ Cerebral angiography outlines blood vessels and pinpoints the occlusion or rupture site.
+ Digital subtraction angiography reveals the occlusion or narrowing of the vessels.

MEDICAL MANAGEMENT

Medical treatment commonly includes physical rehabilitation, dietary and drug regimens to help decrease risk factors, and measures to help the patient adapt to specific deficits, such as speech impairment and paralysis. Percutaneous transluminal angioplasty or stent insertion may be performed to open occluded vessels.

Drugs commonly used for stroke therapy include:
+ thrombolytic therapy, such as tissue plasminogen activator, given within the first 3 hours of an ischemic stroke to restore circulation to the affected brain tissue and limit the extent of brain injury
+ anticonvulsants, such as phenytoin or phenobarbital, to treat or prevent seizures
+ stool softeners, such as docusate sodium, to avoid straining, which increases intracranial pressure
+ corticosteroids, such as dexamethasone, to minimize cerebral edema
+ anticoagulants, such as heparin, warfarin, and ticlopidine, to reduce the risk of thrombotic stroke
+ analgesics, such as codeine, to relieve headache that may follow hemorrhagic stroke.

(continued)

Key facts about stroke
+ Also known as *cerebrovascular accident* or *brain attack*
+ Involves the sudden impairment of cerebral circulation in one or more blood vessels
+ Commonly causes serious damage or necrosis in brain tissue
+ Third most common cause of death in the United States

Causes
+ Thrombosis of the cerebral arteries or the intracranial vessels that occludes blood flow
+ Embolism from a thrombus outside the brain
+ Hemorrhage from an intracranial artery or vein

Management
+ Physical rehabilitation
+ Dietary regimens
+ Drug therapy, including thrombolytics, anticonvulsants, stool softeners, corticosteroids, anticoagulants, and analgesics
+ Measures to help the patient adapt to specific deficits.
+ Percutaneous transluminal angioplasty or stent insertion
+ Craniotomy
+ Carotid endarterectomy
+ Ventricular shunt

Medical causes
(continued)
Transient ischemic attack
+ Aphasia may occur suddenly and resolve within 24 hours of the attack.

Special considerations
+ Help orient the patient by frequently telling him what has happened, where he is and why, and what the date is.
+ Expect periods of depression as the patient recognizes his disability.
+ Help the patient communicate by providing a relaxed environment with minimal stimuli.

Peds points
+ Brain damage associated with aphasia in children most commonly follows anoxia — the result of near drowning or airway obstruction.

Teaching points
+ Alternate means of communication
+ Risk reduction factors for stroke

Key facts about apraxia
+ Inability to perform purposeful movements in the absence of significant weakness, sensory loss, poor coordination, or lack of comprehension or motivation
+ Classified as ideational, ideomotor, or kinetic, or by type of impairment

---

Stroke (continued)

SURGICAL MANAGEMENT
Depending on the stroke's cause and extent, surgery may include:
+ craniotomy to remove a hematoma
+ carotid endarterectomy to remove atherosclerotic plaque
+ ventricular shunt to drain cerebrospinal fluid.

Transient ischemic attack
Transient ischemic attacks can produce any type of aphasia, which occurs suddenly and resolves within 24 hours of the attack. Associated signs and symptoms include transient hemiparesis, hemianopia, and paresthesia (all usually right-sided), dizziness, and confusion.

SPECIAL CONSIDERATIONS
Immediately after aphasia develops, the patient may become confused or disoriented. Help to restore a sense of reality by frequently telling him what has happened, where he is and why, and what the date is. Carefully explain diagnostic tests, such as skull X-rays, computed tomography scan or magnetic resonance imaging, angiography, and EEG. Later, expect periods of depression as the patient recognizes his disability. Help him to communicate by providing a relaxed, accepting environment with a minimum of distracting stimuli.

PEDIATRIC POINTERS
Recognize that the term childhood aphasia is sometimes mistakenly applied to children who fail to develop normal language skills but who aren't considered mentally retarded or developmentally delayed. Aphasia refers solely to loss of previously developed communication skills.

Brain damage associated with aphasia in children most commonly follows anoxia — the result of near drowning or airway obstruction.

PATIENT COUNSELING
Assist the patient with an alternate means of communication, such as a communication board. If aphasia is due to a stroke, teach the patient to reduce risk factors, such as not smoking, eating a healthy diet, and exercising regularly.

APRAXIA
Apraxia is the inability to perform purposeful movements in the absence of significant weakness, sensory loss, poor coordination, or lack of comprehension or motivation. This neurologic sign usually indicates a lesion in the cerebral hemisphere. Its onset, severity, and duration vary.

Apraxia is classified as ideational, ideomotor, or kinetic, depending on the stage at which voluntary movement is impaired. It can also be classified by type of motor or skill impairment. For example, *facial* and *gait apraxia* involve specific motor groups and are easily perceived. *Constructional apraxia* refers to the inability to copy simple drawings or patterns. *Dressing apraxia* refers to the inability to correctly dress oneself. *Callosal apraxia* refers to normal motor function on one side of the body accompanied by the inability to reproduce movements on the other side.

EMERGENCY ACTIONS During your assessment, be alert for signs and symptoms of increased intracranial pressure, such as headache and vomiting. If you detect any, elevate the head of the bed 30 degrees and monitor the patient closely for altered pupil size and reactivity, bradycardia, widened pulse pressure, and irregular respirations. Have emergency resuscitation equipment nearby, and be prepared to give mannitol I.V. to decrease cerebral edema.

If the patient is experiencing seizures, stay with him and have another nurse notify the physician immediately. Avoid restraining the patient. Help him to a lying position, loosen tight clothing, and place a pillow or other soft object beneath his head. If the patient's teeth are clenched, don't force anything into his mouth. If his mouth is open, protect the tongue by placing a soft object, such as a washcloth, between his teeth. Turn the patient's head to provide an open airway.

HISTORY

If you detect apraxia, ask about previous neurologic disease. Ask the patient if he has recently experienced headaches or dizziness. Ask about previous cerebrovascular disease, atherosclerosis, neoplastic disease, infection, or hepatic disease. Then assess the apraxia further to help determine its type.

PHYSICAL ASSESSMENT

Perform a neurologic assessment. First, take the patient's vital signs and assess his level of consciousness. Be alert for any evidence of aphasia or dysarthria. Then test the patient's motor function, observing for weakness and tremors. Next, use a small pin or other pointed object to test sensory function. Check deep tendon reflexes for quality and symmetry. Finally, test the patient for visual field deficits.

MEDICAL CAUSES

Alzheimer's disease

Alzheimer's disease sometimes causes gradual and irreversible ideomotor apraxia. It can also cause amnesia, anomia, decreased attention span, apathy, aphasia, restlessness, agitation, paranoid delusions, incontinence, social withdrawal, ataxia, and tremors.

Brain abscess

Apraxia occasionally results from a large brain abscess but usually resolves spontaneously after the infection subsides. Depending on the location of the abscess, apraxia may be accompanied by headache, fever, drowsiness, decreased mental acuity, aphasia, dysarthria, hemiparesis, hyperreflexia, incontinence, focal or generalized seizures, and ocular disturbances, such as nystagmus, visual field deficits, and unequal pupils.

Brain tumor

With a brain tumor, progressive apraxia may be preceded by decreased mental acuity, headache, dizziness, and seizures. It may occur with or directly after early signs of increased intracranial pressure, such as pupil changes. It may also occur with other localizing signs and symptoms of the tumor, such as aphasia, dysarthria, visual field deficits, weakness, stiffness, and hyperreflexia in the extremities.

Hepatic encephalopathy

Hepatic encephalopathy may cause gradual onset of constructional apraxia, which may be reversible with treatment. Early associated signs and symptoms include disorientation, amnesia, slurred speech, dysarthria, asterixis, and lethargy. Later signs

---

In an emergency

If the patient is having seizures:
- Help the patient to a lying position, loosen tight clothing, and place a pillow or other soft object beneath his head.
- If the patient's teeth are clenched, don't force anything into his mouth.
- Turn the patient's head to provide an open airway.

Key history points

- History of headaches or dizziness
- Medical history, including previous neurologic, cerebrovascular, neoplastic, or hepatic disease; atherosclerosis; or infection

Critical assessment steps

- Take vital signs and assess LOC.
- Test the patient's motor function.
- Check deep tendon reflexes for quality and symmetry.

Medical causes

Alzheimer's disease
- Gradual and irreversible ideomotor apraxia sometimes occurs.

Brain abscess
- Apraxia occasionally results from a large brain abscess; it resolves spontaneously after the infection subsides.

Brain tumor
- Apraxia may occur with or after early signs of increased ICP.

Hepatic encephalopathy
- Onset of constructional apraxia is gradual and may be reversible with treatment.

Medical causes
(continued)

Stroke
+ Onset of apraxia is sudden and commonly resolves spontaneously.

Special considerations
+ Take measures to ensure the patient's safety.

Peds points
+ Sudden inability to perform a previously accomplished movement warrants prompt neurologic evaluation.
+ Developmental apraxia may be caused by brain damage.

Teaching points
+ Explanation of apraxia
+ Demonstration of routine tasks
+ Referral to physical or occupational therapy

Key facts about arm pain
+ Usually results from musculoskeletal disorders
+ May be referred from another area
+ Can be sharp or dull, burning or numbing, and shooting or penetrating

Key history points
+ History of injury, if applicable
+ Onset and description of pain
+ Location of referred pain
+ Factors associated with pain
+ Preexisting illnesses
+ Family history of gout or arthritis
+ Current drug therapy

---

include hyperreflexia, positive Babinski's reflex, agitation, seizures, fetor hepaticus, stupor, and coma.

Stroke
Stroke commonly causes sudden onset of apraxia, which usually resolves spontaneously but may persist. Associated signs and symptoms vary according to the affected artery but can include headache, confusion, coma, hemiplegia, unilateral or bilateral visual field deficits, aphasia, agnosia, dysarthria, and urinary incontinence.

SPECIAL CONSIDERATIONS

Prepare the patient for diagnostic studies, such as computed tomography and radionuclide brain scans. Because weakness, sensory deficits, confusion, and seizures may accompany apraxia, take measures to ensure safety. For example, assist the patient with gait apraxia in walking.

PEDIATRIC POINTERS

Detecting apraxia in children can be difficult. However, any sudden inability to perform a previously accomplished movement warrants prompt neurologic evaluation because brain tumor — the most common cause of apraxia in children — can be treated effectively if detected early.

Brain damage in a young child may cause developmental apraxia, which interferes with the ability to learn activities that require sequential movement, such as hopping, jumping, hitting or kicking a ball, or dancing. When caring for a child with apraxia, be aware of his limitations; yet provide an environment that's conducive to rehabilitation. Provide emotional support because playmates will commonly tease a child who can't perform normal physical activities.

PATIENT COUNSELING

Explain the patient's apraxia to him, and encourage his participation in normal activities. Help him to overcome his frustrations at being unable to perform routine tasks by demonstrating each step in these tasks and giving the patient sufficient time to imitate each step. Avoid giving complex directions, and enlist the help of family members in rehabilitation. Also, refer the patient to a physical or occupational therapist.

ARM PAIN

Arm pain usually results from musculoskeletal disorders, but it can also stem from neurovascular or cardiovascular disorders. In some cases, it may be referred pain from another area, such as the chest, neck, or abdomen. Its location, onset, and character provide clues to its cause. The pain may affect the entire arm or only the upper arm or forearm. It may arise suddenly or gradually and be constant or intermittent. Arm pain can be described as sharp or dull, burning or numbing, and shooting or penetrating. Diffuse arm pain, though, may be difficult to describe, especially if it isn't associated with injury.

HISTORY

If the patient reports arm pain after an injury, take a brief history of the injury from the patient. Then quickly assess him for severe injuries requiring immediate treatment. If you've ruled out severe injuries, check pulses, capillary refill time, sensation, and movement distal to the affected area because circulatory impairment or nerve injury may require immediate surgery. Inspect the arm for deformities, assess the level of pain, and immobilize the arm to prevent further injury.

If the patient reports continuous or intermittent arm pain, ask him to describe it and to relate when it began. Is the pain associated with repetitive or specific movements or positions? Ask him to point out other painful areas because arm pain may be referred. For example, arm pain commonly accompanies the characteristic chest pain of myocardial infarction, and right shoulder pain may be referred from the right-upper-quadrant abdominal pain of cholecystitis. Ask the patient if the pain worsens in the morning or in the evening, if it prevents him from performing his job, and if it restricts any movements. Also ask if heat, rest, or drugs relieve it. Finally, ask about any preexisting illnesses, a family history of gout or arthritis, and current drug therapy.

PHYSICAL ASSESSMENT

Perform a focused examination. Observe the way the patient walks, sits, and holds his arm. Inspect the entire arm, comparing it with the opposite arm for symmetry, movement, and muscle atrophy. (It's important to know if the patient is right- or left-handed.) Palpate the entire arm for swelling, nodules, and tender areas. In both arms, compare active range of motion, muscle strength, and reflexes.

If the patient reports numbness or tingling, check his sensation to vibration, temperature, and pinprick. Compare bilateral hand grasps and shoulder strength to detect weakness.

If a patient has a cast, splint, or restrictive dressing, check for circulation, sensation, and mobility distal to the dressing. Ask the patient about edema and if the pain has worsened within the last 24 hours.

Examine the neck for pain on motion, point tenderness, muscle spasms, or arm pain when the neck is extended with the head toward the involved side.

MEDICAL CAUSES

Angina

Angina may cause inner arm pain as well as chest and jaw pain. Typically, pain follows exertion and persists for a few minutes. Accompanied by dyspnea, diaphoresis, and apprehension, the pain is relieved by rest or vasodilators, such as nitroglycerin.

Cellulitis

Typically, cellulitis affects the legs, but it can also affect the arms. It produces pain as well as redness, tenderness, edema and, at times, fever, chills, tachycardia, headache, and hypotension. Cellulitis usually follows an injury or an insect bite.

Cervical nerve root compression

Compression of the cervical nerves supplying the upper arm produces chronic arm and neck pain, which may worsen with movement or prolonged sitting. The patient may also experience muscle weakness, paresthesia, and decreased reflex response.

Compartment syndrome

Severe pain with passive muscle stretching is the cardinal symptom of compartment syndrome. It may also impair distal circulation and cause muscle weakness, decreased reflex response, paresthesia, and edema. Ominous signs include paralysis and absent pulse.

Fractures

In fractures of the cervical vertebrae, humerus, scapula, clavicle, radius, or ulna, pain can occur at the injury site and radiate throughout the entire arm. Pain at a

---

Critical assessment steps

+ Inspect the arm; compare it with the opposite arm for symmetry, movement, and muscle atrophy.
+ Palpate for swelling, nodules, and tender areas.
+ In both arms, compare active range of motion, muscle strength, and reflexes.
+ If there's numbness or tingling, check sensation to vibration, temperature, and pinprick.
+ Examine the neck for pain, point tenderness, muscle spasms, or arm pain when the neck is extended with the head toward the involved side.

Medical causes

Angina

+ Inner arm, chest, and jaw pain follow exertion.

Cellulitis

+ Leg pain usually occurs, but arms may also be affected.

Cervical nerve root compression

+ If nerves supplying upper arm are affected, chronic arm and neck pain occurs.

Compartment syndrome

+ Severe pain with passive muscle stretching occurs along with muscle weakness, decreased reflex response, paresthesia, and edema.

Fractures

+ Cervical vertebrae, humerus, scapula, clavicle, radius, or ulna fractures cause pain that may radiate throughout the arm.

Medical causes
(continued)

Muscle contusion or strain

✦ Pain occurs in the area of injury.
✦ Local swelling and ecchymosis may occur.

Myocardial infarction

✦ The patient may complain of left arm pain as well as deep, crushing chest pain.

Neoplasms of the arm

✦ Continuous, deep, and penetrating pain develops and worsens at night.

Osteomyelitis

✦ Vague and evanescent localized arm pain and fever occur.

Special considerations

✦ Apply a sling or splint.
✦ Monitor patient for worsening pain, numbness, or decreased circulation distal to injury site.
✦ Promote comfort by elevating the arm and applying ice.

Peds points

✦ Arm pain commonly results from fractures, muscle sprain, muscular dystrophy, or rheumatoid arthritis.
✦ If the child has a fracture or sprain, obtain a complete account of the injury; don't dismiss the possibility of child abuse.

Geri points

✦ Patients with osteoporosis are prone to degenerative joint disease and may experience fractures from simple trauma, heavy lifting, or unexpected movements.

fresh fracture site is intense and worsens with movement. Associated signs and symptoms include crepitus, felt and heard from bone ends rubbing together (don't attempt to elicit this sign); deformity, if bones are misaligned; local ecchymosis and edema; impaired distal circulation; paresthesia; and decreased sensation distal to the injury site. Fractures of the small wrist bones can manifest with pain and swelling several days after the trauma.

Muscle contusion or strain

Muscle contusion may cause generalized pain in the area of injury. It may also cause local swelling and ecchymosis. Acute or chronic muscle strain causes mild to severe pain with movement. The resultant reduction in arm movement may cause muscle weakness and atrophy.

Myocardial infarction

A patient with myocardial infarction, a life-threatening disorder, may complain of left arm pain as well as the characteristic deep and crushing chest pain. He may display weakness, pallor, nausea, vomiting, diaphoresis, altered blood pressure, tachycardia, dyspnea, and feelings of apprehension or impending doom.

Neoplasms of the arm

A neoplasm of the arm produces continuous, deep, and penetrating arm pain that worsens at night. Occasionally, redness and swelling accompany arm pain; later, skin breakdown, impaired circulation, and paresthesia may occur.

Osteomyelitis

Osteomyelitis typically begins with vague and evanescent localized arm pain and fever and is accompanied by local tenderness, painful and restricted movement and, later, swelling. Associated findings include malaise and tachycardia.

SPECIAL CONSIDERATIONS

If you suspect a fracture, apply a sling or a splint to immobilize the arm, and monitor the patient for worsening pain, numbness, or decreased circulation distal to the injury site. Also monitor vital signs, and be alert for tachycardia, hypotension, and diaphoresis. Withhold food, fluids, and analgesics until potential fractures are evaluated. Promote the patient's comfort by elevating his arm and applying ice. Clean abrasions and lacerations and apply dry, sterile dressings, if necessary. Also, prepare the patient for X-rays or other diagnostic tests.

PEDIATRIC POINTERS

In children, arm pain commonly results from fractures, muscle sprain, muscular dystrophy, or rheumatoid arthritis. In young children especially, the exact location of the pain may be difficult to establish. Watch for nonverbal clues, such as wincing or guarding.

    If the child has a fracture or sprain, obtain a complete account of the injury. Closely observe interactions between the child and his family, and don't dismiss the possibility of child abuse.

GERIATRIC POINTERS

Elderly patients with osteoporosis may experience fractures from simple trauma or even from heavy lifting or unexpected movements. They're also prone to degenerative joint disease that can involve several joints in the arm or neck.

Patient counseling

Advise a patient with a cast to notify his physician if he detects any worsening swelling, purple discoloration of fingers, or numbness or tingling because these signs may represent circulatory impairment due to a tight cast. Also advise patients with angina that arm pain, usually left-sided, may represent an ischemic event, especially if accompanied by diaphoresis, nausea, vomiting, and anxiety.

ATAXIA

Classified as cerebellar or sensory, ataxia refers to incoordination and irregularity of voluntary, purposeful movements. Cerebellar ataxia results from disease of the cerebellum and its pathways to and from the cerebral cortex, brain stem, and spinal cord. It causes gait, trunk, limb and, possibly, speech disorders. Sensory ataxia results from impaired position sense (proprioception) due to interruption of afferent nerve fibers in the peripheral nerves, posterior roots, posterior columns of the spinal cord, or medial lemnisci or, occasionally, is caused by a lesion in both parietal lobes. It causes gait disorders. (*See Identifying ataxia, page 66.*)

Ataxia occurs in acute and chronic forms. Acute ataxia may result from stroke, hemorrhage, or a large tumor in the posterior fossa. With this life-threatening condition, the cerebellum may herniate downward through the foramen magnum behind the cervical spinal cord, or upward through the tentorium on the cerebral hemispheres. Herniation may also compress the brain stem. Acute ataxia may also result from drug toxicity or poisoning. Chronic ataxia can be progressive and, at times, can result from acute disease. It can also occur in metabolic and chronic degenerative neurologic disease.

 EMERGENCY ACTIONS If ataxic movements suddenly develop, examine the patient for signs of increased intracranial pressure and impending herniation. Determine his level of consciousness (LOC), and be alert for pupillary changes, motor weakness or paralysis, neck stiffness or pain, and vomiting. Check vital signs, especially respirations; abnormal respiratory patterns may quickly lead to respiratory arrest. Elevate the head of the bed. Have emergency resuscitation equipment readily available. Prepare the patient for computed tomography scanning or surgery.

History

If the patient isn't in distress, review his history. Ask about multiple sclerosis, diabetes, central nervous system infection, neoplastic disease, previous stroke, and a family history of ataxia. Also ask about chronic alcohol abuse or prolonged exposure to industrial toxins such as mercury. Find out if the patient's ataxia developed suddenly or gradually.

Physical assessment

If necessary, perform Romberg's test to help distinguish between cerebellar and sensory ataxia. Instruct the patient to stand with his feet together and his arms at his sides. Note his posture and balance, first with his eyes open, then closed. Test results may indicate normal posture and balance (minimal swaying), cerebellar ataxia (swaying and inability to maintain balance with eyes open or closed), or sensory ataxia (increased swaying and inability to maintain balance with eyes closed). Stand close to the patient during this test to prevent his falling.

Teaching points
+ Signs and symptoms of circulatory impairment to report
+ Signs and symptoms of an ischemic event

Key facts about ataxia
+ Incoordination and irregularity of voluntary, purposeful movements
+ Can be classified as cerebellar (resulting from disease of the cerebellum) or sensory (resulting from proprioception)
+ Has acute and chronic forms

In an emergency
+ Examine for signs of increased ICP and impending herniation.
+ Determine the patient's LOC.
+ Be alert for pupillary changes, motor weakness or paralysis, neck stiffness or pain, and vomiting.
+ Check vital signs, especially respirations.
+ Have emergency resuscitation equipment readily available.

Key history points
+ History of multiple sclerosis, diabetes, CNS infection, neoplastic disease, or stroke
+ Family history of ataxia
+ Alcohol abuse
+ Exposure to industrial toxins
+ Onset (gradual or sudden)

Critical assessment steps
+ Perform Romberg's test to help distinguish between cerebellar and sensory ataxia.
+ If you test for gait and limb ataxia, check motor strength.

Identifying ataxia

TYPE	DESCRIPTION
Speech ataxia	A form of dysarthria, the patient typically speaks slowly and stresses usually unstressed words and syllables. Speech content is unaffected.
Truncal ataxia	A disturbance in equilibrium, the patient can't sit or stand without falling. Also, his head and trunk may bob and sway (titubation). If he can walk, his gait is reeling.
Limb ataxia	The patient loses the ability to gauge distance, speed, and power of movement, resulting in poorly controlled, variable, and inaccurate voluntary movements. He may move too quickly or too slowly, or his movements may break down into component parts, giving him the appearance of a puppet or a robot. Other effects include a coarse, irregular tremor in purposeful movement (but not at rest) and reduced muscle tone.
Gait ataxia	The patient's gait is wide based, unsteady, and irregular.
Cerebellar ataxia	The patient may stagger or lurch in zigzag fashion, turn with extreme difficulty, and lose his balance when his feet are together.
Sensory ataxia	The patient moves abruptly and stomps or taps his feet. This occurs because he throws his feet forward and outward, and then brings them down first on the heels and then on the toes. The patient also fixes his eyes on the ground, watching his steps. However, if he can't watch them, staggering worsens. When he stands with his feet together, he sways or loses balance.

Medical causes

Cerebellar abscess

✦ Limb ataxia occurs on the same side as the lesion, accompanied by gait and truncal ataxia.

✦ Typically, the initial symptom is headache localized behind the ear or in the occipital region.

Cerebellar hemorrhage

✦ Ataxia is usually acute but transient; it may affect the trunk, gait, or limbs.

Creutzfeldt-Jakob disease

✦ Ataxia accompanies other neurologic signs, such as myoclonic jerking and aphasia.

If you test for gait and limb ataxia, be aware that motor weakness may mimic ataxic movements and check motor strength, too. Gait ataxia may be severe, even when limb ataxia is minimal. With gait ataxia, ask the patient if he tends to fall to one side and if falling usually occurs at night. With truncal ataxia, remember that inability to walk or stand, combined with the absence of other signs when lying down, may give the impression of hysteria or drug or alcohol intoxication.

MEDICAL CAUSES

Cerebellar abscess
Cerebellar abscess commonly causes limb ataxia on the same side as the lesion as well as gait and truncal ataxia. Typically, the initial symptom is headache localized behind the ear or in the occipital region, followed by oculomotor palsy, fever, vomiting, altered LOC, and coma.

Cerebellar hemorrhage
With cerebellar hemorrhage, a life-threatening disorder, ataxia is usually acute but transient. Unilateral or bilateral ataxia affects the trunk, gait, or limbs. The patient initially experiences repeated vomiting, occipital headache, vertigo, oculomotor palsy, dysphagia, and dysarthria. Later signs, such as decreased LOC or coma, signal impending herniation.

Creutzfeldt-Jakob disease

Creutzfeldt-Jakob disease is a rapidly progressive dementia accompanied by neurologic signs and symptoms, such as myoclonic jerking, ataxia, aphasia, vision disturbances, and paralysis. It generally affects adults ages 40 to 65.

Diabetic neuropathy

Peripheral nerve damage due to diabetes mellitus may cause sensory ataxia, extremity pain, slight leg weakness, skin changes, and bowel and bladder dysfunction. As neuropathy progresses, the patient may report numbness in the feet. Reduced proprioception and sensation may produce an unsteady gait.

Diphtheria

Within 4 to 8 weeks of the onset of symptoms of diphtheria, a life-threatening neuropathy can produce sensory ataxia. Diphtheria can be accompanied by fever, paresthesia, and paralysis of the limbs and, sometimes, the respiratory muscles.

Hepatocerebral degeneration

Patients who survive hepatic coma are occasionally left with residual neurologic defects, including mild cerebellar ataxia with a wide-based, unsteady gait. Ataxia may be accompanied by altered LOC, dysarthria, rhythmic arm tremors, and choreoathetosis of the face, neck, and shoulders.

Hyperthermia

With hyperthermia, cerebellar ataxia occurs if the patient survives the coma and seizures characteristic of the acute phase. Subsequent findings include spastic paralysis, dementia, and slowly resolving confusion.

Metastatic cancer

Cancer that metastasizes to the cerebellum may cause gait ataxia accompanied by headache, dizziness, nystagmus, decreased LOC, nausea, and vomiting. A cerebellar tumor may produce gait ataxia, dizziness, muscle incoordination, and nystagmus. The patient may fall toward the side with the lesion.

Multiple sclerosis

Nystagmus and cerebellar ataxia commonly occur in multiple sclerosis, but they aren't always accompanied by limb weakness and spasticity. Speech ataxia (especially scanning) may occur as well as sensory ataxia from spinal cord involvement. During remissions, ataxia may subside or even disappear. During exacerbations, it may reappear, worsen, or even become permanent. Multiple sclerosis also causes optic neuritis, optic atrophy, numbness and weakness, diplopia, dizziness, and bladder dysfunction.

Poisoning

Chronic arsenic poisoning may cause sensory ataxia, along with headache, seizures, altered LOC, motor deficits, and muscle aching. Chronic mercury poisoning causes gait ataxia and limb ataxia, principally of the arms. It also causes tremors of the extremities, tongue, and lips; mental confusion; mood changes; and dysarthria.

Polyarteritis nodosa

Acute or subacute polyarteritis nodosa may cause sensory ataxia, abdominal and limb pain, hematuria, fever, and elevated blood pressure. Other findings include myalgia, headache, joint pain, and weakness.

Polyneuropathy

Carcinomatous and myelomatous polyneuropathy may occur before detection of the primary tumor in cancer, multiple myeloma, or Hodgkin's disease. Signs and

Medical causes
(continued)

Diabetic neuropathy
+ Peripheral nerve damage may cause sensory ataxia.

Diphtheria
+ Neuropathy can produce sensory ataxia within 4 to 8 weeks of the onset of symptoms.

Hepatocerebral degeneration
+ Residual neurologic defects, including mild cerebellar ataxia, occur in those who survive hepatic coma.

Hyperthermia
+ Cerebellar ataxia occurs if patient survives the acute phase.

Metastatic cancer
+ Gait ataxia may occur if cancer metastasizes to cerebellum or if a cerebellar tumor develops.

Multiple sclerosis
+ Cerebellar ataxia may occur.
+ Spinal cord involvement may cause speech and sensory ataxia.

Poisoning
+ Chronic arsenic poisoning may cause sensory ataxia.
+ Chronic mercury poisoning causes gait and limb ataxia.

Polyarteritis nodosa
+ Sensory ataxia, abdominal and limb pain, hematuria, and elevated blood pressure may occur

Polyneuropathy
+ Ataxia, severe motor weakness, muscle atrophy, and sensory loss in the limbs occur.

Medical causes
(continued)

Posterior fossa tumor
+ Gait, truncal, or limb ataxia is an early sign; ataxia may worsen as the tumor enlarges.

Spinocerebellar ataxia
+ Fatigue occurs initially, followed by stiff-legged gait ataxia.
+ Eventually, limb ataxia occurs.

Stroke
+ Infarction in medulla, pons, or cerebellum may lead to ataxia, which may remain as residual deficit.
+ Worsening ataxia during acute phase may indicate extension of stroke or severe swelling.

Wernicke's disease
+ Gait ataxia occurs.
+ With severe ataxia, the patient may be unable to stand or walk.

Other causes
+ Aminoglutethimide
+ Toxic levels of anticonvulsants, anticholinergics, and tricyclic antidepressants

Special considerations
+ If toxic drug levels are the cause, discontinue the offending drug.

Peds points
+ Acute ataxia may stem from febrile infection, brain tumors, mumps, and other disorders.
+ Chronic ataxia may stem from Gaucher's disease, Refsum's disease, and other inborn errors of metabolism.
+ If you suspect ataxia, refer the child for a neurologic evaluation to rule out a brain tumor.

symptoms include ataxia, severe motor weakness, muscle atrophy, and sensory loss in the limbs. Pain and skin changes may also occur.

Posterior fossa tumor
Gait, truncal, or limb ataxia is an early sign of a posterior fossa tumor and may worsen as the tumor enlarges. It's accompanied by vomiting, headache, papilledema, vertigo, oculomotor palsy, decreased LOC, and motor and sensory impairments on the same side as the lesion.

Spinocerebellar ataxia
With spinocerebellar ataxia, the patient may initially experience fatigue, followed by stiff-legged gait ataxia. Eventually, limb ataxia, dysarthria, static tremor, nystagmus, cramps, paresthesia, and sensory deficits occur.

Stroke
With stroke, occlusions in the vertebrobasilar arteries halt blood flow to cause infarction in the medulla, pons, or cerebellum that may lead to ataxia. Ataxia may occur at the onset of stroke and remain as a residual deficit. Worsening ataxia during the acute phase may indicate extension of the stroke or severe swelling. Ataxia may be accompanied by unilateral or bilateral motor weakness, possible altered LOC, sensory loss, vertigo, nausea, vomiting, oculomotor palsy, and dysphagia.

Wernicke's disease
The result of thiamine deficiency, Wernicke's disease produces gait ataxia and, rarely, intention tremor or speech ataxia. With severe ataxia, the patient may be unable to stand or walk. Ataxia decreases with thiamine therapy. Associated signs and symptoms include nystagmus, diplopia, ocular palsies, confusion, tachycardia, exertional dyspnea, and orthostatic hypotension.

OTHER CAUSES

Drugs
Toxic levels of anticonvulsants, especially phenytoin, may result in gait ataxia. Toxic levels of anticholinergics and tricyclic antidepressants may also result in ataxia. Aminoglutethimide causes ataxia in about 10% of patients; however, this effect usually disappears 4 to 6 weeks after drug therapy is discontinued.

SPECIAL CONSIDERATIONS
Prepare the patient for laboratory studies such as blood tests for toxic drug levels and radiologic tests. Treatment approaches depend on the underlying cause. For example, physical therapy may improve function following a stroke. Surgery, chemotherapy, and radiation therapy may be necessary to treat a brain tumor. If toxic drug levels are the cause, discontinue the offending drug.

PEDIATRIC POINTERS
In children, ataxia occurs in acute and chronic forms and results from congenital or acquired disease. Acute ataxia may stem from febrile infection, brain tumors, mumps, and other disorders. Chronic ataxia may stem from Gaucher's disease, Refsum's disease, and other inborn errors of metabolism.

When assessing a child for ataxia, consider his level of motor skills and emotional state. Your examination may be limited to observing the child in spontaneous activity and carefully questioning his parents about changes in his motor activity, such as increased unsteadiness or falling. If you suspect ataxia, refer the child for a neurologic evaluation to rule out a brain tumor.

PATIENT COUNSELING

Focus on helping the patient adapt to his condition. Promote rehabilitation goals and help ensure the patient's safety. For example, instruct the patient with sensory ataxia to move slowly, especially when turning or getting up from a chair. Provide a cane or walker for extra support. Ask the patient's family to check his home for hazards, such as uneven surfaces or the absence of handrails on stairs. If appropriate, refer the patient with progressive disease for counseling.

AURA

An aura is a sensory or motor phenomenon, idea, or emotion that marks the initial stage of a seizure or the approach of a classic migraine headache. Auras may be classified as cognitive, affective, psychosensory, or psychomotor. (See *Recognizing types of auras.*)

When associated with a seizure, an aura stems from an irritable focus in the brain that spreads throughout the cortex. Although an aura was once considered a sign of impending seizure, it's now considered the first stage of a seizure. Typically, it occurs seconds to minutes before the ictal phase. Its intensity, duration, and type depend on the origin of the irritable focus. Unfortunately, an aura is difficult to describe because the postictal phase of a seizure temporarily alters the patient's level of consciousness, impairing his memory of the event.

The aura associated with a classic migraine headache results from cranial vasoconstriction. Diagnostically important, it helps distinguish a classic migraine from other types of headaches.

EMERGENCY ACTIONS **When an aura rapidly progresses to the ictal phase of a seizure, quickly evaluate the seizure and be alert for life-threatening complications such as apnea. When an aura heralds a classic migraine, make the patient as comfortable as possible. Place him in a dark, quiet room and administer drugs to prevent the headache, if necessary.**

HISTORY

Obtain a thorough history of the patient's headaches or seizure history, asking him to describe any sensory or motor phenomena that precede each headache or seizure. Find out how long each headache or seizure typically lasts. Does anything make it worse, such as bright lights, noise, or caffeine? Does anything make it better? Ask the patient about drugs he takes for pain relief.

PHYSICAL ASSESSMENT

First, perform a full neurologic examination. Then proceed to a complete physical examination to detect systemic disorders. Be aware that the physical assessment may not reveal abnormalities.

MEDICAL CAUSES

Classic migraine headache

A migraine headache is preceded by a vague premonition and then, usually, a visual aura involving flashes of light. The aura lasts 10 to 30 minutes and may intensify until it completely obscures the patient's vision. A classic migraine may cause

Recognizing types of auras

Determining whether an aura marks the patient's thought processes, emotions, or sensory or motor function usually requires keen observation. An aura is typically difficult to describe and is only dimly remembered when associated with seizure activity. The types of auras the patient may experience are listed below.

AFFECTIVE AURAS
+ Fear
+ Paranoia
+ Other emotions

COGNITIVE AURAS
+ Déjà vu (familiarity with unfamiliar events or environments)
+ Flashback of past events
+ Jamais vu (unfamiliarity with a known event)
+ Time standing still

PSYCHOMOTOR AURAS
+ Automatisms (inappropriate, repetitive movements): lip smacking, chewing, swallowing, grimacing, picking at clothes, climbing stairs

PSYCHOSENSORY AURAS
+ Auditory: buzzing or ringing in the ears
+ Gustatory: acidic, metallic, or bitter tastes
+ Olfactory: foul odors
+ Tactile: numbness or tingling
+ Vertigo
+ Visual: flashes of light (scintillations)

Medical causes
(continued)

Seizure, generalized tonic-clonic
+ An aura may or may not occur at the start of the seizure.

Special considerations
+ Advise the patient to keep a diary of factors that precipitate each headache or seizure as well as their associated symptoms.

Peds points
+ Watch for nonverbal clues possibly associated with aura, such as rubbing the eyes, coughing, and spitting.

Teaching points
+ Ways to prevent headaches
+ Anticonvulsant therapy
+ Importance of follow-up blood studies

---

numbness or tingling of lips, face, or hands; slight confusion; and dizziness before the characteristic unilateral, throbbing headache appears. It slowly intensifies; when it peaks, it may cause photophobia, nausea, and vomiting.

Seizure, generalized tonic-clonic
A generalized tonic-clonic seizure may begin with or without an aura. The patient loses consciousness and falls to the ground. His body stiffens (tonic phase); then he experiences rapid, synchronous muscle jerking and hyperventilation (clonic phase). The seizure usually lasts 2 to 5 minutes.

SPECIAL CONSIDERATIONS
Advise the patient to keep a diary of factors that precipitate each headache or seizure as well as their associated symptoms to help you evaluate the effectiveness of drug therapy. Recommend lifestyle changes such as stress-reduction measures, which may help reduce the frequency of headaches.

PEDIATRIC POINTERS
Watch for nonverbal clues possibly associated with aura, such as rubbing the eyes, coughing, and spitting. When taking the seizure history, recognize that children — like adults — tend to forget the aura. Ask simple, direct questions, such as "Do you see anything funny before the seizure?" and "Do you get a bad taste in your mouth?" Give the child ample time to respond because he may have difficulty describing the aura.

PATIENT COUNSELING
If the patient recognizes the aura as a warning sign, tell him to prevent the headache by taking appropriate drugs. If the patient has a seizure disorder, emphasize the importance of taking anticonvulsants as directed. Stress the importance of regular follow-up appointments for blood studies.

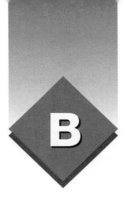

BABINSKI'S REFLEX

Babinski's reflex — dorsiflexion of the great toe with extension and fanning of the other toes — is an abnormal reflex elicited by firmly stroking the lateral aspect of the sole of the foot with a blunt object. (See *How to elicit Babinski's reflex,* page 72.) In some patients, this reflex can be triggered by noxious stimuli, such as pain, noise, or even bumping of the bed. An indicator of corticospinal damage, Babinski's reflex may occur unilaterally or bilaterally. It may also be temporary or permanent. A temporary Babinski's reflex commonly occurs during the postictal phase of a seizure, whereas a permanent Babinski's reflex occurs with corticospinal damage. A positive Babinski's reflex is normal in neonates and in infants up to 24 months old.

HISTORY

Ask the patient about his recent medical history. Has the patient experienced a recent head trauma, spinal cord injury, or an animal bite? Then ask whether he has a personal or family history of neurologic disorders.

PHYSICAL ASSESSMENT

After eliciting a positive Babinski's reflex, evaluate the patient for other neurologic signs. Evaluate muscle strength in each extremity by having the patient push or pull against your resistance. Passively flex and extend the extremity to assess muscle tone. Intermittent resistance to flexion and extension indicates spasticity, and a lack of resistance indicates flaccidity.

Next, check for evidence of incoordination by asking the patient to perform a repetitive activity. Test deep tendon reflexes (DTRs) in the patient's elbow, antecubital area, wrist, knee, and ankle by striking the tendon with a reflex hammer. An exaggerated muscle response indicates hyperactive DTRs; little or no muscle response indicates hypoactivity.

Then evaluate pain sensation and proprioception in the feet. As you move the patient's toes up and down, ask him to identify the direction in which the toes have been moved without looking at his feet.

MEDICAL CAUSES

Amyotrophic lateral sclerosis

With amyotrophic lateral sclerosis (ALS), a progressive motor neuron disorder, bilateral Babinski's reflex may occur with hyperactive DTRs and spasticity. Typically, ALS produces fasciculations accompanied by muscle atrophy and weakness. Incoordination makes carrying out activities of daily living difficult for the patient. As-

How to elicit Babinski's reflex

To elicit Babinski's reflex, also known as the *extensor plantar reflex,* stroke the lateral aspect of the sole of the patient's foot with your thumbnail or another moderately sharp object. Normally, this elicits flexion of all toes (a negative Babinski's reflex), as shown below left. With a positive Babinski's reflex, the great toe dorsiflexes and the other toes fan out, as shown below right.

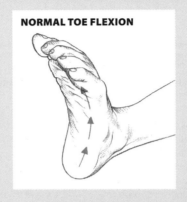

NORMAL TOE FLEXION

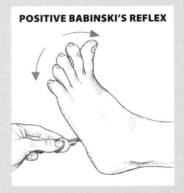

POSITIVE BABINSKI'S REFLEX

Medical causes

ALS

✦ Babinski's reflex may occur with hyperactive DTRs and spasticity.
✦ Fasciculations are accompanied by muscle atrophy and weakness.

Brain tumor

✦ Babinski's reflex may be produced if the tumor involves the corticospinal tract.

Head trauma

✦ Unilateral or bilateral Babinski's reflex may occur because of primary corticospinal damage or secondary injury associated with increased ICP.
✦ Hyperactive DTRs and spasticity commonly occur.

Meningitis

✦ Bilateral Babinski's reflex follows fever, chills, and malaise.
✦ Nausea and vomiting occur.

sociated signs and symptoms include impaired speech; difficulty chewing, swallowing, and breathing; urinary frequency and urgency; and, occasionally, choking and excessive drooling. Although his mental status remains intact, the patient's poor prognosis may cause periodic depression.

Brain tumor

A brain tumor that involves the corticospinal tract may produce Babinski's reflex. The reflex may be accompanied by hyperactive DTRs (unilateral or bilateral), spasticity, seizures, cranial nerve dysfunction, hemiparesis or hemiplegia, decreased pain sensation, unsteady gait, incoordination, headache, emotional lability, and decreased level of consciousness (LOC).

Head trauma

In a patient with head trauma, unilateral or bilateral Babinski's reflex may occur as the result of primary corticospinal damage or secondary injury associated with increased intracranial pressure. Hyperactive DTRs and spasticity commonly occur with Babinski's reflex. The patient may also have weakness and incoordination. Other signs and symptoms vary with the type of head trauma and include headache, vomiting, behavior changes, altered vital signs, and decreased LOC with abnormal pupillary size and response to light.

Meningitis

With meningitis, bilateral Babinski's reflex commonly follows fever, chills, and malaise and is accompanied by nausea and vomiting. As meningitis progresses, it also causes decreased LOC, nuchal rigidity, positive Brudzinski's and Kernig's signs, hyperactive DTRs, and opisthotonos. Associated signs and symptoms include irritability, photophobia, diplopia, delirium, and deep stupor that may progress to coma.

Multiple sclerosis

In most patients with multiple sclerosis, a demyelinating disorder, Babinski's reflex eventually occurs bilaterally. It follows initial signs and symptoms of multiple sclerosis — usually, paresthesia, nystagmus, and blurred or double vision. Associated signs and symptoms include scanning speech (clipped speech with some pauses between syllables), dysphagia, intention tremor, weakness, incoordination, spasticity, gait ataxia, seizures, paraparesis or paraplegia, bladder incontinence and, occasionally, loss of pain and temperature sensation and proprioception. Emotional lability is also characteristic.

Pernicious anemia

Bilateral Babinski's reflex occurs late in pernicious anemia when vitamin B_{12} deficiency affects the central nervous system. Anemia may eventually cause widespread GI, neurologic, and cardiovascular effects. Characteristic GI signs and symptoms include nausea, vomiting, anorexia, weight loss, flatulence, diarrhea, and constipation. Gingival bleeding and a sore, inflamed tongue may make eating painful and intensify anorexia. The lips, gums, and tongue also appear markedly pale. Jaundice may cause pale to bright yellow skin.

Characteristic neurologic signs and symptoms include neuritis, weakness, peripheral paresthesia, disturbed position sense, incoordination, ataxia, positive Romberg's sign, light-headedness, bowel and bladder incontinence, and altered vision (diplopia, blurred vision), taste, and hearing (tinnitus). The disorder may also produce irritability, poor memory, headache, depression, impotence, and delirium. Characteristic cardiovascular signs and symptoms include palpitations, wide pulse pressure, dyspnea, orthopnea, and tachycardia.

Rabies

Bilateral Babinski's reflex — possibly elicited by nonspecific noxious stimuli alone — appears in the excitation phase of rabies. This phase occurs 2 to 10 days after the onset of prodromal signs and symptoms, such as fever, malaise, and irritability (which occur 30 to 40 days after a bite from an infected animal). Rabies is characterized by marked restlessness and extremely painful pharyngeal muscle spasms. Difficulty swallowing causes excessive drooling and hydrophobia in about 50% of affected patients. Seizures and hyperactive DTRs may also occur.

Spinal cord injury

With acute injury, spinal shock temporarily erases all reflexes. As shock resolves, Babinski's reflex occurs — unilaterally when injury affects only one side of the spinal cord (Brown-Séquard's syndrome), bilaterally when injury affects both sides. Rather than signaling the return of neurologic function, this reflex confirms corticospinal damage. It's accompanied by hyperactive DTRs, spasticity, and variable or total loss of pain and temperature sensation, proprioception, and motor function. Horner's syndrome, marked by unilateral ptosis, pupillary constriction, and facial anhidrosis, may occur with lower cervical cord injury.

Spinal cord tumor

With spinal cord tumor, bilateral Babinski's reflex occurs with variable loss of pain and temperature sensation, proprioception, and motor function. Spasticity, hyperactive DTRs, absent abdominal reflexes, and incontinence are also characteristic. Diffuse pain may occur at the level of the tumor.

Stroke

Babinski's reflex varies with the site of a stroke. If it involves the cerebrum, it produces unilateral Babinski's reflex accompanied by hemiplegia or hemiparesis, uni-

Medical causes
(continued)

Multiple sclerosis
+ Babinski's reflex occurs bilaterally following initial signs and symptoms.

Pernicious anemia
+ Bilateral Babinski's reflex occurs late, when vitamin B_{12} deficiency affects the CNS.

Rabies
+ Bilateral Babinski's reflex occurs 2 to 10 days after the onset of prodromal signs and symptoms.

Spinal cord injury
+ Reflex occurs unilaterally if injury affects only one side of the spinal cord; bilaterally if injury affects both sides.

Spinal cord tumor
+ Bilateral Babinski's reflex occurs with variable loss of pain and temperature sensation, proprioception, and motor function.

Stroke
+ Cerebral involvement produces unilateral Babinski's reflex accompanied by hemiplegia or hemiparesis, unilateral hyperactive DTRs, hemianopsia, and aphasia.
+ Brain stem involvement produces bilateral Babinski's reflex accompanied by bilateral weakness or paralysis, bilateral hyperactive DTRs, cranial nerve dysfunction, incoordination, and unsteady gait.

Special considerations

+ Because the patient is at risk for injury, assist him with activity and keep his environment free from obstructions.

Peds points

+ Babinski's reflex occurs normally in infants up to 24 months old, reflecting immaturity of the corticospinal tract.
+ After age 2, Babinski's reflex is pathologic and may result from hydrocephalus or any of the causes more commonly seen in adults.

Teaching points

+ Diagnostic tests
+ Need for assistance when getting out of bed
+ Ways to maintain a safe environment
+ Use of adaptive devices

Key facts about back pain

+ Affects an estimated 80% of the U.S. population
+ May be acute or chronic
+ May be localized or radiate along the spine or legs

Key history points

+ Medical and family history
+ Diet
+ Alcohol use
+ Drug history

lateral hyperactive DTRs, hemianopsia, and aphasia. If it involves the brain stem, it produces bilateral Babinski's reflex accompanied by bilateral weakness or paralysis, bilateral hyperactive DTRs, cranial nerve dysfunction, incoordination, and unsteady gait. Generalized signs and symptoms of stroke include headache, vomiting, fever, disorientation, nuchal rigidity, seizures, and coma.

SPECIAL CONSIDERATIONS

Babinski's reflex usually occurs with incoordination, weakness, and spasticity, all of which increase the patient's risk of injury. To prevent injury, assist the patient with activity and keep his environment free from obstructions.

Diagnostic tests may include a computed tomography scan or magnetic resonance imaging of the brain or spine, angiography or myelography and, possibly, a lumbar puncture to clarify or confirm the cause of Babinski's reflex.

PEDIATRIC POINTERS

Babinski's reflex occurs normally in infants up to 24 months old, reflecting immaturity of the corticospinal tract. After age 2, Babinski's reflex is pathologic and may result from hydrocephalus or any of the causes more commonly seen in adults.

PATIENT COUNSELING

Prepare the patient for diagnostic tests by telling him what to expect before, during, and after the procedure. Reinforce the need for the patient to call for help before getting out of bed. Discuss ways to maintain a safe environment at home with the patient, his family, and caregivers. Teach the patient to use adaptive devices, such as braces or crutches, to maintain independence with activities of daily living.

BACK PAIN

Back pain affects an estimated 80% of the U.S. population; in fact, it's the second leading reason — after the common cold — for lost time from work. Although this symptom may herald a spondylogenic disorder, it may also result from a genitourinary, GI, cardiovascular, or neoplastic disorder. Postural imbalance associated with pregnancy may also cause back pain.

The onset, location, and distribution of pain and its response to activity and rest provide important clues about the cause. Pain may be acute or chronic, constant or intermittent. It may remain localized in the back or radiate along the spine or down one or both legs. Pain may be exacerbated by activity — usually, bending, stooping, or lifting — and alleviated by rest, or it may be unaffected by either.

Intrinsic back pain results from muscle spasm, nerve root irritation, fracture, or a combination of these mechanisms. It usually occurs in the lower back, or lumbosacral area. Back pain may also be referred from the abdomen or flank, possibly signaling a life-threatening perforated ulcer, acute pancreatitis, or dissecting abdominal aortic aneurysm. To learn more about treating life-threatening back pain, see *Managing acute, severe back pain*.

HISTORY

If life-threatening causes of back pain are ruled out, continue with a complete history. Be aware of the patient's expressions of pain as you do so.

EMERGENCY ACTIONS

Managing acute, severe back pain

If the patient reports acute, severe back pain, quickly take his vital signs; then perform a rapid evaluation to rule out life-threatening causes. Ask him when the pain began. Can he relate it to any causes? For example, did the pain occur after eating? After falling on ice? Ask the patient to describe the pain. Is it burning, stabbing, throbbing, or aching? Is it constant or intermittent? Does it radiate to the buttocks or legs? Does he have leg weakness? Does the pain seem to originate in the abdomen and radiate to the back? Has he had a pain like this before? What makes it better or worse? Is it affected by activity or rest? Is it worse in the morning or evening? Does it wake him up? Typically, visceral-referred back pain is unaffected by activity and rest. In contrast, spondylogenic-referred back pain worsens with activity and improves with rest. Pain of neoplastic origin is usually relieved by walking and worsens at night.

If the patient describes deep lumbar pain unaffected by activity, palpate for a pulsating epigastric mass. If this sign is present, suspect dissecting abdominal aortic aneurysm. Withhold food and fluid in anticipation of emergency surgery. Prepare for I.V. fluid replacement and oxygen administration.

If the patient describes severe epigastric pain that radiates through the abdomen to the back, assess him for absent bowel sounds and for abdominal rigidity and tenderness. If these occur, suspect perforated ulcer or acute pancreatitis. Start an I.V. line for fluids and drugs, administer oxygen, and insert a nasogastric tube while withholding food.

CULTURAL CUE *A patient's cultural background may impact his response to pain. For example, a patient of Irish descent may have a stoic response. A Jewish patient or one of Italian descent may be more vocal. The Navajo patient may view pain as a way of life. A patient of Filipino descent may regard pain as a chance to atone for past transgressions.*

Obtain a medical history, including past injuries and illnesses, and a family history. Ask about diet and alcohol intake. Also, take a drug history, including past and present prescriptions and over-the-counter drugs as well as herbal remedies.

PHYSICAL ASSESSMENT

Perform a thorough physical examination. Observe skin color, especially in the patient's legs, and palpate skin temperature. Palpate femoral, popliteal, posterior tibial, and pedal pulses. Ask about unusual sensations in the legs, such as numbness and tingling. Observe the patient's posture if pain doesn't prohibit standing. Does he stand erect or tend to lean toward one side? Observe the level of the shoulders and pelvis and the curvature of the back. Ask the patient to bend forward, backward, and side to side while you palpate for paravertebral muscle spasms. Note rotation of the spine on the trunk. Palpate the dorsolumbar spine for point tenderness. Then ask the patient to walk—first on his heels, then on his toes; protect him from falling as he does so. Weakness may reflect a muscular disorder or spinal nerve root irritation. Place the patient in a sitting position to evaluate and compare patellar tendon (knee), Achilles tendon, and Babinski's reflexes. Evaluate the strength of the extensor hallucis longus by asking the patient to hold up his big toe against resistance. Measure leg length and hamstring and quadriceps muscles bilaterally. Note a difference of more than ⅜″ (1 cm) in muscle size, especially in the calf.

To reproduce leg and back pain, position the patient in a supine position on the examination table. Grasp his heel and slowly lift his leg. If he feels pain, note its ex-

Critical assessment steps

+ Observe skin color, especially in the legs.
+ Palpate skin temperature.
+ Palpate femoral, popliteal, posterior tibial, and pedal pulses.
+ Ask about unusual sensations in the legs.
+ Ask the patient to bend forward, backward, and side to side while you palpate for paravertebral muscle spasms.
+ Palpate the dorsolumbar spine for point tenderness.
+ Ask the patient to walk—first on his heels, then on his toes.
+ Evaluate and compare patellar tendon (knee), Achilles tendon, and Babinski's reflexes.
+ Evaluate the strength of the extensor hallucis longus by asking the patient to hold up his big toe against resistance.
+ Measure leg length and hamstring and quadriceps muscles bilaterally.
+ Position the patient in a supine position on the examination table. Grasp his heel and slowly lift his leg. Note the pain's exact location and the angle between the table and his leg when it occurs. Repeat this maneuver with the opposite leg.
+ Note the range of motion of the hip and knee.
+ Palpate the flanks and percuss with the fingertips or perform fist percussion to elicit costovertebral angle tenderness.

act location and the angle between the table and his leg when it occurs. Repeat this maneuver with the opposite leg. Pain along the sciatic nerve may indicate disk herniation or sciatica. Also, note the range of motion of the hip and knee.

Palpate the flanks and percuss with the fingertips or perform fist percussion to elicit costovertebral angle tenderness.

MEDICAL CAUSES

Abdominal aortic aneurysm (dissecting)

Life-threatening dissection of abdominal aortic aneurysm may initially cause low back pain or dull abdominal pain. More commonly, it produces constant upper abdominal pain. A pulsating abdominal mass may be palpated in the epigastrium; after rupture, though, it no longer pulses. Aneurysmal dissection can also cause mottled skin below the waist, absent femoral and pedal pulses, lower blood pressure in the legs than in the arms, mild to moderate tenderness with guarding, and abdominal rigidity. Signs of shock (such as cool, clammy skin) appear if blood loss is significant.

Ankylosing spondylitis

Ankylosing spondylitis is a chronic, progressive disorder that causes sacroiliac pain, which radiates up the spine and is aggravated by lateral pressure on the pelvis. The pain is usually most severe in the morning or after a period of inactivity and isn't relieved by rest. Abnormal rigidity of the lumbar spine with forward flexion is also characteristic. This disorder can cause local tenderness, fatigue, fever, anorexia, weight loss, and occasional iritis.

Appendicitis

Appendicitis is a life-threatening disorder that causes a vague and dull discomfort in the epigastric or umbilical region, which migrates to McBurney's point in the right lower quadrant. With retrocecal appendicitis, pain may also radiate to the back. The shift in pain is preceded by anorexia and nausea and is accompanied by fever, occasional vomiting, abdominal tenderness (especially over McBurney's point), and rebound tenderness. Some patients also have painful, urgent urination.

Cholecystitis

Cholecystitis produces severe pain in the right upper quadrant of the abdomen that may radiate to the right shoulder, chest, or back. The pain may arise suddenly or may increase gradually over several hours, and patients usually have a history of similar pain after a high-fat meal. Accompanying signs and symptoms include anorexia, fever, nausea, vomiting, right-upper-quadrant tenderness, abdominal rigidity, pallor, and sweating.

Endometriosis

Endometriosis causes deep sacral pain and severe, cramping pain in the lower abdomen. The pain worsens just before or during menstruation and may be aggravated by defecation. It's accompanied by constipation, abdominal tenderness, dysmenorrhea, and dyspareunia.

Intervertebral disk rupture

An intervertebral disk rupture produces gradual or sudden low back pain with or without leg pain (sciatica). It rarely produces leg pain alone. Pain usually begins in the back and radiates to the buttocks and leg. The pain is exacerbated by activity, coughing, and sneezing and is eased by rest. It's accompanied by paresthesia (most commonly, numbness or tingling in the lower leg and foot), paravertebral muscle spasm, and decreased reflexes on the affected side. This disorder also affects posture

---

Medical causes

Abdominal aortic aneurysm (dissecting)
+ Initially, low back pain or dull abdominal pain may occur.
+ Upper abdominal pain is more common.

Ankylosing spondylitis
+ Sacroiliac pain radiates up the spine and is aggravated by lateral pressure on the pelvis.
+ Pain is usually most severe in the morning or after a period of inactivity and isn't relieved by rest.

Appendicitis
+ With retrocecal appendicitis, pain may radiate to the back.
+ Back pain is preceded by anorexia and nausea and is accompanied by fever, occasional vomiting, abdominal tenderness, and rebound tenderness.

Cholecystitis
+ Severe pain in the right upper quadrant of the abdomen may radiate to the right shoulder, chest, or back.

Endometriosis
+ Sacral pain and severe, cramping pain in the lower abdomen occur.

Intervertebral disk rupture
+ Gradual or sudden low back pain occurs with or without sciatica.
+ Pain is exacerbated by activity, coughing, and sneezing and is eased by rest.

and gait. The patient's spine is slightly flexed and he leans toward the painful side. He walks slowly and rises from a sitting to a standing position with extreme difficulty.

Lumbosacral sprain

A lumbosacral sprain causes aching, localized pain and tenderness associated with muscle spasm on lateral motion. The recumbent patient typically flexes his knees and hips to help ease pain. Flexion of the spine intensifies pain, whereas rest helps relieve it. The pain worsens with movement and is relieved by rest.

Myeloma

Myeloma, a primary malignant tumor, causes back pain that usually begins abruptly and worsens with exercise. It may be accompanied by arthritic signs and symptoms, such as achiness, joint swelling, and tenderness. Other signs and symptoms include fever, malaise, peripheral paresthesia, and weight loss.

Pancreatitis (acute)

Acute pancreatitis is a life-threatening disorder that usually produces fulminating, continuous upper abdominal pain that may radiate to both flanks and to the back. To relieve this pain, the patient may bend forward, draw his knees to his chest, or move restlessly about.

Early associated signs and symptoms of acute pancreatitis include abdominal tenderness, nausea, vomiting, fever, pallor, tachycardia and, in some patients, abdominal guarding, rigidity, rebound tenderness, and hypoactive bowel sounds. A late sign may be jaundice. Occurring as inflammation subsides, Turner's sign (ecchymosis of the abdomen or flank) or Cullen's sign (bluish discoloration of skin around the umbilicus and in both flanks) signals hemorrhagic pancreatitis.

Perforated ulcer

In some patients, perforation of a duodenal or gastric ulcer causes sudden, prostrating epigastric pain that may radiate throughout the abdomen and to the back. This life-threatening disorder also causes boardlike abdominal rigidity, tenderness with guarding, generalized rebound tenderness, the absence of bowel sounds, and grunting, shallow respirations. Associated signs include fever, tachycardia, and hypotension.

Prostate cancer

Chronic aching back pain may be the only symptom of prostate cancer. This disorder may also produce hematuria, difficulty initiating a urine stream, dribbling, urine retention, unexplained cystitis as well as decrease in the urine stream. Signs and symptoms of prostate cancer may appear only in the advanced stages.

Pyelonephritis (acute)

Acute pyelonephritis produces progressive flank and lower abdominal pain accompanied by back pain or tenderness (especially over the costovertebral angle). Other signs and symptoms include high fever and chills, nausea and vomiting, flank and abdominal tenderness, and urinary frequency and urgency.

Reiter's syndrome

In some patients, sacroiliac pain is the first sign of Reiter's syndrome. Pain is accompanied by the classic triad of conjunctivitis, urethritis, and arthritis. In 30% of patients, skin lesions develop 4 to 6 weeks after onset of other symptoms and may last for several weeks.

Medical causes
(continued)

Lumbosacral sprain
+ Aching, localized pain and tenderness is associated with muscle spasm on lateral motion.
+ Flexion of the spine intensifies pain; rest helps relieve it.

Myeloma
+ Back pain usually begins abruptly and worsens with exercise.
+ Pain may be accompanied by arthritic signs and symptoms.

Pancreatitis (acute)
+ Upper abdominal pain may radiate to the flanks and the back.
+ Bending forward, drawing the knees to the chest, or moving around may relieve pain.

Perforated ulcer
+ Epigastric pain may radiate throughout the abdomen and to the back.

Prostate cancer
+ Chronic aching back pain may be the only symptom, appearing in the advanced stages.

Pyelonephritis (acute)
+ Progressive flank and lower abdominal pain accompanies back pain or tenderness (especially over the costovertebral angle).

Reiter's syndrome
+ Sacroiliac pain may be the first sign.
+ Pain is accompanied by conjunctivitis, urethritis, and arthritis.

Medical causes
(continued)

Renal calculi
+ Pain travels from the costovertebral angle to the flank, suprapubic region, and external genitalia.
+ Pain resolves or decreases after calculi move to the bladder.

Sacroiliac strain
+ Sacroiliac pain may radiate to the buttock, hip, and lateral aspect of the thigh.

Smallpox
+ High fever, malaise, prostration, severe headache, backache, and abdominal pain occur initially.

Spinal stenosis
+ Back pain occurs with or without sciatica.

Transverse process and vertebral compression fractures
+ Severe localized back pain occurs with muscle spasm and hematoma.

Vertebral osteomyelitis
+ Initially, back pain is insidious.
+ As it progresses, pain may become constant, more pronounced at night, and aggravated by spinal movement.

Vertebral osteoporosis
+ Chronic, aching back pain is aggravated by activity.

Renal calculi
The colicky pain of renal calculi usually results from irritation of the ureteral lining, which increases the frequency and force of peristaltic contractions. The pain travels from the costovertebral angle to the flank, suprapubic region, and external genitalia. Its intensity varies but may become excruciating if calculi travel down a ureter. If calculi are in the renal pelvis and calyces, dull and constant flank pain may occur. Renal calculi also cause nausea, vomiting, urinary urgency (if a calculus lodges near the bladder), hematuria, and agitation due to pain. Pain resolves or significantly decreases after calculi move to the bladder. Encourage the patient to recover the calculi for analysis.

Sacroiliac strain
Sacroiliac strain causes sacroiliac pain that may radiate to the buttock, hip, and lateral aspect of the thigh. The pain is aggravated by weight bearing on the affected extremity and by abduction with resistance of the leg. Associated signs and symptoms include tenderness of the symphysis pubis and a limp or gluteus medius or abductor lurch.

Smallpox
Initial signs and symptoms of smallpox include high fever, malaise, prostration, severe headache, backache, and abdominal pain. A maculopapular rash develops on the mucosa of the mouth, pharynx, face, and forearms and then spreads to the trunk and legs. Within 2 days the rash becomes vesicular and later pustular. The lesions develop at the same time, appear identical, and are more prominent on the face and extremities. The pustules are round, firm, and deeply embedded in the skin. After 8 to 9 days, the pustules form a crust, and later the scab separates from the skin leaving a pitted scar. In fatal cases, death results from encephalitis, extensive bleeding, or secondary infection.

Spinal stenosis
Resembling a ruptured intervertebral disk, spinal stenosis produces back pain with or without sciatica, which commonly affects both legs. The pain may radiate to the toes and may progress to numbness or weakness unless the patient rests.

Transverse process and vertebral compression fractures
A transverse process fracture causes severe localized back pain with muscle spasm and hematoma. Initially, a vertebral compression fracture may be painless. Several weeks later, it causes back pain aggravated by weight bearing and local tenderness. Fracture of a thoracic vertebra may cause referred pain in the lumbar area.

Vertebral osteomyelitis
Initially, vertebral osteomyelitis causes insidious back pain. As it progresses, the pain may become constant, more pronounced at night, and aggravated by spinal movement. Accompanying signs and symptoms include vertebral and hamstring spasms, tenderness of the spinous processes, fever, and malaise.

Vertebral osteoporosis
Vertebral osteoporosis causes chronic, aching back pain that's aggravated by activity and somewhat relieved by rest. Tenderness may also occur. Vertebral collapse, causing a backache with pain that radiates around the trunk, is the most common presenting feature of osteoporosis.

SPECIAL CONSIDERATIONS

Monitor the patient closely if the back pain suggests a life-threatening cause. Be alert for increasing pain, altered neurovascular status in the legs, loss of bowel or bladder control, altered vital signs, sweating, and cyanosis.

Until a tentative diagnosis is made, withhold analgesics, which may mask symptoms. Also withhold food and fluids in case surgery is necessary. Make the patient as comfortable as possible by elevating the head of the bed and placing a pillow under his knees. Encourage relaxation techniques such as deep breathing. Prepare the patient for a rectal or pelvic examination. He may also require routine blood tests, urinalysis, computed tomography scan, appropriate biopsies, and X-rays of the chest, abdomen, and spine.

Fit the patient for a corset or lumbosacral support. Instruct him not to wear this in bed. He may also require heat or cold therapy, a backboard, a convoluted foam mattress, or pelvic traction. Explain these pain-relief measures to the patient. Teach the patient about alternatives to analgesic drug therapy, such as biofeedback and transcutaneous electrical nerve stimulation.

PEDIATRIC POINTERS

Because a child may have difficulty describing back pain, be alert for nonverbal clues, such as wincing or refusal to walk. Closely observe family dynamics during history taking for clues suggesting child abuse.

Back pain in a child may stem from intervertebral disk inflammation (diskitis), neoplasms, idiopathic juvenile osteoporosis, and spondylolisthesis. Disk herniation typically doesn't cause back pain. Scoliosis, a common disorder in adolescents, rarely causes back pain.

GERIATRIC POINTERS

Suspect metastatic cancer — especially of the prostate, colon or breast — in older patients with a recent onset of back pain that usually isn't relieved by rest and worsens at night.

PATIENT COUNSELING

If the patient has chronic back pain, reinforce instructions about bed rest, analgesics, anti-inflammatories, and exercise. Also, suggest that he take daily warm baths to help relieve pain. Help the patient recognize the need to make necessary lifestyle changes, such as losing weight or correcting poor posture. Advise patients with acute back pain secondary to a musculoskeletal problem to continue their daily activities as tolerated, rather than staying on total bed rest.

BATTLE'S SIGN

Battle's sign — ecchymosis over the mastoid process of the temporal bone — is commonly the only outward sign of a basilar skull fracture. Appearing behind one or both ears, Battle's sign is easily overlooked or hidden by the patient's hair. In fact, this type of fracture may go undetected even by skull X-rays. If left untreated, it can be fatal because of associated injury to the nearby cranial nerves and brain stem as well as to blood vessels and the meninges.

A force that's strong enough to fracture the base of the skull causes Battle's sign by damaging supporting tissues of the mastoid area and causing seepage of blood

Special considerations
+ Monitor the patient closely if the cause is life-threatening.
+ Be alert for increasing pain, altered neurovascular status in the legs, loss of bowel or bladder control, altered vital signs, sweating, and cyanosis.
+ Withhold analgesics until a tentative diagnosis is made.
+ Withhold food and fluids in case surgery is necessary.
+ Elevate the head of the bed and place a pillow under the knees.
+ Encourage relaxation.
+ Fit the patient for a corset or lumbosacral support.

Peds points
+ Back pain in a child may stem from diskitis, neoplasms, idiopathic juvenile osteoporosis, and spondylolisthesis.

Geri points
+ Suspect metastatic cancer if back pain is recent, isn't relieved by rest, and worsens at night.

Teaching points
+ Bed rest
+ Anti-inflammatories and analgesics
+ Lifestyle changes, such as losing weight or correcting posture

Key facts about Battle's sign
+ Ecchymosis over the temporal bone's mastoid process
+ Develops 24 to 36 hours after a basilar skull fracture

Key history points

+ Recent head trauma or accidents

Critical assessment steps

+ Perform a complete neurologic examination.
+ Check vital signs; be alert for signs of increased ICP.
+ Assess cranial nerve function in nerves II, III, IV, VI, VII, and VIII.
+ Evaluate pupillary size, response to light, and motor and verbal responses; relate data to the Glasgow Coma Scale.
+ Note CSF leakage from the nose or ears.
+ Look for the halo sign on bed linens or dressings.
+ Test drainage with a glucose reagent strip to confirm that it's CSF.
+ Perform a complete physical examination.

Medical causes

Basilar skull fracture
+ Battle's sign may be the only outward sign.

Special considerations

+ Keep the patient flat to decrease pressure on dural tears and to minimize CSF leakage.
+ Monitor neurologic status.
+ Avoid nasogastric intubation and nasopharyngeal suction.

Peds points

+ Victims of abuse frequently sustain basilar skull fractures.
+ If you suspect abuse, follow protocol for reporting the incident.

from the fracture site to the mastoid. Battle's sign usually develops 24 to 36 hours after the fracture and may persist for several days to weeks.

HISTORY

Ask the patient about recent trauma to the head. Did he sustain a severe blow to the head? Was he involved in a motor vehicle accident? Note the patient's level of consciousness (LOC) as he responds. Does he respond quickly or slowly? Are his answers appropriate, or does he appear confused?

PHYSICAL ASSESSMENT

Perform a complete neurologic examination. Check the patient's vital signs; be alert for widening pulse pressure and bradycardia, signs of increased intracranial pressure. Assess cranial nerve function in nerves II, III, IV, VI, VII, and VIII. Evaluate pupillary size and response to light as well as motor and verbal responses. Relate these data to the Glasgow Coma Scale. Also, note cerebrospinal fluid (CSF) leakage from the nose or ears. Ask about postnasal drip, which may reflect CSF drainage down the throat. Look for the halo sign — a bloodstain encircled by a yellowish ring — on bed linens or dressings. To confirm that drainage is CSF, test it with a glucose reagent strip; CSF is positive for glucose, whereas mucus isn't. Follow up the neurologic examination with a complete physical examination to detect other injuries associated with basilar skull fracture.

MEDICAL CAUSES

Basilar skull fracture

Battle's sign may be the only outward sign of a basilar skull fracture, or it may be accompanied by periorbital ecchymosis (raccoon eyes), conjunctival hemorrhage, nystagmus, ocular deviation, epistaxis, anosmia, a bulging tympanic membrane (from CSF or blood accumulation), visible fracture lines on the external auditory canal, tinnitus, difficulty hearing, facial paralysis, or vertigo.

SPECIAL CONSIDERATIONS

Expect a patient with basilar skull fracture to be on bed rest for several days to weeks. Keep him flat to decrease pressure on dural tears and to minimize CSF leakage. Monitor neurologic status closely. Avoid nasogastric intubation and nasopharyngeal suction, which may cause cerebral infection.

The patient may need skull X-rays and a computed tomography scan to help confirm basilar skull fracture and to evaluate the severity of head injury. Typically, basilar skull fracture and any associated dural tears heal spontaneously within several days to weeks. However, if the patient has a large dural tear, a craniotomy may be necessary to repair the tear with a graft patch.

PEDIATRIC POINTERS

Children who are victims of abuse frequently sustain basilar skull fractures from severe blows to the head. As in adults, Battle's sign may be the only outward sign of fracture and, perhaps, the only clue to child abuse. If you suspect child abuse, follow hospital protocol for reporting the incident.

PATIENT COUNSELING

Explain activity restrictions and the need for bed rest to the patient. Provide emotional support to the patient and his family. Caution the patient against blowing his nose, which may worsen a dural tear.

Before discharge, instruct the patient's family or caregiver to watch closely for changes in mental status, LOC, or respirations. Tell them to give the patient acetaminophen if he experiences headaches.

BLADDER DISTENTION

Bladder distention — abnormal enlargement of the bladder — results from an inability to excrete urine, which results in its accumulation. Distention can be caused by a mechanical or anatomic obstruction, neuromuscular disorder, or the use of certain drugs. Relatively common in all ages and both sexes, it's most common in older men with prostate disorders that cause urine retention.

Distention usually develops gradually, but it occasionally has a sudden onset. Gradual distention usually produces no symptoms until stretching of the bladder produces discomfort. Acute distention produces suprapubic fullness, pressure, and pain. If severe distention isn't corrected promptly by catheterization or massage, the bladder rises within the abdomen, its walls become thin, and renal function can be impaired.

Bladder distention is aggravated by the intake of caffeine, alcohol, large quantities of fluid, and diuretics.

 EMERGENCY ACTIONS If the patient has severe distention, insert an indwelling urinary catheter to help relieve discomfort and prevent bladder rupture. If more than 700 ml is emptied from the bladder, compressed blood vessels dilate and may make the patient feel faint. Typically, the indwelling urinary catheter is clamped for 30 to 60 minutes to permit vessel compensation.

HISTORY

If distention isn't severe, begin by reviewing the patient's voiding patterns. Find out the time and amount of the patient's last voiding and the amount of fluid consumed since then. Ask if he has difficulty urinating. Does he use Valsalva's or Credé's maneuver to initiate urination? Does he urinate with urgency or without warning? Is urination painful or irritating? Ask about the force and continuity of his urine stream and whether he feels that his bladder is empty after voiding.

Explore the patient's history of urinary tract obstruction or infections; venereal disease; neurologic, intestinal, or pelvic surgery; lower abdominal or urinary tract trauma; and systemic or neurologic disorders. Note his drug history, including his use of over-the-counter drugs.

PHYSICAL ASSESSMENT

Take the patient's vital signs, and percuss and palpate the bladder. (Remember that if the bladder is empty, it can't be palpated through the abdominal wall.) Inspect the urethral meatus, and measure its diameter. Describe the appearance and amount of any discharge. Finally, test for perineal sensation and anal sphincter tone; in male patients, digitally examine the prostate gland.

Teaching points

- ✦ Activity restrictions and bed rest
- ✦ Signs and symptoms of changes in mental status, LOC, or respirations
- ✦ Acetaminophen for headaches

Key facts about bladder distention

- ✦ Abnormal bladder enlargement
- ✦ Results from an inability to excrete urine
- ✦ Caused by a mechanical or anatomic obstruction, neuromuscular disorder, or the use of certain drugs

In an emergency

- ✦ Insert an indwelling urinary catheter.
- ✦ Be aware that if more than 700 ml is emptied, compressed blood vessels dilate and may make the patient feel faint.

Key history points

- ✦ Voiding patterns and characteristics
- ✦ Time and amount of last voiding
- ✦ Amount of fluid consumed since last voiding
- ✦ Medical and drug history

Critical assessment steps

- ✦ Take vital signs.
- ✦ Percuss and palpate the bladder.
- ✦ Inspect the urethral meatus, and measure its diameter.
- ✦ Describe the appearance and amount of any discharge.
- ✦ Test for perineal sensation and anal sphincter tone.
- ✦ In males, digitally examine the prostate gland.

Medical causes

BPH
+ Bladder distention develops gradually as the prostate enlarges.

Bladder cancer
+ Neoplasms can cause bladder distention by blocking the urethral orifice.

Multiple sclerosis
+ Urine retention and bladder distention result from interrupted upper motor neuron control of the bladder.

Prostatitis
+ Bladder distention occurs rapidly along with perineal discomfort and suprapubic fullness.

Spinal neoplasms
+ Upper neuron control of the bladder is disrupted, causing neurogenic bladder and distention.

Urethral calculi
+ Urethral obstruction causes bladder distention and radiation pain.

Urethral stricture
+ Urine retention and bladder distention result.
+ Urethral discharge and urinary frequency are common signs.

MEDICAL CAUSES

Benign prostatic hyperplasia

With benign prostatic hyperplasia (BPH), bladder distention gradually develops as the prostate enlarges. Occasionally, its onset is acute. Initially, the patient experiences urinary hesitancy, straining, and frequency; reduced force of and the inability to stop the urine stream; nocturia; and postvoiding dribbling. As the disorder progresses, it produces prostate enlargement, sensations of suprapubic fullness and incomplete bladder emptying, perineal pain, constipation, and hematuria.

Bladder cancer

By blocking the urethral orifice, neoplasms can cause bladder distention. Associated signs and symptoms include hematuria (most common sign); urinary frequency and urgency; nocturia; dysuria; pyuria; pain in the bladder, rectum, pelvis, flank, back, or legs; vomiting; diarrhea; and sleeplessness. A mass may be palpable on bimanual examination.

 CULTURAL CUE *Bladder cancer is twice as common in Whites as in Blacks. It's relatively uncommon among Asians, Hispanics, and Native Americans.*

Multiple sclerosis

With multiple sclerosis, a neuromuscular disorder, urine retention and bladder distention result from interruption of upper motor neuron control of the bladder. Associated signs and symptoms include optic neuritis, paresthesia, impaired position and vibratory senses, diplopia, nystagmus, dizziness, abnormal reflexes, dysarthria, muscle weakness, emotional lability, Lhermitte's sign (transient, electric-like shocks that spread down the body when the head is flexed), Babinski's sign, and ataxia.

Prostatitis

With acute prostatitis, bladder distention occurs rapidly along with perineal discomfort and suprapubic fullness. Other signs and symptoms include perineal pain; tense, boggy, tender, and warm enlarged prostate; decreased libido; impotence; decreased force of the urine stream; dysuria; hematuria; and urinary frequency and urgency. Additional signs and symptoms include fatigue, malaise, myalgia, fever, chills, nausea, and vomiting.

Spinal neoplasms

Disrupting upper neuron control of the bladder, spinal neoplasms cause neurogenic bladder and resultant distention. Associated signs and symptoms include a sense of pelvic fullness, continuous overflow dribbling, back pain that typically mimics sciatica pain, constipation, tender vertebral processes, sensory deficits, and muscle weakness, flaccidity, and atrophy. Signs and symptoms of urinary tract infection (dysuria, urinary frequency and urgency, nocturia, tenesmus, hematuria, and weakness) may also occur.

Urethral calculi

With urethral calculi, urethral obstruction leads to bladder distention. The patient experiences interrupted urine flow. The obstruction causes pain radiating to the penis or vulva and referred to the perineum or rectum. It may also produce a palpable stone and urethral discharge.

Urethral stricture

Urethral stricture results in urine retention and bladder distention with chronic urethral discharge (most common sign), urinary frequency (also common), dysuria, urgency, decreased force and diameter of the urine stream, and pyuria. Urinoma and urosepsis may also develop.

OTHER CAUSES

Catheterization
Using an indwelling urinary catheter can result in urine retention and bladder distention. While the catheter is in place, inadequate drainage due to kinked tubing or an occluded lumen may lead to urine retention. In addition, a misplaced urinary catheter or irritation with catheter removal may cause edema, thereby blocking urine outflow.

Drugs
Parasympatholytics, anticholinergics, ganglionic blockers, sedatives, anesthetics, and opiates can produce urine retention and bladder distention.

SPECIAL CONSIDERATIONS
Monitor the patient's vital signs and the extent of bladder distention. Encourage the patient to change positions to alleviate discomfort. He may require an analgesic.

Prepare the patient for diagnostic tests (such as endoscopy and radiologic studies) to determine the cause of bladder distention. You may need to prepare him for surgery if interventions fail to relieve bladder distention and obstruction prevents catheterization.

PEDIATRIC POINTERS
Look for urine retention and bladder distention in any infant who fails to void normal amounts. (In the first 48 hours of life, an infant excretes about 60 ml of urine; during the next week, he excretes about 300 ml of urine daily.) In males, posterior urethral valves, meatal stenosis, phimosis, spinal cord anomalies, bladder diverticula, and other congenital defects may cause urinary obstruction and resultant bladder distention.

PATIENT COUNSELING
If the patient doesn't require immediate urinary catheterization, provide privacy and suggest that he assume the normal voiding position. Teach him to perform Valsalva's maneuver, or gently perform Credé's maneuver. You can also stroke or intermittently apply ice to the inner thigh, or help him relax in a warm tub or sitz bath. Use the power of suggestion to stimulate voiding. For example, run water in the sink, pour warm water over his perineum, place his hands in warm water, or play tapes of aquatic sounds.

BLOOD PRESSURE DECREASE

Low blood pressure, also known as *hypotension*, refers to inadequate intravascular pressure to maintain the oxygen requirements of the body's tissues. Typically, a reading below 90/60 mm Hg, or a drop of 30 mm Hg from the baseline, is considered low blood pressure. Although commonly linked to shock, this sign may also result from a cardiovascular, respiratory, neurologic, or metabolic disorder. Hypoperfusion states especially affect the kidneys, brain, and heart, and may lead to change in level of consciousness (LOC), or myocardial ischemia. Low blood pres-

Other causes
+ Anesthetics
+ Anticholinergics
+ Catheterization
+ Ganglionic blockers
+ Opiates
+ Parasympatholytics
+ Sedatives

Special considerations
+ Monitor vital signs and the extent of bladder distention.
+ Encourage the patient to change positions to alleviate discomfort.
+ Give analgesics, as ordered, if needed.
+ Prepare the patient for surgery as needed.

Peds points
+ Look for urine retention and bladder distention in any infant who fails to void normal amounts.
+ In males, posterior urethral valves, meatal stenosis, phimosis, spinal cord anomalies, bladder diverticula, and other congenital defects may cause urinary obstruction and resultant bladder distention.

Teaching points
+ Vasalva's maneuver
+ Ways to stimulate voiding

Key facts about decreased blood pressure
+ Inadequate intravascular pressure to maintain oxygen requirements
+ Also called *hypotension*
+ Typically defined as a reading below 90/60 mm Hg or a drop of 30 mm Hg from the baseline

In an emergency

+ Quickly evaluate the patient for decreased LOC.
+ Check the apical pulse for tachycardia; check respirations for tachypnea.
+ Inspect for cool, clammy skin.
+ Elevate the patient's legs above the level of his heart, or place him in Trendelenburg's position.
+ Start an I.V. line using a large-bore needle to replace fluids and blood or to administer drugs.
+ Prepare to administer oxygen with mechanical ventilation if necessary.
+ Monitor intake and output.
+ Prepare for cardiac or hemodynamic monitoring.

Key history points

+ Associated symptoms, such as weakness, nausea, dizziness, and chest pain

Critical assessment steps

+ Inspect the skin for pallor, sweating, and clamminess.
+ Palpate peripheral pulses.
+ Auscultate for abnormal heart sounds, rate, or rhythm.
+ Auscultate for abnormal breath sounds, rate, or rhythm.
+ Look for signs of hemorrhage.
+ Assess for abdominal rigidity and rebound tenderness.
+ Auscultate for abnormal bowel sounds.
+ Assess for possible sources of infection such as open wounds.

sure may be drug-induced or may accompany diagnostic tests — most commonly those using contrast media. It may stem from stress or change of position — specifically, rising abruptly from a supine or sitting position to a standing position (orthostatic hypotension).

Low blood pressure can reflect an expanded intravascular space (as in severe infections, allergic reactions, or adrenal insufficiency), reduced intravascular volume (as in dehydration and hemorrhage), or decreased cardiac output (as in impaired cardiac muscle contractility). Because the body's pressure-regulating mechanisms are complex and interrelated, a combination of these factors usually contributes to low blood pressure.

EMERGENCY ACTIONS If the patient's systolic pressure is less than 80 mm Hg, or 30 mm Hg below his baseline, suspect shock immediately. Quickly evaluate the patient for a decreased LOC. Check his apical pulse for tachycardia and respirations for tachypnea. Also, inspect the patient for cool, clammy skin. Elevate the patient's legs above the level of his heart, or place him in Trendelenburg's position if the bed can be adjusted. Then start an I.V. line using a large-bore needle to replace fluids and blood or to administer drugs. Prepare to administer oxygen with mechanical ventilation, if necessary. Monitor the patient's intake and output and insert an indwelling urinary catheter for the accurate measurement of urine. The patient may also need a central venous line or a pulmonary artery catheter to facilitate monitoring of fluid status. Prepare for cardiac monitoring to evaluate heart rhythm. Be ready to insert a nasogastric tube to prevent aspiration in the comatose patient. Throughout emergency interventions, keep the patient's spinal column immobile until spinal cord trauma is ruled out.

HISTORY

If the patient is conscious, ask him about associated symptoms. For example, does he feel unusually weak or fatigued? Has he had nausea, vomiting, or dark or bloody stools? Is his vision blurred? Gait unsteady? Does he have palpitations? Does he have chest or abdominal pain or difficulty breathing? Has he had episodes of dizziness or fainting? Do these episodes occur when he stands up suddenly? If so, take the patient's blood pressure while he's lying down, sitting, and then standing; compare readings. A drop in systolic or diastolic pressure of 10 to 20 mm Hg or more and an increase in heart rate of more than 15 beats/minute between position changes suggest orthostatic hypotension. (See *Ensuring accurate blood pressure measurement*.)

PHYSICAL ASSESSMENT

Perform a physical examination. Inspect the skin for pallor, sweating, and clamminess. Palpate peripheral pulses. Note paradoxical pulse — an accentuated fall in systolic pressure during inspiration — which suggests pericardial tamponade. Then auscultate for abnormal heart sounds (gallops, murmurs), rate (bradycardia, tachycardia), or rhythm. Auscultate the lungs for abnormal breath sounds (diminished sounds, crackles, wheezing), rate (bradypnea, tachypnea), or rhythm (agonal or Cheyne-Stokes respirations). Look for signs of hemorrhage, including visible bleeding and palpable masses, bruising, and tenderness. Assess the patient for abdominal rigidity and rebound tenderness; auscultate for abnormal bowel sounds. Also, carefully assess the patient for possible sources of infection such as open wounds.

Ensuring accurate blood pressure measurement

To obtain an accurate blood pressure, be sure to follow these guidelines:

✦ Have the patient rest for at least 5 minutes before measuring his blood pressure. Make sure he hasn't had caffeine or smoked cigarettes for at least 30 minutes. If your patient is crying or anxious, delay blood pressure measurement until the patient is calm to avoid false-high readings.

✦ Keep the patient's arm level with his heart. If the artery is below the heart, you may get a false-high reading.

✦ Wrap the cuff snugly around the upper arm above the antecubital area (the inner aspect of the elbow). A cuff that's wrapped too loosely will give a false-high reading.

✦ The cuff bladder width should be about 40% of the circumference of the midpoint of the limb; bladder length should be twice the width. If the arm circumference is less than 13″ (33 cm), select a regular-sized cuff; if it's between 13″ and 16″ (33 to 40.5 cm), a large-sized cuff; if it's more than 16″, a thigh cuff.

✦ Deflate the cuff no faster than 2 to 3 mm Hg/second. Deflating less than 2 mm Hg/ second causes venous congestion and may give you a false-high reading.

✦ Estimate the systolic pressure by palpation first, to avoid missing the top Korotkoff sound. Then inflate the cuff rapidly—at a rate of 2 to 3 mm Hg/second—to about 30 mm Hg above the palpable systolic pressure.

✦ Read the mercury column at eye level. If the column is below eye level, you may record a false-low reading; if it's above eye level, a false-high reading. Make sure the column is straight for your reading.

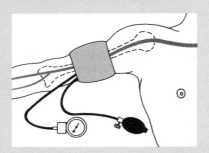

MEDICAL CAUSES

Acute adrenal insufficiency

Orthostatic hypotension is characteristic of acute adrenal insufficiency. It's accompanied by fatigue, weakness, nausea, vomiting, abdominal discomfort, weight loss, fever, and tachycardia. The patient may also have hyperpigmentation of fingers, nails, nipples, scars, and body folds; pale, cool, clammy skin; restlessness; decreased urine output; tachypnea; and coma.

Anaphylactic shock

Following exposure to an allergen, such as penicillin or insect venom, a dramatic fall in blood pressure and narrowed pulse pressure signal anaphylactic shock. Initially, this severe allergic reaction causes anxiety, restlessness, a feeling of doom, intense itching (especially of the hands and feet), and pounding headache. Later, it may also produce weakness, sweating, nasal congestion, coughing, difficulty breathing, nausea, abdominal cramps, involuntary defecation, seizures, flushing, change or loss of voice due to laryngeal edema, urinary incontinence, and tachycardia.

Anthrax (inhalation)

Inhalation anthrax is caused by inhalation of aerosolized spores of the gram-positive bacterium *Bacillus anthracis*. Initial signs and symptoms are flulike and include fever, chills, weakness, cough, and chest pain. The disease generally occurs in

Medical causes

Acute adrenal insufficiency
✦ Orthostatic hypotension is a characteristic sign.
✦ Fatigue, weakness, nausea, vomiting, abdominal discomfort, weight loss, fever, and tachycardia occur.

Anaphylactic shock
✦ Blood pressure falls dramatically and pulse pressure narrows.
✦ Initially, anxiety, restlessness, a feeling of doom, intense itching, and pounding headache occur.

Anthrax (inhalation)
✦ Initial signs and symptoms are flulike.
✦ The second stage is marked by fever, dyspnea, stridor, and hypotension.

Medical causes
(continued)

Cardiac arrhythmia
+ Blood pressure may fluctuate between normal and low readings.
+ Dizziness, chest pain, difficulty breathing, light-headedness, weakness, fatigue, and palpitations may occur.

Cardiac tamponade
+ Systolic pressure falls more than 10 mm Hg during inspiration.

Cardiogenic shock
+ Systolic pressure falls to less than 80 mm Hg or to 30 mm Hg less than baseline.
+ Tachycardia, narrowed pulse pressure, diminished Korotkoff sounds, peripheral cyanosis, and pale, cool, clammy skin occur.

Cholera
+ Watery diarrhea and vomiting occur.
+ Water and electrolyte loss causes hypotension.

Diabetic ketoacidosis
+ Hypovolemia — triggered by osmotic diuresis in hyperglycemia — causes low blood pressure.

Heart failure
+ Blood pressure may fluctuate between normal and low readings.
+ Various types of dyspnea may occur along with fatigue, weight gain, pallor or cyanosis, sweating, and anxiety.

two stages with a period of recovery after the initial signs and symptoms. The second stage develops abruptly with rapid deterioration marked by fever, dyspnea, stridor, and hypotension generally leading to death within 24 hours. Radiologic findings include mediastinitis and symmetric mediastinal widening.

Cardiac arrhythmia
With a cardiac arrhythmia, blood pressure may fluctuate between normal and low readings. Dizziness, chest pain, difficulty breathing, light-headedness, weakness, fatigue, and palpitations may also occur. Auscultation typically reveals an irregular rhythm and a pulse rate greater than 100 beats/minute or less than 60 beats/minute.

Cardiac tamponade
An accentuated fall in systolic pressure (more than 10 mm Hg) during inspiration, known as *paradoxical pulse,* is characteristic in patients with cardiac tamponade. This disorder also causes restlessness, cyanosis, tachycardia, jugular vein distention, muffled heart sounds, dyspnea, and Kussmaul's sign (increased venous distention with inspiration).

Cardiogenic shock
A fall in systolic pressure to less than 80 mm Hg or to 30 mm Hg less than the patient's baseline, because of decreased cardiac contractility, is characteristic in patients with cardiogenic shock. Accompanying low blood pressure are tachycardia, narrowed pulse pressure, diminished Korotkoff sounds, peripheral cyanosis, and pale, cool, clammy skin. Cardiogenic shock also causes restlessness and anxiety, which may progress to disorientation and confusion. Associated signs and symptoms include angina, dyspnea, jugular vein distention, oliguria, ventricular gallop, tachypnea, and weak, rapid pulse.

Cholera
Cholera, an acute infection that's caused by the bacterium *Vibrio cholerae,* may be mild with uncomplicated diarrhea or severe and life-threatening. Signs include abrupt watery diarrhea and vomiting. Severe water and electrolyte loss leads to thirst, weakness, muscle cramps, decreased skin turgor, oliguria, tachycardia, and hypotension. Without treatment, death can occur within hours.

Diabetic ketoacidosis
Hypovolemia triggered by osmotic diuresis in hyperglycemia is responsible for the low blood pressure associated with diabetic ketoacidosis, which is usually present in patients with type 1 diabetes mellitus. It also commonly produces polydipsia, polyuria, polyphagia, dehydration, weight loss, abdominal pain, nausea, vomiting, breath with fruity odor, Kussmaul's respirations, tachycardia, seizures, confusion, and stupor that may progress to coma.

Heart failure
With heart failure, blood pressure may fluctuate between normal and low readings. However, a precipitous drop in blood pressure may signal cardiogenic shock. Other signs and symptoms of heart failure include exertional dyspnea, dyspnea of abrupt or gradual onset, paroxysmal nocturnal dyspnea or difficulty breathing in the supine position (orthopnea), fatigue, weight gain, pallor or cyanosis, sweating, and anxiety. Auscultation reveals ventricular gallop, tachycardia, bilateral crackles, and tachypnea. Dependent edema, jugular vein distention, increased capillary refill time, and hepatomegaly may also occur.

Hypovolemic shock

A fall in systolic pressure to less than 80 mm Hg or 30 mm Hg less than the patient's baseline, secondary to acute blood loss or dehydration, is characteristic in patients with hypovolemic shock. Accompanying it are diminished Korotkoff sounds, narrowed pulse pressure, and rapid, weak, and irregular pulse. Peripheral vasoconstriction causes cyanosis of the extremities and pale, cool, clammy skin. Other signs and symptoms include oliguria, confusion, disorientation, restlessness, and anxiety.

Hypoxemia

Initially, blood pressure may be normal or slightly elevated, but as hypoxemia becomes more pronounced blood pressure drops. The patient may also display tachycardia, tachypnea, dyspnea, and confusion, and may progress from stupor to coma.

Myocardial infarction

With myocardial infarction (MI), a life-threatening disorder, blood pressure may be low or high. However, a precipitous drop in blood pressure may signal cardiogenic shock. Associated signs and symptoms of MI include chest pain that may radiate to the jaw, shoulder, arm, or epigastrium; dyspnea; anxiety; nausea or vomiting; sweating; and cool, pale, or cyanotic skin. Auscultation may reveal an atrial gallop, a murmur and, occasionally, an irregular pulse.

Neurogenic shock

The result of sympathetic denervation due to cervical injury or anesthesia, neurogenic shock produces low blood pressure and bradycardia. However, the patient's skin remains warm and dry because of cutaneous vasodilation and sweat gland denervation. Depending on the cause of shock, there may also be motor weakness of the limbs or diaphragm.

Pulmonary embolism

Pulmonary embolism causes sudden, sharp chest pain and dyspnea accompanied by cough and, occasionally, low-grade fever. Low blood pressure occurs with narrowed pulse pressure and diminished Korotkoff sounds. Associated signs include tachycardia, tachypnea, paradoxical pulse, jugular vein distention, and hemoptysis.

Septic shock

Initially, septic shock produces fever and chills. Low blood pressure, tachycardia, and tachypnea may also develop early, but the patient's skin remains warm. Later, low blood pressure becomes increasingly severe — less than 80 mm Hg, or 30 mm Hg less than the patient's baseline — and is accompanied by narrowed pulse pressure. Other late signs and symptoms include pale skin, cyanotic extremities, apprehension, thirst, oliguria, and coma.

Vasovagal syncope

Vasovagal syncope, a transient attack of loss or near-loss of consciousness, is characterized by low blood pressure, pallor, cold sweats, nausea, palpitations or slowed heart rate, and weakness following stressful, painful, or claustrophobic experiences.

OTHER CAUSES

Diagnostic tests

Diagnostic tests that may cause low blood pressure include the gastric acid stimulation test using histamine and X-ray studies using contrast media. The latter may trigger an allergic reaction, which causes low blood pressure.

Medical causes
(continued)

Hypovolemic shock
+ Systolic pressure falls to less than 80 mm Hg or 30 mm Hg less than the patient's baseline, secondary to acute blood loss or dehydration.

Hypoxemia
+ Initially, blood pressure may be normal or slightly elevated.
+ Blood pressure drops as hypoxemia becomes pronounced.

Myocardial infarction
+ Blood pressure may be low or high.

Neurogenic shock
+ Low blood pressure and bradycardia occur.

Pulmonary embolism
+ Low blood pressure occurs with narrowed pulse pressure and diminished Korotkoff sounds.
+ Sharp chest pain, dyspnea, and cough occur initially.

Septic shock
+ Initially, fever and chills occur.
+ Low blood pressure, tachycardia, and tachypnea may develop early.
+ Blood pressure continues to decrease and occurs with narrowed pulse pressure.

Vasovagal syncope
+ Low blood pressure, pallor, cold sweats, nausea, palpitations or slowed heart rate, and weakness follow stressful, painful, or claustrophobic experiences.

Other causes

- Alpha- and beta-adrenergic blockers
- Anxiolytics
- Calcium channel blockers
- Diuretics
- Gastric acid tests that use histamine
- General anesthetics
- I.V. antiarrhythmics
- MAO inhibitors
- Opioid analgesics
- Tranquilizers
- Vasodilators
- Contrast media

Special considerations

- Check vital signs frequently to determine if low blood pressure is constant or intermittent.
- Place the patient on bed rest.
- Assist ambulatory patients as necessary.
- Don't leave a dizzy patient unattended when he's sitting or walking.

Peds points

- Normal blood pressure in children is lower than that in adults.
- Suspect trauma or shock first as a possible cause of low blood pressure.
- Dehydration may cause low blood pressure in children.

Geri points

- Low blood pressure commonly results from the use of multiple drugs with this potential adverse effect.
- Orthostatic hypotension may occur because of autonomic dysfunction.

Normal pediatric blood pressure

This chart shows the normal systolic and diastolic pressure readings for pediatric patients.

AGE	SYSTOLIC	DIASTOLIC
Birth to 3 months	40 to 80 mm Hg	Not detectable
3 months to 1 year	80 to 100 mm Hg	Not detectable
1 to 4 years	100 to 108 mm Hg	60 mm Hg
4 to 12 years	108 to 124 mm Hg	60 to 70 mm Hg

Drugs

Calcium channel blockers, diuretics, vasodilators, alpha- and beta-adrenergic blockers, general anesthetics, opioid analgesics, monoamine oxidase inhibitors, anxiolytics (such as benzodiazepines), tranquilizers, and most I.V. antiarrhythmics can cause low blood pressure.

SPECIAL CONSIDERATIONS

Check the patient's vital signs frequently to determine if low blood pressure is constant or intermittent. If blood pressure is extremely low, an arterial catheter may be inserted to allow close monitoring of pressures. Alternatively, a Doppler flowmeter may be used.

Place the patient on bed rest. If the patient is ambulatory, assist him as necessary. To avoid falls, don't leave a dizzy patient unattended when he's sitting or walking.

Prepare the patient for laboratory tests, which may include urinalysis, routine blood studies, an electrocardiogram, and chest, cervical, and abdominal X-rays.

PEDIATRIC POINTERS

Normal blood pressure in children is lower than that in adults. (See *Normal pediatric blood pressure.*)

Because accidents occur frequently in children, suspect trauma or shock first as a possible cause of low blood pressure. Remember that low blood pressure typically doesn't accompany head injury in adults because intracranial hemorrhage is insufficient to cause hypovolemia. However, it does accompany head injury in infants and young children; their expandable cranial vaults allow significant blood loss into the cranial space, resulting in hypovolemia.

Another common cause of low blood pressure in children is dehydration, which results from failure to thrive or from persistent diarrhea and vomiting for as little as 24 hours.

GERIATRIC POINTERS

In elderly patients, low blood pressure commonly results from the use of multiple drugs with this potential adverse effect, a problem that needs to be addressed. Orthostatic hypotension due to autonomic dysfunction is another common cause.

PATIENT COUNSELING

If the patient has orthostatic hypotension, instruct him to stand up slowly. Advise patients with vasovagal syncope to avoid situations that trigger the episodes. Evaluate the patient's need for a cane or walker. Remind the patient to call for assistance when getting out of bed. When assisting the patient out of bed, have him first dangle his feet and then rise slowly.

BLOOD PRESSURE INCREASE

Elevated blood pressure—an intermittent or sustained increase in blood pressure exceeding 140/90 mm Hg—strikes more men than women. By itself, this common sign is easily ignored by the patient; after all, he can't see or feel it. However, its causes can be life-threatening.

 CULTURAL CUE *Blacks have a higher incidence of hypertension than Whites. In addition, hypertension occurs at an earlier age, is more severe, and has a higher mortality in Blacks than in Whites.*

Elevated blood pressure may develop suddenly or gradually. A sudden, severe rise in pressure (exceeding 180/110 mm Hg) may indicate life-threatening hypertensive crisis. However, even a less dramatic rise may be equally significant if it heralds a dissecting aortic aneurysm, increased intracranial pressure, myocardial infarction, eclampsia, or thyrotoxicosis. (See *Associated disorder: Hypertension,* page 90.)

Usually associated with essential hypertension, elevated blood pressure may also result from a renal or endocrine disorder, a treatment that affects fluid status such as dialysis, or a drug's adverse effect. Ingestion of large amounts of certain foods, such as black licorice and cheddar cheese, may temporarily elevate blood pressure. (See *Understanding blood pressure regulation,* page 91.)

 EMERGENCY ACTIONS Elevated blood pressure can signal various life-threatening disorders. However, if pressure exceeds 180/110 mm Hg, the patient may be experiencing hypertensive crisis and may require prompt treatment. Maintain a patent airway in case the patient vomits, and institute seizure precautions. Prepare to administer an I.V. antihypertensive and diuretic. You'll also need to insert an indwelling urinary catheter to accurately monitor urine output.

HISTORY

After ruling out life-threatening causes, complete a more leisurely patient history. Determine if the patient has a history of cardiovascular or cerebrovascular disease, diabetes, or renal disease. Ask about a family history of high blood pressure—a likely finding with essential hypertension, pheochromocytoma, or polycystic kidney disease. Then ask about its onset. Did high blood pressure appear abruptly? Ask the patient's age. Sudden onset of high blood pressure in middle-aged or elderly patients suggests renovascular stenosis. Although essential hypertension may begin in childhood, it typically isn't diagnosed until near age 35. Pheochromocytoma and primary aldosteronism usually occur between ages 40 and 60. If you suspect either, check for orthostatic hypotension. Take the patient's blood pressure with him lying down, sitting, and then standing. Normally, systolic pressure falls and diastolic pressure rises on standing. With orthostatic hypotension, both pressures fall.

Note headache, palpitations, blurred vision, and sweating. Ask about wine-colored urine and decreased urine output; these signs suggest glomerulonephritis, which can cause elevated blood pressure.

Teaching points

+ Standing up slowly (for those with orthostatic hypotension)
+ Avoidance of triggers (for those with vasovagal syncope)
+ Need for assistance when getting out of bed

Key facts about increased blood pressure

+ Intermittent or sustained increase in blood pressure exceeding 140/90 mm Hg
+ Affects men more than women

In an emergency

If blood pressure elevates above 180/110 mm Hg:
+ Suspect hypertensive crisis.
+ Maintain a patent airway in case the patient vomits.
+ Institute seizure precautions.
+ Prepare to administer an I.V. antihypertensive and a diuretic.
+ Insert an indwelling urinary catheter to monitor urine output.

Key history points

+ History of cardiovascular, cerebrovascular, or renal disease or diabetes
+ Family history of high blood pressure
+ Onset of high blood pressure
+ Age
+ Associated signs and symptoms, including headache, palpitations, blurred vision, sweating, wine-colored urine, and decreased urine output
+ Drug history
+ Psychosocial or environmental factors impacting blood pressure control

Key facts about hypertension

+ An elevation in diastolic or systolic blood pressure
+ Can be essential (most common) or secondary
+ Major cause of stroke, cardiac disease, and renal failure

Causes and risk factors

Essential hypertension

+ Family history of hypertension
+ Advancing age
+ Black race
+ Obesity
+ Tobacco use
+ High intake of sodium
+ Excessive alcohol consumption
+ Sedentary lifestyle
+ Stress

Secondary hypertension

+ Coarctation of the aorta
+ Renal artery stenosis
+ Brain tumor, quadriplegia, or head injury
+ Pheochromocytoma or thyroid, pituitary, or parathyroid dysfunction
+ Hormonal contraceptives, cocaine, epoetin alfa, sympathetic stimulants, and MAO inhibitors taken with tyramine
+ Pregnancy-induced hypertension

Management

For essential hypertension, use the NIH approach, which includes:
+ lifestyle modifications
+ drug therapy (increasing dosage, substituting one drug with another drug of the same class, or adding a drug from a different class as needed).

ASSOCIATED DISORDER

Hypertension

Hypertension, an elevation in diastolic or systolic blood pressure, affects 15% to 20% of adults in the United States. There are two major types: essential (primary) hypertension, the most common, and secondary hypertension, which results from renal disease or another identifiable cause. Hypertension is a major cause of stroke, cardiac disease, and renal failure.

Essential hypertension usually begins insidiously as a benign disease, slowly progressing to a malignant state. If untreated, even mild cases can cause major complications and death.

CAUSES

Risk factors for essential hypertension include:
+ family history of hypertension
+ advancing age
+ black race
+ sleep apnea
+ obesity
+ tobacco use
+ high intake of sodium
+ high intake of saturated fat
+ excessive alcohol consumption
+ sedentary lifestyle
+ stress
+ excess renin
+ mineral deficiencies (calcium, potassium, and magnesium)
    Causes of secondary hypertension include:
+ coarctation of the aorta
+ renal artery stenosis and parenchymal disease
+ brain tumor, quadriplegia, or head injury
+ pheochromocytoma; Cushing's syndrome; hyperaldosteronism; or thyroid, pituitary, or parathyroid dysfunction
+ hormonal contraceptives, cocaine, epoetin alfa, sympathetic stimulants, monoamine oxidase inhibitors taken with tyramine, estrogen replacement therapy, and nonsteroidal anti-inflammatory drugs
+ pregnancy-induced hypertension
+ excessive alcohol consumption.

DIAGNOSIS

These tests help diagnose hypertension:
+ Blood chemistry tests show elevated blood urea nitrogen and creatinine levels, suggesting renal disease.
+ Serial blood pressure readings are higher than 140/90 mm Hg.
+ Urinalysis shows protein, casts, red blood cells, and white blood cells, suggesting renal disease; catecholamines, associated with pheochromocytoma; or glucose, suggesting diabetes.
+ Electrocardiography and echocardiography may reveal left ventricular hypertrophy.
+ Chest X-ray may show cardiomegaly.

MEDICAL INTERVENTIONS

The National Institutes of Health recommends the following approach for treating primary hypertension:
+ Help the patient initiate lifestyle modifications, including weight reduction, moderation of alcohol intake, regular physical exercise, reduction of sodium intake, and smoking cessation.
+ If the desired blood pressure isn't achieved, continue lifestyle modifications and begin drug therapy with diuretics, angiotensin-converting enzyme (ACE) inhibitors, or beta-adrenergic blockers. If the patient can't take these drugs or they aren't effective, calcium antagonists, alpha$_1$-receptor blockers, or alpha-beta blockers may be used.
+ If the patient's blood pressure isn't responding as desired, increase the drug dosage, substitute a drug in the same class, or add a drug from a different class.
+ If the patient's blood pressure still isn't responding as desired, add a second or third drug (such as vasodilators, alpha$_1$ antagonists, peripherally acting adrenergic neuron antagonists, ACE inhibitors, and calcium channel blockers) or a diuretic.

Understanding blood pressure regulation

Hypertension may result from a disturbance in one of these intrinsic mechanisms.

RENIN-ANGIOTENSIN SYSTEM
The renin-angiotensin system acts to increase blood pressure through these mechanisms:
+ sodium depletion, reduced blood pressure, and dehydration stimulate renin release
+ renin reacts with angiotensin, a liver enzyme, and converts it to angiotensin I, which increases preload and afterload
+ angiotensin I converts to angiotensin II in the lungs; angiotensin II is a potent vasoconstrictor that targets the arterioles
+ angiotensin II works to increase preload and afterload by stimulating the adrenal cortex to secrete aldosterone; this increases blood volume by conserving sodium and water.

AUTOREGULATION
Several intrinsic mechanisms work to change an artery's diameter to maintain tissue and organ perfusion despite fluctuations in systemic blood pressure. These mechanisms include stress relaxation and capillary fluid shifts:
+ in stress relaxation, blood vessels gradually dilate when blood pressure increases to reduce peripheral resistance

+ in capillary fluid shift, plasma moves between vessels and extravascular spaces to maintain intravascular volume.

SYMPATHETIC NERVOUS SYSTEM
When blood pressure drops, baroreceptors in the aortic arch and carotid sinuses decrease their inhibition of the medulla's vasomotor center. The consequent increases in sympathetic stimulation of the heart by norepinephrine increase cardiac output by strengthening the contractile force, raising the heart rate, and augmenting peripheral resistance by vasoconstriction. Stress can also stimulate the sympathetic nervous system to increase cardiac output and peripheral vascular resistance.

ANTIDIURETIC HORMONE
The release of antidiuretic hormone can regulate hypotension by increasing reabsorption of water by the kidney. With reabsorption, blood plasma volume increases, thus raising blood pressure.

Obtain a drug history, including past and present prescriptions, herbal preparations, and over-the-counter drugs (especially decongestants). If the patient is taking an antihypertensive, determine how well he complies with the regimen. Ask about his perception of elevated blood pressure. How serious does he believe it is? Does he expect drug therapy to help? Explore psychosocial or environmental factors that may impact blood pressure control.

PHYSICAL ASSESSMENT

Follow up the history with a thorough physical assessment. Using a funduscope, check for intraocular hemorrhage, exudate, and papilledema, which characterize severe hypertension. Perform a thorough cardiovascular assessment. Check for carotid bruits and jugular vein distention. Assess skin color, temperature, and turgor. Palpate peripheral pulses. Auscultate for abnormal heart sounds (gallops, louder second sound, murmurs), rate (bradycardia, tachycardia), or rhythm. Then auscultate for abnormal breath sounds (crackles, wheezing), rate (bradypnea, tachypnea), or rhythm.

Palpate the abdomen for tenderness, masses, or liver enlargement. Auscultate for abdominal bruits. Renal artery stenosis produces bruits over the upper abdomen or in the costovertebral angles. Easily palpable, enlarged kidneys and a large, tender

Critical assessment steps

+ Perform a cardiovascular assessment; check for carotid bruits and jugular vein distention.
+ Assess skin color, temperature, and turgor.
+ Palpate peripheral pulses.
+ Auscultate for abnormal heart sounds, rate, or rhythm.
+ Auscultate for abnormal breath sounds, rate, or rhythm.
+ Palpate the abdomen for tenderness, masses, or liver enlargement.
+ Auscultate for abdominal bruits.

liver suggest polycystic kidney disease. Obtain a urine specimen to check for microscopic hematuria.

Medical causes

Anemia
+ Systolic pressure is elevated.
+ Pulsations occur in the capillary beds; bounding pulse, tachycardia, systolic ejection murmur, and pale mucous membranes develop.

Aortic aneurysm (dissecting)
+ Initially, a sudden rise in systolic pressure occurs, but diastolic pressure is stable

Atherosclerosis
+ Systolic pressure rises.
+ Diastolic pressure remains normal or slightly elevated.

Cushing's syndrome
+ Blood pressure elevates and pulse pressure widens.

Hypertension
+ *Essential hypertension* develops insidiously; blood pressure increases gradually.
+ *Malignant hypertension* results when diastolic pressure abruptly rises above 120 mm Hg; systolic pressure may exceed 200 mm Hg.

Increased ICP
+ Respiratory rate increases initially, followed by increased systolic pressure and widened pulse pressure.

MEDICAL CAUSES

Anemia
Elevated systolic pressure in anemia is accompanied by pulsations in the capillary beds, bounding pulse, tachycardia, systolic ejection murmur, pale mucous membranes and, in patients with sickle cell anemia, ventricular gallop and crackles.

Aortic aneurysm (dissecting)
Initially, dissecting aortic aneurysm causes a sudden rise in systolic pressure (which may be the precipitating event) but causes no change in diastolic pressure. However, this increase is brief. The body's ability to compensate fails, resulting in hypotension.

Other signs and symptoms of this life-threatening disorder vary, depending on the type of aortic aneurysm. An abdominal aneurysm may cause persistent abdominal and back pain, weakness, sweating, tachycardia, dyspnea, a pulsating abdominal mass, restlessness, confusion, and cool, clammy skin. A thoracic aneurysm may cause a ripping or tearing sensation in the chest, which may radiate to the neck, shoulders, lower back, or abdomen; pallor; syncope; blindness; loss of consciousness; sweating; dyspnea; tachycardia; cyanosis; leg weakness; murmur; and absent radial and femoral pulses.

Atherosclerosis
With atherosclerosis, systolic pressure rises, whereas diastolic pressure commonly remains normal or slightly elevated. The patient may show no other signs, or he may have a weak pulse, flushed skin, tachycardia, angina, and claudication.

Cushing's syndrome
Twice as common in females as in males, Cushing's syndrome causes elevated blood pressure and widened pulse pressure as well as truncal obesity, moon face, and other cushingoid signs. It's usually caused by corticosteroid use.

Hypertension
Essential hypertension develops insidiously and is characterized by a gradual increase in blood pressure from decade to decade. Except for this high blood pressure, the patient may be asymptomatic or (rarely) may complain of suboccipital headache, light-headedness, tinnitus, and fatigue.

With malignant hypertension, diastolic pressure abruptly rises above 120 mm Hg, and systolic pressure may exceed 200 mm Hg. Typically, the patient has pulmonary edema marked by jugular vein distention, dyspnea, tachypnea, tachycardia, and coughing of pink, frothy sputum. Other characteristic signs and symptoms include severe headache, confusion, blurred vision, tinnitus, epistaxis, muscle twitching, chest pain, nausea, and vomiting.

Increased intracranial pressure
Increased intracranial pressure (ICP) causes an increased respiratory rate initially, followed by increased systolic pressure and widened pulse pressure. It affects heart rate last, causing bradycardia (Cushing's reflex). Associated signs and symptoms of increased ICP include headache, projectile vomiting, decreased level of consciousness, and fixed or dilated pupils.

Myocardial infarction

Myocardial infarction is a life-threatening disorder that can cause high or low blood pressure. Common findings include crushing chest pain that may radiate to the jaw, shoulder, arm, or epigastrium. Other findings include dyspnea, anxiety, nausea, vomiting, weakness, diaphoresis, atrial gallop, and murmurs.

Pheochromocytoma

Paroxysmal or sustained elevated blood pressure characterizes pheochromocytoma and may be accompanied by orthostatic hypotension. Associated signs and symptoms include anxiety, diaphoresis, palpitations, tremors, pallor, nausea, weight loss, and headache.

In advanced stages, this disease may cause concurrent hematuria, life-threatening retroperitoneal bleeding, resulting from cyst rupture, proteinuria, and colicky abdominal pain from the ureteral passage of clots of calculi.

Preeclampsia and eclampsia

Potentially life-threatening to the patient and her fetus, preeclampsia and eclampsia characteristically increase blood pressure. They're defined as a reading of 140/90 mm Hg or more in the first trimester, a reading of 130/80 mm Hg or more in the second or third trimester, an increase of 30 mm Hg above the patient's baseline systolic pressure, or an increase of 15 mm Hg above the patient's baseline diastolic pressure. Accompanying elevated blood pressure are generalized edema, sudden weight gain of 3 lb (1.4 kg) or more per week during the second or third trimester, severe frontal headache, blurred or double vision, decreased urine output, proteinuria, midabdominal pain, neuromuscular irritability, nausea and, possibly, seizures (eclampsia).

Renovascular stenosis

Renovascular stenosis produces abruptly elevated systolic and diastolic pressures. Other characteristic signs and symptoms include bruits over the upper abdomen or in the costovertebral angles, hematuria, and acute flank pain.

Thyrotoxicosis

A potentially life-threatening disorder, thyrotoxicosis is accompanied by elevated systolic pressure, widened pulse pressure, tachycardia, bounding pulse, pulsations in the capillary nail beds, palpitations, weight loss, exophthalmos, an enlarged thyroid gland, weakness, diarrhea, fever over 100° F (37.8° C), and warm, moist skin. The patient may appear nervous and emotionally unstable, displaying occasional outbursts or even psychotic behavior. Heat intolerance, exertional dyspnea and, in females, decreased or absent menses may also occur.

OTHER CAUSES

Drugs

Central nervous system stimulants (such as amphetamines), sympathomimetics, corticosteroids, nonsteroidal anti-inflammatories, hormonal contraceptives, monoamine oxidase inhibitors, and over-the-counter cold remedies can increase blood pressure, as can cocaine abuse.

Treatments

Kidney dialysis and transplantation cause transient elevation of blood pressure.

Medical causes
(continued)

Myocardial infarction
- ✦ Blood pressure may be high or low.
- ✦ Crushing chest pain may radiate to the jaw, shoulder, arm, or epigastrium.

Pheochromocytoma
- ✦ Paroxysmal or sustained elevated blood pressure occurs with possible orthostatic hypotension.

Preeclampsia and eclampsia
- ✦ Blood pressure increases to 140/90 mm Hg or more in the first trimester, 130/80 mm Hg or more in the second or third trimester, 30 mm Hg above baseline systolic pressure, or 15 mm Hg above baseline diastolic pressure.

Renovascular stenosis
- ✦ Systolic and diastolic pressure elevate abruptly.

Thyrotoxicosis
- ✦ Elevated systolic pressure, widened pulse pressure, tachycardia, bounding pulse, pulsations in the capillary nail beds, palpitations, weight loss, exophthalmos, an enlarged thyroid gland, weakness, diarrhea, fever, and warm, moist skin develop.

Other causes
- ✦ CNS stimulants, corticosteroids, hormonal contraceptives, MAO inhibitors, NSAIDs, sympathomimetics, OTC cold remedies
- ✦ Cocaine abuse
- ✦ Kidney dialysis
- ✦ Transplantation

Special considerations
+ Stress the need for follow-up diagnostic tests.

Peds points
+ Elevated blood pressure may result from such conditions as lead or mercury poisoning, chronic pyelonephritis, coarctation of the aorta, patent ductus arteriosus, glomerulonephritis, adrenogenital syndrome, or neuroblastoma.

Geri points
+ Atherosclerosis produces isolated systolic hypertension.

Teaching points
+ Weight loss and exercise
+ Sodium restriction
+ Stress management
+ Risk factors for CAD
+ Ways to monitor blood pressure
+ Prescribed antihypertensives
+ Adverse drug reactions to report

SPECIAL CONSIDERATIONS

If routine screening detects elevated blood pressure, stress to the patient the need for follow-up diagnostic tests. Then prepare him for routine blood tests and urinalysis. Depending on the suspected cause of the increased blood pressure, radiographic studies, especially of the kidneys, may be necessary.

PEDIATRIC POINTERS

Normally, blood pressure in children is lower than it is in adults, an essential point to recognize when assessing a patient for elevated blood pressure. (See *Normal pediatric blood pressure,* page 88.)

Elevated blood pressure in children may result from lead or mercury poisoning, essential hypertension, renovascular stenosis, chronic pyelonephritis, coarctation of the aorta, patent ductus arteriosus, glomerulonephritis, adrenogenital syndrome, or neuroblastoma. Treatment typically begins with drug therapy. Surgery may then follow in patients with patent ductus arteriosus, coarctation of the aorta, neuroblastoma, and some cases of renovascular stenosis. Diuretics and antibiotics are used to treat glomerulonephritis and chronic pyelonephritis; hormonal therapy, to treat adrenogenital syndrome.

GERIATRIC POINTERS

Atherosclerosis commonly produces isolated systolic hypertension in elderly patients. Treatment is warranted to prevent long-term complications.

PATIENT COUNSELING

Encourage the patient to lose weight, if necessary, and to restrict sodium intake. Suggest that he participate in an exercise or stress management program as well. In addition, other risk factors for coronary artery disease, such as smoking and elevated cholesterol levels, need to be addressed. Then teach the patient how to monitor his blood pressure so that he can evaluate the effectiveness of drug therapy and lifestyle changes. Have him record blood pressure readings and symptoms, and ask him to share this information on his return visits.

If the patient has essential hypertension, explain the importance of long-term control of elevated blood pressure and the purpose, dosage, schedule, route, and adverse effects of prescribed antihypertensives. Reassure him that there are other drugs he can take if the one he's taking isn't effective or causes intolerable adverse reactions. Encourage him to report adverse reactions; the drug dosage or schedule may simply need adjustment.

Key facts about absent bowel sounds
+ Characterized by an inability to hear bowel sounds with a stethoscope after listening for at least 5 minutes in each abdominal quadrant
+ Occur when when obstruction or neurogenic inhibition halts peristalsis

BOWEL SOUNDS, ABSENT

Absent bowel sounds, or *silent abdomen,* refers to an inability to hear any bowel sounds through a stethoscope after listening for at least 5 minutes in each abdominal quadrant. Bowel sounds cease when mechanical or vascular obstruction or neurogenic inhibition halts peristalsis. When peristalsis stops, gas from bowel contents and fluid secreted from the intestinal walls accumulate and distend the lumen, leading to life-threatening complications (such as perforation, peritonitis, and sepsis) or hypovolemic shock.

Simple mechanical obstruction, resulting from adhesions, hernia, or tumor, causes loss of fluids and electrolytes and induces dehydration. Vascular obstruction cuts off circulation to the intestinal walls, leading to ischemia, necrosis, and shock.

Are bowel sounds really absent?

Before concluding that your patient has absent bowel sounds, ask yourself these three questions:
Did you use the diaphragm of your stethoscope to auscultate for the bowel sounds?
The diaphragm detects high-frequency sounds, such as bowel sounds, whereas the bell detects low-frequency sounds, such as a vascular bruit or a venous hum.

Did you listen in the same spot for at least 5 minutes for the presence of bowel sounds?
Normally, bowel sounds occur every 5 to 15 seconds, but the duration of a single sound may be less than 1 second.
Did you listen for bowel sounds in all quadrants?
Bowel sounds may be absent in one quadrant but present in another.

Neurogenic inhibition, affecting innervation of the intestinal wall, may result from infection, bowel distention, or trauma. It may also follow mechanical or vascular obstruction or metabolic derangement such as hypokalemia.

Abrupt cessation of bowel sounds, when accompanied by abdominal pain, rigidity, and distention, signals a life-threatening crisis requiring immediate intervention. Absent bowel sounds following a period of hyperactive sounds are equally ominous and may indicate strangulation of a mechanically obstructed bowel.

 EMERGENCY ACTIONS If you fail to detect bowel sounds and the patient reports sudden, severe abdominal pain and cramping or exhibits severe abdominal distention, prepare to insert a nasogastric (NG) or intestinal tube to suction lumen contents and decompress the bowel. (See *Are bowel sounds really absent?*) Administer I.V. fluids and electrolytes to offset dehydration and imbalances caused by the dysfunctioning bowel.

Because the patient may require surgery to relieve an obstruction, withhold oral intake. Take the patient's vital signs, and be alert for signs of shock, such as hypotension, tachycardia, and cool, clammy skin. Measure abdominal girth as a baseline for gauging subsequent changes.

HISTORY

If the patient's condition permits, proceed with a brief history. Start with abdominal pain: When did it begin? Has it gotten worse? Where does he feel it? Ask about a sensation of bloating and about flatulence. Find out if the patient has had diarrhea or has passed pencil-thin stools — possible signs of a developing luminal obstruction. The patient may have had no bowel movements at all — a possible sign of complete obstruction or paralytic ileus.

Ask about conditions that commonly lead to mechanical obstruction, such as abdominal tumors, hernias, and adhesions from past surgery. Determine if the patient was involved in an accident — even a seemingly minor one, such as falling off a stepladder — that may have caused vascular clots. Check for a history of acute pancreatitis, diverticulitis, or gynecologic infection, which may have led to intraabdominal infection and bowel dysfunction. Be sure to ask about previous toxic conditions, such as uremia, and about spinal cord injury, which can lead to paralytic ileus.

If the patient's pain isn't severe or accompanied by other life-threatening signs or symptoms, obtain a detailed medical and surgical history.

In an emergency

If absent bowels sounds are accompanied by sudden, severe abdominal pain and cramping or severe abdominal distention:
✦ Prepare to insert an NG or intestinal tube to suction lumen contents and decompress the bowel.
✦ Administer I.V. fluids and electrolytes.
✦ Withhold oral intake in case surgery is needed.
✦ Take the patient's vital signs.
✦ Be alert for signs of shock.
✦ Measure abdominal girth to establish a baseline.

Key history points

✦ Onset and description of abdominal pain
✦ Description of bowel movements
✦ Recent accidents
✦ Medical and surgical history, including abdominal tumors, hernias, adhesions from past surgery, acute pancreatitis, diverticulitis, gynecologic infection, uremia, or spinal cord injury

Critical assessment steps

+ Inspect abdominal contour.
+ Observe for distention.
+ Gently percuss and palpate the abdomen.
+ Listen for dullness over fluid-filled areas and for tympany over pockets of gas.
+ Palpate for abdominal rigidity and guarding.

Medical causes

Complete mechanical intestinal obstruction
+ Absent bowel sounds follow a period of hyperactivity.
+ Colicky abdominal pain that may radiate arises in the quadrant of obstruction.

Mesenteric artery occlusion
+ Bowel sounds disappear after a brief period of hyperactive sounds.
+ Midepigastric or periumbilical pain occurs.

Paralytic ileus
+ Absent bowel sounds are a cardinal sign.

Other causes

+ Abdominal surgery

Special considerations

+ After NG or intestinal tube insertion, elevate the head of the bed at least 30 degrees.
+ Ensure tube patency.
+ Continue to administer I.V. fluids and electrolytes.

PHYSICAL ASSESSMENT

Perform a complete physical examination followed by an abdominal assessment and pelvic examination. Start your assessment by inspecting abdominal contour. Stoop at the recumbent patient's side and then at the foot of his bed to detect localized or generalized distention. Percuss and palpate the abdomen gently. Listen for dullness over fluid-filled areas and tympany over pockets of gas. Palpate for abdominal rigidity and guarding, which suggest peritoneal irritation that can lead to paralytic ileus.

MEDICAL CAUSES

Complete mechanical intestinal obstruction

Absent bowel sounds follow a period of hyperactive bowel sounds in complete mechanical intestinal obstruction, a potentially life-threatening condition. This silence accompanies acute, colicky abdominal pain that arises in the quadrant of obstruction and may radiate to the flank or lumbar regions. Associated signs and symptoms of complete mechanical intestinal obstruction include abdominal distention, and bloating, constipation, and nausea and vomiting (the higher the blockage, the earlier and more severe the vomiting). In late stages, signs of shock may occur with fever, rebound tenderness, and abdominal rigidity.

Mesenteric artery occlusion

With mesenteric artery occlusion, a life-threatening disorder, bowel sounds disappear after a brief period of hyperactive sounds. Sudden, severe midepigastric or periumbilical pain occurs next, followed by abdominal distention, bruits, vomiting, constipation, and signs of shock. Fever is common. Abdominal rigidity may appear later.

Paralytic ileus

The cardinal sign of paralytic (adynamic) ileus is absent bowel sounds. In addition to abdominal distention, associated signs and symptoms of paralytic ileus include generalized discomfort and constipation or passage of small, liquid stools. If paralytic ileus follows acute abdominal infection, the patient may also experience fever and abdominal pain.

OTHER CAUSES

Abdominal surgery

Bowel sounds are normally absent after abdominal surgery—the result of anesthetic use and surgical manipulation.

SPECIAL CONSIDERATIONS

After you've inserted an NG tube or an intestinal tube, elevate the head of the patient's bed at least 30 degrees, and turn the patient to facilitate passage of the tube through the GI tract. (Remember not to tape an intestinal tube to the patient's face.) Ensure tube patency by checking for drainage and properly functioning suction devices, and irrigate accordingly.

Continue to administer I.V. fluids and electrolytes, and make sure that you send a serum specimen to the laboratory for electrolyte analysis at least once per day. The patient may need X-ray studies and further blood work to determine the cause of absent bowel sounds.

After mechanical obstruction and intra-abdominal sepsis have been ruled out, give the patient drugs to control pain and stimulate peristalsis.

PEDIATRIC POINTERS

Absent bowel sounds in children may result from Hirschsprung's disease or intussusception, both of which can lead to life-threatening obstruction.

GERIATRIC POINTERS

Older patients with a bowel obstruction that doesn't respond to decompression should be considered for early surgical intervention to avoid the risk of bowel infarct.

PATIENT COUNSELING

Explain all diagnostic and therapeutic procedures to the patient and answer any questions he may have. Make sure he understands the rationales for food and fluid restrictions. Encourage early ambulation in the postoperative patient.

BOWEL SOUNDS, HYPERACTIVE

Sometimes audible without a stethoscope, hyperactive bowel sounds reflect increased intestinal motility (peristalsis). They're commonly characterized as rapid, rushing, gurgling waves of sounds. (See *Characterizing bowel sounds,* page 98.) They may stem from life-threatening bowel obstruction or GI hemorrhage, or from GI infection, inflammatory bowel disease (which usually follows a chronic course), food allergies, or stress.

 EMERGENCY ACTIONS After detecting hyperactive bowel sounds, quickly check the patient's vital signs and ask him about associated symptoms, such as abdominal pain, vomiting, and diarrhea. If he reports cramping abdominal pain or vomiting, continue to auscultate for bowel sounds. If bowel sounds stop abruptly, suspect complete bowel obstruction. Prepare to assist with GI suction and decompression, to give I.V. fluids and electrolytes, and prepare the patient for surgery.

If he has diarrhea, record its frequency, amount, color, and consistency. If you detect excessive watery diarrhea or bleeding, prepare to administer an antidiarrheal, I.V. fluids and electrolytes and, possibly, blood transfusions.

HISTORY

If you've ruled out life-threatening conditions, obtain a detailed medical and surgical history. Ask the patient if he has had a hernia or abdominal surgery because these may cause mechanical intestinal obstruction. Does he have a history of inflammatory bowel disease? Also, ask about recent eruptions of gastroenteritis among family members, friends, or coworkers. If the patient has traveled recently, even within the United States, was he aware of any endemic illnesses?

In addition, determine whether stress may have contributed to the patient's problem. Ask about food allergies and recent ingestion of unusual foods or fluids.

PHYSICAL ASSESSMENT

Begin your examination by taking your patient's vital signs. Check for fever, which suggests infection. Having already auscultated, now gently inspect, percuss, and palpate the abdomen.

Peds points
+ Absent bowel sounds in children may result from Hirschsprung's disease or intussusception.

Geri points
+ If a bowel obstruction doesn't respond to decompression, early surgical intervention should be considered to avoid the risk of bowel infarct.

Teaching points
+ Diagnostic tests and therapeutic procedures
+ Food and fluid restrictions
+ Postoperative ambulation

Key facts about hyperactive bowel sounds
+ Reflect peristalsis
+ Characterized as rapid, rushing, gurgling waves of sounds

In an emergency
If there's cramping abdominal pain or vomiting:
+ Auscultate for bowel sounds.
+ If bowel sounds stop abruptly, suspect complete bowel obstruction. Prepare to assist with GI suction and decompression.
+ Prepare to give I.V. fluids and electrolytes.
+ Prepare the patient for surgery.
If the patient has diarrhea:
+ Record its frequency, amount, color, and consistency.
+ If you detect excessive watery diarrhea or bleeding, prepare to administer an antidiarrheal, I.V. fluids and electrolytes and, possibly, blood transfusions.

Key history points

✦ Medical and surgical history, including abdominal surgeries or previous inflammatory bowel disease
✦ Exposure to gastroenteritis
✦ Recent travel
✦ Possible stress factors
✦ Allergies and recent food and fluid consumption

Critical assessment steps

✦ Take vital signs.
✦ Check for fever.
✦ Auscultate, inspect, percuss, and palpate the abdomen.

Medical causes

Crohn's disease

✦ Hyperactive bowel sounds arise insidiously.

Gastroenteritis

✦ Hyperactive bowel sounds follow sudden nausea and vomiting.
✦ Patient has "explosive" diarrhea.

GI hemorrhage

✦ Hyperactive bowel sounds indicate upper GI bleeding.

Malabsorption

✦ Lactose intolerance typically results in hyperactive bowel sounds.

Mechanical intestinal obstruction

✦ Hyperactive bowel sounds occur with cramping abdominal pain every few minutes.
✦ Bowel sounds may later become hypoactive and then disappear.

Characterizing bowel sounds

The sounds of swallowed air and fluid moving through the GI tract are known as bowel sounds. These sounds usually occur every 5 to 15 seconds, but their frequency may be irregular. For example, bowel sounds are normally more active just before and after a meal. Bowel sounds may last less than 1 second or up to several seconds.

To accurately assess bowel sounds, you need to be aware of the various types:

✦ *Normal bowel sounds* can be characterized as murmuring, gurgling, or tinkling.
✦ *Hyperactive bowel sounds* can be characterized as loud, gurgling, splashing, and rushing; they're higher pitched and occur more frequently than normal sounds.
✦ *Hypoactive bowel sounds* can be characterized as softer or lower in tone and less frequent than normal sounds.

MEDICAL CAUSES

Crohn's disease

Hyperactive bowel sounds usually arise insidiously in those with Crohn's disease. Associated signs and symptoms include diarrhea, cramping abdominal pain that may be relieved by defecation, anorexia, low-grade fever, abdominal distention and tenderness and, in many cases, a fixed mass in the right lower quadrant. Muscle wasting, weight loss, and signs of dehydration may occur as Crohn's disease progresses.

Gastroenteritis

With gastroenteritis, hyperactive bowel sounds follow sudden nausea and vomiting and accompany "explosive" diarrhea. Abdominal cramping or pain is common, typically after a peristaltic wave. Fever may occur, depending on the causative organism.

GI hemorrhage

Hyperactive bowel sounds provide the most immediate indication of persistent upper GI bleeding. Other findings include hematemesis, coffee-ground vomitus, abdominal distention, bloody diarrhea, rectal passage of bright red clots and jellylike material or melena, and pain during bleeding. Decreased urine output, tachycardia, and hypotension accompany blood loss.

Malabsorption

Malabsorption — typically lactose intolerance — may cause hyperactive bowel sounds. Associated signs and symptoms include diarrhea and, possibly, nausea and vomiting, angioedema, and urticaria.

Mechanical intestinal obstruction

Mechanical intestinal obstruction — a potentially life-threatening disorder — causes hyperactive bowel sounds to occur simultaneously with cramping abdominal pain every few minutes; bowel sounds may later become hypoactive and then disappear. With small-bowel obstruction, nausea and vomiting occur earlier and with greater severity than in large-bowel obstruction. With complete bowel obstruction, hyperactive sounds are also accompanied by abdominal distention and constipation, although the part of the bowel distal to the obstruction may continue to empty for up to 3 days.

Ulcerative colitis (acute)

Hyperactive bowel sounds arise abruptly in patients with acute ulcerative colitis. The hallmark of this disorder is recurrent bloody diarrhea (usually containing pus and mucus) accompanied by anorexia, abdominal pain, nausea and vomiting, fever, and tenesmus. Weight loss, arthralgia, and arthritis may occur.

SPECIAL CONSIDERATIONS

Prepare the patient for diagnostic tests. These may include endoscopy to view a suspected lesion, barium X-rays, or stool analysis.

I.V. fluids and electrolytes may be necessary to replace losses from diarrhea. Oral food and fluid restrictions may be needed to rest the GI tract.

If the patient has GI bleeding, insert an I.V. line for fluid and blood administration. Administer drugs such as vasopressin to manage bleeding. Insert a nasogastric tube to suction and monitor drainage.

PEDIATRIC POINTERS

Hyperactive bowel sounds in children usually result from gastroenteritis, erratic eating habits, excessive ingestion of certain foods (such as unripened fruit), or food allergy.

PATIENT COUNSELING

Explain prescribed dietary changes to the patient. These may range from complete food and fluid restrictions to a liquid or bland diet. Because stress commonly precipitates or aggravates bowel hyperactivity, teach the patient relaxation techniques such as deep breathing. Encourage rest and restrict the patient's physical activity.

BOWEL SOUNDS, HYPOACTIVE

Hypoactive bowel sounds, detected by auscultation, are diminished in regularity, tone, and loudness from normal bowel sounds. They may portend absent bowel sounds, which can indicate a life-threatening disorder.

Hypoactive bowel sounds result from decreased peristalsis, which, in turn, can result from a developing bowel obstruction. The obstruction may be mechanical (as from a hernia, tumor, or twisting), vascular (as from an embolism or thrombosis), or neurogenic (as from mechanical, ischemic, or toxic impairment of bowel innervation). Hypoactive bowel sounds can also result from the use of certain drugs, abdominal surgery, and radiation therapy.

HISTORY

After detecting hypoactive bowel sounds, look for related symptoms. Ask the patient about the location, onset, duration, frequency, and severity of any pain. Cramping or colicky abdominal pain usually indicates a mechanical bowel obstruction, whereas diffuse abdominal pain usually indicates intestinal distention related to paralytic ileus.

Ask the patient about any recent vomiting: When did it begin? How often does it occur? Does the vomitus look bloody? Also ask about any changes in bowel habits: Does he have a history of constipation? When was the last time he had a bowel movement or expelled gas?

Obtain a detailed medical and surgical history of any conditions that may cause mechanical bowel obstruction, such as an abdominal tumor or hernia. Does the

---

Ulcerative colitis (acute)
+ Hyperactive bowel sounds arise abruptly.
+ Bloody diarrhea accompanied by anorexia, abdominal pain, nausea and vomiting, fever, and tenesmus is hallmark.

Special considerations
If the patient has GI bleeding:
+ Insert an I.V. line for fluid and blood administration.
+ Administer drugs such as vasopressin to manage bleeding.
+ Insert an NG tube to suction and monitor drainage.

Peds points
+ Hyperactive bowel sounds in children usually result from gastroenteritis, erratic eating habits, excessive ingestion of certain foods, or food allergy.

Teaching points
+ Dietary changes
+ Physical activity restrictions

Key facts about hypoactive bowel sounds
+ Are diminished in regularity, tone, and loudness
+ Result if peristalsis is decreased

Key history points
+ Location, onset, frequency, and severity of pain
+ Description of any vomiting or constipation
+ Medical and surgical history
+ Treatment history, including radiation and drug therapy

Critical assessment steps

+ Inspect the abdomen for distention, noting surgical incisions and obvious masses.
+ Gently percuss and palpate the abdomen for masses, gas, fluid, tenderness, and rigidity.
+ Measure abdominal girth.
+ Check for signs of dehydration and electrolyte imbalance.

Medical causes

Mechanical intestinal obstruction

+ Bowel sounds may become hypoactive after a period of hyperactivity.

Mesenteric artery occlusion

+ Bowel sounds become hypoactive after a brief period of hyperactivity and then quickly disappear.

Paralytic ileus

+ Bowel sounds are hypoactive and may become absent.
+ Associated signs and symptoms include abdominal distention and constipation or passage of small, liquid stools and flatus.

Other causes

+ Anticholinergics
+ General or spinal anesthetics
+ Opiates
+ Phenothiazines
+ Surgery involving the bowel
+ Vinca alkaloids

patient have a history of severe pain; trauma; conditions that can cause paralytic ileus such as pancreatitis; bowel inflammation or gynecologic infection, which may produce peritonitis; or toxic conditions such as uremia? Has he recently had radiation therapy or abdominal surgery, or ingested a drug such as an opiate, which can decrease peristalsis and cause hypoactive bowel sounds?

PHYSICAL ASSESSMENT

After the history is complete, perform a careful physical examination. Inspect the abdomen for distention, noting surgical incisions and obvious masses. Gently percuss and palpate the abdomen for masses, gas, fluid, tenderness, and rigidity. Measure abdominal girth to detect any subsequent increase in distention. Also check for poor skin turgor, hypotension, narrowed pulse pressure, and other signs of dehydration and electrolyte imbalance, which may result from paralytic ileus.

MEDICAL CAUSES

Mechanical intestinal obstruction

In a patient with a mechanical intestinal obstruction, bowel sounds may become hypoactive after a period of hyperactivity. The patient may also have acute colicky abdominal pain in the quadrant of obstruction, possibly radiating to the flank or lumbar region; nausea and vomiting (the higher the obstruction, the earlier and more severe the vomiting); constipation; and abdominal distention and bloating. If the obstruction becomes complete, signs of shock may occur.

Mesenteric artery occlusion

In cases of mesenteric artery occlusion, bowel sounds become hypoactive after a brief period of hyperactivity and then quickly disappear, signifying a life-threatening crisis. Associated signs and symptoms include fever; a history of colicky abdominal pain leading to sudden and severe midepigastric or periumbilical pain, followed by abdominal distention and possible bruits; vomiting; constipation; and signs of shock. Abdominal rigidity may appear late.

Paralytic ileus

With paralytic (adynamic) ileus, bowel sounds are hypoactive and may become absent. Associated signs and symptoms include abdominal distention, generalized discomfort, and constipation or passage of small, liquid stools and flatus. If the disorder follows acute abdominal infection, fever and abdominal pain may occur.

OTHER CAUSES

Drugs

Certain classes of drugs reduce intestinal motility and thus produce hypoactive bowel sounds. These include opiates such as codeine, anticholinergics such as propantheline, phenothiazines such as chlorpromazine, and vinca alkaloids such as vincristine. General or spinal anesthetics produce transient hypoactive sounds.

Surgery

Hypoactive bowel sounds may occur after surgical manipulation of the bowel. Motility and bowel sounds in the small intestine usually resume within 24 hours; colonic bowel sounds, in 3 to 5 days.

SPECIAL CONSIDERATIONS

Frequently evaluate the patient with hypoactive bowel sounds for indications of shock (thirst; anxiety; restlessness; tachycardia; cool, clammy skin; weak, thready pulse), which can develop if peristalsis continues to diminish and fluid is lost from the circulation.

Be alert for the sudden absence of bowel sounds, especially in postoperative and hypokalemic patients because they're at increased risk for paralytic ileus. Monitor the patient's vital signs and auscultate for bowel sounds every 2 to 4 hours.

Severe pain, abdominal rigidity, guarding, and fever, accompanied by hypoactive bowel sounds, may indicate paralytic ileus from peritonitis. If these signs and symptoms occur, prepare for emergency interventions. (See "Bowel sounds, absent," page 94.)

The patient with hypoactive bowel sounds may require GI suction and decompression, using a nasogastric or intestinal tube. If so, restrict the patient's oral intake. Then elevate the head of the bed at least 30 degrees, and turn the patient to facilitate passage of the tube through the GI tract.

Remember not to tape an intestinal tube to the patient's face. Ensure tube patency by watching for drainage and properly functioning suction devices. Irrigate the tube, and closely monitor drainage.

Continue to administer I.V. fluids and electrolytes, and send a serum specimen to the laboratory for electrolyte analysis at least once per day. Recognize that the patient may need X-ray studies, endoscopic procedures, and further blood work to determine the cause of hypoactive bowel sounds.

PEDIATRIC POINTERS

Hypoactive bowel sounds in a child may simply be due to bowel distention from excessive swallowing of air while the child was eating or crying. However, be sure to observe the child for further signs of illness. As with an adult, sluggish bowel sounds in a child may signal the onset of paralytic ileus or peritonitis.

PATIENT COUNSELING

Encourage the patient to ambulate to stimulate peristalsis. If he can't move, assist him in turning side to side and with range-of-motion exercises. Explain all diagnostic tests and procedures as well as the need to withhold food and fluids until bowel sounds improve.

BRADYCARDIA

Bradycardia refers to a heart rate of less than 60 beats/minute. It occurs normally in young adults, trained athletes, and elderly people as well as during sleep. It's also a normal response to vagal stimulation caused by coughing, vomiting, or straining during defecation. When bradycardia results from these causes, the heart rate rarely drops below 40 beats/minute. However, when it results from pathologic causes (such as cardiovascular disorders), the heart rate may be slower. (See *Managing severe bradycardia,* page 102.)

HISTORY

After detecting bradycardia, check for related signs of life-threatening disorders. If the patient's bradycardia isn't accompanied by unfavorable signs, ask the patient if he or a family member has a history of a slow pulse rate because this may be inherited. Also, find out if he has an underlying metabolic disorder such as hypothyroidism which can precipitate bradycardia. Ask which medications he's taking and if he's complying with the prescribed schedule and dosage.

Special considerations
+ Frequently evaluate for signs and symptoms of shock.
+ Be alert for sudden absence of bowel sounds; monitor vital signs and auscultate for bowel sounds every 2 to 4 hours.
+ Be aware that GI suction and decompression may be required.

Peds points
+ Hypoactive bowel sounds in a child may be due to bowel distention from excessive swallowing of air while eating or crying.
+ Be sure to observe the child for further signs of illness.

Teaching points
+ Diagnostic tests and procedures
+ Food and fluid restrictions

Key facts about bradycardia
+ Refers to a heart rate of less than 60 beats/minute
+ Occurs normally but can also result from pathologic causes

Key history points
+ Family history of slow pulse rate
+ Medical history, including underlying metabolic disorders
+ Drug history

Managing severe bradycardia

Bradycardia can signal a life-threatening disorder when accompanied by pain, shortness of breath, dizziness, syncope, or other symptoms; prolonged exposure to cold; or head or neck trauma. In such patients, quickly take vital signs. Connect the patient to a cardiac monitor, and insert an I.V. line. Depending on the cause of bradycardia, you'll need to administer fluids, atropine, steroids, or thyroid medication. If indicated, insert an indwelling urinary catheter. Intubation and mechanical ventilation may be necessary if the patient's respiratory rate falls. Assist with the placement of a pacemaker if medications don't increase the heart rate.

If appropriate, perform a focused evaluation to help locate the cause of bradycardia. For example, ask about pain. Viselike pressure or crushing or burning chest pain that radi-

ates to the arms, back, or jaw may indicate an acute myocardial infarction (MI); a severe headache, increased intracranial pressure. Also, ask about nausea, vomiting, or shortness of breath — signs and symptoms associated with an acute MI and cardiomyopathy. Observe the patient for peripheral cyanosis, edema, or jugular vein distention, which may indicate cardiomyopathy. Look for a thyroidectomy scar because severe bradycardia may result from hypothyroidism caused by failure to take thyroid hormone replacements.

If the cause of bradycardia is evident, provide supportive care. For example, keep the hypothermic patient warm by applying blankets, and monitor his core temperature until it reaches 99° F (37.2° C); stabilize the head and neck of a trauma patient until cervical spinal injury is ruled out.

Critical assessment steps

+ Monitor vital signs, temperature, pulse, respirations, blood pressure, and oxygen saturation.
+ Perform a cardiac assessment.

Medical causes

Cardiac arrhythmia
+ Bradycardia may be transient or sustained, benign, or life-threatening.
+ Hypotension, palpitations, dizziness, weakness, dyspnea, chest pain, decreased urine output, altered LOC, syncope, and fatigue develop.

Cardiomyopathy
+ Transient or sustained bradycardia may occur.

Cervical spinal injury
+ Bradycardia may be transient or sustained, depending on the severity of the injury.

Hypothermia
+ Bradycardia is accompanied by shivering, peripheral cyanosis, muscle rigidity, bradypnea, and confusion leading to stupor.

PHYSICAL ASSESSMENT

Monitor vital signs, temperature, pulse, respirations, blood pressure, and oxygen saturation. Then perform a complete cardiac assessment.

MEDICAL CAUSES

Cardiac arrhythmia
Depending on the type of cardiac arrhythmia and the patient's tolerance of it, bradycardia may be transient or sustained, benign, or life-threatening. Related findings result from reduced cardiac output and include hypotension, palpitations, dizziness, weakness, dyspnea, chest pain, decreased urine output, altered level of consciousness (LOC), syncope, and fatigue.

Cardiomyopathy
Cardiomyopathy, a potentially life-threatening disorder, may cause transient or sustained bradycardia. Other findings include dizziness, syncope, edema, fatigue, jugular vein distention, orthopnea, dyspnea, and peripheral cyanosis.

Cervical spinal injury
Bradycardia associated with a cervical spinal injury may be transient or sustained, depending on the severity of the injury. Its onset coincides with sympathetic denervation. Associated signs and symptoms of cervical spinal injury include hypotension, decreased body temperature, slowed peristalsis, leg paralysis, and partial arm and respiratory muscle paralysis.

Hypothermia
When core body temperature drops below 89.6° F (32° C), causing hypothermia, bradycardia usually appears. It's accompanied by shivering, peripheral cyanosis, muscle rigidity, bradypnea, and confusion leading to stupor. If the core tempera-

ture drops below 86° F (30° C), the patient may appear dead (in a state of rigor mortis) with no palpable pulse or audible heart sounds.

Hypothyroidism

Hypothyroidism causes severe bradycardia in addition to fatigue, constipation, unexplained weight gain, and sensitivity to cold. Related signs include cool, dry, thick skin; sparse, dry hair; facial swelling; periorbital edema; thick, brittle nails; and confusion leading to stupor.

Myocardial infarction

Sinus bradycardia is the arrhythmia most commonly associated with acute myocardial infarction (MI). Accompanying signs and symptoms of an MI include an aching, burning, or viselike pressure in the chest that may radiate to the jaw, shoulder, arm, back, or epigastric area; nausea and vomiting; cool, clammy, and pale or cyanotic skin; anxiety; and dyspnea. Blood pressure may be elevated or depressed. Auscultation may reveal abnormal heart sounds.

OTHER CAUSES

Diagnostic tests

Cardiac catheterization and electrophysiologic studies can induce temporary bradycardia.

Drugs

Beta-adrenergic blockers and some calcium channel blockers, cardiac glycosides, topical miotics (such as pilocarpine), protamine, quinidine and other antiarrhythmics, and sympatholytics may cause transient bradycardia. Failure to take thyroid replacements may cause bradycardia.

Invasive treatments

Suctioning can induce hypoxia and vagal stimulation, causing bradycardia. Cardiac surgery can cause edema or damage to conduction tissues, causing bradycardia.

SPECIAL CONSIDERATIONS

Continue to monitor vital signs frequently. Be especially alert for changes in cardiac rhythm, respiratory rate, and LOC.

Prepare the patient for laboratory tests, which can include complete blood count; cardiac enzyme, serum electrolyte, blood glucose, blood urea nitrogen, arterial blood gas, and blood drug levels; thyroid function tests; and a 12-lead electrocardiogram. If appropriate, prepare the patient for 24-hour Holter monitoring.

PEDIATRIC POINTERS

Heart rates are normally higher in children than in adults. Fetal bradycardia—a heart rate of less than 120 beats/minute—may occur during prolonged labor or complications of delivery, such as compression of the umbilical cord, partial abruptio placentae, and placenta previa. Intermittent bradycardia, sometimes accompanied by apnea, commonly occurs in premature infants. Bradycardia rarely occurs in full-term infants or children. However, it can result from congenital heart defects, acute glomerulonephritis, and transient or complete heart block associated with cardiac catheterization or cardiac surgery.

Medical causes
(continued)

Hypothyroidism
+ Severe bradycardia is accompanied by fatigue, constipation, unexplained weight gain, and sensitivity to cold.

Myocardial infarction
+ Sinus bradycardia is common.

Other causes
+ Antiarrhythmics, beta-adrenergic blockers, cardiac glycosides, some calcium channel blockers, sympatholytics, and topical miotics
+ Cardiac catheterization
+ Cardiac surgery
+ Electrophysiologic studies
+ Suctioning

Special considerations
+ Be alert for changes in cardiac rhythm, respiratory rate, and LOC.
+ If appropriate, prepare the patient for 24-hour Holter monitoring.

Peds points
+ Fetal bradycardia (heart rate less than 120 beats/minute) may occur during prolonged labor or complications of delivery.
+ Intermittent bradycardia commonly occurs in premature infants.

Geri points

+ Patients with sinus node dysfunction require careful scrutiny of their drug therapy.

Teaching points

+ Signs and symptoms to report
+ Pulse measurement
+ Pacemaker use, if appropriate

Key facts about bradypnea

+ Involves a pattern of regular respirations with a rate of less than 10 breaths/minute
+ Results from neurologic and metabolic disorders and drug overdose

In an emergency

+ Try to arouse the patient by shaking him and instructing him to breathe.
+ Assess neurologic status.
+ Place the patient on an apnea monitor.
+ Keep emergency airway equipment available.
+ Be prepared to assist with intubation.
+ To prevent aspiration, position the patient on his side or keep his head elevated 30 degrees.

Key history points

+ Drugs taken and by what route
+ Medical history

Critical assessment steps

+ Assess vital signs.
+ Perform a complete physical assessment, paying particular attention to the cardiopulmonary assessment.

GERIATRIC POINTERS

Sinus node dysfunction is the most common bradyarrhythmia encountered among elderly patients. Patients with this disorder may have as their chief complaint fatigue, exercise intolerance, dizziness, or syncope. If the patient is asymptomatic, no intervention is necessary. Symptomatic patients, however, require careful scrutiny of their drug therapy. Beta-adrenergic blockers, verapamil, diazepam, sympatholytics, antihypertensives, and some antiarrhythmics have been implicated; symptoms may clear when these drugs are discontinued. Pacing is usually indicated in patients with symptomatic bradycardia lacking a correctable cause.

PATIENT COUNSELING

Discuss signs and symptoms to report, such as light-headedness or syncope. Teach the patient to take his pulse and make sure he knows parameters for calling the physician and seeking emergency care. If the patient had a pacemaker inserted, provide instructions for its use.

BRADYPNEA

Commonly preceding life-threatening apnea or respiratory arrest, bradypnea is a pattern of regular respirations with a rate of less than 10 breaths/minute. This sign results from neurologic and metabolic disorders and drug overdose, which depress the brain's respiratory control centers.

 EMERGENCY ACTIONS Depending on the degree of central nervous system (CNS) depression, the patient with severe bradypnea may require constant stimulation to breathe. If he seems excessively sleepy, try to arouse him by shaking and instructing him to breathe. Quickly take the patient's vital signs. Assess his neurologic status by checking pupil size and reactions and by evaluating his level of consciousness (LOC) and his ability to move his extremities.

Place the patient on an apnea monitor, keep emergency airway equipment available, and be prepared to assist with intubation and mechanical ventilation if spontaneous respirations cease. To prevent aspiration, position the patient on his side or keep the head elevated 30 degrees higher than the rest of the body, and clear his airway with suction or finger-sweeps, if necessary.

HISTORY

Obtain a brief history from the patient if possible. Alternatively, obtain this information from the person who accompanied him to the facility. Ask if he's experiencing a drug overdose and, if so, try to determine what drugs he took, how much, when, and by what route. Check his arms for needle marks, indicating possible drug abuse. You may need to administer I.V. naloxone, an opioid antagonist.

If you rule out a drug overdose, ask about chronic illnesses, such as diabetes and renal failure. Check for a medical identification bracelet or an I.D. card that identifies an underlying condition. Also, ask whether the patient has a history of head trauma, brain tumor, neurologic infection, or stroke.

PHYSICAL ASSESSMENT

Determine the patient's respiratory rate and assess his other vital signs. Then proceed to a complete physical assessment, paying particular attention to the cardiopulmonary assessment.

MEDICAL CAUSES

Diabetic ketoacidosis
Bradypnea occurs late in patients with severe, uncontrolled diabetes. Patients with severe ketoacidosis may experience Kussmaul's respirations. Associated signs and symptoms include decreased LOC, fatigue, weakness, fruity breath odor, and oliguria.

Increased intracranial pressure
A late sign of increased intracranial pressure (ICP) and a life-threatening condition, bradypnea is preceded by decreased LOC, deteriorating motor function, and fixed, dilated pupils. The triad of bradypnea, bradycardia, and hypertension is a classic sign of late medullary strangulation.

Respiratory failure
Bradypnea occurs with end-stage respiratory failure along with cyanosis, diminished breath sounds, tachycardia, and mildly increased blood pressure. The patient may also be restless, confused, irritable, or have a decreased LOC.

OTHER CAUSES

Drugs
Overdose with an opioid analgesic or, less commonly, a sedative, barbiturate, phenothiazine, or other CNS depressant can cause bradypnea. Use of any of these drugs with alcohol can also cause bradypnea.

SPECIAL CONSIDERATIONS
Because a patient with bradypnea may develop apnea, check his respiratory status frequently and be prepared to give ventilatory support if necessary. Don't leave the patient unattended, especially if his LOC is decreased. Obtain blood for arterial blood gas analysis, electrolyte studies, and a possible drug screen. Prepare the patient for chest X-rays and possibly a computed tomography scan of the head.

Administer prescribed drugs and oxygen. Avoid giving the patient a CNS depressant because it can exacerbate bradypnea. Similarly, give oxygen judiciously to a patient with chronic carbon dioxide retention, which may occur with chronic obstructive pulmonary disease, because excess oxygen therapy can have a negative effect.

When dealing with slow breathing in hospitalized patients, always review all drugs and dosages given during the last 24 hours.

PEDIATRIC POINTERS
Because respiratory rates are higher in children than in adults, bradypnea in children is defined according to age. (See *Respiratory rates in children,* page 106.)

GERIATRIC POINTERS
When drugs are prescribed for older patients, keep in mind that these patients have a higher risk of developing bradypnea secondary to drug toxicity. That's because many of these patients take several drugs that can potentiate this effect and typically have other conditions that predispose them to it. Warn older patients about this potentially life-threatening complication.

Medical causes

Diabetic ketoacidosis
- Bradypnea occurs late in patients with severe, uncontrolled diabetes.
- Associated signs and symptoms include decreased LOC, fatigue, weakness, fruity breath odor, and oliguria.

Increased ICP
- Bradypnea is a late sign.
- Sign is preceded by decreased LOC, deteriorating motor function, and fixed, dilated pupils.

Respiratory failure
- Bradypnea occurs during end-stage failure.

Other causes
- Overdose with opioid analgesic, sedative, barbiturate, phenothiazine, or other CNS depressant
- Use of alcohol with above drugs

Special considerations
- Check respiratory status frequently and be prepared to give ventilatory support if necessary.
- Obtain blood for ABG analysis, electrolyte studies, and possible drug screen.
- Prepare patient for chest X-rays and possibly CT scan of head.
- Administer oxygen.
- When dealing with slow breathing in hospitalized patients, review all drugs and dosages given during the last 24 hours.

Peds points
- Bradypnea in children is defined according to age.

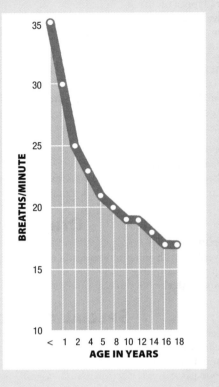

Respiratory rates in children

This graph shows normal respiratory rates in children, which are higher than normal rates in adults. Accordingly, bradypnea in a child is defined by the child's age.

PATIENT COUNSELING

Patients regularly taking an opioid — for example, those with advanced cancer or sickle cell anemia — should be alerted that bradypnea is a serious complication. They should be taught to recognize early signs of toxicity, such as nausea and vomiting. It's also important to identify patients who may be abusing these drugs.

BREAST NODULE

A commonly reported gynecologic sign, a breast nodule (also known as a *breast lump*) has two chief causes: benign breast disease and cancer. Benign breast disease, the leading cause of nodules, can stem from cyst formation in obstructed and dilated lactiferous ducts, hypertrophy or tumor formation in the ductal system, inflammation, or infection.

Although less than 20% of breast nodules are malignant, the signs and symptoms of breast cancer aren't easily distinguished from those of benign breast disease. Breast cancer is a leading cause of death among women but can occur occasionally in men, with signs and symptoms mimicking those found in women. Thus, breast nodules in both sexes should always be evaluated.

A woman who's familiar with the feel of her breasts and performs monthly breast self-examination can detect a nodule 6.4 mm or less in size, considerably smaller than the 1-cm nodule that's readily detectable by an experienced examiner.

HISTORY

If your patient reports a lump, ask her how and when she discovered it. Does the size and tenderness of the lump vary with her menstrual cycle? Has the lump changed since she first noticed it? Has she noticed any other breast signs, such as a change in breast shape, size, or contour; a discharge; or nipple changes?

Is she breast-feeding? Does she have fever, chills, fatigue, or other flulike signs or symptoms? Ask her to describe any pain or tenderness associated with the lump. Is the pain in one breast only? Has she sustained recent trauma to the breast?

Explore the patient's medical and family history for factors that increase her risk of breast cancer. These include a high-fat diet, having a mother or sister with breast cancer, or having a history of cancer, especially cancer in the other breast. Other risk factors include nulliparity and a first pregnancy after age 30.

 CULTURAL CUE *Breast cancer incidence and mortality are about five times higher in North America and northern Europe than in Asia and Africa.*

PHYSICAL ASSESSMENT

Perform a thorough breast examination. Pay special attention to the upper outer quadrant of each breast, where one-half of the ductal tissue is located. This is the most common site of malignant breast tumors.

Carefully palpate a suspected breast nodule, noting its location, shape, size, consistency, mobility, and delineation. Does the nodule feel soft, rubbery, and elastic or hard? Is it mobile, slipping away from your fingers as you palpate it, or firmly fixed to adjacent tissue? Does the nodule seem to limit the mobility of the entire breast? Note the nodule's delineation. Are the borders clearly defined or indefinite? Does the area feel more like a hardness or diffuse induration than a nodule with definite borders?

Do you feel one nodule or several small ones? Is the shape round, oval, lobular, or irregular? Inspect and palpate the skin over the nodule for warmth, redness, and edema. Palpate the lymph nodes of the breast and axilla for enlargement.

Observe the contour of the breasts, looking for asymmetry and irregularities. Be alert for signs of retraction, such as skin dimpling and nipple deviation, retraction, or flattening. (To exaggerate dimpling, have your patient raise her arms over her head or press her hands against her hips.) Gently pull the breast skin toward the clavicle. Is dimpling evident? Mold the breast skin and again observe the area for dimpling.

Be alert for a nipple discharge that's spontaneous, unilateral, and nonmilky (serous, bloody, or purulent). Be careful not to confuse it with the grayish discharge that can be elicited from the nipples of a woman who has been pregnant.

MEDICAL CAUSES

Adenofibroma

The extremely mobile or "slippery" feel of an adenofibroma (a benign neoplasm) helps distinguish it from other breast nodules. The nodule usually occurs singly and characteristically feels firm, elastic, and round or lobular, with well-defined margins. It doesn't cause pain or tenderness, can vary from pinhead size to very

Key history points
+ Description and history of lump
+ Breast-feeding
+ Associated signs and symptoms
+ Medical and family history
+ Breast cancer risk factors

Critical assessment steps
+ Perform a thorough breast examination.
+ Carefully palpate a suspected breast nodule, noting its location, shape, size, consistency, mobility, and delineation.
+ Inspect and palpate the skin over the nodule for warmth, redness, and edema.
+ Palpate the lymph nodes of the breast and axilla for enlargement.
+ Observe the contour of the breasts, looking for asymmetry and irregularities.
+ Be alert for signs of retraction, such as skin dimpling and nipple deviation, retraction, or flattening.
+ Be alert for nipple discharge that's spontaneous, unilateral, and nonmilky.

Medical causes
Adenofibroma
+ The nodule usually occurs singly and feels firm, elastic, and round or lobular, with well-defined margins.

Medical causes
(continued)

Areolar gland abscess
✦ A tender, palpable abscess on the periphery of the areola develops following an inflammation of the sebaceous glands of Montgomery.

Breast abscess
✦ The nodule is localized, hot, tender, and fluctuant with erythema and peau d'orange.

Breast cancer
✦ The nodule is hard, poorly delineated, and fixed to the skin or underlying tissue.
✦ Nodules usually occur singly, developing in the upper outer quadrant 40% to 50% of the time.
✦ Satellite nodules may surround the main one.

Fibrocystic breast disease
✦ Smooth, round, slightly elastic nodules, increase in size and tenderness just before menstruation.
✦ Nodules are mobile, which differentiates them from malignant nodules.

Intraductal papilloma
✦ Nodules are tiny, benign, and usually resist palpation.
✦ Serous or bloody nipple discharge is the primary sign.

Mammary duct ectasia
✦ A rubbery breast nodule lies under the areola.

large, typically grows rapidly, and usually lies around the nipple or on the lateral side of the upper outer quadrant.

Areolar gland abscess
An areolar gland abscess is characterized by a tender, palpable abscess on the periphery of the areola following an inflammation of the sebaceous glands of Montgomery. Fever, local swelling, and drainage may also be present, and the patient may complain of malaise.

Breast abscess
A localized, hot, tender, fluctuant mass with erythema and peau d'orange typifies an acute breast abscess. Associated signs and symptoms include fever, chills, malaise, and generalized discomfort. With a chronic abscess, the nodule is nontender, irregular, and firm and may feel like a thick wall of fibrous tissue. It's commonly accompanied by skin dimpling, peau d'orange, and nipple retraction and sometimes by axillary lymphadenopathy.

Breast cancer
A hard, poorly delineated nodule that's fixed to the skin or underlying tissue suggests breast cancer. Malignant nodules commonly cause breast dimpling, nipple deviation or retraction, or flattening of the nipple or breast contour. Between 40% and 50% of malignant nodules occur in the upper outer quadrant.

Nodules usually occur singly, although satellite nodules may surround the main one. They're usually nontender. Nipple discharge may be serous or bloody. (A bloody nipple discharge in the presence of a nodule is a classic sign of breast cancer.) Additional findings include edema (peau d'orange) of the skin overlying the mass, erythema, tenderness, and axillary lymphadenopathy. A breast ulcer may occur as a late sign. Breast pain, an unreliable symptom, may be present.

Fibrocystic breast disease
The most common cause of breast nodules, fibrocystic breast disease produces smooth, round, slightly elastic nodules, which increase in size and tenderness just before menstruation. The nodules may occur in fine, granular clusters in both breasts or as widespread, well-defined lumps of varying sizes. A thickening of adjacent tissue may be palpable. Cystic nodules are mobile, which helps differentiate them from malignant ones. Because cystic nodules aren't fixed to underlying breast tissue, they don't produce retraction signs, such as nipple deviation or dimpling. A clear, watery (serous), or sticky nipple discharge may appear in one or both breasts. Signs and symptoms of premenstrual syndrome — including headache, irritability, bloating, nausea, vomiting, and abdominal cramping — may also be present.

Intraductal papilloma
The tiny nodules of intraductal papilloma (a benign lesion) usually resist palpation. Nodules large enough to be palpated usually occur singly, but they may be multiple and diffuse. Soft and poorly delineated, the nodules usually lie in the subareolar margin. The primary sign of this disorder is serous or bloody nipple discharge, typically from only one duct. Breast pain and tenderness may occur.

Mammary duct ectasia
The rubbery breast nodule in mammary duct ectasia — a menopausal or postmenopausal disorder — usually lies under the areola. It's commonly accompanied by transient pain, itching, tenderness, and erythema of the areola; thick, sticky, multicolored nipple discharge from multiple ducts; and nipple retraction. The skin overlying the mass may be bluish green or exhibit peau d'orange. Axillary lymphadenopathy is possible.

Mastitis

With mastitis, breast nodules feel firm and indurated or tender, flocculent, and discrete. Gentle palpation defines the area of maximum purulent accumulation. Skin dimpling and nipple deviation, retraction, or flattening may be present, and the nipple may show a crack or abrasion. Accompanying signs and symptoms include breast warmth, erythema, tenderness, and peau d'orange, plus high fever, chills, malaise, and fatigue.

Paget's disease

In Paget's disease, the slow-growing intraductal carcinoma begins as a scaling, eczematoid unilateral nipple lesion. The nipple later becomes reddened and excoriated and may eventually be completely destroyed. The process extends along the skin as well as in the ducts, usually progressing to a deep-seated mass.

SPECIAL CONSIDERATIONS

Although many women regard a breast lump as a sign of breast cancer, most nodules are benign. As a result, try to avoid alarming your patient further. Provide a simple explanation of your examination, and encourage the patient to express her feelings.

Prepare the patient for diagnostic tests, which may include transillumination, mammography, thermography, needle aspiration or open biopsy of the nodule for tissue examination, and cytologic examination of nipple discharge.

Postpone teaching the patient how to perform breast self-examination until she overcomes her initial anxiety at discovering a nodule. Regular breast self-examination is especially important for women who have had a previous cancer, have a family history of breast cancer, are nulliparous, or had their first child after age 30.

Although most nodules occurring in breast-feeding patients result from mastitis, the possibility of cancer demands careful evaluation.

PEDIATRIC POINTERS

Most nodules in children and adolescents reflect the normal response of breast tissue to hormonal fluctuations. For instance, the breasts of young teenage girls may normally contain cordlike nodules that become tender just before menstruation.

A transient breast nodule in young boys (as well as women between ages 20 and 30) may result from juvenile mastitis, which usually affects one breast. Signs of inflammation are present in a firm mass beneath the nipple.

GERIATRIC POINTERS

In women age 70 and older, three-quarters of all breast lumps are malignant.

PATIENT COUNSELING

When teaching patients how to perform breast self-examination, advise them to do the examination 5 to 7 days after the first day of their last menses.

Advise the patient with mastitis to pump her breasts to prevent further milk stasis, to discard the milk, and to substitute formula until the infection responds to antibiotics.

Mastitis
+ Nodules feel firm and indurated or tender, flocculent, and discrete.

Paget's disease
+ A scaling, eczematoid unilateral nipple lesion grows slowly into an intraductal carcinoma.

Special considerations
+ Provide a simple explanation of your examination.
+ Although most nodules occurring in breast-feeding patients result from mastitis, the possibility of cancer demands careful evaluation.

Peds points
+ Most nodules in children and adolescents reflect the normal response of breast tissue to hormonal fluctuations.
+ A transient, firm breast nodule beneath the nipple in young boys (as well as women between ages 20 and 30) may result from juvenile mastitis, which usually affects one breast.

Geri points
+ In women age 70 and older, three-quarters of all breast lumps are malignant.

Teaching points
+ Breast self-examination
+ Tips for dealing with mastitis

Key facts about breast pain

+ Also called *mastalgia*
+ Results from benign breast disease
+ May occur during rest or movement
+ May be aggravated by manipulation or palpation
+ May be unilateral or bilateral

Key history points

+ Onset and description of pain
+ Duration of pain (constant or intermittent)
+ Nursing, pregnant, or menopausal
+ Injury or changes to breast

Critical assessment steps

+ With the patient's arms at her sides, note breast size, symmetry, and contour, and the appearance of the skin.
+ Note the size, shape, and symmetry of the nipples and areolae.
+ Repeat your inspection with the patient's arms raised above her head and then with her hands pressed against her hips.
+ Palpate the breasts with the patient seated and then with her lying down with a pillow placed under her shoulder on the side being examined.
+ Palpate the nipple, noting tenderness and nodules; check for discharge.
+ Palpate axillary lymph nodes, noting any enlargement.

BREAST PAIN

An unreliable indicator of cancer, breast pain commonly results from benign breast disease. Also known as *mastalgia*, breast pain may occur during rest or movement and may be aggravated by manipulation or palpation. (Breast *tenderness* refers to pain elicited by physical contact.) Breast pain may be unilateral or bilateral; cyclic, intermittent, or constant; and dull or sharp. It may result from surface cuts, furuncles, contusions, or similar lesions (superficial pain); nipple fissures or inflammation in the papillary ducts or areolae (severe localized pain); stromal distention in the breast parenchyma; a tumor that affects nerve endings (severe, constant pain); or inflammatory lesions that distend the stroma and irritate sensory nerve endings (severe, constant pain). Breast pain may radiate to the back, the arms and, sometimes, the neck.

Before menstruation, breast pain or tenderness stems from increased mammary blood flow due to hormonal changes. During pregnancy, breast tenderness and throbbing, tingling, or pricking sensations may occur, also from hormonal changes. In men, breast pain may stem from gynecomastia (especially during puberty and senescence), reproductive tract anomalies, or organic disease of the liver or pituitary, adrenal cortex, or thyroid glands.

HISTORY

Begin by asking the patient if breast pain is constant or intermittent. For either type, ask about onset and character. If it's intermittent, determine the relationship of pain to the phase of the menstrual cycle. Is the patient a nursing mother? If not, ask about any nipple discharge and have her describe it. Is she pregnant? Has she reached menopause? Has she recently experienced any flulike symptoms or sustained any injury to the breast? Has she noticed any change in breast shape or contour?

Ask your patient to describe the pain. She may describe it as sticking, stinging, shooting, stabbing, throbbing, or burning. Determine if the pain affects one breast or both, and ask the patient to point to the painful area.

PHYSICAL ASSESSMENT

Instruct the patient to place her arms at her sides, and inspect the breasts. Note their size, symmetry, and contour, and the appearance of the skin. Remember that breast shape and size vary and that breasts normally change during menses, pregnancy, and lactation and with aging. Are the breasts red or edematous? Are the veins prominent?

Note the size, shape, and symmetry of the nipples and areolae. Do you detect ecchymosis, a rash, ulceration, or a discharge? Do the nipples point in the same direction? Do you see signs of retraction, such as skin dimpling or nipple inversion or flattening? Repeat your inspection, first with the patient's arms raised above her head and then with her hands pressed against her hips.

Palpate the breasts, first with the patient seated and then with her lying down and a pillow placed under her shoulder on the side being examined. Use the pads of your fingers to compress breast tissue against the chest wall. Proceed systematically from the sternum to the midline and from the axilla to the midline, noting any warmth, tenderness, nodules, masses, or irregularities. Palpate the nipple, noting tenderness and nodules, and check for discharge. Palpate axillary lymph nodes, noting any enlargement.

MEDICAL CAUSES

Areolar gland abscess

An areolar gland abscess is characterized by a tender, palpable abscess on the periphery of the areola following an inflammation of the sebaceous glands of Montgomery. Fever, local swelling, and drainage may also be present, and the patient may complain of malaise.

Breast abscess (acute)

In the abscessed breast, local pain, tenderness, erythema, peau d'orange, and warmth are associated with a nodule. Malaise, fever, and chills may also occur. Axillary nodes may be enlarged.

Fat necrosis

Local pain and tenderness may develop with fat necrosis—a benign disorder. A history of trauma usually is present. Associated findings include ecchymosis; erythema of the overriding skin; a firm, irregular, fixed mass; and skin retraction signs, such as skin dimpling and nipple retraction. Fat necrosis may be hard to differentiate from cancer.

Fibrocystic breast disease

Fibrocystic breast disease, a common cause of breast pain, is associated with the development of cysts that may cause pain before menstruation and produce no symptoms afterward. Later in the course of the disorder, pain and tenderness may persist throughout the cycle. The cysts feel firm, mobile, and well defined. Many are bilateral and found in the upper outer quadrant of the breast, but others are unilateral and generalized. A clear, serous nipple discharge may be present in one or both breasts. Signs and symptoms of premenstrual syndrome—including headache, irritability, bloating, nausea, vomiting, and abdominal cramping—may also be present.

Intraductal papilloma

Unilateral breast pain or tenderness may accompany intraductal papilloma, although the primary sign is a serous or bloody nipple discharge, usually from only one duct. Intraductal papilloma is the primary cause of nipple discharge in nonpregnant, nonlactating women. Associated signs include a small (usually 1.5-mm to 3-mm), soft, poorly delineated mass in the ducts beneath the areola.

Mammary duct ectasia

With mammary duct ectasia, burning pain and itching around the areola may occur, although ectasia commonly produces no symptoms at first. The history may include one or more episodes of inflammation with pain, tenderness, erythema, and acute fever, or with pain and tenderness alone, which develop and then subside spontaneously in 7 to 10 days. Other findings include a rubbery, subareolar breast nodule; swelling and erythema around the nipple; nipple retraction; a bluish green discoloration or peau d'orange of the skin overlying the nodule; a thick, sticky, multicolored nipple discharge from multiple ducts; and axillary lymphadenopathy. A breast ulcer may occur in late stages.

Mastitis

With mastitis, unilateral pain may be severe, particularly when the inflammation occurs near the skin surface. Breast skin is typically red and warm at the inflammation site; peau d'orange may be present. Palpation reveals a firm area of induration. Skin retraction signs—such as breast dimpling and nipple deviation, inversion, or

Medical causes

Areolar gland abscess

- Sebaceous glands of Montgomery become inflamed.
- Abscess is tender and palpable and is located on the periphery of the areola.

Breast abscess (acute)

- Local pain, tenderness, erythema, peau d'orange, and warmth develop.

Fat necrosis

- Local pain and tenderness may develop.

Fibrocystic breast disease

- Cysts may cause pain before menstruation and produce no symptoms afterward.
- Later, pain may persist throughout the cycle.

Intraductal papilloma

- Unilateral breast pain or tenderness may occur.
- Serous or bloody nipple discharge is the primary sign.

Mammary duct ectasia

- Burning pain and itching around the areola may occur.

Mastitis

- Unilateral pain may be severe.
- Skin is typically red and warm at the inflammation site.

Special considerations
+ Provide emotional support for the patient.
+ When appropriate, emphasize the importance of monthly breast self-examination.

Peds points
+ Transient gynecomastia can cause breast pain in males during puberty.

Geri points
+ Breast pain secondary to benign breast disease is rare in post-menopausal women.
+ Breast pain can be due to trauma from falls or physical abuse.
+ Because of decreased pain perception and decreased cognitive function, elderly patients may not report breast pain.

Teaching points
+ Appropriate type of brassiere
+ Use of warm or cold compresses
+ Breast self-examination

Key facts about fecal breath odor
+ Typically accompanies fecal vomiting associated with a long-standing intestinal obstruction or gastrojejunocolic fistula
+ May indicate a life-threatening GI disorder

Key history points
+ Previous abdominal surgeries
+ Onset, duration, and location of any abdominal pain
+ Normal bowel habits, including time and description of last bowel movement

flattening — may be present. Systemic signs and symptoms — such as high fever, chills, malaise, and fatigue — may also occur.

SPECIAL CONSIDERATIONS

Provide emotional support for the patient and, when appropriate, emphasize the importance of monthly breast self-examination.

Prepare the patient for diagnostic tests, such as mammography, thermography, cytology of nipple discharge, biopsy, or culture of any aspirate.

PEDIATRIC POINTERS

Transient gynecomastia can cause breast pain in males during puberty.

GERIATRIC POINTERS

Breast pain secondary to benign breast disease is rare in postmenopausal women. Breast pain can also be due to trauma from falls or physical abuse. Because of decreased pain perception and decreased cognitive function, elderly patients may not report breast pain.

PATIENT COUNSELING

Advise the patient to wear a brassiere that cups and supports the entire breast with wide shoulder and back straps. Warm or cold compresses may be helpful. Teach the patient how to perform breast self-examination, and instruct her to call the physician immediately if she detects any breast changes.

BREATH WITH FECAL ODOR

Fecal breath odor typically accompanies fecal vomiting associated with a long-standing intestinal obstruction or gastrojejunocolic fistula. It represents an important late diagnostic clue to a potentially life-threatening GI disorder because complete obstruction of any part of the bowel, if untreated, can cause death within hours from vascular collapse and shock.

When the obstructed or adynamic intestine attempts self-decompression by regurgitating its contents, vigorous peristaltic waves propel bowel contents backward into the stomach. When the stomach fills with intestinal fluid, further reverse peristalsis results in vomiting. The odor of feculent vomitus lingers in the mouth.

Fecal breath odor may also occur in patients with a nasogastric (NG) or intestinal tube. The odor is detected only while the underlying disorder persists and abates soon after its resolution. (See *Managing fecal breath odor.*)

HISTORY

If the patient's condition permits, ask about previous abdominal surgery because adhesions can cause an obstruction. Also ask about loss of appetite. Is the patient experiencing abdominal pain? If so, have him describe its onset, duration, and location. Ask if the pain is intense, persistent, or spasmodic. Have the patient describe his normal bowel habits, especially noting constipation, diarrhea, or leakage of stool. Ask when the patient's last bowel movement occurred, and have him describe the stool's color and consistency.

Managing fecal breath odor

Because fecal breath odor signals a potentially life-threatening intestinal obstruction, you'll need to quickly evaluate your patient's condition. Monitor his vital signs, and be alert for signs of shock, such as hypotension, tachycardia, narrowed pulse pressure, and cool, clammy skin. Ask the patient if he's experiencing nausea or has vomited. Find out the frequency of vomiting as well as the color, odor, amount, and consistency of the vomitus. Have an emesis basin nearby to collect and accurately measure the vomitus.

Anticipate possible surgery to relieve an obstruction or repair a fistula, and withhold all food and fluids. Be prepared to insert a nasogastric or intestinal tube for GI tract decompression. Insert a peripheral I.V. line for vascular access, or assist with central line insertion for large-bore access and central venous pressure monitoring. Obtain a blood sample and send it to the laboratory for complete blood count and electrolyte analysis because large fluid losses and shifts can produce electrolyte imbalances. Maintain adequate hydration and support circulatory status with additional fluids. Give a physiologic solution—such as lactated Ringer's or normal saline solution or human plasma protein fraction (Plasmanate)—to prevent metabolic acidosis from gastric losses and metabolic alkalosis from intestinal fluid losses.

PHYSICAL ASSESSMENT

Auscultate for bowel sounds—hyperactive, high-pitched sounds may indicate impending bowel obstruction, whereas hypoactive or absent sounds occur late in obstruction and paralytic ileus. Inspect the abdomen, noting its contour and any surgical scars. Measure abdominal girth to provide baseline data for subsequent assessment of distention. Palpate for tenderness, distention, and rigidity. Percuss for tympany, indicating a gas-filled bowel, and dullness, indicating fluid. Rectal and pelvic examinations should be performed.

MEDICAL CAUSES

Distal small-bowel obstruction

With late small-bowel obstruction, nausea is present although vomiting may be delayed. Vomitus initially consists of gastric contents, then changes to bilious contents, followed by fecal contents with resultant fecal breath odor. Accompanying symptoms include achiness, malaise, drowsiness, and polydipsia. Bowel changes (ranging from diarrhea to constipation) are accompanied by abdominal distention, persistent epigastric or periumbilical colicky pain, and hyperactive bowel sounds and borborygmi. As the obstruction becomes complete, bowel sounds become hypoactive or absent. Fever, hypotension, tachycardia, and rebound tenderness may indicate strangulation or perforation.

Gastrojejunocolic fistula

With gastrojejunocolic fistula, symptoms may be variable and intermittent because of temporary plugging of the fistula. Fecal vomiting with resulting fecal breath odor may occur, but the most common chief complaint is diarrhea, accompanied by abdominal pain. Related GI findings include anorexia, weight loss, abdominal distention and, possibly, marked malabsorption.

Large-bowel obstruction

Vomiting is usually absent at first, but fecal vomiting with resultant fecal breath odor occurs as a late sign of large-bowel obstruction. Typically, symptoms develop

Critical assessment steps

+ Auscultate for bowel sounds.
+ Inspect the abdomen, noting its contour and any surgical scars.
+ Measure abdominal girth to provide a baseline.
+ Palpate for tenderness, distention, and rigidity.
+ Percuss for tympany or dullness.
+ Rectal and pelvic examinations should be performed.

Medical causes

Distal small-bowel obstruction

+ Fecal breath odor results from vomiting of fecal contents following vomiting of gastric contents and bilious contents.

Gastrojejunocolic fistula

+ Fecal vomiting with resulting fecal breath odor may occur.
+ Diarrhea accompanied by abdominal pain is the most common chief complaint.

Large-bowel obstruction

+ Fecal vomiting with resultant fecal breath odor occurs as a late sign.

Special considerations

After an NG or intestinal tube has been inserted:

◆ Keep the head of the bed elevated at least 30 degrees.
◆ Turn the patient to facilitate passage of the intestinal tube through the GI tract.
◆ Don't tape the intestinal tube to the patient's face.
◆ Ensure tube patency. Monitor drainage and watch that suction devices function properly.
◆ Irrigate tube as required.
◆ Monitor GI drainage.
◆ Send serum specimens to the laboratory for electrolyte analysis at least once per day.

Peds points

◆ Carefully monitor the child's fluid and electrolyte status because dehydration can occur rapidly from persistent vomiting.
◆ Clinical signs of dehydration include the absence of tears and dry or parched mucous membranes.

Geri points

◆ Early surgical intervention may be necessary for a bowel obstruction that doesn't respond to decompression because of the high risk of bowel infarct.

Teaching points

◆ Procedures and treatments
◆ Good oral hygiene

Key facts about fruity breath odor

◆ Results from respiratory elimination of excess acetone

more slowly than in small-bowel obstruction. Colicky abdominal pain appears suddenly, followed by continuous hypogastric pain. Marked abdominal distention and tenderness occur, and loops of large bowel may be visible through the abdominal wall. Although constipation develops, defecation may continue for up to 3 days after complete obstruction because of stool remaining in the bowel below the obstruction. Leakage of stool is common with partial obstruction. Explain all procedures and treatments.

SPECIAL CONSIDERATIONS

After an NG or intestinal tube has been inserted, keep the head of the bed elevated at least 30 degrees and turn the patient to facilitate passage of the intestinal tube through the GI tract. Don't tape the intestinal tube to the patient's face. Ensure tube patency by monitoring drainage and watching that suction devices function properly. Irrigate as required. Monitor GI drainage, and send serum specimens to the laboratory for electrolyte analysis at least once per day. Prepare the patient for diagnostic tests, such as abdominal X-rays, barium enema, and proctoscopy.

PEDIATRIC POINTERS

Carefully monitor the child's fluid and electrolyte status because dehydration can occur rapidly from persistent vomiting. The absence of tears and dry or parched mucous membranes are important clinical signs of dehydration.

GERIATRIC POINTERS

In older patients, early surgical intervention may be necessary for a bowel obstruction that doesn't respond to decompression because of the high risk of bowel infarct.

PATIENT COUNSELING

Explain all procedures and treatments. Encourage the patient to brush his teeth and gargle with a flavored mouthwash or half-strength hydrogen peroxide mixture to minimize offensive breath odor. Assure him that the fecal odor is temporary and will abate after treatment of the underlying cause.

BREATH WITH FRUITY ODOR

Fruity breath odor results from respiratory elimination of excess acetone. This sign characteristically occurs with ketoacidosis—a potentially life-threatening condition that requires immediate treatment to prevent severe dehydration, irreversible coma, and death.

Ketoacidosis results from the excessive catabolism of fats for cellular energy in the absence of usable carbohydrates. This process begins when insulin levels are insufficient to transport glucose into the cells, as in diabetes mellitus, or when glucose is unavailable and hepatic glycogen stores are depleted, as in low-carbohydrate diets and malnutrition. Lacking glucose, the cells burn fat faster than enzymes can handle the ketones, the acidic end products. As a result, the ketones (acetone, beta-hydroxybutyric acid, and acetoacetic acid) accumulate in the blood and urine. To compensate for increased acidity, Kussmaul's respirations expel carbon dioxide with enough acetone to flavor the breath. Eventually, this compensatory mechanism fails, producing ketoacidosis. (See *Managing fruity breath odor.*)

Managing fruity breath odor

When you detect fruity breath odor, check for Kussmaul's respirations and examine the patient's level of consciousness. Take vital signs and check skin turgor. Be alert for fruity breath odor that accompanies rapid, deep respirations; stupor; and poor skin turgor. Try to obtain a brief history, noting especially diabetes mellitus, nutritional problems such as anorexia nervosa, and fad diets with little or no carbohydrates. Obtain venous and arterial blood samples for complete blood count and glucose, electrolyte, acetone, and arterial blood gas (ABG) levels. Also obtain a urine specimen to test for glucose and acetone. Administer I.V. fluids and electrolytes to maintain hydration and electrolyte balance and, in patients with diabetic ketoacidosis, give regular insulin to reduce blood glucose levels.

If the patient is obtunded, you'll need to insert endotracheal and nasogastric tubes. Suction as needed. Insert an indwelling urinary catheter, and monitor intake and output. Insert central venous pressure and arterial lines to monitor the patient's fluid status and blood pressure. Place the patient on a cardiac monitor, monitor vital signs and neurologic status, and draw blood hourly to check glucose, electrolyte, acetone, and ABG levels.

HISTORY

If the patient isn't in severe distress, obtain a thorough history. Ask about the onset and duration of fruity breath odor. Find out about any changes in breathing pattern. Ask about increased thirst, frequent urination, weight loss, fatigue, and abdominal pain. Ask the female patient if she has had candidal vaginitis or vaginal secretions with itching. If the patient has a history of diabetes mellitus, ask about stress, infections, and noncompliance with therapy—the most common causes of ketoacidosis in a patient with diabetes. If the patient is suspected of having anorexia nervosa, obtain a dietary and weight history.

PHYSICAL ASSESSMENT

Begin by taking your patient's vital signs. Then proceed with a complete physical assessment.

MEDICAL CAUSES

Anorexia nervosa

Severe weight loss associated with anorexia nervosa may produce fruity breath, usually with nausea, constipation, and cold intolerance as well as dental enamel erosion and scars or calluses in the dorsum of the hand, both related to induced vomiting.

Ketoacidosis

Fruity breath odor accompanies alcoholic ketoacidosis, which is usually seen in poorly nourished alcoholics with vomiting, abdominal pain, and only minimal food intake over several days. Kussmaul's respirations begin abruptly and accompany dehydration, abdominal pain and distention, and absent bowel sounds. Blood glucose levels are normal or slightly decreased.

With diabetic ketoacidosis, fruity breath odor commonly occurs as ketoacidosis develops over 1 to 2 days. Other findings include polydipsia, polyuria, nocturia, weak and rapid pulse, hunger, weight loss, weakness, fatigue, nausea, vomiting, and abdominal pain. Eventually, Kussmaul's respirations, orthostatic hypotension, dehydration, tachycardia, confusion, stupor, and coma may occur.

Key history points
+ Onset and duration of odor
+ Changes in breathing patterns
+ Associated signs and symptoms, including increased thirst, frequent urination, weight loss, fatigue, and abdominal pain
+ History of diabetes mellitus
+ Dietary and weight history (if anorexia nervosa is suspected)

Critical assessment steps
+ Take vital signs.
+ Perform a physical examination.

Medical causes

Anorexia nervosa
+ Severe weight loss may produce fruity breath odor.
+ Nausea, constipation, and cold intolerance may be present.

Ketoacidosis
+ With alcoholic ketoacidosis, fruity breath odor occurs with vomiting and abdominal pain.
+ With diabetic ketoacidosis, fruity breath occurs as it develops over 1 to 2 days.
+ With starvation ketoacidosis, fruity breath onset is gradual.

Other causes
+ Drugs that cause metabolic acidosis, such as nitroprusside and salicylates
+ Low-carbohydrate diets

Special considerations
+ Explain tests and treatments clearly.
+ When the patient is more alert and his condition stabilizes, remove the NG tube and start him on an appropriate diet.
+ Switch his insulin from the I.V. to the subcutaneous route.

Peds points
+ Fruity breath odor in an infant or a child usually stems from uncontrolled diabetes mellitus.

Geri points
+ Consider factors such as poor oral hygiene, increased dental caries, decreased salivary function, poor dietary intake, and use of multiple drugs when evaluating an elderly patient with mouth odor.

Teaching points
+ Signs of hyperglycemia
+ Referral to psychologist or support group, as appropriate

Key facts about Brudzinski's sign
+ Hips and knees go into flexion in response to passive flexion of the neck
+ Signals meningeal irritation

Starvation ketoacidosis is a potentially life-threatening disorder that has a gradual onset. Besides fruity breath odor, typical findings include signs of cachexia and dehydration, decreased level of consciousness, bradycardia, and a history of severely limited food intake (anorexia nervosa).

OTHER CAUSES

Drugs
Any drug known to cause metabolic acidosis, such as nitroprusside and salicylates, can result in fruity breath odor.

Low-carbohydrate diets
Low-carbohydrate diets, which encourage little or no carbohydrate intake, may cause ketoacidosis and a resulting fruity breath odor.

SPECIAL CONSIDERATIONS
Provide emotional support for the patient and his family. Explain tests and treatments clearly. When the patient is more alert and his condition stabilizes, remove the nasogastric tube and start him on an appropriate diet. Switch his insulin from the I.V. to the subcutaneous route.

PEDIATRIC POINTERS
Fruity breath odor in an infant or child usually stems from uncontrolled diabetes mellitus. Ketoacidosis develops rapidly in this age-group because of low glycogen reserves. As a result, prompt administration of insulin and correction of fluid and electrolyte imbalance are necessary to prevent shock and death.

GERIATRIC POINTERS
Elderly patients may have poor oral hygiene, increased dental caries, decreased salivary function with dryness, and poor dietary intake. In addition, many take multiple drugs. Consider all of these factors when evaluating an elderly patient with mouth odor.

PATIENT COUNSELING
Teach the patient and make referrals appropriately. For example, teach the patient with uncontrolled diabetes mellitus to recognize the signs of hyperglycemia and to wear a medical identification bracelet. Refer the patient with starvation ketoacidosis to a psychologist or a support group, and recognize the need for possible long-term follow-up.

BRUDZINSKI'S SIGN

A positive Brudzinski's sign (flexion of the hips and knees in response to passive flexion of the neck) signals meningeal irritation. Passive flexion of the neck stretches the nerve roots, causing pain and involuntary flexion of the knees and hips.

Brudzinski's sign is a common and important early indicator of life-threatening meningitis and subarachnoid hemorrhage. It can be elicited in children as well as adults, although more reliable indicators of meningeal irritation exist for infants.

Testing for Brudzinski's sign isn't part of the routine examination, unless meningeal irritation is suspected. (See *Testing for Brudzinski's sign.*)

Testing for Brudzinski's sign

Here's how to test for Brudzinski's sign when you suspect meningeal irritation:

With the patient in a supine position, place your hands behind her neck and lift her head toward her chest.

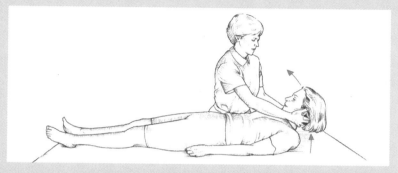

If your patient has meningeal irritation, she'll flex her hips and knees in response to the passive neck flexion.

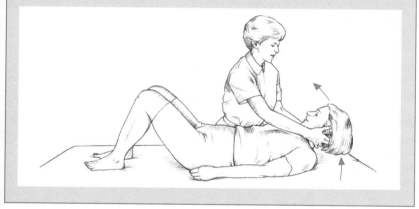

EMERGENCY ACTIONS If the patient is alert, ask him about headache, neck pain, nausea, and vision disturbances (blurred or double vision and photophobia) — all indications of increased intracranial pressure (ICP). Next, observe the patient for altered level of consciousness (LOC) (restlessness, irritability, confusion, lethargy, personality changes, and coma), pupillary changes, bradycardia, widened pulse pressure, irregular respiratory patterns (Cheyne-Stokes or Kussmaul's respirations), vomiting, and moderate fever.

Keep artificial airways, intubation equipment, a handheld resuscitation bag, and suction equipment on hand because your patient's condition may suddenly deteriorate. Elevate the head of his bed 30 to 60 degrees to promote venous drainage. Administer an osmotic diuretic, such as mannitol, to reduce cerebral edema. Monitor and be alert for ICP that continues to rise. You may have to provide mechanical ventilation and administer a barbiturate and additional doses of a diuretic. Also, cerebrospinal fluid (CSF) may have to be drained.

In an emergency

+ Ask the patient about headache, neck pain, nausea, and vision disturbances.
+ Observe the patient for altered LOC, pupillary changes, bradycardia, widened pulse pressure, Cheyne-Stokes or Kussmaul's respirations, vomiting, and moderate fever.
+ Keep artificial airways, intubation equipment, a handheld resuscitation bag, and suction equipment on hand.
+ Elevate the head of the bed 30 to 60 degrees.
+ Administer an osmotic diuretic.
+ Monitor and be alert for ICP that continues to rise. You may have to provide mechanical ventilation and administer a barbiturate and additional doses of a diuretic. Also, CSF may have to be drained.

Key history points

+ History of hypertension, spinal arthritis, head trauma, dental work or abscessed teeth, endocarditis, or I.V. drug abuse
+ Headaches

Critical assessment steps

+ Evaluate the patient's cranial nerve function, noting any motor or sensory deficits.
+ Look for Kernig's sign (resistance to knee extension after flexion of the hip), which is a further indication of meningeal irritation.
+ Look for signs of CNS infection, such as fever and nuchal rigidity.

Medical causes

Meningitis
+ A positive Brudzinski's sign can usually be elicited 24 hours after onset.

Subarachnoid hemorrhage
+ Brudzinski's sign may be elicited within minutes after initial bleeding.

Special considerations

+ Monitor ICP and make frequent neurologic checks.
+ Monitor vital signs, intake and output, and cardiorespiratory status.
+ Maintain low lights and minimal noise and elevate the head of the bed to promote patient comfort.

HISTORY

Ask the patient or his family, if necessary, about a history of hypertension, spinal arthritis, or recent head trauma. Also ask about dental work and abscessed teeth (a possible cause of meningitis), open-head injury, endocarditis, and I.V. drug abuse. Ask about sudden onset of headaches, which may be associated with subarachnoid hemorrhage.

PHYSICAL ASSESSMENT

Continue your neurologic examination by evaluating the patient's cranial nerve function and noting any motor or sensory deficits. Be sure to look for Kernig's sign (resistance to knee extension after flexion of the hip), which is a further indication of meningeal irritation. Also, you should look for signs of central nervous system infection, such as fever and nuchal rigidity.

MEDICAL CAUSES

Meningitis

A positive Brudzinski's sign can usually be elicited 24 hours after the onset of meningitis, a life-threatening disorder. Accompanying findings may include headache, a positive Kernig's sign, nuchal rigidity, irritability or restlessness, deep stupor or coma, vertigo, fever (high or low, depending on the severity of the infection), chills, malaise, hyperalgesia, muscular hypotonia, opisthotonos, symmetrical deep tendon reflexes, papilledema, ocular and facial palsies, nausea and vomiting, photophobia, diplopia, and unequal, sluggish pupils. As ICP rises, arterial hypertension, bradycardia, widened pulse pressure, Cheyne-Stokes or Kussmaul's respirations, and coma may develop.

Subarachnoid hemorrhage

Brudzinski's sign may be elicited within minutes after initial bleeding in subarachnoid hemorrhage, another life-threatening disorder. Accompanying signs and symptoms include sudden onset of severe headache, nuchal rigidity, altered LOC, dizziness, photophobia, cranial nerve palsies (as evidenced by ptosis, pupil dilation, and limited extraocular muscle movement), nausea and vomiting, fever, and a positive Kernig's sign. Focal signs — such as hemiparesis, vision disturbances, or aphasia — may also occur. As ICP rises, arterial hypertension, bradycardia, widened pulse pressure, Cheyne-Stokes or Kussmaul's respirations, and coma may develop.

SPECIAL CONSIDERATIONS

Many patients with a positive Brudzinski's sign are critically ill. They need constant ICP monitoring and frequent neurologic checks, in addition to intensive assessment and monitoring of vital signs, intake and output, and cardiorespiratory status. To promote patient comfort, maintain low lights and minimal noise and elevate the head of the bed. The patient usually won't receive an opioid analgesic because it may mask signs of increased ICP.

Prepare the patient for diagnostic tests. These may include blood, urine, and sputum cultures to identify bacteria; lumbar puncture to assess CSF and relieve pressure; and computed tomography scan, magnetic resonance imaging, cerebral angiography, and spinal X-rays to locate a hemorrhage.

PEDIATRIC POINTERS

Brudzinski's sign may not be useful as an indicator of meningeal irritation in infants because more reliable signs — such as bulging fontanels, a weak cry, fretfulness, vomiting, and poor feeding — appear early.

PATIENT COUNSELING

Explain all tests and procedures to the patient and his family. Teach the patient signs and symptoms of meningitis and recurrent bleeding. Instruct the patient to seek immediate medical attention if they develop.

BRUITS

Commonly an indicator of life- or limb-threatening vascular disease, bruits are swishing sounds caused by turbulent blood flow. They're characterized by location, duration, intensity, pitch, and time of onset in the cardiac cycle. Loud bruits produce intense vibration and a palpable thrill. A thrill, however, doesn't provide any further clue to the causative disorder or to its severity.

Bruits are most significant when heard over the abdominal aorta; the renal, carotid, femoral, popliteal, or subclavian artery; or the thyroid gland. (See *Preventing false bruits,* page 120.) They're also significant when heard consistently despite changes in patient position and when heard during diastole.

HISTORY

Obtain a medical history including past injuries, illnesses, surgeries, and family medical history. Ask about diet and alcohol intake. Take a drug history, including past and present prescriptions, over-the-counter drugs, and herbal remedies. Also obtain a social history.

PHYSICAL ASSESSMENT

If you detect bruits over the abdominal aorta, check for a pulsating mass or a bluish discoloration around the umbilicus (Cullen's sign). Either of these signs — or severe, tearing pain in the abdomen, flank, or lower back — may signal life-threatening dissection of an aortic aneurysm. Also, check peripheral pulses, comparing intensity in the upper versus lower extremities.

If you suspect dissection, monitor the patient's vital signs constantly, and withhold food and fluids until a definitive diagnosis is made. Watch for signs and symptoms of hypovolemic shock, such as thirst; hypotension; tachycardia; weak, thready pulse; tachypnea; altered level of consciousness (LOC); mottled knees and elbows; and cool, clammy skin.

If you detect bruits over the thyroid gland, ask the patient if he has a history of hyperthyroidism or signs and symptoms of it, such as nervousness, tremors, weight loss, palpitations, heat intolerance, and (in females) amenorrhea. Watch for signs and symptoms of life-threatening thyroid storm, such as tremor, restlessness, diarrhea, abdominal pain, and hepatomegaly.

If you detect carotid artery bruits, be alert for signs and symptoms of a transient ischemic attack (TIA), including dizziness, diplopia, slurred speech, flashing lights, and syncope. These findings may indicate an impending stroke. Be sure to evaluate the patient frequently for changes in LOC and muscle function.

If you detect bruits over the femoral, popliteal, or subclavian artery, watch for signs and symptoms of decreased or absent peripheral circulation — edema, weak-

---

Peds points

+ Bulging fontanels, a weak cry, fretfulness, vomiting, and poor feeding appear earlier in infants with meningeal irritation than Brudzinski's sign.

Teaching points

+ Tests and procedures
+ Signs and symptoms of meningitis and recurrent bleeding

Key facts about bruits

+ Swishing sounds caused by turbulent blood flow
+ Characterized by location, duration, intensity, pitch, and time of onset in the cardiac cycle
+ Indicate life- or limb-threatening vascular disease

Key history points

+ Medical history, including past injuries, illnesses, surgeries, and family medical history
+ Diet and alcohol intake
+ Drug history

Critical assessment steps

+ Perform cardiac assessment.

If bruits present over abdominal aorta

+ Check for a pulsating mass, Cullen's sign, or severe, tearing pain in the abdomen, flank, or lower back.
+ Check peripheral pulses, comparing intensity in the upper versus lower extremities.

If bruits present over thyroid gland

+ Ask patient about history of hyperthyroidism.
+ Watch for signs and symptoms of life-threatening thyroid storm.

Critical assessment steps
(continued)

If carotid artery bruits present
+ Be alert for signs and symptoms of a TIA.
+ Evaluate frequently for changes in LOC and muscle function.

If bruits present over femoral, popliteal, or subclavian artery
+ Watch for signs and symptoms of decreased or absent peripheral circulation.
+ Ask if patient has a history of intermittent claudication.
+ Frequently check distal pulses and skin color and temperature.
+ Watch for the sudden absence of pulse, pallor, or coolness.

Medical causes

Abdominal aortic aneurysm
+ A systolic bruit over the aorta accompanies a pulsating periumbilical mass.

Abdominal aortic atherosclerosis
+ Loud systolic bruits in the epigastric and midabdominal areas are common.

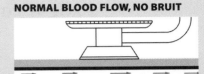

ASSESSMENT TIP

Preventing false bruits

Auscultating bruits accurately requires practice and skill. These sounds typically stem from arterial luminal narrowing or arterial dilation, but they can also result from excessive pressure applied to the stethoscope's bell during auscultation. This pressure compresses the artery, creating turbulent blood flow and a false bruit.

To prevent false bruits, place the bell lightly on the patient's skin. Also, if you're auscultating for a popliteal bruit, help the patient to a supine position, place your hand behind his ankle, and lift his leg slightly before placing the bell behind the knee.

NORMAL BLOOD FLOW, NO BRUIT

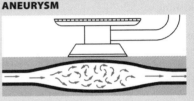

TURBULENT BLOOD FLOW AND RESULTANT BRUIT CAUSED BY ANEURYSM

TURBULENT BLOOD FLOW AND FALSE BRUIT CAUSED BY COMPRESSION OF ARTERY

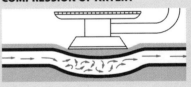

ness, and paresthesia. Ask the patient if he has a history of intermittent claudication. Frequently check distal pulses and skin color and temperature. Also, watch for the sudden absence of pulse, pallor, or coolness, which may indicate a threat to the affected limb.

If you detect a bruit, be sure to check for further vascular damage and perform a thorough cardiac assessment.

MEDICAL CAUSES

Abdominal aortic aneurysm
A pulsating periumbilical mass accompanied by a systolic bruit over the aorta characterizes an abdominal aortic aneurysm. Associated signs and symptoms include a rigid, tender abdomen; mottled skin; diminished peripheral pulses; and claudication. Sharp, tearing pain in the abdomen, flank, or lower back signals imminent dissection.

Abdominal aortic atherosclerosis
Loud systolic bruits in the epigastric and midabdominal areas are common in abdominal aortic atherosclerosis. They may be accompanied by leg weakness, numbness, paresthesia, or paralysis; leg pain; or decreased or absent femoral, popliteal, or pedal pulses. Abdominal pain is rarely present.

Carotid artery stenosis

Systolic bruits can be heard over one or both carotid arteries in a patient with carotid artery stenosis. Other signs and symptoms may be absent. However, dizziness, vertigo, headache, syncope, aphasia, dysarthria, sudden vision loss, hemiparesis, or hemiparalysis signals TIA and may herald a stroke.

Peripheral arteriovenous fistula

With a peripheral arteriovenous fistula, a rough, continuous bruit with systolic accentuation may be heard over the fistula; a palpable thrill is also common. Other signs and symptoms depend on the location of the fistula. For example, there may be claudication or absent pulses distal to the fistula. Skin distal to the fistula may be cool.

Peripheral vascular disease

Peripheral vascular disease characteristically produces bruits over the femoral artery and other arteries in the legs. It can also cause diminished or absent femoral, popliteal, or pedal pulses; intermittent claudication; numbness, weakness, pain, and cramping in the legs, feet, and hips; and cool, shiny skin and hair loss on the affected extremity. It also predisposes the patient to lower extremity ulcers that heal with difficulty.

Renal artery stenosis

With renal artery stenosis, systolic bruits are commonly heard over the abdominal midline and flank on the affected side. Hypertension commonly accompanies stenosis. Headache, palpitations, tachycardia, anxiety, dizziness, retinopathy, hematuria, and mental sluggishness may also appear.

Subclavian steal syndrome

With subclavian steal syndrome, systolic bruits may be heard over one or both subclavian arteries as a result of narrowing of the arterial lumen. They may be accompanied by decreased blood pressure and claudication in the affected arm, hemiparesis, vision disturbances, vertigo, and dysarthria.

Thyrotoxicosis

A systolic bruit heard over the thyroid gland commonly occurs with thyrotoxicosis. Accompanying signs and symptoms appear in all body systems, but the most characteristic ones include thyroid enlargement, fatigue, nervousness, tachycardia, heat intolerance, sweating, tremor, diarrhea, and weight loss despite increased appetite. Exophthalmos may also be present.

SPECIAL CONSIDERATIONS

Because bruits can signal a life-threatening vascular disorder, frequently check the patient's vital signs and auscultate over the affected arteries. Be especially alert for bruits that become louder or develop a diastolic component.

As needed, administer prescribed drugs, such as a vasodilator, an anticoagulant, an antiplatelet drug, or an antihypertensive. Prepare the patient for diagnostic tests, such as blood studies, radiographs, an electrocardiogram, cardiac catheterization, and ultrasonography.

PEDIATRIC POINTERS

Bruits are common in young children but are usually of little significance — for example, cranial bruits are normal until age 4. However, certain bruits may be significant. Because birthmarks commonly accompany congenital arteriovenous fistulas,

Medical causes
(continued)

Carotid artery stenosis
- Systolic bruits can be heard over one or both carotid arteries.
- Other signs and symptoms may be absent.

Peripheral arteriovenous fistula
- A rough, continuous bruit with systolic accentuation may be heard over the fistula.

Peripheral vascular disease
- Bruits may be heard over the femoral artery and other arteries in the legs.

Renal artery stenosis
- Systolic bruits are heard over abdominal midline and flank on affected side.

Subclavian steal syndrome
- Systolic bruits may be heard over subclavian artery.

Thyrotoxicosis
- Systolic bruit is heard over thyroid gland.

Special considerations
- Frequently check vital signs.
- Be alert for bruits that become louder or develop a diastolic component.

Peds points
- Bruits are usually of little significance.
- Auscultate for bruits in a child with port-wine spots or cavernous or diffuse hemangiomas.

Geri points

+ Elderly patients with atherosclerosis may experience bruits over several arteries.
+ Bruits related to carotid artery stenosis are associated with stroke; close follow-up is mandatory as well as prompt surgical referral when indicated.

Teaching points

+ Symptoms of stroke to report
+ Lifestyle modifications, such as smoking cessation, regular exercise, and diet

Key facts about butterfly rash

+ Signals SLE or dermatologic disorders
+ Appears in a malar distribution across the nose and cheeks

Key history points

+ Onset and extent of rash
+ Recent exposure to the sun
+ Recent weight or hair loss
+ Family history of lupus
+ Use of hydralazine or procainamide

Critical assessment steps

+ Inspect the rash, noting any macules, papules, pustules, scaling, hypopigmentation, or hyperpigmentation.
+ Look for blisters or ulcers in the mouth.
+ Note any inflamed lesions.
+ Check for rashes elsewhere on the body.

carefully auscultate for bruits in a child with port-wine spots or cavernous or diffuse hemangiomas.

GERIATRIC POINTERS

Elderly patients with atherosclerosis may experience bruits over several arteries. Those related to carotid artery stenosis are particularly important because of the high incidence of associated stroke. Close follow-up is mandatory as well as prompt surgical referral when indicated.

PATIENT COUNSELING

Instruct the patient to inform the physician if he develops dizziness, pain, or any symptom that suggests a stroke because this may indicate a worsening of his condition. For the patient with atherosclerosis or peripheral vascular disease, discuss lifestyle modifications, such as stopping smoking, exercising regularly (after consulting with the physician), and eating a healthy diet.

BUTTERFLY RASH

The presence of a butterfly rash is typically a sign of systemic lupus erythematosus (SLE), but it can also signal dermatologic disorders. Generally, butterfly rash appears in a malar distribution across the nose and cheeks. (See *Recognizing butterfly rash.*) Similar rashes may appear on the neck, scalp, and other areas. Butterfly rash is sometimes mistaken for sunburn because it can be provoked or aggravated by ultraviolet rays, but it has more substance, is more sharply demarcated, and has a thicker feel in relation to surrounding skin.

HISTORY

Ask the patient when he first noticed the butterfly rash and if he has recently been exposed to the sun. Has he noticed a rash elsewhere on his body? Also, ask about recent weight or hair loss. Does he have a family history of lupus? Is he taking hydralazine or procainamide (common causes of drug-induced lupus erythematosus)?

PHYSICAL ASSESSMENT

Inspect the rash, noting any macules, papules, pustules, or scaling. Is the rash edematous? Are areas of hypopigmentation or hyperpigmentation present? Look for blisters or ulcers in the mouth, and note any inflamed lesions. Check for rashes elsewhere on the body.

MEDICAL CAUSES

Discoid lupus erythematosus

With discoid lupus erythematosus, a localized form of lupus erythematosus, the patient may have a unilateral or butterfly rash that consists of erythematous, raised, sharply demarcated plaques with follicular plugging and central atrophy. The rash may also involve the scalp, ears, chest, or any part of the body exposed to the sun. Telangiectasia, scarring alopecia, and hypopigmentation or hyperpigmentation may occur later. Other accompanying signs include conjunctival redness, dilated capillaries of the nail fold, bilateral parotid gland enlargement, oral lesions, and mottled, reddish blue skin on the legs.

Recognizing butterfly rash

With classic butterfly rash, lesions appear on the cheeks and the bridge of the nose, creating a characteristic butterfly pattern. The rash may vary in severity from malar erythema to discoid lesions (plaques).

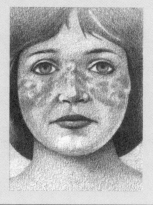

Erysipelas

Occurring primarily in infants and adults older than age 30 following a streptococcal infection, erysipelas causes rosy or crimson swollen lesions, mainly on the neck and head and commonly along the nasolabial fold. It may cause hemorrhagic pus-filled blisters. Other signs and symptoms include fever, chills, cervical lymphadenopathy, and malaise.

Rosacea

Initially, with rosacea, butterfly rash may appear as a prominent, nonscaling, intermittent erythema limited to the lower half of the nose or including the chin, cheeks, and central forehead. As rosacea develops, the duration of the rash increases; instead of disappearing after each episode, the rash varies in intensity and is commonly accompanied by telangiectasia. With advanced rosacea, the skin is oily, with papules, pustules, nodules, and telangiectasis restricted to the central oval of the face. In men with severe rosacea, butterfly rash may be accompanied by rhinophyma—a thickened, lobulated overgrowth of sebaceous glands and epithelial connective tissue on the lower half of the nose and, possibly, the adjacent cheeks. This is more common in elderly patients.

Seborrheic dermatitis

With seborrheic dermatitis, butterfly rash appears as greasy, scaling, slightly yellow macules and papules of varying size on the cheeks and the bridge of the nose, in a "butterfly" pattern. The scalp, beard, eyebrows, portions of the forehead above the bridge of the nose, nasolabial fold, or trunk may also be involved. Associated signs and symptoms include crusts and fissures (particularly when the external ear and scalp are involved), pruritus, redness, blepharitis, styes, severe acne, and oily skin. Severe seborrheic dermatitis of the face occurs in acquired immunodeficiency syndrome.

Systemic lupus erythematosus

Occurring in about 40% of patients with SLE (a connective tissue disorder), butterfly rash appears as a red, commonly scaly, sharply demarcated macular eruption. The rash may be transient in patients with acute SLE or may progress slowly to include the forehead, chin, the area around the ears, and other exposed areas. Com-

Medical causes

Discoid lupus erythematosus
✦ Unilateral or butterfly rash with erythematous, raised, sharply demarcated plaques, follicular plugging, and central atrophy develops.

Erysipelas
✦ Rosy or crimson swollen lesions develop on the neck and head and commonly along the nasolabial fold.
✦ Condition occurs primarily in infants and adults older than age 30.

Rosacea
✦ Rash may appear as a prominent, nonscaling, intermittent erythema limited to the lower half of the nose or including the chin, cheeks, and central forehead.

Seborrheic dermatitis
✦ Rash appears as greasy, scaling, slightly yellow macules and papules of varying size on the cheeks and the bridge of the nose.
✦ The scalp, beard, eyebrows, portions of the forehead above the bridge of the nose, nasolabial fold, or trunk may be involved.

SLE
✦ Rash appears as a red, scaly, sharply demarcated macular eruption.
✦ Rash may progress slowly to include the forehead, chin, the area around the ears, and other exposed areas.

Key facts about lupus

- ✦ Chronic inflammatory disorder of the connective tissues
- ✦ Discoid lupus erythematosus affects the skin; SLE affects skin and organ systems

Causes

- ✦ Physical or mental stress
- ✦ Streptococcal or viral infections
- ✦ Exposure to sunlight or UV light
- ✦ Immunization
- ✦ Pregnancy
- ✦ Abnormal estrogen metabolism
- ✦ Treatment with certain drugs

Management

- ✦ Nonsteroidal anti-inflammatory compounds, including aspirin
- ✦ Topical corticosteroids and systemic corticosteroids
- ✦ Intralesional corticosteroids or antimalarials
- ✦ High-dose steroids and cytotoxic therapy
- ✦ Dialysis or kidney transplant (for renal failure)
- ✦ Antihypertensive drugs

ASSOCIATED DISORDER

Lupus

Lupus erythematosus is a chronic inflammatory disorder of the connective tissues that appears in two forms. Discoid lupus erythematosus affects only the skin. Systemic lupus erythematosus (SLE) affects multiple organ systems as well as the skin and can be fatal. SLE is characterized by recurring remissions and exacerbations, which are especially common during the spring and summer.

The prognosis improves with early detection and treatment but remains poor for patients who develop cardiovascular, renal, or neurologic complications, or severe bacterial infections.

CAUSES

The exact cause of SLE remains a mystery, but evidence points to interrelated immunologic, environmental, hormonal, and genetic factors. These may include:
- ✦ physical or mental stress
- ✦ streptococcal or viral infections
- ✦ exposure to sunlight or ultraviolet light
- ✦ immunization
- ✦ pregnancy
- ✦ abnormal estrogen metabolism
- ✦ treatment with certain drugs, such as procainamide, hydralazine, anticonvulsants and, less commonly, penicillins, sulfa drugs, and hormonal contraceptives.

DIAGNOSIS

These test results may indicate SLE:
- ✦ Antinuclear antibody and lupus erythematosus cell tests are positive in active SLE.
- ✦ Hematology may show anemia, decreased platelet count, elevated erythrocyte sedimentation rate, and a decreased white blood cell count.
- ✦ Serum electrophoresis may show hypergammaglobulinemia.

- ✦ Anti-double-stranded deoxyribonucleic acid antibody, the most specific test for SLE, correlates with disease activity, especially renal involvement, and helps monitor response to therapy; it may be low or absent in remission.
- ✦ Serum complement blood studies show decreased serum complement (C3 and C4) levels, indicating active disease.

Other tests that may be done to detect organ involvement include chest X-ray, electrocardiography, and kidney biopsy.

MEDICAL INTERVENTIONS

Treatment for SLE may include:
- ✦ nonsteroidal anti-inflammatory compounds, including aspirin, to control arthritis symptoms
- ✦ topical corticosteroid creams such as hydrocortisone buteprate or triamcinolone for acute skin lesions
- ✦ intralesional corticosteroids or antimalarials such as hydroxychloroquine to treat refractory skin lesions
- ✦ systemic corticosteroids to reduce systemic symptoms of SLE, for acute generalized exacerbations, or for serious disease related to vital organ systems, such as pleuritis, pericarditis, lupus nephritis, vasculitis, and central nervous system involvement
- ✦ high-dose steroids and cytotoxic therapy (such as cyclophosphamide) to treat diffuse proliferative glomerulonephritis
- ✦ dialysis or kidney transplant for renal failure
- ✦ antihypertensive drugs and dietary changes to minimize effects of renal involvement
- ✦ referral to the Lupus Foundation of America and the Arthritis Foundation as necessary.

---

mon associated skin findings include scaling, patchy alopecia, mucous membrane lesions, mottled erythema of the palms and fingers, periungual erythema with edema, reddish purple macular lesions on the volar surfaces of the fingers, telangiectasia of the base of the nails or eyelids, purpura, petechiae, and ecchymoses.

Butterfly rash may also be accompanied by joint pain, stiffness, and deformities, particularly ulnar deviation of the fingers and subluxation of the proximal interphalangeal joints. Related findings include periorbital and facial edema, dyspnea, low-grade fever, malaise, weakness, fatigue, weight loss, anorexia, nausea, vomiting, lymphadenopathy, photosensitivity, and hepatosplenomegaly. (See *Associated disorder: Lupus.*)

OTHER CAUSES

Drugs
The drugs hydralazine and procainamide can cause a lupus-like syndrome, which is evidenced by the butterfly rash.

SPECIAL CONSIDERATIONS
Prepare the patient for immunologic studies, complete blood count and, possibly, liver studies. Obtain a urine specimen if needed. Withhold photosensitizing drugs, such as phenothiazines, sulfonamides, sulfonylureas, and thiazide diuretics.

PEDIATRIC POINTERS
Rare in pediatric patients, a butterfly rash may occur as part of an infectious disease such as erythema infectiosum, or "slapped cheek syndrome."

PATIENT COUNSELING
Instruct the patient to avoid exposure to the sun or to use a sunscreen. Suggest that he use hypoallergenic makeup to help conceal facial lesions. Provide the patient with contact information for the Lupus Foundation of America.

Other causes
+ Hydralazine
+ Procainamide

Special considerations
+ Prepare the patient for immunologic studies, CBC and, possibly, liver studies.
+ Obtain a urine specimen if needed.
+ Withhold photosensitizing drugs.

Peds points
+ Rarely, butterfly rash may occur as part of an infectious disease such as erythema infectiosum.

Teaching points
+ Use of sunscreen
+ Use of hypoallergenic makeup to conceal facial lesions
+ Sources of support such as Lupus Foundation of America

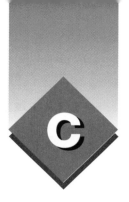

CAPILLARY REFILL TIME, INCREASED

Capillary refill time is the duration required for color to return to the nail bed of a finger or toe after application of slight pressure, which causes blanching. This duration reflects the quality of peripheral vasomotor function. Normal capillary refill time is less than 3 seconds.

Increased refill time isn't diagnostic of any disorder but must be evaluated along with other signs and symptoms. However, this sign usually signals obstructive peripheral arterial disease or decreased cardiac output.

HISTORY

Take a brief medical history, especially noting previous peripheral vascular disease. Find out which medications the patient is taking. Does the patient report pain or any unusual sensations in his fingers or toes, especially after exposure to cold?

PHYSICAL ASSESSMENT

Observe the patient's skin color and check for edema. Then complete the cardiovascular examination. If you detect increased capillary refill time, take the patient's vital signs and check pulses in the affected limb.

MEDICAL CAUSES

Aortic aneurysm (dissecting)

Capillary refill time is increased in the fingers and toes of a patient with a dissecting aneurysm in the thoracic aorta, and is prolonged in just the toes with a dissecting aneurysm in the abdominal aorta. Common accompanying signs and symptoms include a pulsating abdominal mass, systolic bruit, and substernal back or abdominal pain.

Aortic arch syndrome

Increased capillary refill time in the fingers occurs early in patients with aortic arch syndrome. The patient displays absent carotid pulses and possibly unequal radial pulses. Other signs and symptoms usually precede loss of pulses and include fever, night sweats, arthralgia, weight loss, anorexia, nausea, malaise, skin rash, splenomegaly, and pallor.

Arterial occlusion (acute)

With acute arterial occlusion, increased capillary refill time occurs early in the affected limb. Arterial pulses are usually absent distal to the obstruction; the affected limb appears cool and pale or cyanotic. Intermittent claudication, moderate to severe pain, numbness, and paresthesia or paralysis of the affected limb may occur.

Buerger's disease

Capillary refill time is increased in the toes in patients with Buerger's disease. Exposure to low temperatures turns the feet cold, cyanotic, and numb; later, they redden, become hot, and tingle. Other findings include intermittent claudication of the instep and weak peripheral pulses; in later stages the patient may experience ulceration, muscle atrophy, and gangrene. If the disease affects the hands, increased capillary refill time may accompany painful fingertip ulcerations.

 CULTURAL CUE *Be aware that the incidence of Buerger's disease is highest in men of Jewish ancestry who are between ages 20 and 30 and are heavy smokers.*

Hypothermia

Increased capillary refill time may appear early as a compensatory response to hypothermia. Associated signs and symptoms depend on the degree of hypothermia and may include shivering, fatigue, weakness, decreased level of consciousness (LOC), slurred speech, ataxia, muscle stiffness or rigidity, tachycardia or bradycardia, hyporeflexia or areflexia, diuresis, oliguria, bradypnea, decreased blood pressure, and cold, pale skin.

Raynaud's disease

Capillary refill time is prolonged in the fingers, the usual site of Raynaud's disease characteristic episodic arterial vasospasm. Exposure to cold or stress produces blanching in the fingers, then cyanosis, and then erythema before the fingers return to normal temperature. Warmth relieves the symptoms, which may include paresthesia. Chronic disease may produce trophic changes, such as sclerodactyly, ulcerations, or chronic paronychia.

OTHER CAUSES

Diagnostic tests

Cardiac catheterization can cause arterial hematoma or clot formation and increased capillary refill time.

Drugs

Drugs that cause vasoconstriction (particularly alpha-adrenergic blockers) increase capillary refill time.

Treatments

Increased capillary refill time can result from an arterial line or umbilical line (which can cause arterial hematoma and obstructed distal blood flow), or from an improperly fitting cast (which constricts circulation).

SPECIAL CONSIDERATIONS

Frequently assess the patient's vital signs, LOC, and affected extremity, and report any changes, such as progressive cyanosis or loss of an existing pulse. Prepare the patient for diagnostic tests, which may include arteriography or Doppler ultrasonography, to help confirm or rule out arterial occlusion.

PEDIATRIC POINTERS

Capillary refill time may be increased in neonates with acrocyanosis; however, this is a normal finding. Typically, increased capillary refill time is associated with the

Medical causes
(continued)

Aortic arch syndrome
- Increased capillary refill time in the fingers occurs early.

Arterial occlusion (acute)
- Increased capillary refill time occurs early in the affected limb.
- Arterial pulses are usually absent distal to the obstruction.

Buerger's disease
- Capillary refill time is increased in the toes.

Hypothermia
- Increased capillary refill time may appear early as a compensatory response.

Raynaud's disease
- Capillary refill time is prolonged in the fingers.

Other causes
- Arterial or umbilical lines
- Cardiac catheterization
- Drugs that cause vasoconstriction (particularly alpha-adrenergic blockers)
- Improperly fitting casts

Special considerations
- Frequently assess vital signs, LOC, and affected extremity; report any changes.

Peds points
- This sign is normal in neonates with acrocyanosis.
- Cardiac surgery is a common cause.

Teaching points
+ Signs and symptoms to report
+ Ways to modify risk factors
+ Ways to promote circulation

Key facts about carpopedal spasm
+ Violent, painful contraction of muscles in the hands and feet
+ Indicates tetany

In an emergency
+ Examine for signs of respiratory distress or cardiac arrhythmias.
+ Obtain blood samples for electrolyte analysis.
+ Perform an electrocardiogram.
+ Connect the patient to a monitor to watch for arrhythmias.
+ Administer an I.V. calcium preparation.
+ Provide emergency respiratory and cardiac support.
+ If the calcium infusion doesn't control seizures, give a sedative.

Key history points
+ Onset and duration of spasms
+ Extent of pain
+ Related signs and symptoms of hypocalcemia
+ Immunization history
+ History of neck surgery, calcium or magnesium deficiency, tetanus exposure, or hypoparathyroidism
+ Recent puncture wounds

Critical assessment steps
+ Take vital signs.
+ Check for Chvostek's sign.
+ Inspect the patient's skin and fingernails, noting any dryness or scaling or ridged, brittle nails caused by hypocalcemia.

same disorders in children as in adults. However, its most common pediatric cause is cardiac surgery such as the repair of congenital heart defects.

PATIENT COUNSELING

Teach the patient about his disease process and signs and symptoms to report. Help the patient develop a plan to modify risk factors, such as quitting smoking. Discuss measures to promote circulation, such as keeping extremities warm and avoiding cold environments.

CARPOPEDAL SPASM

Carpopedal spasm is the violent, painful contraction of the muscles in the hands and feet. (See *Recognizing carpopedal spasm.*) It's an important sign of tetany, a potentially life-threatening condition characterized by increased neuromuscular excitation and sustained muscle contraction and is commonly associated with hypocalcemia.

Carpopedal spasm requires prompt evaluation and intervention. If the primary event isn't treated promptly, the patient can also develop laryngospasm, seizures, cardiac arrhythmias, and cardiac and respiratory arrest.

 EMERGENCY ACTIONS If you detect carpopedal spasm, quickly examine the patient for signs of respiratory distress (laryngospasm, stridor, loud crowing noises, cyanosis) or cardiac arrhythmias, which indicate hypocalcemia. Obtain blood samples for electrolyte analysis (especially calcium), and perform an electrocardiogram. Connect the patient to a monitor to watch for the appearance of arrhythmias. Administer an I.V. calcium preparation, and provide emergency respiratory and cardiac support. If calcium infusion doesn't control seizures, administer a sedative, such as chloral hydrate or phenobarbital.

HISTORY

If the patient isn't in distress, obtain a detailed history. Ask about the onset and duration of the spasms and the degree of pain they produce. Also ask about related signs and symptoms of hypocalcemia, such as numbness and tingling of the fingertips and feet, other muscle cramps or spasms, and nausea, vomiting, and abdominal pain. Check for previous neck surgery, calcium or magnesium deficiency, tetanus exposure, and hypoparathyroidism. Ask the patient if he had recent puncture wounds, and inquire about his immunizations.

During the history, form a general impression of the patient's mental status and behavior. If possible, ask family members or friends if they have noticed changes in the patient's behavior. Mental confusion or even personality changes may occur with hypocalcemia.

PHYSICAL ASSESSMENT

Take the patient's vital signs. Hypocalcemia may result in hypotension and an irregular heart rhythm. Check for Chvostek's sign, also an indicator of hypocalcemia. Then proceed to perform a complete physical examination. Inspect the patient's skin and fingernails, noting any dryness or scaling or ridged, brittle nails caused by hypocalcemia.

Recognizing carpopedal spasm

In the hand, carpopedal spasm involves adduction of the thumb over the palm, followed by flexion of the metacarpophalangeal joints, extension of the interphalangeal joints (fingers together), adduction of the hyperextended fingers, and flexion of the wrist and elbow joints. Similar effects occur in the joints of the feet.

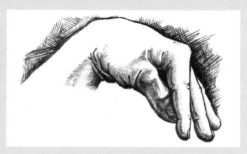

MEDICAL CAUSES

Hypocalcemia

Carpopedal spasm is an early sign of hypocalcemia. It's usually accompanied by paresthesia of the fingers, toes, and perioral area; muscle weakness, twitching, and cramping; hyperreflexia; chorea; fatigue; and palpitations. Positive Chvostek's and Trousseau's signs can be elicited. Laryngospasm, stridor, and seizures may appear in severe hypocalcemia.

Chronic hypocalcemia may be accompanied by mental status changes; cramps; dry, scaly skin; brittle nails; and thin, patchy hair and eyebrows.

Tetanus

With tetanus, an infectious disease caused by *Clostridium tetani,* the patient develops muscle spasms and painful seizures. Difficulty swallowing and a low-grade fever are also present. If the patient isn't treated or treatment is delayed, the mortality rate is very high.

OTHER CAUSES

Treatments

Multiple blood transfusions and parathyroidectomy may cause hypocalcemia, resulting in carpopedal spasm.

Surgical procedures

Surgical procedures that impair calcium absorption, such as ileostomy formation and gastric resection with gastrojejunostomy, may also cause hypocalcemia.

SPECIAL CONSIDERATIONS

Carpopedal spasm can cause severe pain and anxiety, leading to hyperventilation. If this occurs, help the patient slow his breathing through your relaxing touch, reassuring attitude, and clear directions about what he should do. Provide a quiet, dark environment to reduce his anxiety.

Prepare the patient for laboratory tests, such as complete blood count and serum calcium, phosphorus, and parathyroid hormone studies.

Medical causes

Hypocalcemia
+ Carpopedal spasm is an early sign.
+ Paresthesia of the fingers, toes, and perioral area; muscle weakness, twitching, and cramping; hyperreflexia; chorea; fatigue; and palpitations occur.

Tetanus
+ Muscle spasms and seizures develop.
+ Patient has difficulty swallowing and low-grade fever.

Other causes
+ Multiple blood transfusions
+ Parathyroidectomy
+ Surgical procedures that impair calcium absorption

Special considerations
+ If hyperventilation occurs, help the patient slow his breathing.
+ Provide a quiet, dark environment to reduce patient anxiety.

Peds points

+ Monitor children with hypocalcemia caused by idiopathic hypoparathyroidism; carpopedal spasm may herald the onset of epileptiform seizures or generalized tetany.

Geri points

+ Suspect tetanus in anyone with carpopedal spasm, difficulty swallowing, and seizures.
+ Ask elderly patients about their immunization record.

Teaching points

+ Immunization schedule

Key facts about asymmetrical chest expansion

+ Uneven extension of portions of the chest wall during inspiration
+ May develop suddenly or gradually and may affect one or both sides of the chest wall

In an emergency

+ Take the patient's vital signs.
+ Look for signs of acute respiratory distress.
+ Use tape or sandbags to temporarily splint the unstable flail segment.
+ Administer oxygen.
+ Insert an I.V. line to allow fluid replacement and administration of pain medication.
+ Draw a blood sample.
+ Connect the patient to a cardiac monitor.
+ Be alert for signs of respiratory distress.

PEDIATRIC POINTERS

Idiopathic hypoparathyroidism is a common cause of hypocalcemia in children. Carefully monitor children with this condition because carpopedal spasm may herald the onset of epileptiform seizures or generalized tetany followed by prolonged tonic spasms.

GERIATRIC POINTERS

Always ask elderly patients about their immunization record. Suspect tetanus in anyone who comes into your facility with carpopedal spasm, difficulty swallowing, and seizures. Such patients may have incomplete immunizations or may not have had a recent booster shot. Always ask about any recent wound, no matter how inconsequential it may seem.

PATIENT COUNSELING

Teach the patient the importance of receiving immunization against tetanus and of keeping a vaccination record. If you have any doubt about a patient's vaccination record, you must give him the vaccine. Tetanus toxoid booster shots must be given every 10 years after the patient has been properly immunized in childhood.

CHEST EXPANSION, ASYMMETRICAL

Asymmetrical chest expansion is the uneven extension of portions of the chest wall during inspiration. During normal respiration, the thorax uniformly expands upward and outward, then contracts downward and inward. When this process is disrupted, breathing becomes uncoordinated, resulting in asymmetrical chest expansion.

Asymmetrical chest expansion may develop suddenly or gradually and may affect one or both sides of the chest wall. It may occur as delayed expiration (chest lag), as abnormal movement during inspiration (for example, intercostal retractions, paradoxical movement, or chest-abdomen asynchrony), or as unilateral absence of movement. This sign usually results from pleural disorders, such as life-threatening hemothorax or tension pneumothorax. (See *Recognizing life-threatening causes of asymmetrical chest expansion,* page 132.) However, it can also result from a musculoskeletal or neurologic disorder, airway obstruction, or trauma. Regardless of its underlying cause, asymmetrical chest expansion produces rapid and shallow or deep respirations that increase the work of breathing.

EMERGENCY ACTIONS If you detect asymmetrical chest expansion, first consider traumatic injury to the patient's ribs or sternum, which can cause flail chest, a life-threatening emergency characterized by paradoxical chest movement. Quickly take the patient's vital signs and look for signs of acute respiratory distress — rapid and shallow respirations, tachycardia, and cyanosis. Use tape or sandbags to temporarily splint the unstable flail segment.

Depending on the severity of respiratory distress, administer oxygen by nasal cannula, mask, or mechanical ventilator. Insert an I.V. line to allow fluid replacement and administration of pain medication. Draw a blood sample from the patient for arterial blood gas analysis, and connect the patient to a cardiac monitor. Don't leave the patient unattended, and be alert for signs of respiratory distress.

HISTORY

If you don't suspect flail chest and if the patient isn't experiencing acute respiratory distress, obtain a brief history. Asymmetrical chest expansion commonly results from mechanical airflow obstruction, so find out if the patient is experiencing dyspnea or pain during breathing. If so, does he feel short of breath constantly or intermittently? Does the pain worsen his feeling of breathlessness? Does repositioning, coughing, or any other activity relieve or worsen the patient's dyspnea or pain? Is the pain more noticeable during inspiration or expiration? Can he inhale deeply?

Ask if the patient has a history of pulmonary or systemic illness, such as frequent upper respiratory tract infections, asthma, tuberculosis, pneumonia, or cancer. Has he had thoracic surgery? (This typically produces asymmetrical chest expansion on the affected side.) Also, ask about blunt or penetrating chest trauma, which may have caused pulmonary injury. Obtain an occupational history to find out if the patient may have inhaled toxic fumes or aspirated a toxic substance.

PHYSICAL ASSESSMENT

Begin a physical examination by gently palpating the trachea for midline positioning. (Deviation of the trachea usually indicates an acute problem requiring immediate intervention.) Then examine the posterior chest wall for areas of tenderness or deformity. To evaluate the extent of asymmetrical chest expansion, place your hands — fingers together and thumbs abducted toward the spine — flat on both sections of the lower posterior chest wall. Position your thumbs at the 10th rib, and grasp the lateral rib cage with your hands. As the patient inhales, note the uneven separation of your thumbs, and gauge the distance between them. Then repeat this technique on the upper posterior chest wall.

 CULTURAL CUE *Chest size varies with race, ultimately affecting respiratory function. Whites tend to have larger chests and lung capacities than Blacks, Asians, and Native Americans.*

Next, use the ulnar surface of your hand to palpate for vocal or tactile fremitus on both sides of the chest. To check for vocal fremitus, ask the patient to repeat "99" as you proceed. Note any asymmetrical vibrations and areas of enhanced, diminished, or absent fremitus. Then percuss and auscultate to detect air and fluid in the lungs and pleural spaces. Finally, auscultate all lung fields for normal and adventitious breath sounds. Examine the patient's anterior chest wall, using the same assessment techniques.

MEDICAL CAUSES

Bronchial obstruction

With bronchial obstruction, life-threatening loss of airway patency may occur gradually or suddenly. Typically, lack of chest movement indicates complete obstruction; chest lag signals partial obstruction. If air is trapped in the chest, you may detect intercostal bulging during expiration and hyperresonance on percussion. You may also note dyspnea, accessory muscle use, decreased or absent breath sounds, and suprasternal, substernal, or intercostal retractions.

Flail chest

With flail chest, a life-threatening injury to the ribs or sternum, the unstable portion of the chest wall collapses inward during inspiration and balloons outward during expiration (paradoxical movement). The patient may have ecchymoses, severe localized pain, or other signs of traumatic injury to the chest wall. He may also exhibit rapid, shallow respirations, tachycardia, and cyanosis.

Recognizing life-threatening causes of asymmetrical chest expansion

Asymmetrical chest expansion can result from several life-threatening disorders. Two common causes—bronchial obstruction and flail chest—produce distinctive chest wall movements that provide important clues about the underlying disorder.

With *bronchial obstruction*, only the unaffected portion of the chest wall expands during inspiration. Intercostal bulging during expiration may indicate that the air is trapped in the chest.

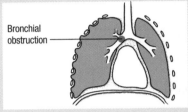

With *flail chest*—a disruption of the thorax due to multiple rib fractures—the unstable portion of the chest wall collapses inward at inspiration and balloons outward at expiration.

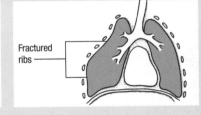

Medical causes
(continued)

Hemothorax
✦ Bleeding into the pleural space causes chest lag during inspiration.

Kyphoscoliosis
✦ Chest wall movement is decreased on the compressed-lung side.
✦ Intercostal muscles expand during inspiration on the opposite side.

Myasthenia gravis
✦ Progressive loss of ventilatory muscle function produces asynchrony of the chest and abdomen during inspiration.

Hemothorax
Hemothorax, life-threatening bleeding into the pleural space, causes chest lag during inspiration. Other findings include signs of traumatic chest injury, stabbing pain at the injury site, anxiety, dullness on percussion, tachypnea, tachycardia, and hypoxemia. If hypovolemia occurs, you'll note signs of shock, such as hypotension and rapid, weak pulse.

Kyphoscoliosis
Abnormal curvature of the thoracic spine in the anteroposterior direction (kyphosis) and the lateral direction (scoliosis) gradually compresses one lung and distends the other causing kyphoscoliosis. This produces decreased chest wall movement on the compressed-lung side and expands the intercostal muscles during inspiration on the opposite side. It can also produce ineffective coughing, dyspnea, back pain, and fatigue.

Myasthenia gravis
With myasthenia gravis, progressive loss of ventilatory muscle function produces asynchrony of the chest and abdomen during inspiration ("abdominal paradox"), which can lead to the onset of acute respiratory distress. Typically, the patient's shallow respirations and increased muscle weakness cause severe dyspnea, tachypnea, and possible apnea.

Phrenic nerve dysfunction

With phrenic nerve dysfunction, the paralyzed hemidiaphragm fails to contract downward, causing asynchrony of the thorax and upper abdomen on the affected side during inspiration ("abdominal paradox"). Its onset may be sudden, as in trauma, or gradual, as in infection or spinal cord disease. If the patient has underlying pulmonary dysfunction that contributes to hyperventilation, his inability to breathe deeply or to cough effectively may cause atelectasis of the affected lung.

Pleural effusion

Chest lag at end-inspiration occurs gradually in pleural effusion, a life-threatening accumulation of fluid, blood, or pus in the pleural space. Usually, some combination of dyspnea, tachypnea, and tachycardia precedes chest lag; the patient may also have pleuritic pain that worsens with coughing or deep breathing. The area of the effusion is delineated by dullness on percussion and by egophony, bronchophony, whispered pectoriloquy, decreased or absent breath sounds, and decreased tactile fremitus. Fever appears if infection causes the effusion.

Pneumonia

Depending on whether fluid consolidation in the lungs develops unilaterally or bilaterally with pneumonia, asymmetrical chest expansion occurs as inspiratory chest lag or as chest-abdomen asynchrony. The patient typically has fever, chills, tachycardia, tachypnea, and dyspnea along with crackles, rhonchi, and chest pain that worsens during deep breathing. He may also be fatigued and anorexic and have a productive cough with rust-colored sputum.

Pneumothorax

Pneumothorax, the entrapment of air in the pleural space, can cause chest lag at end-inspiration. This life-threatening condition also causes sudden, stabbing chest pain that may radiate to the arms, face, back, or abdomen and dyspnea unrelated to the chest pain's severity. Other findings include tachypnea, decreased tactile fremitus, tympany on percussion, decreased or absent breath sounds over the trapped air, tachycardia, restlessness, and anxiety.

With tension pneumothorax, the same signs and symptoms occur as in pneumothorax, but they're much more severe. A tension pneumothorax rapidly compresses the heart and great vessels, causing cyanosis, hypotension, tachycardia, restlessness, and anxiety. The patient may also develop subcutaneous crepitation of the upper trunk, neck, and face and mediastinal and tracheal deviation away from the affected side. You may auscultate a crunching sound over the precordium with each heartbeat; this indicates pneumomediastinum.

OTHER CAUSES

Treatments

Asymmetrical chest expansion can result from treatments such as pneumonectomy and the surgical removal of several ribs. Chest lag or the absence of chest movement may also result from intubation of a mainstem bronchus, a serious complication typically due to incorrect insertion of an endotracheal tube or movement of the tube while it's in the trachea.

SPECIAL CONSIDERATIONS

If you're caring for an intubated patient, regularly auscultate breath sounds in the lung peripheries to help detect a misplaced tube. If this occurs, prepare the patient for a chest X-ray to allow rapid repositioning of the tube. Because asymmetrical chest expansion increases the work of breathing, supplemental oxygen is usually

---

Medical causes
(continued)

Phrenic nerve dysfunction
- The paralyzed hemidiaphragm fails to contract downward.
- Asynchrony of thorax and upper abdomen during inspiration develops on the affected side.

Pleural effusion
- Chest lag at end-inspiration occurs gradually.
- A combination of dyspnea, tachypnea, and tachycardia precedes chest lag.

Pneumonia
- Asymmetrical chest expansion occurs as inspiratory chest lag or as chest-abdomen asynchrony.

Pneumothorax
- Chest lag at end-inspiration can occur.
- Patient has sudden, stabbing chest pain that may radiate to the arms, face, back, or abdomen.

Other causes
- Mainstem bronchi intubation
- Pneumonectomy
- Surgical removal of several ribs

Special considerations
If the patient is intubated:
- Auscultate breath sounds in the lung peripheries to help detect a misplaced tube.
- Be prepared to give supplemental oxygen during acute events.

If the patient has a chest tube:
- Maintain the water seal.
- Check the system for air leaks.
- Monitor drainage.

given during acute events. If the patient has a chest tube, maintain the water seal, check the system for air leaks, and monitor drainage.

PEDIATRIC POINTERS

Children have a greater risk than adults of mainstem bronchi (especially left bronchus) intubation. However, because a child's breath sounds are usually referred from one lung to the other because of the small size of the thoracic cage, use chest wall expansion as an indicator of correct tube position. Children also develop asymmetrical chest expansion, paradoxical breathing, and retractions with acute respiratory illnesses, such as bronchiolitis, asthma, and croup.

Congenital abnormalities, such as cerebral palsy and diaphragmatic hernia, can also cause asymmetrical chest expansion. With cerebral palsy, asymmetrical facial muscles usually accompany chest-abdomen asynchrony. With a life-threatening diaphragmatic hernia, asymmetrical expansion usually occurs on the left side of the chest.

GERIATRIC POINTERS

Asymmetrical chest expansion may be more difficult to determine in elderly patients because of the structural deformities associated with aging.

PATIENT COUNSELING

Teach the patient to recognize early signs and symptoms of respiratory distress. Encourage cough and deep-breathing exercises to promote oxygenation. In flail chest, show the patient how to splint his chest wall so he can perform breathing exercises more effectively. Explain all procedures to the patient and take measures to reduce anxiety.

CHEST PAIN

Chest pain usually results from disorders that affect thoracic or abdominal organs — the heart, pleurae, lungs, esophagus, rib cage, gallbladder, pancreas, or stomach. An important indicator of several acute and life-threatening cardiopulmonary and GI disorders, chest pain can also result from a musculoskeletal or hematologic disorder, anxiety, and drug therapy.

Chest pain can arise suddenly or gradually, and its cause may be difficult to ascertain initially. The pain can radiate to the arms, neck, jaw, or back. It can be steady or intermittent, mild or acute. It can range in character from a sharp shooting sensation to a feeling of heaviness, fullness, or even indigestion. It can be provoked or aggravated by stress, anxiety, exertion, deep breathing, or eating certain foods.

Ask the patient when his chest pain began. Did it develop suddenly or gradually? Is it more severe or frequent now than when it first started? Does anything relieve the pain? Does anything aggravate the pain? Ask the patient about associated symptoms. Sudden, severe chest pain requires prompt evaluation and treatment because it may herald a life-threatening disorder. See *Managing severe chest pain* and *Associated disorder: Myocardial infarction,* page 136.

HISTORY

If the chest pain isn't severe, proceed with the history. Ask if the patient feels diffuse pain or can point to the painful area. Sometimes a patient won't perceive the sensation he's feeling as pain, so ask whether he has any discomfort radiating to his neck,

---

EMERGENCY ACTIONS

Managing severe chest pain

If the patient reports a sudden onset of pleuritic chest pain, described as crushing, shooting, and deep, assess him for diaphoresis, dyspnea, hemoptysis, and tachycardia. If you detect these signs and symptoms, suspect *pulmonary embolism.*

If the patient tells you his pain started suddenly and describes it as tearing, ripping, or stabbing chest pain, question him about syncope and hemiplegia. Check for differences in blood pressure between legs and arms as well as weak or absent femoral or pedal pulses. Begin interventions for *aortic aneurysm* if you assess these signs.

If the patient reports the sudden onset of severe substernal pain that radiates to his left arm, jaw, neck, or shoulder blades that he describes as squeezing, viselike, or burning, have him lie down. Assess for pallor, diaphoresis, nausea, vomiting, apprehension, weakness, fatigue, and dyspnea. If you detect these signs and symptoms, suspect *myocardial infarction (MI).*

If you suspect any of these life-threatening disorders, quickly take the patient's vital signs. Obtain a 12-lead electrocardiogram. Insert an I.V. line to administer fluids and drugs, and give oxygen. Check the patient's vital signs frequently to detect changes from baseline. Begin cardiac monitoring to detect arrhythmias. As appropriate, prepare the patient for emergency surgery.

If the patient reports a sudden onset of chest tightness, assess for wheezing, dry cough, dyspnea, tachycardia, and hyperventilation. The presence of these signs and symptoms suggests an acute *asthmatic attack.* Try to calm the patient to slow his respiratory rate. Ask him if he's ever had this pain before and, if so, what eased it. Give oxygen and insert an I.V. line to administer fluids and drugs. Expect to give epinephrine and a bronchodilator and to begin respiratory therapy.

---

jaw, arms, or back. If he does, ask him to describe it. Is it a dull, aching, pressurelike sensation? A sharp, stabbing, knifelike pain? Does he feel it on the surface or deep inside? Find out whether it's constant or intermittent. If it's intermittent, how long does it last? Ask if movement, exertion, breathing, position changes, or eating certain foods worsens or helps relieve the pain. Does anything in particular seem to bring it on?

Review the patient's history for cardiac or pulmonary disease, chest trauma, intestinal disease, or sickle cell anemia. Find out which medications he's taking, if any, and ask about recent dosage or schedule changes.

PHYSICAL ASSESSMENT

Take the patient's vital signs, noting tachypnea, fever, tachycardia, oxygen saturation, paradoxical pulse, and hypertension or hypotension. Also, look for jugular vein distention and peripheral edema. Observe the patient's breathing pattern, and inspect his chest for asymmetrical expansion. Auscultate his lungs for pleural friction rub, crackles, rhonchi, wheezing, or diminished or absent breath sounds. Next, auscultate for murmurs, clicks, gallops, or pericardial friction rub. Palpate for lifts, heaves, thrills, gallops, tactile fremitus, and abdominal masses or tenderness.

MEDICAL CAUSES

Angina pectoris

With angina pectoris, the patient may experience a feeling of tightness or pressure in the chest that he describes as pain or a sensation of indigestion or expansion. The pain usually occurs in the retrosternal region. It may radiate to the neck, jaw,

Critical assessment steps

+ Take vital signs; note tachypnea, fever, tachycardia, oxygen saturation, paradoxical pulse, and hypertension or hypotension.
+ Look for jugular vein distention and peripheral edema.
+ Observe breathing pattern; inspect the chest for asymmetrical expansion.
+ Auscultate for pleural friction rub, crackles, rhonchi, wheezing, and diminished or absent breath sounds.
+ Auscultate for murmurs, clicks, gallops, and pericardial friction rub.
+ Palpate for lifts, heaves, thrills, gallops, tactile fremitus, and abdominal masses or tenderness.

Medical causes
Angina pectoris
+ Chest discomfort may be described as pain or a sensation of indigestion or expansion.
+ Pain usually occurs in the retrosternal region and typically lasts 2 to 10 minutes.
+ With Prinzmetal's angina, pain occurs at rest.

Key facts about MI
+ Results from reduced blood flow in coronary arteries
+ Causes myocardial ischemia and necrosis

Predisposing factors
+ Family history, gender, and age
+ Hypertension
+ Smoking, high intake of saturated fats, and sedentary lifestyle
+ Stress or type A personality
+ Drug use

Management
+ Morphine or meperidine for pain
+ Continuous cardiac monitoring
+ I.V. fibrinolytic therapy if indicated
+ PTCA
+ I.V. nitroglycerin for 24 to 48 hours
+ Early I.V. beta-adrenergic blocker followed by oral therapy
+ ACE inhibitors
+ Cardiac risk modificiation

ASSOCIATED DISORDER

Myocardial infarction

In myocardial infarction (MI), reduced blood flow through one or more coronary arteries results in myocardial ischemia and necrosis. In cardiovascular disease, death usually results from cardiac damage or complications caused by MI.

Each year, approximately 900,000 people in the United States experience MI. Mortality is high when treatment is delayed, and almost one-half of sudden deaths due to MI occur before hospitalization, within 1 hour of the onset of symptoms. The prognosis improves if vigorous treatment begins immediately.

CAUSES
Predisposing factors for MI include:
+ family history
+ gender (men and postmenopausal women)
+ hypertension
+ smoking
+ elevated serum triglyceride, total cholesterol, and low-density lipoprotein levels
+ excessive intake of saturated fats
+ sedentary lifestyle
+ aging
+ stress or type A personality
+ drug use, especially cocaine and amphetamines.

DIAGNOSIS
These tests help diagnose MI:
+ Serial 12-lead electrocardiography may reveal characteristic changes, such as serial ST-segment depression in non-Q-wave MI and ST-segment elevation in Q-wave MI.
+ Serial cardiac enzymes and proteins may show a characteristic rise and fall, specifically CK-MB, troponin T and I, and myoglobin.
+ Nuclear imaging scanning can identify areas of infarction and viable muscle cells.
+ Cardiac catheterization identifies the involved coronary arteries and reveals ventricular function and pressures and volumes within the heart.
+ Echocardiography may show ventricular wall motion abnormalities.

MEDICAL INTERVENTIONS
The guidelines established by the American College of Cardiology/American Heart Association Task Force on Practice Guidelines recommend these approaches for treating MI:
+ assessment of the patient in the emergency department within 10 minutes of symptom onset because 50% of deaths occur within 1 hour of symptom onset
+ oxygen by nasal cannula for 2 to 3 hours to increase oxygenation
+ nitroglycerin sublingually or I.V. to relieve chest pain, unless systolic blood pressure is less than 90 mm Hg or heart rate is less than 50 or greater than 100 beats/minute
+ morphine or meperidine to relieve pain
+ aspirin every day, indefinitely, to inhibit platelet aggregation
+ continuous cardiac monitoring to detect arrhythmias and ischemia
+ I.V fibrinolytic therapy if chest pain lasts at least 30 minutes and symptoms started within past 12 hours
+ I.V. heparin therapy following fibrinolytic therapy to promote coronary artery patency
+ percutaneous transluminal coronary angioplasty (PTCA) to revascularize narrowed or blocked coronary arteries
+ glycoprotein IIb and IIIa receptor-blocking agents to inhibit platelet aggregation (used as adjunct therapy with PTCA in acute ST-segment elevation MI and as primary therapy in non-ST-segment elevation MI)
+ limited physical activity for the first 12 hours to reduce cardiac workload
+ I.V. nitroglycerin for 24 to 48 hours to reduce afterload and preload and relieve chest pain, unless contraindicated
+ early I.V. beta-adrenergic blockers followed by oral therapy to reduce myocardial oxygen requirements, unless contraindicated
+ angiotensin-converting enzyme inhibitors to reduce afterload and preload and prevent remodeling, unless contraindicated
+ magnesium sulfate for 24 hours to correct hypomagnesemia, if needed
+ angiography and possible PTCA or surgical revascularization for the patient with spontaneous or provoked myocardial ischemia following acute MI

Myocardial infarction *(continued)*

◆ exercise testing before discharge to determine adequacy of medical therapy and provide an exercise prescription
◆ cardiac risk modification program of weight control; a low-fat, low-cholesterol diet; smoking cessation; and regular exercise
◆ lipid-lowering agents, as indicated by the fasting lipid profile.

In addition, be sure to keep these items available in case of an emergency:
◆ drugs to treat arrhythmias
◆ transcutaneous pacing patches or transvenous pacemaker
◆ defibrillator.

---

and arms—classically, to the inner aspect of the left arm. Angina tends to begin gradually, build to its maximum, then slowly subside. Provoked by exertion, emotional stress, or a heavy meal, the pain typically lasts 2 to 10 minutes (usually no longer than 20 minutes). Associated findings include dyspnea, nausea, vomiting, tachycardia, dizziness, diaphoresis, belching, and palpitations. You may hear an atrial gallop (a fourth heart sound [S_4]) or murmur during an anginal episode.

> **CULTURAL CUE** *Not all patients experience angina in the same way. For example, Black and Hispanic patients may not feel chest discomfort. Primary symptoms among these populations may include dyspnea and fatigue.*

With Prinzmetal's angina, caused by vasospasm of coronary vessels, chest pain typically occurs when the patient is at rest—or it may awaken him. It may be accompanied by shortness of breath, nausea, vomiting, dizziness, and palpitations. During an attack, you may hear an atrial gallop.

Anthrax (inhalation)

Inhalation anthrax is caused by inhalation of aerosolized spores of the gram-positive bacterium *Bacillus anthracis*. Initial signs and symptoms are flulike and include fever, chills, weakness, cough, and chest pain. The disease generally occurs in two stages with a period of recovery after the initial signs and symptoms. The second stage develops abruptly with rapid deterioration marked by fever, dyspnea, stridor, and hypotension, generally leading to death within 24 hours. Radiologic findings include mediastinitis and symmetric mediastinal widening.

Anxiety

Acute anxiety—or, more commonly, panic attacks—can produce intermittent, sharp, stabbing pain, commonly located behind the left breast. This pain isn't related to exertion and lasts only a few seconds, but the patient may experience a precordial ache or a sensation of heaviness that lasts for hours or days. Associated signs and symptoms include precordial tenderness, palpitations, fatigue, headache, insomnia, breathlessness, nausea, vomiting, diarrhea, and tremors. Panic attacks may be associated with agoraphobia—fear of leaving home or being in open places with other people.

Aortic aneurysm (dissecting)

The chest pain associated with dissecting aortic aneurysm (a life-threatening disorder) usually begins suddenly and is most severe at its onset. The patient describes an excruciating tearing, ripping, stabbing pain in his chest and neck that radiates to his upper back, abdomen, and lower back. He may also have abdominal tenderness; a palpable abdominal mass; tachycardia; murmurs; syncope; blindness; loss of consciousness; weakness or transient paralysis of the arms or legs; a systolic bruit; sys-

---

Medical causes
(continued)

Anthrax (inhalation)
◆ Initial signs include fever, chills, cough, and chest pain.

Anxiety
◆ Intermittent, sharp pain may occur behind the left breast.

Aortic aneurysm (dissecting)
◆ Stabbing chest and neck pain begin suddenly and radiate to the upper and lower back and abdomen.

Medical causes
(continued)

Asthma
✦ Diffuse and painful chest tightness, dry cough, and mild wheezing arise suddenly.

Bronchitis
✦ The acute form produces a burning chest pain or a sensation of substernal tightness that worsens with cough.

Cardiomyopathy
✦ Hypertrophic cardiomyopathy may cause angina-like chest pain, dyspnea, a cough, dizziness, syncope, gallops, murmurs, and bradycardia associated with tachycardia.

Cholecystitis
✦ Abrupt epigastric or right-upper-quadrant pain occurs.
✦ Pain may be sharp or intensely aching, steady or intermittent.
✦ Pain may radiate to the back or right shoulder.

Costochondritis
✦ Pain and tenderness occur at the costochondral junctions, especially at the second costicartilage.

Distention of colon's splenic flexure
✦ Central chest pain may radiate to the left arm.
✦ Pain may be relieved by defecation or passage of flatus.

Esophageal spasm
✦ Substernal chest pain mimics angina.
✦ Pain may last up to an hour and can radiate to the neck, jaw, arms, or back.

temic hypotension; asymmetrical brachial pulses; lower blood pressure in the legs than in the arms; and weak or absent femoral or pedal pulses. His skin is pale, cool, diaphoretic, and mottled below the waist. Capillary refill time is increased in the toes, and palpation reveals decreased pulsation in one or both carotid arteries.

Asthma
In a life-threatening asthma attack, diffuse and painful chest tightness arises suddenly along with a dry cough and mild wheezing, which progress to a productive cough, audible wheezing, and severe dyspnea. Related respiratory findings include rhonchi, crackles, prolonged expirations, intercostal and supraclavicular retractions on inspiration, accessory muscle use, flaring nostrils, and tachypnea. The patient may also experience anxiety, tachycardia, diaphoresis, flushing, and cyanosis.

Bronchitis
In its acute form, bronchitis produces a burning chest pain or a sensation of substernal tightness. It also produces a cough, initially dry but later productive, that worsens the chest pain. Other findings include a low-grade fever, chills, sore throat, tachycardia, muscle and back pain, rhonchi, crackles, and wheezing. Severe bronchitis causes a fever of 101° to 102° F (38.3° to 38.9° C) and possible bronchospasm with worsening wheezing and increased coughing.

Cardiomyopathy
With hypertrophic cardiomyopathy, angina-like chest pain may occur with dyspnea, a cough, dizziness, syncope, gallops, murmurs, and bradycardia associated with tachycardia. The patient may have a medium-pitched systolic ejection murmur along the left sternal border and apex of the heart. Palpation of peripheral pulses reveals a characteristic double impulse (pulsus biferiens and, with atrial fibrillation, an irregular pulse).

Cholecystitis
Cholecystitis typically produces abrupt epigastric or right-upper-quadrant pain, which may be sharp or intensely aching. Steady or intermittent pain may radiate to the back or the right shoulder. Common associated findings include nausea, vomiting, fever, diaphoresis, and chills. Palpation of the right upper quadrant may reveal an abdominal mass, rigidity, distention, or tenderness. Murphy's sign — inspiratory arrest elicited when the examiner palpates the right upper quadrant as the patient takes a deep breath — may also occur.

Costochondritis
With costochondritis, pain and tenderness occur at the costochondral junctions, especially at the second costicartilage. The pain usually can be elicited by palpating the inflamed joint. It may be described as a sharp pain in the chest wall that worsens with movement.

Distention of colon's splenic flexure
Central chest pain may radiate to the left arm in patients with distention of the colon's splenic flexure. The pain may be relieved by defecation or the passage of flatus. Other signs and symptoms include fever, tachycardia, abdominal pain, and palpable abdominal mass.

Esophageal spasm
With esophageal spasm, substernal chest pain may last up to an hour and can radiate to the neck, jaw, arms, or back. It tends to mimic angina — a squeezing or dull sensation. Associated signs and symptoms include dysphagia for solid foods, bradycardia, and nodal rhythm.

Herpes zoster (shingles)

The pain of preeruptive herpes zoster may mimic that of myocardial infarction (MI). Initially, the pain is characteristically sharp, shooting, and unilateral. About 4 to 5 days after its onset, small, red, nodular lesions erupt on the painful areas—usually the thorax, arms, and legs—and the chest pain becomes burning. Associated findings include fever, malaise, pruritus, and paresthesia or hyperesthesia of the affected areas.

Hiatal hernia

Typically, hiatal hernia produces an angina-like sternal burning (heartburn), ache, or pressure that may radiate to the left shoulder and arm. The discomfort commonly occurs after a meal when the patient bends over or lies down. Other findings include a bitter taste and pain while eating or drinking, especially hot drinks and spicy foods.

Interstitial lung disease

As interstitial lung disease advances, the patient may experience pleuritic chest pain along with progressive dyspnea, cellophane-type crackles, nonproductive cough, fatigue, weight loss, decreased exercise tolerance, clubbing, and cyanosis.

Legionnaires' disease

Legionnaires' disease produces pleuritic chest pain in addition to malaise, headache and, possibly, diarrhea, anorexia, diffuse myalgia, and general weakness. Within 12 to 24 hours, the patient develops a sudden high fever, chills, and a nonproductive cough that progresses to mucoid and then to mucopurulent sputum, possibly with hemoptysis. Patients may also experience flushed skin, mild diaphoresis, prostration, nausea and vomiting, mild temporary amnesia, confusion, dyspnea, crackles, tachypnea, and tachycardia.

Mediastinitis

Mediastinitis produces severe retrosternal chest pain that radiates to the epigastrium, back, or shoulder and may worsen with breathing, coughing, or sneezing. Its accompanying signs and symptoms include chills, fever, and dysphagia.

Mitral valve prolapse

Most patients with mitral valve prolapse are asymptomatic, but some may experience sharp, stabbing precordial chest pain or precordial ache. The pain can last for seconds or for hours, and occasionally mimics the pain of ischemic heart disease. The characteristic sign of mitral valve prolapse is a midsystolic click followed by a systolic murmur at the apex. The patient may experience cardiac awareness, migraine headache, dizziness, weakness, episodic severe fatigue, dyspnea, tachycardia, mood swings, and palpitations.

Muscle strain

Strained chest, arm, or shoulder muscles may cause a superficial and continuous ache or "pulling" sensation in the chest. Lifting, pulling, or pushing heavy objects may aggravate this discomfort. With acute muscle strain, the patient may experience fatigue, weakness, and rapid swelling of the affected area.

Myocardial infarction

The chest pain during an MI lasts from 15 minutes to hours. Typically a crushing substernal pain, unrelieved by rest or nitroglycerin, it may radiate to the patient's left arm, jaw, neck, or shoulder blades. Other findings include pallor, clammy skin, dyspnea, diaphoresis, nausea, vomiting, anxiety, restlessness, a feeling of impending doom, hypotension or hypertension, an atrial gallop, murmurs, and crackles.

Medical causes
(continued)

Herpes zoster (shingles)
- Initially, pain is sharp, shooting, and unilateral; it may mimic MI.
- About 4 to 5 days after onset, chest pain becomes burning.

Hiatal hernia
- Heartburn and sternal ache or pressure occur.
- Eating or drinking may cause pain.

Interstitial lung disease
- Pleuritic chest pain, progressive dyspnea, crackles, nonproductive cough, clubbing, and cyanosis occur.

Legionnaires' disease
- Pleuritic chest pain, malaise, and headache develop.

Mediastinitis
- Severe retrosternal chest pain radiates to the epigastrium, back, or shoulder.
- Pain may worsen with breathing, coughing, or sneezing.

Mitral valve prolapse
- Sharp, stabbing precordial chest pain or precordial ache may occur.
- A midsystolic click is followed by a systolic murmur at the apex.

Muscle strain
- A superficial and continuous ache or "pulling" sensation in the chest may result from strain.

Myocardial infarction
- Crushing substernal pain isn't relieved by nitroglycerin.
- Pain lasts 15 minutes to hours and may radiate.

Medical causes
(continued)

Pancreatitis
+ Acute form causes intense pain in the epigastric area.
+ Pain radiates to the back and worsens in a supine position.

Peptic ulcer
+ Sharp and burning pain arises in the epigastric region hours after food intake.
+ Pain is relieved by food or antacids.

Pericarditis
+ Sharp or cutting precordial or retrosternal pain is aggravated by deep breathing, coughing, and position changes.
+ Pain radiates to the shoulder and neck.

Plague
+ Signs and symptoms include productive cough, chest pain, tachypnea, dyspnea, hemoptysis, increasing respiratory distress, and cardiopulmonary insufficiency.

Pleurisy
+ Sharp, usually unilateral, pain in the lower aspects of the chest arises abruptly, reaching maximum intensity within a few hours.
+ Deep breathing, coughing, or thoracic movement aggravates pain.

Pneumonia
+ Pleuritic chest pain increases with deep inspiration.
+ Shaking chills and fever occur

Pneumothorax
+ Sudden, severe, sharp chest pain that's typically unilateral increases with chest movement.

Pancreatitis
In the acute form, pancreatitis usually causes intense pain in the epigastric area that radiates to the back and worsens when the patient is in a supine position. Nausea, vomiting, fever, abdominal tenderness and rigidity, diminished bowel sounds, and crackles at the lung bases may also occur. A patient with severe pancreatitis may be extremely restless and have mottled skin, tachycardia, and cold, sweaty extremities. Fulminant pancreatitis causes massive hemorrhage, resulting in shock and coma.

Peptic ulcer
With a peptic ulcer, sharp and burning pain usually arises in the epigastric region. This pain characteristically arises hours after food intake, commonly during the night. It lasts longer than angina-like pain and is relieved by food or an antacid. Other findings include nausea, vomiting (sometimes with blood), melena, and epigastric tenderness.

Pericarditis
Pericarditis produces precordial or retrosternal pain aggravated by deep breathing, coughing, position changes, and occasionally by swallowing. The pain is commonly sharp or cutting and radiates to the shoulder and neck. Associated signs and symptoms include pericardial friction rub, fever, tachycardia, and dyspnea. Pericarditis usually follows a viral illness, but several other causes should be considered.

Plague
The pneumonic form of plague, caused by the bacterium *Yersinia pestis,* is characterized by a sudden onset of chills, fever, headache, and myalgia. Pulmonary signs and symptoms include productive cough, chest pain, tachypnea, dyspnea, hemoptysis, increasing respiratory distress and cardiopulmonary insufficiency.

Pleurisy
The chest pain of pleurisy arises abruptly and reaches maximum intensity within a few hours. The pain is sharp, even knifelike, usually unilateral, and located in the lower and lateral aspects of the chest. Deep breathing, coughing, or thoracic movement characteristically aggravates it. Auscultation over the painful area may reveal decreased breath sounds, inspiratory crackles, and a pleural friction rub. Dyspnea, rapid, shallow breathing, cyanosis, fever, and fatigue may also occur.

Pneumonia
Pneumonia produces pleuritic chest pain that increases with deep inspiration and is accompanied by shaking chills and fever. The patient has a dry cough that later becomes productive. Other signs and symptoms include crackles, rhonchi, tachycardia, tachypnea, myalgia, fatigue, headache, dyspnea, abdominal pain, anorexia, cyanosis, decreased breath sounds, and diaphoresis.

Pneumothorax
Spontaneous pneumothorax, a life-threatening disorder, causes sudden sharp chest pain that's severe, typically unilateral, and rarely localized; it increases with chest movement. When the pain is centrally located and radiates to the neck, it may mimic that of an MI. After the pain's onset, dyspnea and cyanosis progressively worsen. Breath sounds are decreased or absent on the affected side with hyperresonance or tympany, subcutaneous crepitation, and decreased vocal fremitus. Asymmetrical chest expansion, accessory muscle use, a nonproductive cough, tachypnea, tachycardia, anxiety, and restlessness also occur.

Pulmonary embolism

Pulmonary embolism produces chest pain or a choking sensation. Typically, the patient first experiences sudden dyspnea with intense angina-like or pleuritic pain aggravated by deep breathing and thoracic movement. Other findings include tachycardia, tachypnea, cough (nonproductive or producing blood-tinged sputum), low-grade fever, restlessness, diaphoresis, crackles, pleural friction rub, diffuse wheezing, dullness to percussion, signs of circulatory collapse (weak, rapid pulse; hypotension), paradoxical pulse, signs of cerebral ischemia (transient unconsciousness, coma, seizures), signs of hypoxia (restlessness) and, particularly in the elderly, hemiplegia and other focal neurologic deficits. Less common signs include massive hemoptysis, chest splinting, and leg edema. A patient with a large embolus may have cyanosis and distended neck veins.

Pulmonary hypertension (primary)

Angina-like pain develops late in patients with primary pulmonary hypertension, usually on exertion. The precordial pain may radiate to the neck but doesn't characteristically radiate to the arms. Typical accompanying signs and symptoms include exertional dyspnea, fatigue, syncope, weakness, cough, and hemoptysis.

Q fever

Signs and symptoms of Q fever, a rickettsial disease caused by *Coxiella burnetti*, include fever, chills, severe headache, malaise, chest pain, nausea, vomiting, and diarrhea. The fever may last up to 2 weeks. In severe cases, the patient may develop hepatitis or pneumonia.

Rib fracture

The chest pain due to fractured ribs is usually sharp, severe, and aggravated by inspiration, coughing, or pressure on the affected area. Besides shallow, splinted respirations, dyspnea, and cough, the patient experiences tenderness and slight edema at the fracture site.

Sickle cell crisis

Chest pain associated with sickle cell crisis typically has a bizarre distribution. It may start as a vague pain, commonly located in the back, hands, or feet. As the pain worsens, it becomes generalized or localized to the abdomen or chest, causing severe pleuritic pain. The presence of chest pain and difficulty breathing requires prompt intervention. The patient may also have abdominal distention and rigidity, dyspnea, fever, and jaundice.

Tuberculosis

In a patient with tuberculosis, pleuritic chest pain and fine crackles occur after coughing. Associated signs and symptoms include night sweats, anorexia, weight loss, fever, malaise, dyspnea, easy fatigability, mild to severe productive cough, occasional hemoptysis, dullness to percussion, increased tactile fremitus, and amphoric breath sounds.

Tularemia

Following inhalation of the gram-negative, non-spore-forming bacterium *Francisella tularensis*, patients with tularemia show signs and symptoms that include the abrupt onset of fever, chills, headache, generalized myalgia, nonproductive cough, dyspnea, and empyema. Pneumonia can develop, causing chest pain and hemoptysis.

Medical causes
(continued)

Pulmonary embolism
+ Patient first experiences sudden dyspnea with intense angina-like or pleuritic pain aggravated by deep breathing and thoracic movement.

Pulmonary hypertension (primary)
+ Angina-like pain develops late.
+ Pain typically occurs on exertion.

Q fever
+ Fever, chills, severe headache, malaise, chest pain, nausea, vomiting, and diarrhea occur.

Rib fracture
+ Chest pain is usually sharp, severe, and aggravated by inspiration, coughing, or pressure on the affected area.

Sickle cell crisis
+ Pain may be vague at first and located in the back, hands, or feet.
+ As pain worsens, it becomes generalized or localized to the abdomen or chest, causing severe pleuritic pain.

Tuberculosis
+ Pleuritic chest pain and fine crackles occur after coughing.

Tularemia
+ Pneumonia can develop, causing chest pain and hemoptysis.

Other causes

+ Abrupt withdrawal from a beta-adrenergic blocker
+ Chinese restaurant syndrome

Special considerations

+ Prepare the patient for cardio-pulmonary studies.
+ Perform a venipuncture to collect a serum specimen for cardiac enzyme and other studies.

Peds points

+ A child may complain of chest pain in an attempt to get attention or to avoid attending school.

Geri points

+ Because older patients have a higher risk of developing life-threatening conditions, carefully evaluate chest pain.

Teaching points

+ Signs and symptoms that require prompt medical attention
+ Diagnostic tests
+ Prescribed drugs

Key facts about chills

+ Also known as *rigors*
+ Extreme, involuntary muscle contractions with characteristic paroxysms of violent shivering and teeth chattering
+ Signal onset of infection

OTHER CAUSES

Chinese restaurant syndrome

This benign condition—a reaction to excessive ingestion of monosodium glutamate, a common additive in Chinese foods—mimics the signs of an acute MI. The patient may complain of retrosternal burning, ache, or pressure; a burning sensation over his arms, legs, and face; a sensation of facial pressure; headache; shortness of breath; and tachycardia.

Drugs

Abrupt withdrawal of a beta-adrenergic blocker can cause rebound angina if the patient has coronary heart disease—especially if he has received high doses for a prolonged period.

SPECIAL CONSIDERATIONS

As needed, prepare the patient for cardiopulmonary studies, such as an electrocardiogram and a lung scan. Perform a venipuncture to collect a serum specimen for cardiac enzyme and other studies.

PEDIATRIC POINTERS

Even children old enough to talk may have difficulty describing chest pain, so be alert for nonverbal clues, such as restlessness, facial grimaces, or holding of the painful area. Ask the child to point to the painful area and then to where the pain goes (to find out if it's radiating). Determine the pain's severity by asking the parents if the pain interferes with the child's normal activities and behavior. Remember, a child may complain of chest pain in an attempt to get attention or to avoid attending school.

GERIATRIC POINTERS

Because older patients have a higher risk of developing life-threatening conditions (such as an MI, angina, and aortic dissection), you must carefully evaluate chest pain in these patients.

PATIENT COUNSELING

Teach patients with coronary artery disease about the typical features of cardiac ischemia as well as the symptoms that should prompt them to seek medical attention. If the pain fails to disappear after sublingual nitroglycerin, lasts more than 20 minutes, or has a different pattern from the usual angina, the patient must be evaluated immediately.

Explain the purpose and procedure of each diagnostic test to the patient to help alleviate his anxiety. Also explain the purpose of any prescribed drugs, and make sure that the patient understands the dosage, schedule, and possible adverse effects.

Keep in mind that a patient with chest pain may deny his discomfort, so stress the importance of reporting symptoms to allow adjustment of his treatment.

CHILLS

Also known as *rigors,* chills are extreme, involuntary muscle contractions with characteristic paroxysms of violent shivering and teeth chattering. Commonly accompanied by fever, chills tend to arise suddenly, usually heralding the onset of infection. Certain diseases, such as pneumococcal pneumonia, produce only a single, shaking chill. Other diseases, such as malaria, produce intermittent chills with recurring high fever. Still others produce continuous chills for up to 1 hour, precipitating a high fever. (See *Why chills accompany fever,* page 144.)

CULTURAL CUE *Malaria infects as many as 500 million people annually in Africa, India, Southeast Asia, the Middle East, Oceania, and Central and South America. If a patient exhibits chills, be sure to ask if he has recently traveled to a foreign country.*

Chills can also result from lymphomas, blood transfusion reactions, and certain drugs. Chills without fever occur as a normal response to exposure to cold.

HISTORY

Ask the patient when the chills began and whether they're continuous or intermittent. Because fever commonly accompanies or follows chills, take his rectal temperature to obtain a baseline reading. Then check his temperature often to monitor fluctuations and to determine his temperature curve. Typically, a localized infection produces a sudden onset of shaking chills, sweats, and high fever. A systemic infection produces intermittent chills with recurring episodes of high fever or continuous chills that may last up to 1 hour and precipitate a high fever.

Ask about related signs and symptoms, such as headache, dysuria, diarrhea, confusion, abdominal pain, cough, sore throat, or nausea. Does the patient have known allergies, an infection, or a recent history of an infectious disorder? Find out which medications he's taking and whether any drug has improved or worsened his symptoms. Has he received treatment that may predispose him to an infection (such as chemotherapy)? Ask about recent exposure to farm animals, guinea pigs, hamsters, dogs, and such birds as pigeons, parrots, and parakeets. Also ask about recent insect or animal bites, travel to foreign countries, and contact with persons who have an active infection.

PHYSICAL ASSESSMENT

Take the patient's other vital signs. Note and record the pattern of the patient's temperature changes. Check his pulse rate. Infection commonly increases the pulse rate, but some infections, notably, typhoid fever and psittacosis, may decrease it. Assess the skin, mucous membranes, liver, spleen, and lymph nodes. Check for drainage from skin lesions. Note skin color, temperature, and turgor. Percuss for costovertebral angle tenderness to determine if cystitis is present. In addition, assess level of consciousness (LOC).

MEDICAL CAUSES

Acquired immunodeficiency syndrome

With acquired immunodeficiency syndrome (AIDS), the patient usually develops lymphadenopathy. He may also experience fatigue, fever and chills, anorexia and weight loss, diarrhea, diaphoresis, skin disorders, and signs of upper respiratory tract infection.

Anthrax (inhalation)

Inhalation anthrax is caused by inhalation of aerosolized spores of the bacterium *Bacillus anthracis.* Initial signs and symptoms are flulike and include fever, chills, weakness, cough, and chest pain. The disease generally occurs in two stages with a period of recovery after the initial signs and symptoms. The second stage develops abruptly with rapid deterioration marked by fever, dyspnea, stridor, and hypotension generally leading to death within 24 hours. Radiologic findings include mediastinitis and symmetric mediastinal widening.

Key history points
+ Onset and duration of chills (continuous or intermittent)
+ Related signs and symptoms
+ History of allergies or infectious disorders
+ Drug history
+ Recent animal exposure, travel, or exposure to infection

Critical assessment steps
+ Take other vital signs.
+ Note and record the pattern of temperature changes.
+ Check pulse rate.
+ Assess the skin, mucous membranes, liver, spleen, and lymph nodes.
+ Check for drainage from skin lesions.
+ Note skin color, temperature, and turgor.
+ Percuss for costovertebral angle tenderness to determine if cystitis is present.
+ Assess LOC.

Medical causes

AIDS
+ The patient may experience fatigue, fever, chills, anorexia, weight loss, diarrhea, diaphoresis, skin disorders, and upper respiratory tract infection.

Anthrax (inhalation)
+ Initial signs and symptoms include fever, chills, weakness, cough, and chest pain.

Why chills accompany fever

Fever usually occurs when exogenous pyrogens activate endogenous pyrogens to reset the body's thermostat to a higher level. At this higher thermostatic set-point, the body feels cold and responds through several compensatory mechanisms, including rhythmic muscle contractions or chills. These muscle contractions in turn generate body heat and help produce fever. This flowchart outlines the events that link chills to fever.

Exogenous pyrogens (infectious organisms, immune complexes, toxins) enter the body.

↓

Phagocytic leukocytes release endogenous pyrogens.

↓

Endogenous pyrogens — possibly with prostaglandins — stimulate temperature-sensitive receptors in the hypothalamus and raise the thermostatic set-point to a higher level.

↓

Descending efferent pathways from the hypothalamus innervate effectors such as skeletal muscles and stimulate them to rhythmically contract.

↓

Rhythmic muscle contractions, or chills, generate body heat, which helps produce fever.

Medical causes
(continued)

Cholangitis
+ Signs and symptoms include Charcot's triad — chills with spiking fever, abdominal pain, and jaundice.

Gram-negative bacteremia
+ Infection causes sudden chills and fever, nausea, vomiting, diarrhea, and prostration.

Hemolytic anemia
+ Fulminating chills occur with fever and abdominal pain.

Hepatic abscess
+ Chills, fever, nausea, vomiting, diarrhea, anorexia, and severe upper abdominal tenderness and pain arise with the abscess.

Hodgkin's disease
+ Several days or weeks of fever and chills alternate with periods of no fever and no chills.

Cholangitis
Charcot's triad — chills with spiking fever, abdominal pain, and jaundice — characterizes cholangitis (the sudden obstruction of the common bile duct). The patient may have associated pruritus, weakness, and fatigue. Dark urine and light-colored stools may also be present.

Gram-negative bacteremia
This infection causes sudden chills and fever, nausea, vomiting, diarrhea, and prostration. The patient may also have tachypnea, hypotension, warm skin, decreased urine output, and an altered LOC.

Hemolytic anemia
With acute hemolytic anemia, fulminating chills occur with fever and abdominal pain. The patient rapidly develops jaundice and hepatomegaly; he may develop splenomegaly. Urine may be brown or red.

Hepatic abscess
Hepatic abscess usually arises abruptly, with chills, fever, nausea, vomiting, diarrhea, anorexia, and severe upper abdominal tenderness and pain that may radiate to the right shoulder. The patient may also report weight loss.

Hodgkin's disease
With Hodgkin's disease, the patient characteristically experiences several days or weeks of fever and chills alternating with periods of no fever and no chills. This disorder commonly produces regional lymphadenopathy that may progress to hepatosplenomegaly. Other findings include diaphoresis, fatigue, and pruritus.

Infective endocarditis

Infective endocarditis produces abrupt onset of intermittent, shaking chills with fever. Petechiae commonly develop. The patient may also have Janeway lesions on his hands and feet and Osler's nodes on his palms and soles. Associated findings include murmur, hematuria, eye hemorrhage, Roth's spots, and signs of cardiac failure (dyspnea, peripheral edema).

Influenza

Initially, influenza causes an abrupt onset of chills, high fever, malaise, headache, myalgia, and nonproductive cough. Some patients may also suddenly develop rhinitis, rhinorrhea, laryngitis, conjunctivitis, hoarseness, and sore throat. Chills generally subside after the first few days, but intermittent fever, weakness, and cough may persist for up to 1 week.

Legionnaires' disease

Within 12 to 48 hours after the onset of legionnaires' disease, the patient suddenly develops chills and a high fever. Prodromal signs and symptoms characteristically include malaise, headache and, possibly, diarrhea, anorexia, diffuse myalgia, and general weakness. An initially nonproductive cough progresses to a productive cough with mucoid or mucopurulent sputum and possibly hemoptysis. Most patients also develop nausea and vomiting, confusion, mild temporary amnesia, pleuritic chest pain, dyspnea, tachypnea, crackles, tachycardia, and flushed and mildly diaphoretic skin.

Lymphangitis

Acute lymphangitis produces chills and other systemic signs and symptoms, such as fever, malaise, and headache. Its characteristic signs are red streaks radiating from a wound and cellulitis draining toward tender, regional lymph nodes. The lymph nodes along the course of drainage may be enlarged, red, and tender.

Malaria

The paroxysmal cycle of malaria begins with a period of chills lasting 1 to 2 hours. This is followed by a high fever lasting 3 to 4 hours and then 2 to 4 hours of profuse diaphoresis. Paroxysms occur every 48 to 72 hours when caused by *Plasmodium malariae* and every 42 to 50 hours when caused by *P. vivax* or *P. ovale*. With benign malaria, the paroxysms may be interspersed with periods of well-being. The patient also has a headache, muscle pain and, possibly, hepatosplenomegaly.

Miliary tuberculosis

With the acute form of miliary tuberculosis, the patient suffers intermittent chills, high fever, and night sweats. Epididymal or testicular nodules and splenomegaly may also occur. Other signs and symptoms may include fatigue, malaise, joint pain, and swollen lymph nodes.

Otitis media

Acute suppurative otitis media produces chills with fever and severe deep, throbbing ear pain. The patient usually displays a mild conductive hearing loss and a bulging, hyperemic tympanic membrane. He may also have dizziness, nausea, and vomiting. When the tympanic membrane ruptures, pus drains externally through the ear canal and the patient feels relief.

Plague

Signs and symptoms of plague, a disease caused by the bacterium *Yersinia pestis*, include fever, chills, and swollen, inflamed, and tender lymph nodes near the site of the flea bite. Septicemic plague develops as a fulminant illness generally with the

Medical causes
(continued)

Infective endocarditis
- Intermittent, shaking chills with fever occur abruptly.

Influenza
- Onset of chills, high fever, malaise, headache, myalgia, and nonproductive cough is abrupt.

Legionnaires' disease
- Chills and high fever develop suddenly within 12 to 48 hours of disease onset.

Lymphangitis
- Chills and other systemic signs and symptoms, (such as fever, malaise, and headache) develop.

Malaria
- The paroxysmal cycle begins with a period of chills lasting 1 to 2 hours.
- Chills are followed by a high fever lasting 3 to 4 hours and then 2 to 4 hours of profuse diaphoresis.

Miliary tuberculosis
- The patient suffers intermittent chills, high fever, and night sweats.

Otitis media
- Acute suppurative otitis media produces chills with fever and severe deep, throbbing ear pain.

Plague
- Fever, chills, and swollen, inflamed, and tender lymph nodes near the site of the flea bite develop.

Medical causes
(continued)

Pneumonia
- A single shaking chill signals the sudden onset of pneumococcal pneumonia.
- Other types of pneumonia cause intermittent chills.

Pyelonephritis
- The patient develops chills, high fever and, possibly, nausea and vomiting over several hours to days.

Q fever
- Fever, chills, severe headache, malaise, chest pain, nausea, vomiting, and diarrhea develop.

Rocky Mountain spotted fever
- Onset of chills, fever, malaise, excruciating headache, and muscle, bone, and joint pain is sudden.

Septic shock
- Chills, fever and, possibly, nausea, vomiting, and diarrhea are produced initially.

Tularemia
- Onset of fever, chills, headache, generalized myalgia, nonproductive cough, dyspnea, pleuritic chest pain, and empyema is abrupt.

bubonic form. The pneumonic form may be contracted through direct person-to-person contact via the respiratory system or through biological warfare from aerosolization and inhalation of the organism. The onset is usually sudden with chills, fever, headache, and myalgia. Pulmonary signs and symptoms include productive cough, chest pain, tachypnea, dyspnea, hemoptysis, increasing respiratory distress, and cardiopulmonary insufficiency.

Pneumonia
A single shaking chill usually heralds the sudden onset of pneumococcal pneumonia; other pneumonias characteristically cause intermittent chills. With any type of pneumonia, related findings may include fever, productive cough with bloody sputum, pleuritic chest pain, dyspnea, tachypnea, and tachycardia. The patient may be cyanotic and diaphoretic, with bronchial breath sounds and crackles, rhonchi, increased tactile fremitus, and grunting respirations. He may also experience achiness, anorexia, fatigue, and headache.

Pyelonephritis
With acute pyelonephritis, the patient develops chills, high fever and, possibly, nausea and vomiting over several hours to days. He generally also has anorexia, fatigue, myalgia, flank pain, costovertebral angle tenderness, hematuria or cloudy urine, and urinary frequency, urgency, and burning.

Q fever
Signs and symptoms of Q fever, a rickettsial disease caused by the bacterium *Coxiella burnetii*, include fever, chills, severe headache, malaise, chest pain, nausea, vomiting, and diarrhea. The fever may last up to 2 weeks. In severe cases, the patient may develop hepatitis or pneumonia.

Rocky Mountain spotted fever
Rocky Mountain spotted fever begins with a sudden onset of chills, fever, malaise, excruciating headache, and muscle, bone, and joint pain. Typically, the patient's tongue is covered with a thick white coating that gradually turns brown. After 2 to 6 days of fever and occasional chills, a macular or maculopapular rash appears on the hands and feet and then becomes generalized; after a few days, the rash becomes petechial.

Septic shock
Initially, septic shock produces chills, fever and, possibly, nausea, vomiting, and diarrhea. The patient's skin is typically flushed, warm, and dry; his blood pressure is normal or slightly low; and he has tachycardia and tachypnea. As septic shock progresses, the patient's arms and legs become cool and cyanotic, and he develops oliguria, thirst, anxiety, restlessness, confusion, and hypotension. Later, his skin becomes cold and clammy; his pulse, rapid and thready. He further develops severe hypotension, persistent oliguria or anuria, signs of respiratory failure, and coma.

Tularemia
Signs and symptoms following inhalation of the gram-negative non-spore-forming bacterium *Francisella tularensis* include the abrupt onset of fever, chills, headache, generalized myalgia, nonproductive cough, dyspnea, pleuritic chest pain, and empyema. Other signs and symptoms of tularemia include a red spot on the skin that ultimately enlarges to an ulcer, enlarged lymph nodes, conjunctivitis, diaphoresis, and joint stiffness.

OTHER CAUSES

Drugs

Amphotericin B is a drug associated with chills. Phenytoin is also a common cause of drug-induced fever that can produce chills. I.V. bleomycin and intermittent administration of an oral antipyretic can also cause chills.

I.V. therapy

Infection at the I.V. insertion site (superficial phlebitis) can cause chills, high fever, and local redness, warmth, induration, and tenderness.

Transfusion reaction

A hemolytic reaction may cause chills during the transfusion or immediately afterward. A nonhemolytic febrile reaction may also cause chills.

SPECIAL CONSIDERATIONS

Check the patient's vital signs often, especially if his chills result from a known or suspected infection. Be alert for such signs of progressive septic shock as hypotension, tachycardia, and tachypnea. If appropriate, obtain samples of blood, sputum, or wound drainage for culture to determine the causative organism. Give the appropriate antibiotic. Radiographic studies and serum samples and urine specimens may be required.

Because chills are an involuntary response to an increased body temperature set by the hypothalamic thermostat, blankets won't stop a patient's chills or shivering. Despite this, keep his room temperature as even as possible. Provide adequate hydration and nutrients, and give an antipyretic to help control fever. Irregular use of an antipyretic can trigger compensatory chills.

PEDIATRIC POINTERS

Infants don't get chills because they have poorly developed shivering mechanisms. In addition, most classic febrile childhood infections, such as measles and mumps, don't typically produce chills. However, older children and teenagers may have chills with mycoplasma pneumonia and acute pyogenic osteomyelitis.

GERIATRIC POINTERS

Chills in an elderly patient usually indicate an underlying infection, such as a urinary tract infection, pneumonia (commonly associated with aspiration of gastric contents), diverticulitis, or skin breakdown in pressure areas. Also, consider an ischemic bowel in an elderly patient who comes into your facility with fever, chills, and abdominal pain.

PATIENT COUNSELING

Advise the patient to measure his temperature with a thermometer when he experiences chills and to document the exact readings and times. This will help reveal patterns that may point to a specific diagnosis. Make sure he understands how to follow his treatment regimen, including taking the full course of antibiotics. Explain signs and symptoms that signal worsening of his condition as well as when to seek medical attention.

Other causes
+ Amphotericin B, I.V. bleomycin, oral antipyretics, phenytoin
+ Infection at the I.V. insertion site
+ Transfusion reaction

Special considerations
+ Check vital signs often.
+ Be alert for signs of progressive septic shock.
+ If appropriate, obtain samples of blood, sputum, or wound drainage for culture to determine the causative organism.
+ Give the appropriate antibiotic.
+ Keep room temperature even.
+ Provide adequate hydration and nutrients.
+ Give an antipyretic.

Peds points
+ Infants don't get chills because they have poorly developed shivering mechanisms.
+ Older children and teenagers may have chills with mycoplasma pneumonia and acute pyogenic osteomyelitis.

Geri points
+ Chills in an elderly patient usually indicate an underlying infection.
+ Consider an ischemic bowel in an elderly patient who comes into your facility with fever, chills, and abdominal pain.

Teaching points
+ Documentation of temperature
+ Treatment regimen and antibiotics
+ Signs and symptoms of worsening condition and when to seek medical attention

Key facts about chorea

✦ Brief, unpredictable bursts of rapid, jerky motion that interrupt normal coordinated movement
✦ Indicates dysfunction of the extrapyramidal system
✦ Usually involves the face, head, lower arms, and hands

Key history points

✦ Onset and description of movements
✦ Family history of choreiform movements or Huntington's disease
✦ Drug history
✦ Occupational history

Critical assessment steps

✦ Ask the patient to stick out his tongue and keep it out. Typically, he'll be unable to do this; instead, his tongue will dart in and out of his mouth.
✦ Observe arms and legs separately for involuntary jerky movements.

Medical causes

Carbon monoxide poisoning
✦ Patient may experience chorea, rigidity, dementia, impaired sensory function, masklike facies, generalized seizures, and myoclonus.

Cerebral infarction
✦ If thalamic area is involved, unilateral or bilateral chorea occurs.

Encephalitis
✦ Chorea may occur in the recovery phase with low-grade fever, athetosis, hemiparesis, hemiplegia, and facial droop.

CHOREA

Chorea—brief, unpredictable bursts of rapid, jerky motion that interrupt normal coordinated movement—indicates dysfunction of the extrapyramidal system. Unlike tics, choreiform movements are seldom repetitive but tend to appear purposeful despite their involuntary nature. Although any muscle can be affected, chorea usually involves the face, head, lower arms, and hands. It can affect both sides of the body or only one side; however, when it affects the face, both sides are usually involved. Chorea may be aggravated by excitement or fatigue and may disappear during sleep. In some patients, it may be difficult to distinguish chorea from athetosis (snakelike, writhing movements), although choreiform movements are generally more rapid than athetoid ones. (See *Distinguishing athetosis from chorea*.)

HISTORY

Ask the patient and his family when they first noticed the choreiform movements. Do the movements disappear when the patient is asleep? Find out if anyone in the patient's family exhibits the same type of movements, and ask about a family history of such diseases as Huntington's disease. Also ask which medications the patient is taking. Obtain an occupational history, noting especially prolonged exposure to manganese or other metals. As you obtain history information, observe the patient for excessive restlessness and periodic facial grimaces that may interrupt his speech.

PHYSICAL ASSESSMENT

Perform a physical examination to evaluate the severity of the patient's chorea. Ask him to stick out his tongue and keep it out. Typically, he'll be unable to do this; instead, his tongue will dart in and out of his mouth. Observe the patient's arms and legs separately for involuntary jerky movements. Ask him to extend and flex his hand as if halting traffic, and note the choreiform movements—they'll be extremely evident in this position. Also, check for such related signs as athetosis, rigidity, or tremor.

To assess the patient for choreoathetotic gait, ask him to walk. He may change the positions of his trunk and upper body parts with each step and jerk and tilt his head to one side. Because of superimposed involuntary movements and postures, the patient's legs may move slowly and awkwardly. (An involuntary movement suspending his leg momentarily with each step may give a dancing quality to his gait.)

MEDICAL CAUSES

Carbon monoxide poisoning

A patient who survives severe carbon monoxide poisoning may have neurologic signs and symptoms, such as chorea, rigidity, dementia, impaired sensory function, masklike facies, generalized seizures, and myoclonus.

Cerebral infarction

A cerebral infarction that involves the thalamic area produces unilateral or bilateral chorea. The patient may also experience dysarthria, tremors, rigidity, weakness, and sensory disturbances such as paresthesia.

Encephalitis

Chorea may occur in the recovery phase of encephalitis. Low-grade fever and athetosis may also be present, in addition to such focal neurologic signs as hemiparesis, hemiplegia, and facial droop. Other signs and symptoms include headache, vomiting, photophobia, stiff neck, confusion, and drowsiness.

Distinguishing athetosis from chorea

In *athetosis*, movements are typically slow, twisting, and writhing. They're associated with spasticity and most commonly involve the face, neck, and distal extremities.

In *chorea*, movements are brief, rapid, jerky, and unpredictable. They can occur at rest or during normal movement. Typically, they involve the hands, lower arm, face, and head.

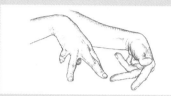
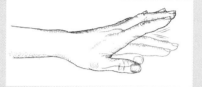

Huntington's disease
In Huntington's disease, an inherited disease, chorea may be the first sign or may occur with the intellectual decline that leads to emotional disturbances and dementia. The patient's movements tend to be choreoathetotic and may be accompanied by dysarthria, dystonia, prancing gait, dysphagia, and facial grimacing.

Lead poisoning
In the later stages of lead poisoning, chorea occurs in addition to seizures, headache, memory lapses, and severe mental impairment. The patient may also develop masklike facies, footdrop, wristdrop, dizziness, ataxia, weakness, lethargy, abdominal pain, anorexia, nausea, vomiting, constipation, lead line on his gums, and a metallic taste in his mouth.

Manganese poisoning
In miners who have been exposed to manganese dioxide for prolonged periods, chorea characteristically occurs with propulsive gait, dystonia, and rigidity. Initially, the patient may have masklike facies, a resting tremor, and personality changes; later, extreme muscle weakness and lethargy occur.

OTHER CAUSES

Drugs
Such drugs as phenothiazines (especially the piperazine derivatives), haloperidol, thiothixene, and loxapine commonly produce chorea. Metoclopramide, metyrosine, hormonal contraceptives, levodopa, and phenytoin may also cause this sign.

SPECIAL CONSIDERATIONS
Because the patient's movements are involuntary and increase his risk of severe injury, pad the side rails of his bed and keep sharp objects out of his environment. Help him minimize physical activity and emotional upset, to avoid aggravating the chorea and ensure adequate periods of rest and sleep.

PEDIATRIC POINTERS
Sydenham's chorea occurs in childhood as a delayed manifestation of rheumatic fever. Chorea can also occur in children with athetoid cerebral palsy.

Medical causes
(continued)

Huntington's disease
- Chorea may be the first sign or may occur with intellectual decline.

Lead poisoning
- Chorea, seizures, headache, memory lapses, and severe mental impairment occur in later stages.

Manganese poisoning
- Chorea occurs with propulsive gait, dystonia, and rigidity.

Other causes
- Haloperidol
- Hormonal contraceptives
- Levodopa
- Loxapine
- Metoclopramide
- Metyrosine
- Phenothiazines
- Phenytoin
- Thiothixene

Special considerations
- Pad the side rails of the bed and keep sharp objects out of the patient's environment.
- Help minimize physical activity and emotional upset.

Peds points
- Sydenham's chorea occurs in childhood as a delayed manifestation of rheumatic fever.
- Chorea can occur in children with athetoid cerebral palsy.

Teaching points

+ Safety measures
+ Genetic counseling (for those with Huntington's disease)

Key facts about Chvostek's sign

+ Indicated by an abnormal spasm of the facial muscles
+ Suggests hypocalcemia
+ Occurs normally in about 25% of patients

In an emergency

+ Test for Trousseau's sign.
+ Monitor for signs of tetany.
+ Act rapidly if a seizure occurs.
+ Perform an ECG to check for changes associated with hypocalcemia, which can predispose the patient to arrhythmias.
+ Place the patient on a cardiac monitor.

Key history points

+ Previous surgical removal of parathyroid glands
+ History of hypoparathyroidism, hypomagnesemia, or malabsorption disorder
+ Mental changes
+ Associated symptoms, including tingling sensations

Critical assessment steps

+ Observe the patient's behavior.
+ Observe for seizures, tetany, and facial spasms.
+ Observe skin for dryness or scaling, brittle nails, and dry hair.
+ Take vital signs.
+ Auscultate the lungs.

PATIENT COUNSELING

Teach the patient and his family safety measures to reduce the risk of falls and poisoning. Discuss genetic counseling if Huntington's disease is the cause of the patient's chorea because each child of a parent with the disease has a 50% chance of inheriting it.

CHVOSTEK'S SIGN

Chvostek's sign is an abnormal spasm of the facial muscles that's elicited by lightly tapping the patient's facial nerve near his lower jaw. (See *Eliciting Chvostek's sign.*) This sign usually suggests hypocalcemia but can occur normally in about 25% of patients. Typically, it precedes other signs of hypocalcemia and persists until the onset of tetany. It can't be elicited during tetany because of strong muscle contractions.

Usually, eliciting Chvostek's sign is attempted only in patients with suspected hypocalcemic disorders. However, because the parathyroid gland regulates calcium balance, Chvostek's sign may also be tested in patients before neck surgery to obtain a baseline.

 EMERGENCY ACTIONS Test for Trousseau's sign, a reliable indicator of hypocalcemia. Closely monitor the patient for signs of tetany, such as carpopedal spasms or circumoral and extremity paresthesia.

Be prepared to act rapidly if a seizure occurs. Perform an electrocardiogram to check for changes associated with hypocalcemia, which can predispose the patient to arrhythmias. Place the patient on a cardiac monitor.

HISTORY

Obtain a brief history. Find out if the patient has had the parathyroid glands surgically removed or if he has a history of hypoparathyroidism, hypomagnesemia, or malabsorption disorder. Ask him or his family if they have noticed any mental changes, such as depression or slowed responses, which can accompany chronic hypocalcemia. Question the patient about tingling around the mouth and in the fingertips and feet.

PHYSICAL ASSESSMENT

During your assessment, observe the patient's behavior. Anxiety and irritability may signal hypocalcemia. Also observe him for seizures, tetany, and facial spasms. Observe his skin for dryness or scaling, brittle nails, and dry hair. Take your patient's vital signs. Be alert for an irregular pulse and hypotension, which suggests low calcium levels. Auscultate the patient's lungs. Note any signs of bronchospasm, laryngospasm, and airway obstruction. Increased GI motility produces hyperactive bowel sounds.

MEDICAL CAUSES

Hypocalcemia

Chvostek's sign may indicate hypocalcemia. The degree of muscle spasm elicited reflects the patient's serum calcium level. Initially, hypocalcemia produces paresthesia in the fingers, toes, and circumoral area that progresses to muscle tension and carpopedal spasms. The patient may also complain of muscle weakness, fatigue, and palpitations. Muscle twitching, hyperactive deep tendon reflexes, choreiform move-

Eliciting Chvostek's sign

Begin by telling the patient to relax his facial muscles. Then stand directly in front of him, and tap the facial nerve either just anterior to the ear-lobe and below the zygomatic arch or between the zygomatic arch and the corner of his mouth. A positive response varies from twitching of the lip at the corner of the mouth to spasm of all facial muscles, depending on the severity of hypocalcemia.

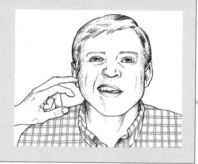

ments, and muscle cramps may also occur. The patient with chronic hypocalcemia may have mental status changes; diplopia; difficulty swallowing; abdominal cramps; dry, scaly skin; brittle nails; and thin, patchy scalp and eyebrow hair.

OTHER CAUSES

Treatments
A massive blood transfusion can lower serum calcium levels and allow Chvostek's sign to be elicited.

SPECIAL CONSIDERATIONS

Collect blood samples for serial calcium studies to evaluate the severity of hypocalcemia and the effectiveness of therapy. Such therapy involves oral or I.V. calcium supplements. Also, look for Chvostek's sign when evaluating a patient postoperatively.

PEDIATRIC POINTERS

Because Chvostek's sign may be observed in healthy infants, it isn't elicited to detect neonatal tetany.

GERIATRIC POINTERS

Always consider malabsorption and poor nutritional status in the elderly patient with Chvostek's sign and hypocalcemia.

PATIENT COUNSELING

Inform patients who will be undergoing thyroidectomy or parathyroidectomy about the early signs and symptoms of hypocalcemia, such as numbness, tingling, and muscle cramps, and tell them to seek immediate medical attention if these occur.

Medical causes
Hypocalcemia
+ The degree of muscle spasm elicited reflects the patient's serum calcium level.
+ Muscle weakness, fatigue, and palpitations may be present.

Other causes
+ Massive blood transfusion

Special considerations
+ Collect blood samples for serial calcium studies.
+ Look for Chvostek's sign postoperatively.

Peds points
+ This sign may be observed in healthy infants, so it isn't used to detect neonatal tetany.

Geri points
+ Always consider malabsorption and poor nutritional status in the elderly patient with Chvostek's sign and hypocalcemia.

Teaching points
+ Early signs and symptoms of hypocalcemia to report

CONFUSION

An umbrella term for puzzling or inappropriate behavior or responses, *confusion* is the inability to think quickly and coherently. Depending on its cause, confusion may arise suddenly or gradually and may be temporary or irreversible. Aggravated by stress and sensory deprivation, confusion commonly occurs in hospitalized patients — especially in elderly patients, in whom it may be mistaken for senility.

When severe confusion arises suddenly and the patient also has hallucinations and psychomotor hyperactivity, his condition is classified as delirium. Long-term, progressive confusion with deterioration of all cognitive functions is classified as dementia.

Confusion can result from fluid and electrolyte imbalance or hypoxemia due to pulmonary disorders. It can also have a metabolic, neurologic, cardiovascular, cerebrovascular, or nutritional origin, or can result from a severe systemic infection or the effects of toxins, drugs, or alcohol. Confusion may signal worsening of an underlying and perhaps irreversible disease.

HISTORY

When you take his history, ask the patient to describe what's bothering him. He may not report confusion as his chief complaint but may complain of memory loss, persistent apprehension, or the inability to concentrate. He may be unable to respond logically to direct questions. Check with a family member or friend about onset and frequency. Find out, too, if the patient has a history of head trauma or a cardiopulmonary, metabolic, cerebrovascular, or neurologic disorder. Find out which medications he's taking, if any. Ask about any changes in eating or sleeping habits and in drug or alcohol use.

PHYSICAL ASSESSMENT

Perform an assessment to determine the presence of systemic disorders. Check vital signs, and assess the patient for changes in blood pressure, temperature, and pulse. Next, perform a neurologic assessment to establish the patient's level of consciousness.

MEDICAL CAUSES

Brain tumor
In the early stages of a brain tumor, confusion is usually mild and difficult to detect. As the tumor impinges on cerebral structures, however, confusion worsens and the patient may exhibit personality changes, bizarre behavior, sensory and motor deficits, visual field deficits, and aphasia.

Decreased cerebral perfusion
Mild confusion is an early symptom of decreased cerebral perfusion. Confusion may be insidious and fleeting, as in a transient ischemic attack, or acute and permanent, as in stroke. Associated findings usually include hypotension, tachycardia or bradycardia, irregular pulse, ventricular gallop, edema, and cyanosis.

Fluid and electrolyte imbalance
A fluid and electrolyte imbalance can cause confusion. The extent of imbalance determines the severity of the patient's confusion. Typically, he'll show signs of dehydration, such as lassitude, poor skin turgor, dry skin and mucous membranes, and oliguria. He may also develop hypotension and a low-grade fever.

Head trauma

Such head trauma as concussions, contusions, and brain hemorrhages may produce confusion at the time of injury, shortly afterward, or months or even years afterward. The patient may be delirious, with periodic loss of consciousness. Vomiting, severe headache, pupillary changes, and sensory and motor deficits are also common.

Heatstroke

Heatstroke causes pronounced confusion that gradually worsens as body temperature rises. Initially, the patient may be irritable and dizzy; later, he may become delirious, have seizures, and lose consciousness.

Heavy metal poisoning

Chronic ingestion or inhalation of heavy metals (such as lead, arsenic, mercury, and manganese) eventually produces confusion and, typically, weakness and drowsiness. The patient may also experience headache, vomiting, seizures, tremors, gait disturbances, and mental deterioration.

Hypothermia

Confusion may be an early sign of hypothermia. Typically, the patient displays slurred speech, cold and pale skin, hyperactive deep tendon reflexes, rapid pulse, and decreased blood pressure and respirations. As his body temperature continues to drop, his confusion progresses to stupor and coma, his muscles develop rigidity, and his respiratory rate decreases.

Hypoxemia

Acute pulmonary disorders that result in hypoxemia produce confusion that can range from mild disorientation to delirium. In advanced stages, chronic pulmonary disorders produce persistent confusion as well as severe dyspnea, disability, cor pulmonale, and severe respiratory failure.

Infection

Severe generalized infection, such as sepsis, commonly produces delirium. Central nervous system (CNS) infections such as meningitis cause varying degrees of confusion along with headache and nuchal rigidity.

Metabolic encephalopathy

Both hyperglycemia and hypoglycemia can produce sudden confusion. A patient with hypoglycemia may also experience transient delirium and seizures. Uremic and hepatic encephalopathies produce gradual confusion that may progress to seizures and coma. Usually, the patient also experiences tremors and restlessness.

Nutritional deficiencies

Inadequate dietary intake of thiamine, niacin, or vitamin B_{12}, which causes nutritional deficiencies, produces insidious, progressive confusion and possible mental deterioration. Associated CNS abnormalities may become severe enough to induce hallucinations and paranoia.

Seizure disorders

Mild to moderate confusion may immediately follow any type of seizure. The confusion usually disappears within several hours. The patient may have difficulty talking and may fall into deep sleep after the seizures.

Thyroid hormone disorders

Hyperthyroidism produces mild to moderate confusion along with nervousness, inability to concentrate, weight loss, flushed skin, and tachycardia. Hypothyroidism

Medical causes
(continued)

Heatstroke
- Confusion gradually worsens as body temperature rises.

Heavy metal poisoning
- Confusion, weakness, and drowsiness occur.

Hypothermia
- Confusion may be an early sign and progresses to stupor and coma as temperature drops.

Hypoxemia
- Confusion ranges from mild disorientation to delirium.

Infection
- Severe generalized infection commonly produces delirium.
- CNS infections cause varying degrees of confusion.

Metabolic encephalopathy
- Hyperglycemia and hypoglycemia can produce sudden confusion.
- Uremic and hepatic encephalopathies produce gradual confusion that may progress to seizures and coma.

Nutritional deficiencies
- Inadequate intake of thiamine, niacin, or vitamin B_{12} produces insidious, progressive confusion.

Seizure disorders
- Mild to moderate confusion may immediately follow a seizure.

Thyroid hormone disorders
- Hyperthyroidism produces mild to moderate confusion.
- Hypothyroidism produces mild, insidious confusion and memory loss.

produces mild, insidious confusion and memory loss; weight gain; bradycardia; and fatigue.

OTHER CAUSES

Alcohol
Intoxication causes confusion and stupor, and alcohol withdrawal may cause delirium and seizures.

Drugs
Large doses of CNS depressants produce confusion that can persist for several days after the drug is discontinued. Opioid and barbiturate withdrawal also causes acute confusion, possibly with delirium. Other drugs that commonly cause confusion include lidocaine, digoxin, indomethacin, cycloserine, chloroquine, atropine, and cimetidine.

SPECIAL CONSIDERATIONS
Never leave a confused patient unattended, to prevent injury to himself and others. Take measures to ensure patient safety. Keep the patient calm and quiet, and plan uninterrupted rest periods. Implement interventions to correct the underlying cause of confusion, such as giving supplemental oxygen to the patient with hypoxemia or withholding the offending drug.

PEDIATRIC POINTERS
Confusion can't be determined in infants and very young children. However, older children with acute febrile illnesses commonly experience transient delirium or acute confusion.

PATIENT COUNSELING
To help the patient stay oriented, keep a large calendar and a clock visible, and make a list of his activities with specific dates and times. Always reintroduce yourself to the patient each time you enter his room.

CONJUNCTIVAL INJECTION

A common ocular sign associated with inflammation, conjunctival injection is nonuniform redness of the conjunctiva from hyperemia. This redness can be diffuse, localized, or peripheral, or it may encircle a clear cornea.

Conjunctival injection usually results from bacterial or viral conjunctivitis, but it can also signal a severe ocular disorder that, if untreated, may lead to permanent blindness. Conjunctival injection can also result from minor eye irritation due to inadequate sleep, overuse of contact lenses, environmental irritants, and excessive eye rubbing.

 CULTURE CUE *Conjunctival injection is an early sign of trachoma, a leading cause of blindness in Third World countries and among Native Americans living in the southwestern United States.*

 EMERGENCY ACTIONS If the patient with conjunctival injection reports a chemical splash to the eye, first remove the contact lenses, and then quickly irrigate the eye with copious amounts of normal saline solution. Evert the lids and wipe the fornices with a cotton-tipped applicator to remove any foreign body particles and as much of the chemical as possible.

Other causes
+ Atropine, chloroquine, cimetidine, cycloserine, digoxin, indomethacin, or lidocaine
+ CNS depressants (large doses)
+ Intoxication
+ Withdrawal from alcohol, opioids, or barbiturates

Special considerations
+ Ensure patient safety.
+ Keep the patient calm and quiet, and plan uninterrupted rest periods.
+ Implement interventions to correct the underlying cause of confusion.

Teaching points
+ Orientation techniques

Key facts about conjunctival injection
+ Presents as nonuniform redness of the conjunctiva
+ May be diffuse, localized, or peripheral or may encircle a clear cornea

In an emergency
In case of chemical splash:
+ Remove contact lenses.
+ Irrigate the eye with normal saline solution.
+ Evert the lids and wipe the fornices with a cotton-tipped applicator.

History

When you take the patient's history, always ask if he has associated pain. If so, when did the pain begin, and where is it located? Is it constant or intermittent? Also, ask about itching, burning, photophobia, blurred vision, halo vision, excessive tearing, or a foreign body sensation in his eye. Does the patient have a history of eye disease or trauma? If he has suffered ocular trauma, avoid touching the affected eye.

Physical assessment

Test the patient's visual acuity and intraocular pressure (IOP) only if his eyelids can be opened without applying pressure. Place a metal shield over the affected eye to protect it if necessary.

If the patient's condition permits, examine the affected eye. First, determine the location and severity of conjunctival injection. Is it circumcorneal or localized? Peripheral or diffuse? Note any conjunctival or lid edema, ocular deviation, conjunctival follicles, ptosis, or exophthalmos. Also note the type and amount of any discharge.

Next, test the patient's visual acuity to establish a baseline. Note if the patient has had vision changes: Is his vision blurred or his visual acuity markedly decreased? Next, test pupillary reaction to light.

Perform IOP measurements. To gauge increased IOP without a tonometer, gently place your index finger over the closed eyelid; if the globe feels rock-hard, IOP is elevated.

Medical causes

Blepharitis

Blepharitis produces diffuse conjunctival injection. Ulcerations appear on the eyelids, which burn, itch, and have no lashes. The patient may report the sensation of a foreign body in his eye. Constant irritation results in rubbing of the eyes causing reddened rims or continuous blinking.

Chemical burns

With chemical burns (an ocular emergency), diffuse conjunctival injection occurs, but severe pain is the most prominent symptom. The patient also displays photophobia, blepharospasm, and decreased visual acuity in the affected eye; the cornea may appear gray, and the pupil may be unilaterally smaller.

Conjunctival foreign bodies and abrasions

Conjunctival foreign bodies and abrasions feature localized conjunctival injection with sudden, severe eye pain. The patient may have increased tearing and photophobia, but usually his visual acuity isn't impaired.

Conjunctivitis

Allergic conjunctivitis produces a milky, diffuse, peripheral conjunctival injection. Related findings include watery, stringy eye discharge; increased tearing; itching; palpebral conjunctival follicles; and (with hay fever) conjunctival edema; photophobia; and a feeling of fullness around the eyes.

Bacterial conjunctivitis causes diffuse peripheral conjunctival injection along with a thick, purulent eye discharge that contains mucus threads. The patient's lids and lashes stick together, and he has excessive tearing, photophobia, burning, and itching. He may have pain and a foreign body sensation if the cornea is involved.

In addition to diffuse peripheral conjunctival injection, the patient with *fungal conjunctivitis* complains of photophobia and increased tearing, itching, and burn-

Key history points

+ Onset, location, and duration of associated pain
+ Associated signs or symptoms

Critical assessment steps

+ Test visual acuity and IOP only if the eyelids can be opened without applying pressure.
+ Determine location and severity of conjunctival injection.
+ Note any discharge, edema, ocular deviation, conjunctival follicles, ptosis, or exophthalmos.

Medical causes

Blepharitis

+ Diffuse conjunctival injection occurs, and ulcerations that burn and itch appear on the eyelids.

Chemical burns

+ Diffuse conjunctival injection occurs with severe pain being the most prominent symptom.

Conjunctival foreign bodies and abrasions

+ Localized conjunctival injection occurs.
+ Eye pain is sudden and severe.

Conjunctivitis

+ With *bacterial conjunctivitis,* diffuse peripheral conjunctival injection occurs along with a thick, purulent eye discharge that contains mucus threads.
+ With *fungal conjunctivitis,* diffuse peripheral conjunctival injection occurs with photophobia and increased tearing, itching, and burning.
+ With *viral conjunctivitis,* the conjunctival injection is brilliant red, diffuse, and peripheral.

Medical causes
(continued)

Corneal abrasion
+ Diffuse conjunctival injection is extremely painful.

Corneal erosion
+ Diffuse conjunctival injection, severe, continuous pain, and photophobia develop.

Corneal ulcer
+ Diffuse conjunctival injection increases in the circumcorneal area.

Dacryoadenitis
+ Diffuse conjunctival injection occurs with constant tearing.

Episcleritis
+ Conjunctival injection is localized and raised and may be purplish.

Glaucoma
+ Conjunctival injection is typically circumcorneal.

Hyphema
+ Diffuse conjunctival injection occurs, possibly with lid and orbital edema.

Iritis
+ Marked conjunctival injection is found mainly around the cornea.

Keratoconjunctivitis sicca
+ Severe diffuse conjunctival injection occurs.

Lyme disease
+ Conjunctival injection occurs with other signs and symptoms of the disease.

ing. The discharge is thick and purulent, making his eyelids crusted, sticky, and swollen. Corneal involvement causes pain.

With *viral conjunctivitis,* the conjunctival injection is brilliant red, diffuse, and peripheral. The patient may also have conjunctival edema, follicles on the palpebral conjunctiva, and lid edema; local viral rash; and signs of upper respiratory tract infection. He complains of itching, increased tearing and, possibly, a foreign body sensation.

Corneal abrasion
With corneal abrasion, diffuse conjunctival injection is extremely painful, especially when the eyelids move over the abrasion. The patient may also report photophobia, excessive tearing, blurred vision, and a foreign body sensation.

Corneal erosion
Recurrent corneal erosion produces diffuse conjunctival injection; severe, continuous pain from rubbing of the eyelid over the eroded area of the cornea; and photophobia. The patient may have reduced vision.

Corneal ulcer
Bacterial, viral, and fungal corneal ulcers produce diffuse conjunctival injection that increases in the circumcorneal area. Accompanying findings include severe photophobia, severe pain in and around the eye, markedly decreased visual acuity, and copious and purulent eye discharge and crusting. If the patient develops associated iritis, a physical examination also reveals corneal opacities and an abnormal pupillary response to light.

Dacryoadenitis
With dacryoadenitis, the patient has large, diffuse conjunctival injection; pain over the temporal part of the eye; considerable lid swelling; and, possibly, purulent eye discharge. The hallmark of this disorder is constant tearing.

Episcleritis
Conjunctival injection is localized and raised and may be violet or purplish pink in patients with episcleritis. The sclera is also inflamed. Associated signs and symptoms include deep pain, photophobia, increased tearing, and conjunctival edema.

Glaucoma
With acute angle-closure glaucoma, conjunctival injection is typically circumcorneal. Signs and symptoms include severe eye pain, nausea and vomiting, severely elevated IOP, blurred vision, and the perception of rainbow-colored halos around lights. Corneas appear steamy because of corneal edema. The pupil of the affected eye is moderately dilated and completely unresponsive to light.

Hyphema
Depending on the type and extent of traumatic injury, a hyphema may produce diffuse conjunctival injection, possibly with lid and orbital edema. The patient may complain of pain in and around the eye. The extent of visual impairment depends on the hyphema's size and location.

Iritis
In acute iritis, marked conjunctival injection is found mainly around the cornea. Other findings include moderate to severe pain, photophobia, blurred vision, constricted pupils, and poor pupillary response to light.

Keratoconjunctivitis sicca

Keratoconjunctivitis sicca produces severe diffuse conjunctival injection. The patient reports generalized eye pain along with burning, itching, a foreign body sensation, excessive mucus secretion from the eye, absence of tears, and photophobia.

Lyme disease

Spread by tick bites, Lyme disease causes conjunctival injection. It may occur with diffuse urticaria, malaise, fatigue, headache, fever, chills, aches, and lymphadenopathy. Other ocular symptoms include pain, photophobia, conjunctivitis, and blurry or double vision.

Ocular lacerations and intraocular foreign bodies

In patients with ocular lacerations and intraocular foreign bodies, diffuse conjunctival injection may be increased in the area of injury. The patient also experiences impaired visual acuity and moderate to severe pain that varies with the type and extent of injury. He may also develop lid edema, photophobia, excessive tearing, and abnormal pupillary response.

Ocular tumors

If an ocular tumor is located in the orbit behind the globe, conjunctival injection may occur together with exophthalmos. With muscle involvement, conjunctival edema, ocular deviation, and diplopia usually occur.

Uveitis

Diffuse conjunctival injection, which may be increased in the circumcorneal area, characterizes uveitis. Accompanying signs and symptoms include constricted, irregularly shaped pupils; blurred vision; tenderness; photophobia; and possibly sudden, severe ocular pain.

SPECIAL CONSIDERATIONS

As indicated, prepare the patient for such diagnostic tests as orbital X-rays, ocular ultrasonography, and fluorescein staining. Obtain cultures of any eye discharge, and record its appearance, consistency, and amount.

PEDIATRIC POINTERS

An infant can develop self-limiting chemical conjunctivitis at birth from the ocular instillation of silver nitrate. He may also develop bacterial conjunctivitis 2 to 5 days after birth, due to contamination of the birth canal. An infant with congenital syphilis has prominent conjunctival injection and grayish pink corneas.

PATIENT COUNSELING

If the patient complains of photophobia, darken the room, or suggest that he wear sunglasses. If the patient's visual acuity is markedly decreased, orient him to his environment to ensure his comfort and safety.

Because most forms of conjunctivitis are contagious, the infection can easily spread to the other eye or to family members. Stress the importance of hand washing and of not touching the affected eye to prevent contagion.

Medical causes
(continued)

Ocular lacerations and intraocular foreign bodies
+ Diffuse conjunctival injection may be increased in the area of injury.

Ocular tumors
+ If tumor is located in the orbit behind the globe, conjunctival injection may be accompanied by exophthalmos.

Uveitis
+ Diffuse conjunctival injection may be increased in the circumcorneal area.

Special considerations
+ Obtain cultures of any eye discharge; record its appearance, consistency, and amount.

Peds points
+ An infant can develop self-limiting chemical conjunctivitis at birth from instillation of silver nitrate.
+ An infant may develop bacterial conjunctivitis 2 to 5 days after birth, due to contamination of the birth canal.
+ An infant with congenital syphilis has prominent conjunctival injection and grayish pink corneas.

Teaching points
+ Techniques for dealing with photophobia
+ Orientation to environment if visual acuity is impaired
+ Ways to avoid spreading the infection

Key facts about constipation

+ Small, infrequent, or difficult bowel movements
+ Can lead to headache, anorexia, and abdominal discomfort
+ Usually occurs when the urge to defecate is suppressed and the muscles associated with bowel movements remain contracted

Key history points

+ Frequency, size, and consistency of bowel movements
+ Onset and location of associated pain
+ Changes in diet, eating habits, drug or alcohol use, or physical activity
+ Recent emotional distress
+ History of GI, rectoanal, neurologic, or metabolic disorders; abdominal surgery; or radiation therapy
+ Drug history

Critical assessment steps

+ Inspect the abdomen for distention or scars from previous surgery.
+ Auscultate for bowel sounds and characterize their motility.
+ Percuss all four quadrants.
+ Gently palpate for abdominal tenderness, a palpable mass, and hepatomegaly.
+ Examine the rectum; inspect for inflammation, lesions, scars, fissures, and external hemorrhoids.
+ Palpate the anal sphincter for laxity or stricture.
+ Palpate for rectal masses and fecal impaction.
+ Obtain a stool specimen and test it for occult blood.

CONSTIPATION

Constipation is defined as small, infrequent, or difficult bowel movements. Because normal bowel movements can vary in frequency and from individual to individual, constipation must be determined in relation to the patient's normal elimination pattern. Constipation may be a minor annoyance or, uncommonly, a sign of a life-threatening disorder such as acute intestinal obstruction. Untreated, constipation can lead to headache, anorexia, and abdominal discomfort and can adversely affect the patient's lifestyle and well-being.

Constipation usually occurs when the urge to defecate is suppressed and the muscles associated with bowel movements remain contracted. Because the autonomic nervous system controls bowel movements — by sensing rectal distention from fecal contents and by stimulating the external sphincter — any factor that influences this system may cause bowel dysfunction. (See *How habits and stress cause constipation*.)

HISTORY

Ask the patient to describe the frequency of his bowel movements and the size and consistency of his stools. How long has he been constipated? Acute constipation usually has an organic cause, such as an anal or rectal disorder. In a patient over age 45, a recent onset of constipation may be an early sign of colorectal cancer. Conversely, chronic constipation typically has a functional cause and may be related to stress.

Does the patient have pain related to constipation? If so, when did he first notice the pain, and where is it located? Cramping abdominal pain and distention suggest obstipation — extreme, persistent constipation due to intestinal tract obstruction. Ask the patient if defecation worsens or helps relieve the pain. Defecation usually worsens pain, but with disorders such as irritable bowel syndrome, it may relieve it.

Ask the patient to describe a typical day's menu; estimate his daily fiber and fluid intake. Ask him, too, about any changes in eating habits, medication or alcohol use, or physical activity. Has he experienced recent emotional distress? Has constipation affected his family life or social contacts? Also, ask about his job. A sedentary or stressful job can contribute to constipation.

Find out whether the patient has a history of GI, rectoanal, neurologic, or metabolic disorders; abdominal surgery; or radiation therapy. Then ask about the medications he's taking, including over-the-counter preparations, such as laxatives, mineral oil, stool softeners, and enemas.

PHYSICAL ASSESSMENT

Inspect the abdomen for distention or scars from previous surgery. Then auscultate for bowel sounds, and characterize their motility. Percuss all four quadrants, and gently palpate for abdominal tenderness, a palpable mass, and hepatomegaly. Next, examine the patient's rectum. Spread his buttocks to expose the anus, and inspect for inflammation, lesions, scars, fissures, and external hemorrhoids. Use a disposable glove and lubricant to palpate the anal sphincter for laxity or stricture. Also, palpate for rectal masses and fecal impaction. Finally, obtain a stool specimen and test it for occult blood.

How habits and stress cause constipation

This flowchart shows how the presence of certain factors can lead to constipation.

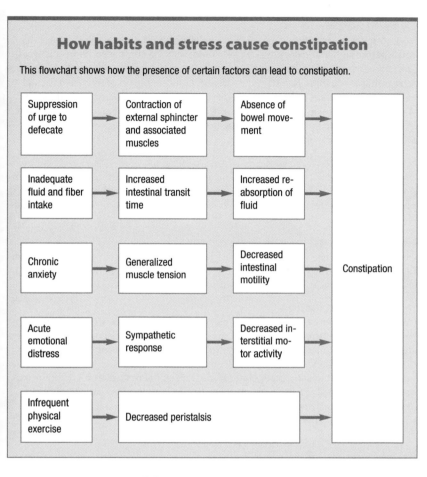

MEDICAL CAUSES

Anal fissure
An anal fissure, a crack or laceration in the lining of the anal wall, can cause acute constipation, usually due to the patient's fear of the severe tearing or burning pain associated with bowel movements. He may notice a few drops of blood streaking toilet tissue or his underwear.

Anorectal abscess
With an anorectal abscess, constipation occurs with severe, throbbing, localized pain and tenderness at the abscess site. The patient may also have localized inflammation, swelling, and purulent drainage and may complain of fever and malaise.

Diverticulitis
With diverticulitis, constipation or diarrhea occurs with left-lower-quadrant pain and tenderness and possibly a palpable, tender, firm, fixed abdominal mass. The patient may develop mild nausea, flatulence, or a low-grade fever.

Hemorrhoids
Thrombosed hemorrhoids cause constipation as the patient tries to avoid the severe pain of defecation. The hemorrhoids may bleed during defecation. The patient may notice bright red blood on stools or toilet tissue.

Medical causes

Anal fissure
✦ Acute constipation usually develops due to the fear of the severe tearing or burning pain associated with bowel movements.

Anorectal abscess
✦ Constipation occurs with severe, throbbing, localized pain and tenderness at the abscess site.

Diverticulitis
✦ Constipation or diarrhea occurs with left-lower-quadrant pain and tenderness.

Hemorrhoids
✦ Constipation occurs as the patient tries to avoid the severe pain of defecation.

Medical causes
(continued)

Hepatic porphyria
✦ Abdominal pain precedes constipation.

Hypercalcemia
✦ Constipation is usually accompanied by anorexia, nausea, vomiting, polyuria, and polydipsia.

Hypothyroidism
✦ Constipation occurs early and insidiously.

Intestinal obstruction
✦ With partial obstruction, constipation may alternate with leakage of liquid stools.
✦ With complete obstruction, obstipation may occur.

Irritable bowel syndrome
✦ Chronic constipation occurs.
✦ Some patients report alternating constipation and diarrhea.

Mesenteric artery ischemia
✦ Constipation is sudden.
✦ The patient fails to expel stools or flatus.

Multiple sclerosis
✦ Constipation occurs with ocular disturbances, vertigo, and sensory disturbances.

Spinal cord lesion
✦ Constipation may occur in addition to urine retention, sexual dysfunction, and pain.

Hepatic porphyria
Abdominal pain, which may be severe, colicky, localized, or generalized, precedes constipation in hepatic porphyria. The patient may also have fever, sinus tachycardia, labile hypertension, excessive diaphoresis, severe vomiting, photophobia, urine retention, nervousness or restlessness, disorientation and, possibly, visual hallucinations. Deep tendon reflexes may be diminished or absent. Some patients have skin lesions causing itching, burning, erythema, altered pigmentation, and edema in areas exposed to light. Severe hepatic porphyria can produce delirium, coma, seizures, paraplegia, or complete flaccid quadriplegia.

Hypercalcemia
With hypercalcemia, constipation usually occurs along with anorexia, nausea, vomiting, polyuria, and polydipsia. The patient may also display arrhythmias, bone pain, muscle weakness and atrophy, hypoactive deep tendon reflexes, and personality changes.

Hypothyroidism
Constipation occurs early and insidiously in patients with hypothyroidism, in addition to fatigue, sensitivity to cold, anorexia with weight gain, menorrhagia, decreased memory, hearing impairment, muscle cramps, and paresthesia.

Intestinal obstruction
Constipation associated with intestinal obstruction varies in severity and onset, depending on the location and extent of the obstruction. With partial obstruction, constipation may alternate with leakage of liquid stools. With complete obstruction, obstipation may occur. Constipation can be the earliest sign of partial colon obstruction, but it usually occurs later if the level of the obstruction is more proximal. Associated findings include episodes of colicky abdominal pain, abdominal distention, nausea, or vomiting. The patient may also develop hyperactive bowel sounds, visible peristaltic waves, a palpable abdominal mass, and abdominal tenderness.

Irritable bowel syndrome
Irritable bowel syndrome, a common disorder, usually produces chronic constipation, although some patients have intermittent, watery diarrhea and others complain of alternating constipation and diarrhea. Stress may trigger nausea and abdominal distention and tenderness, but defecation usually relieves these signs and symptoms. Patients with irritable bowel syndrome commonly have an intense urge to defecate and feelings of incomplete evacuation. Typically, the stools are scybalous and contain visible mucus.

Mesenteric artery ischemia
Mesenteric artery ischemia, a life-threatening disorder, produces sudden constipation with failure to expel stools or flatus. Initially, the abdomen is soft and nontender but soon severe abdominal pain, tenderness, vomiting, and anorexia occur. Later, the patient may develop abdominal guarding, rigidity, and distention; tachycardia; syncope; tachypnea; fever; and signs of shock, such as cool, clammy skin and hypotension. A bruit may be heard.

Multiple sclerosis
Multiple sclerosis (MS) can produce constipation in addition to ocular disturbances, such as nystagmus, blurred vision, and diplopia; vertigo; and sensory disturbances. The patient may also have motor weakness, seizures, paralysis, muscle spasticity, gait ataxia, intention tremor, hyperreflexia, dysarthria, or dysphagia. MS

can also produce urinary urgency, frequency, and incontinence as well as emotional instability. A male patient may experience impotence.

Spinal cord lesion
Constipation may occur with a spinal cord lesion, in addition to urine retention, sexual dysfunction, pain and, possibly, motor weakness, paralysis, or sensory impairment below the level of the lesion.

Ulcerative colitis
Constipation may occur in patients with chronic ulcerative colitis, but bloody diarrhea with pus, mucus, or both is the hallmark of this disorder. Other signs and symptoms include cramping lower abdominal pain, tenesmus, anorexia, low-grade fever and, occasionally, nausea and vomiting. Bowel sounds may be hyperactive. Later, weight loss, weakness, and arthralgia occur.

OTHER CAUSES

Diagnostic tests
Constipation can result from the retention of barium given during certain GI studies.

Drugs
Patients often experience constipation when taking an opioid analgesic or other drugs, including vinca alkaloids, calcium channel blockers, antacids containing aluminum or calcium, anticholinergics, and drugs with anticholinergic effects (such as tricyclic antidepressants). Patients may also experience constipation from excessive use of laxatives or enemas.

Surgery and radiation therapy
Constipation can result from rectoanal surgery, which may traumatize nerves, and abdominal irradiation, which may cause intestinal stricture.

SPECIAL CONSIDERATIONS
As indicated, prepare the patient for diagnostic tests, such as proctosigmoidoscopy, colonoscopy, barium enema, plain abdominal films, and an upper GI series. If the patient is on bed rest, reposition him frequently, and help him perform active or passive exercises, as indicated. Teach abdominal toning exercises if the patient's abdominal muscles are weak and relaxation techniques to help him reduce stress related to constipation.

PEDIATRIC POINTERS
The high content of casein and calcium in cow's milk can produce hard stools and possible constipation in bottle-fed infants. Other causes of constipation in infants include inadequate fluid intake, Hirschsprung's disease, and anal fissures. In older children, constipation usually results from inadequate fiber intake and excessive intake of milk; it can also result from bowel spasm, mechanical obstruction, hypothyroidism, reluctance to stop playing for bathroom breaks, and the lack of privacy in some school bathrooms.

GERIATRIC POINTERS
Acute constipation in elderly patients is usually associated with underlying structural abnormalities. Chronic constipation, however, is chiefly caused by lifelong bowel and dietary habits and laxative use.

Medical causes
(continued)
Ulcerative colitis
+ Constipation may occur in patients with chronic ulcerative colitis
+ Bloody diarrhea with pus, mucus, or both is the hallmark sign.

Other causes
+ Abdominal irradiation
+ Antacids containing aluminum or calcium, anticholinergics, drugs with anticholinergic effects, calcium channel blockers, opioid analesics, and vinca alkaloids
+ Overuse of laxatives or enemas
+ GI studies that use barium
+ Recotanal surgery

Special considerations
+ If the patient is on bed rest, reposition him frequently.
+ Help perform active or passive exercises, as indicated.

Peds points
+ In infants, causes include inadequate fluid intake, anal fissures, Hirschsprung's disease, and casein and calcium in cow's milk.
+ In older children, causes include inadequate fiber intake, excessive intake of milk, bowel spasm, mechanical obstruction, hypothyroidism, reluctance to stop playing for bathroom breaks, and the lack of privacy in some school bathrooms.

Geri points
+ Acute constipation is associated with structural abnormalities.
+ Chronic constipation is chiefly caused by lifelong bowel and dietary habits and laxative use.

Teaching points

+ Avoidance of straining, laxatives, and enemas
+ Diet and fluid intake
+ Exercise
+ Relaxation techniques

Key facts about CVA tenderness

+ Indicates sudden distention of the renal capsule
+ Accompanies unelicited, dull, constant flank pain in the CVA

Key history points

+ Other signs and symptoms
+ Voiding habits and onset and description of any recent changes
+ Personal or family history of urinary tract infections, congenital anomalies, calculi, other obstructive nephropathies or uropathies, or renovascular disorders

Critical assessment steps

+ Take vital signs.
+ If the patient has hypertension and bradycardia, be alert for other autonomic effects of renal pain.
+ Inspect, auscultate, and gently palpate the abdomen for clues to the underlying cause of CVA tenderness.
+ Be alert for abdominal distention, hypoactive bowel sounds, and palpable masses.

PATIENT COUNSELING

Caution the patient not to strain during defecation to prevent injuring rectoanal tissue. Instruct him to avoid using laxatives or enemas. If he has been abusing these products, begin to wean him from them. Use a disposable glove and lubricant to remove impacted fecal contents. (Check if an oil-retention enema can be given first to soften the fecal mass.)

Stress the importance of a high-fiber diet, and encourage the patient to drink plenty of fluids. (Explain that he may experience temporary bloating or flatulence after adding fiber to his diet.) Also, encourage him to exercise at least 1½ hours each week, if possible.

COSTOVERTEBRAL ANGLE TENDERNESS

Costovertebral angle (CVA) tenderness indicates sudden distention of the renal capsule. It almost always accompanies unelicited, dull, constant flank pain in the CVA just lateral to the spine and below the 12th rib. This associated pain typically travels anteriorly in the subcostal region toward the umbilicus.

Percussing the CVA elicits tenderness, if present. (See *Eliciting CVA tenderness*.) A patient who doesn't have this symptom will perceive a thudding, jarring, or pressurelike sensation when tested, but no pain. A patient with a disorder that distends the renal capsule will experience intense pain as the renal capsule stretches and stimulates the afferent nerves which emanate from the spinal cord at levels T11 through L2 and innervate the kidney.

HISTORY

After detecting CVA tenderness, determine the possible extent of renal damage. First, find out if the patient has other symptoms of renal or urologic dysfunction. Ask about voiding habits: How frequently does he urinate, and in what amounts? Has he noticed any change in intake or output? If so, when did he notice the change? (Ask about fluid intake before judging his output as abnormal.) Does he have nocturia? Ask about pain or burning during urination or difficulty starting a stream. Does the patient strain to urinate without being able to do so (tenesmus)? Ask about urine color; brown or bright-red urine may contain blood.

Explore other signs and symptoms. For example, if the patient is experiencing pain in his flank, abdomen, or back, when did he first notice the pain? How severe is it, and where is it located? Find out if the patient or a family member has a history of urinary tract infections, congenital anomalies, calculi, or other obstructive nephropathies or uropathies. Also, ask about a history of renovascular disorders, such as occlusion of the renal arteries or veins.

PHYSICAL ASSESSMENT

Perform a brief physical examination. Begin by taking the patient's vital signs. Fever and chills in a patient with CVA tenderness may indicate acute pyelonephritis. If the patient has hypertension and bradycardia, be alert for other autonomic effects of renal pain, such as diaphoresis and pallor. Inspect, auscultate, and gently palpate the abdomen for clues to the underlying cause of CVA tenderness. Be alert for abdominal distention, hypoactive bowel sounds, and palpable masses.

ASSESSMENT TIP

Eliciting CVA tenderness

To elicit costovertebral angle (CVA) tenderness, have the patient sit upright facing away from you or have him lie in a prone position. Place the palm of your left hand over the left CVA, then strike the back of your left hand with the ulnar surface of your right fist (as shown below). Repeat this percussion technique over the right CVA. A patient with CVA tenderness will experience intense pain.

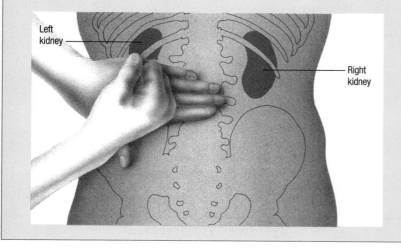

Left kidney

Right kidney

MEDICAL CAUSES

Calculi
Infundibular and ureteropelvic or ureteral calculi produce CVA tenderness and waves of waxing and waning flank pain that may radiate to the groin, testicles, suprapubic area, or labia. The patient may also develop nausea, vomiting, severe abdominal pain, abdominal distention, and decreased bowel sounds.

Perirenal abscess
Causing exquisite CVA tenderness, a perirenal abscess may also produce severe unilateral flank pain, dysuria, persistent high fever, chills, erythema of the skin, and sometimes a palpable abdominal mass. Flank pain may radiate to the groin or down the leg.

Pyelonephritis (acute)
Perhaps the most common cause of CVA tenderness, acute pyelonephritis is commonly accompanied by persistent high fever, chills, flank pain, anorexia, nausea and vomiting, weakness, dysuria, hematuria, nocturia, urinary urgency and frequency, and tenesmus.

Renal artery occlusion
With renal artery occlusion, the patient experiences flank pain as well as CVA tenderness. Other findings include severe, continuous upper abdominal pain; nausea; vomiting; decreased bowel sounds; and high fever. The patient may also report hematuria.

Medical causes

Calculi
✦ CVA tenderness occurs with waves of waxing and waning flank pain that may radiate.

Perirenal abscess
✦ Exquisite CVA tenderness occurs.
✦ Severe unilateral flank pain, dysuria, persistent high fever, chills, erythema of the skin, and a palpable abdominal mass may be present.

Pyelonephritis (acute)
✦ CVA tenderness occurs with persistent high fever, chills, flank pain, anorexia, nausea and vomiting, weakness, dysuria, hematuria, nocturia, urinary urgency and frequency, and tenesmus.

Renal artery occlusion
✦ The patient experiences flank pain and CVA tenderness.

Special considerations
+ Administer pain medication.
+ Collect blood samples and urine specimens.

Peds points
+ An infant won't exhibit CVA tenderness; instead he'll display nonspecific signs and symptoms.

Geri points
+ Advanced age and cognitive impairment reduce an elderly patient's ability to perceive pain.

Teaching points
+ Dietary restrictions
+ Increasing fluid intake
+ Signs and symptoms of kidney infection to report

Key facts about barking cough
+ Resonant, brassy, and harsh cough
+ Indicates edema of the larynx and surrounding tissue

Key history points
+ Onset of cough
+ Associated signs and symptoms
+ Previous episodes of croup syndrome

Critical assessment steps
+ Observe the child for signs of respiratory distress.
+ Note use of sternal or intercostal retractions or nasal flaring.
+ Observe skin for cyanosis and diaphoresis.
+ Take vital signs, noting respiratory rate and depth.
+ Auscultate the lungs.

SPECIAL CONSIDERATIONS

Administer pain medication, and continue to monitor the patient's vital signs and intake and output. Collect blood samples and urine specimens, and then prepare the patient for radiologic studies, such as excretory urography, renal arteriography, and computed tomography scan.

PEDIATRIC POINTERS

An infant with a disorder that distends the renal capsule won't exhibit CVA tenderness. Instead, he'll display nonspecific signs and symptoms, such as vomiting, diarrhea, fever, irritability, poor skin perfusion, and yellow to gray skin. In older children, however, CVA tenderness has the same diagnostic significance as in adults. Vaginal discharge, vulval soreness, and pruritus may occur in girls.

GERIATRIC POINTERS

Advanced age and cognitive impairment reduce an elderly patient's ability to perceive pain or to describe its intensity.

PATIENT COUNSELING

Teach the patient with calculi about dietary restrictions. Explain the importance of increasing fluid intake to prevent and treat renal infection. Reinforce the importance of taking antibiotics for the full prescribed course. Discuss signs and symptoms of kidney infection to report to the physician.

COUGH, BARKING

Resonant, brassy, and harsh, a barking cough is part of a complex of signs and symptoms that characterize croup syndrome, a group of pediatric disorders marked by varying degrees of respiratory distress. Croup syndrome is most common in boys and most prevalent in the fall; it may recur in the same child.

A barking cough indicates edema of the larynx and surrounding tissue. Because children's airways are smaller in diameter than those of adults, edema can rapidly lead to airway occlusion—a life-threatening emergency. (See *Managing a barking cough.*)

HISTORY

Ask the child's parents when the barking cough began and what other signs and symptoms accompanied it. When did the child first appear to be ill? Has he had previous episodes of croup syndrome? Did his condition improve upon exposure to cold air?

Spasmodic croup and epiglottiditis typically occur in the middle of the night. The child with spasmodic croup has no fever, but the child with epiglottiditis has a high fever of sudden onset. An upper respiratory tract infection typically is followed by laryngotracheobronchitis.

PHYSICAL ASSESSMENT

Observe the child for signs of respiratory distress. Note use of sternal or intercostal retractions or nasal flaring. Observe his skin for cyanosis and diaphoresis. Take his vital signs, noting respiratory rate and depth. Although stridor can be heard with-

Managing a barking cough

If the child experiences edema, quickly evaluate his respiratory status. Then take his vital signs. Be particularly alert for tachycardia and signs of hypoxemia. Also, check for a decreased level of consciousness. Try to determine if the child has been playing with a small object that he may have aspirated.

Check for cyanosis in the lips and nail beds. Observe the patient for sternal or intercostal retractions or nasal flaring. Next, note the depth and rate of his respirations; they may become increasingly shallow as respiratory distress increases. Observe the child's body position. Is he sitting up, leaning forward, struggling to breathe? Observe his activity level and facial expression. As respiratory distress increases from airway edema, the child will become restless and have a frightened, wide-eyed expression. As air hunger continues, the child will become lethargic and difficult to arouse.

If the child shows signs of severe respiratory distress, try to calm him, maintain airway patency, and provide oxygen. Endotracheal intubation or a tracheotomy may be necessary.

out a stethoscope, auscultate his lungs. Decreased breath sounds and crackles may be present.

MEDICAL CAUSES

Aspiration of foreign body

Partial obstruction of the upper airway caused by aspiration of foreign body first produces sudden hoarseness, then a barking cough and inspiratory stridor. Other effects of this life-threatening condition include gagging, tachycardia, dyspnea, decreased breath sounds, wheezing and, possibly, cyanosis.

Epiglottiditis

Epiglottiditis, a life-threatening disorder, has become less common since the use of influenza vaccines. It occurs nocturnally, heralded by a barking cough and a high fever. The child is hoarse, dysphagic, dyspneic, and restless and appears extremely ill and panicky. The cough may progress to severe respiratory distress with sternal and intercostal retractions, nasal flaring, cyanosis, and tachycardia. The child will struggle to get sufficient air as epiglottic edema increases. Epiglottiditis is a true medical emergency.

Laryngotracheobronchitis (acute)

Also known as *viral croup*, acute laryngotracheobronchitis is most common in children between 9 and 18 months old and usually occurs in the fall and early winter. It initially produces low to moderate fever, runny nose, poor appetite, and infrequent cough. When the infection descends into the laryngotracheal area, barking cough, hoarseness, and inspiratory stridor occur.

As respiratory distress progresses, substernal and intercostal retractions occur along with tachycardia and shallow, rapid respirations. Sleeping in a dry room worsens these signs. The patient becomes restless, irritable, pale, and cyanotic.

Spasmodic croup

Acute spasmodic croup usually occurs during sleep with the abrupt onset of a barking cough that awakens the child. Typically, he doesn't have a fever but may be hoarse, restless, and dyspneic. As his respiratory distress worsens, the child may exhibit sternal and intercostal retractions, nasal flaring, tachycardia, cyanosis, and an

Medical causes

Aspiration of foreign body
+ Sudden hoarseness occurs initially, followed by barking cough and inspiratory stridor.

Epiglottiditis
+ Condition is heralded by a barking cough and a high fever.

Laryngotracheobronchitis (acute)
+ Fever, runny nose, poor appetite, and infrequent cough occur initially.
+ When infection descends into the laryngotracheal area, barking cough, hoarseness, and inspiratory stridor occur.

Spasmodic croup
+ Onset of a barking cough is abrupt and usually awakens a child from sleep.

Special considerations

+ Don't inspect throat of a child with barking cough unless intubation equipment is available.
+ If the child isn't in severe respiratory distress, a lateral neck X-ray may be done to visualize epiglottal edema.
+ A chest X-ray may be done to rule out lower respiratory tract infection.
+ Depending on child's age and degree of respiratory distress, oxygen may be administered.
+ Rapid-acting epinephrine and a steroid should be considered.
+ Observe the child frequently, and monitor the oxygen level if used.
+ Provide periods of rest.
+ Maintain a calm, quiet environment and offer reassurance.
+ Encourage the parents to stay with the child.

Teaching points

+ Evaluation and treatment of recurrent episodes of croup syndrome

Key facts about nonproductive cough

+ Noisy, forceful expulsion of air from the lungs that doesn't yield sputum
+ Can cause airway collapse or rupture of alveoli or blebs
+ May occur in paroxysms and can worsen by becoming more frequent
+ May be acute (self-limiting) or chronic

anxious, frantic appearance. The signs usually subside within a few hours, but attacks tend to recur.

SPECIAL CONSIDERATIONS

Don't attempt to inspect the throat of a child with a barking cough unless intubation equipment is available. If the child isn't in severe respiratory distress, a lateral neck X-ray may be done to visualize epiglottal edema; a negative X-ray doesn't completely rule out epiglottal edema. A chest X-ray may also be done to rule out lower respiratory tract infection. Depending on the child's age and degree of respiratory distress, oxygen may be administered. Rapid-acting epinephrine and a steroid should be considered.

Be sure to observe the child frequently, and monitor the oxygen level if used. Provide the child with periods of rest with minimal interruptions. Maintain a calm, quiet environment and offer reassurance. Encourage the parents to stay with the child to help alleviate stress.

PATIENT COUNSELING

Teach the parents how to evaluate and treat recurrent episodes of croup syndrome. For example, creating steam by running hot water in a sink or shower and sitting with the child in the closed bathroom may help relieve subsequent attacks. The child may also benefit from being brought outside (properly dressed) to breathe cold night air.

COUGH, NONPRODUCTIVE

A nonproductive cough is a noisy, forceful expulsion of air from the lungs that doesn't yield sputum. It's one of the most common complaints of patients with respiratory disorders.

Coughing is a necessary protective mechanism that clears airway passages. However, a nonproductive cough is ineffective and can cause damage, such as airway collapse or rupture of alveoli or blebs. A nonproductive cough that later becomes productive is a classic sign of progressive respiratory disease.

The cough reflex generally occurs when mechanical, chemical, thermal, inflammatory, or psychogenic stimuli activate cough receptors. (See *Reviewing the cough mechanism*.) However, external pressure — for example, from subdiaphragmatic irritation or a mediastinal tumor — can also induce it, as can voluntary expiration of air, which occasionally occurs as a nervous habit. Certain drugs, such as angiotensin-converting enzyme inhibitors, may also cause a nonproductive cough.

A nonproductive cough may occur in paroxysms and can worsen by becoming more frequent. An acute cough has a sudden onset and may be self-limiting; a cough that persists beyond 1 month is considered chronic and commonly results from cigarette smoking.

HISTORY

Ask the patient when his cough began and whether body position, time of day, or specific activity affects it. How does the cough sound — harsh, brassy, dry, or hacking? Try to determine if the cough is related to smoking or a chemical irritant. If the patient smokes or has smoked, note the number of packs smoked daily multiplied by years ("pack years"). Next, ask about the frequency and intensity of the coughing. If he has pain associated with coughing, breathing, or activity, when did it begin? Where is it located?

Reviewing the cough mechanism

Cough receptors are thought to be located in the nose, sinuses, auditory canals, nasopharynx, larynx, trachea, bronchi, pleurae, diaphragm, and possibly the pericardium and GI tract. When a cough receptor is stimulated, the vagus and glossopharyngeal nerves transmit the impulse to the "cough center" in the medulla. From there, the impulse is transmitted to the larynx and to the intercostal and abdominal muscles. Deep inspiration (1) is followed by closure of the glottis (2), relaxation of the diaphragm, and contraction of the abdominal and intercostal muscles. The resulting increased pressure in the lungs opens the glottis to release the forceful, noisy expiration known as a cough (3).

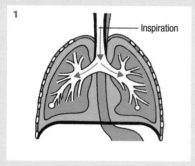

1
Inspiration

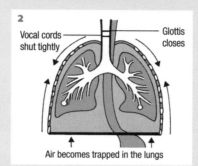

2
Vocal cords shut tightly
Glottis closes
Air becomes trapped in the lungs

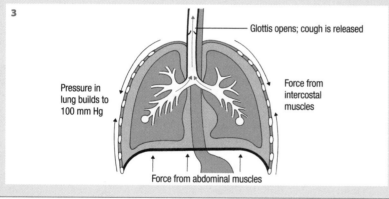

3
Glottis opens; cough is released
Pressure in lung builds to 100 mm Hg
Force from intercostal muscles
Force from abdominal muscles

Ask the patient about recent illness (especially a cardiovascular or pulmonary disorder), surgery, or trauma. Also ask about hypersensitivity to drugs, foods, pets, dust, or pollen. Find out which medications the patient takes, if any, and ask about recent changes in schedule or dosages. Also, ask about recent changes in his appetite, weight, exercise tolerance, or energy level and recent exposure to irritating fumes, chemicals, or smoke.

PHYSICAL ASSESSMENT

As you're taking his history, observe the patient's general appearance and manner: Is he agitated, restless, or lethargic; pale, diaphoretic, or flushed; anxious, confused, or nervous? Also, note whether he's cyanotic or has clubbed fingers or peripheral edema.

Key history points

◆ Onset, frequency, and description of cough
◆ Aggravating factors
◆ Smoking history
◆ Onset and location of associated pain
◆ History of surgery or trauma
◆ Hypersensitivity to drugs, foods, pets, dust, or pollen
◆ Drug history
◆ Recent changes in appetite, weight, exercise tolerance, or energy level
◆ Recent exposure to irritating fumes, chemicals, or smoke

Critical assessment steps

◆ Observe the patient; note cyanosis, clubbed fingers, or edema.
◆ Check the depth and rhythm of respirations; note if wheezing occurs with breathing.
◆ Inspect the neck for distended veins and tracheal deviation.
◆ Examine the chest, looking for abnormal chest wall motion.

Critical assessment steps
(continued)

+ Auscultate for wheezing, crackles, rhonchi, pleural friction rubs, and decreased or absent breath sounds.

Medical causes

Airway occlusion
+ Partial occlusion of the upper airway produces a sudden onset of dry, paroxysmal coughing.

Anthrax (inhalation)
+ Initial signs and symptoms include fever, chills, weakness, cough, and chest pain.

Aortic aneurysm (thoracic)
+ A brassy cough occurs with dyspnea, hoarseness, wheezing, and a substernal ache in the shoulders, lower back, or abdomen.

Asthma
+ Attacks start with a nonproductive cough and mild wheezing.
+ As cough progresses, thick mucus occurs.

Atelectasis
+ As lung tissue deflates, it stimulates cough receptors, causing a nonproductive cough.

Bronchitis (chronic)
+ A nonproductive, hacking cough later becomes productive.

Bronchogenic carcinoma
+ Chronic, nonproductive cough, dyspnea, and vague chest pain are early indicators.

 CULTURAL CUE *Because of the fear of being known as someone with tuberculosis (TB), the patient may be reluctant to provide information about his signs and symptoms such as cough. Ask the patient at risk for TB — those born in another country, those in contact with acute TB, and those with high-risk behaviors — about potential TB exposure.*

Next, perform a physical examination. Start by taking the patient's vital signs. Check the depth and rhythm of his respirations, and note if wheezing or "crowing" noises occur with breathing. Feel the patient's skin: Is it cold or warm; clammy or dry? Check his nose and mouth for congestion, inflammation, drainage, and signs of infection. Inspect his neck for distended veins and tracheal deviation, and palpate for masses or enlarged lymph nodes.

Examine his chest, observing its configuration and looking for abnormal chest wall motion. Do you note any retractions or use of accessory muscles? Percuss for dullness, tympany, or flatness. Auscultate for wheezing, crackles, rhonchi, pleural friction rubs, and decreased or absent breath sounds. Finally, examine his abdomen for distention, tenderness, masses, or abnormal bowel sounds.

MEDICAL CAUSES

Airway occlusion
Partial occlusion of the upper airway produces a sudden onset of dry, paroxysmal coughing. The patient is gagging, wheezing, and hoarse, with stridor, tachycardia, and decreased breath sounds. If the patient has aspirated a foreign body he may exhibit the universal sign for choking — a hand clutched to the throat, with thumb and fingers extended.

Anthrax (inhalation)
Inhalation anthrax is caused by inhalation of aerosolized spores of the gram-positive bacterium *Bacillus anthracis*. Initial signs and symptoms are flulike and include fever, chills, weakness, cough, and chest pain. The disease generally occurs in two stages with a period of recovery after the initial signs and symptoms. The second stage develops abruptly with rapid deterioration marked by fever, dyspnea, stridor, and hypotension generally leading to death within 24 hours. Radiologic findings include mediastinitis and symmetric mediastinal widening.

Aortic aneurysm (thoracic)
A thoracic aortic aneurysm causes a brassy cough with dyspnea, hoarseness, wheezing, and a substernal ache in the shoulders, lower back, or abdomen. The patient may also have facial or neck edema, neck vein distention, dysphagia, prominent veins over his chest, stridor and, possibly, paresthesia or neuralgia.

Asthma
Asthma attacks commonly occur at night, starting with a nonproductive cough and mild wheezing; this progresses to severe dyspnea, audible wheezing, chest tightness, and a cough that produces thick mucus. Other signs include apprehension, rhonchi, prolonged expirations, intercostal and supraclavicular retractions on inspiration, accessory muscle use, flaring nostrils, tachypnea, tachycardia, diaphoresis, and flushing or cyanosis.

Atelectasis
As lung tissue deflates, it stimulates cough receptors, causing a nonproductive cough. The patient with atelectasis may also have pleuritic chest pain, anxiety, dyspnea, tachypnea, and tachycardia. His skin may be cyanotic and diaphoretic, his breath sounds may be decreased, his chest may be dull on percussion, and he may

exhibit inspiratory lag, substernal or intercostal retractions, decreased vocal fremitus, and tracheal deviation toward the affected side.

Bronchitis (chronic)

Chronic bronchitis starts with a nonproductive, hacking cough that later becomes productive. Other findings include prolonged expiration, wheezing, dyspnea, accessory muscle use, barrel chest, cyanosis, tachypnea, crackles, and scattered rhonchi. Clubbing can occur in late stages.

Bronchogenic carcinoma

The earliest indicators of bronchogenic carcinoma can be a chronic, nonproductive cough, dyspnea, and vague chest pain. The patient may also have wheezing, hemoptysis, and stridor.

Common cold

The common cold generally starts with a nonproductive, hacking cough and progresses to some mix of sneezing, headache, malaise, fatigue, rhinorrhea, myalgia, arthralgia, nasal congestion, and sore throat.

Esophageal achalasia

With esophageal achalasia, regurgitation and aspiration produce a dry cough. The patient may also have recurrent pulmonary infections and dysphagia. The patient may report weight loss, heartburn, and chest pain that increases after eating.

Esophageal diverticula

The patient with esophageal diverticula has a nocturnal nonproductive cough, regurgitation and aspiration, dyspepsia, and dysphagia. His neck may appear swollen and have a gurgling sound. He may also exhibit halitosis and weight loss.

Esophageal occlusion

Esophageal occlusion is marked by immediate nonproductive coughing and gagging, with a sensation of something stuck in the throat. Other findings include neck or chest pain, dysphagia, and the inability to swallow.

Esophagitis with reflux

Esophagitis with reflux commonly causes a nonproductive nocturnal cough due to regurgitation and aspiration. The patient may experience chest pain that mimics angina pectoris; heartburn that worsens if he lies down after eating; and increased salivation, dysphagia, hematemesis, and melena.

Hodgkin's disease

Hodgkin's disease may cause a crowing nonproductive cough. However, the earliest sign is usually painless swelling of one of the cervical lymph nodes or, occasionally, of the axillary, mediastinal, or inguinal lymph nodes. Another early sign is pruritus. Other findings depend on the degree and location of systemic involvement and include dyspnea, dysphagia, hepatosplenomegaly, edema, jaundice, nerve pain, and hyperpigmentation.

Hypersensitivity pneumonitis

With hypersensitivity pneumonitis, an acute nonproductive cough, fever, dyspnea, and malaise usually occur 5 to 6 hours after exposure to an antigen. The patient may also report chest tightness and extreme fatigue.

Interstitial lung disease

A patient with interstitial lung disease has a nonproductive cough and progressive dyspnea. He may also be cyanotic and have clubbing, fine crackles, fatigue, variable

Medical causes
(continued)

Common cold
+ Nonproductive, hacking cough progresses to a mix of sneezing, headache, malaise, fatigue, rhinorrhea, myalgia, arthralgia, nasal congestion, and sore throat.

Esophageal achalasia
+ Regurgitation and aspiration produce a dry cough.

Esophageal diverticula
+ Nocturnal nonproductive cough, regurgitation and aspiration, dyspepsia, and dysphagia are characteristic.

Esophageal occlusion
+ Immediate nonproductive coughing and gagging accompanies a sensation of something stuck in the throat.

Esophagitis with reflux
+ Regurgitation and aspiration produce a nonproductive nocturnal cough.

Hodgkin's disease
+ A crowing nonproductive cough may develop.
+ Painless swelling of a cervical lymph node is an early sign.

Hypersensitivity pneumonitis
+ Acute nonproductive cough, fever, dyspnea, and malaise occur 5 to 6 hours after exposure to an antigen.

Interstitial lung disease
+ Nonproductive cough and progressive dyspnea occur.

Medical causes
(continued)

Laryngeal tumor
+ Mild, nonproductive cough; minor throat discomfort; and hoarseness are early signs.

Laryngitis
+ In acute cases, a nonproductive cough occurs with localized pain, fever, and malaise.

Legionnaires' disease
+ After prodromal symptoms develop, a nonproductive cough progresses to a cough that produces mucoid, mucopurulent and, possibly, bloody sputum.

Lung abscess
+ Nonproductive coughing, weakness, dyspnea, and pleuritic chest pain occur initially.
+ Later, cough produces purulent, foul-smelling sputum.

Mediastinal tumor
+ Nonproductive cough, dyspnea, and retrosternal pain occur.

Pleural effusion
+ Nonproductive cough, dyspnea, pleuritic chest pain, and decreased chest motion are characteristic.

Pneumonia
+ Bacterial pneumonia causes nonproductive, hacking, painful cough that becomes productive.
+ With mycoplasma pneumonia, nonproductive cough arises 2 to 3 days after onset of malaise, headache, and sore throat.
+ Viral pneumonia causes a nonproductive, hacking cough and gradual onset of malaise, headache, and low-grade fever.

chest pain, and weight loss. Other findings include dyspnea on exertion and vague chest pain.

Laryngeal tumor

A mild, nonproductive cough is an early sign of a laryngeal tumor, in addition to minor throat discomfort and hoarseness. Later, dysphagia, dyspnea, cervical lymphadenopathy, stridor, and earache may occur.

Laryngitis

In its acute form, laryngitis causes a nonproductive cough with localized pain (especially when the patient is swallowing or speaking) as well as fever and malaise. His hoarseness can range from mild to complete loss of voice.

Legionnaires' disease

After a prodrome of malaise, headache and, possibly, diarrhea, anorexia, diffuse myalgia, and general weakness, legionnaires' disease causes a nonproductive cough that later produces mucoid, mucopurulent and, possibly, bloody sputum.

Lung abscess

Lung abscess typically begins with nonproductive coughing, weakness, dyspnea, and pleuritic chest pain. The patient may also exhibit diaphoresis, fever, headache, malaise, fatigue, crackles, decreased breath sounds, anorexia, and weight loss. Later, his cough produces large amounts of purulent, foul-smelling, possibly bloody sputum.

Mediastinal tumor

A large mediastinal tumor produces a nonproductive cough, dyspnea, and retrosternal pain. The patient may also develop stertorous respirations with suprasternal retraction on inspiration, hoarseness, dysphagia, tracheal shift or tug, neck vein distention, and facial or neck edema.

Pleural effusion

A nonproductive cough along with dyspnea, pleuritic chest pain, and decreased chest motion are characteristic of pleural effusion. Other findings include pleural friction rub, tachycardia, tachypnea, egophony, flatness on percussion, decreased or absent breath sounds, and decreased tactile fremitus.

Pneumonia

Bacterial pneumonia usually starts with a nonproductive, hacking, painful cough that rapidly becomes productive. Other findings include shaking chills, headache, high fever, dyspnea, pleuritic chest pain, tachypnea, tachycardia, grunting respirations, nasal flaring, decreased breath sounds, fine crackles, rhonchi, and cyanosis. The patient's chest may be dull on percussion.

With *mycoplasma pneumonia*, a nonproductive cough arises 2 to 3 days after the onset of malaise, headache, and sore throat. The cough can be paroxysmal, causing substernal chest pain. Fever commonly occurs, but the patient doesn't appear seriously ill.

Viral pneumonia causes a nonproductive, hacking cough and the gradual onset of malaise, headache, anorexia, and low-grade fever.

Pneumothorax

Pneumothorax, a life-threatening disorder, causes a dry cough and signs of respiratory distress, such as severe dyspnea, tachycardia, tachypnea, and cyanosis. The patient experiences sudden, sharp chest pain that worsens with chest movement as well as subcutaneous crepitation, hyperresonance or tympany, decreased vocal fremitus, and decreased or absent breath sounds on the affected side.

Pulmonary edema

Pulmonary edema initially causes a dry cough, exertional dyspnea, paroxysmal nocturnal dyspnea, orthopnea, tachycardia, tachypnea, dependent crackles, and ventricular gallop. If pulmonary edema is severe, the patient's respirations become more rapid and labored, with diffuse crackles and coughing that produces frothy, bloody sputum.

Pulmonary embolism

A life-threatening pulmonary embolism may suddenly produce a dry cough along with dyspnea and pleuritic or anginal chest pain. More commonly, though, the cough produces blood-tinged sputum. Tachycardia and low-grade fever are also common; less common signs and symptoms include massive hemoptysis, chest splinting, leg edema and, with a large embolus, cyanosis, syncope, and distended neck veins. The patient may also have a pleural friction rub, diffuse wheezing, dullness on percussion, and decreased breath sounds.

Sarcoidosis

With sarcoidosis, a nonproductive cough is accompanied by dyspnea, substernal pain, and malaise. The patient may also develop fatigue, arthralgia, myalgia, weight loss, tachypnea, crackles, lymphadenopathy, hepatosplenomegaly, skin lesions, vision impairment, difficulty swallowing, and arrhythmias.

 CULTURAL CUE The risk of sarcoidosis is greatest in young adult Blacks, especially Black women. Others at high risk include those of Scandinavian, German, Irish, or Puerto Rican descent.

Severe acute respiratory syndrome

The incubation period of this acute infectious disease of unknown etiology is 2 to 7 days, and the illness generally begins with a fever (usually greater than 100.4° F [38° C]). Other symptoms of severe acute respiratory syndrome (SARS) include headache, malaise, a dry nonproductive cough, and dyspnea. The severity of the illness is highly variable, ranging from mild illness to pneumonia and, in some cases, progressing to respiratory failure and death.

 CULTURAL CUE Most cases of SARS have been reported in Asia (China, Vietnam, Singapore, Thailand), although some cases have appeared in Europe and North America.

Sinusitis (chronic)

Chronic sinusitis can cause a chronic nonproductive cough due to postnasal drip. The patient's nasal mucosa may appear inflamed, and he may have nasal congestion and profuse drainage. Usually, his breath smells musty.

Tracheobronchitis (acute)

Initially, acute tracheobronchitis produces a dry cough that later becomes productive as secretions increase. Chills, sore throat, slight fever, muscle and back pain, and substernal tightness generally precede the cough's onset. Rhonchi and wheezes are usually heard. Severe illness causes a fever of 101° F to 102° F (38.3° to 38.9° C) and possibly bronchospasm, with severe wheezing and increased coughing.

Tularemia

Following inhalation of the gram-negative, non-spore-forming bacterium *Francisella tularensis,* patients with tularemia show signs and symptoms including the abrupt onset of fever, chills, headache, generalized myalgia, nonproductive cough, dyspnea, pleuritic chest pain, and empyema.

Medical causes
(continued)

Pneumothorax
+ The patient exhibits dry cough and signs of respiratory distress.

Pulmonary edema
+ Dry cough, exertional dyspnea, paroxysmal nocturnal dyspnea, orthopnea, tachycardia, tachypnea, dependent crackles, and ventricular gallop occur initially.

Pulmonary embolism
+ Dry cough, dyspnea, and pleuritic or anginal chest pain may occur suddenly.
+ More commonly, the cough produces blood-tinged sputum.

Sarcoidosis
+ A nonproductive cough is accompanied by dyspnea, substernal pain, and malaise.

SARS
+ Illness begins with fever; headache, malaise, dry nonproductive cough, and dyspnea also occur.

Sinusitis (chronic)
+ Chronic nonproductive cough may develop due to postnasal drip.

Tracheobronchitis (acute)
+ Dry cough becomes productive as secretions increase.
+ Chills, sore throat, slight fever, muscle and back pain, and substernal tightness generally precede the cough's onset.

Tularemia
+ Onset of fever, chills, headache, generalized myalgia, nonproductive cough, dyspnea, pleuritic chest pain, and empyema is abrupt.

Other causes

+ Bronchoscopy
+ Deep endotracheal or tracheal tube placement
+ Inhalants such as pentamidine
+ Intermittent positive-pressure breathing
+ Pulmonary function tests
+ Spirometry
+ Suctioning

Special considerations

+ A nonproductive, paroxysmal cough may induce life-threatening bronchospasm; the patient may need a bronchodilator.
+ Unless the patient has COPD, as ordered, give an antitussive and a sedative to suppress the cough.
+ Humidify the air in the patient's room.

Peds points

+ Sudden onset of paroxysmal nonproductive coughing may indicate aspiration of a foreign body.
+ Nonproductive coughing can result from asthma, bacterial pneumonia, acute bronchiolitis, acute otitis media, measles, cystic fibrosis, airway hyperactivity, or a foreign body in the external auditory canal; it may also be psychogenic.

Geri points

+ Nonproductive cough may indicate serious acute or chronic illness in elderly patients.

OTHER CAUSES

Diagnostic tests

Pulmonary function tests and bronchoscopy may stimulate cough receptors, triggering coughing.

Treatments

Irritation of the carina during suctioning or deep endotracheal or tracheal tube placement can trigger a paroxysmal or hacking cough. Intermittent positive-pressure breathing or spirometry can also cause a nonproductive cough. Some inhalants, such as pentamidine, may stimulate coughing.

SPECIAL CONSIDERATIONS

A nonproductive, paroxysmal cough may induce life-threatening bronchospasm. The patient may need a bronchodilator to relieve his bronchospasm and open his airways. Unless he has chronic obstructive pulmonary disease, you may have to give an antitussive and a sedative to suppress the cough. To relieve mucous membrane inflammation and dryness, humidify the air in the patient's room.

As indicated, prepare the patient for diagnostic tests, such as X-rays, a lung scan, bronchoscopy, and pulmonary function tests.

PEDIATRIC POINTERS

A nonproductive cough can be difficult to evaluate in infants and young children because it can't be voluntarily induced and must be observed.

A sudden onset of paroxysmal nonproductive coughing may indicate aspiration of a foreign body—a common danger in children, especially those between 6 months and 4 years old.

Nonproductive coughing can also result from several disorders that affect infants and children. With asthma, a characteristic nonproductive "tight" cough can arise suddenly or insidiously as an attack begins. The cough usually becomes productive toward the end of the attack. With bacterial pneumonia, a nonproductive, hacking cough arises suddenly and becomes productive in 2 to 3 days. Acute bronchiolitis has a peak incidence at age 6, with paroxysms of nonproductive coughing that become more frequent as the disease progresses. Acute otitis media, which is common in infants and young children because of their short eustachian tubes, also produces nonproductive coughing.

Typically, a child with measles has a slight, nonproductive, hacking cough that increases in severity. The earliest sign of cystic fibrosis may be a nonproductive, paroxysmal cough from retained secretions. Life-threatening pertussis produces a cough that becomes paroxysmal, with an inspiratory "whoop" or crowing sound.

In addition, airway hyperactivity causes a chronic nonproductive cough that increases with exercise or exposure to cold air. Psychogenic coughing may occur when the child is under stress, emotionally stimulated, or seeking attention. A foreign body in a child's external auditory canal may result in a cough, so always examine the child's ears.

GERIATRIC POINTERS

Always ask elderly patients about nonproductive coughing because it may be an indication of serious acute or chronic illness.

PATIENT COUNSELING

Explain to the patient why nonproductive coughs should be suppressed and productive coughs encouraged. Encourage the patient to use a respirator (protective mask) in the presence of airway irritants such as paint fumes and dust. Instruct him to use a humidifier at home. Tell him to avoid using aerosols, powders, or other respiratory irritants — especially cigarettes. Make sure that the patient receives adequate fluids and nutrition.

COUGH, PRODUCTIVE

Productive coughing is the body's mechanism for clearing airway passages of accumulated secretions that normal mucociliary action doesn't remove. It's a sudden, forceful, noisy expulsion of air (from the lungs) that contains sputum or blood (or both). The sputum's color, consistency, and odor provide important clues about the patient's condition. A productive cough can occur as a single cough or as paroxysmal coughing, and it can be voluntarily induced, although it's usually a reflexive response to stimulation of the airway mucosa.

Usually due to a cardiovascular or respiratory disorder, productive coughing commonly results from an acute or chronic infection that causes inflammation, edema, and increased mucus production in the airways. However, this sign can also result from acquired immunodeficiency syndrome. Inhalation of antigenic or irritating substances or foreign bodies is an additional cause. The most common cause of chronic productive coughing is cigarette smoking, which produces mucoid sputum ranging in color from clear to yellow to brown.

EMERGENCY ACTIONS A patient with a productive cough can develop acute respiratory distress from thick or excessive secretions, bronchospasm, or fatigue, so examine him before you take his history. Take vital signs and check the rate, depth, and rhythm of respirations. Keep his airway patent, and be prepared to provide supplemental oxygen if he becomes restless or confused, or if his respirations become shallow, irregular, rapid, or slow. Look for stridor, wheezing, choking, or gurgling. Be alert for nasal flaring and cyanosis.

A productive cough may signal a severe life-threatening disorder. For example, coughing due to pulmonary edema produces thin, frothy, pink sputum, and coughing due to an asthma attack produces thick, mucoid sputum.

HISTORY

When the patient's condition permits, ask when the cough began, and find out how much sputum he's coughing up each day. (The normal tracheobronchial tree can produce up to 3 oz [88.7 ml] of sputum per day.) At what time of day does he cough up the most sputum? Does his sputum production have any relationship to what or when he eats, or to his activities or environment? Ask him if he has noticed an increase in sputum production since his coughing began. This may result from external stimuli or from such internal causes as chronic bronchial infection or a lung abscess. Also ask about the color, odor, and consistency of the sputum. Blood-tinged or rust-colored sputum may result from trauma due to coughing or from an underlying condition, such as a pulmonary infection or a tumor. Foul-smelling sputum may result from an anaerobic infection, such as bronchitis or lung abscess.

How does the cough sound? A hacking cough results from laryngeal involvement, whereas a "brassy" cough indicates major airway involvement. Does the patient feel pain associated with his productive cough? If so, ask about its location

---

Teaching points
+ Use of respirator and humidifier
+ Respiratory irritants

Key facts about productive cough
+ Sudden, forceful, expulsion of air from the lungs that's accompanied by sputum, blood, or both
+ Can result from an acute or chronic infection that causes inflammation, edema, and increased mucus production in the airways

In an emergency
+ Take vital signs.
+ Check the rate, depth, and rhythm of respirations.
+ Keep the airway patent.
+ Be prepared to provide supplemental oxygen as needed.
+ Look for stridor, wheezing, choking, or gurgling.
+ Be alert for nasal flaring and cyanosis.

Key history points
+ Onset of cough
+ Amount and description of sputum
+ Location and severity of associated pain
+ Weight and appetite changes
+ Cigarette, drug, and alcohol use
+ History of asthma, allergies, or respiratory disorders, illnesses, surgery, or trauma
+ Drug history
+ Occupational history

Critical assessment steps

- Examine the mouth and nose for congestion, drainage, or inflammation.
- Note breath odor.
- Inspect the neck for distended veins, and palpate for tenderness and masses or enlarged lymph nodes.
- Observe the chest for accessory muscle use, retractions, and uneven chest expansion.
- Percuss the chest for dullness, tympany, or flatness.
- Auscultate for pleural friction rub and abnormal breath sounds.

Medical causes

Aspiration pneumonitis

- Cough produces pink, frothy, possibly purulent sputum.

Asthma (acute)

- When dry cough progresses to productive cough mucoid sputum and mucus plugs may be produced.

Bronchiectasis

- Cough produces copious, mucopurulent sputum that has characteristic layering (top, frothy; middle, clear; bottom, dense with purulent particles).
- Sputum may smell foul or sickeningly sweet.

Bronchitis (chronic)

- Cough is nonproductive initially.
- Cough progresses to produce mucoid sputum that becomes purulent.
- Coughing usually occurs when the patient is recumbent or rises from sleep.

and severity and whether it radiates to other areas. Does coughing, changing body position, or inspiration increase or help relieve his pain?

Next, ask the patient about his cigarette, drug, and alcohol use and whether his weight or appetite has changed. Find out if he has a history of asthma, allergies, or respiratory disorders, and ask about recent illnesses, surgery, or trauma. What medications is he taking? Does he work around chemicals or respiratory irritants, such as silicone?

PHYSICAL ASSESSMENT

Examine the patient's mouth and nose for congestion, drainage, or inflammation. Note his breath odor: Halitosis can be a sign of pulmonary infection. Inspect his neck for distended veins, and palpate for tenderness and masses or enlarged lymph nodes. Observe his chest for accessory muscle use, retractions, and uneven chest expansion, and percuss for dullness, tympany, or flatness. Finally, auscultate for pleural friction rub and abnormal breath sounds — rhonchi, crackles, or wheezes.

MEDICAL CAUSES

Aspiration pneumonitis

Aspiration pneumonitis causes coughing that produces pink, frothy, possibly purulent sputum. The patient also has marked dyspnea, fever, tachypnea, fatigue, chest pain, halitosis, tachycardia, wheezing, and cyanosis.

Asthma (acute)

A severe asthma attack, which can be life-threatening, may produce mucoid, tenacious sputum and mucus plugs. Such an attack typically starts with a dry cough and mild wheezing, then progresses to severe dyspnea, audible wheezing, chest tightness, and a productive cough. Other findings include apprehension, prolonged expirations, intercostal and supraclavicular retraction on inspiration, accessory muscle use, rhonchi, crackles, flaring nostrils, tachypnea, tachycardia, diaphoresis, and flushing or cyanosis. Attacks commonly occur at night or during sleep.

Bronchiectasis

The chronic cough of bronchiectasis produces copious, mucopurulent sputum that has characteristic layering (top, frothy; middle, clear; bottom, dense with purulent particles). The patient has halitosis: His sputum may smell foul or sickeningly sweet. Other characteristic findings include hemoptysis, persistent coarse crackles over the affected lung area, occasional wheezing, rhonchi, exertional dyspnea, weight loss, fatigue, malaise, weakness, recurrent fever, and late-stage finger clubbing.

Bronchitis (chronic)

Chronic bronchitis causes a cough that may be nonproductive initially. Eventually, however, it produces mucoid sputum that becomes purulent. Secondary infection can also cause mucopurulent sputum, which may become blood-tinged and foul-smelling. The coughing, which may be paroxysmal during exercise, usually occurs when the patient is recumbent or rises from sleep.

The patient also exhibits prolonged expirations, increased use of accessory muscles for breathing, barrel chest, tachypnea, cyanosis, wheezing, exertional dyspnea, scattered rhonchi, coarse crackles (which can be precipitated by coughing), and late-stage clubbing.

Chemical pneumonitis

Chemical pneumonitis causes a cough with purulent sputum. It can also cause dyspnea, wheezing, orthopnea, fever, malaise, and crackles; mucous membrane irritation of the conjunctivae, throat, and nose; laryngitis; or rhinitis. Signs and symptoms may increase for 24 to 48 hours after exposure, then resolve; if severe, however, they may recur 2 to 5 weeks later.

Common cold

When a common cold causes productive coughing, the sputum is mucoid or mucopurulent. Early indications of the common cold include a dry, hacking cough, sneezing, headache, malaise, fatigue, rhinorrhea (watery to tenacious, mucopurulent secretions), nasal congestion, sore throat, myalgia, and arthralgia.

Legionnaires' disease

Legionnaires' disease causes a cough that produces scant mucoid, nonpurulent, possibly blood-streaked sputum. Prodromal signs and symptoms typically include malaise, fatigue, weakness, anorexia, diffuse myalgia and, possibly, diarrhea. Then, within 48 hours, the patient develops a dry cough and a sudden high fever with chills. Many patients also have pleuritic chest pain, headache, tachypnea, tachycardia, nausea, vomiting, dyspnea, crackles, mild temporary amnesia, disorientation, confusion, flushing, mild diaphoresis, and prostration.

Lung abscess (ruptured)

The cardinal sign of ruptured lung abscess is coughing that produces copious amounts of purulent, foul-smelling, possibly blood-tinged sputum. A ruptured abscess can also cause diaphoresis, anorexia, clubbing, weight loss, weakness, fatigue, fever with chills, dyspnea, headache, malaise, pleuritic chest pain, halitosis, inspiratory crackles, and tubular or amphoric breath sounds. The patient's chest is dull on percussion on the affected side.

Lung cancer

One of the earliest signs of bronchogenic carcinoma is a chronic cough that produces small amounts of purulent (or mucopurulent), blood-streaked sputum. In a patient with bronchoalveolar cancer, however, coughing produces large amounts of frothy sputum. Other signs and symptoms include dyspnea, anorexia, fatigue, weight loss, chest pain, fever, diaphoresis, wheezing, and clubbing.

Plague

Signs and symptoms of plague, caused by the bacterium *Yersinia pestis,* include fever, chills, and swollen, inflamed, and tender lymph nodes near the site of the flea bite. Septicemic plague develops as a fulminant illness generally with the bubonic form. The onset of the pneumonic form is usually sudden with chills, fever, headache, and myalgia. Pulmonary signs and symptoms include productive cough, chest pain, tachypnea, dyspnea, hemoptysis, increasing respiratory distress, and cardiopulmonary insufficiency.

Pneumonia

Bacterial pneumonia initially produces a dry cough that becomes productive. Associated signs and symptoms develop suddenly and include shaking chills, high fever, myalgia, headache, pleuritic chest pain that increases with chest movement, tachypnea, tachycardia, dyspnea, cyanosis, diaphoresis, decreased breath sounds, fine crackles, and rhonchi.

Medical causes
(continued)

Chemical pneumonitis
+ Cough produces purulent sputum.

Common cold
+ If present, sputum is mucoid or mucopurulent.

Legionnaires' disease
+ Cough produces scant mucoid, nonpurulent, possibly blood-streaked sputum.

Lung abscess (ruptured)
+ Coughing, a cardinal sign, produces purulent, foul-smelling, possibly blood-tinged sputum.

Lung cancer
+ Chronic cough that produces small amounts of purulent (or mucopurulent), blood-streaked sputum is an early sign.

Plague
+ Pulmonary signs and symptoms include productive cough, chest pain, tachypnea, dyspnea, hemoptysis, increasing respiratory distress, and cardiopulmonary insufficiency.

Pneumonia
+ Dry cough becomes productive.
+ Associated signs and symptoms, such as shaking chills, high fever, and myalgia, develop suddenly.

Medical causes
(continued)

Pulmonary edema

✦ Early signs and symptoms include exertional dyspnea; paroxysmal nocturnal dyspnea, followed by orthopnea; and nonproductive coughing that eventually produces frothy, bloody sputum.

Pulmonary embolism

✦ Cough may be nonproductive or may produce blood-tinged sputum.
✦ Usually, the first symptom is severe dyspnea, which may be accompanied by angina or pleuritic chest pain.

Pulmonary emphysema

✦ Chronic cough produces scant, mucoid, translucent, grayish white sputum that can become mucopurulent.

Pulmonary tuberculosis

✦ Mild to severe productive cough occurs; sputum may be scant and mucoid or copious and purulent.

Silicosis

✦ A productive cough with mucopurulent sputum is the earliest sign.

Tracheobronchitis

✦ After the onset of chills, sore throat, fever, muscle and back pain, and substernal tightness, cough becomes productive.
✦ Sputum is mucoid, mucopurulent, or purulent.

Pulmonary edema

Severe, pulmonary edema is a life-threatening disorder that causes a cough that produces frothy, bloody sputum. Early signs and symptoms of pulmonary edema include exertional dyspnea; paroxysmal nocturnal dyspnea, followed by orthopnea; and coughing, which may be nonproductive initially. Others include fever, fatigue, tachycardia, tachypnea, dependent crackles, and ventricular gallop. As the patient's respirations become increasingly rapid and labored, he develops more diffuse crackles and a productive cough, worsening tachycardia and, possibly, arrhythmias. His skin becomes cold, clammy, and cyanotic; his blood pressure falls; and his pulse becomes thready.

Pulmonary embolism

Pulmonary embolism is a life-threatening disorder that causes a cough that may be nonproductive or may produce blood-tinged sputum. Usually, the first symptom of a pulmonary embolism is severe dyspnea, which may be accompanied by angina or pleuritic chest pain. The patient experiences marked anxiety, a low-grade fever, tachycardia, tachypnea, and diaphoresis. Less common signs include massive hemoptysis, chest splinting, leg edema and, with a large embolus, cyanosis, syncope, and distended neck veins. The patient may also have a pleural friction rub, diffuse wheezing, crackles, chest dullness on percussion, decreased breath sounds, and signs of circulatory collapse.

Pulmonary emphysema

Pulmonary emphysema causes a chronic productive cough with scant, mucoid, translucent, grayish white sputum that can become mucopurulent. The patient is thin and has the characteristic "pink puffer" appearance with weight loss, increased accessory muscle use, tachypnea, grunting expirations through pursed lips, diminished breath sounds, exertional dyspnea, rhonchi, barrel chest, and anorexia. Clubbing is a late sign.

Pulmonary tuberculosis

Pulmonary tuberculosis causes a mild to severe productive cough along with some combination of hemoptysis, malaise, dyspnea, and pleuritic chest pain. Sputum may be scant and mucoid or copious and purulent. Typically, the patient experiences night sweats, easy fatigability, and weight loss. His breath sounds are amphoric. He may have chest dullness on percussion and, after coughing, increased tactile fremitus with crackles.

Silicosis

A productive cough with mucopurulent sputum is the earliest sign of silicosis. The patient also has exertional dyspnea, tachypnea, weight loss, fatigue, general weakness, and recurrent respiratory infections. Auscultation reveals end-inspiratory, fine crackles at the lung bases.

Tracheobronchitis

With tracheobronchitis, inflammation initially causes a nonproductive cough that later — following the onset of chills, sore throat, slight fever, muscle and back pain, and substernal tightness — becomes productive as secretions increase. Sputum is mucoid, mucopurulent, or purulent. The patient typically has rhonchi and wheezes; he may also develop crackles. Severe tracheobronchitis may cause a fever of 101° to 102° F (38.3° to 38.9° C) and bronchospasm.

OTHER CAUSES

Diagnostic tests

Bronchoscopy and pulmonary function tests may increase productive coughing.

Drugs

Expectorants, of course, increase productive coughing. These include guaifenesin, potassium iodide, and terpin hydrate.

Respiratory therapy

Intermittent positive-pressure breathing, nebulizer therapy, and incentive spirometry can help loosen secretions and cause or increase productive coughing.

SPECIAL CONSIDERATIONS

Avoid taking measures to suppress a productive cough because retention of sputum may interfere with alveolar aeration or impair pulmonary resistance to infection. Expect to give a mucolytic and an expectorant, and increase the patient's intake of oral fluids to thin his secretions and increase their flow. In addition, you may give a bronchodilator to relieve bronchospasms and open airways. An antibiotic may be ordered to treat underlying infection.

Humidify the air around the patient; this will relieve mucous membrane inflammation and help loosen dried secretions. Provide pulmonary physiotherapy, such as postural drainage with vibration and percussion, to loosen secretions. Aerosol therapy may be necessary.

Provide the patient with uninterrupted rest periods. Keep him from using respiratory irritants. If he's confined to bed rest, change his position often to promote the drainage of secretions.

Prepare the patient for diagnostic tests, such as chest X-ray, bronchoscopy, a lung scan, and pulmonary function tests. Collect sputum specimens for culture and sensitivity testing.

PEDIATRIC POINTERS

Because his airway is narrow, a child with a productive cough can quickly develop airway occlusion and respiratory distress from thick or excessive secretions. Causes of a productive cough in children include asthma, bronchiectasis, bronchitis, acute bronchiolitis, cystic fibrosis, and pertussis.

When caring for a child with a productive cough, administer expectorants, but don't expect to give a cough suppressant. To soothe inflamed mucous membranes and prevent drying of secretions, provide humidified air or oxygen. Remember, high humidity can induce bronchospasm in a hyperactive child or produce overhydration in an infant.

GERIATRIC POINTERS

Always ask elderly patients about a productive cough because this sign may indicate a serious acute or chronic illness.

PATIENT COUNSELING

Encourage the patient not to smoke because doing so can aggravate his condition. Explain that quitting even after decades of use is helpful. Teach him how to breathe deeply, to cough effectively and, if appropriate, to splint his incision when he coughs. Tell him to sit or stand upright when coughing, if possible, to facilitate

Other causes
- Bronchoscopy
- Expectorants
- Incentive spirometry, intermittent positive-pressure breathing, and nebulizer therapy
- Pulmonary function tests

Special considerations
- Expect to give a mucolytic and an expectorant.
- Increase intake of oral fluids.
- Give a bronchodilator.
- Give antibiotics as ordered.
- Humidify the air.
- Provide pulmonary physiotherapy to loosen secretions.
- Provide rest periods.
- Keep the patient from using respiratory irritants.
- If on bed rest, change the patient's position often.
- Collect sputum specimens for culture and sensitivity testing.

Peds points
- A child with a productive cough can quickly develop airway occlusion and respiratory distress.
- Causes of a productive cough in children include asthma, bronchiectasis, bronchitis, acute bronchiolitis, cystic fibrosis, and pertussis.

Geri points
- Productive cough may indicate a serious acute or chronic illness.

Teaching points
- Stopping smoking
- Coughing and deep-breathing techniques
- Chest percussion
- Protection from secretions

maximum chest expansion. Teach the patient and his family how to use chest percussion to loosen secretions.

Tell the patient to cover his mouth and nose with a tissue when he coughs and to dispose of contaminated tissues properly, to protect himself and others from the cough and secretions. Be sure to provide a container for tissues and sputum.

Key facts about crackles

+ Also known as *rales* or *crepitations*
+ Described as nonmusical clicking or rattling noises heard during auscultation of breath sounds
+ Can be unilateral or bilateral, moist or dry
+ Indicate abnormal movement of air through fluid-filled airways

In an emergency

+ Take vital signs.
+ Examine for signs of respiratory distress or airway obstruction.
+ Check the depth and rhythm of respirations.
+ Check for increased accessory muscle use and chest wall motion, retractions, stridor, or nasal flaring.
+ Provide supplemental oxygen.
+ Be aware that endotracheal intubation may be necessary.

Key history points

+ Onset, duration, and description of associated cough and pain
+ Medical history, including cancer, respiratory or cardiovascular problems, surgery, or trauma
+ Smoking and alcohol use
+ Drug and medical history
+ Recent weight loss, anorexia, nausea, vomiting, fatigue, weakness, vertigo, and syncope
+ Exposure to respiratory irritants

CRACKLES

A common finding in patients with certain cardiovascular and pulmonary disorders, crackles are nonmusical clicking or rattling noises heard during auscultation of breath sounds. Also known as *rales* or *crepitations,* they usually occur during inspiration and recur constantly from one respiratory cycle to the next. They can be unilateral or bilateral, moist or dry. They're characterized by their pitch, loudness, location, persistence, and occurrence during the respiratory cycle.

Crackles indicate abnormal movement of air through fluid-filled airways. They can be irregularly dispersed, as in pneumonia, or localized, as in bronchiectasis. (A few basilar crackles can be heard in normal lungs after prolonged shallow breathing. These normal crackles clear with a few deep breaths.) Usually, crackles indicate the degree of an underlying illness. When crackles result from a generalized disorder, they usually occur in the less distended and more dependent areas of the lungs such as the lung bases when the patient is standing. Crackles due to air passing through inflammatory exudate may not be audible if the involved portion of the lung isn't being ventilated because of shallow respirations. (See *How crackles occur.*)

EMERGENCY ACTIONS

Quickly take the patient's vital signs and examine him for signs of respiratory distress or airway obstruction. Check the depth and rhythm of respirations. Is he struggling to breathe? Check for increased accessory muscle use and chest wall motion, retractions, stridor, or nasal flaring. Provide supplemental oxygen. Endotracheal intubation may be necessary. (See *Associated disorder: Pulmonary edema,* page 180.)

HISTORY

If the patient also has a cough, ask when it began and if it's constant or intermittent. Find out what the cough sounds like and whether he's coughing up sputum or blood. If the cough is productive, determine the sputum's consistency, amount, odor, and color.

Ask the patient if he has pain. If so, where is it located? When did he first notice it? Does it radiate to other areas? Also, ask the patient if movement, coughing, or breathing worsens or helps relieve his pain. Note the patient's position: Is he lying still or moving about restlessly?

Obtain a brief medical history. Does the patient have cancer or any known respiratory or cardiovascular problems? Ask about recent surgery, trauma, or illness. Does he smoke or drink alcohol? Is he experiencing hoarseness or difficulty swallowing? Find out which medications he's taking. Also, ask about recent weight loss, anorexia, nausea, vomiting, fatigue, weakness, vertigo, and syncope. Has the patient been exposed to irritants, such as vapors, fumes, or smoke?

PHYSICAL ASSESSMENT

Perform a physical examination. Examine the patient's nose and mouth for signs of infection, such as inflammation or increased secretions. Note his breath odor: Hali-

How crackles occur

Crackles occur when air passes through fluid-filled airways, causing collapsed alveoli to pop open as the airway pressure equalizes. They can also occur when membranes lining the chest cavity and the lungs become inflamed. The illustrations below show a normal alveolus and two pathologic alveolar changes that cause crackles.

NORMAL ALVEOLUS

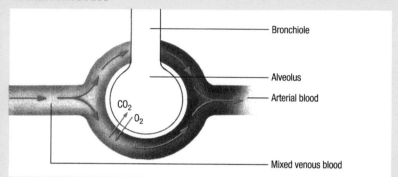

Bronchiole
Alveolus
Arterial blood
Mixed venous blood

ALVEOLUS IN PULMONARY EDEMA

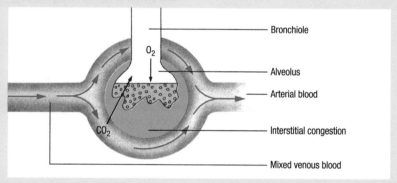

Bronchiole
Alveolus
Arterial blood
Interstitial congestion
Mixed venous blood

ALVEOLUS IN INFLAMMATION

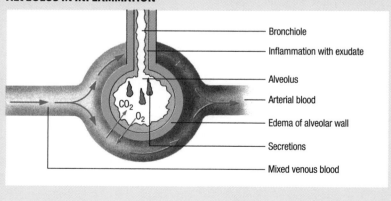

Bronchiole
Inflammation with exudate
Alveolus
Arterial blood
Edema of alveolar wall
Secretions
Mixed venous blood

Critical assessment steps

+ Examine the nose and mouth for signs of infection.
+ Note breath odor.
+ Check the neck for masses, tenderness, lymphadenopathy, swelling, or venous distention.
+ Inspect the chest for abnormal configuration or uneven expansion, and percuss for dullness, tympany, or flatness.
+ Auscultate the lungs for other abnormal, diminished, or absent breath sounds.
+ Listen for abnormal heart sounds.
+ Check the hands and feet for edema or clubbing.

Key facts about pulmonary edema

+ Involves an accumulation of fluid in the extravascular spaces of the lungs
+ Is a complication of cardiac disorders that can develop quickly and rapidly become fatal

Causes

+ Left-sided heart failure

Management

+ High concentrations of oxygen administered by nasal cannula
+ Assisted ventilation
+ Diuretics, positive inotropic agents, pressor agents, antiarrhythmics, arterial vasodilators, morphine

ASSOCIATED DISORDER

Pulmonary edema

Pulmonary edema is an accumulation of fluid in the extravascular spaces of the lungs. It's a common complication of cardiac disorders and may develop quickly and rapidly become fatal.

CAUSES

Pulmonary edema is caused by left-sided heart failure due to:

+ arteriosclerosis
+ cardiomyopathy
+ hypertension
+ valvular heart disease.

Factors that predispose the patient to pulmonary edema include:

+ barbiturate or opiate poisoning
+ cardiac failure
+ excess infusion of I.V. fluids or overly rapid infusion
+ impaired pulmonary lymphatic drainage (from Hodgkin's disease or obliterative lymphangitis after radiation)
+ inhalation of irritating gases
+ mitral stenosis and left atrial myxoma (which impairs left atrial emptying)
+ pneumonia
+ pulmonary venoocclusive disease.

DIAGNOSIS

These test results help diagnose pulmonary edema:

+ Arterial blood gas analysis usually reveals hypoxia with variable partial pressure of arterial carbon dioxide, depending on the patient's degree of fatigue. Respiratory acidosis may occur.
+ Chest X-ray shows diffuse haziness of the lung fields and, usually, cardiomegaly and pleural effusion.
+ Pulse oximetry may reveal decreasing arterial oxygen saturation levels.
+ Pulmonary artery catheterization identifies left-sided heart failure and helps rule out acute respiratory distress syndrome.
+ Electrocardiography may show previous or current myocardial infarction.

MEDICAL INTERVENTIONS

Treatment of pulmonary edema is designed to reduce extravascular fluid, to improve gas exchange and myocardial function and, if possible, to correct underlying pathologic conditions. Correcting this disorder typically involves:

+ high concentrations of oxygen administered by nasal cannula to enhance gas exchange and improve oxygenation
+ assisted ventilation to improve oxygen delivery to the tissues and promote acid-base balance
+ diuretics, such as furosemide, and bumetanide, to increase urination, which helps mobilize extravascular fluid
+ positive inotropic agents, such as digoxin and inamrinone, to enhance contractility in myocardial dysfunction
+ pressor agents to enhance contractility and promote vasoconstriction in peripheral vessels
+ antiarrhythmics for arrhythmias related to decreased cardiac output
+ arterial vasodilators, such as nitroprusside, to decrease peripheral vascular resistance, preload, and afterload
+ morphine to reduce anxiety and dyspnea and to dilate the systemic venous bed, promoting blood flow from pulmonary circulation to the periphery.

tosis could indicate pulmonary infection. Check his neck for masses, tenderness, swelling, lymphadenopathy, or venous distention.

Inspect the patient's chest for abnormal configuration or uneven expansion. Percuss for dullness, tympany, or flatness. Auscultate his lungs for other abnormal, diminished, or absent breath sounds. Listen to his heart for abnormal sounds, and check his hands and feet for edema or clubbing.

MEDICAL CAUSES

Acute respiratory distress syndrome

Acute respiratory distress syndrome (ARDS), a life-threatening disorder, causes diffuse, fine to coarse crackles usually heard in the dependent portions of the lungs. It also produces cyanosis, nasal flaring, tachypnea, tachycardia, grunting respirations, rhonchi, dyspnea, anxiety, and decreased level of consciousness.

Asthma (acute)

A severe asthma attack usually occurs at night or during sleep, causing dry, whistling crackles. An attack typically starts with a dry cough and mild wheezing and progresses to severe dyspnea, audible wheezing, chest tightness, and productive cough. Other findings include apprehension, prolonged expirations, rhonchi, intercostal and supraclavicular retraction on inspiration, accessory muscle use, flaring nostrils, tachypnea, tachycardia, diaphoresis, and flushing or cyanosis.

Bronchiectasis

With bronchiectasis, persistent, coarse crackles are heard over the affected area of the lung. They're accompanied by a chronic cough that produces copious amounts of mucopurulent sputum. Other characteristics include halitosis, occasional wheezes, exertional dyspnea, rhonchi, weight loss, fatigue, malaise, weakness, recurrent fever, and late-stage clubbing.

Bronchitis (chronic)

Chronic bronchitis causes coarse crackles that are usually heard at the lung bases. Prolonged expirations, wheezing, rhonchi, exertional dyspnea, tachypnea, and persistent, productive cough occur because of increased bronchial secretions. Clubbing and cyanosis may occur.

Chemical pneumonitis

With acute chemical pneumonitis, diffuse, fine to coarse, moist crackles accompany a productive cough with purulent sputum, dyspnea, wheezing, orthopnea, fever, malaise, and mucous membrane irritation. Signs and symptoms may worsen for 24 to 48 hours after exposure, then resolve; if severe, however, they may recur 2 to 5 weeks later.

Interstitial fibrosis of the lungs

With interstitial fibrosis of the lungs, cellophane-like crackles can be heard over all lobes. As the disease progresses, a nonproductive cough, dyspnea, fatigue, weight loss, cyanosis, and pleuritic chest pain develop. Nasal flaring and use of accessory muscles may be evident.

Legionnaires' disease

Legionnaires' disease produces diffuse moist crackles and cough productive of scant mucoid, nonpurulent, possibly blood-streaked sputum. Usually, prodromal signs and symptoms occur, including malaise, fatigue, weakness, anorexia, diffuse myalgia and, possibly, diarrhea. Within 12 to 48 hours, the patient develops a dry cough and a sudden high fever with chills. He may also have pleuritic chest pain, headache, tachypnea, tachycardia, nausea, vomiting, dyspnea, mild temporary amnesia, confusion, flushing, mild diaphoresis, and prostration.

Lung abscess

A lung abscess produces fine to medium and moist inspiratory crackles. The onset is insidious; signs and symptoms include sweats, anorexia, weight loss, fever, fatigue, weakness, dyspnea, clubbing, pleuritic chest pain, pleural friction rub, and a cough producing copious amounts of foul-smelling, purulent sputum that may be

Medical causes

ARDS
+ Diffuse, fine to coarse crackles are usually heard in the dependent portions of the lungs.

Asthma (acute)
+ Dry, whistling crackles occur.

Bronchiectasis
+ Persistent, coarse crackles are heard over the affected area of the lung.

Bronchitis (chronic)
+ Coarse crackles are usually heard at the lung base.
+ Prolonged expirations, wheezing, rhonchi, and persistent, productive cough also occur.

Chemical pneumonitis
+ Diffuse, fine to coarse, moist crackles can be heard.

Interstitial fibrosis of the lungs
+ Cellophane-like crackles can be heard over all lobes.

Legionnaires' disease
+ Diffuse moist crackles can be heard.

Lung abscess
+ Fine to medium and moist inspiratory crackles occur.

Medical causes
(continued)

Pneumonia
+ Bacterial pneumonia produces diffuse fine crackles.
+ Mycoplasma pneumonia produces medium to fine crackles.
+ Viral pneumonia causes gradually developing, diffuse crackles.

Pulmonary edema
+ Moist, bubbling crackles on inspiration are one of the first signs.

Pulmonary embolism
+ Fine to coarse crackles occur.
+ Severe dyspnea is usually the first sign.

Pulmonary tuberculosis
+ Fine crackles occur after coughing.

Sarcoidosis
+ Patient has fine, bibasilar, end-inspiratory crackles.

Silicosis
+ End-inspiratory, fine crackles are heard at the lung bases.

Tracheobronchitis
+ Moist or coarse crackles occur.

blood-tinged. The patient's breath sounds are hollow and tubular or amphoric; the affected side of his chest is dull on percussion.

Pneumonia
Bacterial pneumonia produces diffuse fine crackles, sudden onset of shaking chills, high fever, tachypnea, pleuritic chest pain, cyanosis, grunting respirations, nasal flaring, decreased breath sounds, myalgia, headache, tachycardia, dyspnea, cyanosis, diaphoresis, and rhonchi. The patient also has a dry cough that later becomes productive.

Mycoplasma pneumonia produces medium to fine crackles with a nonproductive cough, malaise, sore throat, headache, and fever. The patient may have blood-flecked sputum. *Viral pneumonia* causes gradually developing, diffuse crackles. The patient may also have a nonproductive cough, malaise, headache, anorexia, low-grade fever, and decreased breath sounds.

Pulmonary edema
Moist, bubbling crackles on inspiration are one of the first signs of pulmonary edema, a life-threatening disorder. Other early findings of pulmonary edema include exertional dyspnea; paroxysmal nocturnal dyspnea, then orthopnea; and coughing, which may be initially nonproductive but later produces frothy, bloody sputum. Related clinical effects include tachycardia, tachypnea, and a third heart sound (S_3 gallop). As the patient's respirations become increasingly rapid and labored, he develops more diffuse crackles, worsening tachycardia, hypotension, a rapid and thready pulse, cyanosis, and cold, clammy skin.

Pulmonary embolism
Pulmonary embolism is a life-threatening disorder that can cause fine to coarse crackles and a cough that may be dry or produce blood-tinged sputum. Usually, the first sign of pulmonary embolism is severe dyspnea, which may be accompanied by angina or pleuritic chest pain. The patient has marked anxiety, a low-grade fever, tachycardia, tachypnea, and diaphoresis. Less common signs include massive hemoptysis, chest splinting, leg edema and, with a large embolus, cyanosis, syncope, and distended neck veins. The patient may also have a pleural friction rub, diffuse wheezing, chest dullness on percussion, decreased breath sounds, and signs of circulatory collapse.

Pulmonary tuberculosis
With pulmonary tuberculosis, fine crackles occur after coughing. The patient has some combination of hemoptysis, malaise, dyspnea, and pleuritic chest pain. Sputum may be scant and mucoid or copious and purulent. Typically, the patient is easily fatigued and experiences night sweats, weakness, and weight loss. His breath sounds are amphoric.

Sarcoidosis
Sarcoidosis produces fine, bibasilar, end-inspiratory crackles and, rarely, wheezing. The patient doesn't have a fever but does have malaise, fatigue, weakness, weight loss, cough, dyspnea, and tachypnea.

Silicosis
Silicosis produces end-inspiratory, fine crackles heard at the lung bases. It also causes a productive cough with mucopurulent sputum — the earliest sign of this disorder. The patient also exhibits exertional dyspnea, tachypnea, weight loss, fatigue, general weakness, and recurrent respiratory tract infections.

Tracheobronchitis

In its acute form, tracheobronchitis produces moist or coarse crackles along with a productive cough, chills, sore throat, slight fever, muscle and back pain, and substernal tightness. The patient typically has rhonchi and wheezes. Severe tracheobronchitis may cause moderate fever and bronchospasm.

SPECIAL CONSIDERATIONS

To keep the patient's airway patent and facilitate his breathing, elevate the head of his bed. To liquefy thick secretions and relieve mucous membrane inflammation, administer fluids, humidified air, or oxygen. Diuretics may be needed if crackles result from cardiogenic pulmonary edema. Turn the patient every 1 to 2 hours, and encourage him to breathe deeply.

Plan daily uninterrupted rest periods to help the patient relax and sleep. Prepare the patient for diagnostic tests, such as chest X-rays, a lung scan, and sputum analysis.

PEDIATRIC POINTERS

Crackles in an infant or child may indicate a serious cardiovascular or respiratory disorder. Pneumonias produce diffuse, sudden crackles in children. Esophageal atresia and tracheoesophageal fistula can cause bubbling, moist crackles due to aspiration of food or secretions into the lungs—especially in neonates. Pulmonary edema causes fine crackles at the bases of the lungs, and bronchiectasis produces moist crackles. Cystic fibrosis produces widespread, fine to coarse inspiratory crackles and wheezing in infants. Sickle cell anemia may produce crackles when it causes pulmonary infarction or infection.

GERIATRIC POINTERS

Crackles that clear after deep breathing may indicate mild basilar atelectasis. In older patients, auscultate lung bases before and after auscultating apices.

PATIENT COUNSELING

Teach the patient how to cough effectively and splint incision areas if appropriate. Encourage him to avoid smoking and using aerosols, powders, or other products that might irritate his airways.

CREPITATION, BONY

Bony crepitation, or bony crepitus, is a palpable vibration or an audible crunching sound that results when one bone grates against another. This sign commonly results from a fracture, but it can happen when bones that have been stripped of their protective articular cartilage grind against each other as they articulate—for example, in patients with advanced arthritic or degenerative joint disorders.

Eliciting bony crepitation can help confirm the diagnosis of a fracture, but it can also cause further soft tissue, nerve, or vessel injury. Always evaluate distal pulses and perform neurologic checks distal to the suspected fracture site before manipulation of an extremity. In addition, rubbing fractured bone ends together can convert a closed fracture into an open one if a bone end penetrates the skin. Therefore, after the initial detection of crepitation in a patient with a fracture, avoid subsequent elicitation of this sign.

Special considerations
+ Elevate the head of the bed.
+ Administer fluids, humidified air, or oxygen.
+ Be aware that diuretics may be needed if crackles result from cardiogenic pulmonary edema.
+ Turn the patient every 1 to 2 hours, and encourage deep breathing.
+ Plan daily rest periods.

Peds points
+ Pneumonias produce diffuse, sudden crackles.
+ Esophageal atresia and tracheoesophageal fistula can cause bubbling, moist crackles.
+ Pulmonary edema causes fine crackles.
+ Bronchiectasis produces moist crackles.
+ Cystic fibrosis produces widespread, fine to coarse inspiratory crackles in infants.
+ Sickle cell anemia may produce crackles.

Geri points
+ Crackles that clear after deep breathing may indicate mild basilar atelectasis.

Teaching points
+ Effective coughing techniques
+ Avoiding smoking and irritants

Key facts about bony crepitation
+ Palpable vibration or audible crunching sound that results when one bone grates against another

Key history points

+ History of osteoarthritis or rheumatoid arthritis
+ Drug history
+ Location of pain
+ Details of injury

Critical assessment steps

+ Inspect for abrasions or lacerations.
+ Palpate pulses distal to the injury site.
+ Check skin for pallor or coolness.
+ Test motor and sensory function distal to the injury site.
+ Take vital signs.
+ Test joint ROM only if a fracture isn't suspected.

Medical causes

Fracture
+ Bony crepitation occurs with acute local pain, hematoma, edema, and decreased ROM.

Osteoarthritis
+ Soft fine crepitus on palpation may indicate roughening of the articular cartilage.
+ Coarse grating may indicate badly damaged cartilage.

Rheumatoid arthritis
+ In advanced form, bony crepitation is heard when the affected joint is rotated.

Special considerations

If a fracture is suspected:
+ Prepare the patient for X-rays.
+ Reexamine neurovascular status frequently.
+ Keep the affected part immobilized and elevated.
+ Give an analgesic to relieve pain.

HISTORY

If the patient doesn't have a suspected fracture, ask about a history of osteoarthritis or rheumatoid arthritis. Which medications does he take? Has any medication helped ease arthritic discomfort? If you detect bony crepitation in a patient with a suspected fracture, ask him if he feels pain and if he can point to the painful area. Find out how and when the injury occurred. To prevent lacerating nerves, blood vessels, or other structures, immobilize the affected area by applying a splint that includes the joints above and below the affected area. Elevate the affected area, if possible, and apply cold packs.

PHYSICAL ASSESSMENT

Inspect for abrasions or lacerations. Palpate pulses distal to the injury site; check the skin for pallor or coolness. Test motor and sensory function distal to the injury site. Take the patient's vital signs. Test joint range of motion (ROM) only if a fracture isn't suspected.

MEDICAL CAUSES

Fracture
In addition to bony crepitation, a fracture causes acute local pain, hematoma, edema, and decreased ROM. Other findings may include deformity, point tenderness, discoloration of the limb, and loss of limb function. Neurovascular damage may cause increased capillary refill time, diminished or absent pulses, mottled cyanosis, paresthesia, and decreased sensation (all distal to the fracture site). An open fracture, of course, produces an obvious skin wound.

Osteoarthritis
In the advanced form of osteoarthritis, joint crepitation may be elicited during ROM testing. Soft fine crepitus on palpation may indicate roughening of the articular cartilage; coarse grating may indicate badly damaged cartilage. The cardinal symptom of osteoarthritis is joint pain, especially during motion and weight bearing. Other findings include joint stiffness that typically occurs after resting and subsides within a few minutes after the patient begins moving.

Rheumatoid arthritis
In the advanced form of rheumatoid arthritis, bony crepitation is heard when the affected joint is rotated. However, rheumatoid arthritis usually develops insidiously, producing nonspecific signs and symptoms, such as fatigue, malaise, anorexia, a persistent low-grade fever, weight loss, lymphadenopathy, and vague arthralgia and myalgia. Later, more specific and localized articular signs develop, commonly at the proximal finger joints. These signs usually occur bilaterally and symmetrically and may extend to the wrists, knees, elbows, and ankles. The affected joints stiffen after inactivity. The patient also has increased warmth, swelling, and tenderness of affected joints as well as limited ROM.

SPECIAL CONSIDERATIONS

If a fracture is suspected, prepare the patient for X-rays of the affected area, and reexamine his neurovascular status frequently. Keep the affected part immobilized and elevated until treatment begins. Give an analgesic to relieve pain.

PEDIATRIC POINTERS

Bony crepitation in a child usually occurs after a fracture. Obtain an accurate history of the injury, and be alert for the possibility of child abuse. In a teenager, bony crepitation and pain in the patellofemoral joint help diagnose chondromalacia of the patella.

GERIATRIC POINTERS

Degenerative joint changes, which have usually begun by age 20 or 30, progress more rapidly after age 40 and occur primarily in weight-bearing joints, such as the lumbar spine, hips, knees, and ankles.

PATIENT COUNSELING

Teach the patient about activity limitations. Show him how to perform complete skin and foot care. Discuss proper use of ambulatory aids, such as walkers, canes, and crutches, and body mechanics to prevent injury. Encourage him to perform activities of daily living when possible to maintain independence, muscle strength, and joint ROM. If the patient has a fracture, demonstrate proper cast care.

CREPITATION, SUBCUTANEOUS

When bubbles of air or other gases (such as carbon dioxide) are trapped in subcutaneous tissue, palpation or stroking of the skin produces a crackling sound called *subcutaneous crepitation* or *subcutaneous emphysema.* The bubbles feel like small, unstable nodules and aren't painful, even though subcutaneous crepitation is commonly associated with painful disorders. Usually, the affected tissue is visibly edematous; this can lead to life-threatening airway occlusion if the edema affects the neck or upper chest.

The air or gas bubbles enter the tissues through open wounds from the action of anaerobic microorganisms or from traumatic or spontaneous rupture or perforation of pulmonary or GI organs.

 EMERGENCY ACTIONS If the patient shows signs of respiratory distress — such as severe dyspnea, tachypnea, accessory muscle use, nasal flaring, air hunger, or tachycardia — quickly test for Hamman's sign to detect trapped air bubbles in the mediastinum. (See *Testing for Hamman's sign,* page 186.)

Anticipate endotracheal intubation, an emergency tracheotomy, or chest tube insertion. Administer supplemental oxygen and start an I.V. line to administer fluids and medication. Connect the patient to a cardiac monitor.

If the patient has an open wound with a foul odor and local swelling take his vital signs, checking especially for fever, tachycardia, hypotension, and tachypnea. Next, start an I.V. line to administer fluids and medication, and provide supplemental oxygen. Anticipate emergency surgery to drain and debride the wound or hyperbaric chamber treatment.

HISTORY

Because subcutaneous crepitation can indicate a life-threatening disorder, you'll need to perform a rapid initial evaluation and intervene if necessary. Ask the patient if he's experiencing pain or having difficulty breathing. If he's in pain, find out where the pain is located, how severe it is, and when it began. Ask about recent tho-

Peds points
✦ Bony crepitation usually occurs after a fracture; be alert for child abuse.
✦ In a teenager, bony crepitation and pain in the patellofemoral joint help diagnose chondromalacia of the patella.

Geri points
✦ Degenerative joint changes progress more rapidly after age 40

Teaching points
✦ Activity limitations
✦ Skin, foot, and cast care
✦ Use of ambulatory aids

Key facts about subcutaneous crepitation
✦ Results from trapping of air bubbles and other gases in the subcutaneous tissue
✦ Presents as a crackling sound upon palpation

In an emergency
For signs of respiratory distress:
✦ Test for Hamman's sign.
✦ Anticipate endotracheal intubation or chest tube insertion.
✦ Provide supplemental oxygen.
✦ Start an I.V. line.
✦ Connect the patient to a cardiac monitor.

Key history points
✦ Onset, location, and severity of any associated pain
✦ Medical history

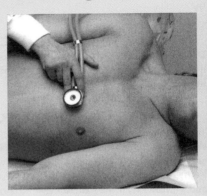

Testing for Hamman's sign

To test for Hamman's sign, help the patient assume a left-lateral recumbent position. Then place your stethoscope over the precordium. If you hear a loud crunching sound that synchronizes with his heartbeat, the patient has a positive Hamman's sign.

Critical assessment steps

+ Palpate the affected skin.
+ Repalpate frequently to determine if the subcutaneous crepitation is increasing.
+ Perform abbreviated cardiac, pulmonary, and GI assessments as the patient's condition allows.
+ When the patient is stabilized, perform a complete physical examination.

Medical causes

Orbital fracture
+ Air from the nasal sinuses escapes into subcutaneous tissue, causing subcutaneous crepitation of the eyelid and orbit.
+ The most common sign is periorbital ecchymosis.

Pneumothorax
+ Subcutaneous crepitation occurs in the upper chest and neck in severe cases.

Rupture of the esophagus
+ Subcutaneous crepitation may be palpable in the neck, chest wall, or supraclavicular fossa, but it doesn't always occur.

racic surgery, diagnostic tests, and respiratory therapy or a history of trauma or chronic pulmonary disease.

PHYSICAL ASSESSMENT

Palpate the affected skin to evaluate the location and extent of subcutaneous crepitation and to obtain baseline information. Repalpate frequently to determine if the subcutaneous crepitation is increasing. Then perform abbreviated cardiac, pulmonary, and GI assessments as the patient's condition allows. When the patient is stabilized, perform a complete physical examination.

MEDICAL CAUSES

Orbital fracture
An orbital fracture allows air from the nasal sinuses to escape into subcutaneous tissue, causing subcutaneous crepitation of the eyelid and orbit. The most common sign of orbital fracture is periorbital ecchymosis. Visual acuity is usually normal, although a swollen lid may prevent accurate testing. The patient has facial edema, diplopia, a hyphema and, occasionally, a dilated or unreactive pupil on the affected side. Extraocular movements may also be affected.

Pneumothorax
Severe pneumothorax produces subcutaneous crepitation in the upper chest and neck. In many cases, the patient has chest pain that's unilateral, rarely localized initially, and increased on inspiration. Dyspnea, anxiety, restlessness, tachypnea, cyanosis, tachycardia, accessory muscle use, asymmetrical chest expansion, and a nonproductive cough can also occur. On the affected side, breath sounds are absent or decreased, hyperresonance or tympany may be heard, and decreased vocal fremitus may be present.

Rupture of the esophagus
A ruptured esophagus usually produces subcutaneous crepitation in the neck, chest wall, or supraclavicular fossa, although this sign doesn't always occur. With a rupture of the cervical esophagus, the patient has excruciating pain in the neck or

supraclavicular area, his neck is resistant to passive motion, and he has local tenderness, soft-tissue swelling, dysphagia, odynophagia, and orthostatic vertigo.

Life-threatening rupture of the intrathoracic esophagus can produce mediastinal emphysema confirmed by a positive Hamman's sign. The patient has severe retrosternal, epigastric, neck, or scapular pain and edema of the chest wall and neck. He may also display dyspnea, tachypnea, asymmetrical chest expansion, nasal flaring, cyanosis, diaphoresis, tachycardia, hypotension, dysphagia, and fever.

Rupture of the trachea or major bronchus

Rupture of the trachea or major bronchus is a life-threatening injury that produces abrupt subcutaneous crepitation of the neck and anterior chest wall. The patient has severe dyspnea with nasal flaring, tachycardia, accessory muscle use, hypotension, cyanosis, extreme anxiety and, possibly, hemoptysis and mediastinal emphysema, with a positive Hamman's sign.

OTHER CAUSES

Diagnostic tests

Endoscopic tests, such as bronchoscopy and upper GI tract endoscopy, can rupture or perforate respiratory or GI organs, producing subcutaneous crepitation.

Respiratory treatments

Mechanical ventilation and intermittent positive-pressure breathing can rupture alveoli, producing subcutaneous crepitation.

Thoracic surgery

If air escapes into the tissue in the area of the incision, subcutaneous crepitation can occur.

SPECIAL CONSIDERATIONS

Monitor the patient's vital signs frequently, especially respirations. Because excessive edema from subcutaneous crepitation in the neck and upper chest can cause airway obstruction, be alert for signs of respiratory distress such as dyspnea. Tell the patient that the affected tissues will eventually absorb the air or gas bubbles, so the subcutaneous crepitation will decrease.

PEDIATRIC POINTERS

Children may develop subcutaneous crepitation in the neck from ingestion of corrosive substances that perforate the esophagus.

PATIENT COUNSELING

Warn patients with asthma or chronic bronchitis to be alert for subcutaneous crepitation, which can signal pneumothorax, a dangerous complication. Explain all tests and procedures to the patient with subcutaneous crepitation. Reassure him frequently to reduce his anxiety.

CYANOSIS

Cyanosis — a bluish or bluish black discoloration of the skin and mucous membranes — results from excessive concentration of unoxygenated hemoglobin in the blood. This common sign may develop abruptly or gradually. It can be classified as central or peripheral, although the two types may coexist.

Medical causes
(continued)

Rupture of trachea or major bronchus
+ Abrupt subcutaneous crepitation of the neck and anterior chest wall occurs.

Other causes
+ Endoscopic tests
+ Intermittent positive-pressure breathing
+ Mechanical ventilation
+ Thoracic surgery

Special considerations
+ Monitor vital signs frequently, especially respirations.
+ Be alert for signs of respiratory distress.
+ Tell the patient that the affected tissues will eventually absorb the air or gas bubbles, decreasing subcutaneous crepitation.

Peds points
+ Children may develop subcutaneous crepitation in the neck from ingestion of corrosive substances that perforate the esophagus.

Teaching points
+ Diagnostic tests and procedures

Key facts about cyanosis
+ Bluish or bluish black discoloration of the skin and mucous membranes
+ Results from excessive concentration of unoxygenated hemoglobin in the blood

Key facts
about cyanosis
(continued)

- Classified as central (inadequate oxygenation of systemic arterial blood) or peripheral (sluggish peripheral circulation)
- Classified as central (inadequate oxygenation of systemic arterial blood) or peripheral (sluggish peripheral circulation)

In an emergency

If localized cyanosis occurs with other signs of arterial occlusion:
- Protect the affected limb from injury, but don't massage it.

If central cyanosis stems from a pulmonary disorder or shock:
- Perform a rapid evaluation.
- Take steps to maintain an airway, assist breathing, and monitor circulation.

Key history points

- Medical history, including cardiac, pulmonary, and hematologic disorders and previous surgery
- Onset and characteristics of sign
- Associated signs and symptoms

Critical
assessment steps

- Evaluate respiratory rate and rhythm.
- Check for nasal flaring and accessory muscle use.
- Inspect the skin and mucous membranes.
- Inspect for asymmetrical chest expansion or barrel chest.
- Note edema.
- Percuss the lungs for dullness or hyperresonance.
- Auscultate for decreased or adventitious breath sounds.

Central cyanosis reflects inadequate oxygenation of systemic arterial blood caused by right-to-left cardiac shunting, pulmonary disease, or hematologic disorders. It may occur anywhere on the skin and on the mucous membranes of the mouth, lips, and conjunctiva.

Peripheral cyanosis reflects sluggish peripheral circulation caused by vasoconstriction, reduced cardiac output, or vascular occlusion. It may be widespread or may occur locally in one extremity; however, it doesn't affect mucous membranes. Typically, peripheral cyanosis appears on exposed areas, such as the fingers, nail beds, feet, nose, and ears.

Although cyanosis is an important sign of cardiovascular and pulmonary disorders, it isn't always an accurate gauge of oxygenation. Several factors contribute to its development: hemoglobin concentration and oxygen saturation, cardiac output, and partial pressure of arterial oxygen (PaO_2). Cyanosis is usually undetectable until the oxygen saturation of hemoglobin falls below 80%. Severe cyanosis is obvious, whereas mild cyanosis is more difficult to detect, even in natural, bright light. In dark-skinned patients, cyanosis is most apparent in the mucous membranes and nail beds.

Transient, nonpathologic cyanosis may result from environmental factors. For example, peripheral cyanosis may result from cutaneous vasoconstriction following a brief exposure to cold air or water. Central cyanosis may result from reduced PaO_2 at high altitudes.

EMERGENCY ACTIONS If the patient displays sudden, localized cyanosis and other signs of arterial occlusion, protect the affected limb from injury; however, don't massage the limb. If you see central cyanosis stemming from a pulmonary disorder or shock, perform a rapid evaluation. Take immediate steps to maintain an airway, assist breathing, and monitor circulation.

HISTORY

Begin with a history, focusing on cardiac, pulmonary, and hematologic disorders. Ask about previous surgery. While taking the patient's history, evaluate his mental status and level of consciousness. Ask the patient when he first noticed the cyanosis. Does it subside and recur? Is it aggravated by cold, smoking, or stress? Is it alleviated by massage or rewarming? Check the skin for coolness, pallor, redness, pain, and ulceration. Also note clubbing. Ask about headaches, dizziness, or blurred vision. Ask the patient about pain in the arms and legs (especially with walking) and about abnormal sensations, such as numbness, tingling, and coldness.

Ask about chest pain and its severity. Can the patient identify any aggravating and alleviating factors? Also, ask about nausea, anorexia, and weight loss. Does the patient have a cough? Is it productive? If so, have the patient describe the sputum. Ask about sleep apnea. Does the patient sleep with his head propped up on pillows?

CULTURAL CUE *The lips of some black people have a bluish hue making it difficult to assess cyanosis. Establishing a baseline color of the patient's skin and mucous membranes will help you detect color changes.*

PHYSICAL ASSESSMENT

Begin the physical assessment by taking vital signs. Evaluate respiratory rate and rhythm. Check for nasal flaring and use of accessory muscles. Inspect the skin and mucous membranes to determine the extent of cyanosis. Check the skin for coolness, pallor, redness, pain, and ulceration. Also note clubbing. Inspect the patient for asymmetrical chest expansion or barrel chest. Inspect the abdomen for ascites and test for shifting dullness or fluid wave. Palpate peripheral pulses, and test capillary refill time. Also, note edema.

Test the patient's motor strength. Percuss the lungs for dullness or hyperresonance, and auscultate for decreased or adventitious breath sounds. Percuss and palpate for liver enlargement and tenderness. Auscultate heart rate and rhythm, especially noting gallops and murmurs. Also auscultate the abdominal aorta and femoral arteries to detect bruits.

MEDICAL CAUSES

Arteriosclerotic occlusive disease (chronic)

With chronic arteriosclerotic occlusive disease, peripheral cyanosis occurs in the legs whenever they're in a dependent position. Associated signs and symptoms include intermittent claudication and burning pain at rest, paresthesia, pallor, muscle atrophy, weak leg pulses, and impotence. Late signs are leg ulcers and gangrene.

Bronchiectasis

Bronchiectasis produces chronic central cyanosis. Its classic sign, though, is chronic productive cough with copious, foul-smelling, mucopurulent sputum or hemoptysis. Auscultation reveals rhonchi and coarse crackles during inspiration. Other signs and symptoms include dyspnea, recurrent fever and chills, weight loss, malaise, clubbing, and signs of anemia.

Buerger's disease

With Buerger's disease, exposure to cold initially causes the feet to become cold, cyanotic, and numb; later, they redden, become hot, and tingle. Intermittent claudication of the instep is characteristic; it's aggravated by exercise and smoking and relieved by rest. Associated signs and symptoms include weak peripheral pulses and, in later stages, ulceration, muscle atrophy, and gangrene.

Chronic obstructive pulmonary disease

Chronic central cyanosis occurs in advanced stages of chronic obstructive pulmonary disease (COPD) and may be aggravated by exertion. Associated signs and symptoms include exertional dyspnea, productive cough with thick sputum, anorexia, weight loss, pursed-lip breathing, tachypnea, and the use of accessory muscles. Examination reveals wheezing and hyperresonant lung fields. Barrel chest and clubbing are late signs. Tachycardia, diaphoresis, and flushing may also accompany COPD.

Heart failure

Acute or chronic cyanosis may occur in patients with heart failure. Typically, it's a late sign and may be central, peripheral, or both. With left-sided heart failure, central cyanosis occurs with tachycardia, fatigue, dyspnea, cold intolerance, orthopnea, cough, ventricular or atrial gallop, bibasilar crackles, and diffuse apical impulse. With right-sided heart failure, peripheral cyanosis occurs with fatigue, peripheral edema, ascites, jugular vein distention, and hepatomegaly.

Peripheral arterial occlusion (acute)

Acute peripheral arterial occlusion produces acute cyanosis of one arm or leg or, occasionally, of both legs. The cyanosis is accompanied by sharp or aching pain that worsens when the patient moves. The affected extremity also exhibits paresthesia, weakness, and pale, cool skin. Examination reveals decreased or absent pulse and increased capillary refill time.

Critical assessment steps
(continued)

✦ Auscultate heart rate and rhythm.

Medical causes

Arteriosclerotic occlusive disease (chronic)

✦ Peripheral cyanosis occurs in the legs whenever they're in a dependent position.

Bronchiectasis

✦ Chronic central cyanosis develops.
✦ The classic sign is chronic productive cough with copious, foul-smelling, mucopurulent sputum or hemoptysis.

Buerger's disease

✦ Exposure to cold initially causes the feet to become cold, cyanotic, and numb.
✦ Intermittent claudication of the instep is characteristic.

COPD

✦ Chronic central cyanosis occurs in advanced stages.
✦ Exertion aggravates cyanosis.

Heart failure

✦ Acute or chronic cyanosis may occur (late sign).
✦ With left-sided failure, central cyanosis occurs.
✦ With right-sided failure, peripheral cyanosis occurs.

Peripheral arterial occlusion (acute)

✦ Acute cyanosis of arm or leg occurs.
✦ Cyanosis is accompanied by sharp or aching pain that worsens with movement.

Medical causes
(continued)

Pneumonia
✦ Acute central cyanosis is usually preceded by fever, shaking chills, cough with purulent sputum, crackles, rhonchi, and pleuritic chest pain that's exacerbated by deep inspiration.

Pneumothorax
✦ Acute central cyanosis is a cardinal sign.

Polycythemia vera
✦ Ruddy complexion that can appear cyanotic is characteristic.

Pulmonary edema
✦ Acute central cyanosis occurs.

Pulmonary embolism
✦ Acute central cyanosis occurs when a large embolus obstructs pulmonary circulation.

Raynaud's disease
✦ Exposure to cold or stress causes the fingers or hands to blanch, turn cold, and become cyanotic.

Shock
✦ Acute peripheral cyanosis develops in the hands and feet.
✦ Feet may be cold, clammy, and pale.

Special considerations
✦ Provide supplemental oxygen.
✦ Position the patient comfortably.
✦ Administer a diuretic, bronchodilator, antibiotic, or cardiac drug as needed.
✦ Provide rest periods.

Pneumonia
With pneumonia, acute central cyanosis is usually preceded by fever, shaking chills, cough with purulent sputum, crackles, rhonchi, and pleuritic chest pain that's exacerbated by deep inspiration. Associated signs and symptoms include tachycardia, dyspnea, tachypnea, diminished breath sounds, diaphoresis, myalgia, fatigue, headache, and anorexia.

Pneumothorax
A cardinal sign of pneumothorax, acute central cyanosis is accompanied by sharp chest pain that's exacerbated by movement, deep breathing, and coughing; asymmetrical chest wall expansion; and shortness of breath. The patient may also exhibit rapid, shallow respirations; weak, rapid pulse; pallor; jugular vein distention; anxiety; and absence of breath sounds over the affected lobe.

Polycythemia vera
A ruddy complexion that can appear cyanotic is characteristic in this chronic myeloproliferative disorder. Other findings in polycythemia vera include hepatosplenomegaly, headache, dizziness, fatigue, aquagenic pruritus, blurred vision, chest pain, intermittent claudication, and coagulation defects.

Pulmonary edema
With pulmonary edema, acute central cyanosis occurs with dyspnea; orthopnea; frothy, blood-tinged sputum; tachycardia; tachypnea; dependent crackles; ventricular gallop; cold, clammy skin; hypotension; weak, thready pulse; and confusion.

Pulmonary embolism
Acute central cyanosis occurs when a large embolus causes significant obstruction of the pulmonary circulation. Syncope and jugular vein distention may also occur. Other common signs and symptoms include dyspnea, chest pain, tachycardia, paradoxical pulse, dry cough or productive cough with blood-tinged sputum, low-grade fever, restlessness, and diaphoresis.

Raynaud's disease
With Raynaud's disease, exposure to cold or stress causes the fingers or hands first to blanch and turn cold, then to become cyanotic, and finally to redden with return of normal temperature. Numbness and tingling may also occur. Raynaud's phenomenon describes the same presentation when associated with other disorders, such as rheumatoid arthritis, scleroderma, or lupus erythematosus.

Shock
With shock, acute peripheral cyanosis develops in the hands and feet, which may also be cold, clammy, and pale. Other characteristic signs and symptoms include lethargy, confusion, increased capillary refill time, and a rapid, weak pulse. Tachypnea, hyperpnea, and hypotension may also be present.

SPECIAL CONSIDERATIONS

Provide supplemental oxygen to relieve shortness of breath, improve oxygenation, and decrease cyanosis. Deliver small doses (2 L/minute) in patients with COPD, who may retain carbon dioxide. Use a low-flow oxygen rate for mild COPD exacerbations. For acute situations, a high-flow oxygen rate may be needed initially. Remember to be attentive to the patient's respiratory drive and adjust the amount of oxygen accordingly. Position the patient comfortably to ease breathing. Administer a diuretic, bronchodilator, antibiotic, or cardiac drug as needed. Make sure that the patient gets sufficient rest between activities to prevent dyspnea.

Prepare the patient for such tests as arterial blood gas analysis and complete blood count to determine the cause of cyanosis.

PEDIATRIC POINTERS

Many pulmonary disorders responsible for cyanosis in adults also cause cyanosis in children. In addition, central cyanosis may result from cystic fibrosis, asthma, airway obstruction by a foreign body, acute laryngotracheobronchitis, or epiglottiditis. It may also result from a congenital heart defect, such as transposition of the great vessels, that causes right-to-left intracardiac shunting.

In children, circumoral cyanosis may precede generalized cyanosis. Acrocyanosis (also called "glove and bootee" cyanosis) may occur in infants because of excessive crying or exposure to cold. Exercise and agitation enhance cyanosis, so provide comfort and regular rest periods. Also, administer supplemental oxygen during cyanotic episodes.

GERIATRIC POINTERS

Because elderly patients have reduced tissue perfusion, peripheral cyanosis can present even with a slight decrease in cardiac output or systemic blood pressure.

PATIENT COUNSELING

Teach patients with chronic cardiopulmonary diseases, such as heart failure, asthma, or COPD, to recognize cyanosis as a sign of severe disease; advise patients to get immediate medical attention when it occurs. If the patient is using oxygen at home, teach him how to use it properly.

Peds points

+ Central cyanosis may result from cystic fibrosis, asthma, airway obstruction, acute laryngotracheobronchitis, epiglottiditis, or congenital heart defects.
+ Circumoral cyanosis may precede generalized cyanosis.
+ Acrocyanosis may occur in infants because of excessive crying or exposure to cold.

Geri points

+ Because of reduced tissue perfusion, peripheral cyanosis can present even with a slight decrease in cardiac output or systemic blood pressure.

Teaching points

+ Importance of seeking medical attention if cyanosis occurs
+ Use of oxygen at home

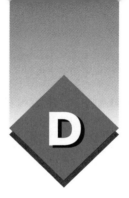

DECEREBRATE POSTURE

Decerebrate posture, also known as *decerebrate rigidity* or *abnormal extensor reflex,* is characterized by adduction (internal rotation) and extension of the arms while the wrists are pronated and the fingers are flexed. In addition, the legs are stiffly extended, with forced plantar flexion of the feet. In severe cases, the back is acutely arched (opisthotonos). This sign indicates upper brain stem damage, which may result from primary lesions, such as infarction, hemorrhage, or tumor; metabolic encephalopathy; head injury; or brain stem compression associated with increased intracranial pressure (ICP).

Decerebrate posture may be elicited by noxious stimuli or may occur spontaneously. It may be unilateral or bilateral. With coancurrent brain stem and cerebral damage, decerebrate posture may affect only the arms, with the legs remaining flaccid. Alternatively, decerebrate posture may affect one side of the body and decorticate posture the other. The two postures may also alternate as the patient's neurologic status fluctuates. Generally, the duration of each posturing episode correlates with the severity of brain stem damage. (See *Comparing decerebrate and decorticate postures.*)

 EMERGENCY ACTIONS Ensuring a patent airway is the priority when caring for a patient who exhibits decerebrate posture. If necessary, insert an artificial airway and institute measures to prevent aspiration. (Don't disrupt spinal alignment if you suspect spinal cord injury.) Suction the patient as necessary.

Next, examine spontaneous respirations. Give supplemental oxygen, and ventilate the patient with a handheld resuscitation bag, if necessary. Intubation and mechanical ventilation may be indicated. Keep emergency resuscitation equipment handy. (Be sure to check the patient's chart for a do-not-resuscitate order.)

HISTORY

Explore the history of the patient's symptoms. If you can't obtain this information, look for clues to the causative disorder, such as hepatomegaly, cyanosis, diabetic skin changes, needle tracks, or obvious trauma. If a family member is available, find out when the patient's level of consciousness (LOC) began deteriorating. Did it occur abruptly? What did the patient complain of before he lost consciousness? Does he have a history of diabetes, liver disease, cancer, blood clots, or aneurysm? Ask about any accident or trauma responsible for the coma.

Comparing decerebrate and decorticate postures

Decerebrate posture results from damage to the upper brain stem. In this posture, the arms are adducted and extended, with the wrists pronated and the fingers flexed. The legs are stiffly extended, with plantar flexion of the feet.

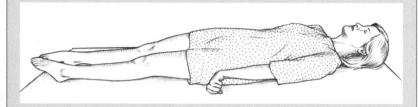

Decorticate posture results from damage to one or both corticospinal tracts. In this posture, the arms are adducted and flexed, with the wrists and fingers flexed on the chest. The legs are stiffly extended and internally rotated, with plantar flexion of the feet.

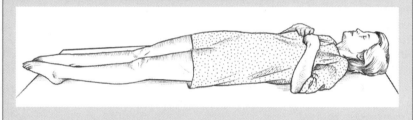

PHYSICAL ASSESSMENT

After taking vital signs, determine the patient's LOC. Use the Glasgow Coma Scale as a reference. Then evaluate the pupils for size, equality, and response to light. Test deep tendon reflexes and cranial nerve reflexes, and check for doll's eye sign. After completing the neurologic examination, perform a full physical assessment.

MEDICAL CAUSES

Brain stem infarction

When brain stem infarction produces a coma, it may be accompanied by decerebrate posture. Associated signs and symptoms vary with the severity of the infarct and may include cranial nerve palsies, bilateral cerebellar ataxia, and sensory loss. With deep coma, all normal reflexes are usually lost, resulting in absence of doll's eye sign, a positive Babinski's reflex, and flaccidity.

Brain stem tumor

Decerebrate posture is a late sign of a brain stem tumor that accompanies coma. Commonly, the posture is preceded by hemiparesis or quadriparesis, cranial nerve palsies, vertigo, dizziness, ataxia, and vomiting.

Cerebral lesion

Whether the cause is trauma, tumor, abscess, or infarction, any cerebral lesion that increases ICP may also produce decerebrate posture. Typically, this posture is a late sign. Associated findings vary with the lesion's site and extent but commonly include coma, abnormal pupil size and response to light, and the classic triad of in-

Critical assessment steps

+ Take vital signs.
+ Determine LOC.
+ Evaluate pupils for size, equality, and response to light.
+ Test deep tendon reflexes and cranial nerve reflexes.
+ Check for doll's eye sign.
+ Perform a physical assessment.

Medical causes

Brain stem infarction
+ Coma may be accompanied by decerebrate posture.

Brain stem tumor
+ Decerebrate posture is a late sign.

Cerebral lesion
+ Increased ICP may produce decerebrate posture, a late sign.

Medical causes
(continued)

Hypoglycemic encephalopathy
✦ Decerebrate posture and coma may occur.
✦ Low blood glucose levels are characteristic.

Hypoxic encephalopathy
✦ Brain stem compression associated with anaerobic metabolism and increased ICP may result in decerebrate posture.

Pontine hemorrhage
✦ Decerebrate posture occurs rapidly along with coma.

Posterior fossa hemorrhage
✦ A subtentorial lesion causes decerebrate posture, vomiting, headache, vertigo, ataxia, stiff neck, drowsiness, papilledema, and cranial nerve palsies.

Other causes
✦ Lumbar puncture

Special considerations
✦ Monitor neurologic status and vital signs as indicated.
✦ Be alert for signs of increased ICP and neurologic deterioration.

Peds points
✦ Children younger than age 2 may not display decerebrate posture because of nervous system immaturity.
✦ In children, the most common cause of decerebrate posture is head injury.

creased ICP: bradycardia, increasing systolic blood pressure, and widening pulse pressure.

Hypoglycemic encephalopathy
Characterized by extremely low blood glucose levels, hypoglycemic encephalopathy may produce decerebrate posture and coma. It also causes dilated pupils, slow respirations, and bradycardia. Muscle spasms, twitching, and seizures eventually progress to flaccidity.

Hypoxic encephalopathy
Severe hypoxia may produce decerebrate posture — the result of brain stem compression associated with anaerobic metabolism and increased ICP. Other findings include coma, a positive Babinski's reflex, absence of doll's eye sign, hypoactive deep tendon reflexes and, possibly, fixed pupils and respiratory arrest.

Pontine hemorrhage
Typically, pontine hemorrhage rapidly leads to decerebrate posture with coma. Accompanying signs of this life-threatening disorder include total paralysis, absence of doll's eye sign, a positive Babinski's reflex, and small, reactive pupils.

Posterior fossa hemorrhage
Posterior fossa hemorrhage is a subtentorial lesion that causes decerebrate posture. Its early signs and symptoms include vomiting, headache, vertigo, ataxia, stiff neck, drowsiness, papilledema, and cranial nerve palsies. The patient eventually slips into a coma and may experience respiratory arrest.

OTHER CAUSES

Diagnostic tests
Relief of high ICP by removal of spinal fluid during a lumbar puncture may precipitate cerebral compression of the brain stem and cause decerebrate posture and coma.

SPECIAL CONSIDERATIONS
Prepare the patient for diagnostic tests that will help determine the cause of his decerebrate posture. Testing may include skull X-rays, computed tomography scanning, magnetic resonance imaging, cerebral angiography, digital subtraction angiography, EEG, brain scanning, and ICP monitoring.

Monitor the patient's neurologic status and vital signs every 30 minutes or as indicated. Also, be alert for signs of increased ICP (bradycardia, increasing systolic blood pressure, and widening pulse pressure) and neurologic deterioration (altered respiratory pattern and abnormal temperature).

PEDIATRIC POINTERS
Children younger than age 2 may not display decerebrate posture because of nervous system immaturity. However, if the posture occurs, it's usually the more severe opisthotonos. In fact, opisthotonos is more common in infants and young children than in adults and is usually a terminal sign. In children, the most common cause of decerebrate posture is head injury. It also occurs with Reye's syndrome — the result of increased ICP causing brain stem compression.

PATIENT COUNSELING

Inform the patient's family that decerebrate posture is a reflex response — not a voluntary response to pain or a sign of recovery. Offer emotional support.

DECORTICATE POSTURE

A sign of corticospinal damage, decorticate posture is characterized by adduction of the arms and flexion of the elbows, with wrists and fingers flexed on the chest. The legs are extended and internally rotated, with plantar flexion of the feet. Decorticate posture, also known as *decorticate rigidity* or *abnormal flexor response*, may occur unilaterally or bilaterally. It usually results from stroke or head injury. It may be elicited by noxious stimuli or may occur spontaneously. The intensity of the required stimulus, the duration of the posture, and the frequency of spontaneous episodes vary with the severity and location of cerebral injury.

Although a serious sign, decorticate posture carries a more favorable prognosis than decerebrate posture. However, if the causative disorder extends lower in the brain stem, decorticate posture may progress to decerebrate posture. (See *Comparing decerebrate and decorticate postures*, page 193.)

EMERGENCY ACTIONS Obtain vital signs and evaluate the patient's level of consciousness (LOC). If consciousness is impaired, insert an oropharyngeal airway and take measures to prevent aspiration (unless spinal cord injury is suspected). Evaluate the patient's respiratory rate, rhythm, and depth. Prepare to assist respirations with a handheld resuscitation bag or with intubation and mechanical ventilation. Also, institute seizure precautions.

HISTORY

Ask about headache, dizziness, nausea, changes in vision, and numbness or tingling. When did the patient first notice these symptoms? Is his family aware of any behavioral changes? Also, ask about a history of cerebrovascular disease, cancer, meningitis, encephalitis, upper respiratory tract infection, bleeding or clotting disorders, or recent trauma.

PHYSICAL ASSESSMENT

Test the patient's motor and sensory functions. Evaluate pupil size, equality, and response to light. Test cranial nerve function and deep tendon reflexes. Then perform a neurologic examination.

MEDICAL CAUSES

Brain abscess

Decorticate posture may occur with a brain abscess. Accompanying findings vary depending on the size and location of the abscess but may include aphasia, hemiparesis, headache, dizziness, seizures, nausea, and vomiting. The patient may also experience behavioral changes, altered vital signs, and decreased LOC.

Brain tumor

A brain tumor may produce decorticate posture that's usually bilateral — the result of increased intracranial pressure (ICP) associated with tumor growth. Related signs and symptoms include headache, behavioral changes, memory loss, diplopia, blurred vision or vision loss, seizures, ataxia, dizziness, apraxia, aphasia, paresis, sensory loss, paresthesia, vomiting, papilledema, and signs of hormonal imbalance.

Teaching points

+ Explanation of posture as a reflex response

Key facts about decorticate posture

+ Signals corticospinal damage
+ Characterized by adducted arms, flexion of the elbows, flexed wrists and fingers on the chest, and extended and internally rotated legs with plantar flexion of the feet

In an emergency

+ Evaluate LOC and maintain a patent airway.
+ Prepare to assist respirations.

Key history points

+ Associated headache, dizziness, nausea, changes in vision, and numbness or tingling
+ History of cerebrovascular disease, cancer, meningitis, encephalitis, upper respiratory tract infection, bleeding or clotting disorders, or recent trauma

Critical assessment steps

+ Evaluate pupil size, equality, and response to light.
+ Perform a neurologic examination.

Medical causes

Brain abscess

+ Decorticate posture may occur along with aphasia, hemiparesis, headache, dizziness, seizures, nausea, and vomiting.

Brain tumor

+ Decorticate posture results from increased ICP.

Medical causes
(continued)

Head injury
✦ Decorticate posture may result depending on the injury.

Stroke
✦ A stroke involving the cerebral cortex produces unilateral decorticate posture.

Special considerations
✦ Assess the patient frequently to detect signs of neurologic deterioration.
✦ Monitor neurologic status and vital signs as indicated.
✦ Be alert for signs of increased ICP.

Peds points
✦ Decorticate posture is an unreliable sign before age 2 because of nervous system immaturity.
✦ In children, decorticate posture usually results from head injury.

Teaching points
✦ Signs and symptoms of decreased LOC and seizures
✦ Quality of life issues
✦ Appropriate referrals
✦ Patient safety measures

Key facts about hyperactive DTRs
✦ Abnormally brisk muscle contractions in response to sudden stretch induced by sharply tapping the muscle's tendon of insertion
✦ Graded as brisk or pathologically hyperactive

Head injury

Decorticate posture may be among the variable features of a head injury, depending on its site and severity. Associated signs and symptoms include headache, nausea and vomiting, dizziness, irritability, decreased LOC, aphasia, hemiparesis, unilateral numbness, seizures, and pupillary dilation.

Stroke

Typically, a stroke involving the cerebral cortex produces unilateral decorticate posture, also called *spastic hemiplegia*. Other signs and symptoms include hemiplegia (contralateral to the lesion), dysarthria, dysphagia, unilateral sensory loss, apraxia, agnosia, aphasia, memory loss, decreased LOC, urine retention, urinary incontinence, and constipation. Ocular effects include homonymous hemianopsia, diplopia, and blurred vision.

SPECIAL CONSIDERATIONS

Assess the patient frequently to detect subtle signs of neurologic deterioration. Also, monitor neurologic status and vital signs every 30 minutes to 2 hours. Be alert for signs of increased ICP, including bradycardia, increasing systolic blood pressure, and widening pulse pressure.

PEDIATRIC POINTERS

Decorticate posture is an unreliable sign before age 2 because of nervous system immaturity. In children, this posture usually results from head injury. It also occurs with Reye's syndrome.

PATIENT COUNSELING

Teach the family to recognize signs and symptoms of decreased LOC and seizures. Discuss quality of life issues with the patient and his family. Make referrals to appropriate resources, such as the National Head Injury Foundation, National Stroke Association, American Cancer Society, or local hospice. Discuss measures to ensure patient safety with the family.

DEEP TENDON REFLEXES, HYPERACTIVE

Hyperactive deep tendon reflexes (DTRs) are abnormally brisk muscle contractions that occur in response to a sudden stretch induced by sharply tapping the muscle's tendon of insertion. This elicited sign may be graded as *brisk* or *pathologically hyperactive*. Hyperactive DTRs are commonly accompanied by clonus.

The corticospinal tract and other descending tracts govern the reflex arc — the relay cycle that produces any reflex response. A corticospinal lesion above the level of the reflex arc being tested may result in hyperactive DTRs. Abnormal neuromuscular transmission at the end of the reflex arc may also cause hyperactive DTRs. For example, a deficiency of calcium or magnesium may cause hyperactive DTRs because these electrolytes regulate neuromuscular excitability.

HISTORY

After eliciting hyperactive DTRs, take the patient's history. Ask about spinal cord injury or other trauma and about prolonged exposure to cold, wind, or water. Also find out if the patient could be pregnant. A positive response to any of these questions requires prompt evaluation to rule out life-threatening autonomic hyper-reflexia, tetanus, preeclampsia, and hypothermia. Ask about the onset and progression of associated signs and symptoms. Also ask about paresthesia, vomiting, and altered bladder habits.

PHYSICAL ASSESSMENT

Perform a neurologic examination. Evaluate level of consciousness, and test motor and sensory function in the limbs. Check for ataxia or tremors and for speech and visual deficits. Test for Chvostek's sign (an abnormal spasm of the facial muscles elicited by light taps on the facial nerve in patients who have hypocalcemia), Trousseau's sign (a carpal spasm induced by inflating a sphygmomanometer cuff on the upper arm to a pressure exceeding systolic blood pressure for 3 minutes in patients who have hypocalcemia or hypomagnesemia), and carpopedal spasm. Be sure to record the patient's vital signs.

MEDICAL CAUSES

Amyotrophic lateral sclerosis

Amyotrophic lateral sclerosis (ALS), which is also known as *Lou Gehrig disease*, produces generalized hyperactive DTRs accompanied by weakness of the hands and forearms and spasticity of the legs. Eventually, the patient develops atrophy of the neck and tongue muscles, fasciculations, weakness of the legs and, possibly, bulbar signs (dysphagia, dysphonia, facial weakness, and dyspnea).

Brain tumor

A cerebral brain tumor causes hyperactive DTRs on the side opposite the lesion. Associated signs and symptoms develop slowly and may include unilateral paresis or paralysis, anesthesia, visual field deficits, spasticity, and a positive Babinski's reflex.

Hepatic encephalopathy

Generalized hyperactive DTRs occur late in the comatose stage of hepatic encephalopathy and are accompanied by a positive Babinski's reflex, fetor hepaticus (a musty, sweet odor to the breath), and coma.

Hypocalcemia

Hypocalcemia may produce sudden or gradual onset of generalized hyperactive DTRs with paresthesia, muscle twitching and cramping, positive Chvostek's and Trousseau's signs, carpopedal spasm, and tetany. Other signs and symptoms include abdominal cramps, muscle cramps, arrhythmias, and diarrhea.

Hypomagnesemia

Hypomagnesemia results in gradual onset of generalized hyperactive DTRs accompanied by muscle cramps, hypotension, tachycardia, paresthesia, ataxia, tetany and, possibly, seizures. Other signs and symptoms include Chvostek's sign, confusion, delusions, hallucinations, arrhythmias, and hypotension.

Hypothermia

Mild hypothermia (90° F to 94° F [32.2° C to 34.4° C]) produces generalized hyperactive DTRs. Other signs and symptoms include shivering, fatigue, weakness, lethargy, slurred speech, ataxia, muscle stiffness, tachycardia, diuresis, bradypnea, hypotension, and cold, pale skin.

Key history points

+ History of spinal cord injury, other trauma, or prolonged exposure to cold, wind, or water
+ Onset and progression of associated signs and symptoms, including paresthesia, vomiting, and altered bladder habits

Critical assessment steps

+ Perform a neurologic examination and evaluate LOC.
+ Test motor and sensory function in the limbs.
+ Check for ataxia or tremors.
+ Test for Chvostek's and Trousseau's signs and carpopedal spasm.

Medical causes

ALS

+ Generalized hyperactive DTRs are accompanied by weakness of the hands and forearms and spasticity of the legs.

Brain tumor

+ Hyperactive DTRs occur on the side opposite the lesion.

Hepatic encephalopathy

+ Generalized hyperactive DTRs occur late in comatose stage.

Hypocalcemia

+ Onset of generalized hyperactive DTRs may be gradual or sudden.

Hypomagnesemia

+ Onset of generalized hyperactive DTRs is gradual.

Hypothermia

+ Mild hypothermia produces generalized hyperactive DTRs.

Medical causes
(continued)

Multiple sclerosis
+ Hyperactive DTRs are preceded by weakness and paresthesia in arms and legs.

Preeclampsia
+ Onset of generalized hyperactive DTRs is gradual.

Spinal cord lesion
+ Incomplete lesions cause hyperactive DTRs below the level of the lesion.
+ In a traumatic lesion, hyperactive DTRs follow resolution of spinal shock.
+ In a neoplastic lesion, hyperactive DTRs gradually replace normal DTRs.

Stroke
+ If the origin of the corticospinal tracts is affected, hyperactive DTRs on the side opposite the lesion suddenly occur.

Tetanus
+ Onset of generalized hyperactive DTRs is sudden.

Special considerations
+ If motor weakness is present, perform ROM exercises.
+ Reposition the patient frequently, provide a special mattress, massage his back, and ensure adequate nutrition.
+ Administer a muscle relaxant and a sedative.
+ Keep emergency resuscitation equipment on hand.
+ Provide a quiet, calm atmosphere and assist with ADLs.

Multiple sclerosis
Typically, hyperactive DTRs are preceded by weakness and paresthesia in one or both arms or legs in patients with multiple sclerosis. Associated signs include clonus and a positive Babinski's reflex. Passive flexion of the patient's neck may cause a tingling sensation down his back. Later, ataxia, diplopia, vertigo, vomiting, urine retention, or urinary incontinence may occur.

Preeclampsia
Occurring in pregnancy of at least 20 weeks' duration, preeclampsia may cause gradual onset of generalized hyperactive DTRs. Accompanying signs and symptoms include increased blood pressure; abnormal weight gain; edema of the face, fingers, and abdomen after bed rest; albuminuria; oliguria; severe headache; blurred or double vision; epigastric pain; nausea and vomiting; irritability; cyanosis; shortness of breath; and crackles. If preeclampsia progresses to eclampsia, the patient develops seizures.

Spinal cord lesion
Incomplete spinal cord lesions cause hyperactive DTRs below the level of the lesion. In a traumatic lesion, hyperactive DTRs follow resolution of spinal shock. In a neoplastic lesion, hyperactive DTRs gradually replace normal DTRs. Other signs and symptoms of spinal cord lesion include paralysis and sensory loss below the level of the lesion, urine retention and overflow incontinence, and alternating constipation and diarrhea. A lesion above T6 may also produce autonomic hyperreflexia with diaphoresis and flushing above the level of the lesion, headache, nasal congestion, nausea, increased blood pressure, and bradycardia.

Stroke
Any stroke that affects the origin of the corticospinal tracts causes sudden onset of hyperactive DTRs on the side opposite the lesion. The patient may also have unilateral paresis or paralysis, anesthesia, visual field deficits, spasticity, and a positive Babinski's reflex.

Tetanus
With tetanus, sudden onset of generalized hyperactive DTRs accompanies tachycardia, diaphoresis, low-grade fever, painful and involuntary muscle contractions, trismus (lockjaw), and risus sardonicus (a masklike grin).

SPECIAL CONSIDERATIONS
Prepare the patient for diagnostic tests to evaluate hyperactive DTRs. These may include laboratory tests for serum calcium magnesium and ammonia levels, spinal X-rays, magnetic resonance imaging, computed tomography, lumbar puncture, and myelography.

If motor weakness accompanies hyperactive DTRs, perform or encourage range-of-motion exercises to preserve muscle integrity and prevent deep vein thrombosis. Also, reposition the patient frequently, provide a special mattress, and massage his back and ensure adequate nutrition to prevent skin breakdown. Administer a muscle relaxant and a sedative to relieve severe muscle contractions. Keep emergency resuscitation equipment on hand. Provide a quiet, calm atmosphere to decrease neuromuscular excitability. Assist with activities of daily living.

PEDIATRIC POINTERS

Hyperreflexia may be a normal sign in neonates. After age 6, reflex responses are similar to those of adults. When testing DTRs in small children, use distraction techniques to promote reliable results.

Cerebral palsy commonly causes hyperactive DTRs in children. Reye's syndrome causes generalized hyperactive DTRs in stage II; in stage V, DTRs are absent. Adult causes of hyperactive DTRs may also appear in children.

PATIENT COUNSELING

Provide emotional support to the patient and his family. Explain all procedures and treatments. Help the patient relax and provide him with quiet activities. Explain safety measures to the patient and his family.

DEEP TENDON REFLEXES, HYPOACTIVE

Hypoactive deep tendon reflexes (DTRs) are abnormally diminished muscle contractions that occur in response to a sudden stretch induced by sharply tapping the muscle's tendon of insertion. Symmetrically reduced reflexes may be normal.

Normally, DTRs depend on intact receptors, intact sensory-motor nerve fibers, intact neuromuscular-glandular junctions, and functional synapses in the spinal cord. Hypoactive DTRs may result from damage to the reflex arc involving the specific muscle, the peripheral nerve, the nerve roots, or the spinal cord at that level. Hypoactive DTRs are an important sign of many disorders, especially when they appear with other neurologic signs and symptoms. (See *Documenting deep tendon reflexes.*)

Peds points

✦ Cerebral palsy commonly causes hyperactive DTRs in children.
✦ Reye's syndrome causes generalized hyperactive DTRs in stage II; in stage V, DTRs are absent.

Teaching points

✦ Procedures and treatments
✦ Safety measures

Key facts about hypoactive DTRs

✦ Abnormally diminished muscle contractions in response to a sudden stretch induced by sharply tapping the muscle's tendon of insertion
✦ May result from damage to the reflex arc involving the specific muscle, the peripheral nerve, the nerve roots, or the spinal cord

Documenting deep tendon reflexes

To record the patient's deep tendon reflex scores, draw a stick figure and enter the grades on this scale at the proper location. The figure shown here indicates hypoactive deep tendon reflexes in the legs; other reflexes are normal.

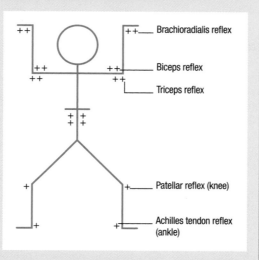

KEY:
0	= absent
+	= hypoactive (diminished)
++	= normal
+++	= brisk (increased)
++++	= hyperactive (clonus may be present)

Key history points

◆ Associated signs and symptoms
◆ Family and drug history

Critical assessment steps

◆ Evaluate LOC.
◆ Test motor function in the limbs.
◆ Palpate for muscle atrophy or increased mass.
◆ Test sensory function.
◆ Evaluate paresthesia.
◆ Observe gait and coordination.
◆ Check for Romberg's sign.
◆ Evaluate speech.
◆ Check for signs of vision and hearing loss.
◆ Take vital signs.
◆ Monitor for increased heart rate and blood pressure.
◆ Inspect the skin for pallor, dryness, flushing, and diaphoresis.
◆ Auscultate for hypoactive bowel sounds.
◆ Palpate for bladder distention.

Medical causes

Botulism
◆ Generalized hypoactive DTRs accompany progressive descending muscle weakness.

Cerebellar dysfunction
◆ An increase in the level of inhibition may produce hypoactive DTRs.

Guillain-Barré syndrome
◆ Bilateral hypoactive DTRs progress rapidly from hypotonia to areflexia.

Peripheral neuropathy
◆ Hypoactive DTRs are progressive.

HISTORY

After eliciting hypoactive DTRs, obtain a thorough history from the patient or a family member. Have him describe current signs and symptoms in detail. Then take a family and drug history.

PHYSICAL ASSESSMENT

Evaluate the patient's level of consciousness. Test motor function in his limbs, and palpate for muscle atrophy or increased mass. Test sensory function, including pain, touch, temperature, and vibration sense. Evaluate paresthesia. To observe gait and coordination, have the patient take several steps. To check for Romberg's sign, ask him to stand with his feet together and his eyes closed. During conversation, evaluate speech. Check for signs of vision and hearing loss. Abrupt onset of hypoactive DTRs accompanied by muscle weakness may occur with life-threatening Guillain-Barré syndrome, botulism, or spinal cord lesions with spinal shock.

Look for autonomic nervous system effects by taking vital signs and monitoring for increased heart rate and blood pressure. Also, inspect the skin for pallor, dryness, flushing, and diaphoresis. Auscultate for hypoactive bowel sounds, and palpate for bladder distention. Ask about nausea, vomiting, constipation, and incontinence.

MEDICAL CAUSES

Botulism

With botulism, generalized hypoactive DTRs accompany progressive descending muscle weakness. Initially, the patient usually complains of blurred and double vision and, occasionally, of anorexia, nausea, and vomiting. Other early bulbar findings include vertigo, hearing loss, dysarthria, and dysphagia. The patient may have signs of respiratory distress and severe constipation marked by hypoactive bowel sounds.

Cerebellar dysfunction

Cerebellar dysfunction may produce hypoactive DTRs by increasing the level of inhibition through long tracts upon spinal motor neurons. Associated clinical findings vary depending on the cause and location of the dysfunction.

Guillain-Barré syndrome

Guillain-Barré syndrome causes bilateral hypoactive DTRs that progress rapidly from hypotonia to areflexia in several days. Guillain-Barré syndrome typically causes muscle weakness that begins in the legs and then extends to the arms and, possibly, to the trunk and neck muscles. Occasionally, weakness may progress to total paralysis. Other signs and symptoms include cranial nerve palsies, pain, paresthesia, and signs of brief autonomic dysfunction, such as sinus tachycardia or bradycardia, flushing, fluctuating blood pressure, and anhidrosis or episodic diaphoresis.

Usually, muscle weakness and hypoactive DTRs peak in severity within 10 to 14 days; then symptoms begin to clear. However, in severe cases, residual hypoactive DTRs and motor weakness may persist.

Peripheral neuropathy

Characteristic of end-stage diabetes mellitus, renal failure, alcoholism, and an adverse effect of various medications, peripheral neuropathy results in progressive hypoactive DTRs. Other effects include motor weakness, sensory loss, paresthesia, tremors, and possible autonomic dysfunction, such as orthostatic hypotension and incontinence.

Polymyositis

With polymyositis, hypoactive DTRs accompany muscle weakness, pain, stiffness, spasms and, possibly, increased size or atrophy. These effects are usually temporary; their location varies with the affected muscles.

Spinal cord lesions

Spinal cord injury or complete transection produces spinal shock, resulting in hypoactive DTRs (areflexia) below the level of the lesion. Associated signs and symptoms include quadriplegia or paraplegia, flaccidity, loss of sensation below the level of the lesion, and dry, pale skin. Also characteristic are urine retention with overflow incontinence, hypoactive bowel sounds, constipation, and genital reflex loss. Hypoactive DTRs and flaccidity are usually transient; reflex activity may return within several weeks.

Syringomyelia

Permanent bilateral hypoactive DTRs occur early in syringomyelia, a slowly progressive disorder. Other signs and symptoms of syringomyelia are muscle weakness and atrophy; loss of sensation, usually extending in a capelike fashion over the arms, shoulders, neck, back, and occasionally the legs; deep, boring pain (despite analgesia) in the limbs; and signs of brain stem involvement (nystagmus, facial numbness, unilateral vocal cord paralysis or weakness, and unilateral tongue atrophy).

OTHER CAUSES

Drugs

Barbiturates and paralyzing drugs, such as pancuronium and curare, may cause hypoactive DTRs.

SPECIAL CONSIDERATIONS

If the patient has sensory deficits, protect him from injury caused by heat, cold, or pressure. Test his bath water, and reposition him frequently, ensuring a soft, smooth bed surface. Keep his skin clean and dry to prevent breakdown. Perform or encourage range-of-motion exercises. Also encourage a balanced diet with plenty of protein and adequate hydration.

PEDIATRIC POINTERS

Hypoactive DTRs commonly occur in patients with muscular dystrophy, Friedreich's ataxia, syringomyelia, and spinal cord injury. They also accompany progressive muscular atrophy, which affects preschoolers and adolescents.

Use distraction techniques to test DTRs; assess motor function by watching the infant or child at play.

GERIATRIC POINTERS

Elderly patients may have reduced DTRs because of a decrease in the number of nerve axons and demyelination of axons. The Achilles tendon reflex may be difficult to elicit in these patients.

Medical causes
(continued)

Polymyositis
+ Hypoactive DTRs accompany muscle weakness, pain, stiffness, spasms and, possibly, increased size or atrophy.

Spinal cord lesions
+ Spinal shock from injury or complete transection results in hypoactive DTRs (areflexia) below the level of the lesion.

Syringomyelia
+ Permanent bilateral hypoactive DTRs occur early.

Other causes
+ Barbiturates
+ Paralyzing drugs (such as pancuronium and curare)

Special considerations
+ If the patient has sensory deficits, protect him from injury caused by heat, cold, or pressure.
+ Keep the skin clean and dry.

Peds points
+ Hypoactive DTRs commonly occur in children with muscular dystrophy, Friedreich's ataxia, syringomyelia, and spinal cord injury.
+ Hypoactive DTRs accompany progressive muscular atrophy, which affects preschoolers and adolescents.

Geri points
+ Elderly patients may have reduced DTRs because of a decrease in the number of nerve axons and demyelination of axons.

Teaching points

+ Ways to perform ADLs
+ Safety measures, including walking with assistance

Key facts about diaphoresis

+ Refers to profuse sweating
+ Can produce more than 1 L of sweat per hour
+ Represents an autonomic nervous system response to physical or psychogenic stress or to fever or high envirnmental temperature

PATIENT COUNSELING

Encourage the patient to perform activities of daily living as independently as possible. Assist the patient when necessary. Try to strike a balance between promoting independence and ensuring the patient's safety. Encourage him to walk with assistance. Make sure personal care articles are within easy reach, and provide an obstacle-free course from his bed to the bathroom.

DIAPHORESIS

Diaphoresis is profuse sweating—at times, amounting to more than 1 L of sweat per hour. This sign represents an autonomic nervous system response to physical or psychogenic stress or to fever or high environmental temperature. When caused by stress, diaphoresis may be generalized or limited to the palms, soles, and forehead. When caused by fever or high environmental temperature, it's usually generalized.

Diaphoresis usually begins abruptly and may be accompanied by other autonomic system signs, such as tachycardia and increased blood pressure. Intermittent diaphoresis may accompany chronic disorders characterized by recurrent fever; isolated diaphoresis may mark an episode of acute pain or fever. Night sweats may characterize intermittent fever because body temperature tends to return to normal between 2 a.m. and 4 a.m. before rising again. (Temperature is usually lowest around 6 a.m.)

When caused by high external temperature, diaphoresis is a normal response. Diaphoresis also commonly occurs during menopause, preceded by a sensation of intense heat (a hot flash). Other causes include exercise or exertion that accelerates

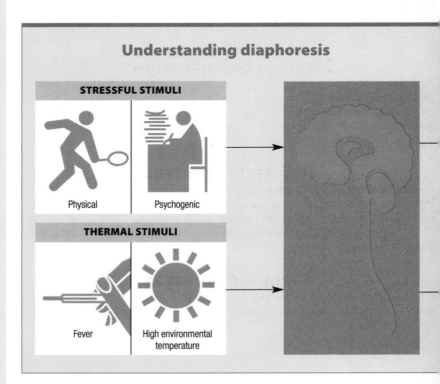

Understanding diaphoresis

STRESSFUL STIMULI

Physical

Psychogenic

THERMAL STIMULI

Fever

High environmental temperature

metabolism, creating internal heat, and mild to moderate anxiety that helps initiate the fight-or-flight response. (See *Understanding diaphoresis*.)

HISTORY

If the patient is diaphoretic, quickly rule out the possibility of a life-threatening cause. (See *When diaphoresis spells crisis*, page 204.) Begin the history by having the patient describe his chief complaint. Then explore associated signs and symptoms. Note general fatigue and weakness. Does the patient have insomnia, headache, and changes in vision or hearing? Is he often dizzy? Does he have palpitations? Ask about pleuritic pain, cough, sputum, difficulty breathing, nausea, vomiting, abdominal pain, and altered bowel or bladder habits. Ask the female patient about amenorrhea and any changes in her menstrual cycle. Is she menopausal? Ask about paresthesia, muscle cramps or stiffness, and joint pain. Has she noticed any changes in elimination habits? Note weight loss or gain. Has the patient had to change her glove or shoe size lately?

Complete the history by asking about travel to tropical countries. Note recent exposure to high environmental temperatures or to pesticides. Did the patient recently experience an insect bite? Check for a history of partial gastrectomy or of drug or alcohol abuse. Finally, obtain a thorough drug history.

PHYSICAL ASSESSMENT

First, determine the extent of diaphoresis by inspecting the trunk and extremities as well as the palms, soles, and forehead. Also, check the patient's clothing and bedding for dampness. Note whether diaphoresis occurs during the day or at night. Observe the patient for flushing, abnormal skin texture or lesions, and an increased

Key history points
+ Chief complaint
+ Associated signs and symptoms
+ Recent travel or exposure to high environmental temperatures or pesticides
+ Recent insect bites
+ History of partial gastrectomy or drug or alcohol abuse
+ Drug history

Sympathetic reactions
+ Increased sweat gland activity
+ Increased metabolic or heart rate and other effects
+ Cutaneous vasoconstriction (pallor)

Parasympathetic reactions
+ Increased sweat gland activity
+ Cutaneous vasodilation (flushing)

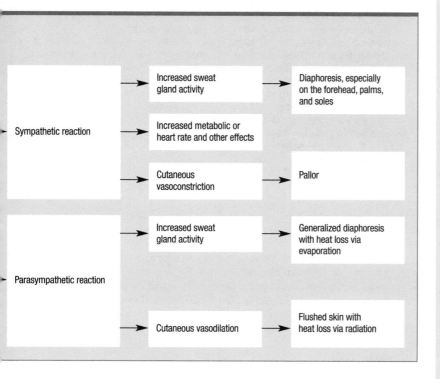

Critical assessment steps

- Inspect the trunk, extremities, palms, soles, and forehead to determine the extent of diaphoresis.
- Check clothing and bedding for dampness.
- Note whether diaphoresis occurs during the day or at night.
- Observe for flushing, abnormal skin texture or lesions, and an increased amount of coarse body hair.
- Note poor skin turgor and dry mucous membranes.
- Check for splinter hemorrhages and Plummer's nails.
- Evaluate mental status.
- Take vital signs.
- Observe for fasciculations and flaccid paralysis.
- Be alert for seizures.
- Note the patient's facial expression; examine the eyes for pupillary dilation or constriction, exophthalmos, and excessive tearing.

When diaphoresis spells crisis

Diaphoresis is an early sign of certain life-threatening disorders. These guidelines will help you promptly detect such disorders and intervene to minimize harm to the patient.

HYPOGLYCEMIA

If you observe diaphoresis in a patient who complains of blurred vision, ask him about increased irritability and anxiety. Has he been unusually hungry lately? Does he have tremors? Take the patient's vital signs, noting hypotension and tachycardia. Then ask about a history of type 2 diabetes or antidiabetic therapy. If you suspect hypoglycemia, evaluate the patient's blood glucose level using a glucose reagent strip, or send a serum sample to the laboratory. Administer I.V. glucose 50% as ordered to return the patient's glucose level to normal. Monitor his vital signs and cardiac rhythm. Ensure a patent airway, and be prepared to assist with breathing and circulation if necessary.

HEATSTROKE

If you observe profuse diaphoresis in a weak, tired, and apprehensive patient, suspect heatstroke, which can progress to circulatory collapse. Take vital signs, noting a normal or subnormal temperature. Check for ashen gray skin and dilated pupils. Was the patient recently exposed to high temperatures and humidity? Was he wearing heavy clothing or performing strenuous physical activity at the time? Also, ask if he takes a diuretic, which interferes with normal sweating.

Then take the patient to a cool room, remove his clothing, and use a fan to direct cool air over his body. Insert an I.V. line, and prepare for electrolyte and fluid replacement. Monitor the patient for signs of shock. Check his urine output carefully along with other sources of output (such as tubes, drains, and ostomies).

AUTONOMIC HYPERREFLEXIA

If you observe diaphoresis in a patient with a spinal cord injury above T6 or T7, ask if he has a pounding headache, restlessness, blurred vision, or nasal congestion. Take the patient's vital signs, noting bradycardia and extremely elevated blood pressure. If you suspect autonomic hyperreflexia, quickly rule out its common complications. Examine the patient for eye pain associated with intraocular hemorrhage and for facial paralysis, slurred speech, or limb weakness associated with intracerebral hemorrhage.

Quickly reposition the patient to remove any pressure stimuli. Also, check for a distended bladder or fecal impaction. Remove any kinks from the urinary catheter if necessary, or administer a suppository or manually remove impacted feces. If you can't locate and relieve the causative stimulus, start an I.V. line. Prepare to administer hydralazine for hypertension.

MYOCARDIAL INFARCTION OR HEART FAILURE

If the patient with diaphoresis complains of chest pain and dyspnea, or has arrhythmias or electrocardiogram changes, suspect a myocardial infarction or heart failure. Connect the patient to a cardiac monitor, ensure a patent airway, and administer supplemental oxygen. Start an I.V. line, and administer an analgesic. Be prepared to begin emergency resuscitation if cardiac or respiratory arrest occurs.

---

amount of coarse body hair. Note poor skin turgor and dry mucous membranes. Check for splinter hemorrhages and Plummer's nails (separation of the fingernail ends from the nail beds).

Then evaluate the patient's mental status and take his vital signs. Observe the patient for fasciculations and flaccid paralysis. Be alert for seizures. Note the patient's facial expression, and examine the eyes for pupillary dilation or constriction, exophthalmos, and excessive tearing. Test visual fields. Also, check for hearing loss and for tooth or gum disease. Percuss the lungs for dullness, and auscultate for crackles, diminished or bronchial breath sounds, and increased vocal fremitus. Look for decreased respiratory excursion. Palpate for lymphadenopathy and hepatosplenomegaly.

MEDICAL CAUSES

Acquired immunodeficiency syndrome

Night sweats may be an early feature of acquired immunodeficiency syndrome (AIDS), occurring either as a manifestation of the disease itself or secondary to an opportunistic infection. The patient also displays fever, fatigue, lymphadenopathy, anorexia, dramatic and unexplained weight loss, diarrhea, and a persistent cough.

Acromegaly

With acromegaly, a slowly progressive disorder, diaphoresis is a sensitive gauge of disease activity, which involves hypersecretion of growth hormone and increased metabolic rate. The patient has a hulking appearance with an enlarged supraorbital ridge and thickened ears and nose. Other signs and symptoms of acromegaly include warm, oily, thickened skin; enlarged hands, feet, and jaw; joint pain; weight gain; hoarseness; and increased coarse body hair. Increased blood pressure, severe headache, and visual field deficits or blindness may also occur.

Anxiety disorders

Acute anxiety characterizes panic, whereas chronic anxiety characterizes phobias, conversion disorders, obsessions, and compulsions. Whether acute or chronic, anxiety may cause sympathetic stimulation, resulting in diaphoresis. The diaphoresis is most dramatic on the palms, soles, and forehead and is accompanied by palpitations, tachycardia, tachypnea, tremors, and GI distress. Psychological signs and symptoms — fear, difficulty concentrating, and behavior changes — also occur.

Autonomic hyperreflexia

Occurring after resolution of spinal shock in a spinal cord injury above T6, autonomic hyperreflexia causes profuse diaphoresis, pounding headache, blurred vision, and dramatically elevated blood pressure. Diaphoresis occurs above the level of the injury, especially on the forehead, and is accompanied by flushing. Other findings include restlessness, nausea, nasal congestion, and bradycardia.

Drug and alcohol withdrawal syndromes

Withdrawal from alcohol or an opioid analgesic may cause generalized diaphoresis, dilated pupils, tachycardia, tremors, and altered mental status (confusion, delusions, hallucinations, agitation). Associated signs and symptoms include severe muscle cramps, generalized paresthesia, tachypnea, increased or decreased blood pressure and, possibly, seizures. Nausea and vomiting are common.

Heart failure

Typically, diaphoresis follows fatigue, dyspnea, orthopnea, and tachycardia in patients with left-sided heart failure. In patients with right-sided heart failure, diaphoresis follows jugular vein distention and dry cough. Other features of heart failure include tachypnea, cyanosis, dependent edema, crackles, ventricular gallop, and anxiety.

Heat exhaustion

Although heat exhaustion is marked by failure of heat to dissipate, it initially may cause profuse diaphoresis, fatigue, weakness, and anxiety. These signs and symptoms may progress to circulatory collapse and shock (confusion, thready pulse, hypotension, tachycardia, and cold, clammy skin). Other features of heat exhaustion include an ashen gray appearance, dilated pupils, and normal or subnormal temperature.

Medical causes

AIDS
+ Night sweats may occur early and may be a manifestation of the disease or secondary to an opportunistic infection.

Acromegaly
+ Diaphoresis gauges disease activity.

Anxiety disorders
+ Anxiety may cause sympathetic stimulation, resulting in diaphoresis, which is most dramatic on the palms, soles, and forehead.

Autonomic hyperreflexia
+ Profuse diaphoresis, pounding headache, blurred vision, and dramatically elevated blood pressure occur.

Drug and alcohol withdrawal syndromes
+ Withdrawal from alcohol or an opioid analgesic may cause generalized diaphoresis, dilated pupils, tachycardia, tremors, and altered mental status.

Heart failure
+ In left-sided heart failure, diaphoresis follows fatigue, dyspnea, orthopnea, and tachycardia.
+ In patients with right-sided heart failure, diaphoresis follows jugular vein distention and dry cough.

Heat exhaustion
+ Profuse diaphoresis, fatigue, weakness, and anxiety may occur initially.

Medical causes
(continued)

Hodgkin's disease
+ Early features may include night sweats, fever, fatigue, pruritus, and weight loss.
+ Initial sign is usually painless swelling of a cervical lymph node.

Hypoglycemia
+ Rapidly induced hypoglycemia may cause diaphoresis, irritability, tremors, hypotension, blurred vision, tachycardia, hunger, and loss of consciousness.

Infective endocarditis (subacute)
+ Generalized night sweats occur early.

Liver abscess
+ Diaphoresis, right-upper-quadrant pain, weight loss, fever, chills, nausea, vomiting, and signs of anemia are common.

Lung abscess
+ Drenching night sweats are common.

Malaria
+ Profuse diaphoresis marks the third stage of paroxysmal malaria.

MI
+ Diaphoresis usually accompanies acute, substernal, radiating chest pain.

Pheochromocytoma
+ Diaphoresis is common.
+ The cardinal sign is persistent or paroxysmal hypertension.

Hodgkin's disease
Especially in elderly patients, early features of Hodgkin's disease may include night sweats, fever, fatigue, pruritus, and weight loss. Usually, however, this disease initially causes painless swelling of a cervical lymph node. Occasionally, a Pel-Ebstein fever pattern is present — several days or weeks of fever and chills alternating with afebrile periods with no chills. Systemic signs and symptoms — such as weight loss, fever, and night sweats — indicate a poor prognosis. Progressive lymphadenopathy eventually causes widespread effects, such as hepatomegaly and dyspnea.

Hypoglycemia
Rapidly induced hypoglycemia may cause diaphoresis accompanied by irritability, tremors, hypotension, blurred vision, tachycardia, hunger, and loss of consciousness. The patient may also experience confusion, motor weakness, hemiplegia, seizures, or coma.

Infective endocarditis (subacute)
Generalized night sweats occur early with subacute infective endocarditis. Accompanying signs and symptoms include intermittent low-grade fever, weakness, fatigue, weight loss, anorexia, and arthralgia. A sudden change in a murmur or the discovery of a new murmur is a classic sign. Petechiae and splinter hemorrhages are also common.

Liver abscess
Signs and symptoms vary, depending on the extent of a liver abscess, but commonly include diaphoresis, right-upper-quadrant pain, weight loss, fever, chills, nausea, vomiting, and signs of anemia. The patient may appear jaundiced and have chalk-colored stools and dark urine.

Lung abscess
Drenching night sweats are common with a lung abscess. Its chief sign, however, is a cough productive of copious purulent, foul-smelling, typically bloody sputum. Associated findings include fever with chills, pleuritic chest pain, dyspnea, weakness, anorexia, weight loss, headache, malaise, clubbing, tubular or amphoric breath sounds, and dullness on percussion.

Malaria
Profuse diaphoresis marks the third stage of paroxysmal malaria; the first two stages are chills (first stage) and high fever (second stage). Headache, arthralgia, and hepatosplenomegaly may also occur. In the benign form of malaria, these paroxysms alternate with periods of well-being. The severe form may progress to delirium, seizures, and coma.

Myocardial infarction
Diaphoresis usually accompanies acute, substernal, radiating chest pain in myocardial infarction (MI), a life-threatening disorder. Associated signs and symptoms of MI include anxiety, dyspnea, nausea, vomiting, tachycardia, irregular pulse, blood pressure change, fine crackles, pallor, and clammy skin.

Pheochromocytoma
Pheochromocytoma commonly produces diaphoresis, but its cardinal sign is persistent or paroxysmal hypertension. Other effects include headache, palpitations, tachycardia, anxiety, tremors, pallor, flushing, paresthesia, abdominal pain, tachypnea, nausea, vomiting, and orthostatic hypotension.

Pneumonia

Intermittent, generalized diaphoresis accompanies fever and chills in patients with pneumonia. They complain of pleuritic chest pain that increases with deep inspiration. Other features are tachypnea, dyspnea, productive cough (with scant and mucoid or copious and purulent sputum), headache, fatigue, myalgia, abdominal pain, anorexia, and cyanosis. Auscultation reveals bronchial breath sounds.

Relapsing fever

Profuse diaphoresis marks resolution of the crisis stage of relapsing fever, which typically produces attacks of high fever accompanied by severe myalgia, headache, arthralgia, diarrhea, vomiting, coughing, and eye or chest pain. Splenomegaly is common, but hepatomegaly and lymphadenopathy may also occur. The patient may develop a transient, macular rash. Between 3 and 10 days after onset, the febrile attack abruptly terminates in chills with increased pulse and respiratory rates. Diaphoresis, flushing, and hypotension may then lead to circulatory collapse and death. Relapse invariably occurs if the patient survives the initial attack.

 CULTURAL CUE *Louse-borne relapsing fever is most common in North and Central Africa, Europe, Asia, and South America. Tick-borne relapsing fever is commonly found in the United States, most prevalently in Texas and other western states.*

Tetanus

Tetanus commonly causes profuse sweating accompanied by low-grade fever, tachycardia, and hyperactive deep tendon reflexes. Early restlessness and pain and stiffness in the jaw, abdomen, and back progress to spasms associated with lockjaw, risus sardonicus, dysphagia, and opisthotonos. Laryngospasm may result in cyanosis or sudden death by asphyxiation.

Thyrotoxicosis

Thyrotoxicosis commonly produces diaphoresis accompanied by heat intolerance, weight loss despite increased appetite, tachycardia, palpitations, an enlarged thyroid, dyspnea, nervousness, diarrhea, tremors, Plummer's nails and, possibly, exophthalmos. Gallops may also occur.

OTHER CAUSES

Drugs

Sympathomimetics, certain antipsychotics, thyroid hormone, corticosteroids, and antipyretics may cause diaphoresis. Aspirin and acetaminophen poisoning also cause this sign.

Dumping syndrome

The result of rapid emptying of gastric contents into the small intestine after partial gastrectomy, dumping syndrome causes diaphoresis, palpitations, profound weakness, epigastric distress, nausea, and explosive diarrhea. This syndrome occurs soon after the patient eats.

Pesticide poisoning

Among the toxic effects of pesticides are diaphoresis, nausea, vomiting, diarrhea, blurred vision, miosis, and excessive lacrimation and salivation. The patient may display fasciculations, muscle weakness, and flaccid paralysis. Signs of respiratory depression and coma may also occur.

Medical causes
(continued)

Pneumonia
+ Intermittent, generalized diaphoresis accompanies fever and chills.

Relapsing fever
+ Profuse diaphoresis marks resolution of the crisis stage of relapsing fever.
+ Febrile attack abruptly terminates in chills with increased pulse and respiratory rates.
+ Diaphoresis, flushing, and hypotension may then lead to circulatory collapse and death.

Tetanus
+ Profuse sweating is accompanied by low-grade fever, tachycardia, and hyperactive DTRs.

Thyrotoxicosis
+ Diaphoresis is accompanied by heat intolerance, weight loss despite increased appetite, tachycardia, palpitations, an enlarged thyroid, dyspnea, nervousness, diarrhea, tremors, Plummer's nails and, possibly, exophthalmos.

Other causes
+ Antipyretics
+ Aspirin or acetaminophen poisoning
+ Certain antipsychotics
+ Corticosteroids
+ Dumping syndrome
+ Pesticide poisoning
+ Sympathomimetics
+ Thyroid hormone

Special considerations

+ Sponge the face and body.
+ Change wet clothes and sheets.
+ To prevent skin irritation, dust skin folds in the groin and axillae and under pendulous breasts with cornstarch.
+ Replace fluids and electrolytes.
+ Monitor urine output.
+ Encourage oral fluids high in electrolytes.
+ Keep the room temperature moderate.

Peds points

+ Diaphoresis in children commonly results from environmental heat, overdressing, drug withdrawal associated with maternal addiction, heart failure, thyrotoxicosis, and the effects of such drugs as antihistamines, ephedrine, haloperidol, and thyroid hormone.

Geri points

+ Older patients may not exhibit diaphoresis because of a decreased sweating mechanism, which puts them at increased risk for developing heatstroke in high temperatures.

Teaching points

+ Proper skin care
+ Disease process

Key facts about diarrhea

+ Increase in the volume of stools
+ May be acute or chronic
+ Can cause life-threatening fluid and electrolyte imbalances

SPECIAL CONSIDERATIONS

After an episode of diaphoresis, sponge the patient's face and body and change wet clothes and sheets. To prevent skin irritation, dust skin folds in the groin and axillae and under pendulous breasts with cornstarch, or tuck gauze or cloth into the folds. Encourage regular bathing.

Replace fluids and electrolytes. Regulate infusions of I.V. saline or lactated Ringer's solution, and monitor urine output. Encourage oral fluids high in electrolytes (such as Gatorade). Enforce bed rest, and maintain a quiet environment. Keep the patient's room temperature moderate to prevent additional diaphoresis.

Prepare the patient for diagnostic tests, such as blood tests, cultures, chest X-rays, immunologic studies, biopsy, computed tomography scan, and audiometry. Monitor the patient's vital signs, including temperature.

PEDIATRIC POINTERS

Diaphoresis in children commonly results from environmental heat or overdressing the child; it's usually most apparent around the head. Other causes include drug withdrawal associated with maternal addiction, heart failure, thyrotoxicosis, and the effects of such drugs as antihistamines, ephedrine, haloperidol, and thyroid hormone. Also, keep in mind that sweat glands function immaturely in infants.

Assess fluid status carefully. Some fluid loss through diaphoresis may precipitate hypovolemia more rapidly in a child than an adult. Monitor input and output, weigh the child daily, and note the duration of each episode of diaphoresis.

GERIATRIC POINTERS

Fever and night sweats, the hallmark of tuberculosis, may not occur in elderly patients, who instead may exhibit a change in activity or weight. Also, keep in mind that older patients may not exhibit diaphoresis because of a decreased sweating mechanism. Therefore, they're at increased risk for developing heatstroke in high temperatures.

PATIENT COUNSELING

Explain to the patient and his family that diaphoresis signals a return to normal body temperature after it has risen for any reason. Explain that diaphoresis can also occur spontaneously, after taking an antipyretic, or as a sympathetic reaction to pain or stress. Be sure to discuss proper skin care to avoid skin breakdown and maceration.

DIARRHEA

Usually a chief sign of an intestinal disorder, diarrhea is an increase in the volume of stools compared with the patient's normal bowel habits. It varies in severity and may be acute or chronic. Acute diarrhea may result from acute infection, stress, fecal impaction, or the effect of a drug. Chronic diarrhea may result from chronic infection, obstructive and inflammatory bowel disease, malabsorption syndrome, an endocrine disorder, or GI surgery. Periodic diarrhea may result from food intolerance or from ingestion of spicy or high-fiber foods or caffeine.

One or more pathophysiologic mechanisms may contribute to diarrhea. (See *What causes diarrhea.*) The fluid and electrolyte imbalances it produces may precipitate life-threatening arrhythmias or hypovolemic shock.

What causes diarrhea

This flowchart shows how certain factors can cause diarrhea.

Ingestion of poorly absorbable material such as a bulk-forming laxative → Excessive osmotic load in the small intestine → Increased fluid drawn into and retained in the small intestine →

Stimulation of mucosal intracellular enzymes (cyclic AMP) by bacterial toxins or other factors → Active transport of electrolytes into the small intestine → Excessive fluid in the small intestine →

Diarrhea

Disrupted integrity of small-intestine mucosa → Impaired intestinal absorption → Excessive fluid in the small intestine →

Increased intestinal motility → Decreased intestinal absorption → Excessive fluid in the small intestine →

Local lymphatic or venous obstruction → Increased intravascular and intracellular hydrostatic pressure → Altered permeability of intestinal mucosa → Passive secretion of fluid and electrolytes into the small intestine →

In an emergency

If diarrhea is profuse and the patient has signs of shock:
- Place the patient in the supine position and elevate his legs 20 degrees.
- Insert an I.V. line for fluid replacement.
- Monitor for electrolyte imbalances.
- Look for an irregular pulse, muscle weakness, anorexia, and nausea and vomiting.
- Keep emergency resuscitation equipment handy.

Key history points

+ Associated signs and symptoms (pain, cramps, difficulty breathing, weakness, fatigue)
+ Drug history
+ Recent GI surgery or radiation therapy
+ Diet and food allergies
+ Possible stress factors

Critical assessment steps

+ Check skin turgor and mucous membranes.
+ Take blood pressure with the patient lying, sitting, and standing.
+ Inspect the abdomen for distention, and palpate for tenderness.
+ Auscultate bowel sounds.
+ Take the patient's temperature.
+ Look for a rash.

Medical causes

Anthrax, GI

+ Later signs and symptoms are severe bloody diarrhea, abdominal pain, and hematemesis.

C. difficile infection

+ Patient may have soft, unformed stools or watery diarrhea that may be foul smelling or bloody.

Crohn's disease

+ Diarrhea is accompanied by abdominal pain, with guarding and tenderness and nausea.

E. coli 0157:H7

+ Watery or bloody diarrhea, nausea, vomiting, fever, and abdominal cramps occur.

Infections

+ Acute viral, bacterial, and protozoal infections cause the sudden onset of watery diarrhea.

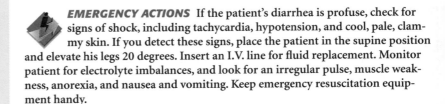

EMERGENCY ACTIONS If the patient's diarrhea is profuse, check for signs of shock, including tachycardia, hypotension, and cool, pale, clammy skin. If you detect these signs, place the patient in the supine position and elevate his legs 20 degrees. Insert an I.V. line for fluid replacement. Monitor patient for electrolyte imbalances, and look for an irregular pulse, muscle weakness, anorexia, and nausea and vomiting. Keep emergency resuscitation equipment handy.

HISTORY

Explore signs and symptoms associated with diarrhea. Does the patient have abdominal pain and cramps? Difficulty breathing? Is he weak or fatigued? Find out his drug history. Has he had GI surgery or radiation therapy recently? Ask the patient to briefly describe his diet. Does he have any known food allergies? Lastly, find out if he's under unusual stress.

PHYSICAL ASSESSMENT

If the patient isn't in shock, proceed with a brief physical examination. Evaluate hydration, check skin turgor and mucous membranes, and take blood pressure with the patient lying, sitting, and standing. Inspect the abdomen for distention, and palpate for tenderness. Auscultate bowel sounds. Check for tympany over the abdomen. Take the patient's temperature, and note any chills. Also, look for a rash. Conduct a rectal examination and a pelvic examination if indicated.

MEDICAL CAUSES

Anthrax, GI

Early signs and symptoms of GI anthrax, an infectious disease caused by eating meat contaminated with the bacterium *Bacillus anthracis*, include decreased appetite, nausea, vomiting, and fever. Later signs and symptoms include severe bloody diarrhea, abdominal pain, and hematemesis.

Clostridium difficile infection

With a *Clostridium difficile* infection, the patient may be asymptomatic or may have soft, unformed stools or watery diarrhea that may be foul smelling or grossly bloody; abdominal pain, cramping, and tenderness; fever; and a white blood cell count as high as 20,000/µl. In severe cases, the patient may develop toxic megacolon, colonic perforation, or peritonitis.

Crohn's disease

Crohn's disease, a recurring inflammatory disorder, produces diarrhea accompanied by abdominal pain with guarding and tenderness, and nausea. The patient may also display fever, chills, weakness, anorexia, and weight loss.

Escherichia coli 0157:H7

Watery or bloody diarrhea, nausea, vomiting, fever, and abdominal cramps occur after the patient eats undercooked beef or other foods contaminated with the *Escherichia coli* 0157:H7 strain of bacteria. Hemolytic uremic syndrome, which causes red blood cell destruction and eventually acute renal failure, is a complication of *E. coli* 0157:H7 in children age 5 and younger and elderly people.

Infections

Acute viral, bacterial, and protozoal infections (such as cryptosporidiosis) cause the sudden onset of watery diarrhea as well as abdominal pain, cramps, nausea, vomiting, and fever. Significant fluid and electrolyte loss may cause signs of dehydration and shock. Chronic tuberculosis and fungal and parasitic infections may produce a less severe but more persistent diarrhea, accompanied by epigastric distress, vomiting, weight loss and, possibly, passage of blood and mucus.

Intestinal obstruction

Partial intestinal obstruction increases intestinal motility, resulting in diarrhea, abdominal pain with tenderness and guarding, nausea and, possibly, distention. Other signs and symptoms may include borborygmi and rushes on auscultation and vomiting of fecal material.

Irritable bowel syndrome

Diarrhea alternates with constipation or normal bowel function. Related findings include abdominal pain, tenderness, and distention; dyspepsia; and nausea. The patient may also report passage of mucus and pasty pencil-like stools.

Ischemic bowel disease

A life-threatening disorder, ischemic bowel disease causes bloody diarrhea with abdominal pain. The patient may also experience abdominal distention, nausea, and vomiting. If severe, shock may occur, requiring surgery.

Lactose intolerance

Diarrhea occurs within several hours of ingesting milk or milk products. It's accompanied by cramps, abdominal pain, borborygmi, bloating, nausea, and flatus.

Large-bowel cancer

With large-bowel cancer, bloody diarrhea is seen with a partial obstruction. Other signs and symptoms include abdominal pain, anorexia, weight loss, weakness, fatigue, exertional dyspnea, and depression.

Lead poisoning

Alternating diarrhea and constipation occur in a patient with lead poisoning. Other GI effects include abdominal pain, anorexia, nausea, and vomiting. The patient complains of a metallic taste, headache, and dizziness and displays a bluish gingival lead line.

Malabsorption syndrome

In a patient with malabsorption syndrome, diarrhea occurs after meals, accompanied by steatorrhea, abdominal distention, and muscle cramps. The patient also displays anorexia, weight loss, bone pain, anemia, weakness, and fatigue. He may bruise easily and have night blindness.

Pseudomembranous enterocolitis

Pseudomembranous enterocolitis, a potentially life-threatening disorder, commonly follows antibiotic administration. It produces copious watery, green, foul-smelling, bloody diarrhea that rapidly precipitates signs of shock. Other signs and symptoms include colicky abdominal pain, distention, fever, and dehydration.

Q Fever

Q Fever is an infection that's caused by the bacterium *Coxiella burnetii* and causes diarrhea along with fever, chills, severe headache, malaise, chest pain, and vomiting. In severe cases, hepatitis or pneumonia may follow. Chronic Q fever may cause prolonged fever, night sweats, chills, fatigue, and dyspnea.

Medical causes
(continued)

Intestinal obstruction
+ Increased intestinal motility results in diarrhea, abdominal pain with tenderness and guarding, nausea and, possibly, distention.

Irritable bowel syndrome
+ Diarrhea alternates with constipation or normal bowel function.

Ischemic bowel disease
+ Bloody diarrhea occurs with abdominal pain.

Lactose intolerance
+ Diarrhea occurs within hours of ingesting milk or milk products.

Large-bowel cancer
+ Bloody diarrhea is seen with a partial obstruction.

Lead poisoning
+ Diarrhea alternates with constipation.

Malabsorption syndrome
+ Diarrhea occurs after meals along with steatorrhea, abdominal distention, and muscle cramps.

Pseudomembranous enterocolitis
+ Copious watery, green, foul-smelling, bloody diarrhea rapidly precipitates signs of shock.

Q Fever
+ Diarrhea occurs along with fever, chills, severe headache, malaise, chest pain, and vomiting.

Medical causes
(continued)
Rotavirus gastroenteritis
✦ Fever, nausea, and vomiting are followed by diarrhea.

Thyrotoxicosis
✦ Diarrhea accompanies such signs and symptomsas diaphoresis, dyspnea, and tachycardia.

Ulcerative colitis
✦ Recurrent bloody diarrhea with pus or mucus is a hallmark sign.

Other causes
✦ Antibiotics, magnesium-containing antacids, colchicine, guanethidine, lactulose, dantrolene, ethacrynic acid, mefenamic acid, methotrexate, metyrosine and, in high doses, cardiac glycosides and quinidine
✦ Gastrectomy, gastroenterostomy, or pyloroplasty
✦ Herbal remedies
✦ High-dose radiation therapy
✦ Laxative abuse

Special considerations
✦ Administer an analgesic and an opiate, unless the patient has a possible or confirmed stool infection.
✦ Clean the perineum thoroughly.
✦ Quantify the amount of liquid stools and carefully observe intake and output.
✦ Monitor electrolyte levels and hematocrit.
✦ Administer I.V. fluid replacements.
✦ Stress the need for medical follow-up to those with inflammatory bowel disease.

Rotavirus gastroenteritis
Rotavirus gastroenteritis commonly starts with a fever, nausea, and vomiting, followed by diarrhea. The illness can range from mild to severe and last from 3 to 9 days. Diarrhea and vomiting may result in dehydration.

Thyrotoxicosis
With thyrotoxicosis, diarrhea is accompanied by nervousness, tremors, diaphoresis, weight loss despite increased appetite, dyspnea, palpitations, tachycardia, enlarged thyroid, heat intolerance and, possibly, exophthalmos.

Ulcerative colitis
The hallmark of ulcerative colitis is recurrent bloody diarrhea with pus or mucus. Other signs and symptoms include tenesmus, hyperactive bowel sounds, cramping lower abdominal pain, low-grade fever, anorexia and, at times, nausea and vomiting. Weight loss, anemia, and weakness are late findings.

OTHER CAUSES
Drugs
Many antibiotics — such as ampicillin, cephalosporins, tetracyclines, and clindamycin — cause diarrhea. Other drugs that may cause diarrhea include magnesium-containing antacids, colchicine, guanethidine, lactulose, dantrolene, ethacrynic acid, mefenamic acid, methotrexate, metyrosine and, in high doses, cardiac glycosides and quinidine. Laxative abuse can cause acute or chronic diarrhea. Herbal remedies — such as ginkgo biloba, ginseng, and licorice — may also cause diarrhea.

Foods
Foods that contain certain oils may inhibit absorption causing acute uncontrollable diarrhea and rectal leakage.

Treatments
Gastrectomy, gastroenterostomy, and pyloroplasty may produce diarrhea. High-dose radiation therapy may produce enteritis, which is associated with diarrhea.

SPECIAL CONSIDERATIONS
Administer an analgesic for pain and an opiate to decrease intestinal motility, unless the patient has a possible or confirmed stool infection. Ensure the patient's privacy during defecation, and empty bedpans promptly. Clean the perineum thoroughly, and apply ointment to prevent skin breakdown. Quantify the amount of liquid stools and carefully observe intake and output. Measure liquid stools, and weigh the patient daily. Monitor electrolyte levels and hematocrit. Accurately administer I.V. fluid replacements.

Stress the need for medical follow-up to patients with inflammatory bowel disease (particularly ulcerative colitis), who have an increased risk of developing colon cancer.

PEDIATRIC POINTERS
Diarrhea in children commonly results from infection, although chronic diarrhea may result from malabsorption syndrome, an anatomic defect, or allergies. Because dehydration and electrolyte imbalance occur rapidly in children, diarrhea can be life-threatening. Diligently monitor all episodes of diarrhea, and immediately replace lost fluids.

GERIATRIC POINTERS

In the elderly patient with new-onset segmental colitis, always consider ischemia before asssuming that the patient has Crohn's disease.

PATIENT COUNSELING

Explain the purpose of diagnostic tests to the patient. These tests may include blood studies, stool cultures, X-rays, and endoscopy.

Help the patient maintain adequate hydration. Remember that dehydration occurs rapidly in elderly people. Encourage the patient to drink plenty of fluids.

Advise the patient to avoid spicy or high-fiber foods (such as fruits), caffeine, high-fat foods, and milk. Suggest smaller, more frequent meals if he has had GI surgery or disease. If appropriate, teach the patient stress-reducing exercises, such as guided imagery and deep-breathing techniques, or recommend counseling.

DIPLOPIA

Diplopia is the clinical term for double vision, or seeing one object as two. This symptom results when extraocular muscles fail to work together, causing images to fall on noncorresponding parts of the retinas. Orbital lesions, the effects of surgery, or impaired function of cranial nerves (CNs) that supply extraocular muscles (oculomotor, CN III; trochlear, CN IV; abducens, CN VI) may be responsible. (See *Testing extraocular muscles,* page 214.)

Diplopia usually begins intermittently and affects near or far vision exclusively. It can be classified as monocular or binocular. More common binocular diplopia may result from ocular deviation or displacement, extraocular muscle palsies, or psychoneurosis, or it may occur after retinal surgery. Monocular diplopia may result from an early cataract, retinal edema or scarring, iridodialysis, a subluxated lens, a poorly fitting contact lens, or an uncorrected refractive error such as astigmatism. Diplopia may also occur in hysteria or malingering.

HISTORY

Briefly ask about associated symptoms, especially a severe headache. Find out about associated neurologic symptoms first because diplopia can accompany serious disorders. Find out when the patient first noticed diplopia. Are the images side-by-side (horizontal), one above the other (vertical), or a combination? Does diplopia affect near or far vision? Does it affect certain directions of gaze? Ask if diplopia has worsened, remained the same, or subsided. Does its severity change throughout the day? Diplopia that worsens or appears in the evening may indicate myasthenia gravis. Find out if the patient can correct diplopia by tilting his head. If so, ask him to show you. (If the patient has a fourth nerve lesion, tilting of the head toward the opposite shoulder causes compensatory tilting of the unaffected eye. If he has incomplete sixth nerve palsy, tilting of the head toward the side of the paralyzed muscle may relax the affected lateral rectus muscle.)

Explore associated symptoms such as eye pain. Ask about hypertension, diabetes mellitus, allergies, and thyroid, neurologic, or muscular disorders. Also, note a history of extraocular muscle disorders, trauma, or eye surgery.

Peds points

+ Diarrhea in children commonly results from infection.
+ Chronic diarrhea may result from malabsorption syndrome, an anatomic defect, or allergies.

Geri points

+ In an elderly patient with new-onset segmental colitis, consider ischemia before assuming Crohn's disease.

Teaching points

+ Ways to maintain adequate hydration
+ Foods to avoid
+ Stress-reducing exercises or referral to counseling

Key facts about diplopia

+ Refers to double vision (seeing one object as two)
+ Results when extraocular muscles fail to work together, causing images to fall on noncorresponding parts of the retinas
+ Can be monocular or binocular

Key history points

+ Associated symptoms, including severe headache, neurologic symptoms, and eye pain
+ Onset and description of diplopia
+ History of hypertension; diabetes mellitus; allergies; thyroid, neurologic, or muscular disorders; extraocular muscle disorders; trauma; or eye surgery

Critical assessment steps

+ Perform a neurologic examination.
+ Evaluate LOC; pupil size, equality, and response to light; and motor and sensory function.
+ Take vital signs.
+ Observe the patient for ocular deviation, ptosis, proptosis, lid edema, and conjunctival injection.
+ Distinguish monocular from binocular diplopia.
+ Test visual acuity and extraocular muscles.

Medical causes

Brain tumor
+ Diplopia may be an early symptom.
+ Other signs and symptoms vary with tumor size and location.

Diabetes mellitus
+ Sudden diplopia due to isolated third cranial nerve palsy may be a long-term effect.

Testing extraocular muscles

The coordinated action of six muscles controls eyeball movements. To test the function of each muscle and the cranial nerve (CN) that innervates it, ask the patient to look in the direction controlled by that muscle. The six directions you can test make up the cardinal fields of gaze. The patient's inability to turn the eye in the designated direction indicates muscle weakness or paralysis.

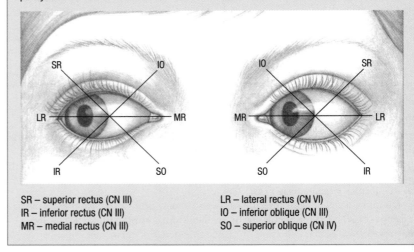

SR – superior rectus (CN III)
IR – inferior rectus (CN III)
MR – medial rectus (CN III)

LR – lateral rectus (CN VI)
IO – inferior oblique (CN III)
SO – superior oblique (CN IV)

PHYSICAL ASSESSMENT

Perform a neurologic examination. Evaluate the patient's level of consciousness (LOC); pupil size, equality, and response to light; and motor and sensory function. Then take his vital signs.

Observe the patient for ocular deviation, ptosis, proptosis, lid edema, and conjunctival injection. Distinguish monocular from binocular diplopia by asking the patient to occlude one eye at a time. If he still sees double out of one eye, he has monocular diplopia. Test visual acuity and extraocular muscles.

MEDICAL CAUSES

Brain tumor

Diplopia may be an early symptom of a brain tumor. Accompanying signs and symptoms vary with the tumor's size and location but may include eye deviation, emotional lability, decreased LOC, headache, vomiting, absence or generalized tonic-clonic seizures, hearing loss, visual field deficits, abnormal pupillary responses, nystagmus, motor weakness, and paralysis.

Diabetes mellitus

Diplopia due to isolated third cranial nerve palsy may be among the long-term effects of diabetes mellitus. It typically begins suddenly and may be accompanied by intense periorbital or head pain. The patient may display the typical signs and symptoms of diabetes to varying degrees.

Encephalitis

Initially, encephalitis may cause a brief episode of diplopia and eye deviation. However, it usually begins with sudden onset of high fever, severe headache, and vomiting. As the inflammation progresses, the patient may display signs of meningeal irritation, decreased LOC, seizures, ataxia, and paralysis.

Head injury

Potentially life-threatening head injuries may cause diplopia, depending on the site and extent of the injury. Associated signs and symptoms include eye deviation, pupillary changes, headache, decreased LOC, altered vital signs, nausea, vomiting, and motor weakness or paralysis.

Intracranial aneurysm

Intracranial aneurysm is a life-threatening disorder that initially produces diplopia and eye deviation, perhaps accompanied by ptosis and a dilated pupil on the affected side. The patient complains of a recurrent, severe, unilateral, frontal headache. After the aneurysm ruptures, the headache becomes violent. Associated signs and symptoms include neck and spinal pain and rigidity, decreased LOC, tinnitus, dizziness, nausea, vomiting, and unilateral muscle weakness or paralysis.

Multiple sclerosis

Diplopia, a common early symptom in multiple sclerosis (MS), is usually accompanied by blurred vision and paresthesia. As MS progresses, signs and symptoms may include nystagmus, constipation, muscle weakness, paralysis, spasticity, hyperreflexia, intention tremor, gait ataxia, dysphagia, dysarthria, impotence, emotional lability, and urinary frequency, urgency, and incontinence.

Myasthenia gravis

Myasthenia gravis initially produces diplopia and ptosis, which worsen throughout the day. It then progressively involves other muscles, resulting in blank facial expression; nasal voice; difficulty chewing, swallowing, and making fine hand movements; and possibly signs of life-threatening respiratory muscle weakness.

Ophthalmologic migraine

Most common in young adults, ophthalmologic migraine results in diplopia that persists for days after the headache. Accompanying signs and symptoms include severe, unilateral pain; ptosis; and extraocular muscle palsies. Irritability, depression, or slight confusion may also occur.

Orbital blowout fracture

An orbital blowout fracture usually causes monocular diplopia affecting the upward gaze. However, with marked periorbital edema, diplopia may affect other directions of gaze. This fracture commonly causes periorbital ecchymosis but doesn't affect visual acuity, although eyelid edema may prevent accurate testing. Subcutaneous crepitation of the eyelid and orbit is typical. Occasionally, the patient's pupil is dilated and unreactive, and he may have a hyphema.

Orbital cellulitis

Orbital cellulitis (inflammation of the orbital tissues and eyelids) causes sudden diplopia. Other findings are eye deviation and pain, purulent drainage, lid edema, chemosis and redness, proptosis, nausea, and fever.

Medical causes
(continued)

Encephalitis
+ A brief episode of diplopia and eye deviation may occur.

Head injury
+ Diplopia may occur depending on the site and extent of injury.

Intracranial aneurysm
+ Diplopia and eye deviation occur initially, possibly with ptosis and a dilated pupil on the affected side.

Multiple sclerosis
+ Diplopia is a common early symptom and is usually accompanied by blurred vision and paresthesia.

Myasthenia gravis
+ Diplopia and ptosis occur initially (may worsen throughout the day).

Ophthalmologic migraine
+ Most common in young adults, diplopia persists for days after the headache.

Orbital blowout fracture
+ Monocular diplopia affecting the upward gaze usually occurs.
+ With marked periorbital edema, diplopia may affect other directions of gaze.

Orbital cellulitis
+ Diplopia develops suddenly.
+ Other findings are eye deviation and pain, purulent drainage, lid edema, chemosis and redness, proptosis, nausea, and fever.

Medical causes
(continued)

Orbital tumors
+ Diplopia can occur, possibly with proptosis and blurred vision.

Stroke
+ Diplopia occurs if stroke affects the vertebrobasilar artery.

Thyrotoxicosis
+ Diplopia beginning in the upper field of gaze accompanies exophthalmos.

Transient ischemic attack
+ Diplopia, dizziness, tinnitus, hearing loss, and numbness usually occur.

Special considerations
+ Continue to monitor vital signs and neurologic status.
+ Provide a safe environment.
+ Institute seizure precautions if indicated.

Peds points
+ School-age children who complain of double vision require a careful examination to rule out serious disorders such as a brain tumor.

Teaching points
+ Safety measures
+ Ambulation assistance

Key facts about dizziness
+ A sensation of imbalance or faintness
+ Typically results from inadequate blood flow and oxygen supply to the cerebrum and spinal cord

Orbital tumors
Orbital tumors can cause diplopia. Proptosis and possibly blurred vision may also occur. One or both eyes may appear prominent. The patient may also report pain and redness and swelling of the lid of the affected eye.

Stroke
Diplopia characterizes stroke when it affects the vertebrobasilar artery. Other signs and symptoms of this life-threatening disorder include unilateral motor weakness or paralysis, ataxia, decreased LOC, dizziness, aphasia, visual field deficits, circumoral numbness, slurred speech, dysphagia, and amnesia.

Thyrotoxicosis
Diplopia accompanies exophthalmos in patients with thyrotoxicosis. It usually begins in the upper field of gaze because of infiltrative myopathy involving the inferior rectus muscle. It's accompanied by impaired eye movement, excessive tearing, lid edema and, possibly, inability to close the lids. Other cardinal findings include tachycardia, palpitations, weight loss, diarrhea, tremors, an enlarged thyroid, dyspnea, nervousness, diaphoresis, and heat intolerance.

Transient ischemic attack
Transient ischemic attack is generally accompanied by diplopia, dizziness, tinnitus, hearing loss, and numbness. It can last for a few seconds or up to 24 hours and may be a warning sign for a future stroke.

SPECIAL CONSIDERATIONS
Continue to monitor the patient's vital signs and neurologic status if you suspect an acute neurologic disorder. Prepare him for neurologic tests such as a computed tomography scan. Provide a safe environment. If the patient has severe diplopia, remove sharp obstacles and assist him with ambulation. Also, institute seizure precautions if indicated.

PEDIATRIC POINTERS
Strabismus, which can be congenital or acquired at an early age, produces diplopia; however, in young children, the brain rapidly compensates for double vision by suppressing one image, so diplopia is a rare complaint. School-age children who complain of double vision require a careful examination to rule out serious disorders such as a brain tumor.

PATIENT COUNSELING
Discuss safety measures with the patient and his family. Stress the importance of ambulating with assistance. Explain all diagnostic tests and procedures to the patient. Encourage the patient to express his concerns regarding diplopia. If necessary, orient the patient to his room and his meal tray.

DIZZINESS

A common symptom, dizziness is a sensation of imbalance or faintness, sometimes associated with giddiness, weakness, confusion, and blurred or double vision. Episodes of dizziness are usually brief; they may be mild or severe with abrupt or gradual onset. Dizziness may be aggravated by standing up quickly and alleviated by lying down and by rest.

Dizziness typically results from inadequate blood flow and oxygen supply to the cerebrum and spinal cord. It may occur with anxiety, respiratory and cardiovascular disorders, and postconcussion syndrome. It's a key symptom in certain serious disorders, such as hypertension and vertebrobasilar artery insufficiency.

Dizziness is commonly confused with vertigo—a sensation of revolving in space or of surroundings revolving about oneself. However, unlike dizziness, vertigo is commonly accompanied by nausea, vomiting, nystagmus, staggering gait, and tinnitus or hearing loss. Dizziness and vertigo may occur together, as in postconcussion syndrome.

EMERGENCY ACTIONS If the patient complains of dizziness, first ensure his safety by preventing falls. Then determine the severity and onset of the dizziness. Ask the patient to describe it. Find out if the dizziness is associated with headache or blurred vision. Next, take the patient's blood pressure while he's lying, sitting, and standing to check for orthostatic hypotension. Ask about a history of high blood pressure. Determine if the patient is at risk for hypoglycemia. Tell him to lie down, and recheck his vital signs every 15 minutes. Start an I.V. line, and prepare to administer medications as ordered.

HISTORY

If the patient's blood pressure is normal, obtain a more complete history. Ask about a history of diabetes and cardiovascular disease. Is the patient taking drugs prescribed for high blood pressure? If so, when did he take his last dose? Also ask about myocardial infarction, heart failure, kidney disease, or atherosclerosis, which may predispose the patient to cardiac arrhythmias, hypertension, and a transient ischemic attack. Does he have a history of anemia, chronic obstructive pulmonary disease, anxiety disorders, or head injury? Obtain a complete drug history.

Next, explore the patient's dizziness. How often does it occur? How long does each episode last? Does the dizziness abate spontaneously? Does it lead to loss of consciousness? Find out if dizziness is triggered by sitting or standing up suddenly or stooping over. Does being in a crowd make the patient feel dizzy? Ask about emotional stress. Has the patient been irritable or anxious lately? Does he have insomnia or difficulty concentrating? Look for fidgeting and eyelid twitching. Does the patient startle easily? Also, ask about palpitations, chest pain, diaphoresis, shortness of breath, and chronic cough.

PHYSICAL ASSESSMENT

Begin the physical examination with a quick check of the patient's neurologic vital signs, including his level of consciousness (LOC), motor and sensory functions, and reflexes. Then inspect for poor skin turgor and dry mucous membranes, signs of dehydration. Auscultate heart rate and rhythm. Inspect for barrel chest, clubbing, cyanosis, and use of accessory muscles. Also auscultate breath sounds. Take the patient's blood pressure while he's lying, sitting, and standing to check for orthostatic hypotension. Test capillary refill time in the extremities, and palpate for edema.

MEDICAL CAUSES

Anemia
Typically, anemia causes dizziness that's aggravated by postural changes or exertion. Other signs and symptoms include pallor, dyspnea, fatigue, tachycardia, and bounding pulse. Capillary refill time is increased.

In an emergency
+ Determine the severity and onset of the dizziness.
+ Check for orthostatic hypotension.
+ Determine if the patient is at risk for hypoglycemia.
+ Have the patient lie down.
+ Recheck vital signs every 15 minutes.
+ Start an I.V. line; prepare to administer medications as ordered.

Key history points
+ Medical history, including diabetes, cardiovascular disease and kidney disease
+ Drug history
+ Onset and characteristics of dizziness
+ Emotional stress factors
+ Associated signs and symptoms (palpitations, chest pain, diaphoresis, shortness of breath, and chronic cough)

Critical assessment steps
+ Check neurologic vital signs.
+ Inspect for poor skin turgor and dry mucous membranes.
+ Auscultate heart rate and rhythm.
+ Inspect for barrel chest, clubbing, cyanosis, and accessory muscle use.
+ Auscultate breath sounds.
+ Check for orthostatic hypotension.
+ Palpate for edema.

Medical causes
Anemia
+ Dizziness is aggravated by postural changes or exertion.

Medical causes
(continued)

Cardiac arrhythmias
✦ Dizziness lasts for several seconds or longer and may precede fainting.

Carotid sinus hypersensitivity
✦ Brief episodes of dizziness usually terminate in fainting.

Generalized anxiety disorder
✦ Continuous dizziness may intensify as the disorder worsens.

Hypertension
✦ Dizziness may precede fainting or may be relieved by rest.

Hyperventilation syndrome
✦ Dizziness lasts a few minutes.
✦ If hyperventilation occurs frequently, dizziness may occur between episodes.

Hypoglycemia
✦ Dizziness, headache, clouding of vision, restlessness, and mental status changes can result from fasting hypoglycemia.

Hypovolemia
✦ Dizziness is caused by a lack of circulating volume.

Orthostatic hypotension
✦ Dizziness may terminate in fainting or disappear with rest.

Panic disorder
✦ Dizziness may accompany acute attacks of panic.

Cardiac arrhythmias
Dizziness lasts for several seconds or longer and may precede fainting in arrhythmias. The patient may experience palpitations; irregular, rapid, or thready pulse; and possibly hypotension. He may also experience weakness, blurred vision, paresthesia, and confusion.

Carotid sinus hypersensitivity
Carotid sinus hypersensitivity is characterized by brief episodes of dizziness that usually terminate in fainting. These episodes are precipitated by stimulation of one or both carotid arteries by seemingly minor sensations or actions, such as wearing a tight collar or moving the head. Associated signs and symptoms include sweating, nausea, and pallor.

Generalized anxiety disorder
Generalized anxiety disorder produces continuous dizziness that may intensify as the disorder worsens. Associated signs and symptoms are persistent anxiety (for at least 1 month), insomnia, difficulty concentrating, and irritability. The patient may show signs of motor tension—for example, twitching or fidgeting, muscle aches, furrowed brow, and a tendency to be startled. He may also display signs of autonomic hyperactivity, such as diaphoresis, palpitations, cold and clammy hands, dry mouth, paresthesia, indigestion, hot or cold flashes, frequent urination, diarrhea, a lump in the throat, pallor, and increased pulse and respiratory rates.

Hypertension
With hypertension, dizziness may precede fainting, but it may also be relieved by rest. Other common signs and symptoms include headache and blurred vision. Retinal changes include hemorrhage, sclerosis of retinal blood vessels, exudate, and papilledema.

Hyperventilation syndrome
Episodes of hyperventilation cause dizziness that usually lasts a few minutes; however, if these episodes occur frequently, dizziness may persist between them. Other effects include apprehension, diaphoresis, pallor, dyspnea, chest tightness, palpitations, trembling, fatigue, and peripheral and circumoral paresthesia.

Hypoglycemia
Dizziness is a central nervous system (CNS) disturbance that can occur due to fasting hypoglycemia. It's generally accompanied by headache, clouding of vision, restlessness, and mental status changes. Other signs and symptoms include irritability, trembling, hunger, cold sweats, and tachycardia.

Hypovolemia
Dizziness is caused by a lack of circulating volume and may be accompanied by other signs of fluid volume deficit (dry mucous membranes, decreased blood pressure, increased heart rate). Other signs and symptoms include orthostatic hypotension, thirst, poor skin turgor, and flattened neck veins.

Orthostatic hypotension
Orthostatic hypotension produces dizziness that may terminate in fainting or disappear with rest. Related findings include dim vision, spots before the eyes, pallor, diaphoresis, hypotension, tachycardia and, possibly, signs of dehydration.

Panic disorder
Dizziness may accompany acute attacks of panic in patients with panic disorder. Other findings include anxiety, dyspnea, palpitations, chest pain, a choking or

smothering sensation, vertigo, paresthesia, hot and cold flashes, diaphoresis, and trembling or shaking. The patient may have the sensation of dying or losing his mind.

Postconcussion syndrome

Occurring 1 to 3 weeks after a head injury, postconcussion syndrome is marked by dizziness, headache (throbbing, aching, bandlike, or stabbing), emotional lability, alcohol intolerance, fatigue, anxiety and, possibly, vertigo. Dizziness and other symptoms are intensified by mental or physical stress. The syndrome may persist for years, but symptoms eventually abate.

Transient ischemic attack

Lasting from a few seconds to 24 hours, a transient ischemic attack (TIA) commonly signals impending stroke and may be triggered by turning the head to the side. Besides dizziness of varying severity, TIAs are accompanied by unilateral or bilateral diplopia, blindness or visual field deficits, ptosis, tinnitus, hearing loss, paresis, and numbness. Other findings include dysarthria, dysphagia, vomiting, hiccups, confusion, decreased LOC, and pallor.

OTHER CAUSES

Drugs

Anxiolytics, CNS depressants, opioids, decongestants, antihistamines, antihypertensives, and vasodilators commonly cause dizziness. Herbal remedies such as St. John's wort can also produce dizziness.

SPECIAL CONSIDERATIONS

Prepare the patient for diagnostic tests, such as blood studies, arteriography, computed tomography scan, EEG, magnetic resonance imaging, and tilt-table studies.

PEDIATRIC POINTERS

Dizziness is less common in children than in adults. Many children have difficulty describing this symptom and instead complain of tiredness, stomachache, or feeling sick. If you suspect dizziness, assess the patient for vertigo as well. A more common symptom in children, vertigo may result from a vision disorder, an ear infection, or antibiotic therapy.

PATIENT COUNSELING

Teach the patient ways to control dizziness. If he's hyperventilating, have him breathe and rebreathe into his cupped hands or a paper bag. If he experiences dizziness in an upright position, tell him to lie down and rest and then to rise slowly. Advise the patient with carotid sinus hypersensitivity to avoid wearing garments that fit tightly at the neck. Instruct the patient who risks a TIA from vertebrobasilar insufficiency to turn his body instead of sharply turning his head to one side.

DYSARTHRIA

Dysarthria, poorly articulated speech, is characterized by slurring and labored, irregular rhythm. It may be accompanied by nasal voice tone caused by palate weakness. Dysarthria is occasionally confused with aphasia, loss of the ability to produce or comprehend speech.

Medical causes
(continued)

Postconcussion syndrome
+ Dizziness, headache, emotional lability, alcohol intolerance, fatigue, anxiety and, possibly, vertigo occur 1 to 3 weeks after a head injury.

Transient ischemic attack
+ Dizziness of varying severity, unilateral or bilateral diplopia, blindness or visual field deficits, ptosis, tinnitus, hearing loss, paresis, and numbness occur.

Other causes
+ Antihistamines, antihypertensives, anxiolytics, CNS depressants, decongestants, opioids, and vasodilators
+ Herbal remedies

Special considerations
+ Prepare the patient for tests.

Peds points
+ If you suspect dizziness, assess for vertigo, a more common symptom in children.

Teaching points
+ Ways to control dizziness

Key facts about dysarthria
+ Poorly articulated speech
+ Characterized by slurring and labored, irregular rhythm
+ Results from damage to brain stem that affects cranial nerves IX, X, or XII

In an emergency

+ Assess for difficulty swallowing and withhold oral fluids if present.
+ Assess respiratory rate and depth.
+ Assess blood pressure and heart rate.
+ Ensure a patent airway.
+ Administer oxygen.
+ Keep emergency resuscitation equipment nearby.
+ Anticipate intubation and mechanical ventilation if progressive respiratory muscle weakness occurs.

Key history points

+ Onset and description
+ Drug and alcohol history

Critical assessment steps

+ Have patient produce a few simple sounds and words.
+ Compare muscle strength and tone in the limbs.
+ Test DTRs, and note gait ataxia.
+ Perform a complete neurologic examination.

Medical causes

Alcoholic cerebellar degeneration
+ Chronic, progressive dysarthria occurs.

ALS
+ Dysarthria occurs when ALS affects the bulbar nuclei.

Basilar artery insufficiency
+ Random, brief episodes of bilateral brain stem dysfunction result in dysarthria.

Dysarthria results from damage to the brain stem that affects cranial nerves IX, X, or XII. Degenerative neurologic disorders and cerebellar disorders commonly cause dysarthria. In fact, dysarthria is a chief sign of olivopontocerebellar degeneration. It may also result from ill-fitting dentures.

 EMERGENCY ACTIONS If the patient displays dysarthria, ask him about associated difficulty swallowing. Then determine his respiratory rate and depth, and measure vital capacity. Assess blood pressure and heart rate. Usually, tachycardia, slightly increased blood pressure, and shortness of breath are early signs of respiratory muscle weakness.

Ensure a patent airway. Place the patient in Fowler's position and suction him if necessary. Administer oxygen, and keep emergency resuscitation equipment nearby. Anticipate intubation and mechanical ventilation in progressive respiratory muscle weakness. Withhold oral fluids in the patient with associated dysphagia.

HISTORY

Explore dysarthria completely. When did it begin? Has it gotten better? Speech improves with resolution of a transient ischemic attack, but not in a completed stroke. Ask if dysarthria worsens during the day. Then obtain a drug and alcohol history. Also, ask about a history of seizures. While taking the patient's history, pay attention to his speech. Dysarthria is usually evident in ordinary conversation. Observe dentures for a proper fit.

PHYSICAL ASSESSMENT

Perform a complete neurologic examination. Ask the patient to produce a few simple sounds and words, such as "ba," "sh," and "cat." Compare muscle strength and tone in the limbs. Then evaluate tactile sensation. Ask the patient about numbness or tingling. Test deep tendon reflexes (DTRs), and note gait ataxia. Assess cerebellar function by observing rapid alternating movement, which should be smooth and coordinated. Next, test visual fields and ask about double vision. Check for signs of facial weakness, such as ptosis. Finally, determine level of consciousness (LOC) and mental status.

MEDICAL CAUSES

Alcoholic cerebellar degeneration
Alcoholic cerebellar degeneration commonly causes chronic, progressive dysarthria along with ataxia, diplopia, ophthalmoplegia, hypotension, and altered mental status.

Amyotrophic lateral sclerosis
Dysarthria occurs when amyotrophic lateral sclerosis (ALS), also known as *Lou Gehrig disease,* affects the bulbar nuclei; it may worsen as the disease progresses. Other signs and symptoms of ALS include dysphagia; difficulty breathing; muscle atrophy and weakness, especially of the hands and feet; fasciculations; spasticity; hyperactive DTRs in the legs; and occasionally excessive drooling. Progressive bulbar palsy may cause crying spells or inappropriate laughter.

Basilar artery insufficiency
Basilar artery insufficiency causes random, brief episodes of bilateral brain stem dysfunction, resulting in dysarthria. Accompanying it are diplopia, vertigo, facial numbness, ataxia, paresis, and visual field loss, all of which last for minutes to hours.

Botulism

The hallmark of botulism is acute cranial nerve dysfunction causing dysarthria, dysphagia, diplopia, and ptosis. Early findings include dry mouth, sore throat, weakness, vomiting, and diarrhea. Later, descending weakness or paralysis of muscles in the extremities and trunk causes hyporeflexia and dyspnea.

Manganese poisoning

Chronic manganese poisoning causes progressive dysarthria accompanied by weakness, fatigue, confusion, hallucinations, drooling, hand tremors, limb stiffness, spasticity, gross rhythmic movements of the trunk and head, and propulsive gait.

Mercury poisoning

Chronic mercury poisoning also causes progressive dysarthria accompanied by weakness, fatigue, depression, lethargy, irritability, confusion, ataxia, and tremors. Changes in vision, hearing, and memory may also occur.

Multiple sclerosis

When demyelination affects the brain stem and cerebellum, the patient displays dysarthria accompanied by nystagmus, blurred or double vision, dysphagia, ataxia, and intention tremor. Exacerbations and remissions of these signs and symptoms are common. Other findings of multiple sclerosis include paresthesia, spasticity, intention tremor, hyperreflexia, muscle weakness or paralysis, constipation, emotional lability, and urinary frequency, urgency, and incontinence.

Myasthenia gravis

Myasthenia gravis is a neuromuscular disorder that causes dysarthria associated with a nasal voice tone. Typically, the dysarthria worsens during the day and may temporarily improve with short rest periods. Other findings include dysphagia, drooling, facial weakness, diplopia, ptosis, dyspnea, and muscle weakness.

Olivopontocerebellar degeneration

Dysarthria, a major sign of olivopontocerebellar degeneration, accompanies cerebellar ataxia and spasticity. The patient may also have abnormal eye movement, sexual dysfunction, bowel and bladder problems, and difficulty swallowing.

Parkinson's disease

Parkinson's disease produces dysarthria and a monotone voice. It also produces muscle rigidity, bradykinesia, involuntary tremor usually beginning in the fingers, difficulty in walking, muscle weakness, and stooped posture. Other findings include masklike facies, dysphagia, and occasionally drooling.

Stroke (brain stem)

Brain stem stroke is characterized by bulbar palsy, resulting in the triad of dysarthria, dysphonia, and dysphagia. The dysarthria is most severe at onset; it may lessen or disappear with rehabilitation and training. Other findings include facial weakness, diplopia, hemiparesis, spasticity, drooling, dyspnea, and decreased LOC.

Stroke (cerebral)

A massive bilateral cerebral stroke causes pseudobulbar palsy. Bilateral weakness produces dysarthria that's most severe at onset. This sign is accompanied by dysphagia, drooling, dysphonia, bilateral hemianopsia, and aphasia. Sensory loss, spasticity, and hyperreflexia may also occur.

Medical causes
(continued)

Botulism
+ Acute cranial nerve dysfunction causes dysarthria, dysphagia, diplopia, and ptosis.

Manganese poisoning
+ Dysarthria is progressive.

Mercury poisoning
+ Progressive dysarthria is accompanied by fatigue, depression, confusion, ataxia, and tremors.

Multiple sclerosis
+ Demyelination affects the brain stem and cerebellum, causing dysarthria.

Myasthenia gravis
+ Dysarthria is associated with a nasal voice tone; it worsens during the day and may temporarily improve with short rest periods.

Olivopontocerebellar degeneration
+ Dysarthria accompanies cerebellar ataxia and spasticity.

Parkinson's disease
+ Dysarthria and a monotone voice occur.

Stroke (brain stem)
+ Dysarthria that's most severe at onset occurs with dysphonia and dysphagia.

Stroke (cerebral)
+ Bilateral weakness produces dysarthria that's most severe at onset.

Other causes
+ Large doses of anticonvulsants and barbiturates

Special considerations
+ Consult with a speech pathologist as needed.
+ Administer medications and treatments as indicated.
+ Assess swallow and gag reflexes before feeding the patient.

Peds points
+ Dysarthria usually results from brain stem glioma; it may also result from cerebral palsy.

Teaching points
+ Communication techniques

Key facts about dyspepsia
+ Feeling of uncomfortable fullness after meals
+ Associated with nausea, belching, heartburn and, possibly, cramping and abdominal distention

Key history points
+ Onset, duration, and description of dyspepsia
+ Alleviating or aggravating factors
+ Associated nausea, vomiting, melena, hematemesis, cough, chest pain, or urine changes
+ Drug and surgical history
+ Medical history, including renal, cardiovascular, or pulmonary disease

OTHER CAUSES

Drugs

Dysarthria can occur when anticonvulsant dosage is too high. Ingestion of large doses of barbiturates may also cause dysarthria.

SPECIAL CONSIDERATIONS

Dysarthria usually requires consultation with a speech pathologist. Administer medications and treatments, as indicated, to treat underlying medical conditions. Assess swallow and gag reflexes before feeding the patient to prevent aspiration.

PEDIATRIC POINTERS

Dysarthria in children usually results from brain stem glioma, a slow-growing tumor that primarily affects children. It may also result from cerebral palsy.

Dysarthria may be difficult to detect, especially in an infant or a young child who hasn't perfected speech. Be sure to look for other neurologic deficits, too. Encourage speech in a child with dysarthria; a child's potential for rehabilitation is typically greater than an adult's.

PATIENT COUNSELING

Encourage the patient with dysarthria to speak slowly so that he can be understood. Give him time to express himself, and encourage him to use gestures. Allow him to express his feelings about his difficulties with verbal communication.

DYSPEPSIA

Dyspepsia refers to an uncomfortable fullness after meals that's associated with nausea, belching, heartburn and, possibly, cramping and abdominal distention. Frequently aggravated by spicy, fatty, or high-fiber foods and by excess caffeine intake, dyspepsia without other pathology indicates impaired digestive function.

Dyspepsia is caused by GI disorders and, to a lesser extent, by cardiac, pulmonary, and renal disorders and the effects of drugs. It apparently results when altered gastric secretions lead to excess stomach acidity. This symptom may also result from emotional upset and overly rapid eating or improper chewing. It usually occurs a few hours after eating and lasts for a variable amount of time. Its severity depends on the amount and type of food eaten and on GI motility. Additional food or an antacid may relieve the discomfort.

HISTORY

If the patient complains of dyspepsia, begin by asking him to describe it in detail. How often and when does it occur, specifically in relation to meals? Do any drugs or activities relieve or aggravate it? Has he had nausea, vomiting, melena, hematemesis, cough, or chest pain? Ask if he's taking prescription drugs and if he has recently had surgery. Does he have a history of renal, cardiovascular, or pulmonary disease? Has he noticed any change in the amount or color of his urine?

Ask the patient if he's experiencing an unusual or overwhelming amount of emotional stress. Determine the patient's coping mechanisms and their effectiveness.

PHYSICAL ASSESSMENT

Focus the physical examination on the abdomen. Inspect for distention, ascites, scars, obvious hernias, jaundice, uremic frost, and bruising. Then auscultate for bowel sounds and characterize their motility. Palpate and percuss the abdomen, noting any tenderness, pain, organ enlargement, or tympany.

Finally, examine other body systems. Auscultate for gallops and crackles. Percuss the lungs to detect consolidation. Note peripheral edema and any swelling of lymph nodes.

MEDICAL CAUSES

Cholelithiasis

Dyspepsia may occur with cholelithiasis (the formation of gallstones), commonly after intake of fatty foods. Biliary colic, a more common symptom of cholelithiasis, causes acute pain that may radiate to the back, shoulders, and chest. The patient may also have diaphoresis, tachycardia, chills, low-grade fever, petechiae, bleeding tendencies, jaundice with pruritus, dark urine, and clay-colored stools.

Cirrhosis

With cirrhosis, dyspepsia varies in intensity and duration and is relieved by ingestion of an antacid. Other GI effects are anorexia, nausea, vomiting, flatulence, diarrhea, constipation, abdominal distention, and epigastric or right-upper-quadrant pain. Weight loss, jaundice, hepatomegaly, ascites, dependent edema, fever, bleeding tendencies, and muscle weakness are also common. Skin changes include severe pruritus, extreme dryness, easy bruising, and lesions, such as telangiectasis and palmar erythema. Gynecomastia or testicular atrophy may also occur.

Duodenal ulcer

A primary symptom of duodenal ulcer, dyspepsia ranges from a vague feeling of fullness or pressure to a boring or aching sensation in the middle or right epigastrium. It usually occurs 1½ to 3 hours after eating and is relieved by intake of food or ingestion of an antacid. The pain may awaken the patient at night with heartburn and fluid regurgitation. Abdominal tenderness and weight gain may occur; vomiting and anorexia are rare.

Gastric dilation (acute)

Epigastric fullness is an early symptom of acute gastric dilation, a life-threatening disorder. Accompanying dyspepsia are nausea and vomiting, upper abdominal distention, succussion splash, and apathy. The patient with acute gastric dilation may display signs and symptoms of dehydration, such as poor tissue turgor and dry mucous membranes, and of electrolyte imbalance, such as irregular pulse and muscle weakness. Gastric bleeding may produce hematemesis and melena.

Gastric ulcer

Typically, dyspepsia and heartburn after eating occur early in a gastric ulcer. The cardinal symptom, however, is epigastric pain that may occur with vomiting, fullness, and abdominal distention and may not be relieved by food. Weight loss and GI bleeding are also characteristic.

Gastritis (chronic)

With chronic gastritis, dyspepsia is relieved by antacids; lessened by smaller, more frequent meals; and aggravated by spicy foods or excessive caffeine. It occurs with anorexia, a feeling of fullness, vague epigastric pain, belching, nausea, and vomiting.

Medical causes
(continued)

GI cancer
✦ Chronic dyspepsia occurs.

Heart failure
✦ In right-sided heart failure, transient dyspepsia may occur with chest tightness and pain or ache in the right upper quadrant.

Hepatitis
✦ The preicteric phase produces moderate to severe dyspepsia.

Hiatal hernia
✦ Dyspepsia results when increased abdominal pressure causes the lower portion of the esophagus and the upper portion of the stomach to rise into the chest.

Pancreatitis (chronic)
✦ A feeling of fullness or dyspepsia may occur with epigastric pain.

Uremia
✦ Dyspepsia may be the earliest and most important GI complaint.

Other causes
✦ Antibiotics, antihypertensives, corticosteroid, diuretics, NSAIDs, and other drugs
✦ GI surgery

GI cancer
GI cancer usually produces chronic dyspepsia. Other features include anorexia, fatigue, jaundice, melena, hematemesis, constipation, and abdominal pain. The patient may also experience pain after eating that isn't relieved by antacids. Syncope, weakness, and weight loss may also occur.

Heart failure
Common with right-sided heart failure, transient dyspepsia may occur with chest tightness and a constant ache or sharp pain in the right upper quadrant. Heart failure also typically causes hepatomegaly, anorexia, nausea, vomiting, bloating, ascites, tachycardia, jugular vein distention, tachypnea, dyspnea, and orthopnea. Other findings include dependent edema, anxiety, fatigue, diaphoresis, hypotension, cough, crackles, ventricular and atrial gallops, nocturia, diastolic hypertension, and cool, pale skin.

Hepatitis
Dyspepsia occurs in two of the three stages of hepatitis. The preicteric phase produces moderate to severe dyspepsia, fever, malaise, arthralgia, coryza, myalgia, nausea, vomiting, an altered sense of taste or smell, and hepatomegaly. Jaundice marks the onset of the icteric phase, along with continued dyspepsia and anorexia, irritability, and severe pruritus. As jaundice clears, dyspepsia and other GI effects also diminish. In the recovery phase, only fatigue remains.

Hiatal hernia
With hiatal hernia, dyspepsia results when increased abdominal pressure causes the lower portion of the esophagus and the upper portion of the stomach to rise into the chest. Other signs and symptoms include heartburn and retrosternal or substernal chest pain. Signs and symptoms of possible complications include dysphagia, bleeding, and severe pain and shock.

Pancreatitis (chronic)
With chronic pancreatitis, a feeling of fullness or dyspepsia is usually accompanied by severe continuous or intermittent epigastric pain that radiates to the back or through the abdomen. Anorexia, nausea, vomiting, jaundice, dramatic weight loss, hyperglycemia, and steatorrhea may also occur. The patient may have Turner's or Cullen's sign.

Uremia
Of the many GI complaints associated with uremia, dyspepsia may be the earliest and most important. Others include anorexia, nausea, vomiting, bloating, diarrhea, abdominal cramps, epigastric pain, and weight gain. As the renal system deteriorates, the patient may experience edema, pruritus, pallor, hyperpigmentation, uremic frost, ecchymoses, sexual dysfunction, poor memory, irritability, headache, drowsiness, muscle twitching, seizures, and oliguria.

OTHER CAUSES

Drugs
Nonsteroidal anti-inflammatories, especially aspirin, commonly cause dyspepsia. Diuretics, antibiotics, antihypertensives, corticosteroids, and many other drugs can cause dyspepsia, depending on the patient's tolerance of the dosage.

Surgery
After GI or other surgery, postoperative gastritis can cause dyspepsia, which usually disappears in a few weeks.

SPECIAL CONSIDERATIONS

Changing the patient's position usually doesn't relieve dyspepsia, but providing food or an antacid may. Have food available at all times, and give an antacid 30 minutes before a meal or 1 hour after it. Because various drugs can cause dyspepsia, give these after meals, if possible.

PEDIATRIC POINTERS

Dyspepsia may occur in adolescents with peptic ulcer disease, but it isn't relieved by food. It may also occur in congenital pyloric stenosis, but projectile vomiting after meals is a more characteristic sign. It may also result from lactose intolerance.

GERIATRIC POINTERS

Most elderly patients with chronic pancreatitis experience less severe pain than do younger adults; some have no pain at all.

PATIENT COUNSELING

Advise patients to eat frequent, small meals. Also, tell them to avoid foods known to cause symptoms as well as coffee, tea, chocolate, alcohol, and tobacco. Explain all diagnostic tests and procedures. Discuss other ways to deal with stress, such as deep breathing and guided imagery. Provide the patient with a calm environment to reduce stress, and make sure the patient gets plenty of rest. In addition, prepare the patient for endoscopy to evaluate the cause of dyspepsia.

DYSPHAGIA

Dysphagia — difficulty swallowing — is a common symptom that's usually easy to localize. It may be constant or intermittent and is classified by the phase of swallowing it affects. (See *Classifying dysphagia*, page 226.) Among the factors that interfere with swallowing are severe pain, obstruction, abnormal peristalsis, impaired gag reflex, and excessive, scanty, or thick oral secretions.

Dysphagia is the most common — and sometimes the only — symptom of esophageal disorders. However, it may also result from oropharyngeal, respiratory, neurologic, and collagen disorders or from the effects of toxins and treatments. Dysphagia increases the risk of choking and aspiration and may lead to malnutrition and dehydration.

 EMERGENCY ACTIONS If the patient suddenly complains of dysphagia and displays signs of respiratory distress, such as dyspnea and stridor, suspect an airway obstruction and quickly perform abdominal thrusts. Prepare to administer oxygen by mask or nasal cannula or to assist with endotracheal intubation.

HISTORY

If the patient's dysphagia doesn't suggest airway obstruction, begin a health history. Ask the patient if swallowing is painful. If so, is the pain constant or intermittent? Have the patient point to where dysphagia feels most intense. Does eating alleviate or aggravate the symptom? Are solids or liquids more difficult to swallow? If the answer is liquids, ask if hot, cold, and lukewarm fluids affect him differently. Does the symptom disappear after he tries to swallow a few times? Is swallowing easier if

Special considerations
✦ Give an antacid 30 minutes before a meal or 1 hour after it.

Peds points
✦ Dyspepsia may occur in adolescents with peptic ulcer disease, congenital pyloric stenosis, and lactose intolerance.

Geri points
✦ Most elderly patients with chronic pancreatitis experience less severe pain than do younger adults; some have no pain at all.

Teaching points
✦ Small, frequent meals
✦ Foods that can cause symptoms

Key facts about dysphagia
✦ Is the most common symptom of esophageal disorders
✦ Classified by three phases: transfer, transport, or entrance

In an emergency
If dysphagia accompanies signs of respiratory distress:
✦ Suspect an airway obstruction.
✦ Perform abdominal thrusts.
✦ Prepare to administer oxygen to assist with endotracheal intubation.

Key history points
✦ Onset and description of accompanying pain
✦ Aggravating and alleviating factors
✦ Recent vomiting, regurgitation, weight loss, anorexia, hoarseness, dyspnea, or cough

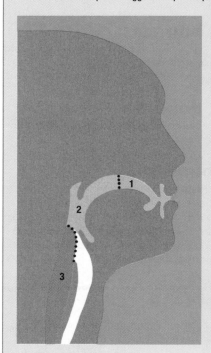

Classifying dysphagia

Because swallowing occurs in three distinct phases, dysphagia can be classified by the phase that it affects. Each phase suggests a specific pathology for dysphagia.

PHASE 1
Swallowing begins in the *transfer phase* with chewing and moistening of food with saliva. The tongue presses against the hard palate to transfer the chewed food to the back of the throat; cranial nerve V then stimulates the swallowing reflex. Phase 1 dysphagia typically results from a neuromuscular disorder.

PHASE 2
In the *transport phase,* the soft palate closes against the pharyngeal wall to prevent nasal regurgitation. At the same time, the larynx rises and the vocal cords close to keep food out of the lungs; breathing stops momentarily as the throat muscles constrict to move food into the esophagus. Phase 2 dysphagia usually indicates spasm or cancer.

PHASE 3
Peristalsis and gravity work together in the *entrance phase* to move food through the esophageal sphincter and into the stomach. Phase 3 dysphagia results from lower esophageal narrowing by diverticula, esophagitis, and other disorders.

he changes position? Ask if he has recently experienced vomiting, regurgitation, weight loss, anorexia, hoarseness, dyspnea, or a cough.

PHYSICAL ASSESSMENT

To evaluate the patient's swallowing reflex, place your finger along his thyroid notch and instruct him to swallow. If you feel his larynx rise, the reflex is intact. Next, have him cough to assess his cough reflex. Check his gag reflex if you're sure he has a good swallow or cough reflex. Listen closely to his speech for signs of muscle weakness. Does he have aphasia or dysarthria? Is his voice nasal, hoarse, or breathy? Assess the patient's mouth carefully. Check for dry mucous membranes and thick, sticky secretions. Observe for tongue and facial weakness and obvious obstructions (for example, enlarged tonsils). Assess the patient for disorientation, which may make him neglect to swallow.

MEDICAL CAUSES

Achalasia

Most common in patients ages 20 to 40, achalasia produces phase 3 dysphagia for solids and liquids. The dysphagia develops gradually and may be precipitated or exacerbated by stress. Occasionally, it's preceded by esophageal colic. Regurgitation of undigested food, especially at night, may cause wheezing, coughing, or choking as well as halitosis. Weight loss, cachexia, hematemesis and, possibly, heartburn are late findings.

Airway obstruction

Life-threatening upper airway obstruction is marked by signs of respiratory distress, such as crowing and stridor. Phase 2 dysphagia occurs with gagging and dysphonia. When hemorrhage obstructs the trachea, dysphagia is usually painless and rapid in onset. When inflammation causes the obstruction, dysphagia may be painful and develop slowly.

Amyotrophic lateral sclerosis

In addition to dysphagia, amyotrophic lateral sclerosis (ALS), which is also known as *Lou Gehrig disease,* causes muscle weakness and atrophy, fasciculations, dysarthria, dyspnea, shallow respirations, tachypnea, slurred speech, hyperactive deep tendon reflexes, and emotional lability.

Botulism

Botulism causes phase 1 dysphagia and dysuria, usually within 36 hours of toxin ingestion. Other early findings include blurred or double vision, dry mouth, sore throat, nausea, vomiting, and diarrhea. Symmetrical descending weakness or paralysis occurs gradually.

Bulbar paralysis

In bulbar paralysis, phase 1 dysphagia occurs along with drooling, difficulty chewing, dysarthria, and nasal regurgitation. Dysphagia for solids and liquids is painful and progressive. Accompanying features may include arm and leg spasticity, hyperreflexia, and emotional lability.

Esophageal cancer

Dysphagia (phases 2 and 3) is the earliest and most common symptom of esophageal cancer. Typically, this painless, progressive symptom is accompanied by rapid weight loss. As the cancer advances, dysphagia becomes painful and constant. In addition, the patient complains of steady chest pain, cough with hemoptysis, hoarseness, and sore throat. He may also develop nausea and vomiting, fever, hiccups, hematemesis, melena, and halitosis.

Esophageal diverticulum

Esophageal diverticulum causes phase 3 dysphagia when the enlarged diverticulum obstructs the esophagus. Associated signs and symptoms include food regurgitation, chronic cough, hoarseness, chest pain, and halitosis.

Esophageal obstruction by foreign body

Esophageal obstruction by foreign body is characterized by sudden onset of dysphagia (phase 2 or 3) as well as gagging, coughing, and esophageal pain. Dyspnea may occur if the obstruction compresses the trachea.

Esophageal spasm

The most striking symptoms of esophageal spasm are phase 2 dysphagia for solids and liquids and dull or squeezing substernal chest pain. The pain may last up to 1 hour; radiate to the neck, arm, back, or jaw; and be relieved by drinking a glass of water. Bradycardia may also occur.

Esophageal stricture

Usually caused by a chemical ingestion or scar tissue, esophageal stricture causes phase 3 dysphagia. Drooling, tachypnea, and gagging also may be evident. In chem-

Medical causes
(continued)

ALS
+ Dysphagia, muscle weakness and atrophy, fasciculations, dysarthria, dyspnea, shallow respirations, tachypnea, slurred speech, hyperactive DTRs, and emotional lability occur.

Botulism
+ Dysphagia (phase 1) and dysuria occur, usually within 36 hours of toxin ingestion.

Bulbar paralysis
+ Painful and progressive phase 1 dysphagia occurs along with drooling, difficulty chewing, dysarthria, and nasal regurgitation.

Esophageal cancer
+ Dysphagia (phases 2 and 3) is the earliest and most common symptom.

Esophageal diverticulum
+ Phase 3 dysphagia occurs when the enlarged diverticulum obstructs the esophagus.

Esophageal obstruction by foreign body
+ Onset of phase 2 or 3 dysphagia is sudden and may be accompanied by gagging, coughing, and esophageal pain.

Esophageal spasm
+ Phase 2 dysphagia for solids and liquids occurs along with substernal chest pain.

Esophageal stricture
+ Phase 3 dysphagia is caused by chemical ingestion or scar tissue.

Medical causes
(continued)

Esophagitis
✦ Corrosive esophagitis, resulting from ingestion of alkalies or acids, causes severe phase 3 dysphagia.
✦ Candidal esophagitis causes phase 2 dysphagia, sore throat and, possibly, retrosternal pain on swallowing.
✦ With reflux esophagitis, phase 3 dysphagia is a late symptom that usually accompanies stricture development.

Hypocalcemia
✦ Neuromuscular irritability may produce phase 1 dysphagia associated with numbness and tingling in the nose, ears, fingertips, and toes and around the mouth.

Laryngeal cancer (extrinsic)
✦ Phase 2 dysphagia and dyspnea develop late.

Lead poisoning
✦ Painless, progressive dysphagia may occur.

Lower esophageal ring
✦ Patient has an attack of phase 3 dysphagia and complains of a foreign body in the lower esophagus, a sensation that may be relieved by drinking water or vomiting.
✦ Attacks may recur several weeks or months later.

Mediastinitis
✦ Insidious or rapid onset of phase 3 dysphagia varies with the extent of esophageal perforation.

ical ingestion, dysphagia may be accompanied by burns, ulcers, or erythema of the lips and mouth.

Esophagitis
Corrosive esophagitis, resulting from ingestion of alkalies or acids, causes severe phase 3 dysphagia. Dysphagia is accompanied by marked salivation, hematemesis, tachypnea, fever, and intense pain in the mouth and anterior chest that's aggravated by swallowing. Signs of shock, such as hypotension and tachycardia, may also occur.

Candidal esophagitis causes phase 2 dysphagia, sore throat and, possibly, retrosternal pain on swallowing.

With reflux esophagitis, phase 3 dysphagia is a late symptom that usually accompanies stricture development. The patient complains of heartburn, which is aggravated by strenuous exercise, bending over, or lying down and is relieved by sitting up or taking an antacid. Other features include regurgitation; frequent, effortless vomiting; a dry, nocturnal cough; and substernal chest pain that may mimic angina pectoris. If the esophagus ulcerates, signs of bleeding, such as melena and hematemesis, may occur along with weakness and fatigue.

Hypocalcemia
Although tetany is its primary sign, severe hypocalcemia may cause neuromuscular irritability, producing phase 1 dysphagia associated with numbness and tingling in the nose, ears, fingertips, and toes and around the mouth. Carpopedal spasms, muscle twitching, and laryngeal spasms also may occur.

Laryngeal cancer (extrinsic)
Phase 2 dysphagia and dyspnea develop late in laryngeal cancer. Accompanying features include muffled voice, stridor, pain, halitosis, weight loss, ipsilateral otalgia, chronic cough, and cachexia. Palpation reveals enlarged cervical lymph nodes.

Lead poisoning
Painless, progressive dysphagia may result from lead poisoning. Related findings include a lead line on the gums, metallic taste, papilledema, ocular palsy, footdrop or wristdrop, and signs of hemolytic anemia, such as abdominal pain and fever. The patient may be depressed and display severe mental impairment and seizures.

Lower esophageal ring
Narrowing of the lower esophagus can cause an attack of phase 3 dysphagia that may recur several weeks or months later. During the attack, the patient complains of a foreign body in the lower esophagus, a sensation that may be relieved by drinking water or vomiting. Esophageal rupture produces severe lower chest pain followed by a feeling of something giving way.

Mediastinitis
Varying with the extent of esophageal perforation, mediastinitis can cause insidious or rapid onset of phase 3 dysphagia. The patient displays chills, fever, and severe retrosternal chest pain that may radiate to the epigastrium, back, or shoulder. The pain may be aggravated by breathing, coughing, or sneezing. Other findings include tachycardia, subcutaneous crepitation in the suprasternal notch, and falling blood pressure.

Myasthenia gravis
Fatigue and progressive muscle weakness characterize myasthenia gravis and account for painless phase 1 dysphagia and possibly choking. Typically, dysphagia follows ptosis and diplopia. Other features include masklike facies, nasal voice, fre-

quent nasal regurgitation, and head bobbing. Shallow respirations and dyspnea may occur with respiratory muscle weakness. Signs and symptoms worsen during menses and with exposure to stress, cold, or infection.

Oral cavity tumor

With an oral cavity tumor, painful phase 1 dysphagia develops along with hoarseness and ulcerating lesions. The patient may report an abnormal taste in the mouth, abnormal bleeding from the mouth, or a feeling that dentures no longer fit properly.

Parkinson's disease

Usually a late symptom of Parkinson's disease, phase 1 dysphagia is painless but progressive and may cause choking. Other signs and symptoms include bradykinesia, tremors, muscle rigidity, dysarthria, masklike facies, muffled voice, increased salivation and lacrimation, constipation, stooped posture, propulsive gait, incontinence, and sexual dysfunction.

Pharyngitis (chronic)

Pharyngitis causes painful phase 2 dysphagia of solids and liquids. Rarely serious, it's accompanied by a dry, sore throat; a cough; and thick mucus in the throat. The patient may report the sensation of a lump in his throat.

Progressive systemic sclerosis

Typically, dysphagia is preceded by Raynaud's phenomenon in patients with progressive systemic sclerosis. The dysphagia may be mild at first and described as a feeling of food sticking behind the breastbone. The patient also complains of heartburn after meals that's aggravated by lying down. As the disease progresses, dysphagia worsens until only liquids can be swallowed. It may be accompanied by other GI effects, including weight loss, abdominal distention, diarrhea, and malodorous, floating stools. Other characteristic late features include joint pain and stiffness and thickening of the skin that progresses to taut, shiny skin. The patient usually has masklike facies.

Rabies

Severe phase 2 dysphagia of liquids results from painful pharyngeal muscle spasms occurring late in this rare, life-threatening disorder. In fact, the patient may become dehydrated and possibly apneic. Dysphagia also causes drooling, and in 50% of patients it's responsible for hydrophobia. Eventually, rabies causes progressive flaccid paralysis that leads to peripheral vascular collapse, coma, and death.

Tetanus

Phase 1 dysphagia usually develops about 1 week after the patient receives a puncture wound. Other characteristics of tetanus include marked muscle hypertonicity, hyperactive deep tendon reflexes, tachycardia, diaphoresis, drooling, and low-grade fever. Painful, involuntary muscle spasms account for lockjaw (trismus), risus sardonicus, opisthotonos, boardlike abdominal rigidity, and intermittent tonic seizures.

OTHER CAUSES

Procedures

Recent tracheostomy or repeated or prolonged intubation may cause temporary dysphagia.

Medical causes
(continued)

Myasthenia gravis
+ Fatigue and progressive muscle weakness account for painless phase 1 dysphagia that typically follows ptosis and diplopia.

Oral cavity tumor
+ Painful phase 1 dysphagia develops along with hoarseness and ulcerating lesions.

Parkinson's disease
+ Phase 1 dysphagia occurs late, is painless, but is progressive and may cause choking.

Pharyngitis (chronic)
+ Painful phase 2 dysphagia occurs.

Progressive systemic sclerosis
+ Preceded by Raynaud's phenomenon, dysphagia may be mild at first but worsens until only liquids can be swallowed.

Rabies
+ Phase 2 dysphagia of liquids results from painful pharyngeal muscle spasms.

Tetanus
+ Phase 1 dysphagia usually develops about 1 week after the patient receives a puncture wound.

Other causes
+ Radiation therapy
+ Repeated or prolonged intubation
+ Tracheostomy

Special considerations

- Stimulate salivation by talking about food, adding a lemon slice or dill pickle to food tray, and providing mouth care.
- Moisten food with a little liquid if the patient has decreased salivation.
- Administer an anticholinergic or antiemetic.
- Consult with the dietitian to select foods with distinct temperatures and textures.
- Consult a therapist to assess the patient's aspiration risk.

Peds points

- Dysphagia in children may result from corrosive esophagitis, esophageal obstruction by a foreign body (most common), and congenital anomalies.

Geri points

- In patients older than age 50, dysphagia is commonly the presenting complaint in cases of head or neck cancer.

Teaching points

- Easy-to-swallow foods
- Measures to reduce the risk of choking and aspiration

Key facts about dysphagia

- The sensation of difficult or uncomfortable breathing (shortness of breath)
- May arise suddenly or slowly
- May subside rapidly or persist for years

Radiation therapy

When directed against oral cancer, radiation therapy may cause scant salivation and temporary dysphagia.

SPECIAL CONSIDERATIONS

Stimulate salivation in a patient with dysphagia by talking with him about food, adding a lemon slice or dill pickle to his tray, and providing mouth care before and after meals. Moisten food with a little liquid if the patient has decreased salivation. Administer an anticholinergic or antiemetic to control excess salivation. If he has a weak or absent cough reflex, begin tube feedings or esophageal drips of special formulas.

Consult with the dietitian to select foods with distinct temperatures and textures. The patient should avoid sticky foods, such as bananas and peanut butter. If the patient is producing mucus, avoid uncooked milk products. Consult a therapist to assess the patient's aspiration risk; swallowing exercises may help decrease this risk.

Prepare the patient for diagnostic evaluation to pinpoint the cause of dysphagia. This may include endoscopy, esophageal manometry, esophagography, and the esophageal acidity test.

PEDIATRIC POINTERS

In assessing for dysphagia in an infant or a small child, be sure to pay close attention to sucking and swallowing ability. Coughing, choking, or regurgitation during feeding suggests dysphagia.

Corrosive esophagitis and esophageal obstruction by a foreign body are more common causes of dysphagia in children than in adults. However, dysphagia may also result from congenital anomalies, such as annular stenosis, dysphagia lusoria, and esophageal atresia.

GERIATRIC POINTERS

In patients older than age 50, dysphagia is commonly the presenting complaint in cases of head or neck cancer. The incidence of such cancers increases markedly in this age-group.

PATIENT COUNSELING

Advise the patient to prepare foods that are easy to swallow. At mealtimes, review measures with the patient to minimize his risk of choking and aspiration. Place the patient in an upright position, and have him flex his neck forward slightly and keep his chin at midline. Instruct the patient to swallow multiple times before taking the next bite or sip. Separate solids from liquids, which are harder to swallow.

DYSPNEA

Typically a symptom of cardiopulmonary dysfunction, dyspnea is the sensation of difficult or uncomfortable breathing. It's usually reported as shortness of breath. Its severity varies greatly and is usually unrelated to the severity of the underlying cause. Dyspnea may arise suddenly or slowly and may subside rapidly or persist for years.

Most people normally experience dyspnea when they exert themselves, and its severity depends on their physical condition. In a healthy person, dyspnea is quickly relieved by rest. Pathologic causes of dyspnea include pulmonary, cardiac, neuro-muscular, and allergic disorders. It may also be caused by anxiety.

 EMERGENCY ACTIONS If a patient complains of shortness of breath, quickly look for signs of respiratory distress, such as tachypnea, cyanosis, restlessness, and accessory muscle use. Prepare to administer oxygen by nasal cannula, mask, or endotracheal tube. Ensure patent I.V. access, and begin cardiac monitoring and oxygen saturation monitoring to detect arrhythmias and low oxygen saturation, respectively. Expect to insert a chest tube for severe pneumothorax and to administer continuous positive airway pressure or apply rotating tourniquets for pulmonary edema.

HISTORY

If the patient can answer questions without increasing his distress, take a complete history. Ask if the shortness of breath began suddenly or gradually. Is it constant or intermittent? Does it occur during activity or while at rest? If the patient has had dyspneic attacks before, ask if they have been increasing in severity. Can the patient identify what aggravates or alleviates these attacks? Does he have a productive or nonproductive cough or chest pain? Ask about recent trauma, and note a history of upper respiratory tract infection, deep vein phlebitis, or other disorders. Ask the patient if he smokes or is exposed to toxic fumes or irritants on the job. Find out if he also has orthopnea, paroxysmal nocturnal dyspnea, or progressive fatigue.

 CULTURAL CUE *Because dyspnea is subjective and is exacerbated by anxiety, patients from cultures that are highly emotional may complain of shortness of breath sooner than those who are more stoic about symptoms of illness.*

PHYSICAL ASSESSMENT

During the physical examination, look for signs of chronic dyspnea, such as accessory muscle hypertrophy (especially in the shoulders and neck). Also look for pursed-lip exhalation, clubbing, peripheral edema, barrel chest, diaphoresis, and jugular vein distention. Check blood pressure and auscultate for crackles, abnormal heart sounds or rhythms, egophony, bronchophony, and whispered pectoriloquy. Finally, palpate the abdomen for hepatomegaly, and assess the patient for edema.

MEDICAL CAUSES

Acute respiratory distress syndrome

Acute respiratory distress syndrome (ARDS) is a life-threatening form of noncardiogenic pulmonary edema that usually produces acute dyspnea as the first complaint. Progressive respiratory distress then develops with restlessness, anxiety, decreased mental acuity, tachycardia, and crackles and rhonchi in both lung fields. Other findings include cyanosis, tachypnea, motor dysfunction, and intercostal and suprasternal retractions. Severe ARDS can produce signs of shock, such as hypotension and cool, clammy skin.

Amyotrophic lateral sclerosis

Also known as *Lou Gehrig disease*, amyotrophic lateral sclerosis (ALS) causes slow onset of dyspnea that worsens with time. Other features include dysphagia, dysarthria, muscle weakness and atrophy, fasciculations, shallow respirations, tachypnea, and emotional lability.

In an emergency

- Look for signs of respiratory distress.
- Prepare to administer oxygen.
- Ensure patent I.V. access.
- Begin cardiac monitoring and oxygen saturation monitoring.

Key history points

- Onset and description
- Aggravating and alleviating factors
- Associated cough
- Medical history, including trauma, upper respiratory tract infection, deep vein phlebitis, orthopnea, paroxysmal nocturnal dyspnea, or progressive fatigue
- Smoking or occupational hazards

Critical assessment steps

- Look for pursed-lip exhalation, clubbing, peripheral edema, barrel chest, diaphoresis, and jugular vein distention.
- Auscultate for crackles, abnormal heart sounds or rhythms, egophony, bronchophony, and whispered pectoriloquy.
- Palpate the abdomen for hepatomegaly.
- Assess for edema.

Medical causes

ARDS

- Acute dyspnea is usually the first complaint.

ALS

- Onset of dyspnea is slow; dyspnea worsens with time.

Medical causes
(continued)

Anemia
✦ Dyspnea develops gradually.

Anthrax (inhalation)
✦ Dyspnea is a symptom of the second stage; it's accompanied by fever, stridor and hypotension (patient usually dies within 24 hours).

Aspiration of foreign body
✦ Acute dyspnea and paroxysmal intercostal, suprasternal, and substernal retractions occur.

Asthma
✦ Dyspneic attacks occur along with audible wheezing, dry cough, and accessory muscle use.

Cardiac arrhythmia
✦ Acute or gradual dyspnea can result from decreased cardiac output.

Cor pulmonale
✦ Chronic dyspnea begins gradually with exertion and progressively worsens until it occurs even at rest.

Emphysema
✦ Progressive exertional dyspnea occurs.

Flail chest
✦ Sudden dyspnea results from multiple rib fractures.
✦ Paradoxical chest movement, severe chest pain, hypotension, tachypnea, tachycardia, and cyanosis occur.

Anemia
Dyspnea usually develops gradually with anemia. Anemia commonly causes fatigue, weakness, and syncope; in severe cases, it may also cause tachycardia, tachypnea, restlessness, anxiety, and thirst. In advanced stages, the patient may develop pallor, inability to concentrate, and irritability. With chronic iron deficiency, nails become spoon-shaped and brittle, the corners of the mouth crack, the tongue becomes smooth, and dysphagia may develop.

Anthrax (inhalation)
Dyspnea is a symptom of the second stage of anthrax inhalation; it's accompanied by fever, stridor and hypotension (the patient usually dies within 24 hours). Initial symptoms of anthrax inhalation, which are caused by the inhalation of aerosolized spores (from infected animals or a result of bioterrorism) from the bacterium *Bacillus anthracis,* are flulike and include fever, chills, weakness, cough, and chest pain.

Aspiration of a foreign body
Aspiration of a foreign body is a life-threatening condition characterized by acute dyspnea and paroxysmal intercostal, suprasternal, and substernal retractions. The patient may also display accessory muscle use, inspiratory stridor, tachypnea, decreased or absent breath sounds, possibly asymmetrical chest expansion, anxiety, cyanosis, diaphoresis, and hypotension.

Asthma
In asthma, a chronic disorder, acute dyspneic attacks occur along with audible wheezing, dry cough, accessory muscle use, nasal flaring, intercostal and supraclavicular retractions, tachypnea, tachycardia, diaphoresis, prolonged expiration, flushing or cyanosis, and apprehension. Medications that block beta receptors can exacerbate asthma attacks.

Cardiac arrhythmia
In a patient with an arrhythmia, acute or gradual dyspnea can result from decreased cardiac output. The patient's pulse rate may be rapid, slow, or irregular, with frequent premature or escape beats. Alternating pulse may be present. Other symptoms include palpitations, chest pain, diaphoresis, light-headedness, weakness, or vertigo.

Cor pulmonale
Chronic dyspnea begins gradually with exertion and progressively worsens until it occurs even at rest. Underlying cardiac or pulmonary disease is usually present. The patient may also have a chronic productive cough, wheezing, tachypnea, jugular vein distention, dependent edema, and hepatomegaly. He may experience increasing fatigue, weakness, and light-headedness.

Emphysema
Emphysema is a chronic disorder that gradually causes progressive exertional dyspnea. The patient may exhibit barrel chest, accessory muscle hypertrophy, diminished breath sounds, anorexia, weight loss, malaise, peripheral cyanosis, tachypnea, pursed-lip breathing, prolonged expiration and, possibly, a chronic productive cough. Clubbing is a late sign.

Flail chest
With flail chest, sudden dyspnea results from multiple rib fractures and is accompanied by paradoxical chest movement, severe chest pain, hypotension, tachypnea,

tachycardia, and cyanosis. Bruising and decreased or absent breath sounds occur over the affected side.

Guillain-Barré syndrome

Usually following a fever and upper respiratory tract infection, Guillain-Barré syndrome causes slowly worsening dyspnea along with fatigue, ascending muscle weakness and, eventually, paralysis. Other clinical features include facial diplegia, dysphagia or dysarthria and, less commonly, weakness of the muscles supplied by cranial nerve XI.

Heart failure

Dyspnea usually develops gradually in patients with heart failure. Chronic paroxysmal nocturnal dyspnea, orthopnea, tachypnea, tachycardia, palpitations, ventricular gallop, fatigue, dependent peripheral edema, hepatomegaly, dry cough, weight gain, and loss of mental acuity may occur. With acute onset, heart failure may produce jugular vein distention, bibasilar rates, oliguria, and hypotension.

Inhalation injury

Dyspnea may develop suddenly or gradually over several hours after inhalation of chemicals or hot gases. Increasing hoarseness, persistent cough, sooty or bloody sputum, and oropharyngeal edema may also be present. The patient may also exhibit thermal burns, singed nasal hairs, and orofacial burns as well as crackles, rhonchi, wheezing, and signs of respiratory distress.

Lung cancer

Dyspnea that develops slowly and progressively worsens occurs with late-stage lung cancer. Other findings include fever, hemoptysis, productive cough, wheezing, clubbing, chest pain, and pleural friction rub. The patient may also report weight loss and anorexia.

 CULTURAL CUE *Among indigenous Arctic populations, the incidence of lung cancer is growing faster than any other cancer. This may be a result of high smoking rates in Native Alaskan adults and children.*

Myasthenia gravis

Myasthenia gravis is a neuromuscular disorder that causes bouts of dyspnea as the respiratory muscles weaken. The patient may have difficulty chewing and swallowing, which may lead to aspiration. With myasthenic crisis, acute respiratory distress may occur, with shallow respirations and tachypnea.

Myocardial infarction

With myocardial infarction, sudden dyspnea occurs with crushing substernal chest pain that may radiate to the back, neck, jaw, and arms. Other signs and symptoms include nausea, vomiting, diaphoresis, vertigo, hypertension or hypotension, tachycardia, anxiety, and pale, cool, clammy skin.

Plague

The pneumonic form of plague, caused by the bacterium *Yersinia pestis,* is characterized by dyspnea, a productive cough, chest pain, tachypnea, hemoptysis, increasing respiratory distress, and cardiopulmonary insufficiency. The onset of this virulent infection is usually sudden and includes such signs and symptoms as chills, fever, headache, and myalgias. If untreated, plague is one of the most potentially lethal diseases known.

Medical causes
(continued)

Guillain-Barré syndrome
- ✦ Dyspnea slowly worsens.
- ✦ Fatigue, ascending muscle weakness and, eventually, paralysis occur.

Heart failure
- ✦ Dyspnea usually develops gradually.

Inhalation injury
- ✦ Dyspnea may develop suddenly or gradually over several hours.

Lung cancer
- ✦ In late stage, dyspnea develops slowly and progressively worsens.

Myasthenia gravis
- ✦ Bouts of dyspnea occur as respiratory muscles weaken.

Myocardial infarction
- ✦ Sudden dyspnea occurs with crushing substernal chest pain that may radiate to the back, neck, jaw, and arms.

Plague
- ✦ Dyspnea, a productive cough, chest pain, tachypnea, hemoptysis, increasing respiratory distress, and cardiopulmonary insufficiency are characteristic.

Medical causes
(continued)

Pleural effusion
+ Dyspnea develops slowly and progressively worsens.
+ Initial findings include pleural friction rub, and pleuritic pain that worsens with coughing or deep breathing.

Pneumonia
+ Dyspnea occurs suddenly and is usually accompanied by fever, shaking chills, pleuritic chest pain, and a productive cough.

Pneumothorax
+ Acute dyspnea that's unrelated to the severity of pain develops.

Pulmonary edema
+ Acute dyspnea is preceded by signs of heart failure.

Pulmonary embolism
+ Acute dyspnea usually accompanies sudden pleuritic chest pain.

Sepsis
+ Dyspnea develops gradually and is accompanied by chills and sudden fever.

SARS
+ Disease generally begins with fever but also involves headache;, malaise; a dry nonproductive cough; and dyspnea.

Pleural effusion

Dyspnea develops slowly and becomes progressively worse with pleural effusion. Initial findings include a pleural friction rub accompanied by pleuritic pain that worsens with coughing or deep breathing. Other findings include dry cough; dullness on percussion; egophony, bronchophony, and whispered pectoriloquy; tachycardia; tachypnea; weight loss; and decreased chest motion, tactile fremitus, and decreased breath sounds. With infection, fever may occur.

Pneumonia

With pneumonia, dyspnea occurs suddenly and is usually accompanied by fever, shaking chills, pleuritic chest pain that worsens with deep inspiration, and a productive cough. Fatigue, headache, myalgia, anorexia, abdominal pain, crackles, rhonchi, tachycardia, tachypnea, cyanosis, decreased breath sounds, and diaphoresis may also occur.

Pneumothorax

Pneumothorax is a life-threatening disorder that causes acute dyspnea unrelated to the severity of pain. Sudden, stabbing chest pain may radiate to the arms, face, back, or abdomen. Other signs and symptoms include anxiety, restlessness, dry cough, cyanosis, decreased vocal fremitus, tachypnea, tympany, decreased or absent breath sounds on the affected side, asymmetrical chest expansion, splinting, and accessory muscle use. In patients with tension pneumothorax, tracheal deviation occurs in addition to these typical findings. Decreased blood pressure and tachycardia may also occur.

Pulmonary edema

Commonly preceded by signs of heart failure, such as jugular vein distention and orthopnea, pulmonary edema causes acute dyspnea. Other features include tachycardia, tachypnea, crackles in both lung fields, a third heart sound (S_3 gallop), oliguria, thready pulse, hypotension, diaphoresis, cyanosis, and marked anxiety. The patient's cough may be dry or may produce copious amounts of pink, frothy sputum.

Pulmonary embolism

Acute dyspnea that's usually accompanied by sudden pleuritic chest pain characterizes pulmonary embolism — a life-threatening disorder. Related findings include tachycardia, low-grade fever, tachypnea, nonproductive or productive cough with blood-tinged sputum, pleural friction rub, crackles, diffuse wheezing, dullness on percussion, decreased breath sounds, diaphoresis, restlessness, and acute anxiety. A massive embolism may cause signs of shock, such as hypotension and cool, clammy skin.

Sepsis

Sepsis, a potentially fatal disorder, gradually causes dyspnea along with chills and sudden fever. As dyspnea worsens, it may be accompanied by tachycardia, tachypnea, restlessness, anxiety, decreased mental acuity, and warm, flushed, dry skin. Late findings include hypotension; oliguria; cool, clammy skin; and rapid, thready pulse.

Severe acute respiratory syndrome

Severe acute respiratory syndrome (SARS) is an infectious disease of unknown etiology that generally begins with a fever (usually greater than 100.4° F [38° C]). Other symptoms include headache; malaise; a dry, nonproductive cough; and dyspnea. The severity of the illness is highly variable, ranging from mild illness to pneumonia and, in some cases, progressing to respiratory failure and death.

CULTURAL CUE *Although most reported SARS cases have been in Asia (particularly China, Vietnam, Singapore, and Thailand), some people in Europe and North America have also been diagnosed with SARS.*

Shock

Dyspnea arises suddenly and worsens progressively in a patient with shock, a life-threatening disorder. Related findings include severe hypotension, tachypnea, tachycardia, decreased peripheral pulses, decreased mental acuity, restlessness, anxiety, and cool, clammy skin.

Tuberculosis

In a patient with tuberculosis, dyspnea is commonly accompanied by chest pain, crackles, and productive cough. Other findings include night sweats, fever, anorexia and weight loss, vague dyspepsia, palpitations on mild exertion, and dullness on percussion.

Tularemia

Also known as *rabbit fever,* tularemia is an infectious disease that causes dyspnea along with fever, chills, headache, generalized myalgia, a nonproductive cough, pleuritic chest pain, and empyema. Other signs and symptoms include diaphoresis, weight loss, and a red spot on the skin that ultimately enlarges to an ulcer.

SPECIAL CONSIDERATIONS

Monitor the patient with dyspnea closely. Be as calm and reassuring as possible to reduce anxiety, and help him into a comfortable position — usually high Fowler's or forward-leaning position. Support him with pillows, loosen his clothing, and administer oxygen if appropriate.

Prepare the patient for diagnostic studies, such as arterial blood gas analysis, chest X-rays, and pulmonary function tests. Administer a bronchodilator, an antiarrhythmic, a diuretic, and an analgesic as needed to dilate bronchioles, correct cardiac arrhythmias, promote fluid excretion, and relieve pain.

PEDIATRIC POINTERS

Normally, an infant's respirations are abdominal, gradually changing to costal by age 7. Suspect dyspnea in an infant who breathes costally, in an older child who breathes abdominally, or in any child who uses his neck or shoulder muscles to help him breathe.

Both acute epiglottiditis and laryngotracheobronchitis (croup) can cause severe dyspnea in a child and may even lead to respiratory or cardiovascular collapse. Expect to administer oxygen, using a hood or cool mist tent.

GERIATRIC POINTERS

Older patients with dyspnea related to chronic illness may not initially be aware of a significant change in their breathing pattern.

PATIENT COUNSELING

Tell the patient that oxygen therapy isn't necessarily indicated for dyspnea. Encourage a patient with chronic dyspnea to pace his daily activities. Teach the patient pursed-lip, diaphragmatic breathing and chest splinting, as indicated. Advise him to avoid exposure to chemical irritants and pollutants and to stay away from people with respiratory infections.

Medical causes
(continued)

Shock
- ✦ Dyspnea arises suddenly and worsens progressively.

Tuberculosis
- ✦ Dyspnea is commonly accompanied by chest pain, crackles, and productive cough.

Tularemia
- ✦ Dyspnea occurs along with fever, chills, headache, generalized myalgia, a nonproductive cough, pleuritic chest pain, and empyema.

Special considerations
- ✦ Monitor the patient closely.
- ✦ Help the patient into a comfortable position.
- ✦ Administer oxygen if needed.

Peds points
- ✦ Suspect dyspnea in an infant who breathes costally, an older child who breathes abdominally, or any child who uses his neck or shoulder muscles to help him breathe.

Geri points
- ✦ Older patients with dyspnea related to chronic illness may not be aware of a significant change in their breathing pattern.

Teaching points
- ✦ Pacing of daily activities
- ✦ Pursed-lip, diaphragmatic breathing, and chest splinting
- ✦ Avoidance of chemical irritants, pollutants, and people with respiratory infections

DYSURIA

Dysuria (painful or difficult urination) is commonly accompanied by urinary frequency, urgency, or hesitancy. This symptom usually reflects lower urinary tract infection (UTI) — a common disorder, especially in women.

Dysuria also results from lower urinary tract irritation or inflammation, which stimulates nerve endings in the bladder and urethra. The onset of pain provides clues to its cause. For example, pain just before voiding usually indicates bladder irritation or distention; whereas pain at the start of urination typically results from bladder outlet irritation. Pain at the end of voiding may signal bladder spasms; in women, it may indicate vaginal candidiasis.

HISTORY

If the patient complains of dysuria, have him describe its severity and location. When did he first notice it? Did anything precipitate it? Does anything aggravate or alleviate it?

Next, ask about previous urinary or genital tract infections. Has the patient recently undergone an invasive procedure, such as cystoscopy or urethral dilatation, or had a urinary catheter placed? Also, ask if he has a history of intestinal disease. Ask the female patient about menstrual disorders and use of products that irritate the urinary tract, such as bubble bath salts, feminine deodorants, contraceptive gels, and perineal lotions. Also ask her about vaginal discharge and pruritus.

PHYSICAL ASSESSMENT

Ask the patient to void before beginning your examination. Inspect the urethral meatus for discharge, irritation, and other abnormalities. Then percuss over the kidneys. Costovertebral angle tenderness indicates kidney inflammation. Percuss the bladder. Start at the symphysis pubis and percuss upward. You should hear tympany; a dull sound signals retained urine. Then palpate the kidneys. Normally, they aren't palpable unless they're enlarged. If the kidneys feel enlarged, the patient may have hydronephrosis, cysts, or tumors. You won't be able to palpate the bladder unless it's distended. (See *Palpating the kidneys*.) A pelvic or rectal examination may be necessary.

MEDICAL CAUSES

Appendicitis
Occasionally, appendicitis causes dysuria that persists throughout voiding and is accompanied by bladder tenderness. Appendicitis is characterized by periumbilical abdominal pain that shifts to McBurney's point, anorexia, nausea, vomiting, constipation, slight fever, abdominal rigidity and rebound tenderness, and tachycardia.

Bladder cancer
In bladder cancer, a predominantly male disorder, dysuria throughout voiding is a late symptom associated with urinary frequency and urgency, nocturia, hematuria, and perineal, back, or flank pain.

 CULTURAL CUE *Bladder cancer is twice as common in White males as in Black males. It's relatively uncommon in Asians, Hispanics, and Native Americans.*

Palpating the kidneys

To palpate the kidneys, first have the patient lie in a supine position. To palpate the right kidney, stand on his right side. Place your left hand under his back and your right hand on his abdomen.

Instruct him to inhale deeply, so his kidney moves downward. As he inhales, press up with your left hand and down with your right, as shown.

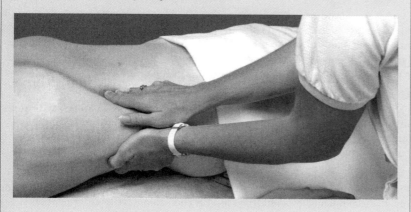

Cystitis

Dysuria throughout voiding is common in all types of cystitis, as are urinary frequency, nocturia, straining to void, and hematuria. Bacterial cystitis, the most common cause of dysuria in women, may also produce urinary urgency, perineal and lower back pain, suprapubic discomfort, fatigue and, possibly, low-grade fever. With chronic interstitial cystitis, dysuria is accentuated at the end of voiding. In tubercular cystitis, symptoms may also include urinary urgency, flank pain, fatigue, and anorexia. With viral cystitis, severe dysuria occurs with gross hematuria, urinary urgency, and fever.

Diverticulitis

Inflammation near the bladder may cause dysuria throughout voiding. Other effects include urinary frequency and urgency, nocturia, hematuria, fever, abdominal pain and tenderness, perineal pain, constipation or diarrhea and, possibly, an abdominal mass.

Paraurethral gland inflammation

Dysuria throughout voiding occurs with urinary frequency and urgency, diminished urine stream, mild perineal pain and, occasionally, hematuria.

Prostatitis

Acute prostatitis commonly causes dysuria throughout or toward the end of voiding. Dysuria may be accompanied by a diminished urine stream, urinary frequency and urgency, hematuria, suprapubic fullness, fever, chills, fatigue, myalgia, nausea, vomiting, and constipation.

With chronic prostatitis, urethral narrowing causes dysuria throughout voiding. Related effects include urinary frequency and urgency; diminished urine stream;

Medical causes
(continued)

Cystitis
+ Dysuria throughout voiding, urinary frequency, nocturia, straining to void, and hematuria are common.
+ Lower back pain and low grade fever may occur with bacterial cystitis.

Diverticulitis
+ Inflammation near the bladder may cause dysuria throughout voiding.

Paraurethral gland inflammation
+ Dysuria throughout voiding occurs with urinary frequency and urgency, diminished urine stream, mild perineal pain and, occasionally, hematuria.

Prostatitis
+ Acute prostatitis causes dysuria throughout or toward the end of voiding.
+ With chronic prostatitis, urethral narrowing causes dysuria throughout voiding.

Medical causes
(continued)

Pyelonephritis (acute)
- Dysuria occurs throughout voiding.
- Associated symtoms include high fever, CVA tenderness, flank pain, urinary urgency and frequency, and hematuria.

Reiter's syndrome
- Dysuria occurs 1 to 2 after ter sexual contact.

Urethral syndrome
- Dysuria throughout voiding may occur with urinary frequency and suprapubic aching and cramping.

Urethritis
- Primarily found in sexually active males.
- Dysuria occurs throughout voiding and is accompanied by a reddened meatus and copious, yellow, purulent discharge (gonorrheal infection) or white or clear mucoid discharge (nongonorrheal infection).

Urinary obstruction
- Outflow obstruction by urethral strictures or calculi produces dysuria throughout voiding.
- With complete obstruction, bladder distention develops and dysuria precedes voiding.

Vaginitis
- Dysuria occurs throughout voiding as urine touches inflamed or ulcerated labia.

Other causes
- Bubble bath salts
- MAO inhibitors
- Metyrosine
- Spermicides

perineal, back, and buttocks pain; urethral discharge; nocturia; and, at times, hematospermia and ejaculatory pain.

Pyelonephritis (acute)
More common in females, acute pyelonephritis causes dysuria throughout voiding. Other features include persistent high fever with chills, costovertebral angle tenderness, unilateral or bilateral flank pain, weakness, urinary urgency and frequency, nocturia, straining on urination, and hematuria. Nausea, vomiting, and anorexia may also occur.

Reiter's syndrome
With Reiter's syndrome, a predominantly male disorder, dysuria occurs 1 to 2 weeks after sexual contact. Initially, the patient has a mucopurulent discharge, urinary urgency and frequency, meatal swelling and redness, suprapubic pain, anorexia, weight loss, and low-grade fever. Hematuria, conjunctivitis, arthritic symptoms, a papular rash, and oral and penile lesions may follow.

Urethral syndrome
Occurring in sexually active women, urethral syndrome mimics urethritis. Dysuria throughout voiding may occur with urinary frequency, diminished urine stream, suprapubic aching and cramping, tenesmus, and lower back and unilateral flank pain. In the absence of pyuria, symptoms usually resolve without intervention.

Urethritis
Primarily found in sexually active males, urethritis causes dysuria throughout voiding. It's accompanied by a reddened meatus and copious, yellow, purulent discharge (gonorrheal infection) or white or clear mucoid discharge (nongonorrheal infection).

Urinary obstruction
Outflow obstruction by urethral strictures or calculi produces dysuria throughout voiding. (With complete obstruction, bladder distention develops and dysuria precedes voiding.) Other features include diminished urine stream, urinary frequency and urgency, and a sensation of fullness or bloating in the lower abdomen or groin.

Vaginitis
Characteristically, dysuria occurs throughout voiding as urine touches inflamed or ulcerated labia. Other findings include urinary frequency and urgency, nocturia, hematuria, perineal pain, and vaginal discharge and odor.

OTHER CAUSES

Chemical irritants
Dysuria may be caused by contact with irritating substances, such as bubble bath salts and feminine deodorants; it's usually most intense at the end of voiding. Spermicides may cause dysuria in both sexes. Other findings include urinary frequency and urgency, a diminished urine stream and, possibly, hematuria.

Drugs
Dysuria can result from monoamine oxidase inhibitor use. Metyrosine can also cause transient dysuria.

SPECIAL CONSIDERATIONS
Monitor the patient's vital signs and intake and output. Administer prescribed drugs, and prepare him for such tests as urinalysis and cystoscopy.

GERIATRIC POINTERS

Be aware that elderly patients tend to underreport their urinary-related symptoms, even though older men have an increased incidence of nonsexually related UTIs and postmenopausal women have an increased incidence of noninfectious dysuria. Although the kidneys typically aren't palpable unless enlarged, you may be able to palpate both kidneys in an elderly patient because of decreased muscle tone and elasticity.

PATIENT COUNSELING

Encourage the patient to increase his fluid intake to 3.2 qt (3 L))/day, unless contraindicated. Explain the importance of frequent urination. Show the female patient how to perform proper perineal care and tell her to avoid tub baths, especially bubble baths, and vaginal deodorants. Explain the importance of taking the full course of prescribed antibiotics, even if symptoms subside.

Special considerations
+ Monitor vital signs and intake and output.
+ Administer prescribed drugs.

Geri points
+ Elderly patients may underreport urinary-related symptoms.
+ Older men have an increased incidence of nonsexually related UTIs.
+ Postmenopausal women have an increased incidence of noninfectious dysuria.

Teaching points
+ Increased fluid intake
+ Importance of frequent urination
+ Proper perineal care
+ Avoidance of bubble baths and vaginal deodorants
+ Compliance with prescribed medications

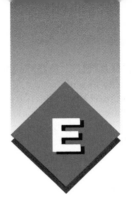

EARACHE

Also known as *otalgia,* earaches usually result from disorders of the external and middle ear that are associated with infection, obstruction, or trauma. Their severity ranges from a feeling of fullness or blockage to deep, boring pain. It may be difficult to determine the precise location of an earache. Earaches can be intermittent or continuous and may develop suddenly or gradually.

HISTORY

Ask the patient to characterize the earache. How long has he had it? Is it intermittent or continuous? Is it painful or slightly annoying? Can he pinpoint the site of the ear pain? Does he have pain in any other areas such as the jaw?

Also ask the patient about recent ear injury or other trauma. Does swimming or showering trigger ear discomfort? Is discomfort associated with itching? If so, find out where the itching is most intense and when it began. Ask about ear drainage and, if present, have the patient characterize it. Does he hear ringing, "swishing," or other noises in his ears? Ask about dizziness or vertigo. Do these symptoms worsen when the patient changes position? Does he have difficulty swallowing, hoarseness, neck pain, or pain when he opens his mouth?

Find out if the patient has recently had a head cold or problems with his eyes, mouth, teeth, jaws, sinuses, or throat. Disorders in these areas may refer pain to the ear along the cranial nerves. Also find out if the patient has recently flown, been to a high altitude location, or been scuba diving.

PHYSICAL ASSESSMENT

Begin your physical examination by inspecting the external ear for redness, drainage, swelling, or deformity. Then apply pressure to the mastoid process and tragus to elicit tenderness. Using an otoscope, examine the external auditory canal for lesions, bleeding or other discharge, impacted cerumen, foreign bodies, tenderness, or swelling. Examine the tympanic membrane. Is it intact? Look for tympanic membrane landmarks: the cone of light, umbo, pars tensa, and the handle and short process of the malleus. (See *Using an otoscope correctly*.) Perform watch tick, whispered voice, Rinne, and Weber's tests to assess for hearing loss.

Key facts about earache

+ Also known as *otalgia*
+ Caused by disorders of the external and middle ear that are associated with infection, obstruction, or trauma
+ Ranges from a feeling of fullness or blockage to deep, boring pain

Key history points

+ Onset and description of pain
+ Recent head cold or problems with mouth, sinuses, or throat
+ Aggravating factors
+ Associated itching, drainage, dizziness, vertigo, and pain when mouth opens
+ Recent airplane travel

Critical assessment steps

+ Inspect external ear for redness, drainage, swelling, or deformity.
+ Apply pressure to mastoid process and tragus to elicit tenderness.
+ Using an otoscope, examine external auditory canal for lesions, bleeding or other discharge, impacted cerumen, foreign bodies, tenderness, or swelling.
+ Examine tympanic membrane.

Using an otoscope correctly

When the patient reports an earache, use an otoscope to inspect ear structures closely. Follow these techniques to obtain the best view and ensure patient safety.

CHILD YOUNGER THAN AGE 3
To inspect an infant's or a young child's ear, grasp the lower part of the auricle and pull it down and back to straighten the upward S curve of the external canal. Then gently insert the speculum into the canal no more than ½" (1.3 cm).

ADULT
To inspect an adult's ear, grasp the upper part of the auricle and pull it up and back to straighten the external canal. Then insert the speculum about 1" (2.5 cm). Also use this technique for children age 3 and older.

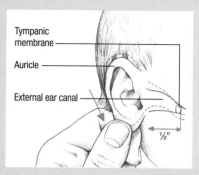

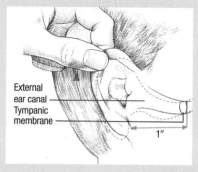

MEDICAL CAUSES

Abscess (extradural)
Severe earache accompanied by persistent ipsilateral headache, malaise, and recurrent mild fever characterizes extradural abscess, a serious complication of middle ear infection. The patient may also experience hearing loss.

Barotrauma (acute)
Earache associated with acute barotrauma ranges from mild pressure to severe pain. Tympanic membrane ecchymosis or bleeding into the tympanic cavity may occur, producing a blue drumhead; the eardrum usually isn't perforated.

Cerumen impaction
Impacted cerumen (earwax) may cause a sensation of blockage or fullness in the ear. Additional features include partial hearing loss, itching and, possibly, dizziness and ringing in the ear.

Chondrodermatitis nodularis chronica
Chondrodermatitis nodularis chronica produces small, painful, indurated areas along the upper rim of the auricle. The lesion may have a central core with scaly discharge.

Frostbite
Prolonged exposure to cold may cause burning or tingling pain in the ear, followed by numbness. The ear appears mottled and gray or white; it turns purplish blue as it's warmed.

Medical causes

Abscess (extradural)
✦ Severe earache is accompanied by persistent ipsilateral headache, malaise, and recurrent mild fever.

Barotrauma (acute)
✦ Earache ranges from mild pressure to severe pain.

Cerumen impaction
✦ Patient may feel blockage or fullness in the ear.

Chondrodermatitis nodularis chronica
✦ Small, painful, indurated areas develop along the upper rim of the auricle.

Frostbite
✦ Burning or tingling pain may occur in the ear, followed by numbness.

Medical causes
(continued)

Furunculosis

◆ Infected hair follicles in the outer ear canal may produce severe, localized ear pain associated with a pus-filled furuncle.

Herpes zoster oticus

◆ Burning or stabbing ear pain (commonly associated with ear vesicles) develops.

Mastoiditis (acute)

◆ Dull ache behind the ear is accompanied by low-grade fever.

Ménière's disease

◆ A sensation of fullness may occur in the affected ear accompanied by severe vertigo, tinnitus, and sensorineural hearing loss.

Middle ear tumor

◆ Deep, boring ear pain and facial paralysis are late signs.

Otitis externa (acute)

◆ Initially, pain is mild to moderate and occurs with tragus manipulation.
◆ Later, ear pain intensifies, causing the side of the head to ache.

Otitis media (acute)

◆ Acute serous otitis media may cause a feeling of fullness in the ear, hearing loss, and a vague sensation of top-heaviness.
◆ Acute suppurative otitis media involves severe, deep, throbbing ear pain, hearing loss, and fever that can reach 102° F (38.9° C).

Petrositis

◆ Infection produces deep ear pain with headache and pain behind the eye.

Furunculosis

Infected hair follicles in the outer ear canal may produce severe, localized ear pain associated with a pus-filled furuncle (boil). The pain is aggravated by jaw movement and relieved by rupture or incision of the furuncle. Pinna tenderness, swelling of the auditory meatus, partial hearing loss, and a feeling of fullness in the ear canal may also occur.

Herpes zoster oticus

Also known as *Ramsay Hunt syndrome,* herpes zoster oticus causes burning or stabbing ear pain, commonly associated with ear vesicles. The patient also complains of hearing loss and vertigo. Associated signs and symptoms include transitory, ipsilateral, facial paralysis; partial loss of taste; tongue vesicles; and nausea and vomiting.

Mastoiditis (acute)

Acute mastoiditis causes a dull ache behind the ear accompanied by low-grade fever (99° F to 100° F [37.2° C to 37.8° C]). The eardrum appears dull and edematous and may perforate, and soft tissue near the eardrum may sag. A purulent discharge is seen in the external canal.

Ménière's disease

Ménière's disease is an inner ear disorder that can produce a sensation of fullness in the affected ear. Its classic effects, however, include severe vertigo, tinnitus, and sensorineural hearing loss. The patient may also experience nausea and vomiting, diaphoresis, and nystagmus.

Middle ear tumor

Deep, boring ear pain and facial paralysis are late signs of a malignant tumor. Hearing loss and facial nerve dysfunction may accompany middle ear tumors.

Otitis externa (acute)

Acute otitis externa begins with mild to moderate ear pain that occurs with tragus manipulation. The pain may be accompanied by low-grade fever, sticky yellow or purulent ear discharge, partial hearing loss, and a feeling of blockage. Later, ear pain intensifies, causing the entire side of the head to ache and throb. Fever may reach 104°F [40° C]. Examination reveals swelling of the tragus, external meatus, and external canal; eardrum erythema; and lymphadenopathy. The patient also complains of dizziness and malaise.

Otitis media (acute)

Acute otitis media is a middle ear inflammation that may be serous or suppurative. Acute serous otitis media may cause a feeling of fullness in the ear, hearing loss, and a vague sensation of top-heaviness. The eardrum may be slightly retracted, amber colored, and marked by air bubbles and a meniscus, or it may be blue-black from hemorrhage.

Severe, deep, throbbing ear pain, hearing loss, and fever that can reach 102° F (38.9° C) characterize acute suppurative otitis media. The pain increases steadily over several hours or days and may be aggravated by pressure on the mastoid antrum. Perforation of the eardrum is possible. Before rupture, the eardrum appears bulging and fiery red. Rupture causes purulent drainage and relieves the pain.

Petrositis

The result of acute otitis media, petrositis is an infection that produces deep ear pain with headache and pain behind the eye. Other findings include diplopia, loss of lateral gaze, vomiting, sensorineural hearing loss, vertigo and, possibly, nuchal rigidity.

Temporomandibular joint infection

Typically unilateral, temporomandibular joint (TMJ) infection produces ear pain that's referred from the jaw joint. The pain is aggravated by pressure on the joint with jaw movement; it commonly radiates to the temporal area or the entire side of the head.

SPECIAL CONSIDERATIONS

Administer an analgesic, and apply heat to relieve the patient's discomfort. Instill eardrops if necessary.

PEDIATRIC POINTERS

Common causes of earache in children are acute otitis media and insertion of foreign bodies that become lodged or cause infection. Be alert for crying or ear tugging in a young child — nonverbal clues to earache.

To examine a child's ears, place him in a supine position with his arms extended and held securely by his parent. Then hold the otoscope with the handle pointing toward the top of the child's head, and brace it against him using one or two fingers. Because an ear examination may upset the child with an earache, perform it at the end of your physical examination.

PATIENT COUNSELING

Teach the patient or his parents how to instill eardrops if they're prescribed for home use. Encourage the patient to complete the full course of antibiotics if prescribed. If the patient experiences vertigo, tell him to rise slowly from a sitting or lying position. Warn the patient not to insert anything into the ear to avoid trauma, infection, and ear pain.

EDEMA, GENERALIZED

A common sign in severely ill patients, generalized edema is the excessive accumulation of interstitial fluid throughout the body. Its severity varies widely; slight edema may be difficult to detect, especially if the patient is obese, whereas massive edema is immediately apparent.

Generalized edema is typically chronic and progressive. It may result from cardiac, renal, endocrine, or hepatic disorders as well as from severe burns, malnutrition, or the effects of certain drugs and treatments.

Common factors responsible for edema are hypoalbuminemia and excess sodium ingestion or retention, both of which influence plasma osmotic pressure. (See *Understanding fluid balance,* page 244.) Cyclic edema associated with increased aldosterone secretion may occur in premenopausal women.

 EMERGENCY ACTIONS Quickly determine the location and severity of edema, including the degree of pitting. (See *Differentiating between pitting and nonpitting edema,* page 245.) If the patient has severe edema, promptly take his vital signs, and check for jugular vein distention and cyanotic lips. Auscultate the lungs and heart. Be alert for signs of heart failure or pulmonary congestion, such as crackles, muffled heart sounds, or ventricular gallop. Unless the patient is hyposensitive, place him in Fowler's position to promote lung expansion. Prepare to administer oxygen and an I.V. diuretic. Have emergency resuscitation equipment nearby.

Medical causes
(continued)

TMJ infection
+ Infection produces ear pain that's referred from the jaw joint.
+ Pain is aggravated by pressure on the joint with jaw movement.

Special considerations
+ Administer an analgesic.
+ Apply heat to relieve discomfort.
+ Instill eardrops if necessary.

Peds points
+ Common causes of earache in children are acute otitis media and insertion of foreign bodies that become lodged or cause infection.

Teaching points
+ Instillation of eardrops
+ Compliance with prescribed antibiotics
+ Ways to avoid vertigo

Key facts about generalized edema
+ Excessive accumulation of interstitial fluid throughout the body
+ Is chronic and progressive

In an emergency
If the patient has severe edema:
+ Take vital signs.
+ Check for jugular vein distention and cyanotic lips.
+ Auscultate the lungs and heart.
+ Place the patient in Fowler's position.
+ Prepare to administer oxygen and an I.V. diuretic.
+ Have emergency resuscitation equipment nearby.

Pressures that control fluid shift

- ✦ Capillary hydrostatic
- ✦ Interstitial fluid
- ✦ Osmotic
- ✦ Interstitial osmotic

Understanding fluid balance

Normally, fluid moves freely between interstitial and intravascular spaces to maintain homeostasis. Four basic pressures control fluid shifts across the capillary membrane that separate these spaces:

- ✦ capillary hydrostatic pressure (the internal fluid pressure on the capillary membrane)
- ✦ interstitial fluid pressure (the external fluid pressure on the capillary membrane)
- ✦ osmotic pressure (the fluid-attracting pressure from protein concentration within the capillary)
- ✦ interstitial osmotic pressure (the fluid-attracting pressure from protein concentration outside the capillary).

Here's how these pressures maintain homeostasis. Normally, capillary hydrostatic pressure is greater than plasma osmotic pressure at the capillary's arterial end, forcing fluid out of the capillary. At the capillary's venous end, the reverse is true: Plasma osmotic pressure is greater than capillary hydrostatic pressure, drawing fluid into the capillary. Normally, the lymphatic system transports excess interstitial fluid back to the intravascular space.

Edema results when this balance is upset by increased capillary permeability, lymphatic obstruction, persistently increased capillary hydrostatic pressure, decreased plasma osmotic or interstitial fluid pressure, or dilation of precapillary sphincters.

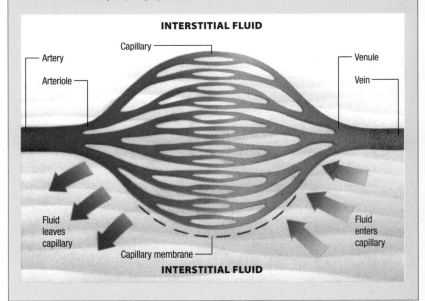

Key history points

- ✦ Onset, location, and description
- ✦ Associated shortness of breath or pain
- ✦ Medical history, including previous burns or cardiac, renal, hepatic, endocrine, or GI disorders
- ✦ Recent weight gain and urine output changes
- ✦ Diet
- ✦ Drug history

HISTORY

When the patient's condition permits, obtain a complete medical history. First, note when the edema began. Does it move throughout the course of the day — for example, from the upper extremities to the lower, periorbitally, or within the sacral area? Is the edema worse in the morning or at the end of the day? Is it affected by position changes? Is it accompanied by shortness of breath or pain in the arms or legs? Find out how much weight the patient has gained. Has his urine output changed in quantity or quality?

Next, ask about previous burns or cardiac, renal, hepatic, endocrine, or GI disorders. Ask the patient to describe his diet so you can determine whether he suffers from protein malnutrition. Explore his drug history, and note recent I.V. therapy.

Differentiating between pitting and nonpitting edema

To distinguish pitting from nonpitting edema, press your finger against a swollen area for 5 seconds, and then quickly remove it.

With *pitting edema,* pressure forces fluid into the underlying tissues, causing an indentation that slowly fills. To determine the severity of pitting edema, estimate the indenta-tion's depth in centimeters: 1+ (1 cm), 2+ (2 cm), 3+ (3 cm), or 4+ (4 cm).

With *nonpitting edema,* pressure leaves no indentation because fluid has coagulated in the tissues. Typically, the skin feels unusually tight and firm.

PITTING EDEMA (4+)

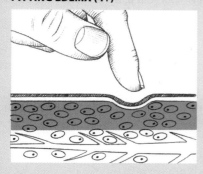

NONPITTING EDEMA

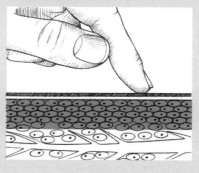

PHYSICAL ASSESSMENT

Begin the physical examination by comparing the patient's arms and legs for symmetrical edema. Also, note ecchymoses and cyanosis. Assess the back, sacrum, and hips of the bedridden patient for dependent edema. Palpate peripheral pulses, noting whether hands and feet feel cold. Finally, perform a complete cardiac and respiratory assessment.

MEDICAL CAUSES

Angioneurotic edema or angioedema
Recurrent attacks of acute, painless, nonpitting edema involving the skin and mucous membranes — especially those of the respiratory tract, face, neck, lips, larynx, hands, feet, genitalia, or viscera — may be the result of a food or drug allergy or emotional stress; they may also be hereditary. Abdominal pain, nausea, vomiting, and diarrhea accompany visceral edema; dyspnea and stridor accompany life-threatening laryngeal edema.

Burns
Edema and associated tissue damage vary with the severity of the burn. Severe generalized edema (4+) may occur within 2 days of a major burn; localized edema may occur with a less severe burn. Depending on the degree of edema, the patient may experience signs and symptoms of reduced or absent circulation and airway obstruction.

Pitting edema
+ Fluid fills slowly
+ Severity assessed by estimating indentation depth in centimeters

Nonpitting edema
+ Fluid coagulates in tissues
+ No indentation

Critical assessment steps
+ Compare the patient's arms and legs for symmetrical edema.
+ Note ecchymoses and cyanosis.
+ Assess the back, sacrum, and hips of a bedridden patient for dependent edema.
+ Palpate peripheral pulses, noting coolness in hands and feet.
+ Perform complete cardiac and respiratory assessments.

Medical causes
Angioneurotic edema or angioedema
+ Recurrent attacks of acute, painless, nonpitting edema involve the skin and mucous membranes.

Burns
+ Severe generalized edema may occur within 2 days of a major burn.

Medical causes
(continued)

Cirrhosis
+ Edema is a late sign.

Heart failure
+ Severe, generalized pitting edema may follow leg edema.
+ Edema may improve with exercise or elevation of limbs and is worst at end of day

Myxedema
+ Generalized nonpitting edema is accompanied by dry, flaky, inelastic, waxy, pale skin; puffy face; and upper eyelid droop.

Nephrotic syndrome
+ Edema is initially localized around the eyes, then becomes generalized and pitting.

Pericardial effusion
+ Generalized pitting edema may be most prominent in arms and legs.

Renal failure
+ Generalized pitting edema occurs as a late sign.
+ With chronic renal failure, edema is less likely to become generalized; its severity depends on the degree of fluid overload.

Other causes
+ Drugs that cause sodium retention (such as antihypertensives, corticosteroids, androgenic and anabolic steroids, estrogens, and NSAIDs)
+ I.V. saline solution infusions
+ Enteral feedings

Cirrhosis
Edema is a late sign of cirrhosis, a chronic disease. Accompanying signs and symptoms include abdominal pain, anorexia, nausea and vomiting, hepatomegaly, ascites, jaundice, pruritus, bleeding tendencies, musty breath, lethargy, mental changes, and asterixis.

Heart failure
Severe, generalized pitting edema — occasionally anasarca — may follow leg edema late in a patient with heart failure. The edema may improve with exercise or elevation of the limbs and tends to be worse at the end of the day. Other classic late findings include hemoptysis, cyanosis, marked hepatomegaly, clubbing, crackles, and a ventricular gallop. Typically, the patient also experiences tachypnea, palpitations, hypotension, weight gain despite anorexia, nausea, slowed mental response, diaphoresis, and pallor. Dyspnea, orthopnea, tachycardia, and fatigue signal left-sided heart failure; jugular vein distention, enlarged liver, and peripheral edema signal right-sided heart failure.

Myxedema
With myxedema, a severe form of hypothyroidism, generalized nonpitting edema is accompanied by dry, flaky, inelastic, waxy, pale skin; a puffy face; and an upper eyelid droop. Observation also reveals masklike facies, hair loss or coarsening, and psychomotor slowing. Associated findings include hoarseness, weight gain, fatigue, cold intolerance, bradycardia, hypoventilation, constipation, abdominal distention, menorrhagia, impotence, and infertility.

Nephrotic syndrome
Although nephrotic syndrome is characterized by generalized pitting edema, the edema is initially localized around the eyes. With severe cases, anasarca develops, increasing body weight by up to 50%. Other common signs and symptoms are ascites, anorexia, fatigue, malaise, depression, and pallor.

Pericardial effusion
With pericardial effusion, generalized pitting edema may be most prominent in the arms and legs. It may be accompanied by chest pain, dyspnea, orthopnea, nonproductive cough, pericardial friction rub, jugular vein distention, dysphagia, and fever.

Renal failure
Generalized pitting edema occurs as a late sign of acute renal failure. With chronic renal failure, edema is less likely to become generalized; its severity depends on the degree of fluid overload. Both forms of renal failure cause oliguria, anorexia, nausea and vomiting, drowsiness, confusion, hypertension, dyspnea, crackles, dizziness, and pallor.

OTHER CAUSES

Drugs
Any drug that causes sodium retention may aggravate or cause generalized edema. Examples include antihypertensives, corticosteroids, androgenic and anabolic steroids, estrogens, and nonsteroidal anti-inflammatory drugs, such as phenylbutazone, ibuprofen, and naproxen.

Treatments

I.V. saline solution infusions and enteral feedings may cause sodium and fluid overload, resulting in generalized edema, especially in patients with cardiac or renal disease.

SPECIAL CONSIDERATIONS

Position the patient with his limbs above heart level to promote drainage. Periodically reposition him to avoid pressure ulcers. If the patient develops dyspnea, lower his limbs, elevate the head of the bed, and administer oxygen. Massage reddened areas, especially where dependent edema has formed (for example, the back, sacrum, hips, buttocks). Prevent skin breakdown in these areas by placing a pressure mattress, lamb's wool pad, or flotation ring on the patient's bed. Restrict fluids and sodium, and administer a diuretic or I.V. albumin.

Monitor intake and output and daily weight. Also monitor serum electrolyte levels — especially sodium and albumin. Prepare the patient for blood and urine tests, X-rays, echocardiography, or an electrocardiogram.

PEDIATRIC POINTERS

Renal failure in children commonly causes generalized edema. Monitor fluid balance closely. Remember that fever and diaphoresis can lead to fluid loss, so promote fluid intake.

Kwashiorkor, a protein-deficiency malnutrition that's more common in children than in adults, causes anasarca.

GERIATRIC POINTERS

Elderly patients are at greater risk for developing edema for several reasons, including decreased cardiac and renal function and, in some cases, poor nutritional status. Use caution when giving older patients I.V. fluids or medications that can raise sodium levels and thereby increase fluid retention.

PATIENT COUNSELING

Teach patients with known heart failure or renal failure to watch for edema; explain that it's an important sign of decompensation that indicates the need for immediate adjustment of therapy. Teach the patient about dietary restrictions as indicated, including modifying sodium, potassium, and fluid intake.

EDEMA OF THE ARM

The result of excess interstitial fluid in the arm, arm edema may be unilateral or bilateral and may develop gradually or abruptly. It may be aggravated by immobility and alleviated by arm elevation and exercise.

Arm edema signals a localized fluid imbalance between the vascular and interstitial spaces. (See *Understanding fluid balance*, page 244.) It commonly results from trauma, venous disorders, toxins, or certain treatments.

 EMERGENCY ACTIONS **Remove rings, bracelets, and watches from the patient's affected arm. These items may act as a tourniquet. Make sure the patient's sleeves don't inhibit drainage of fluid or blood flow. If you detect signs of neurovascular compromise, elevate the arm.**

Key history points

+ Duration of arm edema
+ Associated arm pain, numbness, or tingling
+ Alleviating factors
+ Recent injury, I.V. therapy, surgery, or radiation therapy

Critical assessment steps

+ Compare the size and symmetry of arms and test for pitting.
+ Examine and compare the color and temperature of arms.
+ Look for erythema, ecchymoses, and wounds.
+ Palpate and compare pulses.
+ Look for arm tenderness and decreased sensation or mobility.

Medical causes

Angioneurotic edema
+ Sudden, painless, nonpruritic edema affects hands, feet, eyelids, lips, face, neck, or viscera.

Arm trauma
+ Severe edema may affect the entire arm.

Burns
+ Two days or less after injury, mild to severe edema, pain, and tissue damage may develop.

Envenomation
+ Edema may develop around the bite or sting and spread.

Superior vena cava syndrome
+ Bilateral arm edema usually progresses slowly.

Thrombophlebitis
+ Arm edema, pain, and warmth may occur.

HISTORY

When taking the patient's history, one of the first questions to ask is "How long has your arm been swollen?" Then find out if the patient also has arm pain, numbness, or tingling. Does exercise or arm elevation decrease the edema? Ask about recent arm injury, such as burns or insect stings. Also, note recent I.V. therapy, surgery, or radiation therapy for breast cancer.

PHYSICAL ASSESSMENT

Determine the edema's severity by comparing the size and symmetry of the arms. Use a tape measure to determine the exact girth. Be sure to note whether the edema is unilateral or bilateral, and test for pitting. (See *Differentiating between pitting and nonpitting edema,* page 245.) Next, examine and compare the color and temperature of the arms. Look for erythema and ecchymoses and for wounds that suggest injury. Palpate and compare radial and brachial pulses. Finally, look for arm tenderness and decreased sensation or mobility.

MEDICAL CAUSES

Angioneurotic edema

Angioneurotic edema is a common reaction characterized by sudden onset of painless, nonpruritic edema affecting the hands, feet, eyelids, lips, face, neck, genitalia, or viscera. Although these swellings usually don't itch, they may burn and tingle. If edema spreads to the larynx, signs of respiratory distress may occur.

Arm trauma

Shortly after a crush injury, severe edema may affect the entire arm. Ecchymoses or superficial bleeding, pain or numbness, and paralysis may occur. If a fracture has occurred, deformities may also be present.

Burns

Two days or less after injury, arm burns may cause mild to severe edema, pain, and tissue damage. Depending on the burn degree, the patient may also have erythema; blisters; white, brown, or leathery tissue; or charring.

Envenomation

Envenomation initially may cause edema around the bite or sting that quickly spreads to the entire arm. Pain, erythema, and pruritus at the site are common; paresthesia occurs occasionally. Later, the patient may develop generalized signs and symptoms, such as nausea, vomiting, weakness, muscle cramps, fever, chills, hypotension, headache and, in severe cases, dyspnea, seizures, and paralysis.

Superior vena cava syndrome

With superior vena cava syndrome, bilateral arm edema usually progresses slowly and is accompanied by facial and neck edema. Dilated veins mark these edematous areas. The patient also complains of headache, vertigo, and vision disturbances.

Thrombophlebitis

Thrombophlebitis may cause arm edema, pain, and warmth. Deep vein thrombophlebitis can also produce cyanosis, fever, chills, and malaise. Superficial thrombophlebitis also causes redness, tenderness, and induration along the vein.

OTHER CAUSES

Treatments

Localized arm edema may result from infiltration of I.V. fluid into the interstitial tissue. A radical or modified radical mastectomy that disrupts lymphatic drainage may cause edema of the entire arm, as can axillary lymph node dissection. Also, radiation therapy for breast cancer may produce arm edema immediately after treatment or months later.

SPECIAL CONSIDERATIONS

Treatment of the patient with arm edema varies according to the underlying cause. General care measures include elevation of the arm, frequent repositioning, and appropriate use of bandages and dressings to promote drainage and circulation. Be sure to provide the patient with meticulous skin care to prevent breakdown and formation of pressure ulcers. Also, administer an analgesic and anticoagulant as needed.

PEDIATRIC POINTERS

Arm edema rarely occurs in children, except as part of generalized edema. When it does occur, it may result from such arm trauma as burns and crush injuries.

PATIENT COUNSELING

Warn the patient who has undergone mastectomy or axillary lymph node dissection of the possibility of arm edema, and advise her not to have blood pressure measurements taken or phlebotomies performed on the affected arm. Teach the patient how to perform arm exercises after surgery to prevent lymphedema.

EDEMA OF THE FACE

Facial edema refers to either localized swelling — around the eyes, for example — or more generalized facial swelling that may extend to the neck and upper arms. Occasionally painful, this sign may develop gradually or abruptly. Sometimes it precedes the onset of peripheral or generalized edema. Mild edema may be difficult to detect; the patient or someone who's familiar with his appearance may report it before it's noticed during assessment.

Facial edema may result from venous, inflammatory, and certain systemic disorders; trauma; allergy; malnutrition; or the effects of certain drugs, tests, and treatments.

 EMERGENCY ACTIONS If the patient has facial edema associated with burns or if he reports recent exposure to an allergen, quickly evaluate his respiratory status. Edema may also affect his upper airway, causing life-threatening obstruction. If you detect audible wheezing, inspiratory stridor, or other signs of respiratory distress, administer epinephrine. For patients in severe distress — with absent breath sounds and cyanosis — tracheal intubation, cricothyroidotomy, or tracheotomy may be required. Always administer oxygen.

HISTORY

If the patient isn't in severe distress, take his health history. Ask if facial edema developed suddenly or gradually. Is it more prominent in early morning, or does it worsen throughout the day? Has the patient gained weight? If so, how much and

Other causes
+ Infiltration of I.V. fluid into the interstitial tissue
+ Mastectomy that disrupts lymphatic drainage
+ Radiation for breast cancer

Special considerations
+ Elevate the arm and frequently reposition the patient
+ Use bandages and dressings to provide drainage.
+ Provide meticulous skin care to prevent breakdown and formation of pressure ulcers.
+ Administer analgesic and anticoagulant as needed.

Peds points
+ Arm edema rarely occurs in children, but it may result from burns or crush injuries.

Teaching points
+ Postoperative arm care
+ Arm exercises

Key facts about facial edema
+ Involves localized or generalized facial swelling
+ May extend to neck and upper arms

In an emergency
+ Evaluate respiratory status.
+ If you detect respiratory distress, administer epinephrine.
+ For patients with absent breath sounds and cyanosis, tracheal intubation, cricothyroidotomy, or tracheotomy may be required.
+ Always administer oxygen.

Recognizing angioneurotic edema

Most dramatic in the lips, eyelids, and tongue, angioneurotic edema commonly results from an allergic reaction. It's characterized by rapid onset of painless, nonpitting, subcutaneous swelling that usually resolves in 1 to 2 days. This type of edema may also involve the hands, feet, genitalia, and viscera; laryngeal edema may cause life-threatening airway obstruction.

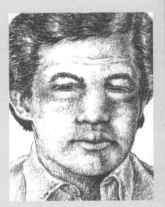

Key history points

+ Onset (sudden or gradual) and description of facial edema
+ Changes in urine color or output
+ Changes in appetite
+ Drug history
+ Recent facial trauma

Critical assessment steps

+ Describe severity, pitting, and location of edema.
+ Take vital signs.
+ Assess neurologic status.
+ Examine the oral cavity.
+ Visualize the oropharynx and look for soft-tissue swelling.

Medical causes

Abscess (periodontal)
+ Edema of the side of the face, pain, warmth, erythema, and purulent discharge around the affected tooth occur.

Abscess (peritonsillar)
+ Facial edema is unilateral.

Allergic reaction
+ Facial edema may develop.
+ With anaphylaxis, angioneurotic facial edema may occur with urticaria and flushing.

over what length of time? Has he noticed a change in his urine color or output? In his appetite? Take a drug history and ask about recent facial trauma.

PHYSICAL ASSESSMENT

Begin the physical examination by characterizing the edema. Is it localized to one part of the face, or does it affect the entire face or other parts of the body? Determine if the edema is pitting or nonpitting, and grade its severity. (See *Differentiating between pitting and nonpitting edema,* page 245.) Next, take the patient's vital signs, and assess neurologic status. Examine the oral cavity to evaluate dental hygiene and look for signs of infection. Visualize the oropharynx and look for soft-tissue swelling.

MEDICAL CAUSES

Abscess (periodontal)

A periodontal abscess can cause edema of the side of the face, pain, warmth, erythema, and purulent discharge around the affected tooth. The gums may be bright red and inflamed.

Abscess (peritonsillar)

A peritonsillar abscess, a complication of tonsillitis, may cause unilateral facial edema. Other key signs and symptoms include severe throat pain, neck swelling, drooling, cervical adenopathy, fever, chills, and malaise.

Allergic reaction

Facial edema may characterize local allergic reactions and anaphylaxis. With life-threatening anaphylaxis, angioneurotic facial edema may occur with urticaria and flushing. (See *Recognizing angioneurotic edema.*) Airway edema causes hoarseness, stridor, and bronchospasm with dyspnea and tachypnea. Signs of shock, such as hypotension and cool, clammy skin, may also occur. A localized reaction produces facial edema, erythema, and urticaria.

Chalazion

A chalazion causes localized swelling and tenderness of the affected eyelid, accompanied by a small red lump on the conjunctival surface. The patient may report increased tearing and photophobia.

Conjunctivitis

Conjunctivitis causes eyelid edema, excessive tearing, and itchy, burning eyes. Inspection reveals a thick purulent discharge, crusty eyelids, and conjunctival injection. Corneal involvement causes photophobia and pain.

Corneal ulcers (fungal)

In patients with fungal corneal ulcers, red, edematous eyelids accompany conjunctival injection, intense pain, photophobia, and severely impaired visual acuity. Copious, purulent eye discharge makes eyelids sticky and crusted. The characteristic dense, central ulcer grows slowly, is whitish gray, and is surrounded by progressively clearer rings.

Dacryocystitis

With dacryocystitis, lacrimal sac inflammation causes prominent eyelid edema and constant tearing. In acute cases, pain and tenderness near the tear sac accompany purulent discharge.

 CULTURAL CUE
Dacryocystitis rarely occurs in blacks because they tend to have a larger nasolacrimal ostium and a shorter, straighter lacrimal canal than whites.

Facial burns

Burns may cause extensive edema that impairs respiration. Additional findings include singed nasal hairs and eyebrows, red mucosa, sooty sputum, and signs of respiratory distress, such as inspiratory stridor.

Facial trauma

With facial trauma, the extent of edema varies with the type of injury. For example, a contusion may cause localized edema, whereas a nasal or maxillary fracture causes more generalized edema. Associated signs and symptoms also depend on the type of injury.

Herpes zoster ophthalmicus

With herpes zoster ophthalmicus (also known as *shingles*), edematous and red eyelids are usually accompanied by excessive tearing and a serous discharge. Severe unilateral facial pain may occur several days before vesicles erupt. Fever and malaise may also occur.

Hordeolum

Typically, localized eyelid edema, erythema, and pain occur with a hordeolum (stye). The patient may report photophobia and a foreign body sensation.

Malnutrition

Severe malnutrition causes facial edema followed by swelling of the feet and legs. Associated signs and symptoms include muscle atrophy and weakness; anorexia; diarrhea; lethargy; dry, wrinkled skin; sparse, brittle, easily plucked hair; and slowed pulse and respiratory rates.

Myxedema

Myxedema eventually causes generalized facial edema; waxy, dry skin; hair loss or coarsening; and other signs of hypothyroidism. Upper eyelid drooping may also be apparent.

Medical causes
(continued)

Chalazion
+ Swelling and tenderness are localized by the affected eyelid.

Conjunctivitis
+ Eyelid edema, excessive tearing, and itchy, burning eyes occur.

Corneal ulcers (fungal)
+ Red, edematous eyelids accompany conjunctival injection, intense pain, photophobia, and severely impaired visual acuity.

Dacryocystitis
+ Lacrimal sac inflammation causes prominent eyelid edema and constant tearing.

Facial burns
+ Extensive edema may develop, impairing respiration.

Facial trauma
+ Extent of edema varies with the type of injury.

Herpes zoster ophthalmicus
+ Edematous and red eyelids are accompanied by excessive tearing and a serous discharge.

Hordeolum
+ Localized eyelid edema, erythema, and pain occur.

Malnutrition
+ Facial edema is followed by swelling of the feet and legs.

Myxedema
+ Generalized facial edema occurs.

Medical causes
(continued)

Nephrotic syndrome
+ Periorbital edema is commonly the first sign.

Orbital cellulitis
+ Onset of periorbital edema is sudden.

Preeclampsia
+ Edema of the face, hands, and ankles is an early sign.

Rhinitis (allergic)
+ Red, edematous eyelids are accompanied by paroxysmal sneezing, itchy nose and eyes, and profuse, watery rhinorrhea.

Sinusitis
+ Frontal sinusitis causes edema of the forehead and eyelids.
+ Maxillary sinusitis produces edema in the maxillary area.

Superior vena cava syndrome
+ Gradually developing facial and neck edema are accompanied by thoracic or jugular vein distention.

Other causes
+ Allergic reactions to drugs, contrast media, or blood transfusion
+ Cranial, nasal, or jaw surgery
+ Fruit pulp of ginkgo biloba
+ Long-term use of glucocorticoids

Special considerations
+ Administer an analgesic for pain.
+ Apply cream to reduce itching.
+ Unless contraindicated, apply cold compresses to the eyes.
+ Elevate the head of the bed to help drain the accumulated fluid.

Nephrotic syndrome

Commonly the first sign of nephrotic syndrome, periorbital edema precedes dependent and abdominal edema. Associated findings include weight gain, nausea, anorexia, lethargy, fatigue, and pallor.

Orbital cellulitis

Sudden onset of periorbital edema marks orbital cellulitis, an inflammatory disorder. It may be accompanied by a unilateral purulent discharge, hyperemia, exophthalmos, conjunctival injection, impaired extraocular movements, fever, and extreme orbital pain.

Preeclampsia

Edema of the face, hands, and ankles is an early sign of preeclampsia. Other characteristics include excessive weight gain, severe headache, blurred vision, hypertension, and midepigastric pain.

Rhinitis (allergic)

With allergic rhinitis, red and edematous eyelids are accompanied by paroxysmal sneezing, itchy nose and eyes, and profuse, watery rhinorrhea. The patient may also develop nasal congestion, excessive tearing, headache, sinus pain, and sometimes malaise and fever.

Sinusitis

Frontal sinusitis causes edema of the forehead and eyelids. Maxillary sinusitis produces edema in the maxillary area as well as malaise, gingival swelling, and trismus. Both types are also accompanied by facial pain, fever, nasal congestion, purulent nasal discharge, and red, swollen nasal mucosa.

Superior vena cava syndrome

Superior vena cava syndrome gradually produces facial and neck edema accompanied by thoracic or jugular vein distention. It also causes central nervous system symptoms, such as headache, vision disturbances, and vertigo.

OTHER CAUSES

Diagnostic tests

An allergic reaction to contrast media used in radiologic tests may produce facial edema.

Drugs

Long-term use of glucocorticoids may produce facial edema. Any drug that causes an allergic reaction (aspirin, antipyretics, penicillin, and sulfa preparations, for example) may have the same effect. Ingestion of the fruit pulp of ginkgo biloba can cause severe erythema and edema and the rapid formation of vesicles.

Surgery and transfusion

Cranial, nasal, or jaw surgery may cause facial edema, as may a blood transfusion that causes an allergic reaction.

SPECIAL CONSIDERATIONS

Administer an analgesic for pain, and apply cream to reduce itching. Unless contraindicated, apply cold compresses to the patient's eyes to decrease edema. Elevate the head of the bed to help drain the accumulated fluid. Urine and blood tests are commonly ordered to help diagnose the cause of facial edema.

PEDIATRIC POINTERS

Normally, periorbital tissue pressure is lower in a child than in an adult. As a result, children are more likely to develop periorbital edema. In fact, periorbital edema is more common than peripheral edema in children with such disorders as heart failure and acute glomerulonephritis. Pertussis may also cause periorbital edema.

PATIENT COUNSELING

Teach the patient with allergies about the risks of delayed symptoms (those that occur up to 24 hours after exposure to an allergen) and the need to report shortness of breath, chest tightness, sweating, angioedema, or other symptoms. Tell him to avoid exposure to known allergens, including all forms of the offending food or drug. Also advise the patient to avoid open fields and wooded areas during the insect season to prevent insect bites or stings. Advise the patient to carry an anaphylaxis kit containing epinephrine. Instruct the patient to wear a medical identification bracelet identifying his allergies and medical conditions.

EDEMA OF THE LEG

Leg edema is a common sign that results when excess interstitial fluid accumulates in one or both legs. It may affect just the foot and ankle or extend to the thigh and may be slight or dramatic, pitting or nonpitting.

Leg edema may result from venous disorders, trauma, and certain bone and cardiac disorders that disturb normal fluid balance. (See *Understanding fluid balance,* page 244.) It may result from nephrotic syndrome, cirrhosis, acute and chronic thrombophlebitis, chronic venous insufficiency (most common), cellulitis, lymphedema, and drugs. However, several nonpathologic mechanisms may also cause leg edema. For example, prolonged sitting, standing, or immobility may cause bilateral orthostatic edema. This pitting edema usually affects the foot and disappears with rest and leg elevation. Increased venous pressure late in pregnancy may cause ankle edema. Constricting garters or pantyhose may mechanically cause lower-extremity edema.

HISTORY

To evaluate the patient, first ask how long he has had the edema. Did it develop suddenly or gradually? Does it decrease if he elevates his legs? Is it painful when touched or when he walks? Is it worse in the morning, or does it get progressively worse during the day? Ask about a recent leg injury, surgery, or illness that may have immobilized the patient. Does he have a history of cardiovascular disease? Finally, obtain a drug history.

PHYSICAL ASSESSMENT

Begin the physical examination by examining each leg for pitting edema. (See *Differentiating between pitting and nonpitting edema,* page 245.) Because leg edema may compromise arterial blood flow, palpate or use Doppler ultrasonography to auscultate peripheral pulses to detect any insufficiency. Observe leg color and look for unusual vein patterns. Then palpate for warmth, tenderness, and cords, and gently squeeze the calf muscle against the tibia to check for deep pain. If leg edema is unilateral, dorsiflex the foot to look for Homans' sign, which is indicated by calf pain. Finally, note skin thickening or ulceration in the edematous areas.

Medical causes

Burns
+ Two days or less after injury, mild to severe edema, pain, and tissue damage may occur.

Cellulitis
+ Pitting edema is caused by a streptococcal or staphylococcal infection.

Envenomation
+ Mild to severe localized edema may develop suddenly at site of bite or sting.

Heart failure
+ Bilateral leg edema is an early sign of right-sided heart failure.
+ Pitting ankle edema signals more advanced heart failure.

Hypoproteinemia
+ Bilateral leg edema is secondary to decreased protein and osmotic pressures.

Leg trauma
+ Localized edema may form.

Nephrotic syndrome
+ Bilateral leg edema is associated with polyuria and eyelid edema.
+ Generalized pitting edema may occur.

Osteomyelitis
+ If the lower leg is affected, localized, mild to moderate edema develops and may spread to the adjacent joint.

Rupture of popliteal cyst
+ Onset of unilateral calf pain and edema is sudden, usually occurring after walking or exercising.

MEDICAL CAUSES

Burns
Two days or less after injury, leg burns may cause mild to severe edema, pain, and tissue damage. Depending on the degree of the burn, the patient may also have erythema; blisters; white, brown, or leathery tissue; or charring.

Cellulitis
With cellulitis, pitting edema and orange peel skin are caused by a streptococcal or staphylococcal infection that most commonly occurs in the lower extremities. Cellulitis is also associated with erythema, warmth, and tenderness in the infected area.

Envenomation
Mild to severe localized edema may develop suddenly at the site of a bite or sting, along with erythema, pain, urticaria, pruritus, and a burning sensation. Later signs include nausea, vomiting, weakness, muscle cramps, fever, chills, hypotension, headache, and, in severe cases, dyspnea, seizures, and paralysis.

Heart failure
Bilateral leg edema is an early sign of right-sided heart failure. Other signs and symptoms include weight gain despite anorexia, nausea, chest tightness, hypotension, pallor, tachypnea, exertional dyspnea, orthopnea, paroxysmal nocturnal dyspnea, palpitations, ventricular gallop, and inspiratory crackles. Pitting ankle edema, hepatomegaly, hemoptysis, and cyanosis signal more advanced heart failure.

Hypoproteinemia
Malnourished patients suffer bilateral leg edema secondary to decreased protein and osmotic pressures. Malnutrition also typically causes muscle weakness; lethargy; anorexia; diarrhea; apathy; dry, wrinkled skin; and signs of anemia, such as dizziness and pallor.

Leg trauma
Mild to severe localized edema may form around the site of leg trauma. Ecchymoses or bleeding, pain or numbness, and paralysis may occur. If a fracture has occurred, deformities may be present.

Nephrotic syndrome
Nephrotic syndrome is commonly seen in children and results in bilateral leg edema. It's associated with polyuria and eyelid swelling. Generalized pitting edema may also occur as well as ascites, fatigue, malaise, depression, and pallor.

Osteomyelitis
When osteomyelitis, a bone infection, affects the lower leg, it usually produces localized, mild to moderate edema, which may spread to the adjacent joint. Edema typically follows fever, localized tenderness, and pain that increases with leg movement.

Rupture of popliteal cyst
A ruptured popliteal (Baker's) cyst can cause sudden onset of unilateral calf pain and edema, usually after walking or exercising. This type of cyst is common in patients with arthritis. It can compress vascular structures and cause severe edema and thrombophlebitis.

Thrombophlebitis

Both deep and superficial vein thrombosis may cause unilateral mild to moderate edema. Deep vein thrombophlebitis may not produce symptoms or may cause mild to severe pain, warmth, and cyanosis in the affected leg as well as fever, chills, and malaise. Superficial thrombophlebitis typically causes pain, warmth, redness, tenderness, and induration along the affected vein.

Venous insufficiency (chronic)

Moderate to severe, unilateral or bilateral leg edema occurs in patients with chronic venous insufficiency. Initially, the edema is soft and pitting; later, it becomes hard as tissues thicken. Other signs include darkened skin and painless, easily infected stasis ulcers around the ankle. Venous insufficiency generally occurs in females.

OTHER CAUSES
Coronary artery bypass surgery
Unilateral venous insufficiency may follow saphenous vein retrieval.

Medications
Estrogen, hormonal contraceptives, lithium, nonsteroidal anti-inflammatory drugs, vasodilators, and drugs that cause sodium retention can cause bilateral leg edema.

SPECIAL CONSIDERATIONS

Provide an analgesic and an antibiotic as needed. Have the patient avoid prolonged sitting or standing, and elevate his legs as necessary. A compression boot (Unna's boot) may be used to help reduce edema. Monitor the patient's intake and output, and check his weight and leg circumference daily to detect any change in the edema. Prepare him for diagnostic tests, such as blood and urine studies and X-rays. Determine the need for dietary modifications, such as water and sodium restrictions. Monitor the affected extremity for skin breakdown.

PEDIATRIC POINTERS

Uncommon in children, leg edema may result from osteomyelitis, leg trauma or, rarely, heart failure.

PATIENT COUNSELING

Show the patient with leg edema how to apply antiembolism stockings or bandages to promote venous return. Encourage him to perform leg exercises. Teach him about any dietary or fluid restrictions.

EPISTAXIS

A common sign, epistaxis (nosebleed) can be spontaneous or induced from the front or back of the nose. Most nosebleeds occur in the anterior-inferior nasal septum (Kiesselbach's area), but they may also occur at the point where the inferior turbinates meet the nasopharynx. Usually unilateral, they seem bilateral when blood runs from the bleeding side behind the nasal septum and out the opposite side. Epistaxis ranges from mild oozing to severe — possibly life-threatening — blood loss.

A rich supply of fragile blood vessels makes the nose particularly vulnerable to bleeding. Air moving through the nose can dry and irritate the mucous mem-

In an emergency

- ✦ Take vital signs; be alert for signs of hypovolemic shock.
- ✦ Insert a large-gauge I.V. line for fluid and blood replacement.
- ✦ Control bleeding by pinching the nares closed or placing gauze under the nose.
- ✦ Have a hypovolemic patient lie down and turn his head to the side.
- ✦ If the patient isn't hypovolemic, have him sit upright and tilt his head forward.
- ✦ Check airway patency.
- ✦ If patient is unstable, begin cardiac monitoring and give oxygen.

Key history points

- ✦ Recent trauma or surgery
- ✦ Description of past nosebleeds
- ✦ Medical history, including hypertension, bleeding or liver disorders, and other recent illnesses
- ✦ Drug history

Critical assessment steps

- ✦ Inspect for other signs of bleeding.
- ✦ Look for associated trauma injuries.

Medical causes

Aplastic anemia

- ✦ Nosebleeds are accompanied by ecchymoses, retinal hemorrhages, menorrhagia, petechiae, and signs of GI bleeding.

Biliary obstruction

- ✦ Bleeding tendencies, including epistaxis, occur.

Cirrhosis

- ✦ Epistaxis and other bleeding tendencies are late signs.

branes, forming crusts that bleed when they're removed. Dry mucous membranes are also more susceptible to infections, which can produce epistaxis as well. Trauma is another common cause of epistaxis. Additional causes include septal deviations; hematologic, coagulation, renal, and GI disorders; and certain drugs and treatments.

 EMERGENCY ACTIONS If your patient has severe epistaxis, quickly take his vital signs. Be alert for tachypnea, hypotension, and other signs of hypovolemic shock. Insert a large-gauge I.V. line for rapid fluid and blood replacement, and attempt to control bleeding by pinching the nares closed. (However, if you suspect a nasal fracture, don't pinch the nares. Instead, place gauze under the patient's nose to absorb the blood.)

Have a hypovolemic patient lie down and turn his head to the side to prevent blood from draining down the back of his throat, which could cause aspiration or vomiting of swallowed blood. If the patient isn't hypovolemic, have him sit upright and tilt his head forward. Constantly check airway patency. If the patient's condition is unstable, begin cardiac monitoring and give supplemental oxygen by mask.

HISTORY

If your patient isn't in distress, take a history. Does he have a history of recent trauma? How often has he had nosebleeds in the past? Have the nosebleeds been long or unusually severe? Has the patient recently had surgery in the sinus area? Ask about a history of hypertension, bleeding or liver disorders, and other recent illnesses. Ask if the patient bruises easily. Find out what drugs he uses, especially anti-inflammatories, such as aspirin, and anticoagulants such as warfarin.

PHYSICAL ASSESSMENT

Begin the physical examination by inspecting the patient's skin for other signs of bleeding, such as ecchymoses and petechiae, and noting any jaundice, pallor, or other abnormalities. When examining a trauma patient, look for associated injuries, such as eye trauma or facial fractures.

MEDICAL CAUSES

Aplastic anemia

Aplastic anemia develops insidiously, eventually producing nosebleeds as well as ecchymoses, retinal hemorrhages, menorrhagia, petechiae, bleeding from the mouth, and signs of GI bleeding. Fatigue, dyspnea, headache, tachycardia, and pallor may also occur.

Biliary obstruction

Biliary obstruction produces bleeding tendencies, including epistaxis. Typical features are colicky right-upper-quadrant pain after eating fatty food, nausea, vomiting, fever, flatulence and, possibly, jaundice.

Cirrhosis

With cirrhosis, epistaxis is a late sign that occurs along with other bleeding tendencies (bleeding gums, easy bruising, hematemesis, melena). Other typical late findings include ascites, abdominal pain, shallow respirations, hepatomegaly or splenomegaly, and fever. The patient may also exhibit muscle atrophy, enlarged superficial abdominal veins, severe pruritus, extremely dry skin, poor tissue turgor, abnormal pigmentation, spider angiomas, palmar erythema and, possibly, jaundice and central nervous system disturbances.

Coagulation disorders

Coagulation disorders, such as hemophilia and thrombocytopenic purpura, can cause epistaxis along with ecchymoses, petechiae, and bleeding from the gums, mouth, and I.V. puncture sites. Menorrhagia and signs of GI bleeding, such as melena and hematemesis, can also occur.

Glomerulonephritis (chronic)

Chronic glomerulonephritis produces nosebleeds as well as hypertension, proteinuria, hematuria, headache, edema, oliguria, hemoptysis, nausea, vomiting, pruritus, dyspnea, malaise, and fatigue.

Hepatitis

When hepatitis interferes with the clotting mechanism, epistaxis and abnormal bleeding tendencies can result. Associated signs and symptoms typically include jaundice, clay-colored stools, pruritus, hepatomegaly, abdominal pain, fever, fatigue, weakness, dark amber urine, anorexia, nausea, and vomiting.

Hypertension

Severe hypertension can produce extreme epistaxis, usually in the posterior nose, with pulsation above the middle turbinate. It may be accompanied by dizziness, a throbbing headache, anxiety, peripheral edema, nocturia, nausea, vomiting, drowsiness, and mental impairment.

Infectious mononucleosis

In patients with infectious mononucleosis, blood may ooze from the nose. Characteristic features include sore throat, cervical lymphadenopathy, and a fluctuating fever that peaks in the evening.

Influenza

When influenza affects the capillaries, a slow, oozing nosebleed results. Other signs and symptoms of influenza include dry cough, chills, fever, malaise, myalgia, sore throat, hoarseness or loss of voice, conjunctivitis, facial flushing, headache, rhinitis, and rhinorrhea.

Leukemia

With acute leukemia, sudden epistaxis is accompanied by a high fever and other types of abnormal bleeding, such as bleeding gums, ecchymoses, petechiae, easy bruising, and prolonged menses. These may follow less-noticeable signs and symptoms, such as weakness, lassitude, pallor, chills, recurrent infections, and low-grade fever. Acute leukemia may also cause dyspnea, fatigue, malaise, tachycardia, palpitations, a systolic ejection murmur, and abdominal or bone pain.

With chronic leukemia, epistaxis is a late sign that may be accompanied by other types of abnormal bleeding, extreme fatigue, weight loss, hepatosplenomegaly, bone tenderness, edema, macular or nodular skin lesions, pallor, weakness, dyspnea, tachycardia, palpitations, and headache.

Maxillofacial injury

With a maxillofacial injury, a pumping arterial bleed usually causes severe epistaxis. Associated signs and symptoms include facial pain, numbness, swelling, asymmetry, open-bite malocclusion or inability to open the mouth, diplopia, conjunctival hemorrhage, lip edema, and buccal, mucosal, and soft-palatal ecchymoses.

Medical causes
(continued)

Coagulation disorders
+ Epistaxis, ecchymoses, petechiae, and bleeding from the gums, mouth, and I.V. puncture sites may occur.

Glomerulonephritis (chronic)
+ Nosebleeds, hypertension, proteinuria, hematuria, headache, edema, oliguria, hemoptysis, nausea, vomiting, pruritus, dyspnea, malaise, and fatigue occur.

Hepatitis
+ Epistaxis and abnormal bleeding tendencies can result if clotting mechanisms are disrupted.

Hypertension
+ Severe hypertension can produce extreme epistaxis, usually in the posterior nose.

Infectious mononucleosis
+ Blood may ooze from the nose.

Influenza
+ If the capillaries are affected, a slow, oozing nosebleed results.

Leukemia
+ With acute leukemia, sudden epistaxis is accompanied by high fever and other types of abnormal bleeding.
+ With chronic leukemia, epistaxis is a late sign.

Maxillofacial injury
+ A pumping arterial bleed usually causes severe epistaxis.

Medical causes
(continued)

Nasal fracture
+ Epistaxis may be unilateral or bilateral.
+ Nasal swelling, periorbital ecchymoses and edema, pain, nasal deformity, and crepitation of the nasal bones may also occur.

Polycythemia vera
+ Spontaneous epistaxis is a common sign.

Renal failure
+ Chronic renal failure may cause epistaxis as well as oliguria or anuria, weight loss, anorexia, abdominal pain, diarrhea, nausea, vomiting, tissue wasting, dry mucous membranes, uremic breath, Kussmaul's respirations, deteriorating mental status, and tachycardia.

Sarcoidosis
+ Oozing epistaxis may occur along with a nonproductive cough, substernal pain, malaise, and weight loss.

Sinusitis (acute)
+ Bloody or blood-tinged nasal discharge may become purulent and copious after 24 to 48 hours.

Skull fracture
+ Epistaxis is direct or indirect, depending on the type of fracture.

Nasal fracture
Unilateral or bilateral epistaxis occurs with nasal swelling, periorbital ecchymoses and edema, pain, nasal deformity, and crepitation of the nasal bones. Skin lacerations and abrasions may be present over the fracture.

Polycythemia vera
A common sign of polycythemia vera, spontaneous epistaxis may be accompanied by bleeding gums; ecchymoses; ruddy cyanosis of the face, nose, ears, and lips; and congestion of the conjunctiva, retina, and oral mucous membranes. Other signs and symptoms vary according to the affected body system but may include headache, dizziness, tinnitus, vision disturbances, hypertension, chest pain, intermittent claudication, early satiety and fullness, marked splenomegaly, epigastric pain, pruritus, and dyspnea.

Renal failure
Chronic renal failure is more likely than acute renal failure to cause epistaxis and a tendency to bruise easily. More common signs and symptoms are oliguria or anuria, weight loss, anorexia, abdominal pain, diarrhea, nausea, vomiting, tissue wasting, dry mucous membranes, uremic breath, Kussmaul's respirations, deteriorating mental status, and tachycardia.

Skin changes include pruritus, pallor, yellow-bronze pigmentation, purpura, excoriation, uremic frost, and brown arcs under the nail margins. Neurologic signs and symptoms may include muscle twitches, fasciculations, asterixis, paresthesia, and footdrop. Cardiovascular effects include hypertension, arrhythmias, signs of heart failure, signs of pericarditis, and peripheral edema.

Sarcoidosis
Oozing epistaxis may occur in sarcoidosis, along with a nonproductive cough, substernal pain, malaise, and weight loss. Related findings include tachycardia, arrhythmias, parotid enlargement, cervical lymphadenopathy, skin lesions, hepatosplenomegaly, and arthritis in the ankles, knees, and wrists.

 CULTURAL CUE *Sarcoidosis occurs predominantly among blacks in the United States. In addition, this condition affects twice as many women as men.*

Sinusitis (acute)
With acute sinusitis, a bloody or blood-tinged nasal discharge may become purulent and copious after 24 to 48 hours. Associated signs and symptoms include nasal congestion, pain, tenderness, malaise, headache, low-grade fever, and red, edematous nasal mucosa.

Skull fracture
Depending on the type of fracture, epistaxis can be direct (when blood flows directly down the nares) or indirect (when blood drains through the eustachian tube and into the nose). Abrasions, contusions, lacerations, or avulsions are common. A severe skull fracture may cause severe headache, decreased level of consciousness, hemiparesis, dizziness, seizures, projectile vomiting, and decreased pulse and respiratory rates.

A basilar fracture may also cause bleeding from the pharynx, ears, and conjunctiva as well as raccoon eyes and Battle's sign. Cerebrospinal fluid or even brain tissue may leak from the nose or ears. A sphenoid fracture may also cause blindness, whereas a temporal fracture may also cause unilateral deafness or facial paralysis.

Systemic lupus erythematosus

Usually affecting women younger than age 50, systemic lupus erythematosus (SLE) causes oozing epistaxis. More characteristic signs and symptoms include butterfly rash, lymphadenopathy, joint pain and stiffness, anorexia, nausea, vomiting, myalgia, and weight loss.

OTHER CAUSES

Chemical irritants

Some chemicals—including phosphorus, sulfuric acid, ammonia, printer's ink, and chromates—irritate the nasal mucosa, producing epistaxis.

Drugs

Anticoagulants, such as warfarin, and anti-inflammatory drugs, such as aspirin, can cause epistaxis. Cocaine use, especially if frequent, can also cause epistaxis.

Vigorous nose blowing

Vigorous nose blowing may rupture superficial blood vessels and cause epistaxis, especially in elderly people and young people.

SPECIAL CONSIDERATIONS

Until the bleeding is completely under control, continue to monitor the patient for signs of hypovolemic shock, such as tachycardia and clammy skin. If external pressure doesn't control the bleeding, insert cotton that has been impregnated with a vasoconstrictor and local anesthetic into the patient's nose.

If bleeding persists, expect to insert anterior or posterior nasal packing. (See *Controlling epistaxis with nasal packing,* page 260.) Administer humidified oxygen by face mask to a patient with posterior packing.

A complete blood count may be ordered to evaluate blood loss and detect anemia. Clotting studies, such as prothrombin time and activated partial thromboplastin time, may be required to test coagulation time. Prepare the patient for X-rays if he has had recent trauma.

PEDIATRIC POINTERS

Children are more likely to experience anterior nosebleeds, usually the result of nose picking or allergic rhinitis. Biliary atresia, cystic fibrosis, hereditary afibrinogenemia, and nasal trauma due to a foreign body can also cause epistaxis. Rubeola may cause an oozing nosebleed along with the characteristic maculopapular rash.

Suspect a coagulation disorder if you see excess umbilical cord bleeding at birth or profuse bleeding during circumcision.

GERIATRIC POINTERS

Elderly patients are more likely to have posterior nosebleeds.

PATIENT COUNSELING

Advise the patient about proper pinching pressure techniques. For prevention, tell him to apply liberal amounts of petroleum jelly to his nostrils to prevent drying, cracking, and picking. Use of a humidifier at night and trimming fingernails are also recommended.

Medical causes
(continued)

SLE
+ Oozing epistaxis occurs.

Other causes
+ Anticoagulants or anti-inflammatory drugs
+ Chemicals
+ Cocaine use
+ Vigorous nose blowing

Special considerations
+ Monitor for signs of hypovolemic shock.
+ If external pressure doesn't control the bleeding, insert cotton that has been impregnated with a vasoconstrictor and local anesthetic into the nose.
+ If bleeding persists, expect to insert anterior or posterior nasal packing.
+ Administer humidified oxygen by face mask to a patient with posterior packing.

Peds points
+ Children are more likely to experience anterior nosebleeds.
+ Causes of epistaxis include nose picking, allergic rhinitis, biliary atresia, cystic fibrosis, hereditary afibrinogenemia, nasal trauma due to foreign body, and rubeola.

Geri points
+ Elderly patients are more likely to have posterior nosebleeds.

Teaching points
+ Pinching pressure techniques
+ Ways to prevent nosebleeds

Controlling epistaxis with nasal packing

When direct pressure and cautery fail to control epistaxis, nasal packing may be required. Anterior packing may be used if the patient has severe bleeding in the anterior nose. Horizontal layers of petroleum jelly gauze strips are inserted into the nostrils near the turbinates.

Posterior packing may be needed if the patient has severe bleeding in the posterior nose or if blood from anterior bleeding starts flowing backward. This type of packing consists of a gauze pack secured by three strong silk sutures. After the nose is anesthetized, sutures are pulled through the nostrils with a soft catheter and the pack is positioned behind the soft palate. Two of the sutures are tied to a gauze roll under the patient's nose, which keeps the pack in place. The third suture is taped to his cheek. Instead of a gauze pack, an indwelling urinary or nasal epistaxis catheter may be inserted through the nose into the area behind the soft palate and inflated with 10 ml of water to compress the bleeding point.

PRECAUTIONS
If the patient has nasal packing, follow these guidelines:
✦ Watch for signs of respiratory distress, such as dyspnea, which may occur if the packing slips and obstructs the airway.
✦ Keep emergency equipment (flashlights, scissors, and hemostat) at the patient's bedside. Expect to cut the cheek suture (or deflate the catheter) and remove the pack at the first sign of airway obstruction.
✦ Avoid tension on the cheek suture, which could cause the posterior pack to slip out of place.
✦ Keep the call bell within easy reach of the patient.
✦ Monitor vital signs frequently. Watch for signs of hypoxia, such as tachycardia and restlessness.
✦ Elevate the head of the patient's bed, and remind him to breathe through his mouth.
✦ Administer humidified oxygen as needed.
✦ Instruct the patient not to blow his nose for 48 hours after the packing is removed.

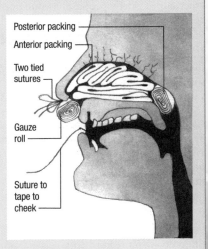

Posterior packing
Anterior packing
Two tied sutures
Gauze roll
Suture to tape to cheek

Key facts about erythema
✦ Also known as *erythroderma*
✦ Refers to red skin caused by dilated or congested blood vessels
✦ Is a common sign of skin inflammation or irritation

ERYTHEMA

Dilated or congested blood vessels produce red skin, or erythema, the most common sign of skin inflammation or irritation. Also known as *erythroderma*, erythema may be localized or generalized and may occur suddenly or gradually. Skin color can range from bright red in patients with acute conditions to pale violet or brown in those with chronic problems. Erythema must be differentiated from purpura, which causes redness from bleeding into the skin. When pressure is applied directly to the skin, erythema blanches momentarily, but purpura doesn't. Moreover, when erythema is caused by inflammation, the skin over the site feels warmer than the rest of the skin.

Erythema usually results from changes in the arteries, veins, and small vessels that lead to increased small-vessel perfusion. Drugs and neurogenic mechanisms can allow extra blood to enter the small vessels. Erythema can also result from trauma and tissue damage; changes in supporting tissues, which increase vessel visibility; and several rare disorders.

EMERGENCY ACTIONS If your patient has sudden progressive erythema with rapid pulse, dyspnea, hoarseness, and agitation, quickly take his vital signs. These may be indications of anaphylactic shock. Provide emergency respiratory support and give epinephrine.

HISTORY

If erythema isn't associated with anaphylaxis, obtain a detailed health history. Find out how long the patient has had the erythema and where it first began. Has he had any associated pain or itching? Has he recently had a fever, upper respiratory tract infection, or joint pain? Does he have a history of skin disease or other illness? Does he or anyone in his family have allergies, asthma, or eczema? Find out if he has been exposed to someone who has had a similar rash or who's now ill. Did he have a recent fall or injury in the area of erythema?

Obtain a complete drug history, including recent immunizations. Ask about food intake and exposure to chemicals.

PHYSICAL ASSESSMENT

Begin the physical examination by assessing the extent, distribution, and intensity of erythema. Look for edema and other skin lesions, such as hives, scales, papules, and purpura. Examine the affected area for warmth, and gently palpate it to check for tenderness or crepitus.

CULTURAL CUE *Dark-skinned patients may have difficulty recognizing erythema; as a result, they may present with associated diseases in a more advanced state.*

MEDICAL CAUSES

Allergic reactions

Foods, drugs, chemicals, and other allergens can cause an allergic reaction and erythema. A localized allergic reaction also produces hivelike eruptions and edema.

Anaphylaxis, a life-threatening condition, produces relatively sudden erythema in the form of urticaria. It also produces flushing; facial edema; diaphoresis; weakness; sneezing; bronchospasm with dyspnea and tachypnea; shock with hypotension and cool, clammy skin; and possibly airway edema with hoarseness and stridor.

Burns

With thermal burns, erythema and swelling appear first, possibly followed by deep or superficial blisters and other signs of damage that vary with the severity of the burn. Burns from ultraviolet rays, such as sunburn, cause delayed erythema and tenderness on exposed areas of the skin.

Candidiasis

When candidiasis, a fungal infection, affects the skin, it produces erythema and a scaly, papular rash under the breasts and at the axillae, neck, umbilicus, and groin, also known as *intertrigo*. Small pustules commonly occur at the periphery of the rash (satellite pustulosis).

Cellulitis

With cellulitis, erythema, tenderness, and edema are a result of a bacterial infection of the skin and subcutaneous tissue. The patient typically feels pain and a warm sensation at the site of the infection.

In an emergency

If erythema accompanies other indicators of anaphylactic shock:
- Provide respiratory support.
- Give epinephrine.

Key history points
- Onset and duration of erythema
- Medical history, including skin disease, allergies, or asthma.
- Associated pain or itching
- Recent fall or injury
- Drug history
- Food intake and exposure to chemicals

Critical assessment steps
- Assess the extent, distribution, and intensity of erythema.
- Look for edema.

Medical causes

Allergic reactions
- Localized reaction produces erythema, hivelike eruptions, and edema.
- With anaphylaxis, erythema is sudden.

Burns
- With thermal burns, erythema and swelling appear first.
- Burns from UV rays cause delayed erythema and tenderness.

Candidiasis
- If the skin is affected, erythema and a scaly, papular rash under breasts and at axillae, neck, umbilicus, and groin develop.

Cellulitis
- Erythema, tenderness, and edema result from a bacterial infection of the skin and subcutaneous tissue.

Medical causes
(continued)

Dermatitis
+ With atopic dermatitis, erythema and intense pruritus precede the development of small papules.
+ Contact dermatitis produces erythema and vesicles, blisters, or ulcerations.
+ With seborrheic dermatitis, erythema appears with dull-red or yellow lesions.

Erysipelas
+ Reddish, well-demarcated, tender, warm areas occur most commonly on face and neck.

Erythema annulare centrifugum
+ Small, pink infiltrated papules appear on the trunk, buttocks, and inner thighs.

Erythema marginatum rheumaticum
+ Lesions are superficial, flat, and slightly hardened.
+ Lesions shift, spread rapidly, and may last for hours or days.

Erythema multiforme
+ In minor form, urticarial red-pink, iris-shaped, localized lesions commonly occur on flexor surfaces of extremities.
+ In major form, blisters on lips, tongue, and buccal mucosa and sore throat precede development of widespread symmetrical, bullous lesions.

Erythema nodosum
+ Tender, bilateral, erythematous nodules develop suddenly on the shins, knees, and ankles.

Dermatitis
Erythema commonly occurs in dermatitis, a group of inflammatory disorders. With atopic dermatitis, erythema and intense pruritus precede the development of small papules that may redden, weep, scale, and lichenify. These occur most commonly at skin folds of the extremities, neck, and eyelids.

Contact dermatitis occurs after exposure to an irritant. It quickly produces erythema and vesicles, blisters, or ulcerations on exposed skin.

With seborrheic dermatitis, erythema appears with dull-red or yellow lesions. Sharply marginated, these lesions are sometimes ring shaped and covered with greasy scales. They usually occur on the scalp, eyebrows, ears, and nasolabial folds, but they may form a butterfly rash on the face or move to the chest or to skin folds on the trunk.

Erysipelas
Erysipelas—a skin infection caused by group A beta-hemolytic streptococci—is characterized by an abrupt onset on reddish, well-demarcated, tender, warm, sometimes elevated areas most commonly on the face and neck, although it may also occur on the extremities. Flaccid bullae that may be filled with pus may occur after 2 to 3 days. Associated signs and symptoms include fever, chills, local adenopathy, malaise, headache, and sore throat.

Erythema annulare centrifugum
With erythema annulare centrifugum, small, pink infiltrated papules appear on the trunk, buttocks, and inner thighs, slowly spreading at the margins and clearing in the center. Itching, scaling, and tissue hardening may also occur.

Erythema marginatum rheumaticum
Associated with rheumatic fever, erythema marginatum rheumaticum causes erythematous lesions that are superficial, flat, and slightly hardened. They shift, spread rapidly, and may last for hours or days, recurring after a time.

Erythema multiforme
Erythema multiform minor has typical urticarial red-pink, iris-shaped, localized lesions with little or no mucous membrane involvement. Most lesions occur on flexor surfaces of the extremities. Burning or itching may occur before or in conjunction with lesion development. Lesions appear in crops and last 2 to 3 weeks. After 1 week individual lesions become flat or hyperpigmented. Early signs and symptoms may include a mild fever, cough, and sore throat.

Erythema multiforme major usually occurs as a drug reaction; has widespread symmetrical, bullous lesions that may become confluent; and includes erosions of the mucous membranes. Erythema is characteristically preceded by blisters on the lips, tongue, and buccal mucosa and a sore throat. Additional signs and symptoms that occur early in the course of the disease include cough, vomiting, diarrhea, coryza, and epistaxis. Later signs and symptoms include fever, prostration, difficulty with oral intake due to mouth and lip lesions, conjunctivitis due to ulceration, vulvitis, and balanitis.

Erythema nodosum
Sudden bilateral eruption of tender erythematous nodules characterizes erythema nodosum. These firm, round, protruding lesions usually appear in crops on the shins, knees, and ankles but may occur on the buttocks, arms, calves, and trunk as well. Other effects include mild fever, chills, malaise, muscle and joint pain and, possibly, swollen feet and ankles. Erythema nodosum is associated with various

diseases, most notably inflammatory bowel disease, sarcoidosis, tuberculosis, and streptococcal and fungal infections.

Frostbite

First-degree frostbite turns the affected body part a lifeless gray color, followed by an intense bluish red flush on rewarming. Blisters, lack of feeling, and tissue necrosis may follow.

Gout

Gout is characterized by tight and erythematous skin over an inflamed, edematous joint. The metatarsophalangeal joint of the great toe usually becomes inflamed first, followed by the instep, ankle, heel, knee, or wrist joints.

Intertrigo

With intertrigo, a superficial fungal infection, skin friction usually causes symmetrical erythema that may be accompanied by soreness or itching. Typically, erythema occurs in skin folds, such as in the groin; in severe cases, the skin may become bright red with erosion and maceration.

Liver disease (chronic)

Any chronic liver disease, such as cirrhosis, can cause local vasodilation and palmar erythema along with jaundice, pruritus, spider angiomas, xanthomas, and characteristic systemic signs.

Lupus erythematosus

Both discoid and systemic lupus erythematosus (SLE) can produce a characteristic butterfly rash. This erythematous eruption may range from a blush with swelling to a scaly, sharply demarcated, macular rash with plaques that may spread to the forehead, chin, ears, chest, and other sun-exposed parts of the body.

Telangiectasia, hyperpigmentation, ear and nose deformity, and mouth, tongue, and eyelid lesions may occur with discoid lupus erythematosus.

With SLE, acute onset of erythema may also be accompanied by photosensitivity and mucous membrane ulcers, especially in the nose and mouth. Mottled erythema may occur on the hands, with edema around the nails and macular reddish purple lesions on the fingers. Telangiectasia occurs at the base of the nails or eyelids, along with purpura, petechiae, ecchymoses, and urticaria. Joint pain and stiffness are common. Other findings vary according to the body systems affected but typically include low-grade fever, malaise, weakness, headache, arthralgias, arthritis, depression, lymphadenopathy, fatigue, weight loss, anorexia, nausea, vomiting, diarrhea, and constipation.

Polymorphous light eruption

Polymorphous light eruption produces erythema, vesicles, plaques, and multiple small papules on sun-exposed areas, which may later eczematize, lichenify, and excoriate. Pruritus may also occur.

Psoriasis

With psoriasis, silvery white scales that occur over a thickened erythematous base usually affect the elbows, knees, chest, scalp, and intergluteal folds. The fingernails may become thick and pitted.

Raynaud's disease

With Raynaud's disease, the skin on the hands and feet typically blanches and cools after exposure to cold and stress. Later, it becomes warm and purplish red. Numbness and tingling may also occur.

Medical causes
(continued)

Frostbite
- Initially, first-degree frostbite turns the affected body part gray; on rewarming, color changes to an intense bluish red flush.

Gout
- Tight, erythematous skin occurs over inflamed, edematous joint.

Intertrigo
- Skin friction causes symmetrical erythema that may be accompanied by soreness or itching.

Liver disease (chronic)
- Local vasodilation and palmar erythema occur.

Lupus erythematosus
- An erythematous butterfly rash develops.
- Acute onset of erythema may be accompanied by photosensitivity and mucous membrane ulcers in SLE.

Polymorphous light eruption
- Erythema, vesicles, plaques, and multiple small papules on sun-exposed areas develop.

Psoriasis
- Silvery white scales with a thickened erythematous base affect the elbows, knees, chest, scalp, and intergluteal folds.

Raynaud's disease
- After blanching in response to cold and stress, skin on the hands and feet becomes warm and purplish red.

Medical causes
(continued)

Rheumatoid arthritis
✦ During flare-ups, erythema, heat, swelling, pain, and stiffness occurs over affected joints.

Rosacea
✦ Scattered erythema develops across the center of the face.

Rubella
✦ Flat solitary lesions form a blotchy pink erythematous rash that spreads rapidly to the trunk and extremities.

Staphylococcal scalded skin syndrome
✦ Occurring mainly in infants and small children, erythema and widespread exfoliation of superficial epidermal layers occur.

Thrombophlebitis
✦ Erythema may develop over the inflamed vein.

Other causes
✦ Drugs
✦ Radiation therapy
✦ Treatments that cause allergic reactions

Special considerations
✦ Monitor and replace fluids and electrolytes, especially in patients with burns or widespread erythema.
✦ Withhold drugs until the cause of erythema has been identified; then expect to administer antibiotic and topical or systemic corticosteroid.

Rheumatoid arthritis
In a flare-up of rheumatoid arthritis, erythema occurs over the affected joints along with heat, swelling, pain, and stiffness. Earlier symptoms include malaise, fatigue, myalgia, prolonged morning stiffness, and clumsiness. As the disease progresses, muscle atrophy, palmar erythema, generalized edema, mottled skin, and structural deformities occur.

Rosacea
With rosacea, scattered erythema initially develops across the center of the face, followed by superficial telangiectases, papules, pustules, and nodules. Rhinophyma may occur on the lower half of the nose.

Rubella
With rubella, flat solitary lesions join to form a blotchy pink erythematous rash that spreads rapidly to the trunk and extremities. Occasionally, small red lesions (Forschheimer spots) occur on the soft palate. Lesions clear in 4 to 5 days. The rash usually follows fever (up to 102° F [38.9° C]), headache, malaise, sore throat, a gritty eye sensation, lymphadenopathy, pain in the joints, and coryza.

Staphylococcal scalded skin syndrome
Also known as *Ritter's disease,* this disease occurs mainly in infants and small children. It's caused by *Staphylococcus aureus* and is characterized by erythema and widespread exfoliation of superficial epidermal layers, resembling scalded skin. Associated signs and symptoms include low-grade fever and irritability. Death may occur, especially in infants with extensive disease.

Thrombophlebitis
Although thrombophlebitis sometimes produces no symptoms, it can produce erythema over the inflamed vein. Fever, chills, and malaise may accompany severe, localized pain, warmth, and induration; distal edema; and a positive Homans' sign.

OTHER CAUSES

Drugs
Many drugs commonly cause erythema. (See *Drugs associated with erythema.*)

Radiation and other treatments
Radiation therapy may produce dull erythema and edema within 24 hours. As the erythema fades, the skin becomes light brown and mildly scaly. Any treatment that causes an allergic reaction can also cause erythema.

SPECIAL CONSIDERATIONS
Because erythema can cause fluid loss, closely monitor and replace fluids and electrolytes, especially in patients with burns or widespread erythema. Be sure to withhold all medications until the cause of the erythema has been identified. Then expect to administer an antibiotic and a topical or systemic corticosteroid.

For the patient with itching skin, expect to give soothing baths or apply open wet dressings containing starch, bran, or sodium bicarbonate; also administer an antihistamine and an analgesic as needed. Advise a patient with leg erythema to keep his legs elevated above heart level. For a burn patient with erythema, immerse the affected area in cold water, or apply a sheet soaked in cold water to reduce pain, edema, and erythema.

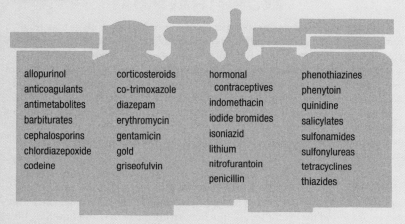

Drugs associated with erythema

Suspect drug-induced erythema in any patient who develops this sign within 1 week of starting a drug. Erythematous lesions can vary in size, shape, type, and amount, but they almost always appear suddenly and symmetrically on the trunk and inner arms. These drugs can produce erythematous lesions:

allopurinol	corticosteroids	hormonal	phenothiazines
anticoagulants	co-trimoxazole	contraceptives	phenytoin
antimetabolites	diazepam	indomethacin	quinidine
barbiturates	erythromycin	iodide bromides	salicylates
cephalosporins	gentamicin	isoniazid	sulfonamides
chlordiazepoxide	gold	lithium	sulfonylureas
codeine	griseofulvin	nitrofurantoin	tetracyclines
		penicillin	thiazides

Some drugs—particularly barbiturates, hormonal contraceptives, salicylates, sulfonamides, and tetracycline—can cause a "fixed" drug eruption. In this type of reaction, lesions can appear in any body part and flake off after a few days, leaving a brownish purple pigmentation. Repeated drug administration causes the original lesions to recur and new ones to develop.

Prepare the patient for diagnostic tests, such as skin biopsy to detect cancerous lesions, cultures to identify infectious organisms, and sensitivity studies to confirm allergies.

PEDIATRIC POINTERS

Typically, neonate rash (erythema toxicum neonatorum), a pink papular rash, develops during the first 4 days after birth and spontaneously disappears by the 10th day. Neonates and infants can also develop erythema from infections and other disorders. For instance, candidiasis can produce thick white lesions over an erythematous base on the oral mucosa as well as diaper rash with beefy red erythema.

Roseola, rubeola, scarlet fever, granuloma annulare, and cutis marmorata also cause erythema in children.

GERIATRIC POINTERS

Elderly patients commonly have well-demarcated purple macules or patches, usually on the back of the hands and on the forearms. Known as *actinic purpura*, this condition results from blood leaking through fragile capillaries. The lesions disappear spontaneously.

Special considerations
(continued)

✦ For the patient with itching skin, expect to give soothing baths or apply open wet dressings containing starch, bran, or sodium bicarbonate; administer an antihistamine and an analgesic as needed.
✦ Advise those with leg erythema to keep the legs elevated above heart level.
✦ For a burn patient with erythema, immerse the affected area in cold water, or apply a sheet soaked in cold water.

Peds points

✦ Neonates may develop a pink papular rash typically during the first 4 days after birth.
✦ Infections and other disorders can cause erythema in neonates and infants.
✦ Roseola, rubeola, scarlet fever, granuloma annulare, and cutis marmorata cause erythema in children.

Geri points

✦ Elderly patients commonly have well-demarcated purple macules or patches, usually on the back of the hands and on the forearms, that result from blood leaking through fragile capillaries.

Teaching points

✦ Signs and symptoms of flare-ups of causative disease
✦ Avoidance of sun exposure and use of sunblock

Key facts about exophthalmos

✦ Also known as *proptosis*
✦ Abnormal protrusion of one or both eyeballs
✦ May be sudden or gradual, mild or dramatic

Key history points

✦ Onset
✦ Associated pain
✦ Recent sinus infection or vision problems

Critical assessment steps

✦ Take vital signs, noting fever.
✦ Evaluate severity of exophthalmos with exophthalmometer.
✦ If eyes bulge severely, look for cloudiness on the cornea, which may indicate ulcer formation.
✦ Describe any eye discharge and observe for ptosis.
✦ Check visual acuity, with and without correction.
✦ Palpate the thyroid for enlargement or goiter.

Medical causes

Foreign body in eye
✦ Exophthalmos may accompany other indicators of ocular trauma, such as eye pain, redness, and tearing.

Hemangioma
✦ Exophthalmos is progressive and may be mild or severe, unilateral or bilateral.

PATIENT COUNSELING

Teach patients with a chronic disease such as SLE or psoriasis about the character of their typical rashes so they can be alert to any flare-ups of their disease. Also, advise such patients to avoid sun exposure and to use sunblock when appropriate.

EXOPHTHALMOS

Exophthalmos — the abnormal protrusion of one or both eyeballs — may result from hemorrhage, edema, or inflammation behind the eye; extraocular muscle relaxation; or space-occupying intraorbital lesions and metastatic tumors. Also known as *proptosis,* this sign may occur suddenly or gradually, causing mild to dramatic protrusion. Occasionally, the affected eye also pulsates. The most common cause of exophthalmos in adults is dysthyroid eye disease.

Exophthalmos is usually easily observed. However, lid retraction may mimic exophthalmos even when protrusion is absent. Similarly, ptosis in one eye may make the other eye appear exophthalmic by comparison. An exophthalmometer can differentiate these signs by measuring ocular protrusion.

HISTORY

Begin by asking when the patient first noticed exophthalmos. Is it associated with pain in or around the eye? If so, ask him how severe the pain is and how long he has had it. Then ask about recent sinus infection or vision problems.

PHYSICAL ASSESSMENT

Begin the assessment by taking the patient's vital signs, noting fever, which may accompany eye infection. Next, evaluate the severity of exophthalmos with an exophthalmometer. (See *Detecting unilateral exophthalmos.*) If the eyes bulge severely, look for cloudiness on the cornea, which may indicate ulcer formation. Describe any eye discharge and observe for ptosis. Then check visual acuity, with and without correction, and evaluate extraocular movements. Palpate the patient's thyroid for enlargement or goiter.

MEDICAL CAUSES

Foreign body in the eye
When a foreign body enters the eye, exophthalmos may accompany other signs and symptoms of ocular trauma, such as eye pain, redness, and tearing. Loss of vision or blurred vision may occur in the affected eye.

Hemangioma
Most common in young adults, hemangioma is an orbital tumor that produces progressive exophthalmos, which may be mild or severe, unilateral or bilateral. Other signs and symptoms include ptosis, limited extraocular movements, and blurred vision.

Lacrimal gland tumor
In patients with a lacrimal gland tumor, exophthalmos usually develops slowly in one eye, causing its downward displacement toward the nose. The patient may also have ptosis, eye deviation, and pain.

Detecting unilateral exophthalmos

If one of the patient's eyes seems more prominent than the other, examine both eyes from above the patient's head. Look down across his face, gently draw his lids up, and compare the relationship of the corneas to the lower lids. Abnormal protrusion of one eye suggests unilateral exophthalmos.

Don't perform this test if you suspect eye trauma.

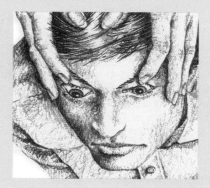

Optic nerve meningioma

An optic nerve meningioma usually produces unilateral exophthalmos and a swollen temple. Impaired visual acuity, visual field deficits, and headache may occur.

Orbital cellulitis

Commonly the result of sinusitis, orbital cellulitis is an ocular emergency that causes sudden onset of unilateral exophthalmos, which may be mild or severe. It may also produce fever, eye pain, headache, malaise, conjunctival injection, tearing, eyelid edema and erythema, purulent discharge, and impaired extraocular movements.

Orbital choristoma

A common sign of orbital choristoma (a benign tumor), progressive exophthalmos may be associated with diplopia and blurred vision. A mass may be visible in the orbital area.

Orbital emphysema

With orbital emphysema, air leaking from the sinus into the orbit usually causes unilateral exophthalmos. Palpation of the globe elicits crepitation. The patient may report orbital pressure.

Parasite infestation

Usually, parasite infestation causes painless, progressive exophthalmos in one eye that may spread to the other eye. Associated findings include limited extraocular movement, diplopia, eye pain, and impaired visual acuity.

Scleritis (posterior)

Gradual onset of mild to severe unilateral exophthalmos is common with scleritis. Other signs and symptoms include severe eye pain, diplopia, papilledema, limited extraocular movement, and impaired visual acuity.

Thyrotoxicosis

Although a classic sign of thyrotoxicosis, exophthalmos is absent in many patients. It's usually bilateral, progressive, and severe. Associated ocular features include pto-

Medical causes
(continued)

Lacrimal gland tumor
✦ Exophthalmos usually develops slowly in one eye, causing its downward displacement toward the nose.

Optic nerve meningioma
✦ Unilateral exophthalmos and a swollen temple are common.

Orbital cellulitis
✦ Onset of unilateral exophthalmos, which may be mild or severe, is sudden.

Orbital choristoma
✦ Progressive exophthalmos is common and may be associated with diplopia and blurred vision.

Orbital emphysema
✦ Air leaking from the sinus into the orbit usually causes unilateral exophthalmos.

Parasite infestation
✦ Painless, progressive exophthalmos develops in one eye and may spread to the other eye.

Scleritis (posterior)
✦ Onset of mild to severe unilateral exophthalmos is gradual.

Thyrotoxicosis
✦ Exophthalmos is usually bilateral, progressive, and severe.

Special considerations

+ Provide privacy and emotional support.
+ Protect the eye from trauma.
+ Don't place a gauze eye pad or other objects over affected eye.
+ If slit-lamp examination is indicated, explain procedure to patient.
+ If necessary, refer patient to ophthalmologist for complete examination.

Peds points

+ Rhabdomyosarcoma produces rapid onset of exophthalmos.
+ In Hand-Schüller-Christian syndrome, exophthalmos typically accompanies signs of diabetes insipidus and bone destruction.

Teaching points

+ Ways to protect eye from trauma, wind, and dust
+ Application of lubricants

Key facts about eye discharge

+ Excretion of any substance other than tears
+ Usually associated with conjunctivitis
+ Characteristics of discharge vary

Key history points

+ Onset and description
+ Location and description of pain
+ Additional signs and symptoms, including burning, tearing, sensitivity to light, and the sensation of something foreign in the eyes

sis, increased tearing, lid lag and edema, photophobia, conjunctival injection, diplopia, and decreased visual acuity. Other findings include an enlarged thyroid, nervousness, heat intolerance, weight loss despite increased appetite, sweating, diarrhea, tremors, palpitations, and tachycardia.

SPECIAL CONSIDERATIONS

Exophthalmos usually makes the patient self-conscious, so provide privacy and emotional support. Protect the affected eye from trauma, especially drying of the cornea. However, *never* place a gauze eye pad or any other object over the affected eye; removal could damage the corneal epithelium. If a slit-lamp examination is indicated, explain the procedure to the patient. If necessary, refer him to an ophthalmologist for a complete examination. The cause of exophthalmos determines the therapy. Prepare the patient for blood tests, such as a thyroid panel and a white blood cell count.

PEDIATRIC POINTERS

Rhabdomyosarcoma usually affects children between ages 4 and 12 and produces rapid onset of exophthalmos. In Hand-Schüller-Christian syndrome, exophthalmos typically accompanies signs of diabetes insipidus and bone destruction.

PATIENT COUNSELING

Teach the patient to protect his eyes from trauma and to avoid exposure to wind and dust. Demonstrate how to apply lubricants to prevent corneal drying. Encourage the patient to verbalize his feelings about changes in body image.

EYE DISCHARGE

Usually associated with conjunctivitis, an eye discharge is the excretion of any substance other than tears. This common sign may occur in one or both eyes, producing scant to copious discharge. The discharge may be purulent, frothy, mucoid, cheesy, serous, or clear, or a stringy white discharge. Sometimes, the discharge can be expressed by applying pressure to the tear sac, punctum, meibomian glands, or canaliculus.

An eye discharge commonly results from inflammatory and infectious eye disorders but may also occur in certain systemic disorders. (See *Sources of eye discharge.*) Because this sign may accompany a disorder that threatens vision, it must be assessed and treated immediately.

HISTORY

Begin your evaluation by finding out when the discharge began. Does it occur at certain times of day or in connection with certain activities? If the patient complains of pain, ask him to show you its exact location and to describe its character. Is the pain dull, continuous, sharp, or stabbing? Do his eyes itch or burn? Do they tear excessively? Are they sensitive to light? Does he feel like something is in them?

PHYSICAL ASSESSMENT

After taking vital signs, carefully inspect the eye discharge. Note its amount, color, and consistency. Then test visual acuity, with and without correction. Examine external eye structures, beginning with the unaffected eye to prevent cross-contamination. Observe for eyelid edema, entropion, crusts, lesions, and trichiasis.

ASSESSMENT TIP

Sources of eye discharge

An eye discharge can come from the tear sac, punctum, meibomian glands, or canaliculi. If the patient reports a discharge that isn't immediately apparent, you can express a sample by pressing your fingertip lightly over these structures. Then characterize the discharge, and note its source.

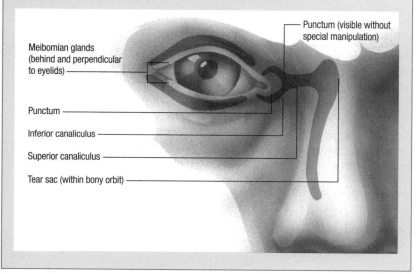

Punctum (visible without special manipulation)

Meibomian glands (behind and perpendicular to eyelids)

Punctum

Inferior canaliculus

Superior canaliculus

Tear sac (within bony orbit)

Next, ask the patient to blink as you watch for impaired lid movement. If the eyes seem to bulge, measure them with an exophthalmometer. Test the six cardinal fields of gaze. Examine for conjunctival injection and follicles and for corneal cloudiness or white lesions.

MEDICAL CAUSES

Conjunctivitis

Five types of conjunctivitis may cause an eye discharge with redness, hyperemia, foreign-body sensation, periocular edema, and tearing.

With *allergic conjunctivitis,* a bilateral ropey discharge is accompanied by itching and tearing.

Bacterial conjunctivitis causes a moderate purulent or mucopurulent discharge that may form sticky crusts on the eyelids during sleep. The discharge is commonly greenish white and usually occurs in one eye. The patient may also experience itching, burning, excessive tearing, and the sensation of a foreign body in the eye. Eye pain indicates corneal involvement.

Viral conjunctivitis is generally more common than the bacterial form. A serous, clear discharge and preauricular adenopathy are usually present. The history includes a runny nose, an upper respiratory tract infection, or recent contact with a person who had these signs. Onset is usually unilateral.

Fungal conjunctivitis produces a copious, thick, purulent discharge that makes the eyelids crusty and sticky. Also characteristic are eyelid edema, itching, burning, and tearing. Pain and photophobia occur only with corneal involvement.

Critical assessment steps

+ Take vital signs.
+ Inspect the eye discharge. Note amount, color, and consistency.
+ Test visual acuity, with and without correction.
+ Examine external eye structures, beginning with unaffected eye to prevent cross-contamination.
+ Observe for eyelid edema, entropion, crusts, lesions, and trichiasis.
+ Ask the patient to blink; watch for impaired lid movement.
+ If eyes seem to bulge, measure them with an exophthalmometer.
+ Test the six cardinal fields of gaze.
+ Examine for conjunctival injection and follicles and for corneal cloudiness or white lesions.

Medical causes
Conjunctivitis

+ *Allergic:* A bilateral ropey discharge is accompanied by itching and tearing.
+ *Bacterial:* Greenish white moderate purulent or mucopurulent discharge may form sticky crusts on the eyelids during sleep.
+ *Viral:* A serous, clear discharge and preauricular adenopathy are usually present.
+ *Fungal:* Copious, thick, purulent discharge makes the eyelids crusty and sticky.
+ *Inclusion:* Scant mucoid discharge in both eyes is accompanied by pseudoptosis and conjunctival follicles.

Medical causes
(continued)

Corneal ulcers
+ Copious, purulent unilateral eye discharge occurs along with crusty, sticky eyelids.

Dacryocystitis
+ Lacrimal sac infection may produce scant but continuous purulent discharge that's easily expressed from the tear sac.

Herpes zoster ophthalmicus
+ Moderate to copious serous eye discharge accompanies excessive tearing.

Keratoconjunctivitis sicca
+ Excessive, continuous mucoid discharge and insufficient tearing occur.

Meibomianitis
+ A continuous frothy eye discharge may be produced.

Orbital cellulitis
+ A unilateral purulent eye discharge may be present but exophthalmos is the obvious sign.

Psoriasis vulgaris
+ Substantial mucus discharge and redness occur in both eyes.

Special considerations
+ Apply warm soaks to soften crusts on the eyelids and lashes.
+ Gently wipe the eyes with a soft gauze pad.
+ Carefully dispose of used dressings, tissues, and cotton swabs.
+ Sterilize ophthalmic equipment after use.

Inclusion conjunctivitis causes scant mucoid discharge — especially in the morning — in both eyes, accompanied by pseudoptosis and conjunctival follicles.

Corneal ulcers
Both bacterial and fungal corneal ulcers produce a copious, purulent unilateral eye discharge. Related findings are crusty, sticky eyelids and, possibly, severe pain, photophobia, and impaired visual acuity.

Bacterial corneal ulcers are also characterized by an irregular gray-white area on the cornea, blurred vision, unilateral pupil constriction, and conjunctival injection.

Fungal corneal ulcers are also characterized by conjunctival injection and eyelid edema and erythema. A painless, dense, whitish gray central ulcer develops slowly and may be surrounded by progressively clearer rings.

Dacryocystitis
With dacryocystitis, lacrimal sac infection may produce scant but continuous purulent discharge that's easily expressed from the tear sac. Additional signs and symptoms include excessive tearing, pain, and tenderness near the tear sac. Eyelid inflammation and edema are most noticeable around the lacrimal punctum.

Herpes zoster ophthalmicus
Herpes zoster ophthalmicus yields a moderate to copious serous eye discharge accompanied by excessive tearing. Examination reveals eyelid edema and erythema, conjunctival injection, and a white, cloudy cornea. The patient also complains of eye pain and severe unilateral facial pain that occurs several days before vesicles erupt.

Keratoconjunctivitis sicca
Better known as *dry eye syndrome,* keratoconjunctivitis sicca typically causes excessive, continuous mucoid discharge and insufficient tearing. Accompanying signs and symptoms include eye pain, itching, burning, a foreign-body sensation, and dramatic conjunctival injection. The patient may also have difficulty closing his eyes.

Meibomianitis
Meibomianitis may produce a continuous frothy eye discharge. Applying pressure on the meibomian glands yields a soft, foul-smelling, cheesy yellow discharge. The eyes also appear chronically red, with inflamed lid margins.

Orbital cellulitis
Although exophthalmos is the most obvious sign of orbital cellulitis, a unilateral purulent eye discharge may also be present. Related findings include eyelid edema, conjunctival injection, headache, orbital pain, impaired visual acuity, limited extraocular movement, and fever.

Psoriasis vulgaris
Usually, psoriasis vulgaris causes a substantial mucus discharge in both eyes, accompanied by redness. The characteristic lesions it produces on the eyelids may extend into the conjunctiva, causing irritation, excessive tearing, and a foreign-body sensation.

SPECIAL CONSIDERATIONS
Apply warm soaks to soften crusts on the eyelids and lashes. Then gently wipe the eyes with a soft gauze pad. Carefully dispose of all used dressings, tissues, and cotton swabs to prevent the spread of infection. Teach the patient how to avoid contaminating the unaffected eye. Also, be sure to sterilize ophthalmic equipment after

use. Explain any ordered diagnostic tests, including culture and sensitivity studies to identify infectious organisms.

PEDIATRIC POINTERS

In infants, prophylactic eye medication (silver nitrate) commonly causes eye irritation and discharge. However, in children, discharges usually result from eye trauma, eye infection, or upper respiratory tract infection.

PATIENT COUNSELING

Inform patients that bacterial and viral conjunctivitis are contagious. Tell those with bacterial conjunctivitis to avoid contact with other people until 24 hours after receiving antibiotic treatment; not to share towels, pillows, or cosmetic eye products; and to stop wearing contact lenses until conjunctivitis resolves. Tell patients with allergic conjunctivitis that this isn't a contagious type of inflammation.

EYE PAIN

Eye pain, or ophthalmalgia, may be described as a burning, throbbing, aching, or stabbing sensation in or around the eye. It may also be characterized as a foreign-body sensation. This sign varies from mild to severe; its duration and exact location provide clues to the causative disorder.

Eye pain usually results from corneal abrasion, but it may also be due to glaucoma or other eye disorders, trauma, and neurologic or systemic disorders. Any of these may stimulate nerve endings in the cornea or external eye, producing pain.

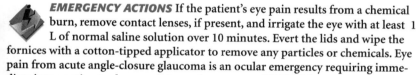 **EMERGENCY ACTIONS** If the patient's eye pain results from a chemical burn, remove contact lenses, if present, and irrigate the eye with at least 1 L of normal saline solution over 10 minutes. Evert the lids and wipe the fornices with a cotton-tipped applicator to remove any particles or chemicals. Eye pain from acute angle-closure glaucoma is an ocular emergency requiring immediate intervention to decrease intraocular pressure (IOP). If drug treatment doesn't reduce IOP, the patient needs laser iridotomy or surgical peripheral iridectomy to save vision.

HISTORY

If the patient's eye pain doesn't result from a chemical burn, take a complete history. Have the patient describe the pain fully. Is it an ache or a sharp pain? How long does it last? Is it accompanied by burning, itching, or discharge? Find out when it began. Is it worse in the morning or late in the evening? Ask about recent trauma or surgery, especially if the patient complains of sudden, severe pain. Does he have headaches? If so, find out how often and at what time of day they occur.

PHYSICAL ASSESSMENT

During the physical examination, don't manipulate the eye if you suspect trauma. Carefully assess the lids and conjunctivae for redness, inflammation, and swelling. Then examine the eyes for ptosis or exophthalmos. Finally, test visual acuity with and without correction, and assess extraocular movements. Characterize any discharge. (See *Examining the external eye*, page 272.)

Peds points
+ In children, eye discharge usually results from eye trauma, eye infection, or upper respiratory tract infection.

Teaching points
+ Measures to prevent spread of bacterial and viral conjunctivitis

Key facts about eye pain
+ Burning, throbbing, aching, stabbing, or foreign body sensation in eye

In an emergency
If patient has a chemical burn:
+ Remove contact lenses, then irrigate eye with at least 1 L of normal saline solution.
+ Evert lids and wipe fornices.
If patient has acute angle-closure glaucoma:
+ Intervene to decrease IOP.
+ If drug treatment doesn't reduce IOP, the patient needs iridotomy to save vision.

Key history points
+ Onset, description and duration of pain and associated symptoms
+ Recent trauma or surgery

Critical assessment steps
+ Don't manipulate the eye if you suspect trauma.
+ Carefully assess the lids and conjunctivae for redness, inflammation, and swelling.
+ Test visual acuity.
+ Characterize any discharge.

Medical causes

Blepharitis
+ Burning pain in both eyelids, itching, sticky discharge, and conjunctival injection occur.

Burns
+ With chemical burns, sudden and severe eye pain may occur.
+ With ultraviolet radiation burns, moderate to severe pain occurs about 12 hours after exposure.

Chalazion
+ Pain is localized.

Conjunctivitis
+ *Allergic conjunctivitis* causes mild, burning, bilateral pain.
+ *Bacterial conjunctivitis* causes pain when it affects the cornea.
+ *Fungal conjunctivitis* may cause pain and photophobia if the cornea is affected.
+ *Viral conjunctivitis* produces itching, red eyes, foreign-body sensation, visible conjunctival follicles, and eyelid edema.

ASSESSMENT TIP

Examining the external eye

For patients with eye pain or other ocular symptoms, examination of the external eye forms an important part of the ocular assessment. Here's how to examine the external eye.

First, inspect the eyelids for ptosis and incomplete closure. Also, observe the lids for edema, erythema, cyanosis, hematoma, and masses. Evaluate skin lesions, growths, swelling, and tenderness by gross palpation. Are the lids everted or inverted? Do the eyelashes turn inward? Have some of them been lost? Do the lashes adhere to one another or contain a discharge? Next, examine the lid margins, noting especially any debris, scaling, lesions, or unusual secretions. Also, watch for eyelid spasms.

Now gently retract the eyelid with your thumb and forefinger, and assess the conjunctiva for redness, cloudiness, follicles, and blisters or other lesions. Check for chemosis by pressing the lower lid against the eyeball and noting any bulging above this compression point. Observe the sclera, noting any change from its normal white color.

Next, shine a light across the cornea to detect scars, abrasions, or ulcers. Note any color changes, dots, or opaque or cloudy areas. Also, assess the anterior eye chamber, which should be clean, deep, shadow-free, and filled with clear aqueous humor.

Inspect the color, shape, texture, and pattern of the iris. Then assess the pupils' size, shape, and equality. Finally, evaluate their response to light. Are they sluggish, fixed, or unresponsive? Does pupil dilation or constriction occur only on one side?

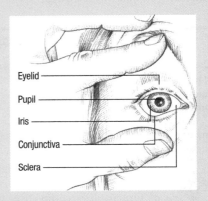

MEDICAL CAUSES

Blepharitis
With blepharitis, burning pain in both eyelids is accompanied by itching, sticky discharge, and conjunctival injection. Related findings include foreign-body sensation, lid ulcerations, and loss of eyelashes.

Burns
With chemical burns, sudden and severe eye pain may occur with erythema and blistering of the face and lids, photophobia, miosis, conjunctival injection, blurring, and inability to keep the eyelids open. With ultraviolet radiation burns, moderate to severe pain occurs about 12 hours after exposure along with photophobia and vision changes.

Chalazion
A chalazion causes localized pain, tenderness, redness, and swelling on the upper or lower eyelid. Eversion of the lid reveals conjunctival injection and a small red lump.

Conjunctivitis
Allergic conjunctivitis causes mild, burning, bilateral pain accompanied by itching, conjunctival injection, and a characteristic ropey discharge.

Bacterial conjunctivitis causes pain only when it affects the cornea. Otherwise, it produces burning and a foreign-body sensation. A purulent discharge and conjunctival injection are also typical.

If the cornea is affected, fungal conjunctivitis may cause pain and photophobia. Even without corneal involvement, it produces itching, burning eyes; a thick, purulent discharge; and conjunctival injection.

Viral conjunctivitis produces itching, red eyes, foreign-body sensation, visible conjunctival follicles, and eyelid edema.

Corneal abrasions

With corneal abrasions, eye pain is characterized by a foreign-body sensation. Excessive tearing, photophobia, and conjunctival injection are also common. The patient commonly reports feeling that "something is in" the eye.

Corneal erosion (recurrent)

With recurrent corneal erosion, severe pain occurs on waking and continues throughout the day. Conjunctival injection and photophobia also occur.

Corneal ulcers

Both bacterial and fungal corneal ulcers cause severe eye pain. They may also cause a purulent eye discharge, sticky eyelids, photophobia, and impaired visual acuity. In addition, bacterial corneal ulcers produce a grayish white, irregularly shaped ulcer on the cornea, unilateral pupil constriction, and conjunctival injection. Fungal corneal ulcers produce conjunctival injection, eyelid edema and erythema, and a dense, cloudy, central ulcer surrounded by progressively clearer rings.

Dacryocystitis

Pain and tenderness near the tear sac characterize acute dacryocystitis. Additional signs include excessive tearing, a purulent discharge, eyelid erythema, and swelling in the lacrimal punctum area.

Foreign body in the cornea or conjunctiva

Sudden severe pain is common but vision usually remains intact. Other findings include excessive tearing, photophobia, miosis, a foreign-body sensation, a dark speck on the cornea, and dramatic conjunctival injection.

Glaucoma

Open-angle glaucoma may cause mild aching in the eyes as well as loss of peripheral vision, halo vision, and reduced visual acuity that isn't corrected by glasses. *Angle-closure* glaucoma is characterized by blurred vision and sudden, excruciating pain in and around the eye. The pain may be so severe that it causes nausea, vomiting, and abdominal pain. Other findings are halo vision, rapidly decreasing visual acuity, and a fixed, nonreactive, moderately dilated pupil.

Herpes zoster ophthalmicus

With herpes zoster ophthalmicus, eye pain occurs with severe unilateral facial pain, usually days before vesicles erupt. Other signs include red, swollen eyelids; excessive tearing; a serous eye discharge; conjunctival injection; and a white, cloudy cornea.

Hordeolum

A hordeolum (stye) usually produces localized eye pain, burning, and discomfort that increases as the stye grows. Eyelid erythema and edema are also common.

Medical causes
(continued)

Corneal abrasions
✦ Eye pain is characterized by a foreign-body sensation.

Corneal erosion (recurrent)
✦ Severe pain occurs on waking and continues during the day.

Corneal ulcers
✦ Severe eye pain may occur with purulent eye discharge, sticky eyelids, photophobia, and impaired visual acuity.

Dacryocystitis
✦ Pain and tenderness occur near the tear sac.

Foreign body in cornea or conjunctiva
✦ Sudden severe pain is common but vision usually remains intact.

Glaucoma
✦ *Open-angle glaucoma* may cause mild aching in the eyes.
✦ *Angle-closure glaucoma* is characterized by blurred vision and sudden, excruciating pain in and around the eye.

Herpes zoster ophthalmicus
✦ Eye pain and unilateral facial pain occur days before vesicles erupt.

Hordeolum
✦ Localized eye pain, burning, and discomfort increases as the stye grows.

Medical causes
(continued)

Hyphema
+ Sudden pain in and around the eye occurs after eye injury or surgery.

Keratoconjunctivitis sicca
+ Chronic burning pain occurs in both eyes.

Lacrimal gland tumor
+ Tumor produces unilateral eye pain, impaired visual acuity, and some degree of exophthalmos.

Ocular laceration and intraocular foreign bodies
+ Penetrating eye injuries usually cause mild to severe eye pain and impaired visual acuity.

Optic cellulitis
+ Dull, aching pain occurs in the affected eye.

Optic neuritis
+ Pain in and around the eye occurs with eye movement.

Orbital floor fracture
+ Eye pain and dramatic eyelid edema occur.

Orbital pseudotumor
+ Deep, boring eye pain and diplopia occur in 50% of patients.

Uveitis
+ With anterior uveitis, onset of severe pain is sudden.
+ With posterior uveitis, onset of pain is insidious.
+ With lens-induced uveitis, moderate eye pain occurs with conjunctival injection, pupil constriction, and impaired visual acuity.

Hyphema
Occurring after eye injury or surgery, hyphema accompanies sudden pain in and around the eye. Orbital and lid edema, conjunctival injection, and visual impairment may occur. The patient may report nausea.

Keratoconjunctivitis sicca
Keratoconjunctivitis sicca, also known as *dry eye syndrome*, causes chronic burning pain in both eyes, itching, a foreign-body sensation, photophobia, dramatic conjunctival injection, and difficulty moving the eyelids. Excessive mucoid discharge and inadequate tearing are typical.

Lacrimal gland tumor
Lacrimal gland tumor is a neoplastic lesion that usually produces unilateral eye pain, impaired visual acuity, and some degree of exophthalmos. The patient may also have ptosis and eye deviation.

Ocular laceration and intraocular foreign bodies
Penetrating eye injuries usually cause mild to severe unilateral eye pain and impaired visual acuity. Eyelid edema, conjunctival injection, and an abnormal pupillary response may also occur.

Optic cellulitis
Optic cellulitis causes dull, aching pain in the affected eye, some degree of exophthalmos, eyelid edema and erythema, purulent discharge, impaired extraocular movement and, occasionally, decreased visual acuity and fever.

Optic neuritis
With optic neuritis, pain in and around the eye occurs with eye movement. Severe vision loss and tunnel vision develop but improve in 2 to 3 weeks. Pupils respond sluggishly to direct light but normally to consensual light.

Orbital floor fracture
Sometimes called a *blowout fracture*, orbital floor fracture causes eye pain, dramatic eyelid edema and, possibly, enophthalmos and diplopia. The patient may report recent eye trauma and reduced vision. Ecchymosis and ptosis may be visible.

Orbital pseudotumor
An orbital pseudotumor causes deep, boring eye pain and diplopia in about 50% of patients. However, prominent exophthalmos and lateral ocular deviation are more characteristic. Eyelid edema and restricted extraocular movement may also occur.

Uveitis
Anterior uveitis causes sudden onset of severe pain, dramatic conjunctival injection, photophobia, and a small, nonreactive pupil. *Posterior* uveitis causes insidious onset of similar features, plus gradual blurring of vision and distorted pupil shape. *Lens-induced uveitis* causes moderate eye pain, conjunctival injection, pupil constriction, and severely impaired visual acuity (the patient usually can perceive only light).

OTHER CAUSES

Treatments
Contact lenses may cause eye pain and a foreign-body sensation. Ocular surgery may also produce eye pain, ranging from a mild ache to a severe pounding or stabbing sensation.

SPECIAL CONSIDERATIONS

To help ease eye pain, have the patient lie down in a darkened, quiet environment and close his eyes. Prepare him for diagnostic studies, including tonometry and orbital X-rays.

PEDIATRIC POINTERS

Trauma and infection are the most common causes of eye pain in children. Be alert for nonverbal clues to pain, such as tightly shutting or frequently rubbing the eyes.

GERIATRIC POINTERS

Glaucoma, which can cause eye pain, is a disease most commonly found in older patients; it becomes clinically significant after age 40. Usually occurring bilaterally, glaucoma can lead to slowly progressive vision loss, especially in peripheral visual fields.

PATIENT COUNSELING

Tell the patient that seeking medical help for eye pain is important. Stress the importance of meticulous compliance with drug therapy to prevent an increase in IOP. Also stress the importance of protecting the eyes when involved in activities that could result in eye injuries.

Other causes
+ Contact lenses
+ Ocular surgery

Special considerations
+ Have the patient lie down in a darkened, quiet environment and close his eyes.

Peds points
+ Trauma and infection are the most common causes of eye pain in children.

Geri points
+ Glaucoma, which can cause eye pain, is a disease most commonly found in older patients.

Teaching points
+ Compliance with drug therapy
+ Eye protection

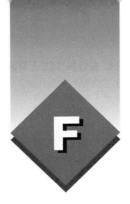

FACIAL PAIN

Facial pain may result from various neurologic, vascular, or infectious disorders. The most common cause of facial pain is trigeminal neuralgia (tic douloureux). Typically paroxysmal and intense, facial pain may occur along the pathway of a specific facial nerve or nerve branch, usually cranial nerve V (trigeminal nerve) or cranial nerve VII (facial nerve). Pain can also be referred to the face in disorders of the ear, nose, paranasal sinuses, teeth, neck, and jaw.

Atypical facial pain is a constant, burning pain with limited distribution at onset; it typically spreads to the rest of the face and may involve the neck or back of the head as well. This type of facial pain is common in middle-age women, especially those who are clinically depressed.

HISTORY

Begin by characterizing the patient's facial pain. Is it stabbing, throbbing, or dull? When did it begin? How long has it lasted? What relieves or worsens it? Ask the patient to point to the painful area. If facial pain is recurrent, have the patient describe a typical episode. Review the patient's medical and dental history, noting especially previous head trauma, dental disease, and infection.

PHYSICAL ASSESSMENT

Carefully examine the face and head. Inspect the ear for vesicles and changes in the tympanic membrane to rule out referred ear pain. Inspect the nose for deformity or asymmetry. Evaluate the condition of the mucous membranes and septum as well as the size and shape of the turbinates. Characterize any secretions. Palpate the frontal, ethmoid, and maxillary sinuses for tenderness and swelling. (See *Associated Disorder: Sinusitis*.)

Evaluate oral hygiene by inspecting the teeth for caries, percussing any diseased teeth for pain, and asking the patient about sensitivity to hot, cold, or sweet liquids or foods. Have him open and close his mouth as you palpate the temporomandibular joint for tenderness, spasm, locking, and crepitus.

Examine the function of cranial nerves V and VII. To evaluate cranial nerve V, instruct the patient to clench his teeth. Then palpate the temporal and masseter muscles and evaluate muscle contraction. Test pain and sensation on his forehead, cheeks, and jaw. Next, test the corneal reflex by lightly touching the cornea with a piece of cotton.

To evaluate cranial nerve VII, inspect the face for symmetry and then have the patient perform facial movements that demonstrate facial muscle strength — have

Key facts about facial pain

+ May result from various neurologic, vascular, or infectious disorders
+ Is typically paroxysmal and intense

Key history points

+ Onset, description, location, and duration of facial pain
+ Alleviating or aggravating factors
+ Medical and dental history

Critical assessment steps

+ Inspect the ear for vesicles and changes in the tympanic membrane.
+ Inspect the nose for deformity or asymmetry. Characterize any secretions.
+ Palpate the sinuses for tenderness and swelling.
+ Ask about sensitivity to hot, cold, or sweet liquids or foods.
+ Have the patient open and close his mouth as you palpate the temporomandibular joint.

ASSOCIATED DISORDER

Sinusitis

Sinusitis — inflammation of the paranasal sinuses — may be acute, subacute, chronic, allergic, or hyperplastic. Acute sinusitis usually results from the common cold and lingers in subacute form in only about 10% of patients. Chronic sinusitis follows persistent bacterial infection; allergic sinusitis accompanies allergic rhinitis; hyperplastic sinusitis is a combination of purulent acute sinusitis and allergic sinusitis or rhinitis. The prognosis is good for all types.

CAUSES
Sinusitis usually results from viral or bacterial infection. The bacteria responsible for acute sinusitis are usually pneumococci, other streptococci, *Haemophilus influenzae,* and *Moraxella catarrhalis.* Staphylococci and gram-negative bacteria are more likely to cause sinusitis in chronic cases or in intensive care patients.

Predisposing factors include any condition that interferes with drainage and ventilation of the sinuses, such as:
+ chronic nasal edema
+ deviated septum
+ viscous mucus
+ nasal polyps
+ allergic rhinitis
+ nasal intubation
+ debilitation due to chemotherapy, malnutrition, diabetes, blood dyscrasias, chronic use of steroids, or immunodeficiency.

Bacterial invasion commonly occurs as a result of the conditions listed above or after viral infection. It may also result from swimming in contaminated water.

DIAGNOSIS
These measures are useful in diagnosing sinusitis:
+ Nasal examination reveals inflammation and pus.
+ Sinus X-rays reveal cloudiness in the affected sinus, air and fluid, and any thickening of the mucosal lining.
+ Ultrasound and computed tomography (CT) scan aid in diagnosing suspected complications. CT scanning is more sensitive than routine X-rays in detecting sinusitis.
+ Transillumination is a simple diagnostic tool that involves shining a light into the patient's mouth with his lips closed around it. Infected sinuses look dark whereas normal sinuses transilluminate.

MEDICAL MANAGEMENT
Treatment may include:
+ decongestants (typically local agents are tried first, followed by systemic decongestants, if necessary) to reduce swelling, congestion, and inflammation of the sinus
+ saline spray, lavage, or steam inhalation to relieve symptoms and promote drainage
+ antibiotics, if indicated, to combat purulent or persistent infection
+ local heat, to relieve pain and congestion
+ if the patient has allergic sinusitis, antihistamines and skin testing to identify allergens and desensitization by immunotherapy
+ epinephrine and corticosteroids, for severe allergic symptoms
+ sinus irrigation, for persistent subacute infection
+ fluids, to promote drainage
+ endoscopic surgery to clean and drain sinuses, repair a deviated septum, or remove nasal polyps, as indicated.

Key facts about sinusitis
+ Inflammation of the paranasal sinuses
+ May be acute, subacute, chronic, allergic, or hyperplastic

Causes
+ Viral or bacterial infection
+ Predisposing factors, such as chronic nasal edema, deviated septum, viscous mucus, nasal polyps, allergic rhinitis, nasal intubation, and debilitation due to various causes

Management
+ Decongestants
+ Saline spray, lavage, or steam inhalation
+ Antibiotics if indicated
+ Local heat
+ Antihistamines and skin testing
+ Epinephrine and corticosteroids
+ Sinus irrigation
+ Fluids
+ Endoscopic surgery as indicated

him raise his eyebrows, frown, show his teeth, close his eyes tightly, and wrinkle his nose. (See *Major nerve pathways of the face,* page 278.)

MEDICAL CAUSES

Angina pectoris
Occasionally, jaw pain may indicate angina pectoris. The pain may be described as burning, squeezing, or tightness and may also radiate to the left arm, neck, and shoulder blade.

Medical causes
Angina pectoris
+ Jaw pain may be described as burning, squeezing, or tightness.

Medical causes
(continued)

Dental caries
+ Caries in the mandibular molars can produce ear, preauricular, and temporal pain.
+ Caries in the maxillary teeth can produce maxillary, orbital, retro-orbital and parietal pain.

Herpes zoster oticus
+ Severe pain localizes around the ear.

Herpetic neuralgia
+ Severe pain localizes around the ear, followed by the appearance of vesicles in the ear.

Multiple sclerosis
+ Facial pain may resemble that of trigeminal neuralgia.
+ Pain is accompanied by jaw and facial weakness.

Ocular glaucoma
+ Pain appears late and is usually located in the periorbital region.

Postherpetic neuralgia
+ Burning, itching, prickly pain that worsens with contact or movement persists along any of the three trigeminal nerve divisions.

Major nerve pathways of the face

Cranial nerve V has three branches. The *ophthalmic branch* supplies sensation to the anterior scalp, forehead, upper nose, and cornea. The *maxillary branch* supplies sensation to the midportion of the face, lower nose, upper lip, and mucous membrane of the anterior palate. The *mandibular branch* supplies sensation to the lower face, lower jaw, mucous membrane of the cheek, and base of the tongue.

Cranial nerve VII innervates the facial muscles. Its motor branch controls the muscles of the forehead, eye orbit, and mouth.

CRANIAL NERVE VII

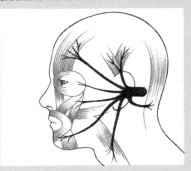

CRANIAL NERVE V

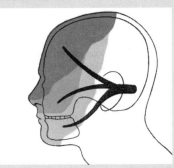

Dental caries
Caries in the mandibular molars can produce ear, preauricular, and temporal pain; caries in the maxillary teeth can produce maxillary, orbital, retro-orbital and parietal pain.

Herpes zoster oticus
With herpes zoster oticus, severe pain localizes around the ear, followed by the appearance of vesicles in the ear and occasionally on the oral mucosa, tonsils, and posterior tongue. Eye pain may occur with corneal and scleral damage and impaired vision.

Herpetic neuralgia
With herpetic neuralgia, severe pain localizes around the ear, followed by the appearance of vesicles in the ear and occasionally on the oral mucosa, tonsils, and posterior tongue. Eye pain may occur with corneal and scleral damage and impaired vision.

Multiple sclerosis
Facial pain may resemble that of trigeminal neuralgia and is accompanied by jaw and facial weakness. Other common findings of multiple sclerosis include visual blurring, diplopia, and nystagmus; sensory impairment such as paresthesia; generalized muscle weakness and gait abnormalities; urinary disturbances; and emotional lability.

Ocular glaucoma

The pain of ocular glaucoma is usually located in the periorbital region. Symptoms appear late in the disease and may also include loss of peripheral vision and reduced visual acuity (especially at night) that isn't correctable with glasses. The patient may also see halos around lights.

Postherpetic neuralgia

With postherpetic neuralgia, burning, itching, prickly pain persists along any of the three trigeminal nerve divisions and worsens with contact or movement. Mild hypoesthesia or paresthesia and vesicles affect the area before the onset of pain.

Sinusitis (acute)

Acute maxillary sinusitis produces unilateral or bilateral pressure, fullness, or burning pain over the cheekbone and upper teeth and around the eyes. Bending over increases the pain. Other findings include nasal congestion and purulent discharge; red, swollen nasal mucosa; tenderness and swelling over the cheekbone; fever; and malaise.

Acute frontal sinusitis commonly produces severe pain above or around the eyes, which worsens when the patient is in a supine position. It also causes nasal obstruction, inflamed nasal mucosa, fever, and tenderness and swelling above the eyes.

Acute ethmoid sinusitis produces pain at or around the inner corner of the eye. Temporal headaches can also occur. Other findings include nasal congestion, purulent rhinorrhea, fever, and tenderness at the medial edge of the eye.

With acute sphenoid sinusitis, a deep-seated pain persists behind the eyes or nose or on the top of the head. Pain increases on bending forward. Fever is common.

Sinusitis (chronic)

Chronic maxillary sinusitis produces a feeling of pressure below the eyes or a chronic toothache. Discomfort typically worsens through the day. Nasal congestion and tenderness over the cheekbone are usually mild.

Chronic ethmoid sinusitis is characterized by nasal congestion, an intermittent and purulent nasal discharge, and low-grade discomfort at the medial corners of the eyes. Also common are recurrent sore throat, halitosis, ear fullness, and involvement of other sinuses.

Chronic frontal sinusitis produces a persistent low-grade pain above the eyes. With chronic sphenoid sinusitis, a low-grade, diffuse headache or retro-orbital discomfort is common.

Sphenopalatine neuralgia

Also called *cluster headaches,* sphenopalatine neuralgia produces unilateral, deep, boring pain below the ear and may radiate to the eye, ear, cheek, nose, palate, maxillary teeth, temple, back of the head, neck, or shoulder. Attacks bring increased tearing and salivation, rhinorrhea, a sensation of fullness in the ear, tinnitus, vertigo, taste disturbances, pruritus, and shoulder stiffness or weakness.

Temporal arteritis

With temporal arteritis, unilateral pain occurs behind the eye or in the scalp, jaw, tongue, or neck. A typical episode consists of a severe throbbing or boring temporal headache with redness, swelling, and nodulation of the temporal artery.

Temporomandibular joint syndrome

Temporomandibular joint (TMJ) syndrome is characterized by intermittent pain, usually unilateral, that's described as a severe, dull ache or intense spasm that radi-

Medical causes
(continued)

Sinusitis (acute)
- Acute maxillary sinusitis produces unilateral or bilateral pressure, fullness, or burning pain over cheekbone and upper teeth and around eyes.
- Acute frontal sinusitis produces severe pain above or around the eyes, which worsens when patient is in supine position.
- Acute ethmoid sinusitis produces pain at or around the inner corner of the eye.
- Acute sphenoid sinusitis produces a persistent, deep-seated pain behind the eyes or nose or on the top of the head.

Sinusitis (chronic)
- Chronic maxillary sinusitis produces a feeling of pressure below the eyes or a toothache.
- Chronic ethmoid sinusitis is characterized by nasal congestion and discharge and discomfort at medial corners of eyes.
- Chronic frontal sinusitis produces a persistent low-grade pain above the eyes.

Sphenopalatine neuralgia
- Unilateral deep, boring pain occurs below ear and may radiate to eye, ear, cheek, nose, palate, maxillary teeth, temple, back of head, neck, or shoulder.

Temporal arteritis
- Unilateral pain occurs behind eye or in scalp, jaw, tongue, or neck.

TMJ syndrome
- Pain is intermittent, usually unilateral, and radiates to cheek, temple, lower jaw, or ear.

Medical causes
(continued)

Trigeminal neuralgia
- ✦ Paroxysms of intense pain shoot along the three branches of the trigeminal nerve.

Special considerations
- ✦ Give pain medications.
- ✦ Apply direct heat or administer a muscle relaxant
- ✦ Provide a humidifier, vaporizer, or decongestant.

Peds points
- ✦ Be alert for subtle signs of pain, such as facial rubbing, irritability, or poor eating habits.

Teaching points
- ✦ Triggers to avoid
- ✦ Signs and symptoms to report

Key facts about fatigue
- ✦ Feeling of excessive tiredness, lack of energy, or exhaustion accompanied by a strong desire to rest or sleep
- ✦ Reflects hypermetabolic and hypometabolic states in which nutrients needed for cellular energy and growth are lacking

Key history points
- ✦ Pattern, onset, and duration
- ✦ Associated symptoms
- ✦ Recent viral or bacterial illness or stress
- ✦ Family and personal history of chronic disorders
- ✦ Drug and alcohol history
- ✦ Carbon monoxide exposure

ates to the cheek, temple, lower jaw, ear, or mastoid area. Associated findings include trismus, malocclusion, and clicking, crepitus, and tenderness in the temporomandibular joint.

Trigeminal neuralgia

With trigeminal neuralgia, paroxysms of intense pain, lasting up to 15 minutes, shoot along any or all of the three branches of the trigeminal nerve. The pain can be triggered by touching the nose, cheek, or mouth; by being exposed to hot or cold weather; by consuming hot or cold foods or beverages; or even by smiling or talking. Between attacks, the pain may diminish to a dull ache or may disappear. This disorder is most common in middle and later life, affecting more women than men.

SPECIAL CONSIDERATIONS

Prepare the patient for diagnostic tests, such as sinus, skull, or dental X-rays; sinus transillumination; and intracranial or sinus computed tomography. Give pain medications, and apply direct heat or administer a muscle relaxant to ease muscle spasms. Provide a humidifier, vaporizer, or decongestant to relieve nasal or sinus congestion.

PEDIATRIC POINTERS

Facial pain may be difficult to assess in a young child if his language skills aren't sufficiently developed for him to describe the pain. Be alert for subtle signs of pain, such as facial rubbing, irritability, or poor eating habits.

PATIENT COUNSELING

If appropriate, instruct the patient with trigeminal neuralgia to avoid stressful situations, hot or cold foods, and sudden jarring movements, which can trigger painful attacks. Tell the patient with a history of coronary artery disease to report episodes of jaw pain.

FATIGUE

Fatigue is a feeling of excessive tiredness, lack of energy, or exhaustion accompanied by a strong desire to rest or sleep. This common symptom is distinct from weakness, which involves the muscles, but may occur with it.

Fatigue is a normal and important response to physical overexertion, prolonged emotional stress, and sleep deprivation. However, it can also be a nonspecific symptom of a psychological or physiologic disorder — especially viral or bacterial infection and endocrine, cardiovascular, or neurologic disease.

Fatigue reflects both hypermetabolic and hypometabolic states in which nutrients needed for cellular energy and growth are lacking because of overly rapid depletion, impaired replacement mechanisms, insufficient hormone production, or inadequate nutrient intake or metabolism.

HISTORY

Obtain a careful history to identify the patient's fatigue pattern. Fatigue that worsens with activity and improves with rest generally indicates a physical disorder; the opposite pattern indicates a psychological disorder. Fatigue lasting longer than 4 months, constant fatigue that's unrelieved by rest, and transient exhaustion that quickly gives way to bursts of energy are other findings associated with psychological disorders.

Ask about related symptoms and any recent viral or bacterial illness or stressful changes in lifestyle. Explore nutritional habits and any appetite or weight changes. Carefully review the patient's medical and psychiatric history for chronic disorders that commonly produce fatigue. Ask about a family history of such disorders.

Obtain a thorough drug history, noting use of any opioid or drug with fatigue as an adverse effect. Ask about alcohol and drug use patterns. Determine the patient's risk of carbon monoxide poisoning, and inquire as to whether the patient has a carbon monoxide detector.

PHYSICAL ASSESSMENT

Begin your physical assessment by observing the patient's general appearance for overt signs of depression or organic illness. Is he unkempt or expressionless? Does he appear tired or sickly, or have a slumped posture? If warranted, evaluate his mental status, noting especially mental clouding, attention deficits, agitation, or psychomotor retardation. Then, take your patient's vital signs and perform a complete physical examination.

MEDICAL CAUSES

Acquired immunodeficiency syndrome

In addition to fatigue, acquired immunodeficiency syndrome (AIDS) may cause fever, night sweats, weight loss, diarrhea, and a cough, followed by several concurrent opportunistic infections. The patient may also show signs of malnutrition.

Adrenocortical insufficiency

Mild fatigue, the hallmark of adrenocortical insufficiency, initially appears after exertion and stress but later becomes more severe and persistent. Weakness and weight loss typically accompany GI disturbances, such as nausea, vomiting, anorexia, abdominal pain, and chronic diarrhea; hyperpigmentation; orthostatic hypotension; and a weak, irregular pulse.

Anemia

Fatigue following mild activity is commonly the first symptom of anemia. Associated findings vary but generally include listlessness, irritability, inability to concentrate, pallor, tachycardia, and dyspnea.

 CULTURAL CUE *To detect anemia-related pallor in the dark-skinned patient, assess his oral mucosa.*

Anxiety

Chronic, unremitting anxiety invariably produces fatigue, commonly characterized as nervous exhaustion. Other persistent findings include apprehension, indecisiveness, restlessness, insomnia, trembling, and increased muscle tension.

Cancer

Unexplained fatigue is commonly the earliest sign of cancer. Related findings reflect the type, location, and stage of the tumor and typically include pain, nausea, vomiting, anorexia, weight loss, abnormal bleeding, and a palpable mass.

Medical causes
(continued)

Chronic fatigue syndrome
+ Fatigue is incapacitating.

COPD
+ Progressive fatigue and dyspnea are the earliest symptoms.

Cirrhosis
+ Severe fatigue occurs late.

Depression
+ Persistent fatigue unrelated to exertion typically accompanies chronic depression.

Diabetes mellitus
+ Fatigue that's insidious or abrupt is the most common symptom.

Heart failure
+ Persistent fatigue and lethargy are characteristic.

Hypercortisolism
+ Fatigue is related in part to accompanying sleep disturbances.

Hypopituitarism
+ Fatigue, lethargy, and weakness usually develop slowly.

Hypothyroidism
+ Fatigue occurs early along with forgetfulness, cold intolerance, weight gain, metrorrhagia, and constipation.

Infection
+ With chronic infection, fatigue is commonly the most prominent symptom.
+ With acute infection, brief fatigue typically accompanies other signs and symptoms.

Chronic fatigue syndrome
Chronic fatigue syndrome, the cause of which is unknown, is characterized by incapacitating fatigue. Other findings are sore throat, myalgia, low-grade fever, painful lymph nodes, sleep disturbances, and cognitive dysfunction.

Chronic obstructive pulmonary disease
The earliest and most persistent symptoms of chronic obstructive pulmonary disease (COPD) are progressive fatigue and dyspnea. The patient may also experience a chronic and usually productive cough, weight loss, barrel chest, cyanosis, slight dependent edema, and poor exercise tolerance.

Cirrhosis
Severe fatigue typically occurs late in cirrhosis, accompanied by weight loss, bleeding tendencies, jaundice, hepatomegaly, ascites, dependent edema, severe pruritus, and decreased level of consciousness (LOC).

Depression
Persistent fatigue unrelated to exertion nearly always accompanies chronic depression. Associated somatic complaints include headache, anorexia (occasionally, increased appetite), constipation, and sexual dysfunction. The patient may also experience insomnia, slowed speech, agitation or bradykinesia, irritability, loss of concentration, feelings of worthlessness, and persistent thoughts of death.

Diabetes mellitus
Fatigue, the most common symptom in diabetes mellitus, may begin insidiously or abruptly. Related findings include weight loss, blurred vision, polyuria, polydipsia, and polyphagia.

Heart failure
Persistent fatigue and lethargy characterize heart failure. Left-sided heart failure produces exertional and paroxysmal nocturnal dyspnea, orthopnea, and tachycardia. Right-sided heart failure produces jugular vein distention and possibly a slight but persistent nonproductive cough. In both types, mental status changes accompany later signs and symptoms, including nausea, anorexia, weight gain and, possibly, oliguria. Cardiopulmonary findings include tachypnea, inspiratory crackles, palpitations and chest tightness, hypotension, narrowed pulse pressure, ventricular gallop, pallor, diaphoresis, clubbing, and dependent edema.

Hypercortisolism
Hypercortisolism typically causes fatigue, related in part to accompanying sleep disturbances. Unmistakable signs include truncal obesity with slender extremities, buffalo hump, moon face, purple striae, acne, and hirsutism; increased blood pressure and muscle weakness are other findings.

Hypopituitarism
With hypopituitarism, fatigue, lethargy, and weakness usually develop slowly. Other insidious effects may include irritability, anorexia, amenorrhea or impotence, decreased libido, hypotension, dizziness, headache, visual disturbances, and cold intolerance.

Hypothyroidism
Fatigue occurs early in hypothyroidism, along with forgetfulness, cold intolerance, weight gain, metrorrhagia, and constipation. Related findings include coarse hair and alopecia; anorexia; edema; dry, flaky skin; and thinning nails.

Infection

With chronic infection (such as acute bacterial endocarditis), fatigue is commonly the most prominent symptom — and sometimes the only one. Low-grade fever and weight loss may accompany signs and symptoms that reflect the type and location of infection, such as burning upon urination or swollen, painful gums.

With acute infection, brief fatigue typically accompanies headache, anorexia, arthralgia, chills, high fever, and such infection-specific signs as cough, vomiting, or diarrhea.

Lyme disease

Besides fatigue and malaise, signs and symptoms of Lyme disease include intermittent headache, fever, chills, expanding red rash, and muscle and joint aches. In later stages of this tick-borne disease, patients may suffer arthritis, fluctuating meningoencephalitis, and cardiac abnormalities, such as a brief, fluctuating atrioventricular heart block.

Malnutrition

Easy fatigability is common in patients with protein-calorie malnutrition, along with lethargy and apathy. Patients may also exhibit weight loss, muscle wasting, sensations of coldness, pallor, edema, and dry, flaky skin.

Myasthenia gravis

The cardinal symptoms of myasthenia gravis are easy fatigability and muscle weakness, which worsen as the day progresses. They also worsen with exertion and abate with rest. Related findings depend on the specific muscles affected.

Myocardial infarction

With myocardial infarction (MI), fatigue can be severe but is typically overshadowed by chest pain. Related findings include dyspnea, anxiety, pallor, cold sweats, increased or decreased blood pressure, and abnormal heart sounds.

Narcolepsy

One or more of the following characterizes narcolepsy: hypersomnia, hypnagogic hallucinations, cataplexy, sleep paralysis, and insomnia. Fatigue is a common symptom as well.

Renal failure

Acute renal failure commonly causes sudden fatigue, drowsiness, and lethargy. Oliguria, an early sign, is followed by severe systemic effects: ammonia breath odor, nausea, vomiting, diarrhea or constipation, and dry skin and mucous membranes. Neurologic findings include muscle twitching and changes in personality and LOC, possibly progressing to seizures and coma.

With chronic renal failure, insidious fatigue and lethargy occur with marked changes in all body systems, including GI disturbances, ammonia breath odor, Kussmaul's respirations, bleeding tendencies, poor skin turgor, severe pruritus, paresthesia, visual disturbances, confusion, seizures, and coma.

Restrictive lung disease

Chronic fatigue may accompany the characteristic signs and symptoms of restrictive lung disease: dyspnea, cough, and rapid, shallow respirations. Cyanosis first appears with exertion; later, even at rest.

Rheumatoid arthritis

With rheumatoid arthritis, fatigue, weakness, and anorexia precede localized articular findings: joint pain, tenderness, warmth, and swelling along with morning

Medical causes
(continued)

Lyme disease
+ Fatigue, malaise, intermittent headache, fever, chills, expanding red rash, and muscle and joint aches occur.

Malnutrition
+ Easy fatigability, lethargy, and apathy are common.

Myasthenia gravis
+ Easy fatigability and muscle weakness, which worsen as the day progresses, are cardinal symptoms.

MI
+ Fatigue can be severe but is typically overshadowed by chest pain.

Narcolepsy
+ Hypersomnia, hypnagogic hallucinations, cataplexy, sleep paralysis, insomnia, and fatigue are common.

Renal failure
+ Acute renal failure causes sudden fatigue, drowsiness, and lethargy.
+ Chronic renal failure causes insidious fatigue and lethargy along with marked changes in all body systems.

Restrictive lung disease
+ Chronic fatigue may accompany dyspnea, cough, and rapid, shallow respirations.

Rheumatoid arthritis
+ Fatigue, weakness, and anorexia precede localized findings.

Medical causes
(continued)

SLE
✦ Fatigue occurs along with generalized aching, malaise, low-grade fever, headache, and irritability.

Thyrotoxicosis
✦ Fatigue may occur.

Valvular heart disease
✦ Progressive fatigue and a cardiac murmur are common.

Other causes
✦ Antihypertensives and sedatives
✦ Carbon monoxide poisoning
✦ Digoxin toxicity

Special considerations
If fatigue is from organic illness:
✦ Help the patient determine which daily activities he may need help with; help him pace himself to ensure sufficient rest.
✦ Alleviate pain and nausea.
If fatigue results from a psychogenic cause:
✦ Refer for psychological counseling.

Peds points
✦ Fatigue occurs normally during accelerated growth phases.
✦ Consider depression as a cause.
✦ In a pubescent child, consider drug abuse.

Geri points
✦ Fatigue may be insidious and mask more serious underlying conditions in this age-group.

stiffness. Assessment findings may include enlarged lymph nodes, fever, leukopenia, anemia, subcutaneous nodules, pericarditis, and Raynaud's phenomenon.

Systemic lupus erythematosus
Fatigue usually occurs in patients with systemic lupus erythematosus (SLE), along with generalized aching, malaise, low-grade fever, headache, and irritability. Primary signs and symptoms include joint pain and stiffness, butterfly rash, and photosensitivity. Also common are Raynaud's phenomenon, patchy alopecia, and mucous membrane ulcers.

Thyrotoxicosis
With thyrotoxicosis, fatigue may occur with characteristic signs and symptoms, including an enlarged thyroid, tachycardia and palpitations, tremors, weight loss despite increased appetite, diarrhea, dyspnea, nervousness, diaphoresis, heat intolerance, amenorrhea and, possibly, exophthalmos.

Valvular heart disease
All types of valvular heart disease commonly produce progressive fatigue and a cardiac murmur. Additional signs and symptoms vary but generally include exertional dyspnea, cough, and hemoptysis.

OTHER CAUSES

Carbon monoxide poisoning
With carbon monoxide poisoning, fatigue occurs along with headache, dyspnea, and confusion, and can eventually progress to unconsciousness and apnea.

Drugs
Fatigue may result from various drugs, notably antihypertensives and sedatives. In persons receiving cardiac glycoside therapy, fatigue may indicate toxicity.

SPECIAL CONSIDERATIONS

If fatigue results from organic illness, help the patient determine which daily activities he may need help with and how he should pace himself to ensure sufficient rest. You can help him reduce chronic fatigue by alleviating pain, which may interfere with rest, or nausea, which may lead to malnutrition. He may benefit from referral to a community health nurse or housekeeping service. If fatigue results from a psychogenic cause, refer him for psychological counseling.

PEDIATRIC POINTERS

When evaluating a child for fatigue, ask his parents if they've noticed any change in his activity level. Fatigue without an organic cause occurs normally during accelerated growth phases in preschool-age and prepubescent children. However, psychological causes of fatigue must be considered—for example, a depressed child may try to escape problems at home or school by taking refuge in sleep. In a pubescent child, consider the possibility of drug abuse, particularly of hypnotics and tranquilizers.

GERIATRIC POINTERS

Always ask elderly patients about fatigue because this symptom may be insidious and mask more serious underlying conditions in this age-group. Temporal arthritis, which is much more common in people older than age 60, is usually characterized by fatigue, weight loss, jaw claudication, proximal muscle weakness, headache, vision disturbances, and associated anemia.

PATIENT COUNSELING

Regardless of the cause of fatigue, you may need to help the patient alter his lifestyle to achieve a balanced diet, a program of regular exercise, and adequate rest. Counsel him about setting priorities, keeping a reasonable schedule, and developing good sleep habits. Teach stress management techniques as appropriate.

FEVER

Fever, or pyrexia, is a common sign that can arise from any one of several disorders. Because these disorders can affect virtually any body system, fever in the absence of other signs usually has little diagnostic significance. A persistent high fever, though, represents an emergency.

Fever can be classified as low (oral reading of 99° to 100.4° F [37.2° to 38° C]), moderate (100.5° to 104° F [38° to 40° C]), or high (above 104° F). Fever over 106° F (41.1° C) causes unconsciousness and, if sustained, leads to permanent brain damage. (See *How fever develops,* page 286.)

Fever may also be classified as remittent, intermittent, sustained, relapsing, or undulant. *Remittent fever,* the most common type, is characterized by daily temperature fluctuations above the normal range. *Intermittent fever* is marked by a daily temperature drop into the normal range and then a rise back to above normal. An intermittent fever that fluctuates widely, typically producing chills and sweating, is called *hectic,* or *septic, fever. Sustained fever* involves persistent temperature elevation with little fluctuation. *Relapsing fever* consists of alternating feverish and afebrile periods. *Undulant fever* refers to a gradual increase in temperature that stays high for a few days and then decreases gradually.

Further classification of fever involves duration—either brief (less than 3 weeks) or prolonged.

EMERGENCY ACTIONS If you detect a fever higher than 106° F (41.1° C), take the patient's other vital signs and determine his level of consciousness (LOC). Administer an antipyretic and begin rapid cooling measures: Apply ice packs to the axillae and groin, give tepid sponge baths, or apply a hypothermia blanket. These methods may evoke a cooling response; to prevent this, constantly monitor the patient's rectal temperature.

HISTORY

If the patient's fever is only mild to moderate, ask him when it began and how high his temperature reached. Did the fever disappear, only to reappear later? Did he experience other symptoms, such as chills, fatigue, or pain?

Obtain a complete medical history, noting especially immunosuppressive treatments or disorders, infection, trauma, surgery, diagnostic testing, and use of anesthesia or other medications. Ask about recent travel because certain diseases are endemic.

PHYSICAL ASSESSMENT

Begin by taking your patient's vital signs. Let the history findings direct your physical examination. Because fever can accompany diverse disorders, the examination

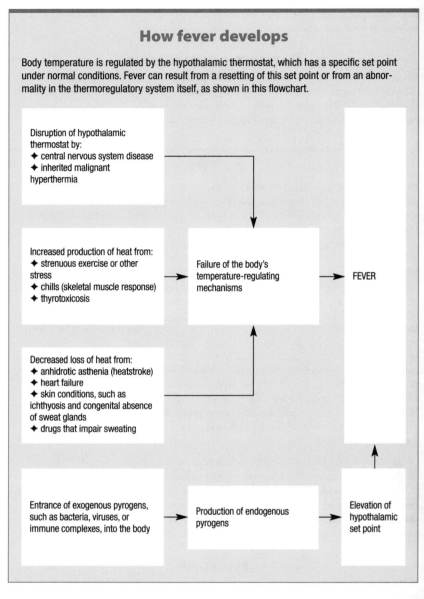

How fever develops

Body temperature is regulated by the hypothalamic thermostat, which has a specific set point under normal conditions. Fever can result from a resetting of this set point or from an abnormality in the thermoregulatory system itself, as shown in this flowchart.

Disruption of hypothalamic thermostat by:
✦ central nervous system disease
✦ inherited malignant hyperthermia

Increased production of heat from:
✦ strenuous exercise or other stress
✦ chills (skeletal muscle response)
✦ thyrotoxicosis

Failure of the body's temperature-regulating mechanisms

FEVER

Decreased loss of heat from:
✦ anhidrotic asthenia (heatstroke)
✦ heart failure
✦ skin conditions, such as ichthyosis and congenital absence of sweat glands
✦ drugs that impair sweating

Entrance of exogenous pyrogens, such as bacteria, viruses, or immune complexes, into the body

Production of endogenous pyrogens

Elevation of hypothalamic set point

may range from a brief evaluation of one body system to a comprehensive review of all systems. (See *Taking an accurate temperature.*)

MEDICAL CAUSES

Anthrax, cutaneous

The patient with cutaneous anthrax may experience a fever along with lymphadenopathy, malaise, and headache. After the bacterium *Bacillus anthracis* enters a cut or abrasion on the skin, the infection begins as a small, painless, or pruritic macular or papular lesion resembling an insect bite. Within 1 to 2 days, the lesion

Medical causes

Anthrax, cutaneous
✦ Patient may have fever along with lymphadenopathy, malaise, and headache.

Taking an accurate temperature

To take a patient's temperature accurately with an electronic thermometer, first verify that the thermometer is set in the correct mode. In the *normal mode,* the thermometer will predict the temperature based on the rate of temperature change; when set in the *monitor mode,* the thermometer obtains an actual temperature.

Also check that the correct probe is being used at the correct site. For example, using an oral probe to obtain a rectal temperature can cause an inaccurate result.

When using a tympanic thermometer, know whether it's set to convert the temperature to rectal, oral, or core temperature. An elevated temperature in the rectal mode may be normal but be considered a fever if obtained in the oral mode.

develops into a vesicle and then into a painless ulcer with a characteristic black, necrotic center.

Anthrax, GI

Following the ingestion of meat contaminated with the bacterium *Bacillus anthracis,* the patient experiences fever, loss of appetite, nausea, and vomiting. The patient may also experience abdominal pain, severe bloody diarrhea, and hematemesis.

Anthrax, inhalation

The initial signs and symptoms of inhalation anthrax are flulike, including fever, chills, weakness, cough, and chest pain. The disease generally occurs in two stages with a period of recovery after the initial symptoms. The second stage develops abruptly with rapid deterioration marked by fever, dyspnea, stridor, and hypotension, generally leading to death within 24 hours.

Escherichia coli 0157:H7

Fever, bloody diarrhea, nausea, vomiting, and abdominal cramps occur after eating foods contaminated with the bacterial strain *Escherichia coli* 0157:H7. In children younger than age 5 and in elderly patients, hemolytic uremic syndrome may develop (in which the red blood cells are destroyed), and this may ultimately lead to acute renal failure.

Immune complex dysfunction

When immune complex dysfunction is present, fever usually remains low, although moderate elevations may accompany erythema multiforme. Fever may be remittent or intermittent, as in acquired immunodeficiency syndrome (AIDS) or systemic lupus erythematosus, or sustained, as in polyarteritis. As one of several vague, prodromal complaints (such as fatigue, anorexia, and weight loss), fever produces nocturnal diaphoresis and accompanies such associated signs and symptoms as diarrhea and a persistent cough (with AIDS) or morning stiffness (with rheumatoid arthritis). Other disease-specific findings include headache and vision loss (temporal arteritis); pain and stiffness in the neck, shoulders, back, or pelvis (ankylosing spondylitis and polymyalgia rheumatica); skin and mucous membrane lesions (erythema multiforme); and urethritis with urethral discharge and conjunctivitis (Reiter's syndrome).

Medical causes
(continued)

Anthrax, GI
✦ Fever, loss of appetite, nausea, and vomiting occur after eating contaminated food.

Anthrax, inhalation
✦ Initially, fever, chills, weakness, cough, and chest pain occur.

E. coli 0157:H7
✦ Fever, bloody diarrhea, nausea, vomiting, and abdominal cramps occur after eating contaminated foods.

Immune complex dysfunction
✦ Fever usually remains low and may be remittent, intermittent, or sustained.

Medical causes
(continued)

Infectious and inflammatory disorders
✦ Fever varies depending on the disorder.

Neoplasms
✦ Prolonged fever of varying elevations occurs.

Plague
✦ Bubonic form causes fever, chills, and swollen, inflamed, and tender lymph nodes near site of bite.
✦ Pneumonic form manifests as a sudden onset of chills, fever, headache, and myalgia.

Rhabdomyolysis
✦ Fever, muscle weakness or pain, nausea, vomiting, malaise, or dark reddish brown urine result.

SARS
✦ Disease generally begins with fever greater than 100.4° F (38° C).
✦ Other symptoms include headache, malaise, a dry nonproductive cough, and dyspnea.

Smallpox
✦ Initial signs and symptoms include high fever, malaise, prostration, severe headache, backache, and abdominal pain.
✦ Characteristic rash occurs.

Infectious and inflammatory disorders
Fever ranges from low (in patients with Crohn's disease or ulcerative colitis) to extremely high (in those with bacterial pneumonia, necrotizing fasciitis, or Ebola virus or Hantavirus). It may be remittent, as in those with infectious mononucleosis or otitis media; hectic as in those with lung abscess, influenza, or endocarditis; sustained, as in those with meningitis; or relapsing, as in those with malaria. Fever may arise abruptly, as in those with toxic shock syndrome or Rocky Mountain spotted fever, or insidiously, as in those with mycoplasmal pneumonia. In patients with hepatitis, fever may represent a disease prodrome; in those with appendicitis, it follows the acute stage. Its sudden late appearance with tachycardia, tachypnea, and confusion heralds life-threatening septic shock in patients with peritonitis or gram-negative bacteremia.

Associated signs and symptoms involve every system. General systemic complaints include weakness, anorexia, and malaise.

Neoplasms
Primary neoplasms and metastases can produce prolonged fever of varying elevations. For instance, acute leukemia may present insidiously with low fever, pallor, and bleeding tendencies, or more abruptly with high fever, frank bleeding, and prostration. Occasionally, Hodgkin's disease produces undulant fever or Pel-Ebstein fever, an irregularly relapsing fever.

In addition to fever and nocturnal diaphoresis, neoplastic disease typically causes anorexia, fatigue, malaise, and weight loss. Examination may reveal lesions, lymphadenopathy, palpable masses, and hepatosplenomegaly.

Plague
Plague is an infection caused by the bacterium *Yersinia pestis.* The bubonic form of plague causes fever, chills, and swollen, inflamed, and tender lymph nodes near the site of the bite. The septicemic form develops as a fulminant illness generally with the bubonic form. The pneumonic form manifests as a sudden onset of chills, fever, headache, and myalgia after person-to-person transmission via the respiratory tract. Other signs and symptoms of the pneumonic form include productive cough, chest pain, tachypnea, dyspnea, hemoptysis, increasing respiratory distress, and cardiopulmonary insufficiency.

Rhabdomyolysis
Rhabdomyolysis produces fever, muscle weakness or pain, nausea, vomiting, malaise, or dark reddish brown urine. Acute renal failure is the most frequently reported complication of the disorder.

Severe acute respiratory syndrome
Severe acute respiratory syndrome (SARS) is an acute infectious disease of unknown etiology that generally begins with a fever (usually greater than 100.4° F [38° C]). Other symptoms include headache, malaise, a dry nonproductive cough, and dyspnea. The severity of the illness is highly variable, ranging from mild illness to pneumonia and, in some cases, progressing to respiratory failure and death.

Smallpox
Initial signs and symptoms of smallpox (also known as *variola major*) include high fever, malaise, prostration, severe headache, backache, and abdominal pain. A maculopapular rash develops on the mucosa of the mouth, pharynx, face, and forearms and then spreads to the trunk and legs. Within 2 days, the rash becomes vesicular and later pustular. The lesions develop at the same time, appear identical, and are more prominent on the face and extremities. The pustules are round, firm, and

deeply embedded in the skin. After about 8 to 9 days, the pustules form a crust, and later the scab separates from the skin, leaving a pitted scar. In fatal cases, death results from encephalitis, extensive bleeding, or secondary infection.

Thermoregulatory dysfunction

Sudden onset of fever that rises rapidly and remains as high as 107° F (41.7° C) occurs in life-threatening disorders, such as heatstroke, thyroid storm, neuroleptic malignant syndrome, and malignant hyperthermia, and in lesions of the central nervous system (CNS). Low or moderate fever appears in dehydrated patients.

Prolonged high fever commonly produces vomiting, anhidrosis, decreased LOC, and hot, flushed skin. Related cardiovascular effects may include tachycardia, tachypnea, and hypotension. Other disease-specific findings include skin changes: dry skin and mucous membranes, poor skin turgor, and oliguria with dehydration; mottled cyanosis with malignant hyperthermia; diarrhea with thyroid storm; and ominous signs of increased intracranial pressure (decreased LOC with bradycardia, widened pulse pressure, and increased systolic pressure) with CNS tumor, trauma, or hemorrhage.

Tularemia

Also known as *rabbit fever*, tularemia is an infectious disease that causes abrupt onset of fever, chills, headache, generalized myalgia, nonproductive cough, dyspnea, pleuritic chest pain, and empyema.

West Nile encephalitis

Mild infection is common from West Nile encephalitis, a mosquito-borne Flavivirus. Signs and symptoms include fever, headache, and body aches, commonly with skin rash and swollen lymph glands. More severe infection is marked by high fever, headache, neck stiffness, stupor, disorientation, coma, tremors, occasional seizures, paralysis and, rarely, death.

 CULTURAL CUE *West Nile encephalitis is commonly found in Africa, West Asia, and the Middle East. It rarely occurs in North America.*

OTHER CAUSES

Drugs

Fever and rash commonly result from hypersensitivity to antifungals, sulfonamides, penicillins, cephalosporins, tetracyclines, barbiturates, phenytoin, quinidine, iodides, phenolphthalein, methyldopa, procainamide, and some antitoxins. Fever can accompany chemotherapy, especially with bleomycin, vincristine, and asparaginase. It can result from drugs that impair sweating, such as anticholinergics, phenothiazines, and monoamine oxidase inhibitors. A drug-induced fever typically disappears after the involved drug is discontinued. Fever can also stem from toxic doses of salicylates, amphetamines, and tricyclic antidepressants.

Inhaled anesthetics and muscle relaxants can trigger malignant hyperthermia in patients with this inherited trait.

SPECIAL CONSIDERATIONS

Regularly monitor the patient's temperature, and record it on a chart for easy follow-up of the temperature curve. Provide increased fluid and nutritional intake. When administering a prescribed antipyretic, minimize resultant chills and diaphoresis by following a regular dosage schedule. Promote patient comfort by maintaining a stable room temperature and providing frequent changes of bedding

Medical causes
(continued)

Thermoregulatory dysfunction

✦ Sudden onset of fever that rises rapidly and remains as high as 107° F (41.7° C) occurs in life-threatening disorders.
✦ Low or moderate fever appears in dehydrated patients.

Tularemia

✦ Onset of fever, chills, headache, generalized myalgia, nonproductive cough, dyspnea, pleuritic chest pain, and empyema is abrupt.

West Nile encephalitis

✦ Fever, headache, body aches, skin rash, and swollen lymph occur.

Other causes

✦ Chemotherapy
✦ Drugs that impair sweating
✦ Hypersensitivity to antifungals, sulfonamides, penicillins, cephalosporins, tetracyclines, barbiturates, phenytoin, quinidine, iodides, phenolphthalein, methyldopa, procainamide, and some antitoxins
✦ Inhaled anesthetics and muscle relaxants
✦ Toxic doses of salicylates, amphetamines, and TCAs

Special considerations

✦ Regularly monitor temperature.
✦ Increase fluid and nutritional intake.
✦ Maintain stable room temperature and provide frequent bedding and clothing changes.

Peds points

+ Infants and young children experience higher and more prolonged fevers, more rapid temperature increases, and greater temperature fluctuations.
+ Common pediatric causes of fever include varicella, croup syndrome, dehydration, meningitis, mumps, otitis media, pertussis, roseola infantum, rubella, rubeola, tonsillitis, and adverse reactions to immunizations and antibiotics.

Geri points

+ Elderly patients may have impaired thermoregulatory mechanisms, making temperature change a much less reliable measure of disease severity.

Teaching points

+ Oral temperature measurement at home
+ Increased fluid intake (unless contraindicated)

Key facts about flank pain

+ Indicates renal and upper urinary tract disease or trauma
+ May range from a dull ache to a severe stabbing or throbbing pain
+ May be unilateral or bilateral, constant or intermittent

In an emergency

+ Insert an I.V. line.
+ Insert an indwelling urinary catheter to monitor urine output and evaluate hematuria.

and clothing. Prepare the patient for laboratory tests, such as complete blood count and cultures of blood, urine, sputum, and wound drainage.

PEDIATRIC POINTERS

Infants and young children experience higher and more prolonged fevers, more rapid temperature increases, and greater temperature fluctuations than older children and adults. Common pediatric causes of fever include varicella, croup syndrome, dehydration, meningitis, mumps, otitis media, pertussis, roseola infantum, rubella, rubeola, and tonsillitis. Fever can also occur as a reaction to immunizations and antibiotics.

Keep in mind that seizures commonly accompany extremely high fever, so take appropriate precautions. Also, instruct parents not to give aspirin to a child with varicella or flulike symptoms because of the risk of precipitating Reye's syndrome.

GERIATRIC POINTERS

Elderly people may have altered sweating mechanisms that predispose them to heatstroke when exposed to high temperatures; they may also have an impaired thermoregulatory mechanism, making temperature change a much less reliable measure of disease severity.

PATIENT COUNSELING

If the patient hasn't been admitted to the hospital, ask him to measure his oral temperature at home and record the time and value. Explain to him that fever is a response to an underlying condition and that it plays an important role in fighting infection. Therefore, advise him not to take an antipyretic until his body temperature reaches 101° F (38.3° C). Encourage the patient with a fever to drink plenty of fluids, unless contraindicated.

FLANK PAIN

Pain in the flank, the area extending from the ribs to the ilium, is a leading indicator of renal and upper urinary tract disease or trauma. Depending on the cause, this symptom may vary from a dull ache to severe stabbing or throbbing pain, and may be unilateral or bilateral and constant or intermittent. It's aggravated by costovertebral angle (CVA) percussion and, in patients with renal or urinary tract obstruction, by increased fluid intake and ingestion of alcohol, caffeine, or diuretics. Unaffected by position changes, flank pain typically responds only to analgesics or, of course, to treatment of the underlying disorder.

 EMERGENCY ACTIONS If the patient has suffered trauma, quickly look for a visible or palpable flank mass, associated injuries, CVA pain, hematuria, Turner's sign, and signs of shock (such as tachycardia and cool, clammy skin). If one or more is present, insert an I.V. line to allow fluid or drug infusion. Insert an indwelling urinary catheter to monitor urine output and evaluate hematuria. Obtain blood samples for typing and crossmatching, complete blood count, and electrolyte levels.

HISTORY

If the patient's condition isn't critical, take a thorough history. Ask about the pain's onset and apparent precipitating events. Have him describe the pain's location, intensity, pattern, and duration. Find out if anything aggravates or alleviates it.

Ask the patient about any changes in his normal pattern of fluid intake and urine output. Explore his history for urinary tract infection (UTI) or obstruction, renal disease, or recent streptococcal infection.

PHYSICAL ASSESSMENT

During the physical examination, palpate the patient's flank area and percuss the CVA to determine the extent of pain.

MEDICAL CAUSES

Bladder cancer

With bladder cancer, dull, constant flank pain may be unilateral or bilateral and may radiate to the leg, back, and perineum. Commonly, the first sign of this cancer is gross, painless, intermittent hematuria, usually with clots. Related effects may include urinary frequency and urgency, nocturia, dysuria, or pyuria; bladder distention; pain in the bladder, rectum, pelvis, back, or legs; diarrhea; vomiting; and sleep disturbances.

Calculi

Renal and ureteral calculi produce intense unilateral, colicky flank pain. Typically, initial CVA pain radiates to the flank, suprapubic region, and perhaps the genitalia; abdominal and lower back pain are also possible. Nausea and vomiting usually accompany severe pain. Associated findings include CVA tenderness, hematuria, hypoactive bowel sounds and, possibly, signs and symptoms of UTI (urinary frequency and urgency, dysuria, nocturia, fatigue, low-grade fever, and tenesmus).

Cystitis (bacterial)

Unilateral or bilateral flank pain occurs secondarily to an ascending UTI. The patient with bacterial cystitis may also report perineal, low back, and suprapubic pain. Other effects include dysuria, nocturia, hematuria, urinary frequency and urgency, tenesmus, fatigue, and low-grade fever.

Glomerulonephritis (acute)

Flank pain in acute glomerulonephritis is bilateral, constant, and moderately intense. The most common findings are moderate facial and generalized edema, hematuria, oliguria or anuria, and fatigue. Other effects include slightly increased blood pressure, low-grade fever, malaise, headache, nausea, and vomiting. Accompanying signs of pulmonary congestion include dyspnea, tachypnea, and crackles.

Obstructive uropathy

With acute obstruction, flank pain may be excruciating; with gradual obstruction, it's typically a dull ache. With both, the pain may also localize in the upper abdomen and radiate to the groin. Nausea and vomiting, abdominal distention, anuria alternating with periods of oliguria and polyuria, and hypoactive bowel sounds may also occur. Additional findings—a palpable abdominal mass, CVA tenderness, and bladder distention—vary with the site and cause of the obstruction.

Medical causes
(continued)

Pancreatitis (acute)
✦ Bilateral flank pain may develop as severe epigastric or left-upper-quadrant pain radiates to the back.

Papillary necrosis (acute)
✦ Intense bilateral flank pain occurs along with renal colic, CVA tenderness, and abdominal pain and rigidity.

Perirenal abscess
✦ Intense unilateral flank pain and CVA tenderness accompany dysuria, persistent high fever, and chills.

Polycystic kidney disease
✦ Dull, aching, bilateral flank pain is an early symptom.

Pyelonephritis (acute)
✦ Intense, constant, unilateral or bilateral flank pain develops.
✦ Typical urinary features include dysuria, nocturia, hematuria, urgency, frequency, and tenesmus.

Renal cancer
✦ Unilateral flank pain that's dull and vague, gross hematuria, and a palpable flank mass are the classic clinical triad.

Renal infarction
✦ Unilateral, constant, severe flank pain and tenderness typically accompany persistent, severe upper abdominal pain.

Renal trauma
✦ Variable bilateral or unilateral flank pain is common.

Pancreatitis (acute)
Bilateral flank pain may develop in patients with acute pancreatitis as severe epigastric or left-upper-quadrant pain radiates to the back. A severe attack causes extreme pain, nausea and persistent vomiting, abdominal tenderness and rigidity, hypoactive bowel sounds and, possibly, restlessness, low-grade fever, tachycardia, hypotension, and positive Turner's and Cullen's signs.

Papillary necrosis (acute)
Intense bilateral flank pain occurs along with renal colic, CVA tenderness, and abdominal pain and rigidity. Urinary signs and symptoms of acute papillary necrosis include oliguria or anuria, hematuria, and pyuria, with associated high fever, chills, vomiting, and hypoactive bowel sounds.

Perirenal abscess
With a perirenal abscess, intense unilateral flank pain and CVA tenderness accompany dysuria, persistent high fever, chills and, in some patients, a palpable abdominal mass.

Polycystic kidney disease
Dull, aching, bilateral flank pain is commonly the earliest symptom of polycystic kidney disease. The pain can become severe and colicky if cysts rupture and clots migrate or cause obstruction. Nonspecific early findings include polyuria, increased blood pressure, and signs of UTI. Later findings include hematuria and perineal, low back, and suprapubic pain.

Pyelonephritis (acute)
With acute pyelonephritis, intense, constant, unilateral or bilateral flank pain develops over a few hours or days along with typical urinary features: dysuria, nocturia, hematuria, urgency, frequency, and tenesmus. Other common findings in acute pyelonephritis include persistent high fever, chills, anorexia, weakness, fatigue, generalized myalgia, abdominal pain, and marked CVA tenderness.

Renal cancer
Unilateral flank pain, gross hematuria, and a palpable flank mass form the classic clinical triad in patients with renal cancer. Flank pain is usually dull and vague, although severe colicky pain can occur during bleeding or passage of clots. Associated signs and symptoms include fever, increased blood pressure, and urine retention. Weight loss, leg edema, nausea, and vomiting are indications of advanced disease.

Renal infarction
With renal infarction, unilateral, constant, severe flank pain and tenderness typically accompany persistent, severe upper abdominal pain. The patient may also develop CVA tenderness, anorexia, nausea and vomiting, fever, hypoactive bowel sounds, hematuria, and oliguria or anuria.

Renal trauma
Variable bilateral or unilateral flank pain is a common symptom of renal trauma. A visible or palpable flank mass may also exist, along with CVA or abdominal pain—which may be severe and radiate to the groin. Other findings include hematuria, oliguria, abdominal distention, Turner's sign, hypoactive bowel sounds, and nausea or vomiting. Severe injury may produce signs of shock, such as tachycardia and cool, clammy skin.

Renal vein thrombosis

Severe unilateral flank and low back pain with CVA and epigastric tenderness typify the rapid onset of venous obstruction. Other features include fever, hematuria, and leg edema. Bilateral flank pain, oliguria, and other uremic signs and symptoms (nausea, vomiting, and uremic fetor) typify bilateral obstruction.

SPECIAL CONSIDERATIONS

Administer pain medication. Continue to monitor the patient's vital signs, and maintain a precise record of the patient's intake and output.

Diagnostic evaluation may involve serial urine and serum analysis, excretory urography, flank ultrasonography, computed tomography scan, voiding cystourethrography, cystoscopy, and retrograde ureteropyelography, urethrography, and cystography.

PEDIATRIC POINTERS

Assessment of flank pain can be difficult if a child can't describe the pain. In such cases, transillumination of the abdomen and flanks may help in assessment of bladder distention and identification of masses. Common causes of flank pain in children include obstructive uropathy, acute poststreptococcal glomerulonephritis, infantile polycystic kidney disease, and nephroblastoma.

PATIENT COUNSELING

Encourage the patient to increase his intake of fluids to 3 qt (3 L)/day, unless contraindicated. Tell him to report such signs and symptoms as hematuria and cloudy, foul smelling urine. Explain the importance of taking all medications as prescribed. Make sure he understands the importance of follow-up appointments to assess renal function.

FLATULENCE

A sensation of gaseous abdominal fullness, flatulence can result from GI disorders, abdominal surgery, excessive intake of certain foods, and stress. It may be accompanied by belching, discomfort, and excessive passage of flatus.

Flatulence reflects slowed intestinal motility, which hampers the passage of gas; excessive swallowing of air (aerophagia), commonly brought on by stress; or increased intraluminal gas production due to an excess of fermentable substrates, such as digested, unabsorbed carbohydrates and proteins.

Although generally not considered a serious symptom, flatulence—and accompanying expulsion of flatus—may cause the patient embarrassment and discomfort.

HISTORY

Determine how long the patient has noticed the flatulence. Find out if he passes an excessive amount of flatus. Also, ask about frequent belching or snoring, and observe for overly rapid speech. These signs are all possible clues to aerophagia.

In addition, be sure to ask the patient if he's undergoing unusual emotional stress because this can cause aerophagia or irritable bowel syndrome. Obtain a medical history, focusing on GI disorders and systemic illnesses such as scleroderma. These can cause malabsorption syndrome.

Critical assessment steps

✦ Inspect abdomen for distention.
✦ Auscultate for abnormal bowel sounds.
✦ Percuss for increased tympany due to gas accumulation.
✦ Palpate for tenderness and masses.

Medical causes

Cirrhosis
✦ Flatulence typically develops early and insidiously.

Colon cancer
✦ Obstruction of the colon by a tumor may cause flatulence.

Crohn's disease
✦ Flatulence accompanies abdominal pain, cramps, and tenderness; diarrhea; low-grade fever; nausea; and melena.

Irritable bowel syndrome
✦ Effects include chronic flatulence, belching, and excessive flatus.

Lactose intolerance
✦ Flatulence develops within several hours after the ingestion of dairy products.

Malabsorption syndromes
✦ Flatulence may occur.
✦ Associated findings include abdominal pain, anorexia, weight loss, and passage of bulky, oily, malodorous, or watery stools.

Other causes
✦ Abdominal surgery

PHYSICAL ASSESSMENT

Inspect the patient's abdomen for distention, and auscultate for abnormal bowel sounds. Percuss for increased tympany due to gas accumulation, and palpate for tenderness and masses.

MEDICAL CAUSES

Cirrhosis
With cirrhosis, flatulence typically develops early and insidiously, along with anorexia, dyspepsia, nausea, vomiting, diarrhea or constipation, dull right-upper-quadrant pain, hepatomegaly, splenomegaly, fatigue, and malaise.

Colon cancer
Obstruction of the colon by a tumor may cause flatulence; acute obstruction also produces abdominal distention and tympany on percussion. Abdominal pain may be present, accompanied by anorexia, weight loss, malaise, and altered bowel habits (constipation, diarrhea, or a change in the timing, frequency, or consistency of stools).

Crohn's disease
With Crohn's disease, flatulence accompanies other acute inflammatory signs and symptoms that mimic those of appendicitis: abdominal pain, cramps, and tenderness; diarrhea; low-grade fever; nausea; and melena.

Irritable bowel syndrome
The effects of irritable bowel syndrome include chronic flatulence, belching, and excessive flatus. Chronic constipation is typical, although the patient may also experience diurnal diarrhea. Intermittent lower abdominal pain characteristically abates with defecation or passage of flatus.

Lactose intolerance
With lactose intolerance, flatulence develops within several hours after the ingestion of dairy products. Accompanying signs and symptoms include cramping, abdominal pain and, possibly, diarrhea.

 CULTURAL CUE *Lactose intolerance is common in many ethnic groups, including Mexican-Americans, Blacks, Native Americans, Asians, and Ashkenazi Jews.*

Malabsorption syndromes
Malabsorption syndromes may cause flatulence. Associated findings vary considerably, depending on which dietary constituent isn't absorbed but may include abdominal pain, anorexia, weight loss, and passage of bulky, oily, malodorous, or slightly watery stools. Severe malabsorption may also cause muscle wasting and weakness as well as skeletal pain, edema, ecchymoses, and ulceration of the tongue.

OTHER CAUSES

Abdominal surgery
When peristalsis returns after postoperative paralytic ileus, gas accumulation in hypomotile areas produces flatulence.

SPECIAL CONSIDERATIONS

Prepare the patient for diagnostic studies, such as blood tests, stool analysis, upper GI series, barium enema, and endoscopy. To aid expulsion of excessive flatus, position the patient on his left side. To prevent gas buildup, encourage frequent repositioning, ambulation, and normal fluid intake, as permitted. If these measures aren't effective, try inserting a rectal tube into his anus to relieve flatus, or administering an enema, suppository, antiflatulent, or anticholinergic. As appropriate, provide the patient with a diet plan that excludes gaseous foods.

PEDIATRIC POINTERS

The common childhood complaint of stomachache commonly results from flatulence. Children may also be more sensitive than adults to flatus-producing foods. They're also generally more prone to aerophagia, especially during eating.

GERIATRIC POINTERS

In elderly patients, increased flatulence may result from poor dentition, leading to poor mastication of food, poor dietary intake, and decreased GI motility. However, disease must first be ruled out.

PATIENT COUNSELING

To reduce flatulence, advise your patient to eat slowly, avoid overeating, and avoid drinking large amounts of liquids with meals. He should also avoid foods and beverages that contain excess air, including souffles, carbonated drinks, and milk shakes. If he's lactose intolerant, tell him to avoid milk, cheese, ice cream, and other dairy products. Flatulence can also be reduced by avoiding gas-forming vegetables and fruits, such as broccoli and prunes, and eliminating fatty foods.

FOOTDROP

Footdrop — plantar flexion of the foot with the toes bent toward the instep — results from weakness or paralysis of the dorsiflexor muscles of the foot and ankle. A characteristic and important sign of certain peripheral nerve or motor neuron disorders, footdrop may also stem from prolonged immobility when inadequate support, improper positioning, or infrequent passive exercise produces shortening of the Achilles tendon. Unilateral footdrop can result from compression of the common peroneal nerve against the head of the fibula.

Footdrop can range in severity from slight to complete, depending on the extent of muscle weakness or paralysis. It develops slowly in progressive muscle degeneration or suddenly in spinal cord injury.

HISTORY

Ask the patient about the sign's onset, duration, and character. Does the footdrop fluctuate in severity or remain constant? Does it worsen with fatigue or improve with rest? Ask the patient if he feels weak or tires easily.

PHYSICAL ASSESSMENT

During the physical examination, assess muscle tone and strength in the patient's feet and legs, and compare findings on both sides. Assess deep tendon reflexes (DTRs) in both legs as well. Have the patient walk; inspect his shoes for wear and observe the patient for steppage gait — a compensatory response to footdrop in which the legs are raised abnormally high.

Special considerations
+ Encourage frequent repositioning, ambulation, and normal fluid intake, as permitted.
+ Insert rectal tube as indicated.
+ As appropriate, provide a diet that excludes gaseous foods.

Peds points
+ Stomachache commonly results from flatulence.
+ Children may be more sensitive to flatus-producing foods.

Geri points
+ Increased flatulence may result from poor dentition, leading to poor mastication of food, poor dietary intake, and decreased GI motility; rule out disease first.

Teaching points
+ Ways to reduce flatulence

Key facts about footdrop
+ Plantar flexion of foot with the toes bent toward the instep
+ Results from weakness or paralysis of dorsiflexor muscles of foot and ankle

Key history points
+ Onset, duration, and character
+ Alleviating or aggravating factors
+ Associated weakness or tiredness

Critical assessment steps
+ Assess muscle tone and strength in feet and legs; compare findings on both sides.
+ Assess DTRs in both legs.

Medical causes

Guillain-Barré syndrome
+ Unilateral or bilateral footdrop and steppage gait may result from profound muscle weakness.

Herniated lumbar disk
+ Footdrop and steppage gait may result from leg muscle weakness and atrophy.

Multiple sclerosis
+ Footdrop may develop suddenly or slowly, producing steppage gait.

Myasthenia gravis
+ Footdrop and related limb weakness are common.

Peroneal muscle atrophy
+ Bilateral footdrop, ankle instability, and steppage gait occur.
+ Foot, peroneal, and ankle dorsiflexor muscles are affected first.

Peroneal nerve trauma
+ Footdrop may occur suddenly, but it's usually temporary, resolving with the release of peroneal nerve compression.

Polyneuropathy
+ Footdrop and steppage gait may accompany muscle weakness, which usually affects distal areas of the extremities and can progress to flaccid paralysis.

MEDICAL CAUSES

Guillain-Barré syndrome

Unilateral or bilateral footdrop and steppage gait may result from profound muscle weakness caused by Guillain-Barré syndrome. This weakness usually begins in the legs and extends to the arms and face within 72 hours. It can progress to total motor paralysis with respiratory failure. The patient may also develop transient paresthesia, hypoactive DTRs, hypernasality, dysphagia, diaphoresis, tachycardia, orthostatic hypotension, and incontinence.

Herniated lumbar disk

In a patient with a herniated lumbar disk, footdrop and steppage gait may result from leg muscle weakness and atrophy. However, the most pronounced symptom is severe low back pain that may radiate to the buttocks, legs, and feet, usually unilaterally. Sciatic pain follows, typically with muscle spasms and sensorimotor loss. Paresthesia, hypoactive DTRs, and fasciculations may occur.

Multiple sclerosis

With multiple sclerosis, footdrop may develop suddenly or slowly, producing steppage gait; it typically fluctuates in severity with this disorder's cycle of periodic exacerbation and remission. Muscle weakness, usually affecting the legs, ranges from minor fatigability to paraparesis with urinary urgency and constipation. Related findings include facial pain, visual disturbances, paresthesia, lack of coordination, and loss of vibration and position sensation in the ankle and toes.

Myasthenia gravis

Footdrop and related limb weakness are common manifestations of myasthenia gravis, which is commonly heralded by weak eye closure, ptosis, and diplopia. Skeletal muscle weakness and fatigability may progress to paralysis. Typically, muscle function worsens through the day and with exercise, and improves with rest. Involvement of respiratory muscles can cause breathing difficulty.

Peroneal muscle atrophy

Bilateral footdrop, ankle instability, and steppage gait occur early with this chronic disorder. Foot, peroneal, and ankle dorsiflexor muscles are affected first. Other early signs and symptoms include paresthesia, aching, and cramping in the feet and legs, along with coldness, swelling, and cyanosis. As the disease progresses, all leg muscles become weak and atrophic, with hypoactive or absent DTRs. Later, atrophy and sensory losses spread to the hands and forearms.

Peroneal nerve trauma

With peroneal nerve trauma, footdrop may occur suddenly, but it's usually temporary, resolving with the release of peroneal nerve compression. It's associated with ipsilateral steppage gait, muscle weakness, and sensory loss over the lateral surface of the calf and foot.

Polyneuropathy

With polyneuropathy, footdrop and steppage gait may accompany muscle weakness, which usually affects distal areas of the extremities and can progress to flaccid paralysis. Muscle atrophy and hypoactive or absent DTRs may occur, along with paresthesia, hyperesthesia, or anesthesia, and loss of vibration sensation in the hands and feet. Cutaneous manifestations include glossy red skin and anhidrosis.

Spinal cord trauma

Unilateral or bilateral footdrop can occur suddenly and may be permanent in patients with spinal cord trauma. In the ambulatory patient, it also produces steppage gait. Other findings vary and may include neck and back pain; paresthesia, sensory loss, and muscle weakness, atrophy, or paralysis distal to the injury; asymmetrical or absent DTRs; and fecal and urinary incontinence.

Stroke

Unilateral footdrop is a common sign of stroke, along with arm and leg weakness or paralysis. Other effects vary according to the site and severity of vascular damage. Sensorimotor disturbances may include paresthesia, dysphagia, visual field deficits, diplopia, and bowel and bladder dysfunction. Personality changes, amnesia, aphasia, dysarthria, and decreased level of consciousness may also occur.

SPECIAL CONSIDERATIONS

Prepare the patient for electromyography to evaluate nerve function. The patient may require physical therapy for gait retraining and possibly in-shoe splints or leg braces to maintain correct foot alignment for walking and standing.

PEDIATRIC POINTERS

Common causes of footdrop in children include spinal birth defects (such as spina bifida) and degenerative disorders (such as muscular dystrophy). To aid ambulation, the child should be fitted with supportive shoes and possibly in-shoe splints or braces.

PATIENT COUNSELING

Instruct the patient in the use of assistive devices such as canes, crutches, or walkers, as necessary. Review the importance of asking for assistance with activities to prevent falls and promote safety. Include the patient's family in this teaching.

Medical causes
(continued)

Spinal cord trauma
- Unilateral or bilateral footdrop can occur suddenly and may be permanent.

Stroke
- Unilateral footdrop is common, along with arm and leg weakness or paralysis.

Special considerations
- Prepare the patient for electromyography to evaluate nerve function.
- The patient may require physical therapy, in-shoe splints, or leg braces.

Peds points
- Common causes of footdrop in children include spinal birth defects and degenerative disorders.

Teaching points
- Use of assistive devices
- Safety measures, such as asking for assistance with activities

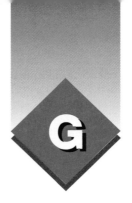

GALLOP, ATRIAL

An atrial, or presystolic, gallop is an extra heart sound (S_4) that's heard or commonly palpated immediately before the first heart sound (S_1), late in diastole. This low-pitched sound is heard best with the bell of the stethoscope pressed lightly against the cardiac apex. Some clinicians say that an S_4 has the cadence of the "Ten" in Tennessee (Ten = S_4; nes = S_1; see = S_2).

An atrial gallop typically results from hypertension, conduction defects, valvular disorders, or other problems such as ischemia. Occasionally, it helps differentiate angina from other causes of chest pain. It results from abnormal forceful atrial contraction caused by augmented ventricular filling or by decreased left ventricular compliance. An atrial gallop usually originates from left atrial contraction, is heard at the apex, and doesn't vary with inspiration. A left-sided S_4 can occur in hypertensive heart disease, coronary artery disease, aortic stenosis, and cardiomyopathy. It may also originate from right atrial contraction. A right-sided S_4 is indicative of pulmonary hypertension and pulmonary stenosis. If so, it's best heard at the lower left sternal border and intensifies with inspiration.

An atrial gallop seldom occurs in normal hearts; however, it may occur in elderly people and in athletes with physiologic hypertrophy of the left ventricle.

 EMERGENCY ACTIONS Suspect myocardial ischemia if you auscultate an atrial gallop in a patient with chest pain. (*Locating heart sounds* and *Interpreting heart sounds,* pages 300 and 301.) Take the patient's vital signs and quickly assess for signs of heart failure, such as dyspnea, crackles, and distended jugular veins. If you detect these signs, connect the patient to a cardiac monitor and obtain an electrocardiogram (ECG). Administer an antianginal and oxygen. If the patient has dyspnea, elevate the head of the bed. Then auscultate for abnormal breath sounds. If you detect coarse crackles, ensure patent I.V. access and give oxygen and diuretics as needed. If the patient has bradycardia, he may require atropine and a pacemaker.

HISTORY

When the patient's condition permits, ask about a history of hypertension, angina, valvular stenosis, or cardiomyopathy. If appropriate, have him describe the frequency and severity of anginal attacks.

PHYSICAL ASSESSMENT

First, take the patient's vital signs. Then perform a complete cardiopulmonary examination.

ASSESSMENT TIP

Locating heart sounds

When auscultating heart sounds, remember that certain sounds are heard best in specific areas. Use the auscultatory points shown below to locate heart sounds quickly and accurately. Then expand your auscultation to nearby areas. Note that the numbers indicate pertinent intercostal spaces.

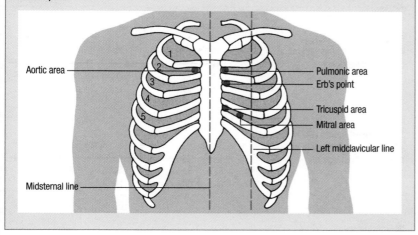

Aortic area

Pulmonic area
Erb's point

Tricuspid area
Mitral area

Left midclavicular line

Midsternal line

MEDICAL CAUSES

Anemia

In anemia, an atrial gallop may accompany increased cardiac output. Associated findings may include fatigue, pallor, dyspnea, tachycardia, bounding pulse, crackles, and a systolic bruit over the carotid arteries.

Angina

An intermittent atrial gallop characteristically occurs during an anginal attack and disappears when angina subsides. This gallop may be accompanied by a paradoxical S_2 or a new murmur. Typically, the patient complains of a feeling of tightness, pressure, aching, or burning that usually radiates from the retrosternal area to the neck, jaws, left shoulder, and arm. He may also exhibit dyspnea, tachycardia, palpitations, increased blood pressure, dizziness, diaphoresis, belching, nausea, and vomiting.

Aortic insufficiency (acute)

Acute aortic insufficiency causes an atrial gallop accompanied by a soft, short diastolic murmur along the left sternal border. S_2 may be soft or absent. Sometimes a soft, short midsystolic murmur may be heard over the second right intercostal space. Related cardiopulmonary findings may include tachycardia, S_3, dyspnea, jugular vein distention, crackles and, possibly, angina. The patient may also be fatigued and have cool extremities.

Aortic stenosis

Aortic stenosis usually causes an atrial gallop, especially when valvular obstruction is severe. Auscultation reveals a harsh, crescendo-decrescendo, systolic ejection murmur that's loudest at the right sternal border near the second intercostal space.

Medical causes

Anemia

✦ An atrial gallop may accompany increased cardiac output.
✦ Other findings may include fatigue, pallor, dyspnea, tachycardia, a bounding pulse, crackles, and a systolic bruit over the carotid arteries.

Angina

✦ An intermittent atrial gallop typically occurs during an attack and disappears when angina subsides.
✦ The gallop may be accompanied by paradoxical S_2 or new murmur.

Aortic insufficiency (acute)

✦ Atrial gallop is accompanied by a soft, short diastolic murmur along the left sternal border.
✦ S_2 may be soft or absent.

Aortic stenosis

✦ Atrial gallop occurs with severe valvular obstruction.
✦ Auscultation reveals a harsh, crescendo-decrescendo, systolic ejection murmur.

ASSESSMENT TIP

Interpreting heart sounds

Detecting subtle variations in heart sounds requires both concentration and practice. After you recognize normal heart sounds, the abnormal sounds become more obvious. To improve your ability to hear heart sounds, be sure to auscultate in a quiet environment.

HEART SOUND AND CAUSE	TIMING AND CADENCE
First heart sound (S_1) Vibrations associated with mitral and tricuspid valve closure	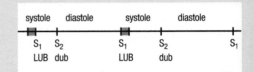
Second heart sound (S_2) Vibrations associated with aortic and pulmonic valve closure	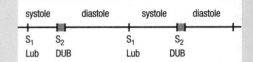
Ventricular gallop (S_3) Vibrations produced by rapid blood flow into the ventricles	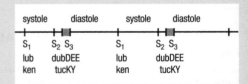
Atrial gallop (S_4) Vibrations produced by an increased resistance to sudden, forceful ejection of atrial blood	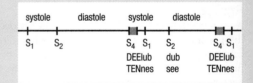
Summation gallop Vibrations produced in middiastole by simultaneous ventricular and atrial gallops, usually caused by tachycardia	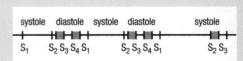

Medical causes
(continued)

AV block
- First-degree AV block may cause an atrial gallop accompanied by a faint S_1.
- Second-degree AV block produces an atrial gallop that's easily heard.
- Third-degree AV block produces an atrial gallop that varies in intensity with S_1.

Dyspnea, anginal chest pain, and syncope are cardinal associated findings. The patient may also display crackles, palpitations, fatigue, and diminished carotid pulses.

Atrioventricular block
First-degree atrioventricular (AV) block may cause an atrial gallop accompanied by a faint first heart sound (S_1). Although the patient may have bradycardia, he's usu-

AUSCULTATION TIPS

Best heard with the diaphragm of the stethoscope at the apex (mitral area)

Best heard with the diaphragm of the stethoscope in the second or third right and left parasternal intercostal spaces with the patient sitting or in a supine position

Best heard through the bell of the stethoscope at the apex with the patient in the left lateral position; may be visible and palpable during early diastole at the midclavicular line between the fourth and fifth intercostal spaces; have the patient cough or raise his legs to augment the sound

Best heard through the bell of the stethoscope at the apex with the patient in the left semilateral position; may be visible in late diastole at the midclavicular line between the fourth and fifth intercostal spaces; may also be palpable in the midclavicular area with the patient in the left lateral decubitus position

Best heard through the bell of the stethoscope at the apex with the patient in the left lateral position; may be louder than S_1 or S_2; may be visible and palpable during diastole

ally asymptomatic. In second-degree AV block, an atrial gallop is easily heard. If bradycardia develops, the patient may also experience hypotension, light-headedness, dizziness, and fatigue. An atrial gallop is also common in third-degree AV block. It varies in intensity with S_1 and is loudest when atrial systole coincides with early, rapid ventricular filling during diastole. The patient may be asymptomatic or have hypotension, light-headedness, dizziness, or syncope, depending on the ven-

Medical causes
(continued)
Cardiomyopathy
+ Atrial gallop occurs along with dyspnea, orthopnea, crackles, fatigue, syncope, chest pain, palpitations, edema, jugular vein distention, S_3, and transient or sustained bradycardia.

Hypertension
+ Atrial gallop is an early sign of systemic arterial hypertension.

Mitral insufficiency
+ Atrial gallop may be accompanied by an S_3.

Myocardial infarction
+ Atrial gallop signifies a life-threatening myocardial infarction and may persist after the infarction heals.

Pulmonary embolism
+ Right-sided atrial gallop is usually heard along the lower left sternal border with a loud pulmonic closure sound.

Thyrotoxicosis
+ Atrial gallop and S_3 may be auscultated.

Special considerations
+ Prepare patient for diagnostic tests.

Peds points
+ Atrial gallop may occur normally in children, especially after exercise, or it may result from congenital heart disease.

tricular rate. Bradycardia may also aggravate or provoke angina or symptoms of heart failure such as dyspnea.

Cardiomyopathy
An atrial gallop is a sign associated with cardiomyopathy, regardless of the type—dilated (most common), hypertrophic, or restrictive (least common). Additional findings may include dyspnea, orthopnea, crackles, fatigue, syncope, chest pain, palpitations, edema, jugular vein distention, S_3, and transient or sustained bradycardia usually associated with tachycardia.

Hypertension
One of the earliest findings in systemic arterial hypertension is an atrial gallop. The patient may be asymptomatic, or he may experience headache, weakness, epistaxis, tinnitus, dizziness, and fatigue.

Mitral insufficiency
In acute mitral insufficiency, auscultation may reveal an atrial gallop accompanied by an S_3, a harsh holosystolic murmur that's heard best at the apex or over the precordium. This murmur radiates to the axilla and back and along the left sternal border. Other features may include fatigue, dyspnea, tachypnea, orthopnea, tachycardia, crackles, and jugular vein distention.

Myocardial infarction
An atrial gallop is a classic sign of life-threatening myocardial infarction; in fact, it may persist even after the infarction heals. Typically, the patient reports crushing substernal chest pain that may radiate to the back, neck, jaw, shoulder, and left arm. Associated signs and symptoms include dyspnea, restlessness, anxiety, a feeling of impending doom, diaphoresis, pallor, clammy skin, nausea, vomiting, and increased or decreased blood pressure.

Pulmonary embolism
Pulmonary embolism—a life-threatening disorder—causes a right-sided atrial gallop that's usually heard along the lower left sternal border with a loud pulmonic closure sound. Other features of pulmonary embolism include tachycardia, tachypnea, fever, chest pain, dyspnea, decreased breath sounds, crackles, a pleural chest rub, apprehension, diaphoresis, syncope, and cyanosis. The patient may have a productive cough with blood-tinged sputum or a nonproductive cough.

Thyrotoxicosis
An atrial gallop and an S_3 may both be auscultated in thyroid hormone overproduction (thyrotoxicosis). Other cardinal features of thyrotoxicosis include tachycardia, bounding pulse, wide pulse pressure, palpitations, weight loss despite increased appetite, diarrhea, tremors, an enlarged thyroid, dyspnea, nervousness, difficulty concentrating, diaphoresis, heat intolerance, exophthalmos, weakness, fatigue, and muscle atrophy.

SPECIAL CONSIDERATIONS
Prepare the patient for diagnostic tests, such as ECG, echocardiography, cardiac catheterization, laboratory tests such as CK-MB and, possibly, a lung scan.

PEDIATRIC POINTERS
An atrial gallop may occur normally in children, especially after exercise. However, it may also result from congenital heart diseases, such as atrial septal defect, ven-

tricular septal defect, patent ductus arteriosus, and severe pulmonary valvular stenosis.

GERIATRIC POINTERS

Because the absolute intensity of an atrial gallop doesn't decrease with age, as it does with an S_1, the relative intensity of S_4 increases compared with S_1. This explains the increased frequency of an audible S_4 in elderly patients as well as why this sound may be considered a normal finding in elderly patients.

PATIENT COUNSELING

Instruct the patient on ways to reduce cardiac risk factors through diet, exercise, weight loss, smoking cessation, and stress reduction. Show the patient how to take his pulse. Tell him to call his physician or seek medical attention for high, low, or irregular heart rates. Explain the importance of keeping all follow-up appointments.

GALLOP, VENTRICULAR

A ventricular gallop is a heart sound (known as S_3) that's associated with rapid ventricular filling in early diastole. Usually palpable, this low-frequency sound occurs about 0.15 second after the second heart sound (S_2). It may originate in either the left or the right ventricle. A right-sided ventricular gallop usually sounds louder on inspiration and is heard best along the lower left sternal border or over the xiphoid region. A left-sided gallop usually sounds louder on expiration and is heard best at the apex.

A physiologic ventricular gallop normally occurs in children and adults younger than age 40; however, most people lose this third heart sound by age 40. This gallop may also occur during the third trimester of pregnancy. Abnormal S_3 in adults older than age 40 can be a sign of decreased myocardial contractility, myocardial failure, and volume overload of the ventricle, as in mitral and tricuspid valve insufficiency. Although the physiologic S_3 has the same timing as the pathologic S_3, its intensity waxes and wanes with respiration. It's also heard more faintly if the patient is sitting or standing.

A pathologic ventricular gallop may be one of the earliest signs of ventricular failure. It may result from one of two mechanisms: rapid deceleration of blood entering a stiff, noncompliant ventricle or rapid acceleration of blood associated with increased flow into the ventricle. A gallop that persists despite therapy indicates a poor prognosis. (See *Associated disorder: Heart failure,* page 304.)

Patients with cardiomyopathy or heart failure may develop both a ventricular gallop and an atrial gallop—a condition known as a *summation gallop.*

HISTORY

Begin the history by asking the patient if he has had any chest pain. If so, have him describe its character, location, frequency, duration, and any alleviating or aggravating factors. Also ask about palpitations, dizziness, or syncope. Does the patient have difficulty breathing after exertion? While lying down? At rest? Does he have a cough? Ask about a history of cardiac disorders. Is the patient currently receiving any treatment for heart failure? If so, which medications is he taking?

Geri points
+ Atrial gallop may be considered a normal finding in elderly patients.

Teaching points
+ Cardiac risk factor reduction
+ Pulse measurement
+ Conditions that require medical attention
+ Importance of follow-up appointments

Key facts about ventricular gallop
+ Refers to an S_3 that occurs about 0.15 second after the S_2
+ May be physiologic or pathologic
+ Best heard along the lower left sternal border or over the xiphoid region on inspiration (right-sided) or at the apex on expiration (left-sided)

Key history points
+ Character, location, frequency, and duration of chest pain (if present)
+ Associated palpitations, dizziness, syncope, difficulty breathing, or cough
+ History of cardiac disorders
+ Drug history

Key facts about heart failure

- ✦ Occurs when the heart can't pump enough blood for the body's metabolic needs
- ✦ Results in intravascular and interstitial volume overload and poor tissue perfusion

Causes

- ✦ Abnormal cardiac muscle function (MI, cardiomyopathy)
- ✦ Abnormal left ventricular volume (valvular insufficiency, high-output states)
- ✦ Abnormal left ventricular pressure (hypertension, pulmonary hypertension, COPD, aortic or pulmonic valve stenosis)
- ✦ Abnormal left ventricular filling (mitral or tricuspid valve stenosis, atrial myxoma, constrictive pericarditis, atrial fibrillation, impaired ventricular relaxation)

Management

- ✦ Treatment of the underlying cause, if known
- ✦ ACE inhibitors, digoxin, beta-adrenergic blockers, diuretics, nitrates, morphine, and oxygen
- ✦ Lifestyle modifications
- ✦ Coronary artery bypass surgery or angioplasty for heart failure due to CAD
- ✦ Heart transplantation
- ✦ Other procedures, such as cardiomyoplasty, intra-aortic balloon pump, partial left ventriculectomy, mechanical ventricular assist device, and implantation of an ICD or biventricular pacemaker

ASSOCIATED DISORDER

Heart failure

A syndrome rather than a disease, heart failure occurs when the heart can't pump enough blood to meet the metabolic needs of the body. Heart failure results in intravascular and interstitial volume overload and poor tissue perfusion. An individual with heart failure experiences reduced exercise tolerance, reduced quality of life, and a shortened life span.

Although the most common cause of heart failure is coronary artery disease, it also results from congenital and acquired heart defects. The incidence of heart failure rises with age: Approximately 1% of people older than age 50 experience heart failure; it occurs in 10% of people older than age 80. About 700,000 Americans die of heart failure each year. Mortality from heart failure is greater for males, blacks, and elderly people.

CAUSES

Causes of heart failure may be divided into four general categories.

Abnormal cardiac muscle function
- ✦ Myocardial infarction
- ✦ Cardiomyopathy

Abnormal left ventricular volume
- ✦ Valvular insufficiency
- ✦ High-output states, such as chronic anemia, arteriovenous fistula, thyrotoxicosis, pregnancy, septicemia, beriberi, and the infusion of large volume of I.V. fluids in a short time

Abnormal left ventricular pressure
- ✦ Hypertension
- ✦ Pulmonary hypertension
- ✦ Chronic obstructive pulmonary disease
- ✦ Aortic or pulmonic valve stenosis

Abnormal left ventricular filling
- ✦ Mitral or tricuspid valve stenosis
- ✦ Atrial myxoma
- ✦ Constrictive pericarditis
- ✦ Atrial fibrillation
- ✦ Impaired ventricular relaxation, such as hypertension, myocardial hibernation, and myocardial stunning

DIAGNOSIS

The following tests are used to help diagnose heart failure:
- ✦ Chest X-rays show increased pulmonary vascular markings, interstitial edema, or pleural effusion and cardiomegaly.
- ✦ Electrocardiography may indicate hypertrophy, ischemic changes, or infarction and may also reveal tachycardia and extrasystoles.
- ✦ Laboratory testing may reveal abnormal liver function tests and elevated blood urea nitrogen and creatinine levels.
- ✦ Echocardiography may reveal left ventricular hypertrophy, dilation, and abnormal contractility.
- ✦ Pulmonary artery monitoring typically demonstrates elevated pulmonary artery and pulmonary artery wedge pressures, left ventricular end-diastolic pressure in left-sided heart failure, and elevated right atrial pressure or central venous pressure in right-sided heart failure.
- ✦ Radionuclide ventriculography may reveal an ejection fraction less than 40%; in diastolic dysfunction, the ejection fraction may be normal.

MEDICAL INTERVENTIONS

Correction of heart failure may involve:
- ✦ treatment of the underlying cause, if known
- ✦ angiotensin-converting enzyme inhibitors for patients with left ventricular dysfunction (to reduce production of angiotensin II, resulting in preload and afterload reduction)
- ✦ digoxin for patients with heart failure due to left ventricular systolic dysfunction to increase myocardial contractility, improve cardiac output, reduce the volume of the ventricle, and decrease ventricular strength
- ✦ diuretics to reduce fluid volume overload and venous return
- ✦ beta-adrenergic blockers in patients with New York Heart Association class II or class III heart failure caused by left ventricular systolic dysfunction to prevent remodeling

Heart failure *(continued)*

- ◆ diuretics, nitrates, morphine, and oxygen to treat pulmonary edema
- ◆ lifestyle modifications to reduce symptoms of heart failure, including weight loss (if obese), limited sodium (to 3 g/day) and alcohol intake, reduced fat intake, smoking cessation (if applicable), stress-reduction techniques, and exercise program development
- ◆ coronary artery bypass surgery or angioplasty for heart failure due to coronary artery disease

- ◆ heart transplantation in patients receiving aggressive medical treatment but still experiencing limitations or repeated hospitalizations
- ◆ other procedures (may be recommended in patients with severe limitations or repeated hospitalizations, despite maximal medical therapy, such as cardiomyoplasty, intra-aortic balloon pump, partial left ventriculectomy, mechanical ventricular assist device, and implantation of an implantable cardioverter-defibrillator or biventricular pacemaker).

PHYSICAL ASSESSMENT

During the physical examination, carefully auscultate for murmurs or abnormalities in the first and second heart sounds. Then listen for pulmonary crackles. Next, assess peripheral pulses, noting an alternating strong and weak pulse. Finally, palpate the liver to detect enlargement or tenderness, and assess for jugular vein distention and peripheral edema. (See *Auscultating the heart,* page 306.)

MEDICAL CAUSES

Aortic insufficiency

Acute and chronic aortic insufficiency may produce an S_3. Typically, acute aortic insufficiency also causes an atrial gallop and a soft, short diastolic murmur over the left sternal border. S_2 may be soft or absent. At times, a soft, short midsystolic murmur may be heard over the second right intercostal space. Related findings include tachycardia, dyspnea, jugular vein distention, and crackles.

Chronic aortic insufficiency produces a ventricular gallop and a high-pitched, blowing, decrescendo diastolic murmur that's best heard over the second or third right intercostal space or the left sternal border. An Austin Flint murmur — an apical, rumbling, mid-diastolic to late-diastolic murmur — may also occur. Typical related findings include palpitations, tachycardia, anginal chest pain, fatigue, dyspnea, orthopnea, and crackles.

Cardiomyopathy

A ventricular gallop is characteristic of cardiomyopathy. When accompanied by an alternating pulse and altered first and second heart sounds, this gallop usually signals advanced heart disease. Other effects may include fatigue, dyspnea, orthopnea, chest pain, palpitations, syncope, crackles, peripheral edema, jugular vein distention, and an atrial gallop.

Heart failure

Ventricular gallop is a cardinal sign of heart failure. When it's loud and accompanied by sinus tachycardia, this gallop may indicate severe heart failure. The patient with left-sided heart failure also exhibits fatigue, exertional dyspnea, paroxysmal nocturnal dyspnea, orthopnea and, possibly, a dry cough; with right-sided heart failure, jugular vein distention occurs. Other late features include tachypnea, chest tightness, palpitations, anorexia, nausea, dependent edema, weight gain, slowed

Auscultating the heart

Follow these tips when you auscultate a patient's heart:

♦ Concentrate as you listen for each sound.
♦ Avoid auscultating through clothing or wound dressings because they can block sound.
♦ Avoid picking up extraneous sounds by keeping the stethoscope tubing off the patient's body and other surfaces.

♦ Until you become proficient at auscultation and can examine a patient quickly, explain to him that even though you may listen to his chest for a long period, it doesn't mean that anything is wrong.
♦ Ask the patient to breathe normally and to hold his breath periodically to enhance sounds that may be difficult to hear.

Medical causes
(continued)

Mitral insufficiency

♦ In acute cases, ventricular gallop may be accompanied by an early or holosystolic decrescendo murmur at the apex, an atrial gallop, and a widely split second heart sound.
♦ In chronic cases, ventricular gallop is progressively severe.

Thyrotoxicosis

♦ Ventricular and atrial gallops may occur.

Special considerations

♦ Watch for and report tachycardia, dyspnea, crackles, and jugular vein distention.
♦ Give oxygen, diuretics, and other drugs, such as digoxin and ACE inhibitors, to prevent pulmonary edema.

Peds points

♦ Ventricular gallop is normally heard in children but may accompany congenital abnormalities associated with heart failure or result from sickle cell anemia.

mental response, diaphoresis, pallor, hypotension, narrowed pulse pressure and, possibly, oliguria. In some patients, inspiratory crackles, clubbing, and a tender, palpable liver may also be present. As heart failure progresses, hemoptysis, cyanosis, severe pitting edema, and marked hepatomegaly may develop.

Mitral insufficiency

In acute mitral insufficiency, auscultation reveals a ventricular gallop and, possibly, an early or holosystolic decrescendo murmur at the apex, an atrial gallop, and a widely split second heart sound. Typically, the patient displays sinus tachycardia, tachypnea, orthopnea, dyspnea, crackles, distended jugular veins, and fatigue.

In chronic mitral insufficiency, a progressively severe ventricular gallop is typical. Auscultation also reveals a holosystolic, blowing, high-pitched apical murmur. The patient may report fatigue, exertional dyspnea, and palpitations, or he may be asymptomatic.

Thyrotoxicosis

Thyrotoxicosis may produce ventricular and atrial gallops, but its cardinal features are an enlarged thyroid gland, weight loss despite increased appetite, heat intolerance, diaphoresis, nervousness, tremors, tachycardia, palpitations, diarrhea, and dyspnea.

SPECIAL CONSIDERATIONS

Monitor the patient with a ventricular gallop; watch for and report tachycardia, dyspnea, crackles, and jugular vein distention. Give oxygen, diuretics, and other drugs, such as digoxin and angiotensin-converting enzyme inhibitors, to prevent pulmonary edema. Prepare the patient for electrocardiography, echocardiography, gated blood pool imaging, and cardiac catheterization.

PEDIATRIC POINTERS

A ventricular gallop is normally heard in children. However, it may accompany congenital abnormalities associated with heart failure, such as a large ventricular septal defect and patent ductus arteriosus. It may also result from sickle cell anemia. This gallop must be correlated with the patient's associated signs and symptoms to be of diagnostic value.

PATIENT COUNSELING

Discuss dietary and fluid restrictions with the patient. Encourage him to incorporate rest into his daily routine. Teach him to recognize and report signs and symptoms of fluid overload. Have him take his weight daily and report an increase of 3 lb (1.36 kg) or more.

GENITAL LESIONS IN THE MALE

Among the diverse lesions that may affect the male genitalia are warts, papules, ulcers, scales, and pustules. These common lesions may be painful or painless, singular or multiple. They may be limited to the genitalia or may also occur elsewhere on the body. (See *Recognizing common male genital lesions,* page 308.)

Genital lesions may result from infection, neoplasms, parasites, allergy, or drug use. These lesions can profoundly affect the patient's self-image and relationships. In fact, the patient may hesitate to seek medical attention because he fears cancer or a sexually transmitted disease (STD).

Genital lesions that arise from an STD could mean that the patient is at risk for other STDs, such as human immunodeficiency virus (HIV). Genital ulcers make HIV transmission between sexual partners more likely.

HISTORY

Begin by asking the patient when he first noticed the lesion. Did it erupt after he began taking a new drug or after a trip out of the country? Has he had similar lesions before? If so, did he get medical treatment for them? Find out if he has been treating the lesion himself. If so, how? Does the lesion itch? If so, is the itching constant or does it bother him only at night? Note whether the lesion is painful. Ask for a description of any drainage from the lesions. Next, take a complete sexual history, noting the frequency of relations, number of sexual partners, and pattern of condom use.

PHYSICAL ASSESSMENT

Before you examine the patient, observe his clothing. Do his pants fit properly? Tight pants or underwear, especially those made of nonabsorbent fabrics, can promote the growth of bacteria and fungi. Examine the entire skin surface, noting the location, size, color, and pattern of the lesions. Do genital lesions resemble lesions on other parts of the body? Palpate for nodules, masses, and tenderness. Also, look for bleeding, edema, or signs of infection, such as purulent drainage or erythema. Finally, take the patient's vital signs.

MEDICAL CAUSES

Balanitis and balanoposthitis

Typically, balanitis (glans infection) and posthitis (prepuce infection) occur together (balanoposthitis), causing painful ulceration on the glans, foreskin, or penile shaft. Ulceration is usually preceded by 2 to 3 days of prepuce irritation and soreness, followed by a foul discharge and edema. The patient may then develop features of acute infection, such as fever with chills, malaise, and dysuria. Without treatment, the ulcers may deepen and multiply. Eventually, the entire penis and scrotum may become gangrenous, resulting in life-threatening sepsis.

Teaching points
+ Dietary and fluid restrictions
+ Scheduled rest periods
+ Signs and symptoms of fluid overload to report
+ Daily weight

Key facts about genital lesions in males
+ Include warts, papules, ulcers, scales, and pustules
+ May be painful or painless, singular or multiple
+ May result from infection, neoplasms, parasites, allergy, or drugs

Key history points
+ Onset and description of lesions
+ Description of associated drainage, itching, or pain
+ Sexual history, including frequency of relations, number of sexual partners, and pattern of condom use

Critical assessment steps
+ Observe patient for tight clothing.
+ Examine the skin, noting location, size, color, and pattern of lesions.
+ Palpate for nodules, masses, and tenderness.
+ Look for bleeding, edema, or signs of infection.
+ Take vital signs.

Medical causes
Balanitis and balanoposthitis
+ Painful ulceration on the glans, foreskin, or penile shaft occurs.

Recognizing common male genital lesions

Various lesions may affect the male genitalia. Some of the more common lesions and their causes appear below.

A **fixed drug eruption** causes a bright red to purplish lesion on the glans penis.

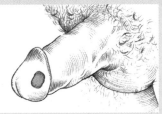

Genital warts are marked by clusters of flesh-colored papillary growths that may be barely visible or several inches in diameter.

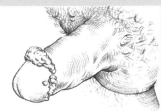

Genital herpes begins as a swollen, slightly pruritic wheal and later becomes a group of small vesicles or blisters on the foreskin, glans, or penile shaft.

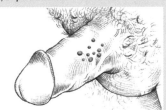

Tinea cruris (commonly known as "jock itch") produces itchy patches of well-defined, slightly raised, scaly lesions that usually affect the inner thighs and groin.

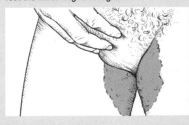

A **chancroid** causes a painful ulcer that's usually less than ¾" (2 cm) in diameter and bleeds easily. The lesion may be deep and covered by a gray or yellow exudate at its base.

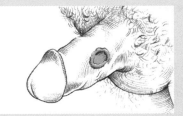

Medical causes
(continued)

Bowen's disease
✦ Painless, premalignant lesion that appears as a brownish red, raised, scaly, indurated plaque with well-defined borders that commonly occurs on penis or scrotum

Candidiasis
✦ Erythematous, weepy, circumscribed lesions usually appear under the prepuce.

Bowen's disease
Bowen's disease, a painless, premalignant lesion, commonly occurs on the penis or scrotum but may also appear elsewhere. It appears as a brownish red, raised, scaly, indurated plaque with well-defined borders, which may ulcerate at its center. When lesions appear on the glans penis, it's called *Queyrat's erythroplasia.*

Candidiasis
When candidiasis involves the anogenital area, it produces erythematous, weepy, circumscribed lesions that usually appear under the prepuce. Vesicles and pustules may also develop.

Chancroid

Chancroid is an STD that's characterized by the eruption of one or more lesions, usually on the groin, inner thigh, or penis. Within 24 hours, the lesion changes from a reddened area to a small papule. (A similar papule may erupt on the tongue, lip, breast, or umbilicus.) It then becomes an inflamed pustule that rapidly ulcerates. This painful—and usually deep—ulcer bleeds easily and often has a purulent gray or yellow exudate covering its base. Rarely more than ¾″ (2 cm) in diameter, it's typically irregular in shape. The inguinal lymph nodes also enlarge, become very tender, and may drain pus.

Folliculitis and furunculosis

Folliculitis (hair follicle infection) may cause red, sharply pointed lesions that are tender and swollen with central pustules. If folliculitis progresses to furunculosis, these lesions become hard, painful nodules that may gradually enlarge and rupture, discharging pus and necrotic material. Rupture relieves the pain, but erythema and edema may persist for days or weeks.

Genital herpes

An STD, genital herpes produces fluid-filled vesicles on the glans penis, foreskin, or penile shaft and, occasionally, on the mouth or anus. Usually painless at first, these vesicles may rupture and become extensive, shallow, painful ulcers accompanied by redness, marked edema, and tender, inguinal lymph nodes. Other findings may include fever, malaise, and dysuria. If the vesicles recur in the same area, the patient usually feels localized numbness and tingling before they erupt. Associated inflammation is typically less marked.

Genital warts

Most common in sexually active males, genital warts initially develop on the subpreputial sac or urethral meatus (less commonly, on the penile shaft); they then spread to the perineum and the perianal area. These painless warts start as tiny red or pink swellings that may grow to 4″ (10.2 cm) and become pedunculated. Multiple swellings are common, giving the warts a cauliflower appearance. Infected warts are also malodorous.

Lichen planus

With lichen planus, small, polygonal, violet papules develop on the glans penis. These papules are shiny and less than 1¼″ (3.2 cm) in diameter and have white, lacy, milky striations. They may be linear or coalesce into plaques. Occasionally, oral lesions precede genital lesions. Also, lesions may affect the lower back, ankles, and lower legs. Accompanying findings may include pruritus, distorted nails, and alopecia.

Pediculosis pubis

Pediculosis pubis, a parasitic infestation, is characterized by erythematous, itching papules in the pubic area and around the anus, abdomen, and thigh. Inspection may detect grayish white specks (lice eggs) attached to hair shafts. Skin irritation from scratching in these areas is common.

Psoriasis

With psoriasis, red, raised, scaly plaques typically affect the scalp, chest, knees, elbows, and lower back. When they occur on the groin or on the shaft and glans of the penis, the plaques are usually redder; on an uncircumcised penis, the characteristic silver scales are absent. The patient commonly reports itching; pain from dry, cracked, encrusted lesions occasionally occurs. Nail pitting and joint stiffness may also occur.

Medical causes
(continued)

Chancroid
+ One or more lesions erupt on the groin, inner thigh, or penis.
+ Lesions progress from a reddened area to a small papule, then to pustule that ulcerates.

Folliculitis and furunculosis
+ Folliculitis may cause red, pointed lesions that are tender and swollen with central pustules.
+ If folliculitis progresses to furunculosis, lesions become hard, painful nodules that may enlarge and rupture.

Genital herpes
+ Fluid-filled vesicles develop on glans penis, foreskin, or shaft.
+ Vesicles are painless at first but may rupture into ulcers.

Genital warts
+ Tiny red or pink swellings develop on subpreputial sac or urethral meatus and spread to perineum and perianal area.
+ Warts may grow and become pedunculated.

Lichen planus
+ Small, shiny, polygonal, violet papules with white, lacy, striations develop on glans penis.
+ Papules may be linear or coalesce into plaques.

Pediculosis pubis
+ Erythematous, itching papules develop in pubic area and around anus, abdomen, and thigh.

Psoriasis
+ Red, raised, scaly plaques develop.

Medical causes
(continued)

Scabies
+ Mites under the skin cause crusted lesions or large papules on the glans and shaft of the penis and on the scrotum.

Seborrheic dermatitis
+ Erythematous, dry or moist scaling papules, and yellow crusts that form annular plaques develop on shaft of penis, scrotum, groin, scalp, chest, eyebrows, back, axillae, and umbilicus.

Syphilis
+ Small, red, fluid-filled chancres may erupt on the genitalia.
+ Chancres erode to form painless, firm, indurated, shallow ulcer with clear base and scant, yellow serous discharge.

Tinea cruris
+ Sharply defined, slightly raised, scaling patches typically develop on the inner thigh or groin.

Urticaria
+ Pruritic hives may appear on genitalia, especially on foreskin or shaft of penis.

Other causes
+ Phenolphthalein
+ Barbiturates
+ Certain broad-spectrum antibiotics

Special considerations
+ Expect to screen every patient with penile lesions for STDs.
+ Provide emotional support, especially if cancer is suspected.

Scabies
Scabies are mites that burrow under the skin and may cause crusted lesions or large papules on the glans and shaft of the penis and on the scrotum. Lesions may also occur on the wrists, elbows, axillae, and waist. They're usually raised, threadlike, ⅜" to 4" (1 to 10 cm) long, and have a swollen nodule or red papule that contains the mite. Nocturnal itching is typical and commonly causes excoriation.

Seborrheic dermatitis
Initially, seborrheic dermatitis causes erythematous, dry or moist greasy scaling papules, and yellow crusts that enlarge to form annular plaques. These itchy plaques may affect the glans and shaft of the penis, scrotum, and groin as well as the scalp, chest, eyebrows, back, axillae, and umbilicus.

Syphilis
Two to four weeks after exposure to the spirochete *Treponema pallidum* (syphilis), one or more primary lesions, or chancres, may erupt on the genitalia; occasionally, they also erupt elsewhere on the body, typically on the mouth or perianal area. The chancre usually starts as a small, red, fluid-filled papule and then erodes to form a painless, firm, indurated, shallow ulcer with a clear base and a scant, yellow serous discharge or, less commonly, a hard papule. This lesion gradually involutes and disappears. Painless, unilateral regional lymphadenopathy is also typical.

Tinea cruris
Also called *jock itch*, tinea cruris is a superficial fungal infection that usually causes sharply defined, slightly raised, scaling patches on the inner thigh or groin (often bilaterally) and, less commonly, on the scrotum and penis. Pruritus may be severe.

Urticaria
Urticaria is a common allergic reaction that's characterized by intensely pruritic hives, which may appear on the genitalia, especially on the foreskin or shaft of the penis. These distinct, raised, evanescent wheals are surrounded by an erythematous flare.

OTHER CAUSES

Drugs
Phenolphthalein, barbiturates, and certain broad-spectrum antibiotics, such as tetracycline and sulfonamides, may cause a fixed drug eruption and a genital lesion.

SPECIAL CONSIDERATIONS
Many disorders produce penile lesions that resemble those of syphilis. Expect to screen every patient with penile lesions for STDs, using the dark-field examination and the Venereal Disease Research Laboratory test. Provide emotional support, especially if cancer is suspected.

To prevent cross-contamination, wash your hands before and after every patient contact. Wear gloves when handling urine or performing catheter care. Dispose of all needles carefully, and double-bag all material contaminated by secretions.

PEDIATRIC POINTERS
In infants, contact dermatitis (also known as *diaper rash*) may produce minor irritation or bright red, weepy, excoriated lesions. Use of disposable diapers and careful cleaning of the penis and scrotum can help reduce diaper rash.

The spirochete that causes syphilis is able to pass through the human placenta, producing congenital syphilis.

In children, impetigo may cause pustules with thick, yellow, weepy crusts. Like adults, children may develop genital warts, but they'll need more reassurance that the treatment (excision) won't hurt or castrate them. Children with STDs must be evaluated for other signs of sexual abuse.

Adolescents ages 15 to 19 have a high incidence of STDs and related genital lesions.

GERIATRIC POINTERS

Elderly adults who are sexually active with multiple partners have as high a risk of developing STDs as do younger adults. However, because of decreased immunity, poor hygiene, poor symptom reporting and, possibly, several concurrent conditions, they may present with different symptoms. Seborrheic dermatitis lasts longer and is more extensive in bedridden patients and those with Parkinson's disease.

PATIENT COUNSELING

Explain to the patient how to use prescribed ointments or creams. Advise him to use a heat lamp to dry moist lesions or to take sitz baths to relieve crusting and itching. Also, instruct him to report any changes in the lesions.

Explain to male patients that condoms effectively prevent many STDs when used correctly. Advise them to use a new condom for each coitus; to avoid damaging the condom with sharp objects, such as fingernails or teeth; to put the condom on the erect penis before any genital contact; to use only water-based lubricants; to hold the condom firmly while withdrawing the penis; to always withdraw the penis while it's still erect to avoid premature condom loss; and to check the expiration date on the individual condom packet. Instruct the patient that hormonal contraceptives, diaphragms, foams, and jellies don't protect against STDs.

GUM BLEEDING

Bleeding gums, or gingival bleeding, usually result from dental disorders; less commonly, they may stem from a blood dyscrasia or the effects of certain drugs. Physiologic causes of this common sign include pregnancy, which can produce gum swelling in the first or second trimester (pregnancy epulis); atmospheric pressure changes, which usually affect divers and aviators; and oral trauma. Bleeding ranges from slight oozing to life-threatening hemorrhage. It may be spontaneous or may follow trauma. Occasionally, direct pressure can control it.

 EMERGENCY ACTIONS If you detect profuse, spontaneous bleeding in the oral cavity, quickly check airway patency and look for signs of cardiovascular collapse, such as tachycardia and hypotension. Suction the patient. Apply direct pressure to the bleeding site. Expect to insert an airway, administer I.V. fluids, and collect serum samples for diagnostic evaluation.

HISTORY

If gum bleeding isn't an emergency, obtain a history. Find out when the bleeding began. Has it been continuous or intermittent? Does it occur spontaneously or when the patient brushes his teeth or flosses? Have the patient show you the site of the bleeding, if possible.

Key history points

+ Onset and description
+ Personal or family history of bleeding tendencies
+ Dental history
+ History of liver or spleen disease
+ Diet and alcohol use
+ Drug history

Critical assessment steps

+ Have patient remove dentures, if applicable.
+ Examine the gums.
+ Check for inflammation, pockets around teeth, swelling, retraction, hypertrophy, discoloration, and gum hyperplasia.
+ Note obvious decay, discoloration, foreign material, and absence of any teeth.

Medical causes

Agranulocytosis

+ Spontaneous gum bleeding and other systemic hemorrhages may occur.

Aplastic anemia

+ Profuse or scant gum bleeding may follow trauma.

Cirrhosis

+ Gum bleeding, epistaxis, and other bleeding tendencies are late signs.

Gingivitis

+ Gingivae between the teeth become bulbous and bleed easily with slight trauma.
+ With acute necrotizing ulcerative gingivitis, bleeding is spontaneous.

Find out if the patient or any family members have bleeding tendencies; for example, ask about easy bruising and frequent nosebleeds. How much does the patient bleed after a tooth extraction? Does he have a history of liver or spleen disease? Next, check the patient's dental history. Find out how often he brushes his teeth, flosses, and goes to the dentist. Also ask the patient what kind of toothbrush and floss he uses. Has he seen a dentist recently? To evaluate nutritional status, have the patient describe his normal diet and intake of alcohol. Finally, note any prescription and over-the-counter drugs he takes.

PHYSICAL ASSESSMENT

Perform a complete oral examination. If the patient wears dentures, have him remove them. Examine the gums to determine the site and amount of bleeding. Gums normally appear pink and rippled with their margins snugly against the teeth. Check for inflammation, pockets around the teeth, swelling, retraction, hypertrophy, discoloration, and gum hyperplasia. Note obvious decay, discoloration, foreign material such as food, and the absence of any teeth.

MEDICAL CAUSES

Agranulocytosis

Spontaneous gum bleeding and other systemic hemorrhages may occur in agranulocytosis, a hematologic disorder that typically causes progressive fatigue and weakness. Bleeding may be followed by signs of infection, such as fever and chills. Inspection may reveal oral and perianal lesions, which are usually rough edged with a gray or black membrane.

Aplastic anemia

In aplastic anemia, profuse or scant gum bleeding may follow trauma. Other signs of bleeding, such as epistaxis and ecchymoses, are also characteristic. The patient exhibits progressive weakness and fatigue, shortness of breath, headache, pallor and, possibly, fever. Eventually, tachycardia and signs of heart failure, such as jugular vein distention and dyspnea, also develop.

Cirrhosis

A late sign of cirrhosis, gum bleeding occurs with epistaxis and other bleeding tendencies. Additional late effects include ascites, hepatomegaly, pruritus, and jaundice. Other signs and symptoms include abdominal pain, anorexia, fatigue, nausea, vomiting, and weakness.

Gingivitis

Reddened and edematous gums are characteristic of gingivitis. The gingivae between the teeth become bulbous and bleed easily with slight trauma. However, with acute necrotizing ulcerative gingivitis, bleeding is spontaneous and the gums become so painful that the patient may be unable to eat. A characteristic grayish yellow pseudomembrane develops over punched-out gum erosions. Offensive halitosis is typical and may be accompanied by headache, malaise, fever, and cervical adenopathy.

Hemophilia

In hemophilia, hemorrhage occurs from many sites in the oral cavity, especially the gums. Mild hemophilia causes easy bruising, hematomas, epistaxis, bleeding gums, and prolonged bleeding during even minor surgery and up to 8 days afterward. Moderate hemophilia produces more frequent episodes of abnormal bleeding and occasional bleeding into the joints, which may cause swelling and pain. Severe hemophilia causes spontaneous or severe bleeding after minor trauma, possibly resulting in large subcutaneous and intramuscular hematomas. Bleeding into joints and muscles causes pain, swelling, and extreme tenderness and may cause permanent deformity. Bleeding near peripheral nerves causes peripheral neuropathies, pain, paresthesia, and muscle atrophy. Signs of anemia and fever may follow bleeding. Severe blood loss may lead to shock and death.

Leukemia

Easy gum bleeding is an early sign of acute monocytic, lymphocytic, or myelocytic leukemia that's accompanied by gum swelling, necrosis, and petechiae. The soft, tender gums appear glossy and bluish. Acute leukemia causes severe prostration marked by high fever and bleeding tendencies, such as epistaxis and prolonged menses. It may also cause dyspnea, tachycardia, palpitations, and abdominal or bone pain. Later effects may include confusion, headaches, vomiting, seizures, papilledema, and nuchal rigidity.

Chronic leukemia usually develops insidiously, producing less-severe bleeding tendencies. Other effects may include anorexia, weight loss, low-grade fever, chills, skin eruptions, and enlarged spleen, tonsils, and lymph nodes. Signs of anemia, such as fatigue and pallor, may also occur.

Periodontal disease

Gum bleeding typically occurs after chewing, toothbrushing, or gum probing but may also occur spontaneously. As gingivae separate from the bone, pus-filled pockets develop around the teeth; occasionally, pus can be expressed. Other findings include unpleasant taste with halitosis, facial pain, loose teeth, and dental calculi and plaque.

Pernicious anemia

Gum bleeding and a sore tongue make eating painful for patients with pernicious anemia. Among other cardinal symptoms are weakness and paresthesia. The patient's lips, gums, and tongue appear markedly pale, and his sclera and skin are jaundiced. Other features are typically widespread, affecting the GI, cardiovascular, and central nervous systems, and include altered bowel and bladder habits, personality changes, ataxia, tinnitus, dyspnea, and tachycardia.

Polycythemia vera

In polycythemia vera, engorged gums ooze blood after even slight trauma. Polycythemia vera usually turns the oral mucosa—especially the gums and tongue—a deep red-violet. Among associated findings are headache, dyspnea, dizziness, fatigue, paresthesia, tinnitus, double or blurred vision, aquagenic pruritus, epigastric distress, weight loss, increased blood pressure, ruddy cyanosis, ecchymosis, and hepatosplenomegaly.

Thrombocytopenia

With thrombocytopenia, blood usually oozes between the teeth and gums; however, severe bleeding may follow minor trauma. Associated signs of hemorrhage include large blood-filled bullae in the mouth, petechiae, ecchymosis, epistaxis, and hematuria. Malaise, fatigue, weakness, and lethargy eventually develop.

Thrombocytopenic purpura (idiopathic)

Profuse gum bleeding occurs in idiopathic thrombocytopenic purpura. Its classic feature, though, is spontaneous hemorrhagic skin lesions that range from pinpoint petechiae to massive hemorrhages. The patient has a tendency to bruise easily, develops petechiae on the oral mucosa, and may exhibit melena, epistaxis, or hematuria.

Medical causes
(continued)

Hemophilia
✦ Mild hemophilia causes easy bruising, hematomas, epistaxis, bleeding gums, and prolonged bleeding during and after surgery.

Leukemia
✦ Easy gum bleeding is an early sign of acute monocytic, lymphocytic, or myelocytic leukemia; it's accompanied by gum swelling, necrosis, and petechiae.

Periodontal disease
✦ Gum bleeding typically occurs after chewing, toothbrushing, or gum probing but may also occur spontaneously.

Pernicious anemia
✦ Gum bleeding and a sore tongue make eating painful.

Polycythemia vera
✦ Engorged gums ooze blood after even slight trauma.
✦ The gums and tongue are a deep red-violet.

Thrombocytopenia
✦ Blood usually oozes between the teeth and gums.
✦ Severe bleeding may follow minor trauma.

Thrombocytopenic purpura (idiopathic)
✦ Profuse gum bleeding occurs.
✦ Spontaneous hemorrhagic skin lesions range from pinpoint petechiae to massive hemorrhages.

Medical causes
(continued)
Vitamin K deficiency
✦ Gums bleed when the teeth are brushed.

Other causes
✦ Abuse of aspirin and NSAIDs
✦ Heparin
✦ Occupational exposure to benzene
✦ Warfarin

Special considerations
✦ Prepare the patient for the possibility of a blood or blood product transfusion, if necessary.
✦ When providing mouth care, avoid using lemon-glycerin swabs, which may burn or dry the gums.

Peds points
✦ In neonates, bleeding gums may result from vitamin K deficiency.
✦ In infants who primarily drink cow's milk and don't receive vitamin supplements, bleeding gums can result from vitamin C deficiency.

Geri points
✦ In patients who have no teeth, constant gum trauma and bleeding may result from using a dental prosthesis.

Teaching points
✦ Proper mouth and gum care
✦ Situations that require medical attention

Vitamin K deficiency
The first sign of vitamin K deficiency is usually gums that bleed when the teeth are brushed. Other signs of abnormal bleeding, such as ecchymosis, epistaxis, and hematuria, may also occur. GI bleeding may produce hematemesis and melena; intracranial bleeding may cause decreased level of consciousness and focal neurologic deficits.

OTHER CAUSES
Chemical irritants
Occupational exposure to benzene may irritate the gums, resulting in bleeding. Other signs of abnormal bleeding may accompany limb weakness and sensory changes.

Drugs
Warfarin and heparin interfere with blood clotting and may cause prolonged gum bleeding. Abuse of aspirin and nonsteroidal anti-inflammatory drugs may alter platelets, producing bleeding gums. Localized gum bleeding may also occur with mucosal "aspirin burn" caused by dissolving aspirin near an aching tooth.

SPECIAL CONSIDERATIONS
Prepare the patient for diagnostic tests, such as blood studies or facial X-rays. Prepare him for the possibility of a blood or blood product (platelets or fresh frozen plasma) transfusion, if necessary. When providing mouth care, avoid using lemon-glycerin swabs, which may burn or dry the gums.

PEDIATRIC POINTERS
In neonates, bleeding gums may result from vitamin K deficiency associated with a lack of normal intestinal flora or poor maternal nutrition. In infants who primarily drink cow's milk and don't receive vitamin supplements, bleeding gums can result from vitamin C deficiency.

Encourage parents to teach proper oral hygiene early. Daily brushing in the morning and before bedtime should begin with eruption of the first tooth. When the child has all of his baby teeth, he should begin receiving regular dental checkups.

GERIATRIC POINTERS
In patients who have no teeth, constant gum trauma and bleeding may result from using a dental prosthesis.

PATIENT COUNSELING
Teach the patient proper mouth and gum care and proper brushing techniques, including use of a soft-bristled toothbrush. Encourage him to seek regular dental care. Make sure patients with chronic disorders that predispose them to bleeding, such as chronic leukemia, cirrhosis, or idiopathic thrombocytopenic purpura, are aware that bleeding gums may indicate a worsening of their condition, requiring immediate medical attention.

GYNECOMASTIA

Occurring only in males, gynecomastia refers to increased breast size due to excessive mammary gland development. Usually bilateral, gynecomastia may be associated with breast tenderness and milk secretion.

Normally, several hormones regulate breast development. Estrogens, growth hormone, and corticosteroids stimulate ductal growth, while progesterone and prolactin stimulate growth of the alveolar lobules. Hormonal imbalance — particularly a change in the estrogen-androgen ratio and an increase in prolactin — is a likely contributing factor. Gynecomastia commonly results from the effects of estrogens and other drugs. It may also result from hormone-secreting tumors and from endocrine, genetic, hepatic, or adrenal disorders. Physiologic gynecomastia may occur in neonatal, pubertal, and geriatric males because of normal fluctuations in hormone levels.

HISTORY

Begin the history by asking the patient when he first noticed his breast enlargement. How old was he at the time? Since then, have his breasts gotten progressively larger, smaller, or stayed the same? Does he also have breast tenderness or discharge? Have him describe the discharge, if any. Ask him if he's ever had his nipples pierced and, if so, did he experience any complications as a result of the piercing? Next, take a thorough drug history, including prescription, over-the-counter, herbal, and street drugs. Then explore associated signs and symptoms, such as a testicular mass or pain, loss of libido, decreased potency, and loss of chest, axillary, or facial hair.

PHYSICAL ASSESSMENT

Focus the physical examination on the breasts, testicles, and penis. As you examine the breasts, note any asymmetry, dimpling, abnormal pigmentation, or ulceration. Observe the testicles for size and symmetry. Then palpate them to detect nodules, tenderness, or unusual consistency. Look for normal penile development after puberty, and note hypospadias.

MEDICAL CAUSES

Breast cancer
Painful unilateral gynecomastia develops rapidly in males with breast cancer. Palpation may reveal a hard or stony breast lump suggesting a malignant tumor. Breast examination may also detect changes in breast symmetry; skin changes, such as thickening, dimpling, peau d'orange, or ulceration; a warm, reddened area; and nipple changes, such as itching, burning, erosion, deviation, flattening, retraction, and a watery, bloody, or purulent discharge.

Cirrhosis
A late sign of cirrhosis, bilateral gynecomastia results from failure of the liver to inactivate circulating estrogens. It's typically accompanied by testicular atrophy, decreased libido, impotence, and loss of facial, chest, and axillary hair. Other late signs and symptoms include mental changes, bleeding tendencies, spider angiomas, palmar erythema, severe pruritus and dry skin, fetor hepaticus, enlarged superficial abdominal veins and, possibly, jaundice and hepatomegaly.

Key facts about gynecomastia
+ Refers to increased breast size in males due to excessive mammary gland development

Key history points
+ Onset of breast enlargement
+ Associated tenderness, discharge, testicular mass or pain, loss of libido, decreased potency, and loss of chest, axillary, or facial hair
+ Complications of any nipple piercing
+ Drug history

Critical assessment steps
+ Examine the breasts for asymmetry, dimpling, abnormal pigmentation, or ulceration.
+ Observe the testicles for size and symmetry; palpate them to detect nodules, tenderness, or unusual consistency.
+ Look for normal penile development after puberty, and note hypospadias.

Medical causes
Breast cancer
+ Painful unilateral gynecomastia develops rapidly.

Cirrhosis
+ Bilateral gynecomastia, a late sign, results from failure of the liver to inactivate circulating estrogens.

Medical causes
(continued)

Hypothyroidism

+ Bilateral gynecomastia occurs along with bradycardia, cold intolerance, weight gain despite anorexia, and mental dullness.

Klinefelter's syndrome

+ Painless bilateral gynecomastia first appears during adolescence.

Malnutrition

+ Painful unilateral gynecomastia may occur when the malnourished patient begins to take nourishment again.

Pituitary tumor

+ Bilateral gynecomastia is accompanied by galactorrhea, impotence, and decreased libido.

Renal failure (chronic)

+ Bilateral gynecomastia may be accompanied by decreased libido and impotence.

Testicular failure (secondary)

+ Bilateral gynecomastia appears after normal puberty.

Testicular tumor

+ Bilateral gynecomastia, nipple tenderness, and decreased libido occur.

Thyrotoxicosis

+ Bilateral gynecomastia may occur with loss of libido and impotence.

Hypothyroidism

Typically, hypothyroidism produces bilateral gynecomastia along with bradycardia, cold intolerance, weight gain despite anorexia, and mental dullness. The patient may display periorbital edema and puffiness in the face, hands, and feet. His hair appears brittle and sparse and his skin is dry, pale, cool, and doughy.

Klinefelter's syndrome

Painless bilateral gynecomastia first appears during adolescence in Klinefelter's syndrome. Before puberty, symptoms also include abnormally small testicles and slight mental deficiency; after puberty, sparse facial hair, a small penis, decreased libido, and impotence.

Malnutrition

Painful unilateral gynecomastia (known as *refeeding gynecomastia*) may occur when the malnourished patient begins to take nourishment again. Other effects of malnutrition include apathy, muscle wasting, weakness, limb paresthesia, anorexia, nausea, vomiting, and diarrhea. Inspection may reveal dull, sparse, dry hair; brittle nails; dark, swollen cheeks and lips; dry, flaky skin; and, occasionally, edema and hepatomegaly.

Pituitary tumor

A pituitary tumor causes bilateral gynecomastia accompanied by galactorrhea, impotence, and decreased libido. Other hormonal effects may include enlarged hands and feet, coarse facial features with prognathism, voice deepening, weight gain, increased blood pressure, diaphoresis, heat intolerance, hyperpigmentation, and thickened, oily skin. Paresthesia or sensory loss and muscle weakness commonly affect the limbs. If the tumor expands, it may cause blurred vision, diplopia, headache, or partial bitemporal hemianopia that may progress to blindness.

Renal failure (chronic)

Chronic renal failure may produce bilateral gynecomastia accompanied by decreased libido and impotence. Among its more characteristic features, however, are ammonia breath odor, oliguria, fatigue, decreased mental acuity, seizures, muscle cramps, and peripheral neuropathy. Common GI effects include anorexia, nausea, vomiting, and constipation or diarrhea. The patient also typically has bleeding tendencies, pruritus, yellow-brown or bronze skin and, occasionally, uremic frost and increased blood pressure.

Testicular failure (secondary)

Commonly associated with mumps and other infectious disorders, secondary testicular failure produces bilateral gynecomastia that appears after normal puberty. This disorder may also cause sparse facial hair, decreased libido, impotence, and testicular atrophy.

Testicular tumor

Choriocarcinomas, Leydig's cell tumors, and other testicular tumors typically cause bilateral gynecomastia, nipple tenderness, and decreased libido. Because these tumors are usually painless, testicular swelling may be the patient's initial complaint. A firm mass and a heavy sensation in the scrotum may occur.

Thyrotoxicosis

With thyrotoxicosis, bilateral gynecomastia may occur with loss of libido and impotence. Cardinal findings include tachycardia, palpitations, weight loss despite increased appetite, diarrhea, tremors, an enlarged thyroid, dyspnea, nervousness, diaphoresis, heat intolerance and, possibly, exophthalmos. An atrial or ventricular gallop may also occur.

OTHER CAUSES

Drugs

When gynecomastia is an effect of drugs, it's typically painful and unilateral. Estrogens used to treat prostate cancer, including diethylstilbestrol, estramustine, and chlorotrianisene, directly affect the estrogen-androgen ratio. Drugs that have an estrogen-like effect, such as cardiac glycosides and human chorionic gonadotropin, may do the same. Regular use of alcohol, marijuana, or heroin reduces plasma testosterone levels, causing gynecomastia. Other drugs — such as flutamide, cyproterone, spironolactone, cimetidine, and ketoconazole — produce this sign by interfering with androgen production or action. Some common drugs, including phenothiazines, tricyclic antidepressants, and antihypertensives, produce gynecomastia in an unknown way.

Treatments

Gynecomastia may develop within weeks of starting hemodialysis for chronic renal failure. It may also follow major surgery or testicular irradiation.

SPECIAL CONSIDERATIONS

To make the patient as comfortable as possible, apply cold compresses to his breasts and administer analgesics. Prepare him for diagnostic tests, including chest and skull X-rays and blood hormone levels.

Some patients are helped by tamoxifen, an antiestrogen, or by testolactone, an inhibitor of testosterone-to-estrogen conversion. Surgical removal of breast tissue may be an option if drug treatment fails.

PEDIATRIC POINTERS

In neonates, gynecomastia may be associated with galactorrhea ("witch's milk"). This sign usually disappears within a few weeks of birth but may persist until age 2.

Most males have physiologic gynecomastia at some time during adolescence, usually around age 14. This gynecomastia is usually asymmetrical and tender; it commonly resolves within 2 years and rarely persists beyond age 20.

PATIENT COUNSELING

Because gynecomastia may alter the patient's body image, provide emotional support. Reassure the patient that treatment can reduce gynecomastia. Be sure to explain all treatments and procedures to the patient.

Other causes
+ Antihypertensives, cyproterone, cimetidine, estrogens and drugs with estrogen-like effects, flutamide, ketoconazole, spironolactone, phenothiazines, and tricyclic antidepressants
+ Hemodialysis
+ Regular use of alcohol, marijuana, or heroin
+ Surgery
+ Testicular irradiation

Special considerations
+ Apply cold compresses to the breasts.
+ Administer analgesics.
+ Some patients are helped by tamoxifen, an antiestrogen, or by testolactone, an inhibitor of testosterone-to-estrogen conversion.
+ Surgical removal of breast tissue may be an option if drug treatment fails.

Peds points
+ In neonates, gynecomastia may be associated with galactorrhea; it usually disappears within a few weeks of birth.
+ Most males have physiologic gynecomastia at some time during adolescence, usually around age 14.

Teaching points
+ Explanation of treatments and procedures

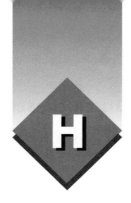

HALITOSIS

Halitosis describes any breath odor that's unpleasant, disagreeable, or offensive. Certain types of halitosis characterize specific disorders — for example, a fruity breath odor typifies ketoacidosis. (See also *specific breath odor types*.) Other types of halitosis include putrid, foul, fetid, and musty breath odors.

Halitosis may result from a disorder of the oral cavity, nasal passages, sinuses, respiratory tract, or esophageal diverticula. It may also stem from a GI disorder and be associated with belching, regurgitation, or vomiting, or it may be an adverse effect of an oral or inhaled drug. Other causes of halitosis include cigarette smoking, ingestion of alcohol and certain foods (such as garlic and onions), and poor oral hygiene — especially in patients with an orthodontic device, dentures, or dental caries. Surprisingly, offensive skin odors — for example, from foot perspiration — may be absorbed locally and later expelled by the lungs, resulting in halitosis.

HISTORY

If you detect halitosis, try to characterize the odor. Does it smell fruity, fecal, or musty? If the patient is aware of it, find out how long he has had it. Does he also have a bad taste in his mouth? Does he have difficulty swallowing or chewing? Does he have reflux or regurgitation? Does he have pain or tenderness? Ask the patient if he has a problem with flatus and about his pattern and description of bowel movements.

Find out if the patient smokes or chews tobacco. Have him describe his diet and daily oral hygiene. Does he wear dentures? Complete the history by asking about chronic disorders and recent respiratory tract infection. If the patient reports a cough, find out if it's productive.

PHYSICAL ASSESSMENT

Begin the physical examination by examining the patient's mouth, throat, and nose. Look for lesions, bleeding, drainage, obstruction, and signs of infection, such as redness and swelling. Check for tenderness by percussing and palpating over the sinuses. Then auscultate the lungs for abnormal breath sounds. Auscultate the abdomen for bowel sounds; percuss, noting any tympany. Finally, take vital signs.

MEDICAL CAUSES

Bowel obstruction

Halitosis is a late sign of both small- and large-bowel obstruction. With a small-bowel obstruction, vomiting of gastric, bilious, and then feculent material produces

---

Key facts about halitosis

♦ Unpleasant, disagreeable, or offensive breath odor

Key history points

♦ Onset and characteristics of halitosis
♦ Associated bad taste, difficulty swallowing or chewing, reflux, regurgitation, pain, tenderness, flatus, or cough
♦ Pattern and description of bowel movements
♦ Smoking or tobacco habits
♦ Diet and daily oral hygiene
♦ History of chronic disorders and respiratory tract infection

Critical assessment steps

♦ Examine the mouth, throat, and nose for lesions, bleeding, drainage, obstruction, and signs of infection.
♦ Percuss and palpate over the sinuses for tenderness.
♦ Auscultate the lungs for abnormal breath sounds.
♦ Auscultate the abdomen for bowel sounds; percuss, noting any tympany.
♦ Take vital signs.

a related breath odor. Other findings include constipation, abdominal distention, and intermittent periumbilical cramping pain. With a large-bowel obstruction, fecal vomiting produces fecal breath odor. Abdominal pain is milder and more constant than that associated with a small-bowel obstruction and is usually located lower in the abdomen.

Bronchiectasis

Bronchiectasis usually produces foul or putrid halitosis, but some patients may have a sickeningly sweet breath odor. The patient typically also has a chronic productive cough with copious, foul-smelling, mucopurulent sputum. The cough is aggravated by lying down and is most productive in the morning. Associated findings commonly include exertional dyspnea, fatigue, malaise, weakness, and weight loss. Auscultation reveals coarse or moist crackles over the affected lung areas during inspiration. Digital clubbing is a late sign.

Common cold

A musty breath odor may accompany a common cold, which usually also causes a dry, hacking cough with sore throat, sneezing, nasal congestion with rhinorrhea, headache, malaise, fatigue, and aching joints and muscles.

Esophageal cancer

With esophageal cancer, halitosis may accompany classic findings of dysphagia, hoarseness, chest pain, and weight loss. Nocturnal regurgitation and cachexia are late signs.

Gastric cancer

Halitosis is a late sign of gastric cancer. Accompanying findings include chronic dyspepsia unrelieved by antacids, a vague feeling of fullness, nausea, anorexia, fatigue, pallor, weakness, altered bowel habits, weight loss, and muscle wasting. Hematemesis and melena are signs of associated gastric bleeding.

Gastrocolic fistula

With gastrocolic fistula, fecal vomiting is responsible for fecal breath odor, which is typically preceded by intermittent diarrhea.

Gingivitis

Characterized by red, edematous gums, gingivitis may also cause halitosis. The gingivae between the teeth become bulbous and bleed easily with slight trauma.

Acute necrotizing ulcerative gingivitis also causes fetid breath, a bad taste in the mouth, and ulcers—especially between the teeth—that may become covered with a gray exudate. Severe ulceration may occur with fever, cervical adenopathy, headache, and malaise.

Hepatic encephalopathy

A characteristic late sign of hepatic encephalopathy is fetor hepaticus, a musty, sweet, or mousy (new-mown hay) breath odor. Major late effects also include coma, asterixis (flapping tremor), and hyperactive deep tendon reflexes.

Lung abscess

A lung abscess typically causes putrid halitosis, but its major sign is a productive cough with copious, purulent, often bloody sputum. Other findings include fever with chills, dyspnea, headache, anorexia, malaise, pleuritic chest pain, asymmetrical chest movement, weight loss, and temporary clubbing.

Medical causes

Bowel obstruction
+ Fecal halitosis is a late sign.

Bronchiectasis
+ Foul or putrid halitosis is typical.
+ Some patients may have a sickeningly sweet breath odor.

Common cold
+ A musty breath odor may occur.

Esophageal cancer
+ Halitosis may accompany dysphagia, hoarseness, chest pain, and weight loss.

Gastric cancer
+ Halitosis is a late sign.

Gastrocolic fistula
+ A fecal breath odor is produced.

Gingivitis
+ Halitosis may occur along with red, edematous gums.
+ Acute necrotizing ulcerative gingivitis causes fetid breath.

Hepatic encephalopathy
+ Musty, sweet, or mousy breath odor is a late sign.

Lung abscess
+ Putrid halitosis develops along with a productive cough.

Medical causes
(continued)

Ozena
✦ Musty or fetid breath odor occurs along with thick, green mucus and progressive anosmia.

Periodontal disease
✦ Halitosis occurs with a bad taste, bleeding gums, and pus-filled pockets around the teeth.

Pharyngitis (gangrenous)
✦ Halitosis occurs with an extremely sore throat.

Renal failure (chronic)
✦ A urinous or ammonia breath odor is produced.

Sinusitis
✦ Acute sinusitis causes purulent nasal discharge that leads to halitosis.
✦ Chronic sinusitis causes continuous mucopurulent discharge and musty breath odor.

Other causes
✦ Drugs known to cause metabolic acidosis such as nitroprusside
✦ Inhaled anesthetics
✦ Triamterene

Special considerations
✦ Prepare the patient for X-rays or endoscopy.

Peds points
✦ In children, halitosis commonly results from physiologic causes.

Geri points
✦ Dental caries, mouth dryness, and poor oral hygiene can cause halitosis in elderly patients.

Ozena
Ozena — a severe, chronic form of rhinitis — causes a musty or fetid breath odor as well as thick, green mucus and progressive anosmia.

Periodontal disease
With periodontal disease, halitosis occurs with an unpleasant taste. Typically, the patient's gums bleed spontaneously or with slight trauma and are marked by pus-filled pockets around the teeth. Related findings include facial pain, headache, and loose teeth covered by calculi and plaque.

Pharyngitis (gangrenous)
Halitosis is a chief sign of gangrenous pharyngitis. The patient also complains of a foul taste in the mouth, an extremely sore throat, and a choking sensation. Examination reveals a swollen, red, ulcerated pharynx, possibly with a grayish membrane. Fever and cervical lymphadenopathy are also common.

Renal failure (chronic)
Chronic renal failure produces a urinous or ammonia breath odor. Among its widespread effects are anemia, emotional lability, lethargy, irritability, decreased mental acuity, coarse muscular twitching, peripheral neuropathies, muscle wasting, anorexia, signs of GI bleeding, ecchymoses, yellow-brown or bronze skin, pruritus, anuria, and increased blood pressure.

Sinusitis
Acute sinusitis causes a purulent nasal discharge that leads to halitosis. Besides a characteristic postnasal drip, the patient may exhibit nasal congestion, sore throat, cough, malaise, headache, facial pain and tenderness, and fever.

Chronic sinusitis causes a continuous mucopurulent discharge that leads to a musty breath odor. Postnasal drip, nasal congestion, and a chronic, nonproductive cough may accompany the musty odor.

OTHER CAUSES

Drugs
Drugs that can cause halitosis include triamterene, inhaled anesthetics, paraldehyde (which is excreted through the lungs), and any drugs known to cause metabolic acidosis such as nitroprusside.

SPECIAL CONSIDERATIONS
If examination of the mouth and sinuses doesn't reveal the cause of halitosis, prepare the patient for upper GI and chest X-rays or endoscopy.

PEDIATRIC POINTERS
In children, halitosis commonly results from physiologic causes, such as continual mouth breathing and thumb or blanket sucking. Phenylketonuria — a metabolic disorder that affects infants — may produce a musty or mousy breath odor.

GERIATRIC POINTERS
Extensive dental caries, mouth dryness, and poor oral hygiene can cause halitosis in elderly patients.

PATIENT COUNSELING

To help control halitosis, encourage good oral hygiene. If halitosis is drug-induced, reassure the patient that it will disappear as soon as his body completely eliminates the drug.

HALO VISION

Halo vision refers to seeing rainbowlike, colored rings around lights or bright objects. Halo vision usually develops suddenly; its duration depends on the causative disorder. This symptom may occur with disorders associated with excessive tearing and corneal epithelial edema. Among these causes, the most common and significant is acute angle-closure glaucoma, which can lead to blindness. With this disorder, increased intraocular pressure (IOP) forces fluid into corneal tissues anterior to Bowman's membrane, causing edema. Halo vision is also an early symptom of cataracts, resulting from dispersion of light by abnormal opacities on the lens.

Nonpathologic causes of excessive tearing associated with halo vision include poorly fitted or overworn contact lenses, emotional extremes, and exposure to intense light, as in snow blindness.

HISTORY

First, ask the patient how long he has been seeing halos around lights and when he usually sees them. Patients with glaucoma usually see halos in the morning, when IOP is most elevated. Ask the patient if light bothers his eyes. Does he have eye pain? If so, have him describe it. Remember that halos associated with excruciating eye pain or a severe headache may point to acute angle-closure glaucoma, an ocular emergency. Note a history of glaucoma or cataracts.

PHYSICAL ASSESSMENT

Examine the patient's eyes, noting conjunctival injection, excessive tearing, and lens changes. Examine pupil size, shape, and response to light. Then test visual acuity by performing an ophthalmoscopic examination.

MEDICAL CAUSES

Cataract
Halo vision may be an early symptom of painless, progressive cataract formation. The glare of headlights may blind the patient, making nighttime driving impossible. Other features include blurred vision, impaired visual acuity, and lens opacity, all of which develop gradually.

Corneal endothelial dystrophy
Typically, halo vision is a late symptom of corneal endothelial dystrophy. Impaired visual acuity may also occur.

Glaucoma
Halo vision characterizes all types of glaucoma. Acute angle-closure glaucoma — an ophthalmic emergency — also causes blurred vision, followed by a severe headache or excruciating pain in and around the affected eye. Examination reveals a moderately dilated fixed pupil that doesn't respond to light, conjunctival injection, a cloudy cornea, impaired visual acuity and, possibly, nausea and vomiting.

Teaching points
+ Good oral hygiene

Key facts about halo vision
+ Refers to seeing rainbowlike, colored rings around lights or bright objects
+ Usually develops suddenly

Key history points
+ Duration and description of halo vision
+ When it occurs
+ Associated eye pain or sensitivity to light
+ History of glaucoma or cataracts

Critical assessment steps
+ Examine the eyes, noting conjunctival injection, excessive tearing, and lens changes.
+ Examine pupil size, shape, and response to light.
+ Perform an ophthalmoscopic examination.

Medical causes

Cataract
+ Halo vision may be an early symptom.

Corneal endothelial dystrophy
+ Halo vision is a late symptom.

Glaucoma
+ Halo vision occurs in all types of glaucoma.
+ With chronic angle-closure glaucoma, halo vision develops slowly.
+ With chronic open-angle glaucoma, halo vision is a late symptom.

Special considerations
+ Remind the patient not to look directly at bright lights.

Peds points
+ Halo vision in a child usually results from congenital cataracts or glaucoma.

Geri points
+ Primary glaucoma is more common in older patients.

Teaching points
+ Proper instillation of prescribed eyedrop.
+ Signs and symptoms to report

Key facts about headache
+ Most common neurologic symptom
+ May be localized or generalized, producing mild to severe pain

Key history points
+ Characteristics and location of headache
+ Precipitating or alleviating factors
+ Drug and alcohol history
+ Recent head trauma, nausea, vomiting, photophobia, or visual changes
+ Associated drowsiness, confusion, dizziness, or seizures

Chronic angle-closure glaucoma is usually asymptomatic until pain and blindness occur in advanced disease. Sometimes, halos and blurred vision develop slowly.

With chronic open-angle glaucoma, halo vision is a late symptom that's accompanied by mild eye ache, peripheral vision loss, and impaired visual acuity.

SPECIAL CONSIDERATIONS

To help minimize halo vision, remind the patient not to look directly at bright lights.

PEDIATRIC POINTERS

Halo vision in a child usually results from congenital cataracts or glaucoma. In a young child, limited verbal ability may make halo vision difficult to assess.

GERIATRIC POINTERS

Primary glaucoma, the most common cause of halo vision, is more common in older patients.

PATIENT COUNSELING

Teach the patient how to properly instill eyedrops, if prescribed, and stress the importance of meticulous compliance. Tell him to report eye discharge, eye watering, blurred or cloudy vision, halos, floaters, flashes of light, or eye pain.

HEADACHE

The most common neurologic symptom, headaches may be localized or generalized, producing mild to severe pain. About 90% of all headaches are benign and can be described as vascular, muscle-contraction, or a combination of both. (See *Comparing benign headaches.*) Occasionally, though, headaches indicate a severe neurologic disorder associated with intracranial inflammation, increased intracranial pressure (ICP), or meningeal irritation. They may also result from an ocular or sinus disorder, tests, drugs, or other treatments.

Other causes of headache include fever, eyestrain, dehydration, and systemic febrile illnesses. Headaches may occur in certain metabolic disturbances—such as hypoxemia, hypercapnia, hyperglycemia, and hypoglycemia—but they aren't a diagnostic or prominent symptom. Some individuals get headaches after seizures or from coughing, sneezing, heavy lifting, or stooping.

HISTORY

If the patient reports a headache, ask him to describe its characteristics and location. How often does he get a headache? How long does a typical headache last? Try to identify precipitating factors, such as certain foods or exposure to bright lights. Ask what helps to relieve the headache. Is the patient under stress? Has he had trouble sleeping?

Take a drug and alcohol history, and ask about head trauma within the last 4 weeks. Has the patient recently experienced nausea, vomiting, photophobia, or visual changes? Does he feel drowsy, confused, or dizzy? Has he recently developed seizures, or does he have a history of seizures?

Comparing benign headaches

Of the many patients who report headaches, only about 10% have an underlying medical disorder. The other 90% suffer from benign headaches, which may be classified as muscle-contraction (tension), vascular (migraine and cluster), or a combination of both.

As you review the chart below, you'll see that the two major types — muscle-contraction and vascular headaches — are quite different. In a combined headache, features of both appear; this type of headache may affect the patient with a severe muscle-contraction headache or a late-stage migraine. Treatment of a combined headache includes analgesics and sedatives.

CHARACTERISTICS	MUSCLE-CONTRACTION HEADACHES	VASCULAR HEADACHES
Incidence	✦ Most common type, accounting for 80% of all headaches	✦ More common in women and those with a family history of migraines ✦ Onset after puberty
Precipitating factors	✦ Stress, anxiety, tension, improper posture, and body alignment ✦ Prolonged muscle contraction without structural damage ✦ Eye, ear, and paranasal sinus disorders that produce reflex muscle contractions	✦ Hormone fluctuations ✦ Alcohol ✦ Emotional upset ✦ Too little or too much sleep ✦ Foods, such as chocolate, cheese, monosodium glutamate, and cured meats; caffeine withdrawal ✦ Weather changes, such as shifts in barometric pressure
Intensity and duration	✦ Produce an aching tightness or a band of pain around the head, especially in the neck and in the occipital and temporal areas ✦ Occur frequently and usually last for several hours	✦ May begin with an awareness of an impending migraine or a 5- to 15-minute prodrome of neurologic deficits, such as visual disturbances, dizziness, unsteady gait, or tingling of the face, lips, or hands ✦ Produce severe, constant, throbbing pain that's typically unilateral and may be incapacitating ✦ Last for 4 to 6 hours
Associated signs and symptoms	✦ Tense neck and facial muscles	✦ Anorexia, nausea, and vomiting ✦ Occasionally, photophobia, sensitivity to loud noises, weakness, and fatigue ✦ Depending on the type (cluster headache or classic, common, or hemiplegic migraine), possibly chills, depression, eye pain, ptosis, tearing, rhinorrhea, diaphoresis, and facial flushing
Alleviating factors	✦ Mild analgesics, muscle relaxants, or other drugs during an attack ✦ Measures to reduce stress, such as biofeedback, relaxation techniques, and counseling ✦ Posture correction to prevent attacks	✦ Methysergide and propranolol to prevent vascular headache ✦ Ergot alkaloids or serotonin-receptor drugs at first sign of migraine ✦ Rest in a quiet, darkened room ✦ Elimination of irritating foods from diet

Key facts about muscle-contraction headaches

✦ Account for 80% of all headaches
✦ Produce an aching tightness or a band of pain around the head, especially in the neck and in the occipital and temporal areas
✦ Usually last for several hours
✦ Treated with mild analgesics, muscle relaxants, or other drugs

Key facts about vascular headaches

✦ Are more common in women and in people with a family history of migraines
✦ Onset after puberty
✦ Produce severe, constant, throbbing pain that's typically unilateral and may be incapacitating
✦ Last for 4 to 6 hours
✦ Associatd with anorexia, nausea, vomiting and, occasionally, photophobia and sensitvity to loud noise
✦ Prevented with methysergide and propranolol
✦ Alleviated by resting in a quiet, darkened room

Critical assessment steps

- ◆ Evaluate LOC.
- ◆ Check vital signs.
- ◆ Be alert for signs of increased ICP.
- ◆ Check pupil size and response to light.
- ◆ Note neck stiffness.

Medical causes

Brain abscess

- ◆ Headache is localized to the abscess site and intensifies over a few days.
- ◆ Straining aggravates headache.

Brain tumor

- ◆ Headache is localized near the tumor site but becomes generalized as the tumor grows.

Cerebral aneurysm (ruptured)

- ◆ Headache is sudden and excruciating and usually peaks within minutes of the rupture.
- ◆ Patient may lose consciousness immediately or display a variably altered LOC.

Encephalitis

- ◆ A severe, generalized headache is characteristic.
- ◆ Within 48 hours, the patient's LOC typically deteriorates.

Epidural hemorrhage (acute)

- ◆ A progressively severe headache is accompanied by nausea, vomiting, bladder distention, confusion, and rapid decrease in LOC.

PHYSICAL ASSESSMENT

Begin the physical examination by evaluating the patient's level of consciousness (LOC). Then check his vital signs. Be alert for signs of increased ICP: widened pulse pressure, bradycardia, altered respiratory pattern, and increased blood pressure. Check pupil size and response to light, and note any neck stiffness.

MEDICAL CAUSES

Brain abscess

With brain abscess, the headache is localized to the abscess site. Usually, it intensifies over a few days and is aggravated by straining. Accompanying the headache may be nausea, vomiting, and focal or generalized seizures. The patient's LOC varies from drowsiness to deep stupor. Depending on the abscess site, associated signs and symptoms may include aphasia, impaired visual acuity, hemiparesis, ataxia, tremors, and personality changes. Signs of infection, such as fever and pallor, usually develop late; however, if the abscess remains encapsulated, these signs may not appear.

Brain tumor

Initially, a brain tumor causes a localized headache near the tumor site; as the tumor grows, the headache eventually becomes generalized. The pain is usually intermittent, deep-seated, and dull, and most intense in the morning. It's aggravated by coughing, stooping, Valsalva's maneuver, and changes in head position, and it's relieved by sitting and rest. Associated signs and symptoms include personality changes, altered LOC, motor and sensory dysfunction, and eventually signs of increased ICP, such as vomiting, increased systolic blood pressure, and widened pulse pressure.

Cerebral aneurysm (ruptured)

Ruptured cerebral aneurysm is a life-threatening disorder that's characterized by a sudden, excruciating headache, which may be unilateral and usually peaks within minutes of the rupture. The patient may lose consciousness immediately or display a variably altered LOC. Depending on the severity and location of the bleeding, he may also exhibit nausea and vomiting; signs and symptoms of meningeal irritation, such as nuchal rigidity and blurred vision; hemiparesis; and other features.

Encephalitis

A severe, generalized headache is characteristic of encephalitis. Within 48 hours, the patient's LOC typically deteriorates — perhaps from lethargy to coma. Associated signs and symptoms include fever, nuchal rigidity, irritability, seizures, nausea and vomiting, photophobia, cranial nerve palsies such as ptosis, and focal neurologic deficits, such as hemiparesis and hemiplegia.

Epidural hemorrhage (acute)

Head trauma and a sudden, brief loss of consciousness usually precede acute epidural hemorrhage, which causes a progressively severe headache that's accompanied by nausea and vomiting, bladder distention, confusion, and then a rapid decrease in LOC. Other signs and symptoms include unilateral seizures, hemiparesis, hemiplegia, high fever, decreased pulse rate and bounding pulse, widened pulse pressure, increased blood pressure, a positive Babinski's reflex, and decerebrate posture.

If the patient slips into coma, his respirations deepen and become stertorous, then shallow and irregular, and eventually they cease. Pupil dilation may occur on the same side as the hemorrhage.

Glaucoma (acute angle-closure)

Acute angle-closure glaucoma is an ophthalmic emergency that may cause an excruciating headache as well as acute eye pain, blurred vision, halo vision, nausea, and vomiting. Assessment reveals conjunctival injection, a cloudy cornea, and a moderately dilated, fixed pupil.

Hypertension

Hypertension may cause a slightly throbbing occipital headache on awakening that decreases in severity during the day. However, if the patient's diastolic blood pressure exceeds 120 mm Hg, the headache remains constant. Associated signs and symptoms include an atrial gallop, restlessness, confusion, nausea and vomiting, blurred vision, seizures, and altered LOC.

Influenza

A severe generalized or frontal headache usually begins suddenly with the flu. Accompanying signs and symptoms may last for 3 to 5 days and include stabbing retro-orbital pain, weakness, diffuse myalgia, fever, chills, coughing, rhinorrhea and, occasionally, hoarseness.

Intracerebral hemorrhage

In some patients, intracerebral hemorrhage produces a severe generalized headache. Signs and symptoms vary with the size and location of the hemorrhage. A large hemorrhage may produce a rapid, steady decrease in LOC, perhaps resulting in coma. Other common findings include hemiplegia, hemiparesis, abnormal pupil size and response, aphasia, dizziness, nausea, vomiting, seizures, decreased sensation, irregular respirations, positive Babinski's reflex, decorticate or decerebrate posture, and increased blood pressure.

Meningitis

Meningitis is marked by the sudden onset of a severe, constant, generalized headache that worsens with movement. Associated signs include nuchal rigidity, positive Kernig's and Brudzinski's signs, hyperreflexia and, possibly, opisthotonos. Fever occurs early with meningitis and may be accompanied by chills. As ICP increases, vomiting and, occasionally, papilledema develop. Other features include altered LOC, seizures, ocular palsies, facial weakness, and hearing loss.

Plague

The pneumonic form of plague, caused by the bacterium *Yersinia pestis,* causes a sudden onset of headache, chills, fever, myalgias, productive cough, chest pain, tachypnea, dyspnea, hemoptysis, respiratory distress, and cardiopulmonary insufficiency.

Postconcussional syndrome

With postconcussional syndrome, a generalized or localized headache may develop 1 to 30 days after head trauma and last for 2 to 3 weeks. This characteristic symptom may be described as an aching, pounding, pressing, stabbing, or throbbing pain. The patient's neurologic examination is normal, but he may experience giddiness or dizziness, blurred vision, fatigue, insomnia, inability to concentrate, and noise and alcohol intolerance.

Signs and symptoms of this disease include severe headache, fever, chills, malaise, chest pain, nausea, vomiting, and diarrhea. The fever may last for up to 2 weeks, and in severe cases, the patient may develop hepatitis or pneumonia.

Medical causes
(continued)

Glaucoma (acute angle-closure)
+ Excruciating headache as well as acute eye pain, blurred vision, halo vision, nausea, and vomiting may occur.

Hypertension
+ A slightly throbbing occipital headache on awakening may occur; severity decreases during the day.

Influenza
+ A severe generalized or frontal headache usually begins suddenly.

Intracerebral hemorrhage
+ A severe generalized headache develops in some patients.

Meningitis
+ Onset of a severe, constant, generalized headache is sudden.
+ Headache worsens with movement.

Plague
+ Pneumonic form results in sudden onset of headache, chills, fever, myalgias, productive cough, chest pain, tachypnea, dyspnea, hemoptysis, respiratory distress, and cardiopulmonary insufficiency.

Postconcussional syndrome
+ A generalized or localized headache may develop 1 to 30 days after head trauma and last for 2 to 3 weeks.
+ Pain may be aching, pounding, pressing, stabbing, or throbbing.

Medical causes
(continued)

SARS
✦ Symptoms include fever, headache, malaise, a dry nonproductive cough, and dyspnea.

Sinusitis (acute)
✦ A dull periorbital headache is usually aggravated by bending over or touching the face and is relieved by sinus drainage.

Smallpox
✦ Initial signs and symptoms include severe headache, backache, abdominal pain, high fever, malaise, prostration, and a maculopapular rash.

Subarachnoid hemorrhage
✦ A sudden, violent headache occurs along with nuchal rigidity, nausea and vomiting, seizures, dizziness, ipsilateral pupil dilation, and altered LOC.

Subdural hematoma
✦ Headache develops and LOC decreases.
✦ In chronic cases, pounding headache fluctuates in severity and is located over the hematoma.

Temporal arteritis
✦ A throbbing unilateral headache in the temporal or frontotemporal region may be accompanied by vision loss, hearing loss, confusion, and fever.

Tularemia
✦ Onset of headache is abrupt.

Severe acute respiratory syndrome

Severe acute respiratory syndrome (SARS) is an acute infectious disease of unknown etiology that generally begins with a fever (usually greater than 100.4° F [38° C]). Other symptoms of SARS include headache, malaise, a dry nonproductive cough, and dyspnea. The severity of the illness is highly variable, ranging from mild illness to pneumonia and, in some cases, progressing to respiratory failure and death.

Sinusitis (acute)

Acute sinusitis is usually marked by a dull periorbital headache that's usually aggravated by bending over or touching the face and is relieved by sinus drainage. Fever, sinus tenderness, nasal turbinate edema, sore throat, malaise, cough, and nasal discharge may accompany the headache.

Smallpox

Initial signs and symptoms of smallpox (variola major) include severe headache, backache, abdominal pain, high fever, malaise, prostration, and a maculopapular rash on the mucosa of the mouth, pharynx, face, and forearms, and then the trunk and legs. The rash becomes vesicular, then pustular and finally forms a crust and scab, leaving a pitted scar. In fatal cases, death results from encephalitis, extensive bleeding, or secondary infection.

Subarachnoid hemorrhage

Subarachnoid hemorrhage commonly produces a sudden, violent headache along with nuchal rigidity, nausea and vomiting, seizures, dizziness, ipsilateral pupil dilation, and altered LOC that may rapidly progress to coma. The patient also exhibits positive Kernig's and Brudzinski's signs, photophobia, blurred vision and, possibly, fever. Focal signs and symptoms (such as hemiparesis, hemiplegia, sensory or vision disturbances, and aphasia) and signs of elevated ICP (such as bradycardia and increased blood pressure) may also occur.

Subdural hematoma

Typically associated with head trauma, both acute and chronic subdural hematomas may cause headache and decreased LOC. With acute subdural hematoma, head trauma also produces drowsiness, confusion, and agitation that may progress to coma. Later findings include signs of increased ICP and focal neurologic deficits such as hemiparesis.

Chronic subdural hematoma produces a dull, pounding headache that fluctuates in severity and is located over the hematoma. Weeks or months after the initial head trauma, the patient may experience giddiness, personality changes, confusion, seizures, and progressively worsening LOC. Late signs may include unilateral pupil dilation, sluggish pupil reaction to light, and ptosis.

Temporal arteritis

A throbbing unilateral headache in the temporal or frontotemporal region may be accompanied by vision loss, hearing loss, confusion, and fever. The temporal arteries are tender, swollen, nodular, and sometimes erythematous.

Tularemia

Signs and symptoms of tularemia (caused by inhalation of the bacterium *Francisella tularensis*) include abrupt onset of headache, fever, chills, generalized myalgias, nonproductive cough, dyspnea, pleuritic chest pain, and empyema.

OTHER CAUSES

Diagnostic tests

A lumbar puncture or myelogram may produce a throbbing frontal headache that worsens on standing.

Drugs

A wide variety of drugs can cause headaches. For example, indomethacin produces headaches—usually in the morning—in many patients. Vasodilators and drugs with a vasodilating effect, such as nitrates, typically cause a throbbing headache. Headaches may also follow withdrawal from vasopressors, such as caffeine, ergotamine, and sympathomimetics.

SPECIAL CONSIDERATIONS

Continue to monitor the patient's vital signs and LOC. Watch for any change in the headache's severity or location. To help ease the headache, administer an analgesic, darken the patient's room, and minimize other stimuli. Explain the rationale of these interventions to the patient.

Prepare the patient for diagnostic tests, such as skull X-rays, computed tomography scan, lumbar puncture, or cerebral arteriography.

PEDIATRIC POINTERS

If a child is too young to describe his symptoms, suspect a headache if you see him banging or holding his head. In an infant, a shrill cry or bulging fontanels may indicate increased ICP and headache. In a school-age child, ask the parents about the child's recent scholastic performance and about any problems at home that may produce a tension headache.

Twice as many young boys have migraine headaches as girls. In children older than age 3, headache is the most common symptom of a brain tumor.

PATIENT COUNSELING

Teach the patient and his family or caregiver how to recognize signs of reduced LOC and seizures. Discuss ways to maintain a safe, quiet environment and reduce environmental stress, if indicated. Discuss the use of analgesics to ease the headache.

HEARING LOSS

Affecting nearly 16 million Americans, hearing loss may be temporary or permanent and partial or complete. This common symptom may involve reception of low-, middle-, or high-frequency tones. If the hearing loss doesn't affect speech frequencies, the patient may be unaware of it. (See *Understanding sound transmission*, page 328.)

Hearing loss can be classified as conductive, sensorineural, mixed, or functional. Conductive hearing loss results from external or middle ear disorders that block sound transmission. Sensorineural hearing loss results from disorders of the inner ear or of the eighth cranial nerve. Mixed hearing loss combines aspects of conductive and sensorineural hearing loss. Functional hearing loss results from psychological factors rather than identifiable organic damage.

Hearing loss may also result from trauma, infection, allergy, tumors, certain systemic and hereditary disorders, and the effects of ototoxic drugs and treatments. In

Other causes

- ✦ Indomethacin, vasodilators, and drugs with a vasodilating effect
- ✦ Lumbar puncture
- ✦ Myelogram
- ✦ Withdrawal from vasopressors

Special considerations

- ✦ Monitor vital signs and LOC.
- ✦ Watch for change in the headache's severity or location.
- ✦ Administer an analgesic, darken the room, and minimize stimuli.
- ✦ Explain the rationale of these interventions to the patient.

Peds points

- ✦ In children older than age 3, headache is the most common symptom of a brain tumor.

Teaching points

- ✦ Signs of reduced LOC and seizures
- ✦ Ways to maintain a safe, quiet environment and reduce environmental stress
- ✦ Use of analgesics

Key facts about hearing loss

- ✦ May be temporary or permanent and partial or complete
- ✦ Classified as conductive (resulting from external or middle ear disorders), sensorineural (resulting from disorders of the inner ear or of the eighth cranial nerve), mixed (resulting from a combination of conductive and sensorineural factors), or functional (resulting from psychological factors)

Sound transmission by air conduction

+ External auditory canal → tympanic membrane and ossicles → cochlea → CN VIII → brain

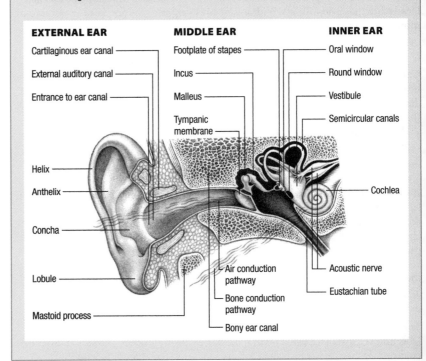

Understanding sound transmission

The ear has three divisions—external, middle, and inner. Normally, sound waves enter the external auditory canal, travel to the middle ear's tympanic membrane and ossicles (incus, malleus, and stapes), and then into the inner ear's cochlea. The cochlear division of the eighth cranial (auditory) nerve carries the sound impulse to the brain. This type of sound transmission is called *air conduction*. Air conduction is normally better than *bone conduction*—sound transmission through bone to the inner ear.

EXTERNAL EAR
- Cartilaginous ear canal
- External auditory canal
- Entrance to ear canal
- Helix
- Anthelix
- Concha
- Lobule
- Mastoid process

MIDDLE EAR
- Footplate of stapes
- Incus
- Malleus
- Tympanic membrane
- Air conduction pathway
- Bone conduction pathway
- Bony ear canal

INNER EAR
- Oral window
- Round window
- Vestibule
- Semicircular canals
- Cochlea
- Acoustic nerve
- Eustachian tube

most cases, though, it results from presbycusis, a type of sensorineural hearing loss that usually affects people older than age 50. Other physiologic causes of hearing loss include cerumen (earwax) impaction; barotitis media (unequal pressure on the eardrum) associated with descent in an airplane or elevator, diving, or close proximity to an explosion; and chronic exposure to noise over 90 decibels, which can occur on the job, with certain hobbies, or from listening to live or recorded music.

History points

+ Description of hearing loss
+ Medical history, including chronic ear infections, ear surgery, ear or head trauma, and recent upper respiratory tract infection
+ Drug history
+ Description of occupational environment
+ Description of associated pain; discharge; ringing, buzzing, hissing, or other noises; dizziness

HISTORY

If the patient reports hearing loss, ask him to describe it fully. Is it unilateral or bilateral? Continuous or intermittent? Ask about a family history of hearing loss. Then obtain the patient's medical history, noting chronic ear infections, ear surgery, and ear or head trauma. Has the patient recently had an upper respiratory tract infection? After taking a drug history, have the patient describe his occupation and work environment.

Next, explore associated signs and symptoms. Does the patient have ear pain? If so, is it unilateral or bilateral, or continuous or intermittent? Ask the patient if he has noticed discharge from one or both ears. If so, have him describe its color and consistency, and note when it began. Does he hear ringing, buzzing, hissing, or other noises in one or both ears? If so, are the noises constant or intermittent? Does he experience any dizziness? If so, when did he first notice it?

PHYSICAL ASSESSMENT

Begin the physical examination by inspecting the external ear for inflammation, boils, foreign bodies, and discharge. Then apply pressure to the tragus and mastoid to elicit tenderness. If you detect tenderness or external ear abnormalities, notify the physician to discuss whether an otoscopic examination should be done. During the otoscopic examination, note any color change, perforation, bulging, or retraction of the tympanic membrane, which normally looks like a shiny, pearl gray cone.

Next, evaluate the patient's hearing acuity, using the ticking watch and whispered voice tests. Then perform the Weber's and Rinne tests to obtain a preliminary evaluation of the type and degree of hearing loss. (See *Differentiating conductive from sensorineural hearing loss*, page 330.)

MEDICAL CAUSES

Acoustic neuroma

An acoustic neuroma is an eighth cranial nerve tumor that causes unilateral, progressive, sensorineural hearing loss. The patient may also develop tinnitus, vertigo and, with cranial nerve compression, facial paralysis.

Adenoid hypertrophy

With adenoid hypertrophy, eustachian tube dysfunction gradually causes conductive hearing loss accompanied by intermittent ear discharge. The patient also tends to breathe through his mouth and may complain of a sensation of ear fullness.

Allergies

Conductive hearing loss may result when an allergy produces eustachian tube and middle ear congestion. Other features include ear pain or a feeling of fullness, nasal congestion, and conjunctivitis.

Cholesteatoma

Gradual hearing loss is characteristic in cholesteatoma. It can be accompanied by vertigo and, at times, facial paralysis. Examination reveals eardrum perforation, pearly white balls in the ear canal and, possibly, a discharge.

External ear canal tumor (malignant)

Progressive conductive hearing loss is characteristic of a malignant external ear canal tumor and is accompanied by deep, boring ear pain; purulent discharge; and eventually facial paralysis. Examination may detect the granular, bleeding tumor.

Furuncle

Reversible conductive hearing loss may occur when a furuncle (a painful, hard nodule) forms in the ear. The patient with a furuncle may report a sense of fullness in the ear and pain on palpation of the tragus or auricle. Boil rupture relieves the pain and produces a purulent, necrotic discharge.

Glomus jugulare tumor

Initially, glomus jugulare (a benign tumor) causes mild, unilateral conductive hearing loss that becomes progressively more severe. The patient may report tinnitus that sounds like his heartbeat. Associated signs and symptoms include gradual congestion in the affected ear, throbbing or pulsating discomfort, bloody otorrhea, fa-

---

Critical assessment steps

+ Inspect the external ear for inflammation, boils, foreign bodies, and discharge.
+ Apply pressure to the tragus and mastoid to elicit tenderness.
+ During otoscopic examination, note color change, perforation, bulging, or retraction of tympanic membrane.

Medical causes

Acoustic neuroma
+ Unilateral, progressive, sensorineural hearing loss occurs.

Adenoid hypertrophy
+ Eustachian tube dysfunction gradually causes conductive hearing loss.

Allergies
+ Conductive hearing loss may result when an allergy produces eustachian tube and middle ear congestion.

Cholesteatoma
+ Gradual hearing loss may be accompanied by vertigo.

External ear canal tumor (malignant)
+ Progressive conductive hearing loss occurs with deep, boring ear pain; purulent discharge; and facial paralysis.

Furuncle
+ Reversible conductive hearing loss may occur when a furuncle forms in the ear.

Glomus jugulare tumor
+ Mild, unilateral conductive hearing loss becomes progressively more severe.

Conductive hearing loss

✦ Abnormal Weber's test result
✦ Negative Rinne test result
✦ Improved hearing in noisy areas
✦ Normal ability to discriminate sounds
✦ Difficulty hearing when chewing
✦ A quiet speaking voice

Sensorineural hearing loss

✦ Positive Rinne test
✦ Poor hearing in noisy areas
✦ Difficulty hearing high-frequency sounds
✦ Complaints that others mumble or shout
✦ Tinnitus

ASSESSMENT TIP

Differentiating conductive from sensorineural hearing loss

The Weber's and Rinne tests can help determine whether the patient's hearing loss is conductive or sensorineural. Weber's test evaluates bone conduction; the Rinne test, bone and air conduction. Using a 512-Hz tuning fork, perform these preliminary tests as described below.

WEBER'S TEST
Place the base of a vibrating tuning fork firmly against the midline of the patient's skull at the forehead. Ask her if she hears the tone equally well in both ears. If she does, the test is graded midline — a normal finding. In an abnormal Weber's test (graded right or left), sound is louder in one ear, suggesting a conductive hearing loss in that ear, or a sensorineural loss in the opposite ear.

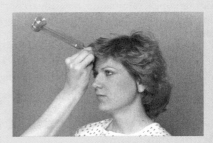

RINNE TEST
Hold the base of a vibrating tuning fork against the patient's mastoid process to test bone conduction. Then quickly move the vibrating fork in front of her ear canal to test air conduction. Ask her to tell you which location has the louder or longer sound. Repeat the procedure for the other ear. In a positive Rinne test, air conduction lasts longer or sounds louder than bone conduction — a normal finding. In a negative test, the opposite is true: Bone conduction lasts longer or sounds louder than air conduction.

After performing both tests, correlate the results with other assessment data.

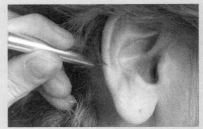

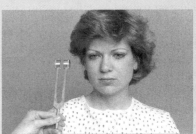

IMPLICATIONS OF RESULTS
Conductive hearing loss produces:
✦ abnormal Weber's test result
✦ negative Rinne test result
✦ improved hearing in noisy areas
✦ normal ability to discriminate sounds
✦ difficulty hearing when chewing
✦ a quiet speaking voice.

Sensorineural hearing loss produces:
✦ positive Rinne test
✦ poor hearing in noisy areas
✦ difficulty hearing high-frequency sounds
✦ complaints that others mumble or shout
✦ tinnitus.

cial nerve paralysis, and vertigo. Although the tympanic membrane is normal, a reddened mass appears behind it.

Head trauma

Sudden conductive or sensorineural hearing loss may result from ossicle disruption, ear canal fracture, tympanic membrane perforation, or cochlear fracture associated with head trauma. Typically, the patient reports a headache and exhibits bleeding from his ear. Neurologic features vary and may include impaired vision and altered level of consciousness.

Hypothyroidism

Hypothyroidism may produce reversible sensorineural hearing loss. Other effects include bradycardia, weight gain despite anorexia, mental dullness, cold intolerance, facial edema, brittle hair, and dry skin that's pale, cool, and doughy.

Ménière's disease

Initially, Ménière's disease produces intermittent, unilateral sensorineural hearing loss that involves only low tones. Later in this inner ear disorder, hearing loss becomes constant and affects other tones. Associated signs and symptoms of Ménière's disease include intermittent severe vertigo, nausea and vomiting, a feeling of fullness in the ear, a roaring or hollow-seashell tinnitus, diaphoresis, and nystagmus.

Osteoma

Commonly affecting women and swimmers, osteoma may cause sudden or intermittent conductive hearing loss. Typically, bony projections are visible in the ear canal, but the tympanic membrane appears normal.

Otitis externa

Conductive hearing loss resulting from debris in the ear canal characterizes both acute and malignant otitis externa. With acute otitis externa, ear canal inflammation produces pain, itching, and a foul-smelling, sticky yellow discharge. Severe tenderness is typically elicited by chewing, opening the mouth, and pressing on the tragus or mastoid. The patient may also develop a low-grade fever, regional lymphadenopathy, headache on the affected side, and mild-to-moderate pain around the ear that may later intensify. Examination may reveal greenish white debris or edema in the canal.

With malignant otitis externa, debris is also visible in the canal. This life-threatening disorder, which most commonly occurs in diabetics, causes sensorineural hearing loss, pruritus, tinnitus, and severe ear pain.

Otitis media

Otitis media is a middle ear inflammation that typically produces unilateral conductive hearing loss. In patients with acute suppurative otitis media, the hearing loss develops gradually over a few hours and is usually accompanied by an upper respiratory tract infection with sore throat, cough, nasal discharge, and headache. Related signs and symptoms include dizziness, a sensation of fullness in the ear, intermittent or constant ear pain, fever, nausea, and vomiting. Rupture of the bulging, swollen tympanic membrane relieves the pain and produces a brief, bloody, purulent discharge. Hearing returns after the infection subsides.

Hearing loss also develops gradually in patients with chronic otitis media. Assessment may reveal a perforated tympanic membrane, purulent ear drainage, earache, nausea, and vertigo.

Commonly associated with an upper respiratory tract infection or nasopharyngeal cancer, serous otitis media commonly produces a stuffy feeling in the ear and

Medical causes
(continued)

Head trauma
+ Sudden conductive or sensorineural hearing loss may result from ossicle disruption, ear canal fracture, tympanic membrane perforation, or cochlear fracture.

Hypothyroidism
+ Reversible sensorineural hearing loss may occur.

Ménière's disease
+ Intermittent, unilateral sensorineural hearing loss that involves only low tones progresses to constant hearing loss that involves other tones.

Osteoma
+ Sudden or intermittent conductive hearing loss occurs.

Otitis externa
+ Conductive hearing loss is characteristic.
+ Acute form produces pain, itching, and discharge.
+ Malignant form involves visible debris in the ear canal.

Otitis media
+ In acute and chronic forms, hearing loss develops gradually.
+ Serous form produces a stuffy feeling in the ear and pain that worsens at night.

Medical causes
(continued)

Otosclerosis
+ Unilateral conductive hearing loss usually begins in early 20s and may gradually progress to bilateral mixed loss.

Skull fracture
+ Auditory nerve injury results in sudden unilateral sensorineural hearing loss.

Temporal arteritis
+ Unilateral sensorineural hearing loss may occur along with throbbing unilateral facial pain, pain behind the eye, temporal or frontotemporal headache and, occasionally, vision loss.

Temporal bone fracture
+ Sudden unilateral sensorineural hearing loss is accompanied by hissing tinnitus.

Tuberculosis
+ Eardrum perforation, mild conductive hearing loss, and cervical lymphadenopathy may occur if infection spreads to the ear.

Tympanic membrane perforation
+ Abrupt hearing loss occurs with ear pain, tinnitus, vertigo, and a sensation of fullness in the ear.

Other causes
+ Ototoxic drugs, such as aminoglycosides, chloroquine, cisplatin, loop diuretics, quinine, quinidine, vancomycin, high doses of erythromycin or salicylates
+ Radiation therapy
+ Myringotomy, myringoplasty, simple or radical mastoidectomy, or fenestrations

pain that worsens at night. Examination reveals a retracted—and perhaps discolored—tympanic membrane and, possibly, air bubbles behind the membrane.

Otosclerosis
In otosclerosis, a hereditary disorder, unilateral conductive hearing loss usually begins when the patient is in his early 20s and may gradually progress to bilateral mixed loss. The patient may report tinnitus and an ability to hear better in a noisy environment. The deafness is usually noticed between ages 11 and 30.

Skull fracture
Auditory nerve injury from a skull fracture causes sudden unilateral sensorineural hearing loss. Accompanying signs and symptoms include ringing tinnitus, blood behind the tympanic membrane, scalp wounds, and other findings.

Temporal arteritis
Temporal arteritis may produce unilateral sensorineural hearing loss accompanied by throbbing unilateral facial pain, pain behind the eye, temporal or frontotemporal headache and, occasionally, vision loss. The hearing loss is usually preceded by a prodrome of malaise, anorexia, weight loss, weakness, and myalgia that lasts for several days. Examination may reveal a nodular, swollen temporal artery. Low-grade fever, confusion, and disorientation may also occur.

Temporal bone fracture
Temporal bone fracture can cause sudden unilateral sensorineural hearing loss accompanied by hissing tinnitus. The tympanic membrane may be perforated, depending on the fracture's location. Loss of consciousness, Battle's sign, and facial paralysis may also occur.

Tuberculosis
Tuberculosis, a pulmonary infection, may spread to the ear, resulting in eardrum perforation, mild conductive hearing loss, and cervical lymphadenopathy. Other signs and symptoms include chest pain, crackles, dyspnea, fatigue, fever, and tachypnea.

Tympanic membrane perforation
Commonly caused by trauma from sharp objects or rapid pressure changes, perforation of the tympanic membrane causes abrupt hearing loss along with ear pain, tinnitus, vertigo, and a sensation of fullness in the ear.

OTHER CAUSES

Drugs
Ototoxic drugs typically produce ringing or buzzing tinnitus and a feeling of fullness in the ear. Chloroquine, cisplatin, vancomycin, and aminoglycosides (especially neomycin, kanamycin, and amikacin) may cause irreversible hearing loss. Loop diuretics, such as furosemide, ethacrynic acid, and bumetanide, usually produce a brief, reversible hearing loss. Quinine, quinidine, and high doses of erythromycin or salicylates (such as aspirin) may also cause reversible hearing loss.

Radiation therapy
Irradiation of the middle ear, thyroid, face, skull, or nasopharynx may cause eustachian tube dysfunction, resulting in hearing loss.

Surgery
Myringotomy, myringoplasty, simple or radical mastoidectomy, or fenestrations may cause scarring that interferes with hearing.

SPECIAL CONSIDERATIONS

When talking with the patient, remember to face him and speak slowly. Don't shout, smoke, eat, or chew gum when talking.

Prepare the patient for audiometry and auditory evoked-response testing. After testing, the patient may require a hearing aid or cochlear implant to improve his hearing.

PEDIATRIC POINTERS

About 3,000 profoundly deaf infants are born in the United States each year. In about half of these infants, hereditary disorders (such as Paget's disease and Alport's, Hurler's, and Klippel-Feil syndromes) cause the hearing loss (typically sensorineural). Nonhereditary disorders associated with congenital sensorineural hearing loss include albinism, cochlear dysplasia, and onychodystrophy, Usher's, Pendred's, Waardenburg's, and Jervell and Lange-Nielsen syndromes. This type of hearing loss may also result from maternal use of ototoxic drugs, birth trauma, and anoxia during or after birth.

Mumps is the most common pediatric cause of unilateral sensorineural hearing loss. Other causes are meningitis, measles, influenza, and acute febrile illness.

Disorders that may produce congenital conductive hearing loss include atresia, ossicle malformation, and other abnormalities. Serous otitis media commonly causes bilateral conductive hearing loss in children. Conductive hearing loss may also occur in children who put foreign objects in their ears.

Hearing disorders in children may lead to speech, language, and learning problems. Early identification and treatment of hearing loss is thus crucial to avoid incorrectly labeling the child as mentally retarded, brain damaged, or a slow learner.

When assessing an infant or a young child for hearing loss, remember that you can't use a tuning fork. Instead, test the startle reflex in infants younger than age 6 months, or have an audiologist test brain stem evoked response in neonates, infants, and young children. Also, obtain a gestational, perinatal, and family history from the parents.

GERIATRIC POINTERS

In older patients, presbycusis may be aggravated by exposure to noise as well as other factors.

PATIENT COUNSELING

Instruct the patient to avoid exposure to loud noise and to use ear protection to arrest loss. If the patient has an upper respiratory tract infection, tell him to avoid flying and driving. Explain the importance of completing the full course of prescribed antibiotics.

HEMATEMESIS

Hematemesis, the vomiting of blood, usually indicates GI bleeding above the ligament of Treitz, which suspends the duodenum at its junction with the jejunum. Bright red or blood-streaked vomitus indicates fresh or recent bleeding. Dark red, brown, or black vomitus (the color and consistency of coffee grounds) indicates that blood has been retained in the stomach and partially digested.

Although hematemesis usually results from a GI disorder, it may stem from a coagulation disorder or from a treatment that irritates the GI tract. Esophageal

In an emergency

◆ Check vital signs.
◆ If you detect signs of shock, place patient in supine position, and elevate feet.
◆ Start a large-bore I.V. line for emergency fluid replacement.
◆ Send a blood sample for typing and crossmatching, hemoglobin level, and hematocrit.
◆ Administer oxygen.

Key history points

◆ Onset, amount, color, and consistency of vomitus
◆ Description of stools
◆ Associated nausea, flatulence, diarrhea, or weakness
◆ History of ulcers or liver or coagulation disorders
◆ Alcohol use
◆ Drug history, including aspirin and other NSAIDs

Critical assessment steps

◆ Check for orthostatic hypotension, an early warning sign of hypovolemia.
◆ Obtain other vital signs.
◆ Inspect the mucous membranes, nasopharynx, and skin for signs of bleeding.
◆ Palpate abdomen for tenderness, pain, or masses.

Medical causes

Anthrax (GI)

◆ Signs and symptoms may progress to hematemesis, abdominal pain, and severe bloody diarrhea.

Coagulation disorders

◆ GI bleeding and moderate to severe hematemesis may occur.

varices may also cause hematemesis. Swallowed blood from epistaxis or oropharyngeal erosion may also cause bloody vomitus. Hematemesis may be precipitated by straining, emotional stress, and the use of an anti-inflammatory or alcohol. In a patient with esophageal varices, hematemesis may be a result of trauma from swallowing hard or partially chewed food.

Hematemesis is always an important sign, but its severity depends on the amount, source, and rapidity of the bleeding. Massive hematemesis (vomiting of 500 to 1,000 ml of blood) may be life-threatening.

 EMERGENCY ACTIONS If the patient has massive hematemesis, check his vital signs. If you detect signs of shock — such as tachypnea, hypotension, and tachycardia — place him in a supine position, and elevate his feet 20 to 30 degrees. Start a large-bore I.V. line for emergency fluid replacement. Also, send a blood sample for typing and crossmatching, hemoglobin level, and hematocrit, and administer oxygen. Emergency endoscopy may be necessary to locate the source of bleeding. Prepare to insert a nasogastric (NG) tube for suction or iced lavage. A Sengstaken-Blakemore tube may be used to compress esophageal varices. (See *Managing hematemesis with intubation.*)

HISTORY

If the patient's hematemesis isn't immediately life-threatening, begin with a thorough history. First, have the patient describe the amount, color, and consistency of the vomitus. When did he first notice this sign? Has he ever had hematemesis before? Find out if he also has bloody or black, tarry stools. Note whether hematemesis is usually preceded by nausea, flatulence, diarrhea, or weakness. Has he recently had bouts of retching with or without vomiting?

Next, ask about a history of ulcers or of liver or coagulation disorders. Find out how much alcohol the patient drinks, if any. Does he regularly take aspirin or another nonsteroidal anti-inflammatory drug (NSAID), such as phenylbutazone or indomethacin? These drugs may cause erosive gastritis or ulcers.

PHYSICAL ASSESSMENT

Begin the physical examination by checking for orthostatic hypotension, an early warning sign of hypovolemia. Take blood pressure and pulse with the patient in supine, sitting, and standing positions. A decrease of 10 mm Hg or more in systolic pressure or an increase of 10 beats/minute or more in pulse rate indicates volume depletion. After obtaining other vital signs, inspect the mucous membranes, nasopharynx, and skin for any signs of bleeding or other abnormalities. Finally, palpate the abdomen for tenderness, pain, or masses. Note lymphadenopathy.

MEDICAL CAUSES

Anthrax (GI)

With GI anthrax, initial signs and symptoms, including loss of appetite, nausea, vomiting, and fever, appear after eating contaminated meat from an animal infected with the gram-positive, spore-forming bacterium *Bacillus anthracis.* Signs and symptoms may progress to hematemesis, abdominal pain, and severe bloody diarrhea.

Coagulation disorders

Any disorder that disrupts normal clotting may result in GI bleeding and moderate to severe hematemesis. Bleeding may occur in other body systems as well, resulting

Managing hematemesis with intubation

A patient with hematemesis will need to have a GI tube inserted to allow blood drainage, to aspirate gastric contents, or to facilitate gastric lavage, if necessary. Here are the most common tubes and their uses.

NASOGASTRIC TUBES

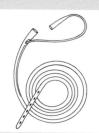

WIDE-BORE GASTRIC TUBES

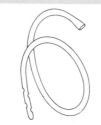

ESOPHAGEAL TUBES

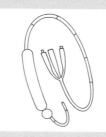

The Salem-Sump tube (shown above), a double-lumen nasogastric (NG) tube, is used to remove stomach fluid and gas or to aspirate gastric contents. It may also be used for gastric lavage, drug administration, or feeding. Its main advantage over the Levin tube—a single-lumen NG device—is that it allows atmospheric air to enter the patient's stomach so the tube can float freely instead of risking adhesion and damage to the gastric mucosa.

The Edlich tube (shown above) has one wide-bore lumen with four openings near the closed distal tip. A funnel or syringe can be connected at the proximal end. Like the other tubes, the Edlich can aspirate a large volume of gastric contents quickly.

The Ewald tube, a wide-bore tube that allows quick passage of a large amount of fluid and clots, is especially useful for gastric lavage in patients with profuse GI bleeding and in those who have ingested poison. Another wide-bore tube, the double-lumen Levacuator, has a large lumen for evacuation of gastric contents and a small one for lavage.

The Sengstaken-Blakemore tube (shown above), a triple-lumen double-balloon esophageal tube, provides a gastric aspiration port that allows drainage from below the gastric balloon. It can also be used to instill medication. A similar tube, the Linton shunt, can aspirate esophageal and gastric contents without risking necrosis because it has no esophageal balloon. The Minnesota esophagogastric tamponade tube, which has four lumina and two balloons, provides pressure-monitoring ports for both balloons without the need for Y-connectors.

in such signs as epistaxis and ecchymosis. Other associated effects vary, depending on the specific coagulation disorder, such as thrombocytopenia or hemophilia.

Esophageal cancer

A late sign of esophageal cancer, hematemesis may be accompanied by steady chest pain that radiates to the back. Other features include substernal fullness, severe dysphagia, nausea, vomiting with nocturnal regurgitation and aspiration, hemoptysis, fever, hiccups, sore throat, melena, and halitosis.

Esophageal injury by caustic substances

Ingestion of corrosive acids or alkalis produces esophageal injury associated with grossly bloody or coffee-ground vomitus. Hematemesis is accompanied by epigastric and anterior or retrosternal chest pain that's intensified by swallowing. With

Medical causes
(continued)

Esophageal cancer

✦ Hematemesis, a late sign, may be accompanied by steady chest pain that radiates to the back.

Esophageal injury by caustic substances

✦ Hematemesis occurs with epigastric and anterior or retrosternal chest pain that's intensified by swallowing.

Medical causes
(continued)

Esophageal rupture
+ Severity of hematemesis depends on the cause of the rupture.
+ Severe retrosternal, epigastric, neck, or scapular pain accompanied by chest and neck edema may occur.

Esophageal varices (ruptured)
+ Coffee-ground or massive, bright red vomitus may occur.

Gastric cancer
+ Painless bright red or dark brown vomitus is a late sign.

Gastritis (acute)
+ Hematemesis and melena are the most common signs.

GI leiomyoma
+ The mucosa or vascular supply erodes to produce hematemesis.

Mallory-Weiss syndrome
+ Hematemesis and melena may occur.

Peptic ulcer
+ Hematemesis may occur when an artery, a vein, or highly vascular tissue is penetrated by the ulcer.

ingestion of alkaline agents, the oral and pharyngeal mucosa may produce a soapy white film. The mucosa becomes brown and edematous with time. Dysphagia, marked salivation, and fever may develop in 3 to 4 weeks and worsen as strictures form.

Esophageal rupture
With esophageal rupture, the severity of hematemesis depends on the cause of the rupture. When an instrument damages the esophagus, hematemesis is usually slight. However, rupture due to Boerhaave's syndrome (increased esophageal pressure from vomiting or retching) or other esophageal disorders typically causes more severe hematemesis. This life-threatening disorder may also produce severe retrosternal, epigastric, neck, or scapular pain accompanied by chest and neck edema. Examination reveals subcutaneous crepitation in the chest wall, supraclavicular fossa, and neck. The patient may also show signs of respiratory distress, such as dyspnea and cyanosis.

Esophageal varices (ruptured)
Life-threatening rupture of esophageal varices may produce coffee-ground or massive, bright red vomitus. Signs of shock, such as hypotension or tachycardia, may follow or even precede hematemesis if the stomach fills with blood before vomiting occurs. Other symptoms may include abdominal distention and melena or painless hematochezia, ranging from slight oozing to massive rectal hemorrhage.

Gastric cancer
Painless bright red or dark brown vomitus is a late sign of gastric cancer, an uncommon cancer that usually begins insidiously with upper-abdominal discomfort. The patient then develops anorexia, mild nausea, and chronic dyspepsia unrelieved by antacids and exacerbated by food. Later symptoms may include fatigue, weakness, weight loss, feelings of fullness, melena, altered bowel habits, and signs of malnutrition, such as muscle wasting and dry skin.

Gastritis (acute)
Hematemesis and melena are the most common signs of acute gastritis. They may even be the only signs, although mild epigastric discomfort, nausea, fever, and malaise may also occur. Massive blood loss precipitates signs of shock. Typically, the patient has a history of alcohol abuse or has used aspirin or some other NSAID. Gastritis may also occur secondary to *Helicobacter pylori* infection.

GI leiomyoma
GI leiomyoma is a benign tumor that occasionally involves the GI tract, eroding the mucosa or vascular supply to produce hematemesis. Other features vary with the tumor's size and location. For example, esophageal involvement may cause dysphagia and weight loss.

Mallory-Weiss syndrome
Characterized by a mucosal tear of the mucous membrane at the junction of the esophagus and the stomach, Mallory-Weiss syndrome may produce hematemesis and melena. It's commonly triggered by severe vomiting, retching, or straining (as from coughing), most commonly in alcoholics or in people whose pylorus is obstructed. Severe bleeding may precipitate signs of shock, such as tachycardia, hypotension, dyspnea, and cool, clammy skin.

Peptic ulcer
Hematemesis may occur when a peptic ulcer penetrates an artery, vein, or highly vascular tissue. Massive—and possibly life-threatening—hematemesis is typical

when an artery is penetrated. Other features include melena or hematochezia, chills, fever, and signs and symptoms of shock and dehydration, such as tachycardia, hypotension, poor skin turgor, and thirst. Most patients have a history of nausea, vomiting, epigastric tenderness, and epigastric pain that's relieved by foods or antacids. The patient may also have a history of habitual use of tobacco, alcohol, or NSAIDs.

OTHER CAUSES

Treatments
Traumatic NG or endotracheal intubation may cause hematemesis associated with swallowed blood. Nose or throat surgery may also cause this sign in the same way.

SPECIAL CONSIDERATIONS
Closely monitor the patient's vital signs, and watch for signs of shock. Check the patient's stools regularly for occult blood, and keep accurate intake and output records. Place the patient on bed rest in a low or semi-Fowler's position to prevent aspiration of vomitus. Keep suctioning equipment nearby, and use it as needed. Provide frequent oral hygiene and emotional support — the sight of bloody vomitus can be extremely frightening. Administer a histamine-2 blocker I.V.; vasopressin may be required for variceal hemorrhage. As the bleeding tapers off, monitor the pH of gastric contents, and give hourly doses of antacids by NG tube as necessary.

PEDIATRIC POINTERS
Hematemesis is much less common in children than in adults and may be related to foreign-body ingestion. Occasionally, neonates develop hematemesis after swallowing maternal blood during delivery or breast-feeding from a cracked nipple. Hemorrhagic disease of the neonate and esophageal erosion may also cause hematemesis in infants; such cases require immediate fluid replacement.

GERIATRIC POINTERS
In elderly patients, hematemesis may be caused by a vascular anomaly, an aortoenteric fistula, or upper GI cancer. In addition, chronic obstructive pulmonary disease, chronic liver or renal failure, and chronic NSAID use all predispose elderly people to hemorrhage secondary to coexisting ulcerative disorders.

PATIENT COUNSELING
Explain diagnostic tests, such as endoscopy, barium swallow, and variceal banding. Explain laboratory tests, such as serum electrolyte levels, complete blood count, prothrombin time, partial thromboplastin time, and International Normalized Ratio. Discuss food or fluid restrictions as needed.

HEMATOCHEZIA

The passage of bloody stools, also known as *hematochezia*, usually indicates — and may be the first sign of — GI bleeding below the ligament of Treitz. However, this sign — usually preceded by hematemesis — may also accompany rapid hemorrhage of 1 L or more from the upper GI tract. Hematochezia ranges from formed, blood-streaked stools to liquid, bloody stools that may be bright red, dark mahogany, or

Other causes
+ Nose or throat surgery
+ Traumatic NG or endotracheal intubation

Special considerations
+ Monitor vital signs; watch for signs of shock.
+ Check stools for occult blood.
+ Place the patient on bed rest.
+ Keep suctioning equipment nearby; use it as needed.
+ Provide frequent oral hygiene.
+ Give a histamine-2 blocker I.V.; vasopressin may be required for variceal hemorrhage.

Peds points
+ Hematemesis may be related to foreign-body ingestion.
+ Hemorrhagic disease and esophageal erosion may cause hematemesis in infants.

Geri points
+ Hematemesis may be caused by a vascular anomaly, an aortoenteric fistula, or upper GI cancer.
+ COPD, chronic liver or renal failure, and chronic NSAID use predispose elderly people to hemorrhage secondary to coexisting ulcerative disorders.

Teaching points
+ Explanation of diagnostic and laboratory tests
+ Food or fluid restrictions

Key facts about hematochezia
+ Passage of bloody stools
+ Usually develops abruptly and indicates bleeding below the ligament of Treitz

In an emergency

+ Check vital signs for signs of shock, place patient in a supine position and elevate his feet.
+ Prepare to administer oxygen.
+ Start a large-bore I.V. line for emergency fluid replacement.
+ Obtain a blood sample for typing and crossmatching, hemoglobin level, and hematocrit.
+ Insert an NG tube.

Key history points

+ Onset, amount, color, and consistency of stools
+ Associated signs and symptoms
+ Medical history, including GI and coagulation disorders
+ Use of GI irritants, such as alcohol, aspirin, and other NSAIDs

Critical assessment steps

+ Check for orthostatic hypotension.
+ Examine the skin for petechiae or spider angiomas.
+ Palpate the abdomen for tenderness, pain, or masses. Note lymphadenopathy.

Medical causes

Anal fissure
+ Slight hematochezia occurs; blood may streak the stools or appear on toilet tissue.

Anorectal fistula
+ Blood, pus, mucus, and occasionally stools may drain from an anorectal fistula.

Coagulation disorders
+ GI bleeding marked by moderate to severe hematochezia may occur.

maroon in color. This sign usually develops abruptly and is heralded by abdominal pain.

Although hematochezia is commonly associated with GI disorders, it may result from a coagulation disorder, exposure to toxins, or certain diagnostic tests. Always a significant sign, hematochezia may precipitate life-threatening hypovolemia.

 EMERGENCY ACTIONS If the patient has severe hematochezia, check his vital signs. If you detect signs of shock, such as hypotension and tachycardia, place him in a supine position and elevate his feet 20 to 30 degrees. Prepare to administer oxygen, and start a large-bore I.V. line for emergency fluid replacement. Next, obtain a blood sample for typing and crossmatching, hemoglobin level, and hematocrit. Insert a nasogastric tube. Iced lavage may be indicated to control bleeding. Endoscopy may be necessary to detect the source of the bleeding.

HISTORY

If the hematochezia isn't immediately life-threatening, ask the patient to fully describe the amount, color, and consistency of his bloody stools. (If possible, also inspect and characterize the stools yourself.) How long have the stools been bloody? Do they always look the same, or does the amount of blood seem to vary? Ask about associated signs and symptoms.

Explore the patient's medical history, focusing on GI and coagulation disorders. Ask about use of GI irritants, such as alcohol, aspirin, and other nonsteroidal anti-inflammatory drugs.

 CULTURAL CUE In the Chinese culture, discomfort isn't usually displayed openly. Direct questioning and vigilant assessment skills are necessary to ensure that a Chinese patient's quiet nature doesn't mask signs and symptoms that may be life-threatening.

PHYSICAL ASSESSMENT

Begin the physical examination by checking for orthostatic hypotension, an early sign of shock. Take the patient's blood pressure and pulse while he's lying down, sitting, and standing. If systolic pressure decreases by 10 mm Hg or more, or pulse rate increases by 10 beats/minute or more when he changes position, suspect volume depletion and impending shock.

Examine the skin for petechiae or spider angiomas. Palpate the abdomen for tenderness, pain, or masses. Also, note lymphadenopathy. Finally, a digital rectal examination must be done to rule out rectal masses or hemorrhoids.

MEDICAL CAUSES

Anal fissure

Slight hematochezia characterizes an anal fissure; blood may streak the stools or appear on toilet tissue. Accompanying hematochezia is severe rectal pain that may make the patient reluctant to defecate, thereby causing constipation.

Anorectal fistula

Blood, pus, mucus, and occasionally stools may drain from an anorectal fistula. Other effects include rectal pain and pruritus. If an abscess is present, the patient may have a fever.

Coagulation disorders

Patients with a coagulation disorder (such as thrombocytopenia and disseminated intravascular coagulation) may experience GI bleeding marked by moderate to severe hematochezia. Bleeding may also occur in other body systems, producing such signs as epistaxis and purpura. Associated findings vary with the specific coagulation disorder.

Colitis

Ischemic colitis commonly causes hematochezia, especially in elderly patients. The hematochezia may be slight or massive and is usually accompanied by severe, cramping lower abdominal pain and hypotension. Other effects include abdominal tenderness, distention, and absent bowel sounds. Severe colitis may cause life-threatening hypovolemic shock and peritonitis.

Ulcerative colitis typically causes hematochezia that may also contain mucus. The hematochezia is preceded by mild to severe abdominal cramps and may cause slight to massive blood loss. Associated signs and symptoms include fever, tenesmus, anorexia, nausea, vomiting, hyperactive bowel sounds and, occasionally, tachycardia. Weight loss and weakness occur late.

Colon cancer

Bright red rectal bleeding with or without pain is a telling sign, especially in cancer of the left colon. Usually, a left colon tumor causes early signs of obstruction, such as rectal pressure, bleeding, and intermittent fullness or cramping. As the disease progresses, the patient also develops obstipation, diarrhea, or ribbon-shaped stools, and pain, which is typically relieved by passage of stools or flatus. Stools are grossly bloody.

Early tumor growth in the right colon may cause melena, abdominal aching, pressure, and dull cramps. As the disease progresses, the patient develops weakness and fatigue. Later, he may also experience diarrhea, anorexia, weight loss, anemia, vomiting, abdominal mass, and signs of obstruction, such as abdominal distention and abnormal bowel sounds.

Colorectal polyps

Colorectal polyps are the most common cause of intermittent hematochezia in adults younger than age 60; however, sometimes such polyps produce no symptoms. When located high in the colon, polyps may cause blood-streaked stools. The stools yield a positive response when tested with guaiac. If the polyps are located closer to the rectum, they may bleed freely.

Crohn's disease

Hematochezia isn't a common sign of Crohn's disease unless the perineum is involved. If rectal bleeding occurs, it's likely to be massive. The chief clinical features of Crohn's disease include fever, abdominal distention and pain with guarding, diarrhea, hyperactive bowel sounds, anorexia, nausea, and fatigue. A palpable mass in the colon area may be present.

Diverticulitis

Most common in elderly patients, diverticulitis can suddenly cause mild to moderate rectal bleeding after the patient feels the urge to defecate. The bleeding may end abruptly or may progress to life-threatening blood loss with signs of shock. Associated signs and symptoms may include left-lower-quadrant pain that's relieved by defecation, alternating episodes of constipation and diarrhea, anorexia, nausea and vomiting, rebound tenderness, and a distended tympanic abdomen.

Dysentery

Bloody diarrhea is common in infection with *Shigella*, *Amoeba*, and *Campylobacter*, but rare with *Salmonella*. In addition, abdominal pain or cramps, tenesmus, fever, and nausea may occur. Signs and symptoms of dehydration may also be present.

Medical causes
(continued)

Colitis
+ Ischemic colitis commonly causes slight or massive hematochezia; severe, cramping lower abdominal pain, and hypotension.
+ Ulcerative colitis typically causes hematochezia that may also contain mucus.

Colon cancer
+ Bright red rectal bleeding with or without pain occurs.

Colorectal polyps
+ Intermittent hematochezia occurs.

Crohn's disease
+ Hematochezia isn't common unless the perineum is involved.
+ If rectal bleeding occurs, it's likely to be massive.

Diverticulitis
+ Moderate rectal bleeding occurs after the patient feels the urge to defecate.

Dysentery
+ Bloody diarrhea is common in infection with *Shigella*, *Amoeba*, and *Campylobacter*.

Medical causes
(continued)

Esophageal varices (ruptured)

+ Hematochezia may range from slight rectal oozing to grossly bloody stools.

Food poisoning (staphylococcal)

+ Bloody diarrhea may occur 1 to 6 hours after ingesting food toxins.

Hemorrhoids

+ Hematochezia may accompany external hemorrhoids, which typically cause painful defecation, resulting in constipation.
+ Internal hemorrhoids usually produce chronic bleeding with bowel movements.

Peptic ulcer

+ Hematochezia, hematemesis, or melena may occur.

Small-intestine cancer

+ Slight hematochezia or blood-streaked stools may result.

Ulcerative proctitis

+ Patient has an intense urge to defecate, but passes only bright red blood, pus, or mucus.

Other causes

+ Certain procedures, especially colonoscopy, polypectomy, and proctosigmoidoscopy
+ Heavy metal poisoning

Esophageal varices (ruptured)

When an esophageal varix ruptures (a life-threatening condition), hematochezia may range from slight rectal oozing to grossly bloody stools and may be accompanied by mild to severe hematemesis or melena. This painless but massive hemorrhage may precipitate signs of shock, such as tachycardia and hypotension. In fact, signs of shock occasionally precede overt signs of bleeding. Typically, the patient with esophageal varices has a history of chronic liver disease.

Food poisoning (staphylococcal)

The patient with staphylococcal food poisoning may have bloody diarrhea 1 to 6 hours after ingesting food toxins. Accompanying signs and symptoms include severe, cramping abdominal pain, nausea and vomiting, and prostration, all of which last a few hours.

Hemorrhoids

Hematochezia may accompany external hemorrhoids, which typically cause painful defecation, resulting in constipation. Less painful internal hemorrhoids usually produce more chronic bleeding with bowel movements, which may eventually lead to signs of anemia, such as weakness and fatigue.

Peptic ulcer

Upper GI bleeding is a common complication in peptic ulcer. The patient may display hematochezia, hematemesis, or melena, depending on the rapidity and amount of bleeding. If the peptic ulcer penetrates an artery or vein, massive bleeding may precipitate signs of shock, such as hypotension and tachycardia. Other findings may include chills, fever, nausea and vomiting, and signs of dehydration, such as dry mucous membranes, poor skin turgor, and thirst. The patient typically has a history of epigastric pain that's relieved by foods or antacids; he may also have a history of habitual use of tobacco, alcohol, or nonsteroidal anti-inflammatory drugs.

Small-intestine cancer

Small-intestine cancer occasionally produces slight hematochezia or blood-streaked stools. Its characteristic features include colicky pain and postprandial vomiting. Other common signs and symptoms include weight loss, anorexia, and fever. Palpation may reveal abdominal masses.

Ulcerative proctitis

Ulcerative proctitis typically causes an intense urge to defecate, but the patient passes only bright red blood, pus, or mucus. Other common signs and symptoms include acute constipation and tenesmus.

OTHER CAUSES

Diagnostic tests

Certain procedures, especially colonoscopy, polypectomy, and proctosigmoidoscopy, may cause rectal bleeding. Bowel perforation is rare.

Heavy metal poisoning

Bloody diarrhea is accompanied by cramping abdominal pain, nausea, and vomiting. Other signs may include tachycardia, hypotension, seizures, paresthesia, depressed or absent deep tendon reflexes, and an altered level of consciousness.

SPECIAL CONSIDERATIONS

Place the patient on bed rest and check his vital signs frequently, watching for signs of shock, such as hypotension, tachycardia, weak pulse, and tachypnea. Monitor the patient's intake and output hourly.

Prepare the patient for blood tests and GI procedures, such as endoscopy and GI X-rays. Visually examine the patient's stools and test them for occult blood. If necessary, send a stool sample to the laboratory to check for parasites.

PEDIATRIC POINTERS

Hematochezia is much less common in children than in adults. It may result from structural disorders, such as intussusception and Meckel's diverticulum, and from inflammatory disorders, such as peptic ulcer disease and ulcerative colitis.

In children, ulcerative colitis typically produces chronic, rather than acute, signs and symptoms and may also cause slow growth and maturation related to malnutrition. Suspect sexual abuse in all cases of rectal bleeding in children.

GERIATRIC POINTERS

Because older people have an increased risk of colon cancer, hematochezia should be evaluated with colonoscopy after perirectal lesions have been ruled out as the cause of bleeding.

PATIENT COUNSELING

Provide emotional support because hematochezia may frighten the patient. Tell the patient to report changes in bowel habits and blood in the stool to his health care provider. Show him how to perform ostomy self-care if indicated. Discuss proper bowel elimination habits and dietary recommendations and restrictions.

HEMATURIA

A cardinal sign of renal and urinary tract disorders, hematuria is the abnormal presence of blood in the urine. Microscopic hematuria is confirmed by an occult blood test, whereas macroscopic hematuria is immediately visible. However, macroscopic hematuria must be distinguished from pseudohematuria. (See *Confirming hematuria*, page 342.) Macroscopic hematuria may be continuous or intermittent, is often accompanied by pain, and may be aggravated by prolonged standing or walking.

Hematuria may be classified by the stage of urination it predominantly affects. Bleeding at the start of urination — *initial hematuria* — usually indicates a urethral disorder; bleeding at the end of urination — *terminal hematuria* — usually indicates a disorder of the bladder neck, posterior urethra, or prostate; bleeding throughout urination — *total hematuria* — usually indicates a disorder above the bladder neck.

Hematuria may result from one of two mechanisms: rupture or perforation of vessels in the renal system or urinary tract, or impaired glomerular filtration, which allows red blood cells to seep into the urine. The color of the bloody urine provides a clue to the source of the bleeding. Generally, dark or brownish blood indicates renal or upper urinary tract bleeding, whereas bright red blood indicates lower urinary tract bleeding.

Although hematuria usually results from renal and urinary tract disorders, it may also result from certain GI, prostate, vaginal, or coagulation disorders, or from

Special considerations
+ Place the patient on bed rest.
+ Check vital signs frequently, watching for signs of shock.
+ Monitor intake and output hourly.
+ Visually examine stools and test them for occult blood. If necessary, send a stool sample to the laboratory to check for parasites.

Peds points
+ Hematochezia may result from structural and inflammatory disorders.
+ In children, ulcerative colitis typically produces chronic signs and symptoms.
+ Suspect sexual abuse in all cases of rectal bleeding in children.

Geri points
+ Hematochezia should be evaluated using colonoscopy after ruling out perirectal lesions as the cause of bleeding.

Teaching points
+ Signs and symptoms to report
+ Ostomy self-care
+ Proper bowel elimination habits
+ Dietary recommendations and restrictions

Key facts about hematuria
+ Abnormal presence of blood in urine
+ May be microscopic or macroscopic
+ Classified as initial (occurring at the start of urination), terminal (occurring at the end of urination), or total (occurring throughout urination)

Key history points

+ Onset, description, and severity of hematuria
+ Associated pain or burning
+ Recent abdominal or flank trauma
+ History of renal, urinary, prostatic, or coagulation disorders
+ Drug history

Critical assessment steps

+ Palpate and percuss the abdomen and flanks.
+ Percuss the CVA to elicit tenderness.
+ Check the urinary meatus for bleeding or other abnormalities.
+ Using a chemical reagent strip, test a urine specimen for protein.
+ A vaginal or digital rectal examination may be necessary.

Medical causes

Appendicitis

+ About 15% of patients with appendicitis have either microscopic or macroscopic hematuria accompanied by bladder tenderness, dysuria, and urinary urgency.

the effects of certain drugs. Invasive therapy and diagnostic tests that involve manipulative instrumentation of the renal and urologic systems may also cause hematuria. Nonpathologic hematuria may result from fever and hypercatabolic states. Transient hematuria may follow strenuous exercise.

HISTORY

After detecting hematuria, take a pertinent health history. If hematuria is macroscopic, ask the patient when he first noticed blood in his urine. Does it vary in severity between voidings? Is it worse at the beginning, middle, or end of urination? Has it occurred before? Is the patient passing any clots? To rule out artifactitious hematuria, ask about bleeding hemorrhoids or the onset of menses, if appropriate. Ask if there's any pain or burning with the episodes of hematuria.

Ask about recent abdominal or flank trauma. Has the patient been exercising strenuously? Note a history of renal, urinary, prostatic, or coagulation disorders. Then obtain a drug history, noting any anticoagulants or aspirin.

PHYSICAL ASSESSMENT

Begin the physical examination by palpating and percussing the abdomen and flanks. Next, percuss the costovertebral angle (CVA) to elicit tenderness. Check the urinary meatus for bleeding or other abnormalities. Using a chemical reagent strip, test a urine specimen for protein. A vaginal or digital rectal examination may be necessary.

MEDICAL CAUSES

Appendicitis

About 15% of patients with appendicitis have either microscopic or macroscopic hematuria accompanied by bladder tenderness, dysuria, and urinary urgency. More typical findings include constant right-lower-quadrant pain (especially over McBurney's point), nausea and vomiting, anorexia, abdominal rigidity, rebound tenderness, constipation, tachycardia, and low-grade fever.

Bladder cancer

A primary cause of gross hematuria in men, bladder cancer may also produce pain in the bladder, rectum, pelvis, flank, back, or leg. Other common features are nocturia, dysuria, urinary frequency and urgency, vomiting, diarrhea, and insomnia.

Bladder trauma

Gross hematuria is characteristic in traumatic rupture or perforation of the bladder. Typically, the hematuria is accompanied by lower abdominal pain and, occasionally, anuria despite a strong urge to void. The patient may also develop swelling of the scrotum, buttocks, or perineum and signs of shock, such as tachycardia and hypotension.

Calculi

Bladder and renal calculi produce hematuria, which may be associated with signs of urinary tract infection, such as dysuria and urinary frequency and urgency. Bladder calculi usually cause gross hematuria, referred pain to the lower back or penile or vulvar area and, in some patients, bladder distention.

More common in women, chronic interstitial cystitis occasionally causes grossly bloody hematuria. Associated features include urinary frequency, dysuria, nocturia, and tenesmus. Both microscopic and macroscopic hematuria may occur with tubercular cystitis, which may also cause urinary urgency and frequency, dysuria, tenesmus, flank pain, fatigue, and anorexia. Viral cystitis usually produces hematuria, urinary urgency and frequency, dysuria, nocturia, tenesmus, and fever.

Renal calculi may produce microscopic or gross hematuria. The cardinal symptom, though, is colicky pain that travels from the CVA to the flank, suprapubic region, and external genitalia when a calculus is passed. The pain may be excruciating at its peak. Other signs and symptoms may include nausea and vomiting, restlessness, fever, chills, abdominal distention and, possibly, decreased bowel sounds.

Coagulation disorders

Macroscopic hematuria is typically the first sign of hemorrhage in coagulation disorders, such as thrombocytopenia or disseminated intravascular coagulation. Among other features are epistaxis, purpura (petechiae and ecchymoses), and signs of GI bleeding.

Cystitis

Hematuria is a telling sign in all types of cystitis. Bacterial cystitis usually produces macroscopic hematuria with urinary urgency and frequency, dysuria, nocturia, and tenesmus. The patient complains of perineal and lumbar pain, suprapubic discomfort, and fatigue and occasionally has a low-grade fever.

Diverticulitis

When diverticulitis involves the bladder, it usually causes microscopic hematuria, urinary frequency and urgency, dysuria, and nocturia. Characteristic findings include left-lower-quadrant pain, abdominal tenderness, constipation or diarrhea and, at times, a palpable, firm, fixed, and tender abdominal mass. The patient may also develop mild nausea, flatulence, and a low-grade fever.

Endocarditis (subacute infective)

Occasionally, subacute infective endocarditis produces embolization, resulting in renal infarction and microscopic or gross hematuria. Among common related findings are constant fever, chills, night sweats, fatigue, pallor, anorexia, weight loss, polyarthralgia, petechiae, flank pain, severe back pain, stiff neck, cardiac murmurs, tachycardia, and splenomegaly.

Medical causes
(continued)

Bladder cancer
+ Gross hematuria may be accompanied by pain in bladder, rectum, pelvis, flank, back, or leg.

Bladder trauma
+ Hematuria is accompanied by lower abdominal pain.

Calculi
+ Bladder calculi usually cause gross hematuria.
+ Renal calculi may produce microscopic or gross hematuria.

Coagulation disorders
+ Macroscopic hematuria is typically first sign of hemorrhage.

Cystitis
+ Bacterial cystitis usually produces macroscopic hematuria with urinary urgency and frequency, dysuria, and nocturia.
+ Chronic interstitial cystitis occasionally causes grossly bloody hematuria.
+ Microscopic and macroscopic hematuria may occur with tubercular cystitis.
+ Viral cystitis usually produces hematuria, urinary urgency and frequency, dysuria, nocturia, tenesmus, and fever.

Diverticulitis
+ When the bladder is involved, microscopic hematuria, urinary frequency and urgency, dysuria, and nocturia occur.

Endocarditis (subacute infective)
+ Embolization occasionally results in renal infarction and microscopic or gross hematuria.

Medical causes
(continued)

Glomerulonephritis
✦ With acute form, gross hematuria tapers off to microscopic hematuria and red cell casts.
✦ Chronic form causes hematuria accompanied by proteinuria, generalized edema, and increased blood pressure.

Nephritis (interstitial)
✦ Microscopic hematuria is typical, but some patients may develop gross hematuria.

Nephropathy (obstructive)
✦ Microscopic or macroscopic hematuria may occur, but rarely is urine grossly bloody.

Polycystic kidney disease
✦ Microscopic or gross hematuria may occur.

Prostatic hyperplasia (benign)
✦ About 20% of patients with enlarged prostates have macroscopic hematuria, usually when a significant obstruction is present.

Prostatitis
✦ Macroscopic hematuria may occur, usually at the end of urination.

Pyelonephritis (acute)
✦ Microscopic or macroscopic hematuria progresses to grossly bloody hematuria.
✦ After the infection resolves, microscopic hematuria may persist for a few months.

Glomerulonephritis

Acute glomerulonephritis usually begins with gross hematuria that tapers off to microscopic hematuria and red cell casts, which may persist for months. It may also produce oliguria or anuria, proteinuria, mild fever, fatigue, flank and abdominal pain, generalized edema, increased blood pressure, nausea, vomiting, and signs of lung congestion, such as crackles and a productive cough.

Chronic glomerulonephritis usually causes microscopic hematuria accompanied by proteinuria, generalized edema, and increased blood pressure. Signs and symptoms of uremia may also occur in advanced disease.

Nephritis (interstitial)

Typically, this infection causes microscopic hematuria. However, some patients with acute interstitial nephritis may develop gross hematuria. Other findings are fever, maculopapular rash, and oliguria or anuria. In chronic interstitial nephritis, the patient has dilute — almost colorless — urine that may be accompanied by polyuria and increased blood pressure.

Nephropathy (obstructive)

Obstructive nephropathy may cause microscopic or macroscopic hematuria, but rarely is urine grossly bloody. The patient may report colicky flank and abdominal pain, CVA tenderness, and anuria or oliguria that alternates with polyuria.

Polycystic kidney disease

Polycystic kidney disease, a hereditary disorder, may cause recurrent microscopic or gross hematuria. Although usually asymptomatic before age 40, it may cause increased blood pressure, polyuria, dull flank pain, and signs of urinary tract infection, such as dysuria and urinary frequency and urgency. Later, the patient develops a swollen, tender abdomen and lumbar pain that's aggravated by exertion and relieved by lying down. He may also have proteinuria and colicky abdominal pain from the ureteral passage of clots or stones.

Prostatic hyperplasia (benign)

About 20% of patients with enlarged prostates have macroscopic hematuria, usually when a significant obstruction is present. The hematuria is usually preceded by diminished urinary stream, tenesmus, and a feeling of incomplete voiding. It may be accompanied by urinary hesitancy, frequency, and incontinence; nocturia; perineal pain; and constipation. Inspection reveals a midline mass representing the distended bladder; rectal palpation reveals an enlarged prostate.

Prostatitis

Whether acute or chronic, prostatitis may cause macroscopic hematuria, usually at the end of urination. It may also produce urinary frequency and urgency and dysuria followed by visible bladder distention.

Acute prostatitis also produces fatigue, malaise, myalgia, polyarthralgia, fever with chills, nausea, vomiting, perineal and low back pain, and decreased libido. Rectal palpation reveals a tender, swollen, firm prostate.

Chronic prostatitis commonly follows an acute attack. It may cause persistent urethral discharge, dull perineal pain, ejaculatory pain, and decreased libido.

Pyelonephritis (acute)

Acute pyelonephritis typically produces microscopic or macroscopic hematuria that progresses to grossly bloody hematuria. After the infection resolves, microscopic hematuria may persist for a few months. Related signs and symptoms include persistent high fever, unilateral or bilateral flank pain, CVA tenderness, shaking chills, weakness, fatigue, dysuria, urinary frequency and urgency, nocturia, and tenesmus. The patient may also exhibit nausea, anorexia, vomiting, and signs of paralytic ileus, such as hypoactive or absent bowel sounds and abdominal distention.

Renal cancer

The classic triad of signs and symptoms of renal cancer includes grossly bloody hematuria; dull, aching flank pain; and a smooth, firm, palpable flank mass. Colicky pain may accompany the passage of clots. Other findings include fever, CVA tenderness, and increased blood pressure. In advanced disease, the patient may develop weight loss, nausea and vomiting, and leg edema with varicoceles.

Renal infarction

Typically, this disorder produces gross hematuria. The patient may complain of constant, severe flank and upper abdominal pain accompanied by CVA tenderness, anorexia, and nausea and vomiting. Other findings include oliguria or anuria, proteinuria, hypoactive bowel sounds and, a day or two after infarction, fever and increased blood pressure.

Renal papillary necrosis (acute)

Acute renal papillary necrosis usually produces grossly bloody hematuria, which may be accompanied by intense flank pain, CVA tenderness, abdominal rigidity and colicky pain, oliguria or anuria, pyuria, fever, chills, vomiting, and hypoactive bowel sounds. Arthralgia and hypertension are common.

Renal trauma

About 80% of patients with renal trauma have microscopic or gross hematuria. Accompanying signs and symptoms may include flank pain, a palpable flank mass, oliguria, hematoma or ecchymoses over the upper abdomen or flank, nausea and vomiting, and hypoactive bowel sounds. Severe trauma may precipitate signs of shock, such as tachycardia and hypotension.

Renal tuberculosis

Gross hematuria is often the first sign of renal tuberculosis. It may be accompanied by urinary frequency, dysuria, pyuria, tenesmus, colicky abdominal pain, lumbar pain, and proteinuria.

Renal vein thrombosis

Grossly bloody hematuria usually occurs in renal vein thrombosis. In abrupt venous obstruction, the patient experiences severe flank and lumbar pain as well as epigastric and CVA tenderness. Other features include fever, pallor, proteinuria, peripheral edema and, when the obstruction is bilateral, oliguria or anuria and other uremic signs. The kidneys are easily palpable. Gradual venous obstruction causes signs of nephrotic syndrome, proteinuria and, occasionally, peripheral edema.

Sickle cell anemia

In this hereditary disorder, gross hematuria may result from congestion of the renal papillae. Associated signs and symptoms of sickle cell anemia may include pallor, dehydration, chronic fatigue, polyarthralgia, leg ulcers, dyspnea, chest pain, impaired growth and development, hepatomegaly and, possibly, jaundice. Auscultation reveals tachycardia and systolic and diastolic murmurs.

Systemic lupus erythematosus

Gross hematuria and proteinuria may occur when systemic lupus erythematosus (SLE) involves the kidneys. Cardinal associated features include nondeforming joint pain and stiffness, a butterfly rash, photosensitivity, Raynaud's phenomenon,

---

Medical causes
(continued)

Renal cancer
✦ Grossly bloody hematuria; dull, aching flank pain; and a smooth, firm, palpable flank mass are the classic triad of this disorder.

Renal infarction
✦ Gross hematuria is typical.
✦ Patient may complain of constant, severe flank and upper abdominal pain accompanied by CVA tenderness, anorexia, nausea, and vomiting.

Renal papillary necrosis (acute)
✦ Grossly bloody hematuria may be accompanied by intense flank pain, CVA tenderness, abdominal rigidity and colicky pain, oliguria or anuria, pyuria, fever, chills, vomiting, and hypoactive bowel sounds.

Renal trauma
✦ About 80% of patients with renal trauma have microscopic or gross hematuria.

Renal tuberculosis
✦ Gross hematuria is often the first sign.

Renal vein thrombosis
✦ Grossly bloody hematuria usually occurs.

Sickle cell anemia
✦ Gross hematuria may result from congestion of the renal papillae.

SLE
✦ Gross hematuria and proteinuria may occur if the kidneys are involved.

Medical causes
(continued)

Urethral trauma
+ Initial hematuria may occur, possibly with blood at the urinary meatus, local pain, and penile or vulvar ecchymoses.

Vaginitis
+ Macroscopic hematuria may occur if vaginitis spreads to the urinary tract.

Vasculitis
+ Microscopic hematuria usually occurs.

Other causes
+ Anticoagulants, aspirin toxicity, analgesics, cyclophosphamide, metyrosine, phenylbutazone, penicillin, rifampin, and thiabendazole
+ Biopsy or manipulative instrumentation of the urinary tract
+ Kidney transplant
+ Renal biopsy

Special considerations
+ Check vital signs frequently.
+ Monitor the amount and pattern of hematuria.
+ If the patient has an indwelling urinary catheter in place, ensure its patency; irrigate if necessary.

Peds points
+ Common causes of hematuria in children include congenital anomalies, birth trauma, hematologic disorders, certain neoplasms, allergies, and foreign bodies in the urinary tract.

seizures or psychoses, recurrent fever, lymphadenopathy, oral or nasopharyngeal ulcers, anorexia, and weight loss.

Urethral trauma
With urethral trauma, initial hematuria may occur, possibly with blood at the urinary meatus, local pain, and penile or vulvar ecchymoses.

Vaginitis
When vaginitis spreads to the urinary tract, it may produce macroscopic hematuria. Related signs and symptoms may include urinary frequency and urgency, dysuria, nocturia, perineal pain, pruritus, and a malodorous vaginal discharge.

Vasculitis
Hematuria is usually microscopic in vasculitis. Associated signs and symptoms include malaise, myalgia, polyarthralgia, fever, increased blood pressure, pallor and, occasionally, anuria. Other features, such as urticaria and purpura, may reflect the etiology of vasculitis.

OTHER CAUSES

Diagnostic tests
Renal biopsy is the diagnostic test most often associated with hematuria. This sign may also result from biopsy or manipulative instrumentation of the urinary tract, as in cystoscopy.

Drugs
Drugs that commonly cause hematuria are anticoagulants, aspirin toxicity, analgesics, cyclophosphamide, metyrosine, phenylbutazone, penicillin, rifampin, and thiabendazole.

Treatments
Any therapy that involves manipulative instrumentation of the urinary tract, such as transurethral prostatectomy, may cause microscopic or macroscopic hematuria. Following a kidney transplant a patient may experience hematuria with or without clots, which may require indwelling urinary catheter irrigation.

SPECIAL CONSIDERATIONS

Because hematuria may frighten and upset the patient, be sure to provide emotional support. Check his vital signs at least every 4 hours and monitor intake and output, including the amount and pattern of hematuria. If the patient has an indwelling urinary catheter in place, ensure its patency and irrigate it if necessary to remove clots and tissue that may impede urine drainage. Administer prescribed analgesics, and enforce bed rest as indicated. Prepare the patient for diagnostic tests, such as blood and urine studies, cystoscopy, and renal X-rays or biopsy.

PEDIATRIC POINTERS

Many of the causes described above also produce hematuria in children. However, cyclophosphamide is more likely to cause hematuria in children than in adults.

Common causes of hematuria that chiefly affect children include congenital anomalies, such as obstructive uropathy and renal dysplasia; birth trauma; hematologic disorders, such as vitamin K deficiency, hemophilia, and hemolytic-uremic syndrome; certain neoplasms, such as Wilms' tumor, bladder cancer, and rhabdomyosarcoma; allergies; and foreign bodies in the urinary tract. Artifactual hematuria may result from recent circumcision.

GERIATRIC POINTERS

Evaluation of hematuria in elderly patients should include a urine culture, excretory urography or sonography, and consultation with a urologist.

PATIENT COUNSELING

Teach the patient how to collect serial urine specimens using the three-glass technique. This technique helps determine whether hematuria marks the beginning, end, or entire course of urination. Encourage the patient to drink plenty of fluids, unless contraindicated.

HEMIANOPSIA

Hemianopsia is loss of vision in one-half the normal visual field (usually the right or left half) of one or both eyes. However, if the visual field defects are identical in both eyes but affect less than half the field of vision in each eye (incomplete homonymous hemianopsia), the lesion may be in the occipital lobe; otherwise, it probably involves the parietal or temporal lobe. (See *Recognizing visual field defects,* page 348.)

Hemianopsia is caused by a lesion affecting the optic chiasm, tract, or radiation. Defects in visual perception due to cerebral lesions are usually associated with impaired color vision.

HISTORY

Ask the patient if he has recently experienced headache, dysarthria, or seizures. When did neurologic symptoms start? Obtain a medical history, noting especially eye disorders, hypertension, diabetes mellitus, and recent head trauma. Suspect a visual field defect if the patient seems startled when you approach him from one side or if he fails to see objects placed directly in front of him. To help determine the type of defect, compare the patient's visual fields with your own—assuming that yours are normal. First, ask the patient to cover his right eye while you cover your left eye. Then move a pen or similarly shaped object from the periphery of his (and your) uncovered eye into his field of vision. Ask the patient to indicate when he first sees the object. Does he see it at the same time you do? After you do? Repeat this test in each quadrant of both eyes. Then, for each eye, plot the defect by shading the area of a circle that corresponds to the area of vision loss.

PHYSICAL ASSESSMENT

Evaluate the patient's level of consciousness (LOC), take his vital signs, and check his pupillary reaction and motor response. Does he have ptosis or facial or extremity weakness? Hallucinations or loss of color vision?

MEDICAL CAUSES

Carotid artery aneurysm

An aneurysm in the internal carotid artery can cause contralateral or bilateral defects in the visual fields. It can also cause hemiplegia, decreased LOC, headache, aphasia, behavior disturbances, and unilateral hypoesthesia.

Occipital lobe lesion

The most common symptoms arising from a lesion of one occipital lobe are incomplete homonymous hemianopsia, scotomas, and impaired color vision. The

Geri points
+ Evaluation of hematuria should include a urine culture, excretory urography or sonography, and consultation with a urologist.

Teaching points
+ Three-glass technique for collecting serial urine specimens
+ Increasing fluids

Key facts about hemianopsia
+ Vision loss in one-half the visual field of one or both eyes
+ Caused by a lesion affecting the optic chiasm, tract, or radiation

Key history points
+ Associated headache, dysarthria, seizures, hallucinations, or loss of color vision
+ Onset of neurologic symptoms
+ Medical history

Critical assessment steps
+ Evaluate LOC.
+ Check pupillary reaction.
+ Evaluate for ptosis or facial or extremity weakness.

Medical causes
Carotid artery aneurysm
+ Contralateral or bilateral defects in visual fields may occur with hemiplegia, decreased LOC, headache, aphasia, behavior disturbances, and unilateral hypoesthesia.

Occipital lobe lesion
+ Incomplete homonymous hemianopsia, scotomas, and impaired color vision are the most common symptoms.

ASSESSMENT TIP

Recognizing visual field defects

The examples shown here illustrate visual field defects. The black areas represent visual loss.

LEFT   **RIGHT**

A: Blindness of right eye

LEFT   **RIGHT**

C: Left homonymous hemianopsia

B: Bitemporal hemianopsia or loss of half the visual field

D: Left homonymous hemianopsia, superior quadrant

Medical causes
(continued)

Parietal lobe lesion
+ Homonymous hemianopsia and sensory deficits occur.

Pituitary tumor
+ Complete or partial bitemporal hemianopsia first occurs in the upper visual fields but later can progress to blindness.

Stroke
+ Hemianopsia can result when stroke affects any part of the optic pathway.

Special considerations
+ To avoid startling the patient, approach him from the unaffected side; position his bed so that his unaffected side faces the door.
+ Remove objects that could cause falls, and alert the patient to other possible hazards.
+ Place personal objects within field of vision; avoid putting dangerous objects where patient can't see them.

patient may also experience visual hallucinations: flashes of light or color, or visions of objects, people, animals, or geometric forms. These may appear in the defective field or may move toward it from the intact field.

Parietal lobe lesion
A parietal lobe lesion produces homonymous hemianopsia and sensory deficits, such as an inability to perceive body position or passive movement or to localize tactile, thermal, or vibratory stimuli. It may also cause apraxia and visual or tactile agnosia.

Pituitary tumor
A tumor that compresses nerve fibers supplying the nasal half of both retinas causes complete or partial bitemporal hemianopsia that first occurs in the upper visual fields but later can progress to blindness. Related findings include blurred vision, diplopia, and headache.

Stroke
Hemianopsia can result when stroke affects any part of the optic pathway. Associated signs and symptoms vary according to the location and size of the stroke but may include decreased LOC; intellectual deficits, such as memory loss and poor judgment; personality changes; emotional lability; headache; and seizures. The patient may also develop contralateral hemiplegia, dysarthria, dysphagia, ataxia, a unilateral sensory loss, apraxia, agnosia, aphasia, blurred vision, decreased visual acuity, and diplopia. He may also experience urine retention or incontinence, constipation, and vomiting.

SPECIAL CONSIDERATIONS

If the patient's visual field defect is significant, further visual field testing, such as perimetry or a tangent screen examination, may be indicated.

To avoid startling the patient, approach him from the unaffected side and position his bed so that his unaffected side faces the door. If he's ambulatory, remove objects that could cause falls, and alert him to other possible hazards. Place his clock and other personal objects within his field of vision, and avoid putting dangerous objects (such as hot dishes) where he can't see them.

PEDIATRIC POINTERS

In children, a brain tumor is the most common cause of hemianopsia. To help detect this sign, look for nonverbal clues, such as the child reaching for a toy but missing it. To help the child compensate for hemianopsia, place objects within his visual field; teach his parents to do this as well.

PATIENT COUNSELING

Explain to the patient the extent of his defect so that he can learn to compensate for it. Advise him to scan his surroundings frequently, turning his head in the direction of the defective visual field so that he can directly view objects he would normally notice only peripherally.

HEMOPTYSIS

Frightening to the patient, hemoptysis is the expectoration of blood or bloody sputum from the lungs or tracheobronchial tree. It's sometimes confused with bleeding from the mouth, throat, nasopharynx, or GI tract. (See *Identifying hemoptysis,* page 350.) Expectoration of 200 ml of blood in a single episode suggests severe bleeding, whereas expectoration of 400 ml in 3 hours or more than 600 ml in 16 hours signals a life-threatening crisis.

Hemoptysis usually results from chronic bronchitis, lung cancer, or bronchiectasis. However, it may also result from inflammatory, infectious, cardiovascular, or coagulation disorders and, rarely, from a ruptured aortic aneurysm. In up to 15% of patients, the cause is unknown. The most common causes of *massive hemoptysis* are lung cancer, bronchiectasis, active tuberculosis, and cavitary pulmonary disease from necrotic infections or tuberculosis.

A number of pathophysiologic processes can cause hemoptysis. (See *What happens in hemoptysis,* page 351.)

EMERGENCY ACTIONS If the patient coughs up copious amounts of blood, endotracheal intubation may be required. Suction frequently to remove blood. Lavage may be necessary to loosen tenacious secretions or clots. Massive hemoptysis can cause airway obstruction and asphyxiation. Insert an I.V. line to allow fluid replacement, drug administration, and blood transfusions, if needed. An emergency bronchoscopy should be performed to identify the bleeding site. Monitor blood pressure and pulse to detect hypotension and tachycardia, and draw an arterial blood sample for laboratory analysis to monitor respiratory status.

HISTORY

If the hemoptysis is mild, ask the patient when it began. Has he ever coughed up blood before? About how much blood is he coughing up now and about how often? Ask about a history of cardiac, pulmonary, or bleeding disorders. If he's receiving anticoagulant therapy, find out the drug, its dosage and schedule, and the duration of therapy. Is he taking other prescription drugs? Does he smoke? Ask the patient if he has had any recent infections. Has he been exposed to tuberculosis? When was his last tine test and what were the results?

PHYSICAL ASSESSMENT

Take the patient's vital signs and examine his nose, mouth, and pharynx for sources of bleeding. Inspect the configuration of his chest and look for abnormal move-

Peds points
+ The most common cause of hemianopsia in children is brain tumors.

Teaching points
+ Compensation techniques

Key facts about hemoptysis
+ Expectoration of blood or bloody sputum from the lungs or tracheobronchial tree
+ Usually results from chronic bronchitis, lung cancer, or bronchiectasis

In an emergency
+ Endotracheal intubation may be required.
+ Suction frequently; lavage may be necessary to loosen tenacious secretions or clots.
+ Insert an I.V. line, if needed.
+ Bronchoscopy should be performed to identify the bleeding site.
+ Monitor vital signs.
+ Draw an arterial blood sample for laboratory analysis.

Key history points
+ Onset and extent of hemoptysis
+ History of cardiac, pulmonary, or bleeding disorders
+ Drug history, including anticoagulants
+ Recent infections or exposure to tuberculosis
+ Smoking history
+ Tine test results

Critical assessment steps

+ Take vital signs.
+ Examine the nose, mouth, and pharynx for sources of bleeding.
+ Inspect the chest; look for abnormal movement during breathing, use of accessory muscles, and retractions.
+ Observe respiratory rate, depth, and rhythm.
+ Examine skin for lesions.
+ Palpate the chest for diaphragm level and for tenderness, respiratory excursion, fremitus, and abnormal pulsations.
+ Percuss the chest for flatness, dullness, resonance, hyperresonance, and tympany.
+ Auscultate the lungs.
+ Auscultate for heart murmurs, bruits, and pleural friction rubs.
+ Obtain sputum sample, examine it for overall quantity, amount of blood, and color, odor, and consistency.

Medical causes

Bronchial adenoma
+ Recurring hemoptysis occurs along with a chronic cough and local wheezing.

Bronchiectasis
+ Inflamed bronchial surfaces and eroded bronchial blood vessels cause hemoptysis, which can vary from blood-tinged sputum to blood.

Bronchitis (chronic)
+ A productive cough leads to production of blood-streaked sputum.

ASSESSMENT TIP

Identifying hemoptysis

These guidelines will help you distinguish hemoptysis from epistaxis, hematemesis, and brown, red, or pink sputum.

HEMOPTYSIS
Often frothy because it's mixed with air, hemoptysis is typically bright red with an alkaline pH (tested with nitrazine paper). It's strongly suggested by the presence of respiratory signs and symptoms, including a cough, a tickling sensation in the throat, and blood produced from repeated coughing episodes. (You can rule out epistaxis because the patient's nasal passages and posterior pharynx are usually clear.)

HEMATEMESIS
The usual site of hematemesis is the GI tract; the patient vomits or regurgitates coffee-ground material that contains food particles, tests positive for occult blood, and has an acid pH. However, he may vomit bright red blood or swallowed blood from the oral cavity and nasopharynx. After an episode of hematemesis, the patient may have stools with traces of blood. Many patients with hematemesis also complain of dyspepsia.

BROWN, RED, OR PINK SPUTUM
Brown, red, or pink sputum can result from oxidation of inhaled bronchodilators. Sputum that looks like old blood may result from rupture of an amebic abscess into the bronchus. Red or brown sputum may occur in a patient with pneumonia caused by the enterobacterium *Serratia marcescens*. Currant-jelly sputum occurs with *Klebsiella* infections.

ment during breathing, use of accessory muscles, and retractions. Observe his respiratory rate, depth, and rhythm. Finally, examine his skin for lesions.

Next, palpate the patient's chest for diaphragm level and for tenderness, respiratory excursion, fremitus, and abnormal pulsations; then percuss for flatness, dullness, resonance, hyperresonance, and tympany. Finally, auscultate the lungs, noting especially the quality and intensity of breath sounds. Also auscultate for heart murmurs, bruits, and pleural friction rubs.

Obtain a sputum sample and examine it for overall quantity, for the amount of blood it contains, and for its color, odor, and consistency.

MEDICAL CAUSES

Bronchial adenoma
Bronchial adenoma is an insidious disorder that causes recurring hemoptysis along with a chronic cough and local wheezing. The patient with bronchial adenoma may also have recurrent infection, dyspnea, and wheezing.

Bronchiectasis
With bronchiectasis, inflamed bronchial surfaces and eroded bronchial blood vessels cause hemoptysis, which can vary from blood-tinged sputum to blood (in about 20% of patients). The patient's sputum may also be copious, foul-smelling, and purulent. He may exhibit a chronic cough, coarse crackles, clubbing (a late sign), fever, weight loss, fatigue, weakness, malaise, and dyspnea on exertion.

Bronchitis (chronic)
The first sign of chronic bronchitis is typically a productive cough that lasts at least 3 months. Eventually this leads to production of blood-streaked sputum; massive hemorrhage is unusual. Other respiratory effects include dyspnea, prolonged expi-

---

What happens in hemoptysis

Hemoptysis results from bleeding into the respiratory tract by bronchial or pulmonary vessels. Bleeding reflects alterations in the vascular walls and in blood-clotting mechanisms. It can result from any of these pathophysiologic processes:
+ hemorrhage and diapedesis of red blood cells from the pulmonary microvasculature into the alveoli
+ necrosis of lung tissue that causes inflammation and rupture of blood vessels or hemorrhage into the alveolar spaces

+ rupture of an aortic aneurysm into the tracheobronchial tree
+ rupture of distended endobronchial blood vessels from pulmonary hypertension due to mitral stenosis
+ rupture of a pulmonary arteriovenous fistula or of bronchial or pulmonary artery/pulmonary venous collateral channels
+ sloughing of a caseous lesion into the tracheobronchial tree
+ ulceration and erosion of the bronchial epithelium.

---

rations, wheezing, scattered rhonchi, accessory muscle use, barrel chest, tachypnea, and clubbing (a late sign).

Coagulation disorders

Such coagulation disorders as thrombocytopenia and disseminated intravascular coagulation can cause hemoptysis. In addition to their specific related findings, coagulation disorders may share such general signs as multisystem hemorrhaging (for example, GI bleeding or epistaxis) and purpuric lesions.

Laryngeal cancer

Hemoptysis occurs in laryngeal cancer, but hoarseness is the usual early sign. Other findings may include dysphagia, dyspnea, stridor, cervical lymphadenopathy, and neck pain.

Lung abscess

In about 50% of patients, a lung abscess produces blood-streaked sputum resulting from bronchial ulceration, necrosis, and granulation tissue. Common associated findings include a cough with large amounts of purulent, foul-smelling sputum; fever with chills; diaphoresis; anorexia; weight loss; headache; weakness; dyspnea; pleuritic or dull chest pain; and clubbing. Auscultation reveals tubular or cavernous breath sounds and crackles. Percussion reveals dullness on the affected side.

Lung cancer

In patients with lung cancer, ulceration of the bronchus commonly causes recurring hemoptysis (an early sign), which can vary from blood-streaked sputum to blood. Related findings include a productive cough, dyspnea, fever, anorexia, weight loss, wheezing, and chest pain (a late symptom).

Pneumonia

In up to 50% of patients, *Klebsiella* pneumonia produces dark brown or red (currant-jelly) sputum, which is so tenacious that the patient has difficulty expelling it from his mouth. This type of pneumonia begins abruptly with chills, fever, dyspnea, a productive cough, and severe pleuritic chest pain. Associated findings may include cyanosis, prostration, tachycardia, decreased breath sounds, and crackles.

Pneumococcal pneumonia causes pinkish or rusty mucoid sputum. It begins with sudden shaking chills; a rapidly rising temperature; and, in over 80% of patients, tachycardia and tachypnea. Within a few hours, the patient typically experiences a productive cough along with severe, stabbing, pleuritic pain. The agonizing

Medical causes
(continued)

Coagulation disorders
+ Hemoptysis is accompanied by such general signs as multisystem hemorrhaging and purpuric lesions.

Laryngeal cancer
+ Hemoptysis occurs, but hoarseness is the usual early sign.

Lung abscess
+ Blood-streaked sputum resulting from bronchial ulceration, necrosis, and granulation tissue occurs in about 50% of patients.

Lung cancer
+ Ulceration of the bronchus commonly causes recurring hemoptysis (an early sign).

Pneumonia
+ *Klebsiella* pneumonia produces dark brown or red (currant-jelly) sputum that the patient has difficulty expelling from his mouth.
+ Pneumococcal pneumonia causes pinkish or rusty mucoid sputum.

Medical causes
(continued)

Pulmonary contusion
+ Cough and hemoptysis occur after blunt chest trauma.

Pulmonary edema
+ Frothy, blood-tinged pink sputum accompanies severe dyspnea, orthopnea, gasping, anxiety, cyanosis, diffuse crackles, a ventricular gallop, and cold, clammy skin.

Pulmonary embolism with infarction
+ Hemoptysis is common.
+ Typically initial symptoms include dyspnea and anginal or pleuritic chest pain.

Pulmonary hypertension (primary)
+ Hemoptysis, exertional dyspnea, and fatigue are common, but generally develop late.

Pulmonary tuberculosis
+ Blood-streaked or blood-tinged sputum commonly occurs.
+ Massive hemoptysis may occur in advanced cavitary tuberculosis.

Silicosis
+ Initially, silicosis causes cough with mucopurulent sputum.
+ Sputum becomes blood-streaked and, occasionally, massive hemoptysis may occur.

SLE
+ Pleuritis and pneumonitis cause hemoptysis in about 50% of patients.

chest pain leads to rapid, shallow, grunting respirations with splinting. Examination reveals respiratory distress with dyspnea and accessory muscle use, crackles, and dullness on percussion over the affected lung. Malaise, weakness, myalgia, and prostration accompany high fever.

Pulmonary contusion
Pulmonary contusion, resulting from blunt chest trauma, commonly causes a cough with hemoptysis. Other signs and symptoms appear gradually within several hours after the injury and include dyspnea, tachypnea, chest pain, tachycardia, hypotension, crackles, and decreased or absent breath sounds over the affected area. Severe respiratory distress — with oppressive dyspnea, nasal flaring, use of accessory muscles, extreme anxiety, cyanosis, and diaphoresis — may develop at any time.

Pulmonary edema
Severe pulmonary edema commonly causes frothy, blood-tinged pink sputum, which accompanies severe dyspnea, orthopnea, gasping, anxiety, cyanosis, diffuse crackles, a ventricular gallop, and cold, clammy skin. This life-threatening condition may also cause tachycardia, lethargy, cardiac arrhythmias, tachypnea, hypotension, and a thready pulse.

Pulmonary embolism with infarction
Hemoptysis is a common finding in this life-threatening disorder, although massive hemoptysis is infrequent. Typical initial symptoms are dyspnea and anginal or pleuritic chest pain. Other common clinical features include tachycardia, tachypnea, low-grade fever, and diaphoresis. Less commonly, splinting of the chest, leg edema, and — with a large embolus — cyanosis, syncope, and distended jugular veins may occur. Examination reveals decreased breath sounds, pleural friction rub, crackles, diffuse wheezing, dullness on percussion, and signs of circulatory collapse (weak, rapid pulse; hypotension), cerebral ischemia (transient loss of consciousness, convulsions), and hypoxemia (restlessness and, particularly in elderly patients, hemiplegia and other focal neurologic deficits).

Pulmonary hypertension (primary)
Features of primary pulmonary hypertension generally develop late. Hemoptysis, exertional dyspnea, and fatigue are common. Angina-like pain usually occurs with exertion and may radiate to the neck but not to the arms. Other findings include arrhythmias, syncope, cough, and hoarseness.

Pulmonary tuberculosis
Blood-streaked or blood-tinged sputum commonly occurs in pulmonary tuberculosis; massive hemoptysis may occur in advanced cavitary tuberculosis. Accompanying respiratory findings include a chronic productive cough, fine crackles after coughing, dyspnea, dullness to percussion, increased tactile fremitus, and possible amphoric breath sounds. The patient may also develop night sweats, malaise, fatigue, fever, anorexia, weight loss, and pleuritic chest pain.

Silicosis
Initially, silicosis causes a productive cough with mucopurulent sputum. Subsequently, the sputum becomes blood-streaked and, occasionally, massive hemoptysis may occur. Other findings include fine, end-inspiratory crackles at lung bases, exertional dyspnea, tachypnea, weight loss, fatigue, and weakness.

Systemic lupus erythematosus
In 50% of patients with systemic lupus erythematosus (SLE), pleuritis and pneumonitis cause hemoptysis, cough, dyspnea, pleuritic chest pain, and crackles. Relat-

ed findings are a butterfly rash in the acute phase, nondeforming joint pain and stiffness, photosensitivity, Raynaud's phenomenon, convulsions or psychoses, anorexia with weight loss, and lymphadenopathy.

OTHER CAUSES

Diagnostic tests

Lung or airway injury from bronchoscopy, laryngoscopy, mediastinoscopy, or lung biopsy can cause bleeding and hemoptysis.

SPECIAL CONSIDERATIONS

If necessary to protect the nonbleeding lung, place the patient in the lateral decubitus position, with the suspected bleeding lung facing down. Perform this maneuver with caution because hypoxemia may worsen with the healthy lung facing up.

Prepare the patient for diagnostic tests to determine the cause of bleeding. These may include a complete blood count, a sputum culture and smear, chest X-rays, coagulation studies, bronchoscopy, lung biopsy, pulmonary arteriography, and a lung scan.

PEDIATRIC POINTERS

Hemoptysis in children may stem from Goodpasture's syndrome, cystic fibrosis, or (rarely) idiopathic primary pulmonary hemosiderosis. Sometimes, no cause can be found for pulmonary hemorrhage occurring within the first 2 weeks of life; in such cases, the prognosis is poor.

GERIATRIC POINTERS

If the patient is receiving anticoagulants, determine any changes that need to be made in diet or medications (including over-the-counter and natural supplements) because these factors may affect clotting.

PATIENT COUNSELING

Comfort and reassure the patient, who may react to this alarming sign with anxiety and apprehension. Hemoptysis generally ceases (but not abruptly) during treatment of the causative disorder. Many chronic disorders, however, cause recurrent hemoptysis. Instruct the patient to report recurring episodes and to bring a sputum specimen containing blood if he returns for treatment or reevaluation.

HEPATOMEGALY

Hepatomegaly (an enlarged liver) indicates potentially reversible primary or secondary liver disease. This sign may stem from diverse pathophysiologic mechanisms, including dilated hepatic sinusoids (in heart failure), persistently high venous pressure leading to liver congestion (in chronic constrictive pericarditis), dysfunction and engorgement of hepatocytes (in hepatitis), fatty infiltration of parenchymal cells causing fibrous tissue (in cirrhosis), distention of liver cells with glycogen (in diabetes), and infiltration of amyloid (in amyloidosis).

Hepatomegaly may be confirmed by palpation, percussion, or radiologic tests. It may be mistaken for displacement of the liver by the diaphragm, in a respiratory disorder; by an abdominal tumor; by a spinal deformity such as kyphosis; by the gallbladder; or by fecal material or a tumor in the colon.

Other causes
+ Lung or airway injury from bronchoscopy, laryngoscopy, mediastinoscopy, or lung biopsy

Special considerations
+ If necessary to protect the nonbleeding lung, place the patient in the lateral decubitus position, with the suspected bleeding lung facing down.

Peds points
+ Hemoptysis in children may stem from Goodpasture's syndrome, cystic fibrosis, or (rarely) idiopathic primary pulmonary hemosiderosis.

Geri points
+ If the patient is receiving anticoagulants, determine any changes that need to be made in diet or medications because these factors may affect clotting.

Teaching points
+ Importance of reporting recurrent episodes
+ Sputum sample instructions

Key facts about hepatomegaly
+ Enlargement of the liver
+ Indicates potentially reversible primary or secondary liver disease
+ May be confirmed by palpation, percussion, or radiologic tests

Key history points

+ Alcohol use
+ Exposure to hepatitis
+ Drug history
+ Location and description of any associated abdominal pain

Critical assessment steps

+ Inspect the skin and sclerae for jaundice, dilated veins, scars from previous surgery, and spider angiomas.
+ Inspect the contour of the abdomen and measure abdominal girth.
+ Percuss the liver.
+ During deep inspiration, palpate the liver's edge.
+ Take baseline vital signs.
+ Assess nutritional status.
+ Evaluate LOC.
+ Watch for personality changes, irritability, agitation, memory loss, inability to concentrate, poor mentation, and — in a severely ill patient — coma.

Medical causes

Cirrhosis
+ In late cirrhosis, liver becomes enlarged, nodular, and hard.

Diabetes mellitus
+ Poorly controlled diabetes in overweight patients can produce fatty infiltration of liver, hepatomegaly, and right-upper-quadrant tenderness along with polydipsia, polyphagia, and polyuria.

HISTORY

Hepatomegaly is seldom a patient's chief complaint. It's usually discovered during palpation and percussion of the abdomen.

If you suspect hepatomegaly, ask the patient about his use of alcohol and exposure to hepatitis. Also ask if he's currently ill or taking any prescribed drugs. If he complains of abdominal pain, ask him to locate and describe it.

PHYSICAL ASSESSMENT

Inspect the patient's skin and sclerae for jaundice, dilated veins (suggesting generalized congestion), scars from previous surgery, and spider angiomas (often occurring in cirrhosis). Next, inspect the contour of his abdomen. Is it protuberant over the liver or distended (possibly from ascites)? Measure his abdominal girth.

Percuss the liver, but be careful to identify structures and conditions that can obscure dull percussion notes, such as the sternum, ribs, breast tissue, pleural effusions, and gas in the colon (See *Percussing for liver size and position.*) Next, during deep inspiration, palpate the liver's edge; it's tender and rounded in hepatitis and cardiac decompensation, rocklike in carcinoma, and firm in cirrhosis.

Take the patient's baseline vital signs, and assess his nutritional status. An enlarged liver that's functioning poorly causes muscle wasting, exaggerated skeletal prominences, weight loss, thin hair, and edema.

Evaluate the patient's level of consciousness. When an enlarged liver loses its ability to detoxify waste products, the result is accumulation of metabolic substances toxic to brain cells. As a result, watch for personality changes, irritability, agitation, memory loss, inability to concentrate and poor mentation, and — in a severely ill patient — coma.

MEDICAL CAUSES

Cirrhosis

In late cirrhosis, the liver becomes enlarged, nodular, and hard. Other late signs and symptoms affect all body systems. Respiratory findings include limited thoracic expansion due to abdominal ascites, leading to hypoxia. Central nervous system findings include signs and symptoms of hepatic encephalopathy, such as lethargy, slurred speech, asterixis, peripheral neuritis, paranoia, hallucinations, extreme obtundation, and coma. Hematologic signs include epistaxis, easy bruising, and bleeding gums. Endocrine findings include testicular atrophy, gynecomastia, loss of chest and axillary hair, or menstrual irregularities. Integumentary effects include abnormal pigmentation, jaundice, severe pruritus, extreme dryness, poor tissue turgor, spider angiomas, and palmar erythema.

The patient may also develop fetor hepaticus, enlarged superficial abdominal veins, muscle atrophy, right-upper-quadrant pain that worsens when he sits up or leans forward, and a palpable spleen. Portal hypertension — elevated pressure in the portal vein — causes bleeding from esophageal varices.

Diabetes mellitus

Poorly controlled diabetes in overweight patients can produce fatty infiltration of the liver, hepatomegaly, and right-upper-quadrant tenderness along with polydipsia, polyphagia, and polyuria. These features are more common in type 2 than in type 1 diabetes. A chronically enlarged fatty liver typically produces no symptoms except for slight tenderness.

ASSESSMENT TIP

Percussing for liver size and position

With your patient in a supine position, begin at the right iliac crest to percuss up the right midclavicular line (MCL), as shown here. The percussion note becomes dull when you reach the liver's inferior border—usually at the costal margin but sometimes at a lower point in a patient with liver disease. Mark this point and then percuss down from the right clavicle, again along the right MCL. The liver's superior border usually lies between the fifth and seventh intercostal spaces. Mark the superior border.

The distance between the two marked points represents the approximate span of the liver's right lobe, which normally ranges from 2¼" to 4¾" (5.5 to 12 cm).

Next, assess the liver's left lobe similarly, percussing along the sternal midline. Again,

mark the points where you hear dull percussion notes. Also, measure the span of the left lobe, which normally ranges from 1½" to 3⅛" (4 to 8 cm). Record your findings for use as a baseline.

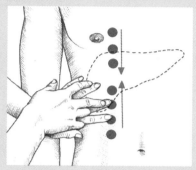

Heart failure

Heart failure produces hepatomegaly along with jugular vein distention, cyanosis, nocturia, dependent edema of the legs and sacrum, steady weight gain, confusion and, possibly, nausea, vomiting, abdominal discomfort, and anorexia due to visceral edema. Ascites is a late sign. Massive right-sided heart failure may cause anasarca, oliguria, severe weakness, and anxiety. If left-sided heart failure precedes right-sided heart failure, the patient exhibits dyspnea, orthopnea, paroxysmal nocturnal dyspnea, tachypnea, arrhythmias, tachycardia, and fatigue.

Hepatitis

In viral hepatitis, early signs and symptoms include nausea, anorexia, vomiting, fatigue, malaise, photophobia, sore throat, cough, and headache. Hepatomegaly occurs in the icteric phase and continues during the recovery phase. Also, during the icteric phase, the early signs and symptoms diminish and others appear: liver tenderness, slight weight loss, dark urine, clay-colored stools, jaundice, pruritus, right-upper-quadrant pain, and splenomegaly.

Leukemia and lymphomas

Leukemia and lymphomas are proliferative blood cell disorders that commonly cause moderate to massive hepatomegaly and splenomegaly as well as abdominal discomfort. General signs and symptoms include malaise, low-grade fever, fatigue, weakness, tachycardia, weight loss, bleeding disorders, and anorexia.

Liver cancer

Primary tumors commonly cause irregular, nodular, firm hepatomegaly, with pain or tenderness in the right upper quadrant and a friction rub or bruit over the liver. Common related findings are weight loss, anorexia, cachexia, nausea, and vomiting. Peripheral edema, ascites, jaundice, and a palpable right-upper-quadrant mass may also develop. When metastatic liver tumors cause hepatomegaly, the patient's accompanying signs and symptoms reflect his primary cancer.

Medical causes
(continued)

Heart failure
✦ Heart failure produces hepatomegaly, jugular vein distention, cyanosis, nocturia, dependent edema of the legs and sacrum, steady weight gain, confusion and, possibly, nausea, vomiting, abdominal discomfort, and anorexia.

Hepatitis
✦ Hepatomegaly occurs in the icteric phase and continues during the recovery phase.

Leukemia and lymphomas
✦ Moderate to massive hepatomegaly, splenomegaly, and abdominal discomfort are common.

Liver cancer
✦ Primary tumors cause irregular, nodular, firm hepatomegaly, with pain or tenderness in the right upper quadrant and a friction rub or bruit over the liver.
✦ Metastatic liver tumors cause hepatomegaly, but accompanying signs and symptoms reflect the primary cancer.

Medical causes
(continued)
Mononucleosis (infectious)
+ Hepatomegaly may occur.

Obesity
+ Hepatomegaly can result from fatty infiltration of the liver.

Pancreatic cancer
+ Hepatomegaly accompanies anorexia, weight loss, abdominal or back pain, and jaundice.

Special considerations
+ Provide bed rest, relief from stress, and adequate nutrition.
+ Monitor and restrict dietary protein as needed.
+ Give hepatotoxic drugs or drugs metabolized by the liver in very small doses, if at all.
+ Explain treatment measures to the patient.

Peds points
+ Childhood hepatomegaly may stem from Reye's syndrome, biliary atresia, rare disorders, or poorly controlled type 1 diabetes mellitus.

Teaching points
+ Explanation of treatment plan for underlying disorder
+ Avoidance of alcohol and people with infections
+ Personal hygiene
+ Importance of pacing activities and rest periods

Mononucleosis (infectious)
Occasionally, infectious mononucleosis causes hepatomegaly. Prodromal symptoms include headache, malaise, and fatigue. After 3 to 5 days, the patient typically develops sore throat, cervical lymphadenopathy, and temperature fluctuations. He may also develop stomatitis, palatal petechiae, periorbital edema, splenomegaly, exudative tonsillitis, pharyngitis and, possibly, a maculopapular rash.

Obesity
Hepatomegaly can result from fatty infiltration of the liver. Weight loss reduces the liver's size. Obesity may also produce findings related to respiratory difficulties, hypertension, cardiovascular disease, diabetes, renal disease, gallbladder disease, and psychological difficulties.

Pancreatic cancer
In pancreatic cancer, hepatomegaly accompanies such classic signs and symptoms as anorexia, weight loss, abdominal or back pain, and jaundice. Other findings include nausea, vomiting, fever, fatigue, weakness, pruritus, and skin lesions (usually on the legs).

SPECIAL CONSIDERATIONS
Prepare the patient for hepatic enzyme, alkaline phosphatase, bilirubin, albumin, and globulin studies to evaluate liver function, and for X-rays, liver scan, celiac arteriography, computed tomography scan, and ultrasonography to confirm hepatomegaly.

Bed rest, relief from stress, and adequate nutrition are important for the patient with hepatomegaly to help protect liver cells from further damage and to allow the liver to regenerate functioning cells. Dietary protein may need to be monitored and possibly restricted. Ammonia, a major cause of hepatic encephalopathy, is a byproduct of protein metabolism. Hepatotoxic drugs or drugs metabolized by the liver should be given in very small doses, if at all. These treatment measures should be explained to the patient.

PEDIATRIC POINTERS
Assess hepatomegaly in children the same way you do in adults. Childhood hepatomegaly may stem from Reye's syndrome; biliary atresia; rare disorders, such as Wilson's disease, Gaucher's disease, and Niemann-Pick disease; or poorly controlled type 1 diabetes mellitus.

PATIENT COUNSELING
Instruct the patient to avoid alcohol. Explain the importance of following the treatment plan to correct or control the underlying disorder as needed. Tell the patient to avoid exposure to people with infections and to maintain good personal hygiene. Explain the importance of pacing activities and having frequent rest periods.

HIRSUTISM

Hirsutism is the excessive growth of coarse body hair in females. Excessive androgen (male hormone) production stimulates hair growth on the pubic region, axillae, chin, upper lip, cheeks, anterior neck, sternum, linea alba, forearms, abdomen, back, and upper arms. This condition may also occur with normal levels of androgens when there's an increased sensitivity of the skin to the hormones. In mild hirsutism, fine and pigmented hair appears on the sides of the face and the chin (but doesn't form a complete beard) and on the extremities, chest, abdomen, and perineum. In moderate hirsutism, coarse and pigmented hair appears on the same areas. In severe hirsutism, coarse hair covers the whole beard area, the proximal interphalangeal joints, and the ears and nose.

Depending on the degree of excess androgen production, hirsutism may be associated with acne and increased skin oiliness, increased libido, and menstrual irregularities (including anovulation and amenorrhea). Extremely high androgen levels cause further virilization, including such signs as breast atrophy, loss of female body contour, frontal balding, and deepening of the voice. (See *Recognizing signs of virilization,* page 358.)

Hirsutism may result from endocrine abnormalities and idiopathic causes. It may also occur in pregnancy from transient androgen production by the placenta or corpus luteum and in menopause from increased androgen and decreased estrogen production.

 CULTURAL CUE *Some patients have a strong familial predisposition to hirsutism, which may be considered normal in the context of their genetic background, culture, and race. Although hirsutism is a female characteristic, excessive hair growth may be present in female and male family members.*

HISTORY

Begin by asking the patient where on her body she first noticed excessive hair. How old was she then? Where and how quickly did other hirsute areas develop? Does she use any hair removal technique? If so, how often does she use it, and when did she use it last? Next, obtain a menstrual history: the patient's age at menarche, the duration of her menses, the usual amount of blood flow, and the number of days between menses.

Also ask about medications. If the patient is taking a drug containing an androgen or progestin compound, or another drug that can cause hirsutism, find out its name, dosage, schedule, and therapeutic aim. Does she sometimes miss doses or take extra ones?

PHYSICAL ASSESSMENT

Examine the hirsute areas. Does excessive hair appear only on the upper lip or on other body parts as well? Is the hair fine but pigmented, or dense and coarse? Is the patient obese? Observe the patient for signs of virilization.

MEDICAL CAUSES

Acromegaly

About 15% of patients with acromegaly (a chronic, progressive disorder) display hirsutism. Acromegaly also causes enlarged hands and feet, coarsened facial features, prognathism, increased diaphoresis and need for sleep, oily skin, fatigue, weight gain, heat intolerance, and lethargy.

Adrenocortical carcinoma

Adrenocortical carcinoma produces rapidly progressive hirsutism along with truncal obesity, buffalo hump, moon face, oligomenorrhea, amenorrhea, muscle wasting, and thin skin with purple striae. The patient also exhibits muscle weakness, excessive diaphoresis, poor wound healing, weakness, fatigue, hypertension, hyperpigmentation, and personality changes.

Recognizing signs of virilization

Excessive androgen levels produce severe hirsutism and other marked signs of virilization. As you examine your patient, be alert for the signs of virilization shown in the figure below.

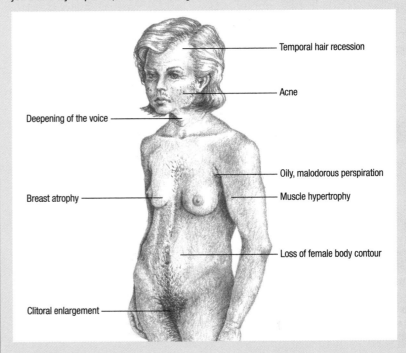

Temporal hair recession

Acne

Deepening of the voice

Oily, malodorous perspiration

Breast atrophy

Muscle hypertrophy

Loss of female body contour

Clitoral enlargement

Medical causes
(continued)

Androgen overproduction by ovaries
✦ Hirsutism and anovulation occur with other signs of virilization.

Cushing's syndrome
✦ Hair growth increases on the face, abdomen, breasts, chest, or upper thighs.

Hyperprolactinemia
✦ Hirsutism, hypogonadism, galactorrhea, amenorrhea, and acne are produced.

Androgen overproduction by ovaries

The most common cause of hirsutism, androgen overproduction is associated with anovulation that progresses slowly over several years. Other signs of virilization may also become apparent, such as deepening of the voice, acne, and clitoral enlargement.

Cushing's syndrome

Cushing's syndrome commonly causes increased hair growth on the face, abdomen, breasts, chest, or upper thighs. Other findings include truncal obesity, buffalo hump, moon face, thin skin, purple striae, ecchymoses, petechiae, muscle wasting and weakness, poor wound healing, hypertension, weakness, fatigue, excessive diaphoresis, hyperpigmentation, menstrual irregularities, and personality changes.

Hyperprolactinemia

Hyperprolactinemia produces hirsutism, hypogonadism, galactorrhea, amenorrhea, and acne. The patient may also have a history of infertility. If a pituitary tumor is the cause of elevated prolactin levels, visual field defects may also be present.

Idiopathic hirsutism

In patients with normal-sized ovaries, normal menses, and no evidence of adrenal hyperplasia or adrenal or ovarian tumors, excess hair appears at puberty and increases into early adulthood. It's accompanied by acne, obesity, infrequent menses or anovulation, and thick, oily skin. Idiopathic hirsutism with regular ovulation and no menstrual abnormalities may be hereditary or related to certain ethnic groups who are hypersensitive to androgens.

Ovarian tumor

An ovarian tumor can cause rapidly progressing hirsutism — but only if the tumor produces androgens. Amenorrhea and rapidly developing virilization are additional findings. However, some ovarian tumors produce no symptoms.

Polycystic ovary disease

Ovarian cysts, particularly chronic ones, can cause hirsutism. This hirsutism usually occurs after the onset of menstrual irregularities, which may begin at puberty. The patient may also be obese and have amenorrhea, oligomenorrhea, menometrorrhagia, infertility, and acne.

OTHER CAUSES

Drugs

Hirsutism can result from drugs containing androgens or progestins or from aminoglutethimide, glucocorticoids, metoclopramide, cyclosporine, and minoxidil.

SPECIAL CONSIDERATIONS

Prepare the patient for tests to determine blood levels of luteinizing hormone, follicle-stimulating hormone (FSH), prolactin, and other hormones. Other tests may include computed tomography scan and ultrasonography.

PEDIATRIC POINTERS

Childhood hirsutism can stem from congenital adrenal hyperplasia. This disorder is usually detected at birth because affected infants have ambiguous genitalia. Hirsutism that occurs at or after puberty commonly results from polycystic ovary disease.

GERIATRIC POINTERS

Hirsutism can occur after menopause if peripheral conversion of estrogen is poor.

PATIENT COUNSELING

Help relieve the patient's anxiety by explaining the cause of excessive hair growth and by encouraging her to talk about her self-image problems or fears. Involve the family in your discussions.

Tell the patient that hormonal treatment stops further hair growth but doesn't always reverse hair growth that has already occurred. Treatment requires a minimum of 6 to 24 months and may be lifelong.

At the patient's request, provide information on hair removal methods, such as bleaching, tweezing, hot wax treatments, chemical depilatories, shaving, and electrolysis. Advise the patient that electrolysis should be done only by a licensed professional.

Idiopathic hirsutism
+ Excess hair appears at puberty and increases into early adulthood.

Ovarian tumor
+ If tumor produces androgens, rapidly progressing hirsutism may occur.

Polycystic ovary disease
+ Hirsutism usually occurs after onset of menstrual irregularities.

Other causes
+ Aminoglutethimide
+ Cyclosporine
+ Drugs containing androgens or progestins
+ Glucocorticoids
+ Metoclopramide
+ Minoxidil

Special considerations
+ Prepare patient for tests to determine blood levels of luteinizing hormone, FSH, prolactin, and other hormones.

Peds points
+ Hirsutism can stem from congenital adrenal hyperplasia.
+ Hirsutism that occurs at or after puberty commonly results from polycystic ovary disease.

Geri points
+ Hirsutism can occur after menopause if peripheral conversion of estrogen is poor.

Teaching points
+ Cause of hirsutism
+ Explanation of treatment
+ Hair removal techniques

HOARSENESS

Hoarseness—a rough or harsh sound to the voice—can result from infections or inflammatory lesions or exudates of the larynx, from laryngeal edema, and from compression or disruption of the vocal cords or recurrent laryngeal nerve. This common sign can also result from a thoracic aortic aneurysm, vocal cord paralysis, and systemic disorders, such as Sjögren's syndrome and rheumatoid arthritis. It's characteristically worsened by excessive alcohol intake, smoking, inhalation of noxious fumes, excessive talking, and shouting.

Hoarseness can be acute or chronic. For example, chronic hoarseness and laryngitis result when irritating polyps or nodules develop on the vocal cords. Gastroesophageal reflux into the larynx should also be considered as a possible cause of chronic hoarseness. Hoarseness may also result from progressive atrophy of the laryngeal muscles and mucosa due to aging, which leads to diminished control of the vocal cords.

HISTORY

Obtain a patient history. First, consider his age and sex; laryngeal cancer is most common in men between ages 50 and 70. Be sure to ask about the onset of hoarseness. Has the patient been overusing his voice? Has he experienced shortness of breath, a sore throat, dry mouth, a cough, or difficulty swallowing dry food? In addition, ask if he has been in or near a fire within the past 48 hours. Be aware that inhalation injury can cause sudden airway obstruction.

Next, explore associated symptoms. Does the patient have a history of cancer, rheumatoid arthritis, or aortic aneurysm? Does he regularly drink alcohol or smoke?

PHYSICAL ASSESSMENT

Inspect the oral cavity and pharynx for redness or exudate, possibly indicating an upper respiratory infection. Palpate the neck for masses and the cervical lymph nodes and the thyroid for enlargement. Palpate the trachea—is it midline? Ask the patient to stick out his tongue; if he can't, he may have paralysis from cranial nerve involvement. Examine the eyes for corneal ulcers and enlarged lacrimal ducts (signs of Sjögren's syndrome). Dilated jugular and chest veins may indicate compression by an aortic aneurysm.

Take the patient's vital signs, noting especially fever and bradycardia. Inspect for asymmetrical chest expansion or signs of respiratory distress—nasal flaring, stridor, and intercostal retractions. Then auscultate for crackles, rhonchi, wheezing, and tubular sounds, and percuss for dullness.

MEDICAL CAUSES

Gastroesophageal reflux

Irritation of the larynx by reflux of gastric juices may result in hoarseness as well as sore throat, cough, throat clearing, and a sensation of a lump in the throat. The arytenoid tissue and the vocal cords may appear red and swollen.

Hypothyroidism

Hoarseness may be an early sign of hypothyroidism. Other signs and symptoms include fatigue, cold intolerance, weight gain despite anorexia, and menorrhagia. Assessment may also reveal coarse hair and alopecia as well as dry, flaky skin and thinning nails.

Laryngeal cancer

Hoarseness is an early sign of vocal cord cancer but may not occur until later in cancer of other laryngeal areas. The patient usually has a long history of smoking. Other common findings include a mild, dry cough; minor throat discomfort; otalgia; and, sometimes, hemoptysis.

Laryngeal leukoplakia

Leukoplakia is a common cause of hoarseness, especially in smokers. Histologic examination from direct laryngoscopy usually reveals mild, moderate, or severe dysphagia.

Laryngitis

Persistent hoarseness may be the only sign of chronic laryngitis. With acute laryngitis, hoarseness or a complete loss of voice develops suddenly. Related findings include pain (especially during swallowing or speaking), cough, fever, profuse diaphoresis, sore throat, and rhinorrhea.

Tracheal trauma

Torn tracheal mucosa may cause hoarseness, hemoptysis, dysphagia, neck pain, airway occlusion, and respiratory distress. The patient with tracheal trauma may also have manifestations of cervical spine injuries.

Vocal cord paralysis

Unilateral vocal cord paralysis causes hoarseness and vocal weakness. Paralysis may accompany signs of trauma, such as pain and swelling of the head and neck. The patient may also experience dysphagia.

Vocal cord polyps or nodules

Raspy hoarseness, the chief complaint, accompanies a chronic cough and a crackling voice. Typically, this condition is painless.

OTHER CAUSES

Inhalation injury

Inhalation injury from a fire or explosion produces hoarseness and coughing, singed nasal hairs, orofacial burns, and soot-stained sputum. Subsequent signs and symptoms include crackles, rhonchi, and wheezing, which rapidly deteriorate to respiratory distress.

Treatments

Occasionally, surgical trauma to the laryngeal nerve results in temporary or permanent unilateral vocal cord paralysis, leading to hoarseness. Prolonged intubation may cause temporary hoarseness.

SPECIAL CONSIDERATIONS

Carefully observe the patient for stridor, which may indicate bilateral vocal cord paralysis. When hoarseness lasts for longer than 2 weeks, indirect or fiber-optic laryngoscopy is indicated to observe the larynx at rest and during phonation.

PEDIATRIC POINTERS

In children, hoarseness may result from congenital anomalies, such as laryngocele and dysphonia plicae ventricularis. In prepubescent boys, it can stem from juvenile papillomatosis of the upper respiratory tract.

Medical causes
(continued)

Laryngeal cancer
- Hoarseness is an early sign of vocal cord cancer but may not occur until later in cancer of other laryngeal areas.

Laryngeal leukoplakia
- Hoarseness is common, especially in smokers.

Laryngitis
- Persistent hoarseness may be the only sign of chronic form.
- With acute laryngitis, hoarseness or complete loss of voice develops suddenly.

Tracheal trauma
- Torn tracheal mucosa may cause hoarseness, hemoptysis, dysphagia, neck pain, airway occlusion, and respiratory distress.

Vocal cord paralysis
- Hoarseness and vocal weakness occur.

Vocal cord polyps or nodules
- Raspy hoarseness accompanies chronic cough and crackling voice.

Other causes
- Inhalation injury
- Prolonged intubation
- Surgical trauma to the laryngeal nerve

Special considerations
- Observe for stridor.
- When hoarseness lasts for longer than 2 weeks, indirect or fiber-optic laryngoscopy is indicated.

Peds points

+ In children, hoarseness may result from congenital anomalies.
+ In prepubescent boys, hoarseness can stem from juvenile papillomatosis of the upper respiratory tract.
+ In infants and young children, hoarseness commonly stems from croup.

Teaching points

+ Importance of resting voice
+ Alternative ways to communicate
+ Avoidance of alcohol and smoking

Key facts about Homans' sign

+ Deep calf pain results from strong and abrupt dorsiflexion of ankle
+ Results from venous thrombosis or inflammation of calf muscles

Key history points

+ Signs and symptoms of deep vein thrombosis or thrombophlebitis
+ Associated shortness of breath or chest pain
+ Predisposing events

Critical assessment steps

+ Inspect and palpate calf for warmth, tenderness, redness, swelling, and a palpable vein.
+ Measure circumferences of both calves.

Medical causes

Deep vein thrombophlebitis
+ Positive Homans' sign and calf tenderness may be the only signs.

In infants and young children, hoarseness commonly stems from acute laryngotracheobronchitis (croup). Acute laryngitis in children younger than age 5 may cause respiratory distress since the larynx is small, and if irritated or infected, subject to spasm. This may cause partial or total obstruction of the larynx. Temporary hoarseness commonly results from laryngeal irritation due to aspiration of liquids, foreign bodies, or stomach contents.

PATIENT COUNSELING

Stress to the patient the importance of resting his voice: Talking — even whispering — further traumatizes the vocal cords. Suggest other ways to communicate, such as writing or using body language. Urge the patient to avoid alcohol, smoking, and the company of smokers. If he has laryngitis, advise him to use a humidifier.

HOMANS' SIGN

Homans' sign is positive when deep calf pain results from strong and abrupt dorsiflexion of the ankle. This pain results from venous thrombosis or inflammation of the calf muscles. However, because a positive Homans' sign appears in only 35% of patients with these conditions, it's an unreliable indicator. (See *Eliciting Homans' sign.*) Even when accurate, a positive Homans' sign doesn't indicate the extent of the venous disorder.

This elicited sign may be confused with continuous calf pain, which can result from strains, contusions, cellulitis, or arterial occlusion, or with pain in the posterior ankle or Achilles tendon (for example, in a woman with Achilles tendons shortened from wearing high heels).

HISTORY

When you detect a positive Homans' sign, focus your patient history on signs and symptoms that can accompany deep vein thrombosis or thrombophlebitis. These include throbbing, aching, heavy, or tight sensations in the calf and leg pain during or after exercise or routine activity. Also, ask about shortness of breath or chest pain, which may indicate pulmonary embolism. Be sure to ask about predisposing events, such as leg injury, recent surgery, childbirth, use of contraceptive pills, associated diseases (cancer, nephrosis, hypercoagulable states), and prolonged inactivity or bed rest.

PHYSICAL ASSESSMENT

Inspect and palpate the patient's calf for warmth, tenderness, redness, swelling, and the presence of a palpable vein. If you strongly suspect deep vein thrombosis, elicit Homans' sign very carefully to avoid dislodging the clot, which could cause pulmonary embolism, a life-threatening condition. (See *Associated disorder: Thrombophlebitis,* page 364.)

In addition, measure the circumferences of both of the patient's calves. The calf with the positive Homans' sign may be larger because of edema and swelling.

MEDICAL CAUSES

Deep vein thrombophlebitis
A positive Homans' sign and calf tenderness may be the only clinical features of deep vein thrombophlebitis. However, the patient may also have severe pain, heavi-

ASSESSMENT TIP

Eliciting Homans' sign

To elicit Homans' sign, first support the patient's thigh with one hand and his foot with the other. Bend his leg slightly at the knee; then firmly and abruptly dorsiflex the ankle. Resulting deep calf pain indicates a positive Homans' sign. (The patient may also resist ankle dorsiflexion or flex the knee involuntarily if Homans' sign is positive.)

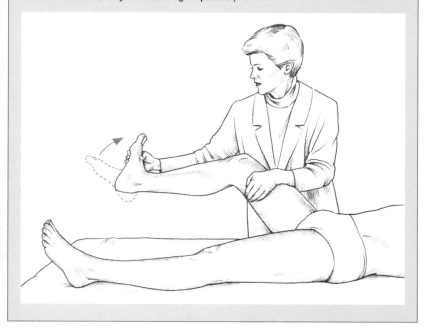

ness, warmth, and swelling of the affected leg; visible, engorged superficial veins or palpable, cordlike veins; and fever, chills, and malaise.

Deep vein thrombosis

Deep vein thrombosis (DVT) causes a positive Homans' sign along with tenderness over the deep calf veins, slight edema of the calves and thighs, a low-grade fever, and tachycardia. If DVT affects the femoral and iliac veins, you'll notice marked local swelling and tenderness. If DVT causes venous obstruction, you'll notice cyanosis and possibly cool skin in the affected leg.

Popliteal cyst (ruptured)

Rupture of this synovial cyst may produce a positive Homans' sign as well as sudden onset of calf tenderness, swelling, and redness. Bruising may be observed on the popliteal space and calf.

SPECIAL CONSIDERATIONS

Place the patient on bed rest, with the affected leg elevated above the heart level. Apply warm, moist compresses to the affected area, and administer mild oral analgesics. In addition, prepare the patient for further diagnostic tests, such as Doppler studies and venograms.

Medical causes
(continued)

Deep vein thrombosis
✦ Positive Homans' sign occurs with tenderness over the deep calf veins, slight edema of the calves and thighs, a low-grade fever, and tachycardia.

Popliteal cyst (ruptured)
✦ Positive Homans' sign and sudden onset of calf tenderness, swelling, and redness are produced.

Special considerations
✦ Place patient on bed rest, with affected leg elevated above heart level.
✦ Keep affected leg elevated while sitting and avoid crossing legs at the knees.

Key facts about thrombophlebitis

- Characterized by inflammation and thrombus formation
- May occur in deep or superficial veins
- May lead to pulmonary embolism

Causes

Deep vein
- Endothelial damage
- Accelerated blood clotting
- Reduced blood flow

Superficial
- Trauma
- Infection
- Chemical irritation due to extensive use of the I.V. route.

Management

- Heparin, followed by oral warfarin or low-molecular-weight heparin
- Thrombolytic therapy
- Bed rest with elevation of affected limb
- Warm, moist soaks
- Embolectomy, venous ligation, or insertion of a vena caval umbrella or filter, if indicated
- ROM exercises during bed rest
- Pneumatic compression devices during lengthy procedures
- Early ambulation to prevent thrombophlebitis
- Analgesics

ASSOCIATED DISORDER

Thrombophlebitis

An acute condition characterized by inflammation and thrombus formation, thrombophlebitis may occur in deep (intermuscular or intramuscular) or superficial (subcutaneous) veins. Deep vein thrombophlebitis affects small veins, such as the soleal venous sinuses, or large veins, such as the vena cava and the femoral, iliac, and subclavian veins, causing venous insufficiency.

This disorder may be progressive, leading to pulmonary embolism, a potentially lethal condition. Superficial thrombophlebitis is usually self-limiting and seldom leads to pulmonary embolism. Thrombophlebitis typically begins with localized inflammation alone (phlebitis), but such inflammation rapidly provokes thrombus formation.

CAUSES

Deep vein thrombophlebitis may be idiopathic, but it usually results from endothelial damage, accelerated blood clotting, and reduced blood flow. Predisposing factors include:
- prolonged bed rest
- trauma
- surgery
- pregnancy and childbirth
- hormonal contraceptives, such as estrogens.

Causes of superficial thrombophlebitis include:
- trauma
- infection
- chemical irritation due to extensive use of the I.V. route for medications and diagnostic tests.

DIAGNOSTIC TESTS

These essential tests help diagnose thrombophlebitis:
- Doppler ultrasonography shows reduced blood flow to a specific area and any obstruction to venous flow, particularly in iliofemoral deep vein thrombophlebitis.
- Plethysmography shows decreased circulation distal to the affected area; it's more sensitive than ultrasonography in detecting deep vein thrombophlebitis.
- Phlebography is usually used to confirm the diagnosis and shows filling defects and diverted blood flow.

MEDICAL INTERVENTIONS

Treatment of superficial thrombophlebitis requires no specific therapy other than symptom relief. Treatment of thrombophlebitis may include:
- heparin, followed by oral warfarin or low-molecular-weight heparin to prolong clotting times
- thrombolytic therapy (such as streptokinase) for acute, extensive deep vein thrombophlebitis
- bed rest with elevation of the affected limb to reduce edema
- warm, moist soaks to improve circulation and relieve pain and inflammation
- embolectomy, venous ligation, or insertion of a vena caval umbrella or filter if anticoagulation is contraindicated, risk of pulmonary embolism is high, or condition persists despite medical therapy
- range-of-motion exercises while the patient is on bed rest, pneumatic compression devices during lengthy surgical or diagnostic procedures, and early ambulation to prevent thrombophlebitis in high-risk patients
- analgesics for pain relief.

When the patient is ambulatory, advise him to wear elastic support stockings after his discomfort decreases (usually in 5 to 10 days) and to continue wearing them for at least 3 months. In addition, instruct the patient to keep the affected leg elevated while sitting and to avoid crossing his legs at the knees.

PEDIATRIC POINTERS

Homans' sign is seldom assessed in children, who rarely have DVT or thrombophlebitis.

PATIENT COUNSELING

If the patient is prescribed long-term anticoagulant therapy, instruct him to report signs of prolonged clotting time. These include black, tarry stools; brown or red urine; bleeding gums; and bruises. Also, stress the importance of keeping follow-up appointments so that prothrombin time can be monitored.

Instruct the patient to avoid alcohol and restrict green leafy vegetables (spinach and parsley), which are high in vitamin K. Also instruct him to review all medications he's taking with his physician because some drugs may enhance or inhibit the effects of the anticoagulant. The patient should also verify with his physician that any future prescriptions and over-the-counter medications are safe to take.

HYPERPNEA

The typical patient with hyperpnea breathes at a normal or increased rate and inhales deeply, displaying marked chest expansion. He may complain of shortness of breath if a respiratory disorder is causing hypoxemia, or he may not be aware of his breathing if a metabolic, psychiatric, or neurologic disorder is causing involuntary hyperpnea. Other causes of hyperpnea include profuse diarrhea or dehydration, loss of pancreatic juice or bile from GI drainage, and ureterosigmoidostomy. All these conditions and procedures cause a loss of bicarbonate ions, resulting in metabolic acidosis. Hyperpnea may also accompany strenuous exercise, and voluntary hyperpnea can promote relaxation in patients experiencing stress or pain — for example, women in labor.

Hyperventilation, a consequence of hyperpnea, is characterized by alkalosis (arterial pH above 7.45 and PCO_2 below 35 mm Hg). In central neurogenic hyperventilation, brain stem dysfunction (such as results from a severe cranial injury) increases the rate and depth of respirations. In acute intermittent hyperventilation, the respiratory pattern may be a response to hypoxemia, anxiety, fear, pain, or excitement. Hyperpnea may also be a compensatory mechanism to metabolic acidosis; under these conditions, it's known as *Kussmaul's respirations.* (See *Kussmaul's respirations: A compensatory mechanism,* page 366.)

HISTORY

If you observe hyperpnea in a patient whose other signs and symptoms signal a life-threatening emergency, you must intervene quickly. (See *Managing hyperpnea,* page 367.) If the patient's condition isn't grave, first determine his level of consciousness (LOC). If he's alert (and if his hyperpnea isn't interfering with speaking), ask about recent illnesses or infections, the ingestion of aspirin or other drugs or chemicals, and the inhalation of drugs or chemicals. Find out if the patient has diabetes mellitus, renal disease, or any pulmonary conditions. Is he excessively thirsty or hungry? Has he recently had severe diarrhea or an upper respiratory tract infection?

PHYSICAL ASSESSMENT

Observe the patient for clues to his abnormal breathing pattern. Is he unable to speak, or does he speak only in brief, choppy phrases? Is his breathing abnormally

Peds points
+ Homans' sign is seldom assessed in children.

Teaching points
+ Signs of prolonged clotting time to report
+ Importance of follow-up appointments
+ Avoidance of alcohol
+ Dietary restrictions (green leafy vegetables)
+ Explanation of drugs

Key facts about hyperpnea
+ Breathing at normal or increased rate with marked chest expansion during inhalation
+ May result in hyperventilation

Key history points
+ Recent illnesses or infections
+ Ingestion of aspirin or other drugs or inhalation of drugs or chemicals
+ Medical history, including diabetes mellitus, renal disease, or pulmonary conditions
+ Associated thirst or hunger

Kussmaul's respirations: A compensatory mechanism

Kussmaul's respirations—fast, deep breathing without pauses—characteristically sound labored, with deep breaths that resemble sighs. This breathing pattern develops when respiratory centers in the medulla detect decreased blood pH, thereby triggering compensatory fast and deep breathing to remove excess carbon dioxide and restore pH balance.

Disorders (such as diabetes mellitus and renal failure), drug effects, and other conditions cause metabolic acidosis (loss of bicarbonate ions and retention of acid).

↓

Blood pH decreases.

↓

Kussmaul's respirations develop to blow off excess carbon dioxide.

↓

Blood pH rises.

↓

Respiratory rate and depth decrease (corrected pH) in effective compensation.

Critical assessment steps

♦ Observe for clues to abnormal breathing pattern.
♦ Examine for cyanosis, restlessness, and anxiety.
♦ Observe for intercostal and abdominal retractions, accessory muscle use, and diaphoresis.
♦ Inspect for draining wounds or signs of infection.
♦ Take vital signs, including oxygen saturation.
♦ Auscultate the heart and lungs.
♦ Assess for dehydration.

Medical causes

Head injury
♦ Hyperpnea can occur.
♦ Other signs and symptoms depend on site and extent of injury.

Hyperventilation syndrome
♦ Acute anxiety triggers episodic hyperpnea, resulting in respiratory alkalosis.

rapid? Examine the patient for cyanosis (especially of the mouth, lips, mucous membranes, and earlobes), restlessness, and anxiety—all signs of decreased tissue oxygenation, as occurs in shock. In addition, observe the patient for intercostal and abdominal retractions, use of accessory muscles, and diaphoresis, all of which may indicate deep breathing related to an insufficient supply of oxygen. Next, inspect for draining wounds or signs of infection, and ask about nausea and vomiting. Take the patient's vital signs, including oxygen saturation, noting fever, and examine his skin and mucous membranes for turgor, possibly indicating dehydration. Auscultate the patient's heart and lungs.

MEDICAL CAUSES

Head injury
Hyperpnea can occur with severe head injury. Other clinical manifestations depend on the site and extent of injury and can include loss of consciousness; soft-tissue injury or bony deformity of the face, head, or neck; facial edema; clear or bloody drainage from the mouth, nose, or ears; raccoon eyes; Battle's sign; an absent doll's eye sign; and motor and sensory disturbances.

Signs of increased intracranial pressure include decreased response to painful stimulation, loss of pupillary reaction, bradycardia, increased systolic pressure, and widening pulse pressure.

Hyperventilation syndrome
Acute anxiety triggers episodic hyperpnea, resulting in respiratory alkalosis. Other findings may include agitation, vertigo, syncope, pallor, circumoral and peripheral paresthesia, muscle twitching, carpopedal spasm, weakness, and arrhythmias.

Managing hyperpnea

Carefully examine the patient with hyperpnea for related signs of life-threatening conditions, such as increased intracranial pressure (ICP), metabolic acidosis, diabetic ketoacidosis, and uremia. Be prepared for rapid interventions.

INCREASED ICP

If you observe hyperpnea in a patient who has signs of head trauma (soft-tissue injury, edema, or ecchymoses on the face or head) from a recent accident and has lost consciousness, act quickly to prevent further brain stem injury and irreversible deterioration. Take the patient's vital signs, noting bradycardia, increased systolic blood pressure, and widening pulse pressure — signs of increased ICP.

Examine his pupillary reaction. Elevate the head of the bed 30 degrees (unless you suspect spinal cord injury), insert an artificial airway, and administer oxygen. Connect the patient to a cardiac monitor, and continuously observe his respiratory pattern. (Irregular respirations signal deterioration.) Start an I.V. line at a slow infusion rate and prepare to administer an osmotic diuretic, such as mannitol, to decrease cerebral edema. Obtain a blood sample for arterial blood gas analysis to help guide treatments.

METABOLIC ACIDOSIS

If the patient with hyperpnea doesn't have a head injury, his increased respiratory rate probably indicates metabolic acidosis. Suspect shock if the patient has cold, clammy skin. Palpate for a rapid, thready pulse and take his blood pressure, noting hypotension. Elevate the patient's legs 30 degrees, apply pressure dressings to any obvious hemorrhage, start several large-bore I.V. lines, and prepare to administer fluids, vasopressors, and blood transfusions.

A patient with hyperpnea who has a history of alcohol abuse, is vomiting profusely, has diarrhea or profuse abdominal drainage, has ingested an overdose of aspirin, or is cachectic and has a history of starvation may also have metabolic acidosis. Inspect his skin for dryness and poor turgor, indicating dehydration. Take his vital signs, looking for low-grade fever and hypotension. Start an I.V. line for fluid replacement. Draw blood for electrolyte studies, and prepare to administer sodium bicarbonate.

DIABETIC KETOACIDOSIS

If the patient has a history of diabetes mellitus, is vomiting, and has a fruity breath odor (acetone breath), suspect diabetic ketoacidosis. Catheterize him to monitor increased urine output, and infuse normal saline solution. Perform a fingerstick to estimate blood glucose levels with a reagent strip. Obtain a urine specimen to test for glucose and acetone, and draw blood for glucose and ketone tests. Also, administer fluids, insulin, potassium, and sodium bicarbonate I.V.

UREMIA

If the patient has a history of renal disease, an ammonia breath odor (uremic fetor), and a fine, white powder on his skin (uremic frost), suspect uremia. Start an I.V. line at a slow rate, and prepare to administer sodium bicarbonate. Monitor his electrocardiogram for arrhythmias due to hyperkalemia. Monitor his serum electrolyte, blood urea nitrogen, and creatinine levels as well until hemodialysis or peritoneal dialysis begins.

In an emergency
+ Examine the patient for related signs of such life-threatening conditions as increased ICP, metabolic acidosis, diabetic ketoacidosis, and uremia.
+ Be prepared for rapid intervention.

Hypoxemia

Many pulmonary disorders that cause hypoxemia — for example, pneumonia, pulmonary edema, chronic obstructive pulmonary disease, and pneumothorax — may cause hyperpnea and episodes of hyperventilation with chest pain, dizziness, and paresthesia. Other effects include dyspnea, cough, crackles, rhonchi, wheezing, and decreased breath sounds.

Medical causes
(continued)

Hypoxemia
+ Many pulmonary disorders that cause hypoxemia may cause hyperpnea and episodes of hyperventilation with chest pain, dizziness, and paresthesia.

Medical causes
(continued)

Ketoacidosis
+ Alcoholic, diabetic, and starvation ketoacidosis can cause Kussmaul's respirations.

Renal failure
+ Life-threatening acidosis and Kussmaul's respirations can occur.

Sepsis
+ Severe infection may cause acidosis, resulting in Kussmaul's respirations.

Shock
+ Kussmaul's respirations, hypotension, tachycardia, narrowed pulse pressure, weak pulse, dyspnea, oliguria, anxiety, restlessness, stupor that can progress to coma, and cool, clammy skin develop.

Other causes
+ Toxic levels of salicylates, ammonium chloride, acetazolamide, and other carbonic anhydrase inhibitors
+ Ingestion of methanol and ethylene glycol

Ketoacidosis

Alcoholic ketoacidosis typically follows cessation of drinking after a marked increase in alcohol consumption has caused severe vomiting. Kussmaul's respirations begin abruptly and are accompanied by vomiting for several days, fruity breath odor, slight dehydration, abdominal pain and distention, and absent bowel sounds. The patient is alert and has a normal blood glucose level, unlike the patient with diabetic ketoacidosis.

Diabetic ketoacidosis is potentially life-threatening and typically produces Kussmaul's respirations. The patient usually experiences polydipsia, polyphagia, and polyuria before the onset of acidosis; he may or may not have a history of diabetes mellitus. Other clinical features include fruity breath odor; orthostatic hypotension; rapid, thready pulse; generalized weakness; decreased LOC (lethargy to coma); nausea; vomiting; anorexia; and abdominal pain.

Starvation ketoacidosis is also potentially life-threatening and can cause Kussmaul's respirations. Its onset is gradual; typical findings include signs of cachexia and dehydration, decreased LOC, bradycardia, and a history of severely limited food intake.

Renal failure

Acute or chronic renal failure can cause life-threatening acidosis with Kussmaul's respirations. Signs and symptoms of severe renal failure include oliguria or anuria, uremic fetor, and yellow, dry, scaly skin. Other cutaneous signs include severe pruritus, uremic frost, purpura, and ecchymoses. The patient may complain of nausea and vomiting, weakness, burning pain in the legs and feet, and diarrhea or constipation.

As acidosis progresses, corresponding clinical features include frothy sputum, pleuritic chest pain, and signs of heart failure and pleural or pericardial effusion. Neurologic signs include altered LOC (lethargy to coma), twitching, and seizures. Hyperkalemia and hypertension, if present, require rapid intervention to prevent cardiovascular collapse.

Sepsis

A severe infection may cause lactic acidosis, resulting in Kussmaul's respirations. Other findings in sepsis include tachycardia, fever or a low temperature, chills, headache, lethargy, profuse diaphoresis, anorexia, cough, wound drainage, burning on urination, confusion or change in mental status, and other signs of local infection.

Shock

Potentially life-threatening metabolic acidosis produces Kussmaul's respirations, hypotension, tachycardia, narrowed pulse pressure, weak pulse, dyspnea, oliguria, anxiety, restlessness, stupor that can progress to coma, and cool, clammy skin. Other clinical features may include external or internal bleeding (in hypovolemic shock); chest pain or arrhythmias and signs of heart failure (in cardiogenic shock); high fever, chills and, rarely, hypothermia (in septic shock); or stridor due to laryngeal edema (in anaphylactic shock). Onset is usually acute in hypovolemic, cardiogenic, or anaphylactic shock, but it may be gradual in septic shock.

OTHER CAUSES

Drugs

Toxic levels of salicylates, ammonium chloride, acetazolamide, and other carbonic anhydrase inhibitors can cause Kussmaul's respirations. So can ingestion of methanol and ethylene glycol, found in antifreeze solutions.

SPECIAL CONSIDERATIONS

Monitor vital signs including oxygen saturation in all patients with hyperpnea, and observe for increasing respiratory distress or an irregular respiratory pattern signaling deterioration. Prepare for immediate intervention to prevent cardiovascular collapse: Start an I.V. line for administration of fluids, blood transfusions, and vasopressor drugs for hemodynamic stabilization, as ordered, and prepare to give ventilatory support. Prepare the patient for arterial blood gas analysis and blood chemistry studies.

PEDIATRIC POINTERS

Hyperpnea in a child indicates the same metabolic or neurologic causes as in an adult and requires the same prompt intervention. The most common cause of metabolic acidosis in a child is diarrhea, which can cause a life-threatening crisis. In an infant, Kussmaul's respirations may accompany acidosis due to inborn errors of metabolism.

PATIENT COUNSELING

Teach the patient with diabetes to monitor blood glucose levels. Encourage strict adherence to the therapy prescribed for his diabetes. Encourage the patient with renal disease to limit fluids and maintain a low-protein, low-sodium, low-potassium, low-phosphorus, high-calorie, high-carbohydrate diet. For the patient with pulmonary disease, discuss how to maintain pulmonary hygiene and avoid respiratory infections.

Special considerations
+ Monitor vital signs.
+ Observe for increasing respiratory distress or an irregular respiratory pattern.
+ Start an I.V. line for administration of fluids, blood transfusions, and vasopressor drugs, as ordered.
+ Prepare to give ventilatory support.

Peds points
+ Hyperpnea in a child indicates the same metabolic or neurologic causes as in an adult.

Teaching points
+ Blood glucose level monitoring
+ Importance of compliance with diabetes therapy, if applicable
+ Fluid and dietary restrictions
+ Pulmonary hygiene
+ Avoidance of respiratory infections

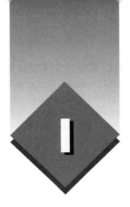

INSOMNIA

Insomnia is the inability to fall asleep, remain asleep, or feel refreshed by sleep. Acute and transient during periods of stress, insomnia may become chronic, causing constant fatigue, extreme anxiety as bedtime approaches, and psychiatric disorders. This common complaint is experienced occasionally by about 25% of Americans and chronically by another 10%.

Physiologic causes of insomnia include jet lag, arguing, and lack of exercise. Pathophysiologic causes range from medical and psychiatric disorders to pain, adverse effects of a drug, and idiopathic factors. Complaints of insomnia are subjective and require close investigation.

HISTORY

Take a thorough sleep and health history. Find out when the patient's insomnia began and the circumstances surrounding it. Is the patient trying to stop using a sedative? Does he take a central nervous system (CNS) stimulant, such as an amphetamine, pseudoephedrine, a theophylline derivative, phenylpropanolamine, cocaine, or a drug that contains caffeine, or does he drink caffeinated beverages?

Find out if the patient has a chronic or acute condition, the effects of which may be disturbing his sleep, particularly cardiac or respiratory disease or painful or pruritic conditions. Ask if he has an endocrine or neurologic disorder or a history of drug or alcohol abuse. Is he a frequent traveler who suffers from jet lag? Does he use his legs a lot during the day and then feel restless at night? Ask about daytime fatigue and regular exercise. Also ask if he often finds himself gasping for air, experiencing apnea, or frequently repositioning his body. If possible, consult the patient's spouse or sleep partner because the patient may be unaware of his own behavior. Ask how many pillows the patient uses to sleep.

Assess the patient's emotional status, and try to estimate his level of self-esteem. Ask about personal and professional problems and psychological stress. Also ask if he experiences hallucinations, and note behavior that may indicate alcohol withdrawal.

PHYSICAL ASSESSMENT

To detect an underlying disorder that may affect sleep, perform a complete physical assessment. Pay close attention to findings that suggest a neurologic, cardiac, respiratory, or endocrine disorder.

Key facts
about insomnia

✦ Inability to fall asleep, remain asleep, or feel refreshed by sleep
✦ May have physiologic or pathophysiologic cause

Key history points

✦ Sleep and health history
✦ Onset of insomnia
✦ Drug history
✦ Current chronic or acute conditions
✦ History of drug and alcohol use
✦ Emotional status and stress factors

Critical
assessment steps

✦ Perform a complete physical assessment.
✦ Pay close attention to findings that suggest neurologic, cardiac, respiratory, or endocrine disorder.

MEDICAL CAUSES

Alcohol withdrawal syndrome

Abrupt cessation of alcohol intake after long-term use causes insomnia that may persist for up to 2 years. Other early effects of this acute syndrome include excessive diaphoresis, tachycardia, hypertension, tremors, restlessness, irritability, headache, nausea, flushing, and nightmares. Progression to delirium tremens produces confusion, disorientation, paranoia, delusions, hallucinations, and seizures.

Depression

Depression commonly causes chronic insomnia with difficulty falling asleep, waking and being unable to fall back to sleep, or waking early in the morning. Related findings include dysphoria (a primary symptom), decreased appetite with weight loss or increased appetite with weight gain, and psychomotor agitation or retardation. The patient experiences loss of interest in his usual activities, feelings of worthlessness and guilt, fatigue, difficulty concentrating, indecisiveness, and recurrent thoughts of death.

Generalized anxiety disorder

Anxiety can cause chronic insomnia as well as symptoms of tension, such as fatigue and restlessness; signs of autonomic hyperactivity, such as diaphoresis, dyspepsia, and high resting pulse and respiratory rates; and signs of apprehension.

Nocturnal myoclonus

With nocturnal myoclonus, a seizure disorder, involuntary and fleeting muscle jerks of the legs occur every 20 to 40 seconds, disturbing sleep. The patient typically reports poor sleep and daytime somnolence.

Pain

Almost any condition that causes pain can also cause insomnia. Related findings reflect the specific cause. Behavioral responses that may accompany pain include altered body position, moaning, grimacing, withdrawal, crying, restlessness, muscle twitching, and immobility. With mild or moderate pain the patient may have pallor, elevated blood pressure, dilated pupils, skeletal muscle tension, dyspnea, tachycardia, and diaphoresis. Severe, deep pain may produce pallor, decreased blood pressure, bradycardia, nausea and vomiting, weakness, dizziness, and loss of consciousness.

Pruritus

Localized skin infections and systemic disorders, such as liver failure, can cause pruritus, resulting in insomnia. The patient may report scratching as a way to relieve the itching.

Sleep apnea syndrome

Apneic periods begin with the onset of sleep, continue for 10 to 90 seconds, and end with a series of gasps and arousal. With central sleep apnea, respiratory movement ceases for the apneic period; with obstructive sleep apnea, upper airway obstruction blocks incoming air, although breathing movements continue. Repeated possibly hundreds of times during the night, this cycle alternates with bradycardia and tachycardia. Associated findings include morning headache, daytime fatigue, hypertension, ankle edema, and personality changes, such as hostility, paranoia, and agitated depression.

Medical causes

Alcohol withdrawal syndrome
+ Insomnia may persist for up to 2 years.

Depression
+ Chronic insomnia occurs with difficulty falling asleep, waking and being unable to fall back to sleep, or waking early in the morning.

Generalized anxiety disorder
+ Chronic insomnia occurs with symptoms of tension, signs of autonomic hyperactivity, and signs of apprehension.

Nocturnal myoclonus
+ Involuntary and fleeting muscle jerks of the legs occur every 20 to 40 seconds, disturbing sleep.

Pain
+ Conditions that cause pain can also cause insomnia.

Pruritus
+ Insomnia results becuase of scratching.

Sleep apnea syndrome
+ Sleep is disturbed by apneic periods that end with a series of gasps and arousal.

Medical causes
(continued)

Thyrotoxicosis
+ Difficulty falling asleep and then sleeping for only a brief period is a characteristic symptom.

Other causes
+ Use of, abuse of, or withdrawal from sedatives or hypnotics
+ CNS stimulants

Special considerations
+ Prepare the patient for tests to evaluate his insomnia.

Peds points
+ Insomnia in early childhood may develop along with separation anxiety (ages 2 to 3), after a stressful or tiring day, or during illness or teething.
+ In children ages 6 to 11, insomnia usually reflects residual excitement from the day's activities.
+ Sleep problems are common in foster children.

Geri points
+ Sleep patterns of older people are marked by frequent awakenings, diminished stage III and stage IV non-rapid eye movement time, increased time spent awake at night, and more frequent daytime naps.

Teaching points
+ Comfort and relaxation techniques
+ Appropriate use of tranquilizers or sedatives
+ Referral to counseling or sleep disorder clinic as needed

Thyrotoxicosis

Difficulty falling asleep and then sleeping for only a brief period is one of the characteristic symptoms of thyrotoxicosis. Cardiopulmonary features include dyspnea, tachycardia, palpitations, and atrial or ventricular gallop. Other findings include weight loss despite increased appetite, diarrhea, tremors, nervousness, diaphoresis, hypersensitivity to heat, an enlarged thyroid, and exophthalmos.

OTHER CAUSES

Drugs

Use of, abuse of, or withdrawal from sedatives or hypnotics may produce insomnia. CNS stimulants—including amphetamines, theophylline derivatives, pseudoephedrine, phenylpropanolamine, cocaine, and caffeinated beverages—may also produce insomnia.

SPECIAL CONSIDERATIONS

Prepare the patient for tests to evaluate his insomnia, such as blood and urine studies for 17-hydroxycorticosteroids and catecholamines, polysomnography (including an EEG, electro-oculography, and electrocardiography), and sleep EEG.

PEDIATRIC POINTERS

Insomnia in early childhood may develop along with separation anxiety at ages 2 to 3, after a stressful or tiring day, or during illness or teething. In children ages 6 to 11, insomnia usually reflects residual excitement from the day's activities; a few children continue to have bedtime fears. Sleep problems are common in foster children.

GERIATRIC POINTERS

Older people who are deprived of sleep may become forgetful, disoriented, or confused. Those who are cognitively impaired exhibit increased restlessness, wandering behavior, and "sundowner syndrome" (confusion, agitation, and disruptive behavior during late afternoon and early evening hours).

Sleep patterns of older people are marked by frequent awakenings, diminished stage III and stage IV non-rapid eye movement time, increased time spent awake at night, and more frequent daytime naps. Most healthy older adults report no symptoms related to these changes other than not getting enough sleep or sleeping poorly.

PATIENT COUNSELING

Teach the patient comfort and relaxation techniques to promote natural sleep. (See *Tips for relieving insomnia.*) Advise him to awaken and retire at the same time each day and to exercise regularly. When he can't sleep, advise him to get up but remain inactive. Urge him to use his bed only for sleeping, not for relaxation or watching TV.

Advise the patient to use tranquilizers or sedatives for acute insomnia only when relaxation techniques fail. If appropriate, refer him for counseling or to a sleep disorder clinic for biofeedback training or other interventions.

Tips for relieving insomnia

COMMON PROBLEMS	CAUSES	INTERVENTIONS
Acroparesthesia	Improper positioning may compress superficial (ulnar, radial, and peroneal) nerves, disrupting circulation to the compressed nerve. This causes numbness, tingling, and stiffness in an arm or leg.	Teach the patient to assume a comfortable position in bed, with his limbs unrestricted. If he tends to awaken with a numb arm or leg, tell him to massage and move it until sensation returns completely and then to assume an unrestricted position.
Anxiety	Physical and emotional stress produces anxiety, which causes autonomic stimulation.	Encourage the patient to discuss his fears and concerns, and teach him relaxation techniques, such as guided imagery and deep breathing. If ordered, administer a mild sedative, such as temazepam or another sedative hypnotic, before bedtime. Emphasize that these medications are to be used for the short-term only.
Dyspnea	With many cardiac and pulmonary disorders, a recumbent position and inactivity cause restricted chest expansion, secretion pooling, and pulmonary vascular congestion, leading to coughing and shortness of breath.	Elevate the head of the bed, or provide at least two pillows or a reclining chair to help the patient sleep. Suction him when he awakens, and encourage deep breathing and incentive spirometry every 2 to 4 hours. Also, provide supplementary oxygen by nasal cannula. If the patient is pregnant, encourage her to sleep on her left side at a comfortable elevation.
Pain	Chronic or acute pain from any cause can prevent or disrupt sleep.	Administer pain medication, as ordered, 20 minutes before bedtime, and teach deep, even, slow breathing to promote relaxation. If the patient has back pain, help him lie on his side with his legs flexed. If he has epigastric pain, encourage him to take an antacid before bedtime and to sleep with the head of the bed elevated. If he has incisions, instruct him to splint during coughing or movement.
Pruritus	A localized skin infection or a systemic disorder, such as liver failure, may produce intensely annoying itching, even during the night.	Wash the patient's skin with a mild soap and water, and dry the skin thoroughly. Apply moisturizing lotion on dry, unbroken skin and an antipruritic such as calamine lotion on pruritic areas. Administer diphenhydramine or hydroxyzine, as ordered, to help minimize itching.
Restless leg	Excessive exercise during the day may cause tired, aching legs at night, requiring movement for relief.	Help the patient exercise his legs gently by slowly walking with him around the room and down the hall. If ordered, administer a muscle relaxant such as diazepam.

INTERMITTENT CLAUDICATION

Most common in the legs, intermittent claudication is cramping limb pain brought on by exercise and relieved by 1 to 2 minutes of rest. This pain may be acute or chronic; when acute, it may signal acute arterial occlusion. Intermittent claudication is most common in men ages 50 to 60 with a history of diabetes mellitus, hyperlipidemia, hypertension, or tobacco use. Without treatment, it may progress to pain at rest. With chronic arterial occlusion, limb loss is uncommon because collateral circulation usually develops.

With occlusive artery disease, intermittent claudication results from an inadequate blood supply. Pain in the calf (the most common area) or foot indicates disease of the femoral or popliteal arteries; pain in the buttocks and upper thigh, disease of the aortoiliac arteries. During exercise, the pain typically results from the release of lactic acid due to anaerobic metabolism in the ischemic segment, secondary to obstruction. When exercise stops, the lactic acid clears and the pain subsides.

Intermittent claudication may also have a neurologic cause: narrowing of the vertebral column at the level of the cauda equina. This condition creates pressure on the nerve roots to the lower extremities. Walking stimulates circulation to the cauda equina, causing increased pressure on those nerves and resultant pain.

 EMERGENCY ACTIONS If the patient has sudden intermittent claudication with severe or aching leg pain at rest, check leg temperature and color and palpate femoral, popliteal, posterior tibial, and dorsalis pedis pulses. Ask about numbness and tingling. Suspect acute arterial occlusion if pulses are absent; if the leg feels cold and looks pale, cyanotic, or mottled; and if paresthesia and pain are present. Mark the area of pallor, cyanosis, or mottling, and reassess it frequently, noting an increase in the area. Don't elevate the leg. Protect it, allowing nothing to press on it. Prepare the patient for preoperative blood tests, urinalysis, electrocardiography, chest X-rays, lower-extremity Doppler studies, and angiography. Start an I.V. line, and administer an anticoagulant and analgesics.

HISTORY

If the patient has chronic intermittent claudication, ask how far he can walk before pain occurs and how long he must rest before it subsides. Can he walk less distance now than before, or does he need to rest longer? Does the pain-rest pattern vary? Has this symptom affected his lifestyle?

Obtain a history of risk factors for atherosclerosis, such as smoking, diabetes, hypertension, and hyperlipidemia. Next, ask about associated signs and symptoms, such as paresthesia in the affected limb and visible changes in the color of the fingers (white to blue to pink) when he's smoking, exposed to cold, or under stress. If the patient is male, does he experience impotence?

PHYSICAL ASSESSMENT

Focus the physical examination on the cardiovascular system. Palpate for femoral, popliteal, dorsalis pedis, and posterior tibial pulses. Note character, amplitude, and bilateral equality. Diminished or absent popliteal and pedal pulses with the femoral pulse present may indicate atherosclerotic disease of the femoral artery. Diminished femoral and distal pulses may indicate disease of the terminal aorta or iliac branches. Absent pedal pulses with normal femoral and popliteal pulses may indicate Buerger's disease.

Listen for bruits over the major arteries. Note color and temperature differences between his legs or compared with his arms; also note where on his leg the changes in temperature and color occur. Elevate the affected leg for 2 minutes; if it becomes pale or white, blood flow is severely decreased. When the leg hangs down, how long does it take for color to return? (Thirty seconds or longer indicates severe disease.) If possible, check the patient's deep tendon reflexes after exercise; note if they're diminished in his lower extremities.

Examine his feet, toes, and fingers for ulceration, and inspect his hands and lower legs for small, tender nodules and erythema along blood vessels. Note the quality of his nails and the amount of hair on his fingers and toes.

If the patient has arm pain, inspect his arms for a change in color (to white) on elevation. Next, palpate for changes in temperature, muscle wasting, and a pulsating mass in the subclavian area. Palpate and compare the radial, ulnar, brachial, axillary, and subclavian pulses to identify obstructed areas.

MEDICAL CAUSES

Aortic arteriosclerotic occlusive disease

With aortic arteriosclerotic occlusive disease, intermittent claudication occurs in the buttock, hip, thigh, and calf, along with absent or diminished femoral pulses. Bruits can be auscultated over the femoral and iliac arteries. Examination reveals pallor of the affected limb on elevation and profound limb weakness. The leg may be cool to the touch.

Arterial occlusion (acute)

Acute arterial occlusion produces intense intermittent claudication. A saddle embolus may affect both legs. Associated findings include paresthesia, paresis, and a sensation of cold in the affected limb. The limb is cool, pale, and cyanotic (mottled) with absent pulses below the occlusion. Capillary refill time is increased.

Arteriosclerosis obliterans

Arteriosclerosis obliterans usually affects the femoral and popliteal arteries, causing intermittent claudication (the most common symptom) in the calf. Typical associated findings include diminished or absent popliteal and pedal pulses, coolness in the affected limb, pallor on elevation, and profound limb weakness with continuing exercise. Other possible findings include numbness, paresthesia and, in severe disease, pain in the toes or foot while at rest, ulceration, and gangrene.

Buerger's disease

Buerger's disease typically produces intermittent claudication of the instep. Early signs include migratory superficial nodules and erythema along extremity blood vessels (nodular phlebitis) as well as migratory venous phlebitis. With exposure to cold, the feet initially become cold, cyanotic, and numb; later, they redden, become hot, and tingle. Occasionally, Buerger's disease also affects the hands and can cause painful ulcerations on the fingertips. Other characteristic findings include impaired peripheral pulses, paresthesia of the hands and feet, and migratory superficial thrombophlebitis.

 CULTURAL CUE *Buerger's disease is common in patients from the Orient, southeast Asia, India, and the Middle East. It rarely occurs in blacks.*

Leriche's syndrome

With Leriche's syndrome, arterial occlusion causes intermittent claudication of the hip, thigh, buttocks, and calf as well as impotence in men. Examination reveals bruits, global atrophy, absent or diminished pulses, and gangrene of the toes. The leg becomes cool and pale when elevated.

Neurogenic claudication

Neurospinal disease causes pain from neurogenic intermittent claudication that requires a longer rest time than the 2 to 3 minutes needed in vascular claudication. Associated findings include paresthesia, weakness and clumsiness when walking, and hypoactive deep tendon reflexes after walking. Pulses are unaffected.

SPECIAL CONSIDERATIONS

Encourage the patient to exercise to improve collateral circulation and increase venous return, and advise him to avoid prolonged sitting or standing as well as crossing his legs at the knees. If intermittent claudication interferes with the patient's lifestyle, he may require diagnostic tests (Doppler flow studies, arteriography, and digital subtraction angiography) to determine the location and degree of occlusion.

PEDIATRIC POINTERS

Intermittent claudication rarely occurs in children. Although it sometimes develops in patients with coarctation of the aorta, extensive compensatory collateral circulation typically prevents manifestation of this sign. Muscle cramps from exercise and growing pains may be mistaken for intermittent claudication in children.

PATIENT COUNSELING

Counsel the patient with intermittent claudication about risk factors. Encourage him to stop smoking, and refer him to a support group, if appropriate. Teach him to inspect his legs and feet for ulcers; to keep his extremities warm, clean, and dry; and to avoid injury.

Urge the patient to immediately report skin breakdown that doesn't heal. Also urge him to report any chest discomfort when circulation is restored to his legs. Increased exercise tolerance may lead to angina if the patient has coronary artery disease that was previously asymptomatic because of exercise limitations.

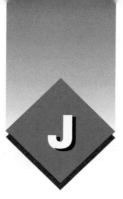

JAUNDICE

A yellow discoloration of the skin, mucous membranes, or sclerae of the eyes, jaundice indicates excessive levels of conjugated or unconjugated bilirubin in the blood. Also known as *icterus,* jaundice is most apparent in natural sunlight. In fact, it may be undetectable in artificial or poor light. It's commonly accompanied by pruritus (because bile pigment damages sensory nerves), dark urine, and clay-colored stools.

 CULTURAL CUE *In fair-skinned patients, jaundice is most noticeable on the face, trunk, and sclerae; in dark-skinned patients, it's noticeable on the hard palate, sclerae, and conjunctivae.*

Jaundice may result from any of three pathophysiologic processes. (See *Jaundice: Impaired bilirubin metabolism,* page 378.) It may be the only warning sign of certain disorders such as pancreatic cancer.

HISTORY

Begin by asking the patient when he first noticed the jaundice. Does he also have pruritus, clay-colored stools, or dark urine? Ask about past episodes or a family history of jaundice. Does he have nonspecific signs or symptoms, such as fatigue, fever, or chills; GI signs or symptoms, such as anorexia, abdominal pain, nausea, weight loss, or vomiting; or cardiopulmonary symptoms, such as shortness of breath or palpitations? Ask about alcohol use and a history of cancer or liver or gallbladder disease. Has the patient lost weight recently? Also, obtain a drug history. Ask about a history of hepatitis, gallstones, or pancreatic disease.

PHYSICAL ASSESSMENT

Perform the physical examination in a room with natural light. Make sure that the orange-yellow hue is jaundice and not due to hypercarotenemia, which is more prominent on the palms and soles and doesn't affect the sclerae. Inspect the patient's skin for texture and dryness and for hyperpigmentation and xanthomas. Look for spider angiomas or petechiae, clubbed fingers, and gynecomastia. If the patient has heart failure, auscultate for arrhythmias, murmurs, and gallops. For all patients, auscultate for crackles and abnormal bowel sounds. Palpate the lymph nodes for swelling and the abdomen for tenderness, pain, and swelling. Palpate and percuss the liver and spleen for enlargement, and test for ascites with the shifting dullness and fluid wave techniques. Obtain baseline data on the patient's mental status: Slight changes in sensorium may be an early sign of deteriorating hepatic function.

Key facts about jaundice
+ Yellow discoloration of skin, mucous membranes, or sclerae of eyes
+ Indicates excessive levels of bilirubin in the blood

Key history points
+ Onset of jaundice
+ Associated pruritus, clay-colored stools, dark urine, fatigue, fever, chills, GI signs or symptoms, cardiopulmonary symptoms
+ History of cancer; liver, pancreatic or gallbladder disease; hepatitis; or gallstones
+ Drug and alcohol use

Critical assessment steps
+ Perform the physical examination in a room with natural light.
+ Rule out hypercarotenemia.
+ Inspect patient's skin for texture, dryness, hyperpigmentation, and xanthomas.
+ Palpate abdomen for tenderness, pain, and swelling.
+ Palpate and percuss the liver and spleen for enlargement.
+ Test for ascites.
+ Obtain baseline data on mental status.

Jaundice: Impaired bilirubin metabolism

Jaundice occurs in three forms: prehepatic, hepatic, and posthepatic. In all three, bilirubin levels in the blood increase due to impaired metabolism.

With *prehepatic jaundice,* certain conditions and disorders, such as transfusion reactions and sickle cell anemia, cause massive hemolysis. Red blood cells rupture faster than the liver can conjugate bilirubin, so large amounts of unconjugated bilirubin pass into the blood, causing increased intestinal conversion of this bilirubin to water-soluble urobilinogen for excretion in urine and stools. (Unconjugated bilirubin is insoluble in water, so it can't be directly excreted in urine.)

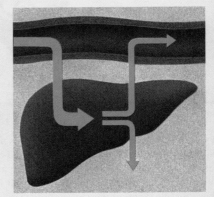

Hepatic jaundice results from the liver's inability to conjugate or excrete bilirubin, leading to increased blood levels of conjugated and unconjugated bilirubin. This occurs with such disorders as hepatitis, cirrhosis, and metastatic cancer and during the prolonged use of drugs metabolized by the liver.

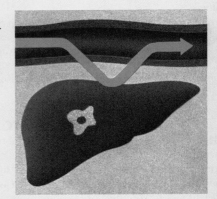

With *posthepatic jaundice,* which occurs in patients with a biliary or pancreatic disorder, bilirubin forms at its normal rate, but inflammation, scar tissue, a tumor, or gallstones block the flow of bile into the intestine. This causes an accumulation of conjugated bilirubin in the blood. Water-soluble, conjugated bilirubin is excreted in the urine.

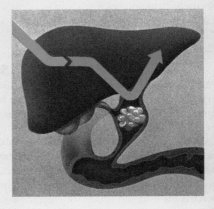

MEDICAL CAUSES

Carcinoma

Cancer of the ampulla of Vater initially produces fluctuating jaundice, mild abdominal pain, recurrent fever, and chills. Occult bleeding may be its first sign. Other findings include weight loss, pruritus, and back pain.

Hepatic cancer (primary liver cancer or metastases to the liver) may cause jaundice by causing obstruction of the bile duct. Even advanced cancer causes nonspecific signs and symptoms, such as right-upper-quadrant discomfort and tenderness, nausea, weight loss, and slight fever. Examination may reveal irregular, nodular, firm hepatomegaly, ascites, peripheral edema, a bruit heard over the liver, and a right-upper-quadrant mass.

With pancreatic cancer, progressive jaundice—possibly with pruritus—may be the only sign. Related early findings are nonspecific, such as weight loss and back or abdominal pain. Other signs and symptoms include anorexia, nausea and vomiting, fever, steatorrhea, fatigue, weakness, diarrhea, pruritus, and skin lesions (usually on the legs).

Cholangitis

Obstruction and infection in the common bile duct cause Charcot's triad: jaundice, right-upper-quadrant pain, and high fever with chills. The patient may also report pruritus. Acholic or hypocholic stools may be present.

Cholecystitis

Cholecystitis produces nonobstructive jaundice in about 25% of patients. Biliary colic typically peaks abruptly, persisting for 2 to 4 hours. The pain then localizes to the right upper quadrant and becomes constant. Local inflammation or passage of stones to the common bile duct causes jaundice. Other findings include nausea, vomiting (usually indicating the presence of a stone), fever, profuse diaphoresis, chills, tenderness on palpation, a positive Murphy's sign and, possibly, abdominal distention and rigidity.

Cholelithiasis

Cholelithiasis commonly causes jaundice and biliary colic. It's characterized by severe, steady pain in the right upper quadrant or epigastrium that radiates to the right scapula or shoulder and intensifies over several hours. Accompanying signs and symptoms include nausea and vomiting, tachycardia, and restlessness. Occlusion of the common bile duct causes fever, chills, jaundice, clay-colored stools, and abdominal tenderness. After consuming a fatty meal, the patient may experience vague epigastric fullness and dyspepsia.

Cholestasis

With benign, recurrent intrahepatic cholestasis, the patient experiences prolonged attacks of jaundice (sometimes spaced several years apart) accompanied by pruritus. Other signs and symptoms are similar to those of hepatitis—fatigue, nausea, weight loss, anorexia, pale stools, and right-upper-quadrant pain.

Cirrhosis

With Laënnec's cirrhosis, mild to moderate jaundice with pruritus usually signals hepatocellular necrosis or progressive hepatic insufficiency. Common early findings include ascites, weakness, leg edema, nausea and vomiting, diarrhea or constipation, anorexia, weight loss, and right-upper-quadrant pain. Massive hematemesis and other bleeding tendencies may also occur. Other findings include an enlarged liver and parotid gland, clubbed fingers, Dupuytren's contracture, mental changes, asterixis, fetor hepaticus, spider angiomas, and palmar erythema. Males may exhib-

Medical causes

Carcinoma
+ With cancer of the ampulla of Vater, jaundice fluctuates.
+ With hepatic cancer, jaundice may result from obstruction of the bile duct.
+ With pancreatic cancer, progressive jaundice may be the only sign.

Cholangitis
+ Obstruction and infection in the common bile duct cause Charcot's triad: jaundice, right-upper-quadrant pain, and high fever with chills.

Cholecystitis
+ Nonobstructive jaundice occurs in about 25% of patients.
+ Local inflammation or passage of stones to the common bile duct causes jaundice.

Cholelithiasis
+ Jaundice and biliary colic are common.

Cholestasis
+ Prolonged attacks of jaundice (sometimes spaced several years apart) are accompanied by pruritus.

Cirrhosis
+ With Laënnec's cirrhosis, mild to moderate jaundice with pruritus usually signals hepatocellular necrosis or progressive hepatic insufficiency.
+ With primary biliary cirrhosis, fluctuating jaundice may appear years after the onset of other signs and symptoms.

it gynecomastia, scanty chest and axillary hair, and testicular atrophy; females may experience menstrual irregularities.

With primary biliary cirrhosis, fluctuating jaundice may appear years after the onset of other signs and symptoms, such as pruritus that worsens at bedtime (commonly the first sign), weakness, fatigue, weight loss, and vague abdominal pain. Itching may lead to skin excoriation. Associated findings include hyperpigmentation; indications of malabsorption, such as nocturnal diarrhea, steatorrhea, purpura, and osteomalacia; hematemesis from esophageal varices; ascites; edema; xanthelasmas; xanthomas on the palms, soles, and elbows; and hepatomegaly.

Glucose-6-phosphate dehydrogenase deficiency

Acute intravascular hemolysis following ingestion of such drugs as quinine or aspirin causes jaundice, pallor, dyspnea, tachycardia, and malaise. Palpation may reveal splenomegaly and hepatomegaly.

Heart failure

Jaundice due to liver dysfunction occurs in patients with severe right-sided heart failure. Other effects include jugular vein distention, cyanosis, dependent edema of the legs and sacrum, steady weight gain, confusion, hepatomegaly, nausea and vomiting, abdominal discomfort, and anorexia due to visceral edema. Ascites is a late sign. Oliguria, marked weakness, and anxiety may also occur. If left-sided heart failure develops first, other findings may include fatigue, dyspnea, orthopnea, paroxysmal nocturnal dyspnea, tachypnea, arrhythmias, and tachycardia.

Hemolytic anemia (acquired)

Acquired hemolytic anemia may produce prominent jaundice along with dyspnea, fatigue, pallor, tachycardia, and palpitations. Rapid hemolysis causes chills, fever, irritability, headache, and abdominal pain; severe hemolysis causes signs of shock.

Hepatitis

Dark urine and clay-colored stools usually develop before jaundice in the late stages of acute viral hepatitis. Early systemic signs and symptoms vary and include fatigue, nausea, vomiting, malaise, arthralgias, myalgias, headache, anorexia, photophobia, pharyngitis, cough, diarrhea or constipation, and a low-grade fever associated with liver and lymph node enlargement. During the icteric phase (which subsides within 2 to 3 weeks unless complications occur), systemic signs subside, but an enlarged, palpable liver may be present along with weight loss, anorexia, and right-upper-quadrant pain and tenderness.

Pancreatitis (acute)

Pancreatitis can cause jaundice; however, this disorder's primary symptom is usually severe epigastric pain that commonly radiates to the back. Lying with the knees flexed on the chest or sitting up and leaning forward brings relief. Early associated signs and symptoms include nausea, persistent vomiting, abdominal distention, and Turner's or Cullen's sign. Other findings include fever, tachycardia, abdominal rigidity and tenderness, hypoactive bowel sounds, and crackles.

Severe pancreatitis produces extreme restlessness; mottled skin; cold, diaphoretic extremities; paresthesia; and tetany—the last two being symptoms of hypocalcemia. Fulminant pancreatitis causes massive hemorrhage.

Sickle cell anemia

Hemolysis produces jaundice in patients with sickle cell anemia. Other findings include impaired growth and development, increased susceptibility to infection, life-threatening thrombotic complications and, commonly, leg ulcers, swollen joints (sometimes painful), fever, and chills. Bone aches and chest pain may also occur.

Medical causes
(continued)

Glucose-6-phosphate dehydrogenase deficiency
✦ Acute intravascular hemolysis following ingestion of such drugs as quinine or aspirin causes jaundice, pallor, dyspnea, tachycardia, and malaise.

Heart failure
✦ Jaundice due to liver dysfunction occurs in patients with severe right-sided heart failure.

Hemolytic anemia (acquired)
✦ Jaundice may be prominent and appears with dyspnea, fatigue, pallor, tachycardia, and palpitations.

Hepatitis
✦ Jaundice occurs late and is preceded by dark urine and clay-colored stools.

Pancreatitis (acute)
✦ Jaundice may occur.
✦ Primary symptom is usually severe epigastric pain that commonly radiates to the back.

Sickle cell anemia
✦ Hemolysis produces jaundice.

Severe hemolysis may cause hematuria and pallor, chronic fatigue, weakness, dyspnea (or dyspnea on exertion), and tachycardia. The patient may also have splenomegaly. During a sickle cell crisis, the patient may have severe bone, abdominal, thoracic, and muscular pain; low-grade fever; and increased weakness, jaundice, and dyspnea.

OTHER CAUSES

Drugs
Many drugs may cause hepatic injury and resultant jaundice. Examples include acetaminophen, phenylbutazone, I.V. tetracycline, isoniazid, hormonal contraceptives, sulfonamides, mercaptopurine, erythromycin estolate, niacin, troleandomycin, androgenic steroids, HMG-CoA reductase inhibitors, phenothiazines, ethanol, methyldopa, rifampin, and dilantin.

Treatments
Upper abdominal surgery may cause postoperative jaundice, which occurs secondary to hepatocellular damage from the manipulation of organs. Postoperative jaundice may lead to edema and obstructed bile flow from the administration of halothane or from prolonged surgery resulting in shock, blood loss, or blood transfusion. A surgical shunt used to reduce portal hypertension (such as a portacaval shunt) may also produce jaundice.

SPECIAL CONSIDERATIONS
To help decrease pruritus, frequently bathe the patient, apply an antipruritic lotion such as calamine, and administer diphenhydramine or hydroxyzine. Prepare the patient for diagnostic tests to evaluate biliary and hepatic function. Laboratory studies include urine and fecal urobilinogen, serum bilirubin, hepatic enzyme, and cholesterol levels; prothrombin time; and a complete blood count. Other tests include ultrasonography, cholangiography, liver biopsy, and exploratory laparotomy.

PEDIATRIC POINTERS
Physiologic jaundice is common in neonates, developing 3 to 5 days after birth. In infants, obstructive jaundice usually results from congenital biliary atresia. A choledochal cyst—a congenital cystic dilation of the common bile duct—may also cause jaundice in children, particularly in those of Japanese descent.

The list of other causes of jaundice is extensive and includes, but isn't limited to, Crigler-Najjar syndrome, Gilbert's disease, Rotor's syndrome, thalassemia major, hereditary spherocytosis, erythroblastosis fetalis, Hodgkin's disease, infectious mononucleosis, Wilson's disease, amyloidosis, and Reye's syndrome.

GERIATRIC POINTERS
In patients older than age 60, jaundice is usually caused by cholestasis resulting from extrahepatic obstruction.

PATIENT COUNSELING
Encourage the patient with a hepatic disorder to decrease his protein intake sharply and increase his intake of carbohydrates. If he has obstructive jaundice, encourage a nutritious, balanced diet (avoiding high-fat foods) and frequent small meals. Teach the patient ways to reduce pruritus.

Other causes
+ Drugs causing hepatic injury, such as acetaminophen, phenylbutazone, and I.V. tetracycline
+ Upper abdominal surgery
+ Surgical shunts used to reduce portal hypertension

Special considerations
+ To decrease pruritus, frequently bathe the patient, apply an antipruritic lotion such as calamine, and administer diphenhydramine or hydroxyzine.
+ Prepare the patient for diagnostic tests to evaluate biliary and hepatic function.

Peds points
+ Physiologic jaundice is common in neonates, developing 3 to 5 days after birth.
+ In infants, obstructive jaundice usually results from congenital biliary atresia.

Geri points
+ In patients older than age 60, jaundice is usually caused by cholestasis resulting from extrahepatic obstruction.

Teaching points
+ Appropriate dietary changes
+ Ways to reduce pruritus

Key facts about jaw pain

+ May arise from the maxilla, mandible, or TMJ
+ Usually results from disorders of the teeth, soft tissue, or glands of the mouth or throat or from local trauma or infection

In an emergency

If jaw pain occurs with chest pain, shortness of breath, or arm pain:
+ Perform an ECG.
+ Obtain blood samples for cardiac enzyme levels.
+ Administer oxygen, morphine sulfate, and a vasodilator as indicated.

Key history points

+ Onset, character, intensity, and frequency of jaw pain
+ Recent trauma, surgery, or procedures
+ Associated signs and symptoms, such as joint or chest pain, dyspnea, palpitations, fatigue, headache, malaise, anorexia, weight loss, intermittent claudication, diplopia, and hearing loss
+ Aggravating or alleviating factors

Critical assessment steps

+ Inspect the painful area for redness; palpate for edema or warmth.
+ Look for facial asymmetry.
+ Check the TMJs.
+ Palpate the parotid area for pain and swelling.
+ Inspect and palpate the oral cavity for lesions, elevation of the tongue, or masses.

JAW PAIN

Jaw pain may arise from either of the two bones that hold the teeth in the jaw—the maxilla (upper jaw) and the mandible (lower jaw). Jaw pain also includes pain in the temporomandibular joint (TMJ), where the mandible meets the temporal bone. (See *Associated disorder: Temporomandibular joint disorders.*)

Jaw pain may develop gradually or abruptly and may range from barely noticeable to excruciating, depending on its cause. It usually results from disorders of the teeth, soft tissue, or glands of the mouth or throat or from local trauma or infection. Systemic causes include musculoskeletal, neurologic, cardiovascular, endocrine, immunologic, metabolic, and infectious disorders. Life-threatening disorders, such as myocardial infarction (MI) and tetany, also produce jaw pain, as do certain drugs (especially phenothiazines) and dental or surgical procedures.

Jaw pain is seldom a primary indicator of any one disorder; however, some causes are medical emergencies.

 EMERGENCY ACTIONS Sudden severe jaw pain, especially when associated with chest pain, shortness of breath, or arm pain, requires prompt evaluation because it may herald a life-threatening disorder. Perform an electrocardiogram and obtain blood samples for cardiac enzyme levels. Administer oxygen, morphine sulfate, and a vasodilator as indicated.

HISTORY

Begin the patient history by asking the patient to describe the pain's character, intensity, and frequency. When did he first notice the jaw pain? Did it arise suddenly or gradually? Where on the jaw does he feel pain? Does the pain radiate to other areas?

Sharp or burning pain arises from the skin or subcutaneous tissues. Causalgia, an intense burning sensation, usually results from damage to the fifth cranial, or trigeminal, nerve. This type of superficial pain is easily localized, unlike dull, aching, boring, or throbbing pain, which originates in muscle, bone, or joints.

Ask about recent trauma, surgery, or procedures, especially dental work. Ask about associated signs and symptoms, such as joint or chest pain, dyspnea, palpitations, fatigue, headache, malaise, anorexia, weight loss, intermittent claudication, diplopia, and hearing loss. Also ask about aggravating or alleviating factors.

PHYSICAL ASSESSMENT

Focus your physical examination on the jaw. Inspect the painful area for redness, and palpate for edema or warmth. Facing the patient directly, look for facial asymmetry indicating swelling. Check the TMJs by placing your fingertips just anterior to the external auditory meatus and asking the patient to open and close, and to thrust out and retract his jaw. Note the presence of crepitus, an abnormal scraping or grinding sensation in the joint. (Clicks heard when the jaw is widely spread apart are normal.) How wide can the patient open his mouth? Less than 1⅛″ (2.9 cm) or more than 2⅜″ (6 cm) between upper and lower teeth is abnormal. Next, palpate the parotid area for pain and swelling, and inspect and palpate the oral cavity for lesions, elevation of the tongue, or masses.

Temporomandibular joint disorders

The temporomandibular joint (TMJ) is a hinge joint that connects the mandible to the temporal bone of the skull. The bony surfaces of the joint are separated by a disk that keeps the bones from rubbing together. The TMJ is stabilized by the muscles that allow the mouth to open and close.

TMJ disorders are a group of disorders of the jaw, TMJ, and surrounding muscles that result in pain, a popping sensation in the jaw, and headaches. These disorders affect approximately 10 million Americans. They appear in twice as many women as men, especially young women. TMJ disorders can be acute or chronic, and the pain can range from minor to severe. Conservative therapy, such as inserting a mouth splint or resting the jaw, relieves TMJ pain in the majority of people.

The three main categories of TMJ disorders are:

- myofascial pain (pain in the muscles of the jaw, neck, and shoulders)
- internal joint derangement (dislocated jaw, displaced disk, or condyle injury)
- degenerative joint disease (such as rheumatoid arthritis and osteoarthritis).

CAUSES

Possible causes of TMJ disorders include:

- trauma to the jaw, TMJ, or muscles of the head and neck
- malocclusion
- grinding or clenching of the teeth (bruxism)
- stress
- poor posture
- osteoarthritis or rheumatoid arthritis of the TMJ
- congenital anomalies.

DIAGNOSTIC TESTING

TMJ disorders cause symptoms similar to other disorders. These tests may help confirm diagnosis:

- X-ray of the face may reveal bone and joint abnormalities.
- Magnetic resonance imaging may determine whether the TMJ is in proper alignment.
- A computed tomography scan can study the bones of the TMJ for defects.

MEDICAL INTERVENTIONS

Conservative treatment of TMJ disorders may include:

- stress management to reduce the patient's tendency to grind and clench her teeth
- stretching and range-of-motion exercises of the jaw to stretch and relax jaw muscles
- moist heat to the face to relieve muscle spasm and pain
- dietary changes, such as eating soft foods, cutting food into small pieces, and avoiding hard, crunchy, and chewy foods, to keep the jaw in alignment and reduce pain
- mouth splints and night guards to reduce the harmful effects of grinding and clenching the teeth and to position the teeth and jaw in proper alignment
- nonsteroidal anti-inflammatory drugs to reduce muscle pain and swelling
- muscle relaxants to relieve tight jaw muscles in people who clench and grind their teeth
- anti-anxiety medications if stress is a factor in the patient's TMJ disorder
- antidepressants, in low doses, to help reduce and control chronic pain
- correction of dental problems, such as replacing missing teeth and getting fitted for braces, crowns, or bridges
- avoiding extreme jaw movements, such as yawning, chewing ice, and yelling, to keep the jaw in alignment and reduce pain
- using proper posture to reduce jaw pain
- avoiding cradling the telephone between the shoulder and ear and resting the chin on the hands to maintain proper alignment
- transcutaneous electrical nerve stimulation to relax the jaw and facial muscles
- ultrasonography to reduce pain and enhance joint mobility
- trigger point injections to relieve pain.

These surgeries may be considered if conservative therapies fail to relieve TMJ pain:

- arthrocentesis (to relieve restricted jaw opening)
- arthroscopy (to remove inflamed or scarred tissue or realign structures such as the disk or condyle)
- open joint surgery (to remove tumors, scar tissue, bone chips, and deteriorating bone).

Key facts about TMJ disorders

- Include disorders of the jaw, TMJ, and surrounding muscles
- Result in pain, a popping sensation in the jaw, and headaches
- Categorized as myofascial pain, internal joint derangement, or degenerative joint disease

Causes

- Trauma to the jaw, TMJ, or muscles of the head and neck
- Malocclusion
- Bruxism
- Stress
- Poor posture
- Osteoarthritis or rheumatoid arthritis of the TMJ
- Congenital anomalies

Management

- Stress management
- Stretching and ROM exercises
- Moist heat to the face
- Dietary changes
- Mouth splints and night guards
- NSAIDs, muscle relaxants, anti-anxiety drugs, or antidepressants
- Correction of dental problems
- Avoidance of extreme jaw movements
- Proper posture
- TENS to relax muscles
- Ultrasonography
- Trigger point injections
- Surgery

Medical causes

Angina pectoris
+ Substernal area pain may radiate to the jaw.
+ Pain may also radiate to the left arm and may be accompanied by shortness of breath, tachycardia, dizziness, diaphoresis, and palpitations.

Arthritis
+ With osteoarthritis, aching jaw pain increases with activity.
+ Rheumatoid arthritis causes symmetrical pain in all joints, including the jaw.

Head and neck cancer
+ Jaw pain has an insidious onset.

Hypocalcemic tetany
+ Painful muscle contractions of the jaw and mouth occur with paresthesia and carpopedal spasms.

Ludwig's angina
+ Severe jaw pain in the mandibular area occurs with tongue elevation, sublingual edema, and drooling.

Myocardial infarction
+ Curshing substernal pain may radiate to the lower jaw, left arm, neck, back, or shoulder blades.

MEDICAL CAUSES

Angina pectoris
Angina may produce jaw pain (usually radiating from the substernal area) and left arm pain. Angina is less severe than the pain of an MI. It's commonly triggered by exertion, emotional stress, or ingestion of a heavy meal and usually subsides with rest and the administration of nitroglycerin. Other signs and symptoms include shortness of breath, nausea and vomiting, tachycardia, dizziness, diaphoresis, belching, and palpitations.

Arthritis
With osteoarthritis, aching jaw pain increases with activity (talking, eating) and subsides with rest. Other features are crepitus heard and felt over the TMJ, enlarged joints with a restricted range of motion, and stiffness on awakening that improves with a few minutes of activity. Redness and warmth are usually absent.

Rheumatoid arthritis causes symmetrical pain in all joints, including the jaw. The joints display limited range of motion and are tender, warm, swollen, and stiff after inactivity, especially in the morning. Myalgia is common. Systemic signs and symptoms include fatigue, weight loss, malaise, anorexia, lymphadenopathy, and mild fever. Painless, movable rheumatoid nodules may appear on the elbows, knees, and knuckles. Progressive disease causes deformities, crepitation with joint rotation, muscle weakness and atrophy around the involved joint, and multiple systemic complications.

Head and neck cancer
Many types of head and neck cancer, especially those of the oral cavity and nasopharynx, produce aching jaw pain of insidious onset. Other findings include a history of leukoplakia ulcers of the mucous membranes; palpable masses in the jaw, mouth, and neck; dysphagia; bloody discharge; drooling; lymphadenopathy; and trismus.

Hypocalcemic tetany
Besides painful muscle contractions of the jaw and mouth, this life-threatening disorder produces paresthesia and carpopedal spasms. The patient may complain of weakness, fatigue, and palpitations. Examination reveals hyperreflexia and positive Chvostek's and Trousseau's signs. Muscle twitching, choreiform movements, and muscle cramps may also occur. With severe hypocalcemia, laryngeal spasm may occur with stridor, cyanosis, seizures, and cardiac arrhythmias.

Ludwig's angina
Ludwig's angina is an acute streptococcal infection of the sublingual and submandibular spaces that produces severe jaw pain in the mandibular area with tongue elevation, sublingual edema, and drooling. Fever is a common sign. Progressive disease produces dysphagia, dysphonia, and stridor and dyspnea due to laryngeal edema and obstruction by an elevated tongue.

Myocardial infarction
Initially, this life-threatening disorder causes intense, crushing substernal pain that's unrelieved by rest or nitroglycerin. The pain may radiate to the lower jaw, left arm, neck, back, or shoulder blades. (Rarely, jaw pain occurs without chest pain.) Other findings in MI include pallor, clammy skin, dyspnea, excessive diaphoresis, nausea and vomiting, anxiety, restlessness, a feeling of impending doom, low-grade fever, decreased or increased blood pressure, arrhythmias, an atrial gallop, new murmurs (in many cases from mitral insufficiency), and crackles.

Osteomyelitis

Bone infection after trauma, sinus infection, dental injury, or surgery (dental or facial) may produce diffuse, aching jaw pain along with warmth, swelling, tenderness, erythema, and restricted jaw movement. Acute osteomyelitis may also cause tachycardia, sudden fever, nausea, and malaise. Chronic osteomyelitis may recur after minor trauma.

Sinusitis

Maxillary sinusitis produces intense boring pain in the maxilla and cheek that may radiate to the eye. This type of sinusitis also causes a feeling of fullness, increased pain on percussion of the first and second molars and, in those with nasal obstruction, the loss of the sense of smell. Sphenoid sinusitis causes scanty nasal discharge and chronic pain at the mandibular ramus and vertex of the head and in the temporal area. Other signs and symptoms of both types of sinusitis include fever, halitosis, headache, malaise, cough, sore throat, and fever.

Suppurative parotitis

With suppurative parotitis, bacterial infection of the parotid gland by *Staphylococcus aureus* produces abrupt onset of jaw pain, high fever, and chills. Other findings include erythema and edema of the overlying skin; a tender, swollen gland; and pus at the second top molar (Stensen's ducts). Infection may lead to disorientation; shock and death are common.

Temporal arteritis

Temporal arteritis produces sharp jaw pain after chewing or talking. Nonspecific signs and symptoms include low-grade fever, generalized muscle pain, malaise, fatigue, anorexia, and weight loss. Vascular lesions produce jaw pain; throbbing, unilateral headache in the frontotemporal region; swollen, nodular, tender and, possibly, pulseless temporal arteries; and, at times, erythema of the overlying skin.

Temporomandibular joint disorders

TMJ disorders produce jaw pain at the TMJ; spasm and pain of the masticating muscle; clicking, popping, or crepitus of the TMJ; and restricted jaw movement. Unilateral, localized pain may radiate to other head and neck areas. The patient typically reports teeth clenching, bruxism, and emotional stress. He may also experience ear pain, headache, deviation of the jaw to the affected side upon opening the mouth, and jaw subluxation or dislocation, especially after yawning.

Trauma

Injury to the face, head, or neck — particularly fracture of the maxilla or mandible — may produce jaw pain and swelling and decreased jaw mobility. Associated findings include hypotension and tachycardia (indicating shock), lacerations, ecchymoses, and hematomas. Rhinorrhea or otorrhea indicates the leakage of cerebrospinal fluid; blurred vision indicates orbital involvement.

Trigeminal neuralgia

Trigeminal neuralgia is marked by paroxysmal attacks of intense unilateral jaw pain (stopping at the facial midline) or rapid-fire shooting sensations in one division of the trigeminal nerve (usually the mandibular or maxillary division). This superficial pain, felt mainly over the lips and chin and in the teeth, lasts from 1 to 15 minutes. Mouth and nose areas may be hypersensitive. Involvement of the ophthalmic branch of the trigeminal nerve causes a diminished or absent corneal reflex on the same side. Attacks can be triggered by mild stimulation of the nerve (for example, lightly touching the cheeks), exposure to heat or cold, or consumption of hot or cold foods or beverages.

Medical causes
(continued)

Osteomyelitis
+ Aching jaw pain may occur along with warmth, swelling, tenderness, erythema, and restricted jaw movement.

Sinusitis
+ Maxillary sinusitis produces intense boring pain in the maxilla and cheek that may radiate to the eye.

Suppurative parotitis
+ Onset of jaw pain, high fever, and chills is abrupt.

Temporal arteritis
+ Sharp jaw pain occurs after chewing or talking.

TMJ disorders
+ Jaw pain at the TMJ; spasm and pain of the masticating muscle; clicking, popping, or crepitus of the TMJ; and restricted jaw movement may occur.

Trauma
+ Injury to the face, head, or neck may produce jaw pain and swelling and decreased jaw mobility.

Trigeminal neuralgia
+ Paroxysmal attacks of intense unilateral jaw pain (stopping at the facial midline) or rapid-fire shooting sensations in one division of the trigeminal nerve (usually the mandibular or maxillary division) occur.

Other causes

+ Drugs affecting extrapyramidal tract
+ Drugs that cause tetany of jaw secondary to hypocalcemia

Special considerations

+ If patient is in severe pain, withhold food, liquids, and oral medications until diagnosis is confirmed.
+ Administer an analgesic.
+ Apply ice pack if jaw is swollen.
+ Discourage patient from talking or moving the jaw.

Peds points

+ Mumps causes unilateral or bilateral swelling from the lower mandible to the zygomatic arch.
+ Parotiditis due to cystic fibrosis causes jaw pain.
+ When trauma causes jaw pain in children, always consider the possibility of abuse.

Teaching points

+ Explanation of the disorder and treatments
+ Proper insertion of mouth splints
+ Ways to reduce stress
+ Identification and avoidance of triggers

Key facts about jugular vein distention

+ Abnormal fullness and height of pulse waves in internal or external jugular veins
+ Involves a pulse wave height greater than 1¼" to 1½"
+ Occurs in cardiovascular disorders

OTHER CAUSES

Drugs

Some drugs, such as phenothiazines, affect the extrapyramidal tract, causing dyskinesias; others cause tetany of the jaw secondary to hypocalcemia.

SPECIAL CONSIDERATIONS

If the patient is in severe pain, withhold food, liquids, and oral medications until the diagnosis is confirmed. Administer an analgesic. Prepare the patient for diagnostic tests such as jaw X-rays. Apply an ice pack if the jaw is swollen, and discourage the patient from talking or moving his jaw.

PEDIATRIC POINTERS

Be alert for nonverbal signs of jaw pain, such as rubbing the affected area or wincing while talking or swallowing. In infants, initial signs of tetany from hypocalcemia include episodes of apnea and generalized jitteriness progressing to facial grimaces and generalized rigidity. Finally, seizures may occur.

Jaw pain in children sometimes stems from disorders uncommon in adults. Mumps, for example, causes unilateral or bilateral swelling from the lower mandible to the zygomatic arch. Parotiditis due to cystic fibrosis also causes jaw pain. When trauma causes jaw pain in children, always consider the possibility of abuse.

PATIENT COUNSELING

Teach the patient about his disorder and its treatments. Demonstrate how to insert mouth splints and discuss ways to reduce stress. Help the patient identify and avoid factors that may trigger an attack.

JUGULAR VEIN DISTENTION

Jugular vein distention is the abnormal fullness and height of the pulse waves in the internal or external jugular veins. For a patient in a supine position with his head elevated 45 degrees, a pulse wave height greater than 1¼" to 1½" (3 to 4 cm) above the angle of Louis indicates distention. Engorged, distended veins reflect increased venous pressure in the right side of the heart, which in turn, indicates an increased central venous pressure. This common sign characteristically occurs in heart failure and other cardiovascular disorders, such as constrictive pericarditis, tricuspid stenosis, and obstruction of the superior vena cava.

 EMERGENCY ACTIONS Evaluation of jugular vein distention involves visualizing and assessing venous pulsations. (See *Evaluating jugular vein distention.*) If you detect jugular vein distention in a patient with pale, clammy skin who suddenly appears anxious and dyspneic, take his blood pressure. If you note hypotension and paradoxical pulse, suspect cardiac tamponade. Elevate the foot of the bed 20 to 30 degrees, give supplemental oxygen, and monitor cardiac status and rhythm, oxygen saturation, and mental status. Start an I.V. line for medication administration, and keep cardiopulmonary resuscitation equipment close by. Assemble the needed equipment for emergency pericardiocentesis (to relieve pressure on the heart). Throughout the procedure, monitor the patient's blood pressure, heart rhythm, and respirations.

Evaluating jugular vein distention

With the patient in a supine position, elevate the head of the bed 45 to 90 degrees. (In the normal patient, veins distend only when the patient lies flat.)

Next, locate the angle of Louis (sternal notch)—the reference point for measuring venous pressure. To do so, palpate the clavicles where they join the sternum (the suprasternal notch). Place your first two fingers on the suprasternal notch. Then, without lifting them from the skin, slide them down the sternum until you feel a bony protuberance—this is the angle of Louis.

Find the internal jugular vein (which indicates venous pressure more reliably than the external jugular vein). Shine a flashlight across the patient's neck to create shadows that highlight his venous pulse. Be sure to distinguish jugular vein pulsations from carotid artery pulsations. One way to do this is to palpate the vessel: Arterial pulsations continue, whereas venous pulsations disappear with light finger pressure. Also, venous pulsations increase or decrease with changes in body position; arterial pulsations remain constant.

Next, locate the highest point along the vein where you can see pulsations. Using a centimeter ruler, measure the distance between that high point and the sternal notch. Record this finding as well as the angle at which the patient was lying. A finding greater than 1¼″ to 1½″ (3 to 4 cm) above the sternal notch, with the head of the bed at a 45-degree angle, indicates jugular vein distention.

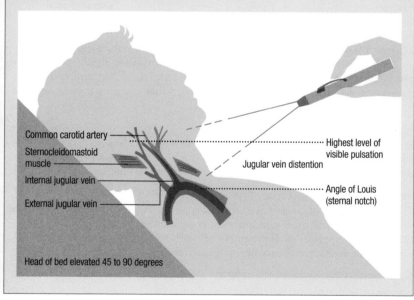

Common carotid artery

Sternocleidomastoid muscle

Internal jugular vein

External jugular vein

Highest level of visible pulsation

Jugular vein distention

Angle of Louis (sternal notch)

Head of bed elevated 45 to 90 degrees

HISTORY

If the patient isn't in severe distress, obtain a personal history. Has he recently gained weight? Does he have difficulty putting on shoes? Are his ankles swollen? Ask about chest pain, shortness of breath, paroxysmal nocturnal dyspnea, anorexia, nausea or vomiting, and a history of cancer or cardiac, pulmonary, hepatic, or renal disease. Obtain a drug history, noting diuretic use and dosage. Is the patient taking drugs as prescribed? Ask the patient about his regular diet patterns, noting a high sodium intake.

In an emergency
+ Take blood pressure.
+ If you note hypotension and paradoxical pulse, suspect cardiac tamponade.
+ Elevate the foot of the bed 20 to 30 degrees.
+ Give supplemental oxygen.
+ Monitor cardiac status and rhythm, oxygen saturation, and mental status.
+ Start an I.V. line for medication administration.
+ Keep cardiopulmonary resuscitation equipment close by.
+ Assemble equipment for emergency pericardiocentesis.

Key history points
+ Recent weight gain or swelling
+ Associated chest pain, shortness of breath, paroxysmal nocturnal dyspnea, anorexia, nausea, or vomiting
+ History of cancer or cardiac, pulmonary, hepatic, or renal disease
+ Drug history
+ Diet history, especially sodium intake

PHYSICAL ASSESSMENT

Begin the physical examination by checking the patient's vital signs. Tachycardia, tachypnea, and increased blood pressure indicate fluid overload that's stressing the heart. Inspect and palpate the patient's extremities and face for edema. Then weigh the patient and compare that weight to his baseline.

Auscultate his lungs for crackles and his heart for gallops, a pericardial friction rub, and muffled heart sounds. Inspect his abdomen for distention, and palpate and percuss for an enlarged liver. Finally monitor urine output and note any decrease.

MEDICAL CAUSES

Cardiac tamponade

Cardiac tamponade, a life-threatening condition, produces jugular vein distention along with anxiety, restlessness, cyanosis, chest pain, dyspnea, hypotension, and clammy skin. It also causes tachycardia, tachypnea, muffled heart sounds, a pericardial friction rub, weak or absent peripheral pulses or pulses that decrease during inspiration (pulsus paradoxus), and hepatomegaly. The patient may sit upright or lean forward to ease breathing.

Heart failure

Right-sided heart failure commonly causes jugular vein distention, along with weakness, anxiety, cyanosis, dependent edema of the legs and sacrum, steady weight gain, confusion, and hepatomegaly. Other findings include nausea and vomiting, abdominal discomfort, and anorexia due to visceral edema. Ascites is a late sign. Massive right-sided heart failure may produce anasarca and oliguria.

If left-sided heart failure precedes right-sided heart failure, jugular vein distention is a late sign. Other signs and symptoms include fatigue, dyspnea, orthopnea, paroxysmal nocturnal dyspnea, tachypnea, tachycardia, and arrhythmias. Auscultation reveals crackles and a ventricular gallop.

Hypervolemia

Markedly increased intravascular fluid volume causes jugular vein distention, along with rapid weight gain, elevated blood pressure, bounding pulse, peripheral edema, dyspnea, and crackles. An S_3 gallop may be heard on auscultation.

Pericarditis (chronic constrictive)

Progressive signs and symptoms of chronic constrictive pericarditis include jugular vein distention that's more prominent on inspiration (Kussmaul's sign). The patient usually complains of chest pain. Other signs and symptoms include fluid retention with dependent edema, hepatomegaly, ascites, and pericardial friction rub.

Superior vena cava obstruction

An obstruction, such as a tumor or, rarely, thrombosis, may gradually lead to jugular vein distention when the veins of the head, neck, and arms fail to empty effectively, causing facial, neck, and upper arm edema. Metastasis of a malignant tumor to the mediastinum may cause dyspnea, cough, substernal chest pain, and hoarseness.

SPECIAL CONSIDERATIONS

If the patient has cardiac tamponade, prepare him for pericardiocentesis. If he doesn't have cardiac tamponade, restrict fluids and monitor his intake and output. Insert an indwelling urinary catheter if necessary. If the patient has heart failure, administer a diuretic. Routinely change his position to avoid skin breakdown from peripheral edema. Prepare the patient for a central venous or pulmonary artery catheter insertion in order to measure right- and left-sided heart pressure.

PEDIATRIC POINTERS

Jugular vein distention is difficult (sometimes impossible) to evaluate in most infants and toddlers because of their short, thick necks. Even in school-age children, measurement of jugular vein distention can be unreliable because the sternal angle may not be the same distance (2″ to 2¾″ [5 to 7 cm]) above the right atrium as it is in adults.

PATIENT COUNSELING

Teach the patient with heart failure about appropriate treatments, including dietary restrictions (such as a low-sodium diet). Explain the importance of monitoring daily weight and reporting a gain of 1 to 2 lb (0.5 to 1 kg)/day. Have the patient slowly resume daily activities, but make sure he schedules rest periods into his routine.

Special considerations

✦ If patient has cardiac tamponade, prepare him for pericardiocentesis.
✦ If patient doesn't have cardiac tamponade, restrict fluids and monitor intake and output. Insert indwelling urinary catheter if necessary.
✦ If patient has heart failure, administer a diuretic.
✦ Routinely change patient's position to avoid skin breakdown from peripheral edema.
✦ Prepare patient for central venous or pulmonary artery catheter insertion.

Peds points

✦ Jugular vein distention is difficult to evaluate in infants, toddlers, and children.

Teaching points

✦ Dietary restrictions
✦ Daily weight monitoring
✦ Weight gain to report
✦ Scheduled rest periods

KERNIG'S SIGN

A reliable early indicator and tool used to diagnose meningeal irritation, Kernig's sign elicits resistance and hamstring muscle pain when the examiner attempts to extend the knee while the hip and knee are both flexed 90 degrees. However, when the patient's thigh isn't flexed on the abdomen, he's usually able to completely extend his leg. (See *Eliciting Kernig's sign.*) This sign is usually elicited in meningitis or subarachnoid hemorrhage. With these potentially life-threatening disorders, hamstring muscle resistance results from stretching the blood- or exudate-irritated meninges surrounding spinal nerve roots.

Kernig's sign can also indicate a herniated disk or spinal tumor. With these disorders, sciatic pain results from disk or tumor pressure on spinal nerve roots.

HISTORY

If you elicit a positive Kernig's sign and suspect life-threatening meningitis or subarachnoid hemorrhage, immediately prepare for emergency intervention. (See *When Kernig's sign signals CNS crisis,* page 392.)

If you don't suspect meningeal irritation, ask the patient if he feels back pain that radiates down one or both legs. Does he also feel leg numbness, tingling, or weakness? Ask about other signs and symptoms, and find out if he has a history of cancer or back injury.

PHYSICAL ASSESSMENT

Perform a physical examination, concentrating on motor and sensory function. Assessing motor function includes inspecting the muscles and testing muscle tone and strength. Cerebellar testing is also done because the cerebellum plays a role in smooth muscle movements such as tics, tremors, or fasciculations. Sensory system evaluation involves checking the patient's sensitivity to pain, light touch, vibration, position, and discrimination.

MEDICAL CAUSES

Lumbosacral herniated disk
A positive Kernig's sign may be elicited in patients with a herniated disk, but the cardinal and earliest feature is sciatic pain on the affected side or on both sides. Associated findings include postural deformity (lumbar lordosis or scoliosis), paresthesia, hypoactive deep tendon reflexes in the involved leg, and dorsiflexor muscle weakness.

Eliciting Kernig's sign

To elicit Kernig's sign, place the patient in a supine position. Flex her leg at the hip and knee, as shown below. Then try to extend the leg while you keep the hip flexed. If the patient experiences pain and, possibly, spasm in the hamstring muscle and resists further extension, you can assume that meningeal irritation has occurred.

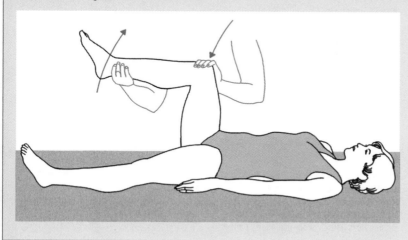

Meningitis

A positive Kernig's sign usually occurs early with meningitis, along with fever and, possibly, chills. Other signs and symptoms of meningeal irritation include nuchal rigidity, hyperreflexia, Brudzinski's sign, and opisthotonos. As intracranial pressure (ICP) increases, headache and vomiting may occur. In severe meningitis, the patient may experience stupor, coma, and seizures. Cranial nerve involvement may produce ocular palsies, facial weakness, deafness, and photophobia. An erythematous maculopapular rash may occur in viral meningitis; a purpuric rash may be seen in those with meningococcal meningitis.

Spinal cord tumor

Kernig's sign can be elicited occasionally, but the earliest symptom of a spinal cord tumor is typically pain felt locally or along the spinal nerve, commonly in the leg. Associated findings include weakness or paralysis distal to the tumor, paresthesia, urine retention, urinary or fecal incontinence, and sexual dysfunction.

Subarachnoid hemorrhage

Kernig's sign and Brudzinski's sign can both be elicited within minutes after the initial bleed. The patient experiences a sudden onset of severe headache that begins in a localized area and then spreads, pupillary inequality, nuchal rigidity, and decreased level of consciousness. Photophobia, fever, nausea and vomiting, dizziness, and seizures are possible. Focal signs include hemiparesis or hemiplegia, aphasia, and sensory or visual disturbances. Increasing ICP may produce bradycardia, increased blood pressure, respiratory pattern change, and rapid progression to coma.

Medical causes
(continued)

Meningitis
✦ Positive Kernig's sign usually occurs early, along with fever and, possibly, chills.

Spinal cord tumor
✦ Kernig's sign can be elicited occasionally.
✦ Earliest symptom of spinal cord tumor is pain felt locally or along the spinal nerve, commonly in the leg.

Subarachnoid hemorrhage
✦ Kernig's sign and Brudzinski's sign can be elicited within minutes after the initial bleed.

Special considerations

+ Closely monitor vital signs, ICP, and cardiopulmonary and neurologic status.
+ Ensure bed rest, quiet, and minimal stress.
+ For those with subarachnoid hemorrhage, darken the room and elevate the head of the bed at least 30 degrees to reduce ICP.
+ If patient has a herniated disk or spinal tumor, he may require pelvic traction.

Peds points

+ Kernig's sign is considered ominous in children because of their greater potential for rapid deterioration.

Teaching points

+ Signs and symptoms of meningitis
+ Ways to prevent meningitis
+ Activities to avoid with a herniated disk
+ Application of back brace or cervical collar, as needed

EMERGENCY ACTIONS

When Kernig's sign signals CNS crisis

Because Kernig's sign may signal meningitis or subarachnoid hemorrhage — both life-threatening central nervous system (CNS) disorders — take the patient's vital signs at once to obtain baseline information. Then test for Brudzinski's sign to obtain further evidence of meningeal irritation. Next, ask the patient or his family to describe the onset of illness. Typically, the progressive onset of headache, fever, nuchal rigidity, and confusion suggests meningitis. Conversely, the sudden onset of a severe headache, nuchal rigidity, photophobia and, possibly, loss of consciousness usually indicates subarachnoid hemorrhage.

MENINGITIS

If a diagnosis of meningitis is suspected, ask about recent infections, especially tooth abscesses. Ask about exposure to infected persons or places where meningitis is endemic. Meningitis is usually a complication of another bacterial infection, so draw blood for culture studies to determine the causative organism. Prepare the patient for a lumbar puncture (if a tumor or abscess can be ruled out). Also, find out if the patient has a history of I.V. drug abuse, an open-head injury, or endocarditis. Insert an I.V. line, and immediately begin administering an antibiotic.

SUBARACHNOID HEMORRHAGE

If subarachnoid hemorrhage is the suspected diagnosis, ask about a history of hypertension, cerebral aneurysm, head trauma, or arteriovenous malformation. Also ask about sudden withdrawal of an antihypertensive.

Check the patient's pupils for dilation, and assess him for signs of increasing intracranial pressure, such as bradycardia, increased systolic blood pressure, and widened pulse pressure. Insert an I.V. line, and administer supplemental oxygen.

SPECIAL CONSIDERATIONS

Prepare the patient for diagnostic tests, such as a computed tomography scan, magnetic resonance imaging, spinal X-ray, myelography, and lumbar puncture. Closely monitor his vital signs, ICP, and cardiopulmonary and neurologic status. Ensure bed rest, quiet, and minimal stress.

If the patient has a subarachnoid hemorrhage, darken the room and elevate the head of the bed at least 30 degrees to reduce ICP. If he has a herniated disk or spinal tumor, he may require pelvic traction.

PEDIATRIC POINTERS

Kernig's sign is considered ominous in children because of their greater potential for rapid deterioration.

PATIENT COUNSELING

Teach the patient how to recognize signs and symptoms of meningitis as well as measures to prevent this infection. If the patient has a herniated disk, tell him to avoid activities such as lifting, sleeping prone, climbing stairs, and riding in a car. Show the patient how to apply a back brace or cervical collar, as needed, then have him give a return demonstration.

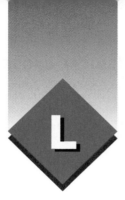

LEG PAIN

Although leg pain commonly signifies a musculoskeletal disorder, it can also result from a more serious vascular or neurologic disorder. The pain may arise suddenly or gradually and may be localized or affect the entire leg. Constant or intermittent, it may feel dull, burning, sharp, shooting, or tingling. Leg pain may affect locomotion, limiting weight bearing. Severe leg pain that follows cast application for a fracture may signal limb-threatening compartment syndrome. Sudden onset of severe leg pain in a patient with underlying vascular insufficiency may signal acute deterioration, possibly requiring an arterial graft or amputation.

 EMERGENCY ACTIONS If the patient has acute leg pain and a history of trauma, quickly take his vital signs and determine the leg's neurovascular status. Observe the patient's leg position, and check for swelling, gross deformities, or abnormal rotation. Also be sure to check distal pulses and note skin color and temperature. A pale, cool, and pulseless leg may indicate impaired circulation, which may require emergency surgery.

HISTORY

If the patient's condition permits, ask him when the pain began and have him describe its intensity, character, and pattern. Is the pain worse in the morning, at night, or with movement? If it doesn't prevent him from walking, must he rely on a crutch or other assistive device? Also ask him about the presence of other signs and symptoms.

Find out if the patient has a history of leg injury or surgery and if he or a family member has a history of joint, vascular, or back problems. Also ask which medications he's taking and whether they have helped to relieve his leg pain.

PHYSICAL ASSESSMENT

Begin the physical examination by watching the patient walk, if his condition permits. Observe how he holds his leg while standing and sitting. Palpate the legs, buttocks, and lower back to determine the extent of pain and tenderness. If a fracture has been ruled out, test the patient's range of motion (ROM) in the hip and knee. Also, check reflexes with the patient's leg straightened and raised, noting any action that causes pain. Then compare both legs for symmetry, movement, and active ROM. Additionally, assess sensation and strength. If the patient wears a leg cast, splint, or restrictive dressing, carefully check distal circulation, sensation, and mobility, and stretch his toes to elicit any associated pain.

Key facts about leg pain
+ May be gradual or sudden, localized or affect the entire leg
+ May feel dull, burning, sharp, shooting, or tingling

In an emergency
+ Take vital signs and determine the leg's neurovascular status.
+ Check for position, swelling, gross deformities, or abnormal rotation.
+ Check distal pulses and note skin color and temperature.

Key history points
+ Onset and description of pain
+ History of injury, surgery, or joint, vascular, or back problems

Critical assessment steps
+ Observe leg while patient walks (if possible), stands, and sits.
+ If leg isn't fractured, test hip and knee ROM; check reflexes.
+ Compare both legs for symmetry, movement, and active ROM.
+ If leg is immobilized, check distal circulation, sensation, and mobility; stretch the toes to elicit associated pain.

Medical causes

Bone cancer
✦ Continuous deep or boring pain worsens at night.

Compartment syndrome
✦ Progressive, intense lower leg pain increases with passive muscle stretching.

Fracture
✦ Acute leg pain accompanies swelling and ecchymosis.

Infection
✦ Leg pain, erythema, swelling, streaking, and warmth are local.

Occlusive vascular disease
✦ Continuous cramping pain may worsen with walking.

Sciatica
✦ Shooting, aching, or tingling pain radiates down the back of the leg along the sciatic nerve.

Strain or sprain
✦ Acute strain causes sharp, transient pain and rapid swelling.
✦ Chronic strain produces stiffness, soreness, and generalized leg tenderness.
✦ A sprain causes local pain, especially during joint movement.

Thrombophlebitis
✦ Discomfort ranges from calf tenderness to severe pain and swelling, warmth, and heaviness.

MEDICAL CAUSES

Bone cancer
Continuous deep or boring pain, commonly worse at night, may be the first symptom of bone cancer. Later, skin breakdown and impaired circulation may occur, along with cachexia, fever, and impaired mobility.

Compartment syndrome
Progressive, intense lower leg pain that increases with passive muscle stretching is a cardinal sign of compartment syndrome, a limb-threatening disorder. Restrictive dressings or traction may aggravate the pain, which typically worsens despite analgesic administration. Other findings include muscle weakness and paresthesia, but apparently normal distal circulation. With irreversible muscle ischemia, paralysis and absent pulse also occur.

Fracture
With a fracture, severe, acute pain accompanies swelling and ecchymosis in the affected leg. Movement produces extreme pain, and the leg may be unable to bear weight. Neurovascular status distal to the fracture may be impaired, causing paresthesia, absent pulse, mottled cyanosis, and cool skin. Deformity, muscle spasms, and bony crepitation may also occur.

Infection
Local leg pain, erythema, swelling, streaking, and warmth characterize soft-tissue and bone infections. Fever and tachycardia may be present with other systemic signs. The patient may also experience a loss of function of the affected limb.

Occlusive vascular disease
With occlusive vascular disease, continuous cramping pain in the legs and feet may worsen with walking, inducing claudication. The patient may report increased pain at night, cold feet, cold intolerance, numbness, and tingling. Examination may reveal ankle and lower leg edema, decreased or absent pulses, and increased capillary refill time.

Sciatica
Patients with sciatica experience shooting, aching, or tingling pain that radiates down the back of the leg along the sciatic nerve. Typically, activity exacerbates the pain and rest relieves it. The patient may limp to avoid exacerbating the pain and may have difficulty moving from a sitting to a standing position.

Strain or sprain
Acute strain causes sharp, transient pain and rapid swelling, followed by leg tenderness and ecchymosis. Chronic strain produces stiffness, soreness, and generalized leg tenderness several hours after the injury; active and passive motion may be painful or impossible. A sprain causes local pain, especially during joint movement; ecchymosis and, possibly, local swelling and loss of mobility develop.

Thrombophlebitis
Discomfort caused by thrombophlebitis may range from calf tenderness to severe pain accompanied by swelling, warmth, and a feeling of heaviness in the affected leg. The patient may also develop fever, chills, malaise, muscle cramps, and a positive Homans' sign. Assessment may reveal superficial veins that are visibly engorged, sensitive to pressure, and palpable, hard, thready, and cordlike.

Varicose veins

Mild to severe leg symptoms may develop in patients with varicose veins, including nocturnal cramping; a feeling of heaviness; diffuse, dull aching after prolonged standing or walking; and aching during menses. Assessment may reveal palpable nodules, orthostatic edema, and stasis pigmentation of the calves and ankles.

Venous stasis ulcers

Localized pain and bleeding arise from infected ulcerations on the lower extremities. Mottled, bluish pigmentation is characteristic, and local edema may occur.

SPECIAL CONSIDERATIONS

If the patient has acute leg pain, closely monitor his neurovascular status by frequently checking distal pulses and evaluating both legs for temperature, color, and sensation. Also monitor his thigh and calf circumference to evaluate bleeding into tissues from a possible fracture site. Prepare him for X-rays. Use sandbags to immobilize his leg; apply ice and, if needed, skeletal traction. If a fracture isn't suspected, prepare the patient for laboratory tests to detect an infectious agent or for venography, Doppler ultrasonography, plethysmography, or angiography to determine vascular competency. Withhold food and fluids until the need for surgery has been ruled out. Administer an anticoagulant and antibiotic as needed.

PEDIATRIC POINTERS

Common pediatric causes of leg pain include fracture, osteomyelitis, and bone cancer. If parents fail to give an adequate explanation for a leg fracture, consider the possibility of child abuse.

PATIENT COUNSELING

If the patient has chronic leg pain, instruct him to take an anti-inflammatory and teach him to perform ROM exercises and, if necessary, to use a cane, walker, or other assistive device. Discuss with the patient and his family any lifestyle changes that may be necessary until leg pain resolves. If physical therapy is necessary, stress the importance of establishing a daily exercise regimen. Based on the cause of the leg pain, discuss the appropriate positioning of the lower extremity to enhance blood flow and venous return.

LEVEL OF CONSCIOUSNESS, DECREASED

A decrease in level of consciousness (LOC), which can range from lethargy to stupor to coma, usually results from a neurologic disorder and may signal a life-threatening complication, such as hemorrhage, trauma, or cerebral edema. However, this sign can also result from metabolic, GI, musculoskeletal, urologic, or cardiopulmonary disorders; severe nutritional deficiency; effects of toxins; or drug use. LOC can deteriorate suddenly or gradually and can remain altered temporarily or permanently.

Consciousness is affected by the reticular activating system (RAS), an intricate network of neurons with axons extending from the brain stem, thalamus, and hypothalamus to the cerebral cortex. A disturbance in any part of this integrated system prevents the intercommunication that makes consciousness possible. Loss of consciousness can result from a bilateral cerebral disturbance, an RAS disturbance, or both. Cerebral dysfunction characteristically produces the least dramatic decrease in a patient's LOC. In contrast, dysfunction of the RAS produces the most dramatic decrease in LOC — coma.

Medical causes
(continued)

Varicose veins
- Nocturnal cramping; heaviness; diffuse, dull aching after prolonged standing or walking; and aching during menses occur.

Venous stasis ulcers
- Localized pain and bleeding occur.

Special considerations
- Check distal pulses and evaluate legs for temperature, color, and sensation.
- Monitor thigh and calf circumference.
- Administer anticoagulant and antibiotic as needed.

Peds points
- Common pediatric causes of leg pain include fracture, osteomyelitis, and bone cancer.
- If parents fail to give adequate explanation for leg fracture, consider child abuse.

Teaching points
- Use of anti-inflammatories, ROM exercises, and assistive devices
- Lifestyle changes
- Appropriate positioning to enhance blood flow and venous return

Key facts about decreased LOC
- Ranges from lethargy to stupor to coma
- Involves bilateral cerebral disturbance or disturbance in the reticular activating system

Glasgow Coma Scale

The Glasgow Coma Scale provides an easy way to describe a patient's mental status and to detect and interpret changes.

    To use the Glasgow Coma Scale, test the patient's ability to respond to verbal, motor, and sensory stimulation. The scoring system doesn't determine exact level of consciousness, but it does provide an easy way to describe the patient's basic status and helps to detect and interpret changes from baseline findings. A decreased reaction score in one or more categories may signal an impending neurologic crisis. A score of 7 or lower indicates severe neurologic damage.

TEST	REACTION	SCORE
Eyes	Open spontaneously	4
	Open to verbal command	3
	Open to pain	2
	No response	1
Best motor response	Obeys verbal command	6
	Localizes painful stimulus	5
	Flexion — withdrawal	4
	Flexion — abnormal (decorticate rigidity)	3
	Extension (decerebrate rigidity)	2
	No response	1
Best verbal response	Oriented and converses	5
	Disoriented and converses	4
	Inappropriate words	3
	Incomprehensible sounds	2
	No response	1
Total		3 to 15

In an emergency

+ Evaluate airway, breathing, and circulation.
+ Use the Glasgow Coma Scale to determine LOC and to obtain baseline data.
+ Insert an artificial airway.
+ Elevate the head of the bed 30 degrees.
+ If spinal cord injury has been ruled out, turn the patient's head to the side.
+ Prepare to suction the patient, if necessary.
+ Determine the rate, rhythm, and depth of spontaneous respirations.
+ Support breathing with a handheld resuscitation bag if necessary.
+ If Glasgow Coma Scale score is 7 or lower, intubation and resuscitation may be necessary.
+ Continue to monitor vital signs, being alert for signs of increasing ICP.

The most sensitive indicator of decreased LOC is a change in the patient's mental status. The Glasgow Coma Scale, which measures a patient's ability to respond to verbal, sensory, and motor stimulation, can be used to quickly evaluate a patient's LOC.

 EMERGENCY ACTIONS After evaluating the patient's airway, breathing, and circulation, use the Glasgow Coma Scale to quickly determine his LOC and to obtain baseline data. (See *Glasgow Coma Scale.*) Insert an artificial airway, elevate the head of the bed 30 degrees and, if spinal cord injury has been ruled out, turn the patient's head to the side. Prepare to suction the patient, if necessary. You may need to hyperventilate him to reduce carbon dioxide levels and decrease intracranial pressure (ICP). Then determine the rate, rhythm, and depth of spontaneous respirations. Support his breathing with a handheld resuscitation bag if necessary. If the patient's Glasgow Coma Scale score is 7 or lower, intubation and resuscitation may be necessary. Continue to monitor the patient's vital signs, being alert for signs of increasing ICP, such as bradycardia and widening pulse pressure. When his airway, breathing, and circulation are stabilized, perform a neurologic examination.

HISTORY

Try to obtain history information from the patient, if he's lucid, and from his family. Did the patient complain of headache, dizziness, nausea, visual or hearing disturbances, weakness, fatigue, or any other problems before his LOC decreased? Has his family noticed any changes in the patient's behavior, personality, memory, or temperament? Also ask about a history of neurologic disease or cancer; recent trauma or infection; drug and alcohol use; and the development of other signs and symptoms.

PHYSICAL ASSESSMENT

Decreased LOC can result from a disorder affecting virtually any body system. After performing a complete neurologic examination, let the results of your history guide the rest of your physical assessment.

MEDICAL CAUSES

Adrenal crisis

Decreased LOC, ranging from lethargy to coma, may develop within 12 hours of adrenal crisis onset. Early associated findings include progressive weakness, irritability, anorexia, headache, nausea and vomiting, diarrhea, abdominal pain, and fever. Later signs and symptoms include hypotension; rapid, thready pulse; oliguria; cool, clammy skin; and flaccid extremities. The patient with chronic adrenocortical hypofunction may have hyperpigmented skin and mucous membranes.

Brain abscess

Decreased LOC varies from drowsiness to deep stupor, depending on abscess size and site. Early signs and symptoms—constant intractable headache, nausea, vomiting, and seizures—reflect increasing ICP. Typical later features include ocular disturbances (nystagmus, vision loss, and pupillary inequality) and signs of infection such as fever. Other findings may include personality changes, confusion, abnormal behavior, dizziness, facial weakness, aphasia, ataxia, tremor, and hemiparesis.

Brain tumor

In patients with brain tumors, LOC decreases slowly, from lethargy to coma. The patient may also experience apathy, behavior changes, memory loss, decreased attention span, morning headache, dizziness, vision loss, ataxia, and sensorimotor disturbances. Aphasia and seizures are possible, along with signs of hormonal imbalance, such as fluid retention or amenorrhea. Signs and symptoms vary according to the location and size of the tumor. In later stages, papilledema, vomiting, bradycardia, and widening pulse pressure also appear. In the final stages, the patient may exhibit decorticate or decerebrate posture.

Cerebral aneurysm (ruptured)

Somnolence, confusion and, at times, stupor characterize a moderate bleed; deep coma occurs with severe bleeding, which can be fatal. Onset of a ruptured cerebral aneurysm is usually abrupt, with sudden, severe headache, nausea, and vomiting. Nuchal rigidity, back and leg pain, fever, restlessness, irritability, occasional seizures, and blurred vision point to meningeal irritation. The type and severity of other findings vary with the site and severity of the hemorrhage and may include hemiparesis, hemisensory defects, dysphagia, and visual defects.

Key history points

- ✦ Associated headache, dizziness, nausea, visual or hearing disturbances, weakness, and fatigue
- ✦ Changes in behavior, personality, memory, or temperament
- ✦ History of neurologic disease or cancer; recent trauma or infection
- ✦ Drug and alcohol use

Critical assessment steps

- ✦ Perform a complete neurologic examination.
- ✦ Perform a physical assessment.

Medical causes

Adrenal crisis
- ✦ Decreased LOC, ranging from lethargy to coma, may develop within 12 hours of onset.

Brain abscess
- ✦ Decreased LOC varies from drowsiness to deep stupor.
- ✦ Intractable headache, nausea, vomiting, and seizures occur.

Brain tumor
- ✦ LOC decreases slowly, from lethargy to coma.
- ✦ Apathy, behavior changes, memory loss, decreased attention span, morning headache, dizziness, vision loss, ataxia, and sensorimotor disturbances may occur.

Cerebral aneurysm (ruptured)
- ✦ Somnolence, confusion and, at times, stupor characterize a moderate bleed.
- ✦ Deep coma occurs with severe bleeding.

Medical causes
(continued)

Cerebral contusion
+ Unconscious patients may have dilated, nonreactive pupils and decorticate or decerebrate posture.
+ Conscious patients may be drowsy, confused, disoriented, agitated, or violent.

Diabetic ketoacidosis
+ Decrease in LOC is rapid and ranges from lethargy to coma.
+ Polydipsia, polyphagia, and polyuria precede decreased LOC.

Encephalitis
+ Decreased LOC may range from lethargy to coma within 24 to 48 hours of onset.

Encephalopathy
+ With hepatic encephalopathy, decreased LOC ranges from slight personality changes to coma depending on the stage.
+ With hypertensive encephalopathy, LOC progressively decreases from lethargy to stupor to coma.
+ With hypoglycemic encephalopathy, LOC rapidly deteriorates from lethargy to coma.
+ Hypoxic encephalopathy produces a sudden or gradual decrease in LOC, leading to coma and brain death.
+ With uremic encephalopathy, LOC decreases gradually from lethargy to coma.

Cerebral contusion
Usually unconscious for a prolonged period, the patient may develop dilated, nonreactive pupils and decorticate or decerebrate posture. If he's conscious or recovers consciousness, he may be drowsy, confused, disoriented, agitated, or even violent. Associated findings include blurred or double vision, fever, headache, pallor, diaphoresis, tachycardia, altered respirations, aphasia, and hemiparesis. Residual effects include seizures, impaired mental status, slight hemiparesis, and vertigo.

Diabetic ketoacidosis
Diabetic ketoacidosis produces a rapid decrease in LOC that ranges from lethargy to coma. It's commonly preceded by polydipsia, polyphagia, and polyuria. The patient may complain of weakness, anorexia, abdominal pain, nausea, and vomiting. He may also exhibit orthostatic hypotension; fruity breath odor; Kussmaul's respirations; warm, dry skin; and a rapid, thready pulse. Untreated, this condition invariably leads to coma and death.

Encephalitis
Within 48 hours of onset, the patient with encephalitis may develop LOC changes ranging from lethargy to coma. Other possible findings include abrupt onset of fever, headache, nuchal rigidity, nausea, vomiting, irritability, personality changes, seizures, aphasia, ataxia, hemiparesis, nystagmus, photophobia, myoclonus, and cranial nerve palsies.

Encephalopathy
With hepatic encephalopathy, signs and symptoms develop in four stages: in the *prodromal* stage, slight personality changes (disorientation, forgetfulness, slurred speech) and slight tremor; in the *impending* stage, tremor progressing to asterixis (the hallmark of hepatic encephalopathy), lethargy, aberrant behavior, and apraxia; in the *stuporous* stage, stupor and hyperventilation, with the patient noisy and abusive when aroused; in the *comatose* stage, coma with decerebrate posture, hyperactive reflexes, positive Babinski's reflex, and fetor hepaticus.

With life-threatening hypertensive encephalopathy, LOC progressively decreases from lethargy to stupor to coma. Besides markedly elevated blood pressure, the patient may experience severe headache, vomiting, seizures, visual disturbances, transient paralysis, and eventually Cheyne-Stokes respirations.

With hypoglycemic encephalopathy, LOC rapidly deteriorates from lethargy to coma. Early signs and symptoms include nervousness, restlessness, agitation, and confusion; hunger; alternate flushing and cold sweats; and headache, trembling, and palpitations. Blurred vision progresses to motor weakness, hemiplegia, dilated pupils, pallor, decreased pulse rate, shallow respirations, and seizures. Flaccidity and decerebrate posture appear late.

Depending on its severity, hypoxic encephalopathy produces a sudden or gradual decrease in LOC, leading to coma and brain death. Early on, the patient appears confused and restless, with cyanosis and increased heart and respiratory rates and blood pressure. Later, his respiratory pattern becomes abnormal, and assessment reveals decreased pulse, blood pressure, and deep tendon reflexes (DTRs); Babinski's reflex; absent doll's eye sign; and fixed pupils.

With uremic encephalopathy, LOC decreases gradually from lethargy to coma. Early on, the patient may appear apathetic, inattentive, confused, and irritable and may complain of headache, nausea, fatigue, and anorexia. Other findings include vomiting, tremors, edema, papilledema, hypertension, cardiac arrhythmias, dyspnea, crackles, oliguria, and Kussmaul's and Cheyne-Stokes respirations.

Epidural hemorrhage (acute)

Acute epidural hemorrhage, a life-threatening posttraumatic disorder, produces momentary loss of consciousness, sometimes followed by a lucid interval. While lucid, the patient has a severe headache, nausea, vomiting, and bladder distention. Rapid deterioration in consciousness follows, possibly leading to coma. Other findings include irregular respirations, seizures, decreased and bounding pulse, increased pulse pressure, hypertension, unilateral or bilateral fixed and dilated pupils, unilateral hemiparesis or hemiplegia, decerebrate posture, and Babinski's reflex.

Heatstroke

As body temperature increases, LOC gradually decreases from lethargy to coma. Early signs and symptoms of heatstroke include malaise, tachycardia, tachypnea, orthostatic hypotension, muscle cramps, rigidity, and syncope. The patient may be irritable, anxious, and dizzy and may report a severe headache. At the onset of heatstroke, the patient's skin is hot, flushed, and diaphoretic with blotchy cyanosis; later, when his fever exceeds 105° F (40.6° C), his skin becomes hot, flushed, and anhidrotic. Pulse and respiratory rate increase markedly, and blood pressure drops precipitously. Other findings include vomiting, diarrhea, dilated pupils, and Cheyne-Stokes respirations.

Hypernatremia

Hypernatremia, life-threatening if acute, causes LOC to deteriorate from lethargy to coma. The patient is irritable and exhibits twitches progressing to seizures. Other associated signs and symptoms include a weak, thready pulse; nausea; malaise; fever; thirst; flushed skin; and dry mucous membranes.

Hyperosmolar hyperglycemic nonketotic syndrome

LOC decreases rapidly from lethargy to coma in hyperosmolar hyperglycemic nonketotic syndrome (HHNS). Early findings include polyuria, polydipsia, weight loss, and weakness. Later, the patient may develop hypotension, poor skin turgor, dry skin and mucous membranes, tachycardia, tachypnea, oliguria, and seizures.

Hypokalemia

With hypokalemia, LOC gradually decreases to lethargy; coma is rare. Other findings include confusion, nausea, vomiting, diarrhea, polyuria, weakness, decreased reflexes, malaise, dizziness, hypotension, arrhythmias, and abnormal electrocardiogram results.

Hyponatremia

Hyponatremia, life-threatening if acute, produces decreased LOC in late stages. Early nausea and malaise may progress to behavior changes, confusion, lethargy, incoordination and, eventually, seizures and coma.

Hypothermia

With severe hypothermia (temperature below 90° F [32.2° C]), LOC decreases from lethargy to coma. DTRs disappear, and ventricular fibrillation occurs, possibly followed by cardiopulmonary arrest. With mild to moderate hypothermia, the patient may experience memory loss and slurred speech as well as shivering, weakness, fatigue, and apathy. Other early signs and symptoms include ataxia, muscle stiffness, and hyperactive DTRs; diuresis; tachycardia and decreased respiratory rate and blood pressure; and cold, pale skin. Later, muscle rigidity and decreased reflexes may develop, along with peripheral cyanosis, bradycardia, arrhythmias, severe hypotension, decreased respiratory rate with shallow respirations, and oliguria.

Medical causes
(continued)

Intracerebral hemorrhage

+ A rapid, steady loss of consciousness occurs within hours and is accompanied by severe headache, dizziness, nausea, and vomiting.

Meningitis

+ Confusion and irritability occur.
+ Stupor, coma, and seizures may occur in severe cases.

Myxedema crisis

+ Decline in LOC may be swift.

Pontine hemorrhage

+ A sudden, rapid decrease in LOC to the point of coma occurs within minutes.
+ Death occurs within hours.

Seizure disorders

+ A complex partial seizure causes decreased LOC, manifested as a blank stare, purposeless behavior, and unintelligible speech.
+ An absence seizure involves a brief change in LOC, indicated by blinking or eye rolling, blank stare, and slight mouth movements.
+ A generalized tonic-clonic seizure typically begins with a loud cry and sudden loss of consciousness; consciousness returns after the seizure.
+ An atonic seizure produces sudden unconsciousness for a few seconds.
+ Status epilepticus involves rapidly recurring seizures.

Shock

+ Decreased LOC occurs late.

Intracerebral hemorrhage

Intracerebral hemorrhage, a life-threatening disorder, produces a rapid, steady loss of consciousness within hours, commonly accompanied by severe headache, dizziness, nausea, and vomiting. Associated signs and symptoms vary and may include increased blood pressure, irregular respirations, Babinski's reflex, seizures, aphasia, decreased sensations, hemiplegia, decorticate or decerebrate posture, and dilated pupils.

Meningitis

Confusion and irritability are expected; however, stupor, coma, and seizures may occur in those with severe meningitis. Fever develops early, possibly accompanied by chills. Associated findings include severe headache, nuchal rigidity, hyperreflexia and, possibly, opisthotonos. The patient exhibits Kernig's and Brudzinski's signs and, possibly, ocular palsies, photophobia, facial weakness, and hearing loss.

Myxedema crisis

The patient experiencing myxedema crisis may exhibit a swift decline in LOC. Other findings include severe hypothermia, hypoventilation, hypotension, bradycardia, hypoactive reflexes, periorbital and peripheral edema, impaired hearing and balance, and seizures.

Pontine hemorrhage

With pontine hemorrhage, a sudden, rapid decrease in LOC to the point of coma occurs within minutes; death occurs within hours. The patient may also exhibit total paralysis, decerebrate posture, Babinski's reflex, absent doll's eye sign, and bilateral miosis (however, the pupils remain reactive to light).

Seizure disorders

A complex partial seizure produces decreased LOC, manifested as a blank stare, purposeless behavior (picking at clothing, wandering, lip smacking or chewing motions), and unintelligible speech. The seizure may be heralded by an aura and followed by several minutes of mental confusion.

An absence seizure usually involves a brief change in LOC, indicated by blinking or eye rolling, blank stare, and slight mouth movements.

A generalized tonic-clonic seizure typically begins with a loud cry and sudden loss of consciousness. Muscle spasm alternates with relaxation. Tongue biting, incontinence, labored breathing, apnea, and cyanosis may also occur. Consciousness returns after the seizure, but the patient remains confused and may have difficulty talking. He may complain of drowsiness, fatigue, headache, muscle aching, and weakness and may fall into deep sleep.

An atonic seizure produces sudden unconsciousness for a few seconds.

Status epilepticus, rapidly recurring seizures without intervening periods of physiologic recovery and return of consciousness, can be life-threatening.

Shock

Decreased LOC—lethargy progressing to stupor and coma—occurs late in shock. Associated findings include confusion, anxiety, and restlessness; hypotension; tachycardia; weak pulse with narrowing pulse pressure; dyspnea; oliguria; and cool, clammy skin.

Hypovolemic shock is generally the result of massive or insidious bleeding, either internally or externally. Cardiogenic shock may produce chest pain or arrhythmias and signs of heart failure, such as dyspnea, cough, edema, jugular vein distention, and weight gain. Septic shock may be accompanied by high fever and chills. Anaphylactic shock usually involves stridor.

Stroke

With stroke, LOC changes vary in degree and onset, depending on the lesion's size and location and the presence of edema. A thrombotic stroke usually follows multiple transient ischemic attacks (TIAs). LOC changes may be abrupt or take several minutes, hours, or days. An embolic stroke occurs suddenly, and deficits reach their peak almost at once. Deficits associated with a hemorrhagic stroke usually develop over minutes or hours.

Associated findings vary with stroke type and severity and may include disorientation; intellectual deficits, such as memory loss and poor judgment; personality changes; and emotional lability. Other possible findings include dysarthria, dysphagia, ataxia, aphasia, apraxia, agnosia, unilateral sensorimotor loss, and visual disturbances. In addition, urine retention, incontinence, constipation, headache, vomiting, and seizures may occur.

 CULTURAL CUE *The incidence of stroke is higher in Blacks than Whites. In fact, Blacks have a 60% higher risk for stroke than Whites or Hispanics of the same age. This is believed to be the result of an increased prevalence of hypertension in Blacks.*

Subdural hematoma (chronic)

LOC deteriorates slowly in patients with chronic subdural hematomas. Other signs and symptoms include confusion, decreased ability to concentrate, and personality changes accompanied by headache, light-headedness, seizures, and a dilated ipsilateral pupil with ptosis.

Subdural hemorrhage (acute)

With acute subdural hemorrhage, a potentially life-threatening disorder, agitation and confusion are followed by progressively decreasing LOC from somnolence to coma. The patient may also experience headache, fever, unilateral pupil dilation, decreased pulse and respiratory rates, widening pulse pressure, seizures, hemiparesis, and Babinski's reflex.

Thyroid storm

LOC decreases suddenly and can progress to coma. Irritability, restlessness, confusion, and psychotic behavior precede the deterioration. Associated signs and symptoms of a thyroid storm include tremors and weakness; visual disturbances; tachycardia, arrhythmias, angina, and acute respiratory distress; warm, moist, flushed skin; and vomiting, diarrhea, and fever to 105° F (40.6° C).

TIA

LOC decreases abruptly (with varying severity) and gradually returns to normal within 24 hours of a TIA. Site-specific findings may include vision loss, nystagmus, aphasia, dizziness, dysarthria, unilateral hemiparesis or hemiplegia, tinnitus, paresthesia, dysphagia, or staggering or incoordinated gait.

West Nile encephalitis

Signs and symptoms of this brain infection caused by the West Nile virus include fever, headache, and body aches, commonly with skin rash and swollen lymph glands. More severe infection is marked by high fever, headache, neck stiffness, stupor, disorientation, coma, tremors, occasional seizures, paralysis and, rarely, death.

Medical causes
(continued)

Stroke
✦ LOC changes vary in degree and onset.
✦ LOC changes may be abrupt or take several minutes, hours, or days.

Subdural hematoma (chronic)
✦ LOC deteriorates slowly.

Subdural hemorrhage (acute)
✦ Agitation and confusion are followed by progressively decreasing LOC from somnolence to coma.

Thyroid storm
✦ LOC decreases suddenly and can progress to coma.
✦ Irritability, restlessness, confusion, and psychotic behavior precede the deterioration.

TIA
✦ LOC decreases abruptly (with varying severity) and gradually returns to normal within 24 hours.

West Nile encephalitis
✦ Severe infection is marked by high fever, headache, neck stiffness, stupor, disorientation, coma, tremors, occasional seizures, paralysis and, rarely, death.

Other causes

+ Alcohol
+ Overdose of barbiturates, other CNS depressants, or aspirin
+ Poisoning

Special considerations

+ Reassess LOC and neurologic status at least hourly.
+ Monitor ICP and intake and output.
+ Ensure airway patency and proper nutrition.
+ Keep patient on bed rest with the side rails up.
+ Keep the head of the bed elevated to at least 30 degrees.
+ Don't give an opioid or a sedative.

Peds points

+ The primary cause of decreased LOC in children is head trauma.
+ Other causes include poisoning, hydrocephalus, meningitis, or brain abscess following an ear or a respiratory infection.

Teaching points

+ Explanation of treatments and procedures
+ Explanation of safety and seizure precautions
+ Referrals to sources of support

Key facts about light flashes

+ Involve seeing spots, stars, or lightning-type streaks
+ Can occur locally or throughout the visual field
+ Signal the splitting of the posterior vitreous membrane into two layers

OTHER CAUSES

Alcohol

Alcohol use causes varying degrees of sedation, irritability, and incoordination; intoxication commonly causes stupor.

Drugs

Sedation and other degrees of decreased LOC can result from an overdose of a barbiturate, another central nervous system depressant, or aspirin.

Poisoning

Toxins, such as lead, carbon monoxide, and snake venom, can cause varying degrees of decreased LOC. Confusion is common, as are headache, nausea, and vomiting. Other general features include hypotension, cardiac arrhythmias, dyspnea, sensorimotor loss, and seizures.

SPECIAL CONSIDERATIONS

Reassess the patient's LOC and neurologic status at least hourly. Carefully monitor ICP and intake and output. Ensure airway patency and proper nutrition. Take precautions to help ensure the patient's safety. Keep him on bed rest with the side rails up, and maintain seizure precautions. Keep emergency resuscitation equipment at the patient's bedside. Prepare the patient for a computed tomography scan of the head, magnetic resonance imaging of the brain, EEG, and lumbar puncture. Keep the head of the bed elevated at least 30 degrees. Don't administer an opioid or a sedative because either may further decrease the patient's LOC and hinder an accurate, meaningful neurologic examination. Apply restraints only if necessary because their use may increase his agitation and confusion.

PEDIATRIC POINTERS

The primary cause of decreased LOC in children is head trauma, which usually results from physical abuse or a motor vehicle accident. Other causes include accidental poisoning, hydrocephalus, and meningitis or brain abscess following an ear or a respiratory infection. To reduce the parents' anxiety, include them in the child's care. Offer them support and realistic explanations of their child's condition.

PATIENT COUNSELING

Talk to the patient even if he appears comatose; your voice may help reorient him to reality. Explain all treatments and procedures to the patient and his family. Explain all safety and seizure precautions. Discuss quality-of-life decisions with the patient and his family, and make the appropriate referrals to other sources of support such as hospice care.

LIGHT FLASHES

A cardinal symptom of vision-threatening retinal detachment, light flashes can occur locally or throughout the visual field. The patient usually reports seeing spots, stars, or lightning-type streaks. Also known as *photopsias,* flashes can occur suddenly or gradually and can indicate temporary or permanent vision impairment.

In most cases, light flashes signal the splitting of the posterior vitreous membrane into two layers; the inner layer detaches from the retina, and the outer layer remains fixed to it. The sensation of light flashes may result from vitreous traction on the retina, hemorrhage caused by a tear in the retinal capillary, or strands of solid vitreous floating in a local pool of liquid vitreous.

 EMERGENCY ACTIONS Until retinal detachment is ruled out, restrict the patient's eye and body movement.

HISTORY

Ask the patient when the light flashes began. Can he pinpoint their location, or do they occur throughout the visual field? If the patient is experiencing eye pain or headache, have him describe it. Ask if the patient wears or has ever worn corrective lenses and if he or a family member has a history of eye or vision problems. Also ask if the patient has other medical problems — especially hypertension or diabetes mellitus, which can cause retinopathy and, possibly, retinal detachment. Obtain an occupational history because light flashes may be related to job stress or eye strain.

PHYSICAL ASSESSMENT

Perform a complete eye and vision assessment, especially if trauma is apparent or suspected. Begin by inspecting the external eye, lids, lashes, and tear puncta for abnormalities and the iris and sclera for signs of bleeding. Observe pupillary size and shape; check for reaction to light, accommodation, and consensual light response. Then test visual acuity in each eye. Also test visual fields; document any light flashes that the patient reports during this test.

MEDICAL CAUSES

Head trauma

A patient who has sustained minor head trauma may report "seeing stars" when the injury occurs. He may also complain of localized pain at the injury site, generalized headache, and dizziness. Later, he may develop nausea, vomiting, and decreased level of consciousness.

Migraine headache

Light flashes — possibly accompanied by an aura — may herald a classic migraine headache. As these symptoms subside, the patient typically experiences a severe, throbbing, unilateral headache that usually lasts 1 to 12 hours and may be accompanied by paresthesia of the lips, face, or hands; slight confusion; dizziness; photophobia; nausea; and vomiting.

Retinal detachment

Light flashes described as floaters or spots are localized in the portion of the visual field where the retina is detaching. With macular involvement, the patient may experience painless visual impairment resembling a curtain covering the visual field.

Vitreous detachment

With vitreous detachment, visual floaters may accompany a sudden onset of light flashes. Usually, one eye is affected at a time. These floaters may move with the eye and settle when the eye rests.

SPECIAL CONSIDERATIONS

If the patient has retinal detachment, prepare him for reattachment surgery. For the patient with a migraine headache, maintain a quiet, darkened environment; encourage sleep; and administer an analgesic as ordered.

In an emergency
✦ Until retinal detachment is ruled out, restrict eye and body movement.

Key history points
✦ Onset and location of light flashes
✦ Description of associated eye pain or headache
✦ Medical history

Critical assessment steps
✦ Inspect the external eye, lids, lashes, iris, sclera, and tear puncta.
✦ Observe pupillary size and shape; check for reaction to light.

Medical causes

Head trauma
✦ Patient may "see stars" when minor head trauma occurs.

Migraine headache
✦ Light flashes may be accompanied by an aura.

Retinal detachment
✦ Light flashes described as floaters or spots are localized where the retina is detaching.

Vitreous detachment
✦ Visual floaters may accompany a sudden onset of light flashes.

Special considerations
✦ If patient has retinal detachment, prepare him for surgery.
✦ For patient with a migraine headache, maintain a quiet, darkened environment and administer an analgesic as ordered.

Peds points

+ Children may experience light flashes after minor head trauma.

Teaching points

+ Postoperative restrictions

Key facts about lymphadenopathy

+ Refers to enlargement of one or more lymph nodes
+ May be generalized or localized
+ Are cause for concern if more than ⅜″ in diameter

Key history points

+ Onset, location, and description of swelling
+ Recent infections or health problems
+ Previous biopsies or personal or family history of cancer

Critical assessment steps

+ If you detect enlarged nodes, note their size and whether they're fixed or mobile, tender or nontender, and erythematous.
+ If you detect tender, erythematous lymph nodes, check the area drained by that part of the lymph system for signs of infection.

Medical causes

AIDS

+ Lymphadenopathy occurs with a history of fatigue, night sweats, afternoon fevers, diarrhea, weight loss, and cough with several concurrent infections.

PEDIATRIC POINTERS

Children may experience light flashes after minor head trauma.

PATIENT COUNSELING

Explain to the patient that after retinal surgery he may need to continue wearing bilateral eye patches and may have activity and position restrictions until the retina heals completely. If the patient doesn't have retinal detachment, reassure him that his light flashes are temporary and don't indicate eye damage.

LYMPHADENOPATHY

Lymphadenopathy — enlargement of one or more lymph nodes — may result from increased production of lymphocytes or reticuloendothelial cells, or from infiltration of cells that aren't normally present. This sign may be generalized (involving three or more node groups) or localized. Generalized lymphadenopathy may be caused by an inflammatory process, such as bacterial or viral infection, connective tissue disease, an endocrine disorder, or neoplasm. Localized lymphadenopathy most commonly results from infection or trauma affecting a specific area. (See *Areas of localized lymphadenopathy*.)

Normally, lymph nodes are discrete, mobile, soft, nontender and, except in children, nonpalpable. (However, palpable nodes may be normal in adults.) Nodes that are more than ⅜″ (1 cm) in diameter are cause for concern. They may be tender, and the skin overlying the lymph node may be erythematous, suggesting a draining lesion. Alternatively, they may be hard and fixed, and tender or nontender, suggesting a malignant tumor.

HISTORY

Ask the patient when he first noticed the swelling and whether it's located on one side of his body or both. Are the swollen areas sore, hard, or red? Ask the patient if he has recently had an infection or other health problem. Also ask if a biopsy has ever been done on any node because this may indicate a previously diagnosed cancer. Find out if the patient has a family history of cancer.

PHYSICAL ASSESSMENT

Palpate the entire lymph node system to determine the extent of lymphadenopathy and to detect other areas of local enlargement. Use the pads of your index and middle fingers to move the skin over underlying tissues at the nodal area. If you detect enlarged nodes, note their size in centimeters and whether they're fixed or mobile, tender or nontender, and erythematous. Note their texture: Is the node discrete, or does the area feel matted? If you detect tender, erythematous lymph nodes, check the area drained by that part of the lymph system for signs of infection, such as erythema and swelling. Also, palpate for and percuss the spleen.

MEDICAL CAUSES

Acquired immunodeficiency syndrome

Besides lymphadenopathy, acquired immunodeficiency syndrome (AIDS) findings include a history of fatigue, night sweats, afternoon fevers, diarrhea, weight loss, and cough with several concurrent infections appearing soon afterward.

Areas of localized lymphadenopathy

When you detect an enlarged lymph node, palpate the entire lymph node system to determine the extent of lymphadenopathy. Include the lymph nodes indicated below in your assessment.

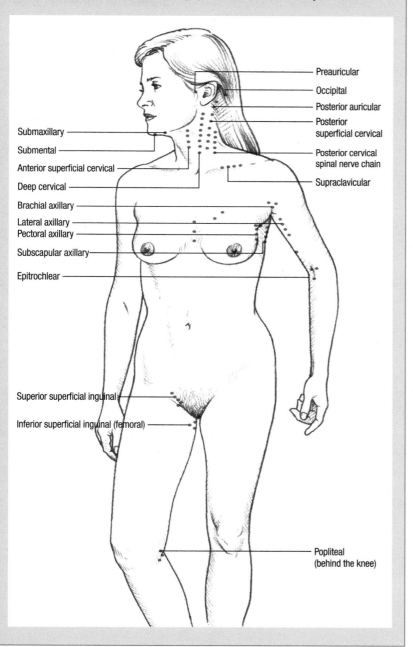

Medical causes
(continued)

Anthrax (cutaneous)
✦ Lymphadenopathy, malaise, headache, and fever may develop along with lesions.

Chronic fatigue syndrome
✦ Lymphadenopathy may occur with incapacitating fatigue, sore throat, low-grade fevers, myalgia, cognitive dysfunction, and sleep disturbances.

Cytomegalovirus infection
✦ Generalized lymphadenopathy is accompanied by fever, malaise, and hepatosplenomegaly.

Hodgkin's disease
✦ Extent of lymphadenopathy reflects stage of malignancy.

Leukemia
✦ In acute lymphocytic leukemia, generalized lymphadenopathy is accompanied by fatigue, malaise, pallor, and low fever.
✦ In chronic lymphocytic leukemia, generalized lymphadenopathy appears early.

Lyme disease
✦ As disease progresses, lymphadenopathy, constant malaise and fatigue, and intermittent headache, fever, chills, and aches develop.

Mononucleosis (infectious)
✦ Painful lymphadenopathy involves cervical, axillary, and inguinal nodes.

Anthrax (cutaneous)
With cutaneous anthrax, lymphadenopathy, malaise, headache, and fever may develop along with a small, elevated, itchy lesion resembling an insect bite that progresses into a painless, necrotic-centered ulcer.

Chronic fatigue syndrome
Lymphadenopathy may occur with incapacitating fatigue, sore throat, low-grade fevers, myalgia, cognitive dysfunction, and sleep disturbances. The patient may also experience arthralgia with arthritis, headache, and memory deficits.

Cytomegalovirus infection
Generalized lymphadenopathy is accompanied by fever, malaise, and hepatosplenomegaly in a patient infected with cytomegalovirus. The patient also develops a pruritic rash of small, erythematous macules that progresses to papules and then to vesicles.

Hodgkin's disease
In Hodgkin's disease, the extent of lymphadenopathy reflects the stage of malignancy, from stage I involvement of a single lymph node region to stage IV — generalized lymphadenopathy. Common early signs and symptoms include pruritus and, in older patients, fatigue, weakness, night sweats, malaise, weight loss, and unexplained fever (usually to 101° F [38.3° C]). Also, if mediastinal lymph nodes enlarge, tracheal and esophageal pressure produces dyspnea and dysphagia.

Leukemia
In acute lymphocytic leukemia, generalized lymphadenopathy is accompanied by fatigue, malaise, pallor, and low fever. The patient also experiences prolonged bleeding time, swollen gums, weight loss, bone or joint pain, and hepatosplenomegaly.

In chronic lymphocytic leukemia, generalized lymphadenopathy appears early, along with fatigue, malaise, and fever. As the disease progresses, hepatosplenomegaly, severe fatigue, and weight loss occur. Other late findings include bone tenderness, edema, pallor, dyspnea, tachycardia, palpitations, bleeding, anemia, and macular or nodular lesions.

Lyme disease
Spread by the bite of certain ticks, Lyme disease begins with a skin lesion called erythema chronicum migrans. As the disease progresses, the patient may suffer from lymphadenopathy, constant malaise and fatigue, and intermittent headache, fever, chills, and aches. He may go on to develop arthralgia and, eventually, neurologic and cardiac abnormalities.

Mononucleosis (infectious)
Patients with mononucleosis develop painful lymphadenopathy that involves the cervical, axillary, and inguinal nodes. Posterior cervical adenopathy is also common. Typically, prodromal symptoms — such as headache, malaise, and fatigue — occur 3 to 5 days before the appearance of the classic triad of lymphadenopathy, sore throat, and temperature fluctuations with an evening peak of about 102° F (38.9° C). Hepatosplenomegaly may develop, along with findings of stomatitis, exudative tonsillitis, or pharyngitis.

Non-Hodgkin's lymphoma

Painless enlargement of one or more peripheral lymph nodes is the most common sign of non-Hodgkin's lymphoma, with generalized lymphadenopathy characterizing stage IV. Dyspnea, cough, and hepatosplenomegaly occur, along with systemic complaints of fever to 101° F (38.3° C), night sweats, fatigue, malaise, and weight loss.

Rheumatoid arthritis

Lymphadenopathy is an early, nonspecific finding of rheumatoid arthritis that's associated with fatigue, malaise, continuous low fever, weight loss, and vague arthralgia and myalgia. Later, the patient develops joint tenderness, swelling, and warmth; joint stiffness after inactivity (especially in the morning); and subcutaneous nodules on the elbows. Eventually joint deformity, muscle weakness, and atrophy may occur.

Sarcoidosis

Generalized, bilateral hilar and right paratracheal forms of lymphadenopathy (seen on chest X-ray) with splenomegaly are common in sarcoidosis. Initial findings are arthralgia, fatigue, malaise, weight loss, and pulmonary symptoms. Other findings vary with the site and extent of fibrosis. Typical cardiopulmonary findings include breathlessness, cough, substernal chest pain, and arrhythmias. Musculoskeletal and cutaneous features may include muscle weakness and pain, phalangeal and nasal mucosal lesions, and subcutaneous skin nodules. Common ophthalmic findings include eye pain, photophobia, and nonreactive pupils. Central nervous system involvement may produce cranial or peripheral nerve palsies and seizures.

Syphilis

Localized lymphadenopathy and a painless ulcer (canker) with an indurated border and relatively smooth base at the site of sexual exposure characterize a primary syphilis infection. The ulcer is usually single, but more than one may be present. In the second stage of syphilis, generalized lymphadenopathy occurs and may be accompanied by a macular, papular, pustular, or nodular rash on the arms, trunk, palms, soles, face, and scalp. A palmar rash is a significant diagnostic sign. Headache, malaise, anorexia, weight loss, nausea, vomiting, sore throat, and low fever may occur.

Systemic lupus erythematosus

Generalized lymphadenopathy typically accompanies the hallmark butterfly rash, photosensitivity, Raynaud's phenomenon, and joint pain and stiffness associated with systemic lupus erythematosus (SLE). Pleuritic chest pain and cough may appear with systemic findings, such as fever, anorexia, and weight loss.

Tuberculous lymphadenitis

With tuberculous lymphadenitis, lymphadenopathy may be generalized or restricted to superficial lymph nodes. Affected lymph nodes may become fluctuant and drain to surrounding tissue. They may be accompanied by fever, chills, weakness, and fatigue.

OTHER CAUSES

Drugs

Phenytoin may cause generalized lymphadenopathy.

Immunizations

Typhoid vaccination may cause generalized lymphadenopathy.

Medical causes
(continued)

Non-Hodgkin's lymphoma
+ Painless enlargement of one or more peripheral lymph nodes is the most common sign.
+ Generalized lymphadenopathy characterizes stage IV.

Rheumatoid arthritis
+ Lymphadenopathy is an early, nonspecific finding.

Sarcoidosis
+ Generalized, bilateral hilar and right paratracheal forms of lymphadenopathy with splenomegaly are common.

Syphilis
+ Localized lymphadenopathy occurs with painless canker that develops at site of sexual exposure.

SLE
+ Generalized lymphadenopathy typically accompanies butterfly rash, photosensitivity, Raynaud's phenomenon, and joint pain and stiffness.

Tuberculous lymphadenitis
+ Lymphadenopathy may be generalized or restricted to superficial lymph nodes.
+ Lymph nodes may become fluctuant and drain to surrounding tissue.

Other causes
+ Phenytoin
+ Typhoid vaccination

Special considerations

✦ Provide antipyretic, tepid sponge bath, or a hypothermia blanket if patient is uncomfortable.
✦ Expect to obtain blood.
✦ If diagnostic tests reveal infection, check your facility's policy regarding infection control.

Peds points

✦ Infection is the most common cause of lymphadenopathy in children.

Teaching points

✦ Ways to prevent infection
✦ Signs and symptoms of infection to report
✦ Reasons for isolation (as needed)
✦ Importance of healthy diet and rest

SPECIAL CONSIDERATIONS

If the patient has a fever above 101° F (38.3° C), don't automatically assume that the temperature should be lowered. A patient with a bacterial or viral infection must tolerate the fever, which may assist recovery. Provide an antipyretic if the patient is uncomfortable. Tepid sponge baths or a hypothermia blanket may also be used.

Expect to obtain blood for routine blood work, platelet and white blood cell counts, liver and renal function studies, erythrocyte sedimentation rate, and blood cultures. Prepare the patient for other scheduled diagnostic tests, such as chest X-ray, liver and spleen scan, lymph node biopsy, or lymphography, to visualize the lymphatic system. If tests reveal infection, check your facility's policy regarding infection control.

PEDIATRIC POINTERS

Infection is the most common cause of lymphadenopathy in children. The condition is commonly associated with otitis media and pharyngitis.

Provide an antipyretic if the child has a history of febrile seizures.

PATIENT COUNSELING

Explain the importance of avoiding crowds and washing hands properly to prevent infection. Teach the patient the signs and symptoms of infection he needs to report to the health care provider. If isolation is required, explain its purpose and associated interventions to the patient and his family. Encourage the patient to eat a healthy diet and get plenty of rest.

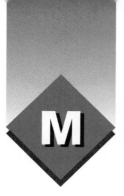

MELENA

A common sign of upper GI bleeding, melena is the passage of black, tarry stools containing digested blood. Characteristic color results from bacterial degradation and hydrochloric acid acting on the blood as it travels through the GI tract. At least 60 ml of blood is needed to produce this sign. (See *Comparing melena to hematochezia,* page 410.)

Severe melena can signal acute bleeding and life-threatening hypovolemic shock. Usually, melena indicates bleeding from the esophagus, stomach, or duodenum, although it can also indicate bleeding from the jejunum, ileum, or ascending colon. This sign can also result from swallowing blood, as in epistaxis; from taking certain drugs; or from ingesting alcohol. Because false melena may be caused by ingestion of lead, iron, bismuth, or licorice (which produces black stools without the presence of blood), all black stools should be tested for occult blood.

EMERGENCY ACTIONS If the patient is experiencing severe melena, quickly take orthostatic vital signs to detect hypovolemic shock. A decline of 10 mm Hg or more in systolic pressure or an increase of 10 beats/minute or more in pulse rate indicates volume depletion. Quickly examine the patient for other signs of shock, such as tachycardia, tachypnea, and cool, clammy skin. Insert a large-bore I.V. line to administer replacement fluids and allow blood transfusion. Obtain a hematocrit, prothrombin time, International Normalized Ratio, and partial thromboplastin time. Place the patient flat with his head turned to the side and his feet elevated. Administer supplemental oxygen as needed.

HISTORY

If the patient's condition permits, ask when he discovered his stools were black and tarry. Ask about the frequency and quantity of bowel movements. Has he had melena before? Ask about other signs and symptoms, notably hematemesis or hematochezia, and about use of anti-inflammatories, alcohol, or other GI irritants. Also, find out if he has a history of GI lesions. Ask if the patient takes iron supplements, which may also cause black stools. Obtain a drug history, noting the use of warfarin or other anticoagulants.

PHYSICAL ASSESSMENT

Inspect the patient's mouth and nasopharynx for evidence of bleeding. Perform an abdominal assessment that includes auscultation, palpation, and percussion. Perform a cardiovascular assessment to detect signs and symptoms of shock.

Key facts about melena
+ Passage of black, tarry stools containing digested blood
+ Commonly indicates upper GI bleeding

In an emergency
+ Take orthostatic vital signs, and look for other signs of shock.
+ Administer replacement fluids and allow blood transfusion.
+ Obtain hematocrit, PT, INR, and PTT.

Key history points
+ Onset of melena
+ Frequency and quantity of bowel movements
+ Associated hematemesis or hematochezia
+ Use of anti-inflammatories, alcohol, other GI irritants, or iron supplements

Critical assessment steps
+ Perform an abdominal assessment that includes auscultation, palpation, and percussion.
+ Perform a cardiovascular assessment to detect signs and symptoms of shock.

ASSESSMENT TIP

Comparing melena to hematochezia

With GI bleeding, the site, amount, and rate of blood flow through the GI tract determine if a patient will develop melena (black, tarry stools) or hematochezia (bright red, bloody stools). Usually, melena indicates upper GI bleeding, and hematochezia indicates lower GI bleeding. However, with some disorders, melena may alternate with hematochezia. This chart helps differentiate these two commonly related signs.

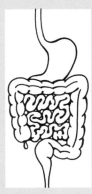

SIGN	SITES	CHARACTERISTICS
Melena	Esophagus, stomach, duodenum; rarely, jejunum, ileum, ascending colon.	Black, loose, tarry stools. Delayed or minimal passage of blood through GI tract.
Hematochezia	Usually distal to or affecting the colon; rapid hemorrhage of 1 L or more is associated with esophageal, stomach, or duodenal bleeding.	Bright red or dark, mahogany-colored stools; pure blood; blood mixed with formed stool; or bloody diarrhea. Reflects lower GI bleeding or rapid blood loss and passage of undigested blood through GI tract.

Medical causes

Colon cancer
✦ Right-sided tumor growth may cause melena and abdominal aching, pressure, or cramps.
✦ With left-sided tumor growth, melena is rare until late in the disease.

Esophageal cancer
✦ Melena is a late sign.

Esophageal varices (ruptured)
✦ Melena, hematochezia, and hematemesis may occur.
✦ Melena is preceded by signs of shock.

MEDICAL CAUSES

Colon cancer

On the right side of the colon, early tumor growth may cause melena accompanied by abdominal aching, pressure, or cramps. As the disease progresses, the patient develops weakness, fatigue, and anemia. Eventually, he also experiences diarrhea or obstipation, anorexia, weight loss, vomiting, and other signs and symptoms of intestinal obstruction.

With a tumor on the left side, melena is a rare sign until late in the disease. Early tumor growth commonly causes rectal bleeding with intermittent abdominal fullness or cramping and rectal pressure. As the disease progresses, the patient may develop obstipation, diarrhea, or pencil-shaped stools. At this stage, bleeding from the colon is signaled by melena or bloody stools.

 CULTURAL CUE Ask your patient about his religious and ethnic background to determine if they put him at risk for colon cancer. Colon cancer is more prevalent in Jewish people of Eastern European descent.

Esophageal cancer

Melena is a late sign of esophageal cancer, a malignant neoplastic disease. Increasing obstruction first produces painless dysphagia, then rapid weight loss. The patient may experience steady chest pain with substernal fullness, nausea, vomiting, and hematemesis. Other findings include hoarseness, persistent cough (possibly hemoptysis), hiccups, sore throat, and halitosis. In the later stages, signs and symptoms include painful dysphagia, anorexia, and regurgitation.

Esophageal varices (ruptured)

This life-threatening disorder can produce melena, hematochezia, and hematemesis. Melena is preceded by signs of shock, such as tachycardia, tachypnea, hypotension, and cool, clammy skin. Agitation or confusion signals developing hepatic encephalopathy.

Gastric cancer

Melena and altered bowel habits may occur late with gastric cancer. More common findings include insidious onset of upper abdominal or retrosternal discomfort and chronic dyspepsia that are unrelieved by antacids and are exacerbated by food. Anorexia and slight nausea usually occur, along with hematemesis, pallor, fatigue, weight loss, and a feeling of abdominal fullness.

 CULTURAL CUE *Asian countries, such as Korea, China, Taiwan, and Japan, have higher rates of gastric cancer than the United States.*

Gastritis

Melena and hematemesis are common in gastritis. The patient may also experience mild epigastric or abdominal discomfort that's exacerbated by eating, belching, nausea, vomiting, and malaise.

Mallory-Weiss syndrome

Mallory-Weiss syndrome is characterized by massive bleeding from the upper GI tract due to a tear in the mucous membrane of the esophagus or the junction of the esophagus and the stomach. Melena and hematemesis follow vomiting. Severe upper abdominal bleeding leads to signs and symptoms of shock, such as tachycardia, tachypnea, hypotension, and cool, clammy skin. The patient may also report epigastric or back pain.

Mesenteric vascular occlusion

Mesenteric vascular occlusion is a life-threatening disorder that produces slight melena with 2 to 3 days of persistent, mild abdominal pain. Later, abdominal pain becomes severe and may be accompanied by tenderness, distention, guarding, and rigidity. The patient may also experience anorexia, vomiting, fever, and profound shock.

Peptic ulcer

Melena may signal life-threatening hemorrhage from vascular penetration in patients with peptic ulcers. The patient may also develop decreased appetite, nausea, vomiting, hematemesis, hematochezia, and left epigastric pain that's gnawing, burning, or sharp and may be described as heartburn or indigestion. With hypovolemic shock come tachycardia, tachypnea, hypotension, dizziness, syncope, and cool, clammy skin.

Small-bowel tumors

Small-bowel tumors may bleed and produce melena. Other signs and symptoms include abdominal pain, distention, and increasing frequency and pitch of bowel sounds.

Thrombocytopenia

With thrombocytopenia, melena or hematochezia may accompany other manifestations of bleeding tendency: hematemesis, epistaxis, petechiae, ecchymoses, hematuria, vaginal bleeding, and characteristic blood-filled oral bullae. Typically, the patient displays malaise, fatigue, weakness, and lethargy.

Other causes
+ Aspirin and other NSAIDs
+ Alcohol

Special considerations
+ Monitor vital signs; look closely for signs of hypovolemic shock.
+ An NG tube may be necessary to assist with drainage of gastric contents and decompression.
+ Prepare patient for blood transfusions as indicated by hematocrit.

Peds points
+ Neonates may experience melena neonatorum.
+ In older children, melena usually results from peptic ulcer, gastritis, or Meckel's diverticulum.

Geri points
+ Patients with recurrent intermittent GI bleeding without clear etiology should be considered for angiography or exploratory laparotomy.

Teaching points
+ Importance of reporting changes in bowel elimination, undergoing colorectal cancer screening, and avoiding aspirin, other NSAIDs, and alcohol

Key facts about mouth lesions
+ Include ulcers (most common), cysts, firm nodules, hemorrhagic lesions, papules, vesicles, bullae, and erythematous lesions
+ May occur anywhere on the lips, cheeks, hard and soft palate, salivary glands, tongue, gingivae, or mucous membranes

OTHER CAUSES

Drugs and alcohol
Aspirin, other nonsteroidal anti-inflammatory drugs (NSAIDs), or alcohol can cause melena as a result of gastric irritation.

SPECIAL CONSIDERATIONS

Monitor vital signs, and look closely for signs of hypovolemic shock. For general comfort, encourage bed rest and keep the patient's perianal area clean and dry to prevent skin irritation and breakdown. A nasogastric tube may be necessary to assist with drainage of gastric contents and decompression. Prepare the patient for diagnostic tests, including blood studies, gastroscopy or other endoscopic studies, barium swallow, and upper GI series. Prepare the patient for blood transfusions as indicated by his hematocrit.

PEDIATRIC POINTERS

Neonates may experience melena neonatorum due to extravasation of blood into the alimentary canal. In older children, melena usually results from peptic ulcer, gastritis, or Meckel's diverticulum.

GERIATRIC POINTERS

In elderly patients with recurrent intermittent GI bleeding without a clear etiology, angiography or exploratory laparotomy should be considered when the risk from continued anemia is deemed to outweigh the risk associated with the procedures.

PATIENT COUNSELING

Teach the patient the importance of reporting changes in bowel elimination and to undergo screening for colorectal cancer as recommended by his health care provider. Discuss the importance of avoiding aspirin, other NSAIDs, and alcohol.

MOUTH LESIONS

Mouth lesions include ulcers (the most common type), cysts, firm nodules, hemorrhagic lesions, papules, vesicles, bullae, and erythematous lesions. They may occur anywhere on the lips, cheeks, hard and soft palate, salivary glands, tongue, gingivae, or mucous membranes. Many are painful and can be readily detected. Some, however, don't produce symptoms; when they occur deep in the mouth, they may be discovered only through a complete oral examination. (See *Common mouth lesions.*)

Mouth lesions can result from trauma, infection, systemic disease, drug use, or radiation therapy.

HISTORY

Begin your evaluation with a thorough history. Ask the patient when the lesions appeared and whether he has noticed any pain, odor, or drainage. Also ask about associated complaints, particularly skin lesions. Obtain a complete drug history, including drug allergies and antibiotic use, and a complete medical history. Note especially any malignancy, sexually transmitted disease, I.V. drug use, recent infection, or trauma. Ask about his dental history, including oral hygiene habits, frequency of dental examinations, and the date of his most recent dental visit.

Common mouth lesions

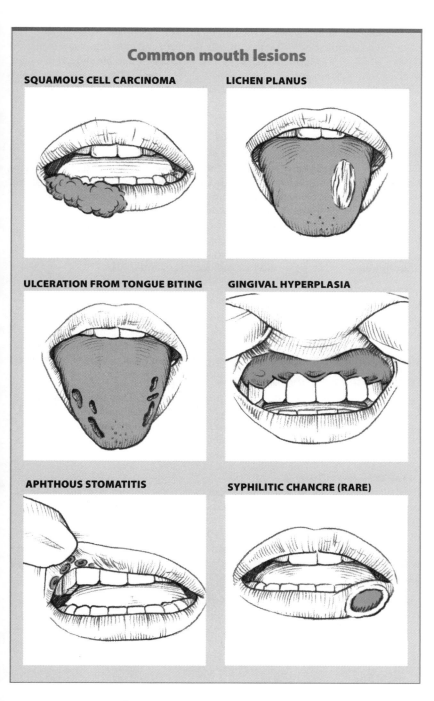

SQUAMOUS CELL CARCINOMA

LICHEN PLANUS

ULCERATION FROM TONGUE BITING

GINGIVAL HYPERPLASIA

APHTHOUS STOMATITIS

SYPHILITIC CHANCRE (RARE)

Key history points
- Onset of lesions
- Associated pain, odor, drainage, or skin lesions
- Drug history
- Medical history, including malignancies, STDs, I.V. drug use, recent infection, or trauma
- Dental history

Critical assessment steps
- Note lesion sites and character.
- Examine the lips for color and texture.
- Inspect and palpate the buccal mucosa and tongue for color, texture, and contour; especially note any painless ulcers on the sides or base of the tongue.
- Examine the oropharynx.
- Inspect the teeth and gums.
- Palpate the neck for adenopathy, especially in patients who smoke tobacco or use alcohol excessively.

PHYSICAL ASSESSMENT

Perform a complete oral examination, noting lesion sites and character. Examine the patient's lips for color and texture. Inspect and palpate the buccal mucosa and tongue for color, texture, and contour; especially note any painless ulcers on the sides or base of the tongue. Hold the tongue with a piece of gauze, lift it, and examine its underside and the floor of the mouth. Depress the tongue with a tongue blade, and examine the oropharynx. Inspect the teeth and gums, noting missing, broken, or discolored teeth; dental caries; excessive debris; and bleeding, inflamed, swollen, or discolored gums.

Palpate the neck for adenopathy, especially in patients who smoke tobacco or use alcohol excessively.

MEDICAL CAUSES

Acquired immunodeficiency syndrome

Oral lesions may be an early indication of the immunosuppression that's characteristic of acquired immunodeficiency syndrome (AIDS). Fungal infections can occur, with oral candidiasis being the most common. Bacterial or viral infections of oral mucosa, tongue, gingivae, and periodontal tissue may also occur.

The primary oral neoplasm associated with AIDS is Kaposi's sarcoma. The tumor is usually found on the hard palate. Initially producing no symptoms, it may appear as a flat or raised lesion, ranging in color from red to blue to purple. As these tumors grow, they may ulcerate and become painful.

Candidiasis

Candidiasis, a common fungal infection, characteristically produces soft, elevated plaques on the buccal mucosa, tongue, and sometimes the palate, gingivae, and floor of the mouth; the plaques may be wiped away. The lesions of acute atrophic candidiasis are red and painful. The lesions of chronic hyperplastic candidiasis are white and firm. Localized areas of redness, pruritus, and foul odor may be present.

Discoid lupus erythematosus

Oral lesions are common in discoid lupus erythematosus. They typically appear on the tongue, buccal mucosa, and palate as erythematous areas with white spots and radiating white striae. Associated findings include skin lesions on the face, possibly extending to the neck, ears, and scalp; if the scalp is involved, alopecia may result. Hair follicles are enlarged and filled with scale.

Erythema multiforme

Erythema multiforme, an acute inflammatory skin disease, produces sudden onset of vesicles and bullae on the lips and buccal mucosa. Also, erythematous macules and papules form symmetrically on the hands, arms, feet, legs, face, and neck and, possibly, in the eyes and on the genitalia. Lymphadenopathy may also occur. With visceral involvement, other findings include fever, malaise, cough, throat and chest pain, vomiting, diarrhea, myalgia, arthralgia, fingernail loss, blindness, hematuria, and signs of renal failure.

Gingivitis (acute necrotizing ulcerative)

Gingivitis, a recurring periodontal condition, causes a sudden onset of gingival ulcers covered with a grayish white pseudomembrane. Other findings include tender or painful gingivae, intermittent gingival bleeding, halitosis, enlarged lymph nodes in the neck, and fever.

Gonorrhea

With gonorrhea, painful lip ulcerations may occur, along with rough, reddened, bleeding gingivae (possibly necrotic and covered by a yellowish pseudomembrane), and a swollen, ulcerated tongue. Related effects vary. Most men develop dysuria, purulent urethral discharge, and a reddened, edematous urinary meatus. Most women remain asymptomatic, but others develop inflammation and a greenish yellow cervical discharge.

Medical causes

AIDS
+ Oral lesions may be an early sign of immunosuppression.
+ Kaposi's sarcoma may appear on the hard palate.

Candidiasis
+ Soft, elevated plaques usually develop on the buccal mucosa and tongue.
+ In acute atrophic form, lesions are red and painful.
+ In chronic hyperplastic form, lesions are white and firm.

Discoid lupus erythematosus
+ Erythematous areas with white spots and radiating white striae appear on the tongue, buccal mucosa, and palate.

Erythema multiforme
+ Onset of vesicles and bullae on the lips and buccal mucosa is sudden.

Gingivitis (acute necrotizing ulcerative)
+ Gingival ulcers have a grayish white pseudomembrane.

Gonorrhea
+ Painful lip ulcerations may occur, along with rough, reddened, bleeding gingivae and a swollen, ulcerated tongue.

Herpes simplex 1

With primary herpes simplex infection, a brief period of prodromal tingling and itching, which is accompanied by fever and pharyngitis, is followed by eruption of small and irritating vesicles on any part of the oral mucosa, especially the tongue, gums, and cheeks. Vesicles form on an erythematous base and then rupture, leaving a painful ulcer, followed by a yellowish crust. Other findings include submaxillary lymphadenopathy, increased salivation, halitosis, anorexia, and keratoconjunctivitis.

Herpes zoster

Herpes zoster is a common viral infection that may produce painful vesicles on the buccal mucosa, tongue, uvula, pharynx, and larynx. Small, red nodules usually erupt unilaterally around the thorax or vertically on the arms and legs and rapidly become vesicles filled with clear fluid or pus; vesicles dry and form scabs about 10 days after eruption. Fever and general malaise accompany pruritus, paresthesia or hyperesthesia, and tenderness along the course of the involved sensory nerve.

Leukoplakia, erythroplakia

Leukoplakia is a white lesion that can't be removed simply by rubbing the mucosal surface — unlike candidiasis. It may occur in response to chronic irritation from dentures or tobacco or pipe smoking, or it may represent dysplasia or early squamous cell carcinoma.

Erythroplakia is red and edematous and has a velvety surface. About 90% of erythroplakia cases are either dysplasia or cancer.

Lichen planus

With lichen planus, oral lesions develop on the buccal mucosa or, less commonly, on the tongue as painless, white or gray, velvety, threadlike papules. These precede the eruption of violet papules with white lines or spots, usually on the genitalia, lower back, ankles, and anterior lower legs; pruritus; nails with longitudinal ridges; and alopecia.

Squamous cell carcinoma

A squamous cell carcinoma is typically a painless ulcer with an elevated, indurated border. It may erupt in areas of leukoplakia and is most common on the lower lip, but it may also occur on the edge of the tongue or the floor of the mouth. High risk factors include chronic smoking and alcohol intake.

Stomatitis (aphthous)

Aphthous stomatitis is a common disease characterized by painful ulcerations of the oral mucosa, usually on the dorsum of the tongue, gingivae, and hard palate.

With recurrent aphthous stomatitis minor, the ulcer begins as one or more erosions covered by a gray membrane and surrounded by a red halo. It's commonly found on the buccal and lip mucosa and junction, tongue, soft palate, pharynx, gingivae, and all places not bound to the periosteum.

With recurrent aphthous stomatitis major, large, painful ulcers commonly occur on the lips, cheek, tongue, and soft palate; they may last up to 6 weeks and leave a scar.

Syphilis

Primary syphilis typically produces a solitary painless, red ulcer (chancre) on the lip, tongue, palate, tonsil, or gingivae. The ulcer appears as a crater with undulated, raised edges and a shiny center; lip chancres may develop a crust. Similar lesions may appear on the fingers, breasts, or genitals, and regional lymph nodes may become enlarged and tender.

Medical causes
(continued)

Herpes simplex 1
✦ Small vesicles develop on the oral mucosa.

Herpes zoster
✦ Painful vesicles develop on the buccal mucosa, tongue, uvula, pharynx, and larynx.

Leukoplakia, erythroplakia
✦ Leukoplakia is a white lesion that can't be removed by rubbing the mucosal surface.
✦ Erythroplakia is red and edematous and has a velvety surface.

Lichen planus
✦ White or gray, velvety, threadlike papules develop on the buccal mucosa or the tongue.

Squamous cell carcinoma
✦ A painless ulcer with an elevated, indurated border most commonly appears on the lower lip.

Stomatitis (aphthous)
✦ In minor form, one or more erosions covered by a gray membrane and surrounded by a red halo appear on the mucosa.
✦ In major form, large, painful ulcers occur on the lips, cheek, tongue, and soft palate.

Syphilis
✦ Primary syphilis typically produces a solitary painless, red ulcer on the lip or mouth.
✦ Secondary syphilis may produce multiple painless ulcers covered by grayish plaque on mouth.
✦ At tertiary stage, lesions develop on skin and mucous membranes, especially tongue and palate.

Medical causes
(continued)

SLE

+ Oral lesions appear as erythematous areas associated with edema, petechiae, and superficial ulcers with a red halo and a tendency to bleed.

Other causes

+ Allergic reactions to penicillin, sulfonamides, gold, quinine, streptomycin, phenytoin, aspirin, and barbiturates
+ Inhaled steroids used for pulmonary disorders
+ Radiation therapy
+ Chemotherapeutic agents

Special considerations

+ Provide a topical anesthetic such as lidocaine.

Peds points

+ Causes of mouth ulcers in children include chickenpox, measles, scarlet fever, diphtheria, and hand-foot-and-mouth disease.
+ In neonates, mouth ulcers can result from candidiasis or congenital syphilis.

Geri points

+ Ill-fitting dentures can cause irritation, leading to inflammation and ulcers.

Teaching points

+ Irritants to avoid
+ Proper mouth care and oral hygiene

During the secondary stage, multiple painless ulcers covered by a grayish white plaque may erupt on the tongue, gingivae, or buccal mucosa. A macular, papular, pustular, or nodular rash appears, usually on the arms, trunk, palms, soles, face, and scalp; genital lesions usually subside. Other findings include generalized lymphadenopathy, headache, malaise, anorexia, weight loss, nausea, vomiting, sore throat, low fever, metrorrhagia, and postcoital bleeding.

At the tertiary stage, lesions (usually gummas — chronic, painless, superficial nodules or deep granulomatous lesions) develop on the skin and mucous membranes, especially the tongue and palate.

Systemic lupus erythematosus

Oral lesions are common with systemic lupus erythematosus (SLE) and appear as erythematous areas associated with edema, petechiae, and superficial ulcers with a red halo and a tendency to bleed. Primary effects include nondeforming arthritis, butterfly rash across the nose and cheeks, and photosensitivity.

OTHER CAUSES

Drugs

Various chemotherapeutic agents can directly produce stomatitis. Also, allergic reactions to penicillin, sulfonamides, gold, quinine, streptomycin, phenytoin, aspirin, and barbiturates commonly cause lesions to develop and erupt. Inhaled steroids used for pulmonary disorders can also cause oral lesions.

Treatments

Radiation therapy may cause oral lesions.

SPECIAL CONSIDERATIONS

If the patient's mouth ulcers are painful, provide a topical anesthetic such as lidocaine.

PEDIATRIC POINTERS

Causes of mouth ulcers in children include chickenpox, measles, scarlet fever, diphtheria, and hand-foot-and-mouth disease. In neonates, mouth ulcers can result from candidiasis or congenital syphilis.

GERIATRIC POINTERS

Ill-fitting dentures can cause irritation, leading to inflammation and ulcers (inflammatory fibrous hyperplasia).

PATIENT COUNSELING

Instruct the patient to avoid irritants, such as highly seasoned foods, citrus fruits, alcohol, tobacco, and foods that contain salt or vinegar. For mouth care, warn against using lemon-glycerin swabs because these can dry and irritate the lesions.

As appropriate, teach the patient proper oral hygiene. If toothbrushing is contraindicated, instruct him to use a mouth rinse, such as normal saline solution or half-strength hydrogen peroxide, and to avoid commercial mouthwashes that contain alcohol. Stress the importance of frequently changing to a new toothbrush. If the patient uses an inhaled steroid, instruct him to rinse his mouth after each use. Also tell him to report any mouth lesions that don't heal within 2 weeks.

MURMURS

Murmurs are auscultatory sounds heard within the heart chambers or major arteries. They're classified by their timing and duration in the cardiac cycle, auscultatory location, loudness, configuration, pitch, and quality. (See *Classifying murmurs.*)

Murmurs can reflect accelerated blood flow through normal or abnormal valves; forward blood flow through a narrowed or irregular valve or into a dilated vessel; blood backflow through an incompetent valve, septal defect, or patent ductus arteriosus; or decreased blood viscosity. Commonly the result of organic heart disease, murmurs occasionally may signal an emergency situation — for example, a loud holosystolic murmur after an acute myocardial infarction (MI) may signal papillary muscle rupture or ventricular septal defect. Murmurs may also result from surgical implantation of a prosthetic valve.

Some murmurs are innocent, or functional. An *innocent systolic murmur* is generally soft, medium-pitched, and loudest along the left sternal border at the second or third intercostal space. It's exacerbated by physical activity, excitement, fever, pregnancy, anemia, or thyrotoxicosis. (See *Detecting common congenital murmurs,* page 418.)

 EMERGENCY ACTIONS Although not usually a sign of an emergency, murmurs — especially newly developed ones — may signal a serious complication in patients with bacterial endocarditis or a recent acute MI. When caring for a patient with known or suspected bacterial endocarditis, carefully auscultate for any new murmurs. Their development along with crackles, distended jugular veins, orthopnea, and dyspnea may signal heart failure.

ASSESSMENT TIP

Classifying murmurs

After you've auscultated a murmur, determine its timing in the cardiac cycle, auscultatory location, loudness, configuration, pitch, and quality. Identifying these qualities will help you establish the type of murmur your patient has.

Timing can be characterized as systolic (between S_1 and S_2), holosystolic (continuous throughout systole), diastolic (between S_2 and S_1), or continuous throughout systole and diastole; systolic and diastolic murmurs can be further characterized as early, middle, or late.

Location refers to the area of maximum loudness, such as the apex, the lower left sternal border, or an intercostal space.

Loudness is graded on a scale of 1 to 6. A grade 1 murmur is very faint, detected only after careful auscultation. A grade 2 murmur is a soft, evident murmur. Murmurs considered to be grade 3 are moderately loud. A grade 4 murmur is a loud murmur with a possible intermittent thrill. Grade 5 murmurs are loud and associated with a palpable precordial thrill. Grade 6 murmurs are loud and, like grade 5 murmurs, are associated with a thrill. A grade 6 murmur is audible even when the stethoscope is lifted from the thoracic wall.

Configuration, or shape, refers to the nature of loudness — crescendo (grows louder), decrescendo (grows softer), crescendo-decrescendo (first rises, then falls), decrescendo-crescendo (first falls, then rises), plateau (even intensity), or variable (uneven intensity).

The murmur's *pitch* may be high or low. Its *quality* may be described as harsh, rumbling, blowing, scratching, buzzing, musical, or squeaking.

Key facts about murmurs

+ Auscultatory sounds heard within the heart chambers or major arteries
+ Classified by their timing and duration in the cardiac cycle, auscultatory location, loudness, configuration, pitch, and quality
+ Reflect accelerated, forward, or backward blood flow or decreased blood viscosity

In an emergency

In patients with bacterial endocarditis:
+ Auscultate for any new murmurs, which may signal heart failure if they develop along with crackles, distended jugular veins, orthopnea, and dyspnea.

In patients with recent acute MI:
+ Auscultate regularly.
+ Watch for signs of acute pulmonary edema.

Murmur characteristics

+ Timing — systolic, holosystolic, diastolic, or continuous
+ Location — area of maximum loudness
+ Loudness — scale of 1 to 6
+ Configuration — crescendo, decrescendo, plateau, or variable
+ Pitch — high or low
+ Quality — harsh, musical, or squeaking

Detecting common congenital murmurs

HEART DEFECT	TYPE OF MURMUR
Aortopulmonary septal defect	*Small defect:* a continuous rough or crackling murmur best heard at the upper left sternal border and below the left clavicle, possibly accompanied by a systolic ejection click. *Large defect:* a harsh systolic murmur heard at the left sternal border.
Atrial septal defect	A midsystolic, spindle-shaped murmur of grade II or III intensity heard at the upper left sternal border, with a fixed splitting of S_2. Large shunts may also produce a low- to medium-pitched early diastolic murmur over the lower left sternal border.
Bicuspid aortic valve	An early systolic, loud, high-pitched ejection sound or click that's best heard at the apex and is commonly accompanied by a soft, early or midsystolic murmur at the upper right sternal border. The aortic component of S_2 is usually accentuated at the apex. This murmur may not be recognized until early childhood.
Coarctation of the aorta	Usually a systolic ejection click at the base of the heart, at the apex, and occasionally over the carotid arteries, commonly accompanied by a systolic ejection murmur at the base. This disorder may also produce a blowing diastolic murmur of aortic insufficiency or an apical pansystolic murmur of unknown origin.
Ebstein's anomaly	A soft, high-pitched holosystolic blowing murmur that increases with inspiration (Carvallo's sign); best heard over the lower left sternal border and the xiphoid area; possibly accompanied by a low-pitched diastolic rumbling murmur at the apex. Fixed splitting of S_2 and a loud split S_4 also occur.
Patent ductus arteriosus	A continuous rough or crackling murmur best heard at the upper left sternal border and below the left clavicle. The murmur is accentuated late in systole.
Pulmonic stenosis	An early systolic, harsh, crescendo-decrescendo murmur of grades IV to VI intensity heard at the second left intercostal space, possibly radiating along the left sternal border.
Tetralogy of Fallot	A midsystolic murmur with a systolic thrill palpable at the left midsternal border; softer murmurs occurring earlier in systole generally indicate a more severe obstruction.
Ventricular septal defect	*Small defect:* usually a holosystolic (but may be limited to early or midsystole), grades II to IV decrescendo murmur heard along the lower left sternal border, accompanied by a normal S_2. *Large defect:* a holosystolic murmur at the lower left sternal border and a midsystolic rumbling murmur at the apex, accompanied by an increased S_1 at the lower left sternal border and an increased pulmonic component of S_2.

ASSESSMENT TIP

Identifying common murmurs

The timing and configuration of a murmur can help you identify its underlying cause. Learn to recognize the characteristics of these common murmurs.

AORTIC INSUFFICIENCY (CHRONIC)
Thickened valve leaflets fail to close correctly, permitting backflow of blood into the left ventricle.

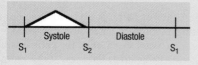

AORTIC STENOSIS
Thickened, scarred, or calcified valve leaflets impede ventricular systolic ejection.

MITRAL PROLAPSE
Incompetent mitral valve bulges into the left atrium because of an enlarged posterior leaflet and elongated chordae tendineae.

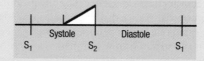

MITRAL INSUFFICIENCY (CHRONIC)
Incomplete mitral valve closure permits backflow of blood into the left atrium.

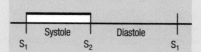

MITRAL STENOSIS
Thickened or scarred valve leaflets cause valve stenosis and restrict blood flow.

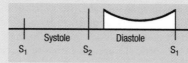

Regular auscultation is also important in a patient who has experienced an acute MI. A loud decrescendo holosystolic murmur at the apex that radiates to the axilla and left sternal border or throughout the chest is significant, particularly in association with a widely split S_2 and an atrial gallop (S_4). This murmur, when accompanied by signs of acute pulmonary edema, usually indicates the development of acute mitral insufficiency due to rupture of the chordae tendineae — a medical emergency.

HISTORY

If you discover a murmur, try to determine its type through careful auscultation. (See *Identifying common murmurs*.) Use the bell of your stethoscope for low-pitched murmurs; the diaphragm for high-pitched murmurs.

Next, obtain a patient history. Ask if the murmur is a new discovery or if it has been known since birth or childhood. Find out if the patient has experienced any associated symptoms, particularly palpitations, dizziness, syncope, chest pain, dyspnea, and fatigue. Explore the patient's medical history, noting especially any incidence of rheumatic fever, recent dental work, heart disease, or heart surgery, particularly prosthetic valve replacement.

Key history points
✦ Whether murmur is new or existing
✦ Associated symptoms, including palpitations, dizziness, syncope, chest pain, dyspnea, and fatigue
✦ Medical history, including any incidence of rheumatic fever, recent dental work, heart disease, or heart surgery

Critical assessment steps

✦ Note the presence of cardiac arrhythmias, jugular vein distention, dyspnea, orthopnea, and crackles.

Medical causes

Aortic insufficiency

✦ In acute form, a soft, short diastolic murmur is heard over the left sternal border.
✦ In chronic form, a high-pitched, blowing, decrescendo diastolic murmur is heard over the second or third right intercostal space or the left sternal border.

Aortic stenosis

✦ Murmur is systolic, harsh and grating, medium-pitched, and crescendo-decrescendo; it begins after S_1 and ends at or before aortic valve closure.

Cardiomyopathy (hypertrophic)

✦ A harsh late systolic murmur, ends at S_2; it's commonly accompanied by audible S_3 or S_4.

Mitral insufficiency

✦ Acute form produces medium-pitched blowing, early systolic or holosystolic decrescendo murmur at apex, along with a widely split S_2 and, commonly, S_4.
✦ Chronic form produces high-pitched, blowing, holosystolic plateau murmur that's loudest at apex and may radiate to axilla or back.

Mitral prolapse

✦ Midsystolic to late-systolic click with high-pitched late-systolic crescendo murmur occurs.

PHYSICAL ASSESSMENT

Perform a systematic physical assessment. Note especially the presence of cardiac arrhythmias, jugular vein distention, and such pulmonary signs and symptoms as dyspnea, orthopnea, and crackles. Is the patient's liver tender or palpable? Does he have peripheral edema?

MEDICAL CAUSES

Aortic insufficiency

Acute aortic insufficiency typically produces a soft, short diastolic murmur over the left sternal border that's best heard when the patient sits and leans forward and at the end of a forced held expiration. S_2 may be soft or absent. Sometimes, a soft, short midsystolic murmur may also be heard over the second right intercostal space. Associated findings include tachycardia, dyspnea, jugular vein distention, crackles, increased fatigue, and pale, cool extremities.

Chronic aortic insufficiency causes a high-pitched, blowing, decrescendo diastolic murmur that's best heard over the second or third right intercostal space or the left sternal border with the patient sitting, leaning forward, and holding his breath after deep expiration. An Austin Flint murmur—a rumbling, mid-to-late diastolic murmur best heard at the apex—may also occur. Findings include palpitations, tachycardia, angina, increased fatigue, dyspnea, orthopnea, and crackles.

Aortic stenosis

With aortic stenosis, the murmur is systolic, beginning after S_1 and ending at or before aortic valve closure. It's harsh and grating, medium-pitched, and crescendo-decrescendo. Loudest over the second right intercostal space when the patient is sitting and leaning forward, this murmur may also be heard at the apex, at the suprasternal notch (Erb's point), and over the carotid arteries.

If the patient has advanced disease, S_2 may be heard as a single sound, with inaudible aortic closure. An early systolic ejection click at the apex is typical but is absent when the valve is severely calcified. Associated signs and symptoms may include dizziness, syncope, dyspnea on exertion, paroxysmal nocturnal dyspnea, fatigue, and angina.

Cardiomyopathy (hypertrophic)

Hypertrophic cardiomyopathy generates a harsh late systolic murmur, ending at S_2. Best heard over the left sternal border and at the apex, the murmur is commonly accompanied by an audible S_3 or S_4. The murmur decreases with squatting and increases with sitting down. Major associated symptoms are dyspnea and chest pain; palpitations, dizziness, and syncope may also occur.

Mitral insufficiency

Acute mitral insufficiency is characterized by a medium-pitched blowing, early systolic or holosystolic decrescendo murmur at the apex, along with a widely split S_2 and commonly an S_4. This murmur doesn't get louder on inspiration as with tricuspid insufficiency. Associated findings typically include tachycardia and signs of acute pulmonary edema.

Chronic mitral insufficiency produces a high-pitched, blowing, holosystolic plateau murmur that's loudest at the apex and usually radiates to the axilla or back. Fatigue, dyspnea, and palpitations may also occur.

Mitral prolapse

Mitral prolapse generates a midsystolic to late-systolic click with a high-pitched late-systolic crescendo murmur, best heard at the apex. Occasionally, multiple clicks may be heard, with or without a systolic murmur. Associated findings include cardiac awareness, migraine headaches, dizziness, weakness, syncope, palpitations, chest pain, dyspnea, severe episodic fatigue, mood swings, and anxiety.

Mitral stenosis

With mitral stenosis, the murmur is soft, low-pitched, rumbling, crescendo-decrescendo, and diastolic, accompanied by a loud S_1 or an opening snap — a cardinal sign. It's best heard at the apex with the patient in the left lateral position. Mild exercise will help make this murmur audible.

With severe stenosis, the murmur of mitral insufficiency may also be heard. Other findings include hemoptysis, exertional dyspnea and fatigue, and signs of acute pulmonary edema.

Papillary muscle rupture

Papillary muscle rupture, a life-threatening complication of an acute MI, produces a loud holosystolic murmur that can be auscultated at the apex. Related findings include severe dyspnea, chest pain, syncope, hemoptysis, tachycardia, and hypotension.

Rheumatic fever with pericarditis

A pericardial friction rub along with murmurs and gallops is heard best with the patient leaning forward on his hands and knees during forced expiration. The most common murmurs heard in patients with rheumatic fever are the systolic murmur of mitral insufficiency, a midsystolic murmur due to swelling of the leaflet of the mitral valve, and the diastolic murmur of aortic insufficiency. Other signs and symptoms include fever, joint and sternal pain, edema, and tachypnea.

Tricuspid insufficiency

Tricuspid insufficiency is a valvular abnormality that's characterized by a soft, high-pitched, holosystolic blowing murmur that increases with inspiration (Carvallo's sign) and decreases with exhalation and Valsalva's maneuver. This murmur is best heard over the lower left sternal border and the xiphoid area. Following a lengthy period without symptoms, exertional dyspnea and orthopnea may develop, along with jugular vein distention, ascites, peripheral cyanosis and edema, muscle wasting, fatigue, weakness, and syncope.

Tricuspid stenosis

Tricuspid stenosis is a valvular disorder that produces a diastolic murmur similar to that of mitral stenosis, but louder with inspiration and decreased with exhalation and Valsalva's maneuver. S_1 may also be louder. Associated signs and symptoms include fatigue, syncope, peripheral edema, jugular vein distention, ascites, hepatomegaly, and dyspnea.

OTHER CAUSES

Treatments

Prosthetic valve replacement may cause variable murmurs, depending on the location, valve composition, and method of operation.

SPECIAL CONSIDERATIONS

Prepare the patient for diagnostic tests, such as electrocardiography, echocardiography, and angiography. Administer an antibiotic and an anticoagulant as appropriate.

Medical causes
(continued)

Mitral stenosis
+ Murmur is soft, low-pitched, rumbling, crescendo-decrescendo, and diastolic and is accompanied by loud S_1 or opening snap.
+ With severe stenosis, murmur of mitral insufficiency may also be heard.

Papillary muscle rupture
+ Loud holosystolic murmur can be auscultated at apex.

Rheumatic fever with pericarditis
+ Systolic murmur of mitral insufficiency, midsystolic murmur due to swelling of leaflet of mitral valve, and diastolic murmur of aortic insufficiency are common.

Tricuspid insufficiency
+ Soft, high-pitched, holosystolic blowing murmur increases with inspiration and decreases with exhalation and Valsalva's maneuver.

Tricuspid stenosis
+ A diastolic murmur similar to that of mitral stenosis, but louder with inspiration and decreased with exhalation and Valsalva's maneuver, is produced.

Other causes
+ Prosthetic valve replacement

Special considerations
+ Administer an antibiotic and an anticoagulant as appropriate.

Peds points

+ Innocent murmurs are commonly heard in young children.
+ Pathognomonic heart murmurs in infants and young children usually result from congenital heart disease.
+ Other murmurs can be acquired.

Teaching points

+ Possible need for prophylactic antibiotics before procedures or dental work

Key facts about muscle spasms

+ Involve strong, painful contractions of the muscle
+ Most commonly occur in the calf and foot

In an emergency

+ Attempt to elicit Chvostek's and Trousseau's signs.
+ Evaluate respiratory function.
+ Insert an I.V. line for administration of a calcium supplement.
+ Monitor cardiac status.

Key history points

+ Onset and description of spasms
+ Precipitating, alleviating, or aggravating factors
+ Associated weakness, sensory loss, or paresthesia
+ Drug and diet history

Critical assessment steps

+ Check muscle strength and tone.
+ Check all major muscle groups and note whether movements precipitate spasms.
+ Test peripheral pulses.
+ Examine limbs for color and temperature changes.

PEDIATRIC POINTERS

Innocent murmurs, such as Still's murmur, are commonly heard in young children and typically disappear in puberty. Pathognomonic heart murmurs in infants and young children usually result from congenital heart disease, such as atrial and ventricular septal defects. Other murmurs can be acquired, as with rheumatic heart disease.

PATIENT COUNSELING

Instruct the patient to contact his physician before undergoing invasive procedures or dental work because prophylactic antibiotics may be necessary. Because any cardiac abnormality is frightening to the patient, provide emotional support.

MUSCLE SPASMS

Muscle spasms, or muscle cramps, are strong, painful contractions. They can occur in virtually any muscle but are most common in the calf and foot. Muscle spasms typically occur from simple muscle fatigue, after exercise, and during pregnancy. However, they may also develop in electrolyte imbalances and neuromuscular disorders, or as the result of certain drugs. They're typically precipitated by movement, especially a quick or jerking movement, and can usually be relieved by slow stretching.

 EMERGENCY ACTIONS If the patient complains of frequent or unrelieved spasms in many muscles, accompanied by paresthesia in his hands and feet, quickly attempt to elicit Chvostek's and Trousseau's signs. If these signs are present, suspect hypocalcemia. Evaluate respiratory function, watching for the development of laryngospasm. Provide supplemental oxygen as necessary, and prepare to intubate the patient and provide mechanical ventilation. Draw blood for calcium and electrolyte levels and arterial blood gas analysis, and insert an I.V. line for administration of a calcium supplement. Monitor cardiac status, and prepare to begin resuscitation, if necessary.

HISTORY

If the patient isn't in distress, ask when the spasms began. Is there any particular activity that precipitates them? How long did they last? How painful were they? Did anything worsen or lessen the pain? Ask about other symptoms, such as weakness, sensory loss, or paresthesia. Obtain a thorough drug and diet history. Ask the patient if he has had recent vomiting or diarrhea.

PHYSICAL ASSESSMENT

Evaluate muscle strength and tone. Then check all major muscle groups and note whether any movements precipitate spasms. Test the presence and quality of all peripheral pulses, and examine the limbs for color and temperature changes. Test capillary refill time (normal is less than 3 seconds), and inspect for edema, especially in the involved area. Observe for signs and symptoms of dehydration such as dry mucous membranes. Finally, test reflexes and sensory function in all extremities.

MEDICAL CAUSES

Amyotrophic lateral sclerosis

With amyotrophic lateral sclerosis (ALS), muscle spasms may accompany progressive muscle weakness and atrophy that typically begin in one hand, spread to the arm, and then spread to the other hand and arm. Eventually, muscle weakness and atrophy affect the trunk, neck, tongue, larynx, pharynx, and legs; progressive respiratory muscle weakness leads to respiratory insufficiency. Other findings include muscle flaccidity progressing to spasticity, coarse fasciculations, hyperactive deep tendon reflexes, dysphagia, impaired speech, excessive drooling, and depression.

Arterial occlusive disease

Arterial occlusion typically produces spasms and intermittent claudication in the leg, with residual pain. Associated findings are usually localized to the legs and feet and include loss of peripheral pulses, pallor or cyanosis, decreased sensation, hair loss, dry or scaling skin, edema, and ulcerations.

Dehydration

Sodium loss may produce limb and abdominal cramps. Other findings in dehydration include a slight fever, decreased skin turgor, dry mucous membranes, tachycardia, orthostatic hypotension, muscle twitching, seizures, nausea, vomiting, and oliguria.

Fracture

Localized spasms and pain are mild if the fracture is nondisplaced, intense if it's severely displaced. Other findings include swelling, limited mobility and, possibly, bony crepitation.

Hypocalcemia

The classic feature of hypocalcemia is tetany — a syndrome of muscle cramps and twitching, carpopedal and facial muscle spasms, and seizures, possibly with stridor. Both Chvostek's and Trousseau's signs may be elicited. Related findings include paresthesia of the lips, fingers, and toes; choreiform movements; hyperactive deep tendon reflexes; fatigue; palpitations; and cardiac arrhythmias.

Hypothyroidism

Muscle involvement may produce spasms and stiffness, along with leg muscle hypertrophy or proximal limb weakness and atrophy. Other findings include forgetfulness and mental instability; fatigue; cold intolerance; dry, pale, cool, doughy skin; puffy face, hands, and feet; periorbital edema; dry, sparse, brittle hair; bradycardia; and weight gain despite anorexia.

Muscle trauma

Excessive muscle strain may cause mild to severe spasms. The injured area may be painful, swollen, reddened, or warm. The patient may report hearing a snapping sound at the time of injury.

Respiratory alkalosis

With respiratory alkalosis, acute onset of muscle spasms may be accompanied by twitching and weakness, carpopedal spasms, circumoral and peripheral paresthesia, vertigo, syncope, pallor, and extreme anxiety. With severe alkalosis, cardiac arrhythmias may occur.

Medical causes

ALS

+ Muscle spasms may accompany progressive muscle weakness and atrophy that typically begin in one hand and then spread.

Arterial occlusive disease

+ Spasms and intermittent claudication occur in the leg.

Dehydration

+ Limb and abdominal cramps and muscle twitching may occur.

Fracture

+ Localized spasms and pain are mild if fracture is nondisplaced; intense if severely displaced.

Hypocalcemia

+ Tetany occurs.

Hypothyroidism

+ Spasms and stiffness occur with leg muscle hypertrophy or proximal limb weakness and atrophy.

Muscle trauma

+ Excessive muscle strain may cause mild to severe spasms.

Respiratory alkalosis

+ Acute onset of muscle spasms may be accompanied by twitching and weakness, carpopedal spasms, circumoral and peripheral paresthesia, vertigo, syncope, pallor, and anxiety.

Medical causes
(continued)

Spinal injury or disease
✦ Resulting muscle spasms worsen with movement.

Other causes
✦ Corticosteroids, diuretics, and estrogens

Special considerations
✦ Help alleviate spasms by slowly stretching the affected muscle in the direction opposite the contraction.
✦ If necessary, administer a mild analgesic.

Peds points
✦ Muscle spasms may indicate hypoparathyroidism, osteomalacia, rickets or, rarely, congenital torticollis.

Teaching points
✦ Immobilization and wrapping the injured area
✦ Pain relief measures
✦ Use of assistive devices

Key facts about muscle spasticity
✦ State of excessive muscle tone manifested by increased resistance to stretching and heightened reflexes

In an emergency
If you suspect tetanus:
✦ Look for signs of respiratory distress; provide ventilatory support if necessary.
✦ Monitor the patient closely.

Spinal injury or disease

Muscle spasms can result from spinal injury, such as cervical extension injury or spinous process fracture, or from spinal disease such as infection. The patient may report that the muscle spasms worsen with movement.

OTHER CAUSES

Drugs

Common spasm-producing drugs include diuretics, corticosteroids, and estrogens.

SPECIAL CONSIDERATIONS

Depending on the cause, help alleviate your patient's spasms by slowly stretching the affected muscle in the direction opposite the contraction. If necessary, administer a mild analgesic.

Diagnostic studies may include serum calcium, sodium and carbon dioxide levels, thyroid function tests, and blood flow studies or arteriography.

PEDIATRIC POINTERS

Muscle spasms rarely occur in children. However, their presence may indicate hypoparathyroidism, osteomalacia, rickets or, rarely, congenital torticollis.

PATIENT COUNSELING

Teach the patient how to immobilize or wrap the injured area. Explain that taking analgesics and using treatments such as heat or cold can help relieve pain. If the patient requires traction or immobilization, suggest such diversionary activities as books, television, board games, and conversation. Demonstrate how to use assistive devices, if necessary.

MUSCLE SPASTICITY

Spasticity is a state of excessive muscle tone manifested by increased resistance to stretching and heightened reflexes. Also known as *muscle hypertonicity,* it's commonly detected by evaluating a muscle's response to passive movement; a spastic muscle offers more resistance when the passive movement is performed quickly. Caused by an upper-motor-neuron lesion, spasticity usually occurs in the arm and leg muscles. Long-term spasticity results in muscle fibrosis and contractures. (See *How spasticity develops.*)

 EMERGENCY ACTIONS Keep in mind that generalized spasticity and trismus in a patient with a recent skin puncture or laceration indicates tetanus. If you suspect this rare disorder, look for signs of respiratory distress. Provide ventilatory support, if necessary, and monitor the patient closely.

HISTORY

If you detect spasticity, ask the patient about its onset, duration, and progression. What, if any, events precipitate onset? Has he experienced other muscular changes or related symptoms? Does his medical history reveal any incidence of trauma or degenerative or vascular disease?

How spasticity develops

Motor activity is controlled by pyramidal and extrapyramidal tracts that originate in the motor cortex, basal ganglia, brain stem, and spinal cord. Nerve fibers from the various tracts converge and synapse at the anterior horn in the spinal cord. Together, they maintain segmental muscle tone by modulating the stretch reflex arc. This arc, shown in simplified form below, is basically a negative feedback loop in which muscle stretch (stimulation) causes reflexive contraction (inhibition), thus maintaining muscle length and tone.

Damage to certain tracts results in loss of inhibition and disruption of the stretch reflex arc. Uninhibited muscle stretch produces exaggerated, uncontrolled muscle activity, accentuating the reflex arc and eventually resulting in spasticity.

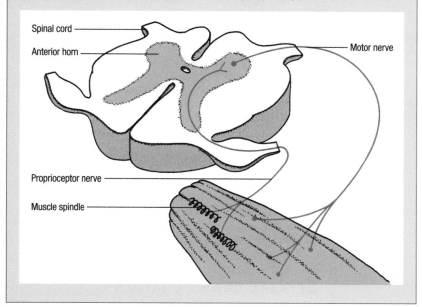

Spinal cord
Anterior horn
Motor nerve
Proprioceptor nerve
Muscle spindle

PHYSICAL ASSESSMENT

Take the patient's vital signs, and perform a complete neurologic assessment. Test reflexes and evaluate motor and sensory function in all limbs. Evaluate muscles for wasting and contractures.

MEDICAL CAUSES

Amyotrophic lateral sclerosis

Amyotrophic lateral sclerosis (ALS) commonly produces spasticity, spasms, coarse fasciculations, hyperactive deep tendon reflexes (DTRs), and a positive Babinski's sign. Earlier effects include progressive muscle weakness and flaccidity that typically begin in the hands and arms and eventually spread to the trunk, neck, larynx, pharynx, and legs. Progressive respiratory muscle weakness leads to respiratory insufficiency. Other findings include dysphagia, dysarthria, excessive drooling, and depression.

Epidural hemorrhage

Bilateral limb spasticity is a late and ominous sign of epidural hemorrhage. Other findings include a momentary loss of consciousness after head trauma, followed by

Key history points

+ Onset, duration, and progression of spasticity
+ Precipitating factors
+ Muscular changes or related symptoms
+ History of trauma or degenerative or vascular disease

Critical assessment steps

+ Take vital signs and perform a neurologic assessment.
+ Test reflexes and evaluate motor and sensory function in all limbs.
+ Evaluate muscles for wasting and contractures.

Medical causes

ALS

+ Spasticity, spasms, coarse fasciculations, hyperactive DTRs, and a positive Babinski's sign result.

Epidural hemorrhage

+ Bilateral limb spasticity is a late and ominous sign.

Medical causes
(continued)

Multiple sclerosis
+ Muscle spasticity, hyperreflexia, and contractures may eventually develop.
+ Progressive weakness and atrophy occur early.

Spinal cord injury
+ Spastic paralysis in the affected limbs follows initial flaccid paralysis.
+ Spasticity and muscle atrophy increase for up to 2 years after the injury, then gradually regress to flaccidity.

Stroke
+ Spastic paralysis may develop on the affected side following the acute stage.

Special considerations
+ Administer pain medication and an antispasmodic.
+ Passive ROM exercises, splinting, traction, and application of heat may help relieve spasms and prevent contractures.
+ Maintain a calm, quiet environment, and encourage bed rest.
+ In cases of prolonged, uncontrollable spasticity, nerve blocks or surgical transection may be necessary.

Peds points
+ In children, muscle spasticity may be a sign of cerebral palsy.

Teaching points
+ Use of assistive devices

a lucid interval and then a rapid deterioration in level of consciousness (LOC). The patient may also develop unilateral hemiparesis or hemiplegia; seizures; fixed, dilated pupils; high fever; decreased and bounding pulse; widened pulse pressure; elevated blood pressure; irregular respiratory pattern; and decerebrate posture. A positive Babinski's sign can be elicited.

Multiple sclerosis
Muscle spasticity, hyperreflexia, and contractures may eventually develop in patients with multiple sclerosis; earlier muscle changes include progressive weakness and atrophy. Associated signs and symptoms typically wax and wane and may include diplopia, blurring or loss of vision, nystagmus, sensory loss or paresthesia, dysarthria, dysphagia, incoordination, ataxic gait, intention tremors, emotional lability, impotence, and urinary dysfunction.

Spinal cord injury
Spasticity commonly results from cervical and high thoracic spinal cord injury, especially from incomplete lesions. Spastic paralysis in the affected limbs follows initial flaccid paralysis; typically, spasticity and muscle atrophy increase for up to 2 years after the injury, then gradually regress to flaccidity. Associated signs and symptoms vary with the level of injury but may include respiratory insufficiency or paralysis, sensory losses, bowel and bladder dysfunction, hyperactive DTRs, positive Babinski's sign, sexual dysfunction, priapism, hypotension, anhidrosis, and bradycardia.

Stroke
Spastic paralysis may develop on the affected side following the acute stage of a stroke. Associated findings vary with the site and extent of vascular damage and may include dysarthria, aphasia, ataxia, apraxia, agnosia, ipsilateral paresthesia or sensory loss, visual disturbance, altered LOC, amnesia and poor judgment, personality changes, emotional lability, bowel and bladder dysfunction, headache, vomiting, and seizures.

SPECIAL CONSIDERATIONS
Prepare the patient for diagnostic tests, which may include electromyography, muscle biopsy, or intracranial or spinal magnetic resonance imaging or computed tomography. Administer pain medication and an antispasmodic. Passive range-of-motion exercises, splinting, traction, and application of heat may help relieve spasms and prevent contractures. Maintain a calm, quiet environment to help relieve spasms and prevent recurrence, and encourage bed rest. In cases of prolonged, uncontrollable spasticity, as with spastic paralysis, nerve blocks or surgical transection may be necessary for permanent relief.

PEDIATRIC POINTERS
In children, muscle spasticity may be a sign of cerebral palsy.

PATIENT COUNSELING
Teach the patient how to use assistive devices to perform activities of daily living. Encourage him to be as independent as possible. Also encourage him to verbalize his feelings about changes in his body image and issues of control.

MUSCLE WEAKNESS

Muscle weakness is detected by observing and measuring the strength of an individual muscle or muscle group. It can result from a malfunction in the cerebral hemispheres, brain stem, spinal cord, nerve roots, peripheral nerves, or myoneural junctions and within the muscle itself. Muscle weakness occurs with certain neurologic, musculoskeletal, metabolic, endocrine, and cardiovascular disorders; as a response to certain drugs; and after prolonged immobilization.

HISTORY

Determine the location of the patient's muscle weakness. Ask if he has difficulty with specific movements such as rising from a chair. Find out when he first noticed the weakness; ask him whether it worsens with exercise or as the day progresses. Also ask about related symptoms, especially muscle or joint pain, altered sensory function, and fatigue.

Obtain a medical history, noting especially chronic disease such as hyperthyroidism; musculoskeletal or neurologic problems, including recent trauma; family history of chronic muscle weakness, especially in males; and alcohol and drug use.

PHYSICAL ASSESSMENT

Focus your physical assessment on evaluating muscle strength. Test all major muscles bilaterally. (See *Testing muscle strength,* pages 428 and 429.)

When testing, make sure the patient's effort is constant; if it isn't, suspect pain or other reluctance to make the effort. If the patient complains of pain, ease or discontinue testing and have him try the movements again. Remember that the patient's dominant arm, hand, and leg are somewhat stronger than their nondominant counterparts. Besides testing individual muscle strength, test for range of motion (ROM) at all major joints (shoulder, elbow, wrist, hip, knee, and ankle). Also test sensory function in the involved areas, and test deep tendon reflexes (DTRs) bilaterally.

MEDICAL CAUSES

Amyotrophic lateral sclerosis

Amyotrophic lateral sclerosis (ALS) typically begins with muscle weakness and atrophy in one hand that rapidly spread to the arm and then to the other hand and arm. Eventually, these effects spread to the trunk, neck, tongue, larynx, pharynx, and legs; progressive respiratory muscle weakness leads to respiratory insufficiency.

Brain tumor

Signs and symptoms of muscle weakness vary with the tumor's location and size. Associated findings include headache, vomiting, diplopia, decreased visual acuity, decreased level of consciousness (LOC), pupillary changes, decreased motor strength, hemiparesis, hemiplegia, diminished sensations, ataxia, seizures, and behavioral changes.

Guillain-Barré syndrome

With Guillain-Barré syndrome, rapidly progressive, symmetrical weakness and pain ascends from the feet to the arms and facial nerves and may progress to total motor paralysis and respiratory failure. Associated findings include sensory loss or paresthesia, muscle flaccidity, loss of DTRs, tachycardia or bradycardia, fluctuating hypertension and orthostatic hypotension, diaphoresis, bowel and bladder incontinence, facial diplegia, dysphagia, dysarthria, and hypernasality.

Key facts about muscle weakness

- Detected by observing and measuring the strength of an individual muscle or muscle group

Key history points

- Onset and location of weakness
- Aggravating factors
- Related symptoms, including muscle or joint pain, altered sensory function, and fatigue
- Medical history, including hyperthyroidism, musculoskeletal or neurologic problems, recent trauma, and family history of chronic muscle weakness
- Alcohol and drug use

Critical assessment steps

- Test major muscles bilaterally.
- Test for ROM at all major joints.
- Test sensory function in the involved areas.
- Test DTRs bilaterally.

Medical causes

ALS

- Muscle weakness and atrophy in one hand rapidly spread to the arm and then to the other hand and arm.

Brain tumor

- Weakness varies with the tumor's location and size.

Guillain-Barré syndrome

- Rapidly progressive, symmetrical weakness and pain ascends from the feet to the arms and facial nerves.

Testing muscle strength

Obtain an overall picture of your patient's motor function by testing strength in 10 selected muscle groups. Ask the patient to attempt normal range-of-motion movements against your resistance. If the muscle group is weak, vary the amount of resistance as needed to permit accurate assessment. If necessary, position the patient so his limbs don't have to resist gravity, and repeat the test.

ARM MUSCLES

Biceps. With your hand on the patient's hand, have him flex his forearm against your resistance. Watch for biceps contraction.

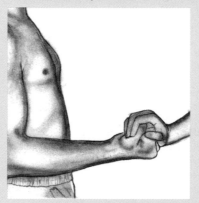

Triceps. Have the patient abduct and hold his arm midway between flexion and extension. Hold and support his arm at the wrist, and ask him to extend it against your resistance. Watch for triceps contraction.

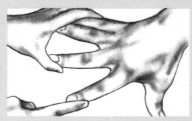

Dorsal interossei. Have the patient extend and spread his fingers, and tell him to try to resist your attempt to squeeze them together.

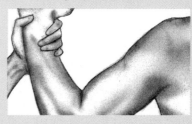

Deltoid. With the patient's arm fully extended, place one hand over his deltoid muscle and the other on his wrist. Ask him to abduct his arm to a horizontal position against your resistance; as he does so, palpate for deltoid contraction.

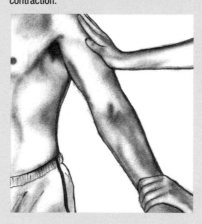

Forearm and hand (grip). Have the patient grasp your middle and index fingers and squeeze as hard as he can. To prevent pain or injury to the examiner, the examiner should cross his fingers.

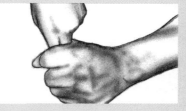

Rate muscle strength on a scale from 0 to 5:
0 = Total paralysis
1 = Visible or palpable contraction, but no movement
2 = Full muscle movement with force of gravity eliminated
3 = Full muscle movement against gravity, but no movement against resistance
4 = Full muscle movement against gravity; partial movement against resistance
5 = Full muscle movement against both gravity and resistance — normal strength.

LEG MUSCLES

Anterior tibial. With the patient's leg extended, place your hand on his foot and ask him to dorsiflex his ankle against your resistance. Palpate for anterior tibial contraction.

Extensor hallucis longus. With your finger on the patient's great toe, have him dorsiflex the toe against your resistance. Palpate for extensor hallucis contraction.

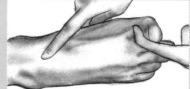

Quadriceps. Have the patient bend his knee slightly while you support his lower leg. Then ask him to extend the knee against your resistance; as he's doing so, palpate for quadriceps contraction.

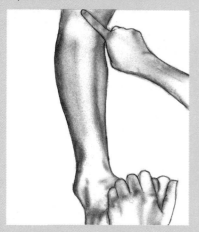

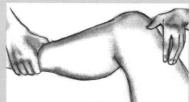

Psoas. While you support his leg, have the patient raise his knee and then flex his hip against your resistance. Watch for psoas contraction.

Gastrocnemius. With the patient on his side, support his foot and ask him to plantarflex his ankle against your resistance. Palpate for gastrocnemius contraction.

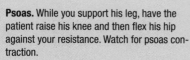

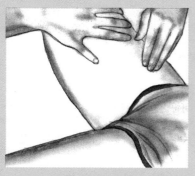

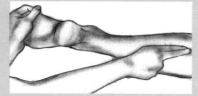

Medical causes
(continued)

Head trauma
◆ Varying degrees of muscle weakness occur.

Herniated disk
◆ Pressure on nerve roots from a herniated disk leads to muscle weakness, disuse and, ultimately, atrophy.

Hodgkin's lymphoma
◆ Muscle weakness may accompany painless, progressive lymphadenopathy.

Hypercortisolism
◆ Limb weakness and atrophy occur.

Hypothyroidism
◆ Reversible weakness and atrophy of proximal limb muscles may occur.

Multiple sclerosis
◆ Muscle weakness in one or more limbs may progress to atrophy, spasticity, and contractures.

Myasthenia gravis
◆ Gradually progressive skeletal muscle weakness and fatigue are the cardinal symptoms.

Osteoarthritis
◆ Progressive muscle disuse and weakness lead to atrophy.

Paget's disease
◆ Muscle weakness, paralysis, paresthesia, and pain may develop.

Head trauma
Severe head trauma can cause varying degrees of muscle weakness. Other findings include decreased LOC, otorrhea or rhinorrhea, raccoon eyes and Battle's sign, sensory disturbances, and signs of increased intracranial pressure.

Herniated disk
Pressure on nerve roots from a herniated disk leads to muscle weakness, disuse and, ultimately, atrophy. The primary symptom is severe low back pain, possibly radiating to the buttocks, legs, and feet — usually on one side. Diminished reflexes and sensory changes may also occur.

Hodgkin's lymphoma
With Hodgkin's lymphoma, muscle weakness may accompany the classic sign of painless, progressive lymphadenopathy. Other findings include paresthesia, fatigue, persistent fever, night sweats, and weight loss.

Hypercortisolism
Hypercortisolism may cause limb weakness and, eventually, atrophy. Related cushingoid features include buffalo hump, moon face, truncal obesity, purple striae, thin skin, acne, elevated blood pressure, fatigue, hyperpigmentation, easy bruising, poor wound healing, and diaphoresis. The male patient may be impotent; the female patient may exhibit hirsutism and menstrual irregularities.

Hypothyroidism
Reversible weakness and atrophy of proximal limb muscles may occur in hypothyroidism. Accompanying findings commonly include muscle cramps; cold intolerance; weight gain despite anorexia; mental dullness; dry, pale, doughy skin; puffy face, hands, and feet; impaired hearing and balance, and bradycardia.

Multiple sclerosis
With multiple sclerosis, muscle weakness in one or more limbs may progress to atrophy, spasticity, and contractures. Other findings typically wax and wane and may include diplopia and blurred vision, vision loss, nystagmus, hyperactive deep tendon reflexes, sensory loss or paresthesia, dysarthria, dysphagia, incoordination, ataxic gait, intention tremors, emotional lability, impotence, and urinary dysfunction.

Myasthenia gravis
Gradually progressive skeletal muscle weakness and fatigue are the cardinal symptoms of myasthenia gravis. Typically, weakness is mild upon awakening but worsens during the day. Early signs include weak eye closure, ptosis, and diplopia; a blank, masklike facies; difficulty chewing and swallowing; nasal regurgitation of fluid with hypernasality; and a hanging jaw and bobbing head. Respiratory muscle involvement may eventually lead to respiratory failure.

Osteoarthritis
Osteoarthritis is a chronic disorder that causes progressive muscle disuse and weakness that lead to atrophy. Other findings include crepitation; enlarged edematous joints; Heberden's nodes; increased pain in damp, cold weather; joint stiffness; limited range of motion; pain relieved by resting joints; and smooth, taunt, shiny skin.

Paget's disease

As Paget's disease progresses, muscle weakness or paralysis may develop, along with paresthesia and pain. The patient may also have bowed tibias, frequent fractures, and kyphosis.

Parkinson's disease

Muscle weakness accompanies rigidity in patients with Parkinson's disease. Related findings include a unilateral pill-rolling tremor, propulsive gait, dysarthria, bradykinesia, drooling, dysphagia, a masklike facies, and a high-pitched, monotonic voice.

Peripheral nerve trauma

Prolonged pressure on or injury to a peripheral nerve causes muscle weakness and atrophy. Other findings include paresthesia or sensory loss, pain, and loss of reflexes supplied by the damaged nerve.

Peripheral neuropathy

With peripheral neuropathy, muscle weakness progresses slowly to flaccid paralysis, generally affecting distal extremities first. It may be accompanied by loss of vibration sense; paresthesia, hyperesthesia, or anesthesia in the hands and feet; hypoactive or absent DTRs; mild to sharp burning pain; anhidrosis; and glossy red skin.

Potassium imbalance

With hypokalemia, temporary generalized muscle weakness may be accompanied by nausea, vomiting, diarrhea, decreased mentation, leg cramps, diminished reflexes, malaise, polyuria, dizziness, hypotension, and arrhythmias.

With hyperkalemia, weakness may progress to flaccid paralysis accompanied by irritability and confusion, hyperreflexia, paresthesia or anesthesia, oliguria, anorexia, nausea, diarrhea, abdominal cramps, tachycardia or bradycardia, and arrhythmias.

Rhabdomyolysis

Signs and symptoms of rhabdomyolysis include muscle weakness or pain, fever, nausea, vomiting, malaise, and dark urine. Acute renal failure due to renal structure obstruction and injury from the kidneys' attempt to filter the myoglobin from the bloodstream is a common complication.

Rheumatoid arthritis

With rheumatoid arthritis, symmetric muscle weakness may accompany increased warmth, swelling, and tenderness in involved joints; pain; and stiffness that restrict motion. These findings typically occur bilaterally.

Seizure disorder

Temporary generalized muscle weakness may occur after a generalized tonic-clonic seizure; other postictal findings include headache, muscle soreness, and profound fatigue. The patient may experience an aura before the seizure.

Spinal trauma and disease

Spinal trauma can cause severe muscle weakness, leading to flaccidity or spasticity and, eventually, paralysis. Infection, tumor, and cervical spondylosis or stenosis can also cause muscle weakness.

Stroke

Depending on the site and extent of damage, a stroke may produce contralateral or bilateral weakness of the arms, legs, face, and tongue, possibly progressing to hemiplegia and atrophy. Associated effects include dysarthria, aphasia, ataxia, apraxia,

Medical causes
(continued)

Thyrotoxicosis
+ Insidious, generalized muscle weakness and atrophy may occur.

Other causes
+ Aminoglycoside antibiotics (may worsen weakness in patients with myasthenia gravis)
+ Digoxin
+ Excessive doses of dantrolene.
+ Immobilization
+ Prolonged corticosteroid use

Special considerations
+ Provide assistive devices as necessary.
+ Protect patient from injury.
+ If sensory loss occurs, guard against pressure ulcer formation and thermal injury.
+ With chronic weakness, provide ROM exercises or splint limbs as necessary.
+ Allow for adequate rest periods.
+ Administer pain medications as needed.

Peds points
+ Muscular dystrophy is a major cause of muscle weakness in children.

Teaching points
+ Use of assistive devices
+ Importance of frequent position changes and rest periods

Key facts about mydriasis
+ Pupillary dilation caused by contraction of the dilator of the iris
+ May be a normal response to stimuli or drugs

agnosia, ipsilateral paresthesia or sensory loss, visual disturbance, altered level of consciousness, amnesia and poor judgment, personality changes, bowel and bladder dysfunction, headache, vomiting, and seizures.

Thyrotoxicosis
Thyrotoxicosis may produce insidious, generalized muscle weakness and atrophy. Other effects include anxiety, fatigue, heat intolerance, diaphoresis, tremors, tachycardia, palpitations, ventricular or atrial gallop, dyspnea, weight loss, an enlarged thyroid, and warm, flushed skin. Exophthalmos may be present.

OTHER CAUSES

Drugs
Generalized muscle weakness can result from prolonged corticosteroid use, digoxin, and excessive doses of dantrolene. Aminoglycoside antibiotics may worsen weakness in patients with myasthenia gravis.

Immobility
Immobilization in a cast, a splint, or traction can lead to muscle weakness in the involved extremity; prolonged bed rest or inactivity results in generalized muscle weakness.

SPECIAL CONSIDERATIONS
Provide assistive devices as necessary, and protect the patient from injury. If he has concomitant sensory loss, guard against pressure ulcer formation and thermal injury. With chronic weakness, provide ROM exercises or splint limbs as necessary. Arrange therapy sessions to allow for adequate rest periods, and administer pain medications as needed.

Prepare the patient for blood tests, muscle biopsy, electromyography, nerve conduction studies, and X-rays or computed tomography scans.

PEDIATRIC POINTERS
Muscular dystrophy, usually the Duchenne type, is a major cause of muscle weakness in children.

PATIENT COUNSELING
Teach the patient how to safely use assistive devices. Make sure he understands the importance of frequent position changes to reduce the risk of pressure ulcer formation. Encourage him to plan frequent rest periods throughout the day.

MYDRIASIS

Mydriasis — pupillary dilation caused by contraction of the dilator of the iris — is a normal response to decreased light, strong emotional stimuli, and topical administration of mydriatic and cycloplegic drugs. It can also result from ocular and neurologic disorders, eye trauma, and disorders that decrease level of consciousness (LOC). Mydriasis may be an adverse effect of antihistamines or other drugs.

HISTORY
Begin by asking the patient about any other eye problems, such as pain, blurring, diplopia, or visual field defects. Obtain a health history, focusing on eye or head

Grading pupil size

To ensure accurate evaluation of pupillary size, compare your patient's pupils to the scale shown at right. Keep in mind that maximum constriction may be less than 1 mm and maximum dilation greater than 9 mm.

1 MM	2 MM	3 MM
4 MM	5 MM	6 MM
7 MM	8 MM	9 MM

trauma, glaucoma and other ocular problems, and neurologic and vascular disorders. In addition, obtain a complete drug history.

PHYSICAL ASSESSMENT

Perform a thorough eye and pupil examination. Inspect and compare the pupils' size, color, and shape—many people normally have unequal pupils. (See *Grading pupil size*.) Also, test each pupil for light reflex, consensual response, and accommodation. Perform a swinging flashlight test to evaluate a decreased response to direct light coupled with a normal consensual response (Marcus Gunn pupil). Be sure to check the eyes for ptosis, swelling, and ecchymosis. Test visual acuity in both eyes with and without correction. Evaluate extraocular muscle function by checking the six cardinal fields of gaze.

CULTURAL CUE *When examining the eyes, keep in mind that not all cultures consider maintaining eye contact socially acceptable. For example, some Asian and Native American groups view eye contact as an invasion of privacy. The Navajo consider eye contact rude. Certain Indian cultures regard eye contact as an indicator of social status.*

Keep in mind that mydriasis appears in two ocular emergencies: acute angle-closure glaucoma and traumatic iridoplegia.

MEDICAL CAUSES

Aortic arch syndrome

Bilateral pupillary mydriasis commonly occurs late in aortic arch syndrome. Other ocular findings include visual blurring, transient vision loss, and diplopia. Related findings include dizziness and syncope; neck, shoulder, and chest pain; bruits; loss of radial and carotid pulses; paresthesia; and intermittent claudication. Blood pressure may be decreased in the arms.

Key history points

+ Associated pain, blurring, diplopia, visual field defects, or other eye problems
+ Health history, including eye or head trauma, glaucoma and other ocular problems, and neurologic and vascular disorders
+ Drug history

Critical assessment steps

+ Inspect and compare the pupils' size, color, and shape.
+ Test each pupil for light reflex, consensual response, and accommodation.
+ Perform a swinging flashlight test.
+ Check the eyes for ptosis, swelling, and ecchymosis.
+ Test visual acuity in both eyes with and without correction.
+ Check the six cardinal fields of gaze.

Medical causes

Aortic arch syndrome

+ Bilateral pupillary mydriasis commonly occurs late.
+ Visual blurring, transient vision loss, and diplopia may occur.

Medical causes
(continued)
Carotid artery aneurysm
+ Unilateral mydriasis may occur.

Glaucoma (acute angle-closure)
+ Moderate mydriasis and loss of pupillary reflex occur with excruciating pain, redness, decreased visual acuity, visual blurring, halo vision, conjunctival injection, and a cloudy cornea.

Oculomotor nerve palsy
+ Unilateral mydriasis is commonly the first sign.

Traumatic iridoplegia
+ Mydriasis and loss of pupillary reflex caused by paralysis of sphincter of iris is usually transient.

Other causes
+ Anesthesia induction
+ Anticholinergics, antihistamines, sympathomimetics, barbiturates (overdose), estrogens, and tricyclic antidepressants
+ Ocular surgery
+ Topical mydriatics and cycloplegics

Peds points
+ Mydriasis occurs in children as a result of ocular trauma, drugs, Adie's syndrome and, most commonly, increased ICP.

Teaching points
+ Effects of mydriatic drugs and coping mechanisms

Carotid artery aneurysm
With carotid artery aneurysm, unilateral mydriasis may be accompanied by bitemporal hemianopsia, decreased visual acuity, hemiplegia, decreased LOC, headache, aphasia, behavioral changes, and hypoesthesia.

Glaucoma (acute angle-closure)
Acute angle-closure glaucoma is an ocular emergency characterized by moderate mydriasis and loss of pupillary reflex in the affected eye, accompanied by abrupt onset of excruciating pain, redness, decreased visual acuity, visual blurring, halo vision, conjunctival injection, and a cloudy cornea. Without treatment, permanent blindness occurs in 2 to 5 days.

Oculomotor nerve palsy
Unilateral mydriasis is commonly the first sign of oculomotor nerve palsy. It's soon followed by ptosis, diplopia, decreased pupillary reflexes, exotropia, and complete loss of accommodation. Focal neurologic signs may accompany signs of increased intracranial pressure (ICP).

Traumatic iridoplegia
Eye trauma can paralyze the sphincter of the iris, causing mydriasis and loss of pupillary reflex; usually, this is transient. Associated findings include a quivering iris (iridodonesis), ecchymosis, pain, and swelling.

OTHER CAUSES
Drugs
Mydriasis can be caused by anticholinergics, antihistamines, sympathomimetics, barbiturates (overdose), estrogens, and tricyclic antidepressants; it also commonly occurs early in anesthesia induction. Topical mydriatics and cycloplegics, such as phenylephrine, atropine, homatropine, scopolamine, cyclopentolate, and tropicamide, are administered specifically for their mydriatic effects.

Surgery
Traumatic mydriasis commonly results from ocular surgery.

SPECIAL CONSIDERATIONS
Diagnostic tests may vary, depending on your findings, but may include a complete ophthalmologic examination and a thorough neurologic workup. Explain any diagnostic tests to the patient.

PEDIATRIC POINTERS
Mydriasis occurs in children as a result of ocular trauma, drugs, Adie's syndrome and, most commonly, increased ICP.

PATIENT COUNSELING
If the patient's mydriasis is the result of mydriatic drugs received during an eye examination, explain that he'll likely experience some photophobia and loss of accommodation. Instruct him to wear dark glasses and to avoid bright light, and reassure him that the condition is only temporary.

MYOCLONUS

Myoclonus — sudden, shocklike contractions of a single muscle or muscle group — occurs with various neurologic disorders and may herald onset of a seizure. These contractions may be isolated or repetitive, rhythmic or arrhythmic, symmetrical or asymmetrical, synchronous or asynchronous, and generalized or focal. They may be precipitated by bright flickering lights, a loud sound, or unexpected physical contact. *Intention myoclonus,* is evoked by intentional muscle movement.

Myoclonus occurs normally just before falling asleep and as a part of the natural startle reaction. It also occurs with some poisonings.

 EMERGENCY ACTIONS If you observe myoclonus, check for seizure activity. Take vital signs to rule out arrhythmias or a blocked airway. Have resuscitation equipment on hand. If the patient has a seizure, gently help him lie down. Place a pillow or a rolled-up towel under his head to prevent concussion. Loosen any constrictive clothing, especially around the neck, and turn his head (gently, if possible) to one side to prevent airway occlusion or aspiration of secretions.

HISTORY

If the patient is stable, evaluate level of consciousness (LOC) and mental status. Ask about the frequency, severity, location, and circumstances of myoclonus. Has he ever had a seizure? If so, did myoclonus precede it? Is the myoclonus ever precipitated by a sensory stimulus?

PHYSICAL ASSESSMENT

Check for muscle rigidity and wasting, and test deep tendon reflexes. Then complete the neurologic and musculoskeletal assessments.

MEDICAL CAUSES

Alzheimer's disease

Generalized myoclonus may occur in advanced stages of this slowly progressive dementia. Other late findings in Alzheimer's disease include mild choreoathetoid movements, muscle rigidity, bowel and bladder incontinence, delusions, and hallucinations.

Creutzfeldt-Jakob disease

Diffuse myoclonic jerks appear early in Creutzfeldt-Jakob disease — a rapidly progressive dementia. Initially random, they gradually become more rhythmic and symmetrical, typically occurring in response to sensory stimuli. Associated effects include ataxia, aphasia, hearing loss, muscle rigidity and wasting, fasciculations, hemiplegia, and vision disturbances or, possibly, blindness.

Encephalitis (viral)

With viral encephalitis, myoclonus is usually intermittent and either localized or generalized. Associated findings vary but may include rapidly decreasing LOC, fever, headache, irritability, nuchal rigidity, vomiting, seizures, aphasia, ataxia, hemiparesis, facial muscle weakness, nystagmus, ocular palsies, and dysphagia.

Encephalopathy

Hepatic encephalopathy occasionally produces myoclonic jerks in association with asterixis and focal or generalized seizures.

Medical causes
(continued)

Epilepsy
+ With idiopathic epilepsy, localized myoclonus usually occurs singly or in short bursts in an arm or leg upon awakening.
+ With myoclonic epilepsy, myoclonus is initially infrequent and localized but becomes more frequent and generalized over a period of months.

Other causes
+ Acute intoxication with methyl bromide, bismuth, or strychnine
+ Alcohol, opioid, or sedative withdrawal

Special considerations
+ If myoclonus is progressive, take seizure precautions.
+ Keep an oral airway and suction equipment at the bedside.
+ Pad side rails and remove potentially harmful objects.
+ Remain with the patient while he walks.
+ Give drugs that suppress myoclonus as needed.

Peds points
+ Myoclonus may result from subacute sclerosing panencephalitis, severe meningitis, progressive poliodystrophy, childhood myoclonic epilepsy, and encephalopathies.

Teaching points
+ Safety measures, especially for seizures
+ Referral to social service or community resources as needed

Hypoxic encephalopathy may produce generalized myoclonus or seizures almost immediately after restoration of cardiopulmonary function. The patient may also have a residual intention myoclonus.

Uremic encephalopathy commonly produces myoclonic jerks and seizures. Other signs and symptoms include apathy, fatigue, irritability, headache, confusion, gradually decreasing LOC, nausea, vomiting, oliguria, edema, and papilledema. The patient may also exhibit elevated blood pressure, dyspnea, arrhythmias, and abnormal respirations.

Epilepsy

With idiopathic epilepsy, localized myoclonus is usually confined to an arm or leg and occurs singly or in short bursts, usually upon awakening. It's usually more frequent and severe during the prodromal stage of a major generalized seizure, after which it diminishes in frequency and intensity.

Myoclonic jerks are usually the first signs of myoclonic epilepsy, the most common cause of progressive myoclonus. At first, myoclonus is infrequent and localized, but over a period of months, it becomes more frequent and involves the entire body, disrupting voluntary movement (intention myoclonus). As the disease progresses, myoclonus is accompanied by generalized seizures and dementia.

OTHER CAUSES

Drug withdrawal

Myoclonus may be seen in patients with alcohol, opioid, or sedative withdrawal, or delirium tremens.

Poisoning

Acute intoxication with methyl bromide, bismuth, or strychnine may produce an acute onset of myoclonus and confusion.

SPECIAL CONSIDERATIONS

If your patient's myoclonus is progressive, take seizure precautions. Keep an oral airway and suction equipment at his bedside, and pad the side rails. Because myoclonus may cause falls, remove potentially harmful objects from the patient's environment, and remain with him while he walks.

As needed, administer drugs that suppress myoclonus: ethosuximide, L-5-hydroxytryptophan, phenobarbital, clonazepam, or carbidopa. An EEG may be needed to evaluate myoclonus and related brain activity.

PEDIATRIC POINTERS

Although myoclonus is relatively uncommon in infants and children, it can result from subacute sclerosing panencephalitis, severe meningitis, progressive poliodystrophy, childhood myoclonic epilepsy, and encephalopathies such as Reye's syndrome.

PATIENT COUNSELING

Instruct the patient and his family about the need for safety and seizure precautions. Discuss with the family safety measures to perform during a seizure. Provide support to the family and caregivers during end-stage Alzheimer's disease and encephalopathy. Educate them about the disease involved, and refer them to social service and community resources as needed.

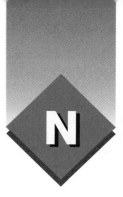

NASAL OBSTRUCTION

Nasal obstruction may result from an allergic, inflammatory, neoplastic, endocrine, or metabolic disorder; a structural abnormality; a traumatic injury; or a mechanical obstruction (foreign objects). It may cause discomfort, alter a person's sense of taste and smell, and cause voice changes. Although a common and typically benign symptom, nasal obstruction may herald certain life-threatening disorders, such as a basilar skull fracture or malignant tumor.

HISTORY

Begin the history by asking the patient about the duration and frequency of the obstruction. Did it begin suddenly or gradually? Is it intermittent or persistent? Unilateral or bilateral? Inquire about the presence and character of drainage. Is it watery, purulent, or bloody? Does the patient have nasal or sinus pain or headaches? Ask about recent travel, the use of drugs or alcohol, and previous trauma or surgery.

PHYSICAL ASSESSMENT

Examine the patient's nose; assess airflow and the condition of the turbinates and nasal septum. Evaluate the orbits for any evidence of dystopia, decreased vision, excess tearing, or abnormal appearance of the eye. Palpate over the frontal and maxillary sinuses for tenderness. Examine the ears for signs of middle ear effusions. Inspect the oral cavity, pharynx, nasopharynx, and larynx to detect inflammation, ulceration, excessive mucosal dryness, and neurologic deficits. Last, palpate the neck for adenopathy.

MEDICAL CAUSES

Basilar skull fracture
A tear in the dura can lead to cerebrospinal rhinorrhea, which increases when the patient lowers his head. Associated findings may include epistaxis, otorrhea, and a bulging tympanic membrane from blood or fluid. A fracture may also cause headache, facial paralysis, nausea, vomiting, impaired eye movement, ocular deviation, vision and hearing loss, depressed level of consciousness, Battle's sign, and raccoon eyes.

Common cold
Onset of the common cold is typified by a watery discharge along with sneezing and nasal obstruction. Edema of the nasal mucosa may lead to sinus pain and in-

Key facts about nasal obstruction
♦ Typically benign, but may cause discomfort or voice changes or alter sense of taste and smell

Key history points
♦ Onset, duration, frequency, and description of obstruction
♦ Associated drainage, sinus pain, or headaches
♦ Drug and alcohol use
♦ Previous trauma or surgery
♦ Recent travel

Critical assessment steps
♦ Assess airflow.
♦ Palpate over the frontal and maxillary sinuses for tenderness.
♦ Examine the ears for effusions.
♦ Inspect the oral cavity.
♦ Palpate the neck for adenopathy.

Medical causes
Basilar skull fracture
♦ A tear in the dura can lead to cerebrospinal rhinorrhea.

Common cold
♦ Watery discharge, sneezing, and nasal obstruction occur.

Medical causes
(continued)

Hypothyroidism
✦ Vascular dilation in the nasal mucosa may occur, resulting in nasal obstruction.

Nasal deformities
✦ A deviated nasal septum may cause nasal obstruction.
✦ A perforated nasal septum may cause a sensation of nasal congestion due to altered air flow.

Nasal fracture
✦ Mucosal swelling, epistaxis, abscess, or a septal deviation caused by trauma results in nasal obstruction.

Nasal polyps
✦ Nasal obstruction, anosmia, and clear, watery drainage develop.

Nasal tumors
✦ Nasal obstruction, rhinorrhea, epistaxis, pain, foul discharge, and cheek swelling may occur.

Nasopharyngeal tumors
✦ Nasal obstruction, rhinorrhea, epistaxis, otitis media, and nasal speech may occur.

Pregnancy
✦ High estrogen levels may cause vascular engorgement of the mucosa, resulting in obstruction.

Rhinitis
✦ Nasal obstruction and watery discharge occur in allergic and vasomotor rhinitis; obstruction is chronic in atrophic rhinitis.

fection as well as loss of smell and taste. Related findings include sore throat, malaise, myalgia, arthralgia, and mild headache.

Hypothyroidism
An underactive thyroid gland may lead to a generalized hypoactive state. This can lead to vascular dilation in the nasal mucosa, resulting in nasal obstruction. Associated findings include fatigue, weight gain despite anorexia, cold intolerance, facial edema, impaired memory, brittle hair, thick skin and tongue, bradycardia, and a hoarse voice.

Nasal deformities
Deviation of the nasal septum may cause unilateral or bilateral nasal obstruction, snoring, and postnasal drip. Perforation of the nasal septum may result in a sensation of nasal congestion due to altered air flow.

Nasal fracture
Nasal obstruction develops because of trauma that results in nasal mucosal swelling, epistaxis, abscess, or a septal deviation. Periorbital ecchymoses and edema, nasal deformity and pain, and crepitation of the nasal bones may also occur.

Nasal polyps
The most common signs and symptoms of nasal polyps are nasal obstruction, anosmia, and clear, watery drainage. The patient may have a history of allergies, chronic sinusitis, trauma, cystic fibrosis, or asthma. Translucent, pear-shaped polyps that are unilateral or bilateral occur.

Nasal tumors
Benign and malignant nasal tumors may cause unilateral or bilateral nasal obstruction, rhinorrhea, epistaxis, pain, foul discharge, and cheek swelling. Most of these tumors are benign papillomas and minor salivary gland tumors; malignant ones are rare. Kaposi's sarcoma of the nose may occur in acquired immunodeficiency syndrome.

Nasopharyngeal tumors
Benign and malignant tumors of the nasopharynx may cause nasal obstruction, rhinorrhea, epistaxis, otitis media, and nasal speech. Tumors usually reach a considerable size before symptoms develop. Cancer of the nasopharynx is the most common malignancy of the nasopharynx and may present first with a neck mass or conductive hearing loss.

Pregnancy
High levels of estrogen during pregnancy may cause vascular engorgement of the nasal mucosa, resulting in nasal obstruction. Associated findings include clear or blood-tinged drainage, sneezing, and edematous and bluish turbinates.

Rhinitis
Allergic rhinitis produces intermittent watery discharge and nasal obstruction. Common signs and symptoms include sneezing, increased lacrimation, decreased sense of smell, postnasal drip, and itching of the eyes, nose, or ears. The mucosa is edematous and pale.

Vasomotor rhinitis produces a profuse watery nasal discharge in addition to nasal obstruction. Sneezing, postnasal drip, and swollen turbinates occur as well.

With atrophic rhinitis, nasal obstruction is chronic and continuous. Associated findings include intermittent, purulent drainage, foul drainage odor, and nasal crusts that bleed on removal. The mucosa is pale pink and shiny.

Sinusitis

With acute sinusitis, the usual findings are marked nasal obstruction along with thick, purulent drainage and severe pain over the involved sinuses. Fever, inflamed nasal mucosa with purulent mucus, and facial tenderness and pressure occur.

With chronic sinusitis, nasal obstruction can be persistent or recurrent. Thick, intermittently purulent rhinorrhea and low-grade discomfort over the involved sinuses are also seen.

Chronic fungal sinusitis is clinically similar to chronic bacterial sinusitis. However, in immunocompromised patients the disease may rapidly progress to proptosis, blindness, and death.

OTHER CAUSES

Drugs

Topical nasal vasoconstrictors may cause rebound rhinorrhea and nasal obstruction if used longer than 5 days. Antihypertensives may cause nasal congestion as well.

Surgery

Nasal obstruction may occur after sinus or cranial surgery or even after rhinoplasty.

SPECIAL CONSIDERATIONS

Prepare the patient for X-rays or computed tomography scans of the nose, sinuses, or skull. Promote fluid intake to thin secretions as needed. Give an antihistamine, a decongestant, an analgesic, or an antipyretic.

PEDIATRIC POINTERS

Acute nasal obstruction in children commonly results from the common cold. In infants and children, especially between ages 3 and 6, chronic nasal obstruction typically results from large adenoids. In neonates, choanal atresia is the most common congenital cause of nasal obstruction and can be unilateral or bilateral. Cystic fibrosis may cause nasal polyps in children, resulting in nasal obstruction. However, if the child has unilateral nasal obstruction and rhinorrhea, you should assume that a foreign body is in the nose until proven otherwise.

PATIENT COUNSELING

Tell the patient not to use over-the-counter nasal vasoconstrictor sprays for more than 5 days. If the patient requires nasal surgery, advise him to limit such activities, as bending at the waist, exercising vigorously, and sneezing with his mouth open.

NAUSEA

Nausea is a sensation of profound revulsion to food or of impending vomiting. Commonly accompanied by such autonomic signs as hypersalivation, diaphoresis, tachycardia, pallor, and tachypnea, it's closely associated with both anorexia and vomiting.

Nausea, a common symptom of GI disorders, also occurs with fluid and electrolyte imbalance; infection; and metabolic, endocrine, labyrinthine, and cardiac disorders; and as a result of drug therapy, surgery, and radiation. Nausea is commonly present during the first trimester of pregnancy. It may also arise from severe

Medical causes
(continued)

Sinusitis
+ Acute sinusitis produces marked nasal obstruction.
+ Chronic sinusitis produces persistent or recurrent nasal obstruction.

Other causes
+ Antihypertensives
+ Rhinoplasty
+ Sinus or cranial surgery
+ Topical nasal vasoconstrictors

Special considerations
+ Promote fluid intake as needed.
+ Give an antihistamine, a decongestant, an analgesic, or an antipyretic.

Peds points
+ Acute nasal obstruction in children commonly results from the common cold; chronic obstruction typically results from large adenoids.
+ In neonates, choanal atresia is the most common congenital cause of nasal obstruction.
+ Cystic fibrosis may cause nasal polyps, resulting in obstruction.

Teaching points
+ Proper use of OTC nasal vasoconstrictor sprays
+ Activity restrictions (for those requiring surgery)

Key facts about nausea
+ Involves a sensation of profound revulsion to food or of impending vomiting

Key history points

+ Onset and description of nausea
+ Aggravating or alleviating factors
+ Medical history, including GI, endocrine, and metabolic disorders; cancer; and infections
+ Associated vomiting, abdominal pain, changes in bowel habits, or other complaints
+ Drug and alcohol use
+ Possibility of pregnancy

Critical assessment steps

+ Inspect for abdominal distention, auscultate for bowel sounds and bruits, palpate for rigidity and tenderness, and test for rebound tenderness.
+ Palpate and percuss the liver.

Medical causes

Adrenal insufficiency
+ Nausea, vomiting, anorexia, and diarrhea are common.

Anthrax (GI)
+ Initial signs and symptoms include nausea, vomiting, loss of appetite, and fever.

Appendicitis
+ A brief period of nausea may accompany onset of abdominal pain.

Cholecystitis (acute)
+ Nausea typically follows severe right-upper-quadrant pain that may radiate to the back or shoulders, commonly after meals.

Cholelithiasis
+ Nausea accompanies severe right-upper-quadrant or epigastric pain after eating fatty foods.

pain, anxiety, alcohol intoxication, overeating, or ingestion of distasteful food or liquids.

HISTORY

Begin by obtaining a complete medical history. Focus on GI, endocrine, and metabolic disorders; recent infections; and cancer and its treatment. Ask about drug use and alcohol consumption. If the patient is a female of childbearing age, ask if she is or could be pregnant. Have the patient describe the onset, duration, and intensity of the nausea as well as what causes or relieves it. Ask about related complaints, particularly vomiting (color, amount), abdominal pain, anorexia and weight loss, changes in bowel habits or stool character, excessive belching or flatus, and a sensation of bloating.

PHYSICAL ASSESSMENT

Inspect the skin for jaundice, bruises, and spider angiomas, and assess skin turgor. Next, inspect the abdomen for distention, auscultate for bowel sounds and bruits, palpate for rigidity and tenderness, and test for rebound tenderness. Palpate and percuss the liver for enlargement. Assess other body systems as appropriate.

MEDICAL CAUSES

Adrenal insufficiency
Common GI findings in adrenal insufficiency include nausea, vomiting, anorexia, and diarrhea. Other findings include weakness, fatigue, weight loss, bronze skin, hypotension, vitiligo, depression, and a weak, irregular pulse.

Anthrax (GI)
Initial signs and symptoms of GI anthrax include nausea, vomiting, loss of appetite, and fever. Signs and symptoms may progress to abdominal pain, severe bloody diarrhea, and hematemesis.

Appendicitis
With acute appendicitis, a brief period of nausea may accompany onset of abdominal pain. Pain typically begins as vague epigastric or periumbilical discomfort and rapidly progresses to severe stabbing pain localized in the right lower quadrant (McBurney's sign). Associated findings usually include abdominal rigidity and tenderness, cutaneous hyperalgesia, fever, constipation or diarrhea, tachycardia, anorexia, moderate malaise, and positive psoas (increased abdominal pain occurs when the examiner places his hand above the patient's right knee and the patient flexes his right hip against resistance) and obturator signs (internal rotation of the right leg with the leg flexed to 90 degrees at the hip and knee with a resulting tightening of the internal obturator muscle that causes abdominal discomfort).

Cholecystitis (acute)
With acute cholecystitis, nausea typically follows severe right-upper-quadrant pain that may radiate to the back or shoulders, commonly following meals. Associated findings include mild vomiting, flatulence, abdominal tenderness and, possibly, rigidity and distention, fever with chills, diaphoresis, and a positive Murphy's sign.

Cholelithiasis
With cholelithiasis, nausea accompanies attacks of severe right-upper-quadrant or epigastric pain after ingestion of fatty foods. Other associated findings include vomiting, abdominal tenderness and guarding, flatulence, belching, epigastric

burning, tachycardia, and restlessness. Occlusion of the common bile duct may cause jaundice, clay-colored stools, fever, and chills.

Cirrhosis

Insidious early signs and symptoms of cirrhosis typically include nausea and vomiting, anorexia, abdominal pain, and constipation or diarrhea. As the disease progresses, jaundice and hepatomegaly may occur with abdominal distention, spider angiomas, palmar erythema, severe pruritus, dry skin, fetor hepaticus, enlarged superficial abdominal veins, mental changes, and bilateral gynecomastia and testicular atrophy or menstrual irregularities.

Diverticulitis

Besides nausea, diverticulitis causes intermittent crampy abdominal pain, constipation or diarrhea, low-grade fever and, in many cases, a palpable, tender, firm, fixed mass. Signs and symptoms may also include anorexia, bloody stools, and flatulence.

Electrolyte imbalances

Electrolyte imbalances such as hyponatremia or hypernatremia, hypokalemia, and hypercalcemia commonly cause nausea and vomiting. Other effects include cardiac arrhythmias, tremors or seizures, anorexia, malaise, and weakness.

Escherichia coli 0157:H7

Signs and symptoms of *E. coli* 0157:H7 include nausea, watery or bloody diarrhea, vomiting, fever, and abdominal cramps. In children under age 5 and in elderly people, hemolytic uremic syndrome may develop, which may ultimately lead to acute renal failure.

Gastritis

Nausea is common with gastritis, especially after ingestion of alcohol, aspirin, spicy foods, or caffeine. Vomiting of mucus or blood, epigastric pain, belching, fever, and malaise may also occur.

Gastroenteritis

Usually viral, gastroenteritis causes nausea, vomiting, diarrhea, and abdominal cramping. Fever, malaise, hyperactive bowel sounds, abdominal pain and tenderness, and possible dehydration and electrolyte imbalances may also develop.

Heart failure

Heart failure may produce nausea and vomiting, particularly with right-sided heart failure. Associated findings include tachycardia, ventricular gallop, profound fatigue, dyspnea, crackles, peripheral edema, jugular vein distention, ascites, nocturia, and diastolic hypertension.

Hepatitis

Nausea is an insidious early symptom of viral hepatitis. Vomiting, fatigue, myalgia and arthralgia, headache, anorexia, photophobia, pharyngitis, cough, and fever also occur early in the preicteric phase.

Hyperemesis gravidarum

In hyperemesis gravidarum, unremitting nausea and vomiting that persist beyond the first trimester of pregnancy are characteristic. Vomitus ranges from undigested food, mucus, and bile in the early stages of the disorder to a coffee-ground appearance in later stages. Associated findings include weight loss, signs of dehydration, headache, and delirium.

Medical causes
(continued)

Cirrhosis
+ Nausea and vomiting, anorexia, abdominal pain, and constipation or diarrhea occur.

Diverticulitis
+ Nausea, intermittent crampy abdominal pain, constipation or diarrhea, low-grade fever and, in many cases, a palpable, fixed mass occur.

Electrolyte imbalances
+ Nausea and vomiting occur with cardiac arrhythmias, tremors or seizures, anorexia, malaise, and weakness.

E. coli 0157:H7
+ Nausea, watery or bloody diarrhea, vomiting, fever, and abdominal cramps occur.

Gastritis
+ Nausea is common, especially after ingestion of alcohol, aspirin, spicy foods, or caffeine.

Gastroenteritis
+ Nausea, vomiting, diarrhea, and abdominal cramping occur.

Heart failure
+ Nausea and vomiting may occur, particularly with right-sided heart failure.

Hepatitis
+ Nausea is an early symptom.

Hyperemesis gravidarum
+ Unremitting nausea and vomiting persist beyond the first trimester of pregnancy.

Medical causes
(continued)

Inflammatory bowel disease
✦ Nausea, vomiting, abdominal pain, and anorexia may occur.

Intestinal obstruction
✦ Nausea, vomiting, constipation, and abdominal pain.

Irritable bowel syndrome
✦ Nausea, dyspepsia, and abdominal distention may result, especially with increased stress.

Labyrinthitis
✦ Nausea and vomiting occur with vertigo, progressive hearing loss, nystagmus, and tinnitus.

Lactose intolerance
✦ Nausea, diarrhea, cramps, bloating, and gas occur after eating dairy products.

Ménière's disease
✦ Sudden, brief, recurrent attacks of nausea, vomiting, vertigo, tinnitus, and nystagmus occur.

Metabolic acidosis
✦ Nausea, vomiting, anorexia, diarrhea, Kussmaul's respirations, and decreased LOC may develop.

Migraine headache
✦ Nausea and vomiting may occur.

Motion sickness
✦ Nausea and vomiting are brought on by motion.

Myocardial infarction
✦ Nausea and vomiting may occur.
✦ Severe substernal chest pain that may radiate.

Inflammatory bowel disease
The most common symptom of inflammatory bowel disease is recurrent diarrhea with blood, pus, and mucus. Nausea, vomiting, abdominal pain, and anorexia may also occur. The patient may report abdominal cramps and spasms after meals.

Intestinal obstruction
Nausea commonly occurs, especially with high small-intestinal obstruction. Vomiting may be bilious or fecal; abdominal pain is usually episodic and colicky but can become severe and steady with strangulation. Constipation occurs early in large-intestinal obstruction and later in small-intestinal obstruction; obstipation may signal complete obstruction. Bowel sounds are typically hyperactive in partial obstruction and hypoactive or absent in complete obstruction. Abdominal distention and tenderness occur, possibly with visible peristaltic waves and a palpable abdominal mass.

Irritable bowel syndrome
Nausea, dyspepsia, and abdominal distention may occur with irritable bowel syndrome, especially during periods of increased stress. Other findings include lower abdominal pain and abdominal tenderness, which is generally relieved by moving the bowels; diurnal diarrhea alternating with constipation or normal bowel function; and small stools with visible mucus and a feeling of incomplete evacuation.

Labyrinthitis
Nausea and vomiting commonly occur with labyrinthitis (acute inner ear inflammation). More significant findings in this disorder include severe vertigo, progressive hearing loss, nystagmus, tinnitus and, possibly, otorrhea.

Lactose intolerance
Depending on the individual, signs and symptoms of lactose intolerance may include nausea, diarrhea, cramps, bloating, and gas that occurs after eating dairy products. Borborygmi may be heard on auscultation.

Ménière's disease
Ménière's disease causes sudden, brief, recurrent attacks of nausea, vomiting, vertigo, tinnitus, diaphoresis, and nystagmus. It also causes hearing loss and ear fullness.

Metabolic acidosis
Metabolic acidosis is an acid-base imbalance that may produce nausea and vomiting, anorexia, diarrhea, Kussmaul's respirations, and decreased level of consciousness. The patient may also exhibit central nervous system depression, drowsiness, lethargy, and stupor.

Migraine headache
Nausea and vomiting may occur in the prodromal stage, along with photophobia, light flashes, increased sensitivity to noise, light-headedness and, possibly, partial vision loss and paresthesia of the lips, face, and hands.

Motion sickness
With motion sickness, nausea and vomiting are brought on by motion or rhythmic movement. Headache, dizziness, fatigue, diaphoresis, hypersalivation, and dyspnea may also occur.

Myocardial infarction
Nausea and vomiting may occur, but the cardinal symptom of myocardial infarction is severe substernal chest pain that may radiate to the left arm, jaw, or neck.

Dyspnea, pallor, clammy skin, diaphoresis, altered blood pressure, and arrhythmias also occur.

Pancreatitis (acute)

Nausea, usually followed by vomiting, is an early symptom of pancreatitis. Other common findings include steady, severe pain in the epigastrium or left upper quadrant that may radiate to the back; abdominal tenderness and rigidity; anorexia; diminished bowel sounds; and fever. Tachycardia, restlessness, hypotension, skin mottling, and cold, sweaty extremities may occur in severe cases.

Peptic ulcer

With a peptic ulcer, nausea and vomiting may follow attacks of sharp or gnawing, burning epigastric pain. Attacks typically occur when the stomach is empty or after ingesting alcohol, caffeine, or aspirin; they're relieved by eating food or taking an antacid or an antisecretory. Hematemesis or melena may also occur.

Peritonitis

Nausea and vomiting usually accompany acute abdominal pain localized to the area of inflammation. Other findings in peritonitis include high fever with chills; tachycardia; hypoactive or absent bowel sounds; abdominal distention, rigidity, and tenderness (including rebound tenderness); positive obturator sign and obturator weakness; pale, cold skin; diaphoresis; hypotension; shallow respirations; and hiccups.

Preeclampsia

Nausea and vomiting commonly occur with this disorder of pregnancy, along with rapid weight gain, epigastric pain, oliguria, severe frontal headache, hyperreflexia, and blurred or double vision. The classic diagnostic triad of signs includes hypertension, proteinuria, and edema.

Renal and urologic disorders

Cystitis, pyelonephritis, calculi, uremia, and other disorders of the renal system can cause nausea. Related findings reflect the specific disorder.

Rhabdomyolysis

Signs and symptoms of rhabdomyolysis include nausea, vomiting, fever, malaise, and dark urine. The patient may also report tenderness, swelling, and muscle weakness that's caused by muscle trauma and pressure.

Thyrotoxicosis

With thyrotoxicosis, nausea and vomiting may accompany the classic findings of severe anxiety, heat intolerance, weight loss despite increased appetite, diaphoresis, diarrhea, tremor, tachycardia, and palpitations. Other signs include exophthalmos, ventricular or atrial gallop, and an enlarged thyroid gland.

OTHER CAUSES

Drugs

Common nausea-producing drugs include antineoplastics, opiates, ferrous sulfate, levodopa, oral potassium chloride replacements, estrogens, sulfasalazine, antibiotics, quinidine, anesthetics, cardiac glycosides, theophylline (upon overdose), and nonsteroidal anti-inflammatories.

Radiation and surgery

Radiation therapy can cause nausea and vomiting. Postoperative nausea and vomiting are common, especially after abdominal surgery.

Medical causes
(continued)

Pancreatitis (acute)
+ Nausea, usually followed by vomiting, is an early symptom.

Peptic ulcer
+ Nausea and vomiting may follow attacks of epigastric pain.

Peritonitis
+ Nausea and vomiting accompany acute abdominal pain localized to the area of inflammation.

Preeclampsia
+ Nausea and vomiting occur.
+ Classic diagnostic triad is hypertension, proteinuria, and edema.

Renal and urologic disorders
+ Cystitis, pyelonephritis, calculi, uremia, and other disorders can cause nausea.

Rhabdomyolysis
+ Nausea, vomiting, fever, malaise, and dark urine are common.

Thyrotoxicosis
+ Nausea and vomiting may accompany severe anxiety, heat intolerance, diaphoresis, diarrhea, tremor, tachycardia, palpitations.

Other causes
+ Antineoplastics, opiates, ferrous sulfate, levodopa, oral potassium chloride replacements, estrogens, sulfasalazine, antibiotics, quinidine, anesthetics, cardiac glycosides, theophylline (upon overdose), and NSAIDS
+ Radiation therapy
+ Abdominal surgery

Special considerations

- ✦ Evaluate fluid and electrolyte status and acid-base balance.
- ✦ Elevate the head or position the patient on his side.
- ✦ Give pain medications as needed.
- ✦ Be alert for abdominal distention and hypoactive bowel sounds when giving an antiemetic.
- ✦ Consult the nutritionist to determine metabolic demands.

Peds points

- ✦ Nausea typically results from overeating but can be part of various disorders ranging from acute infections to conversion reaction caused by fear.

Geri points

- ✦ Conditions causing mouth dryness, reduced gastric acid output and motility, and decreased senses of taste and smell can lead to nonpathologic nausea.

Teaching points

- ✦ Avoidance of aggravating factors
- ✦ Proper oral hygiene
- ✦ Foods to avoid

Key facts about neck pain

- ✦ May originate from any neck structure
- ✦ May be referred from other areas of the body

SPECIAL CONSIDERATIONS

If your patient is experiencing severe nausea, prepare him for blood tests to determine fluid and electrolyte status and acid-base balance. Have him breathe deeply to ease his nausea; keep the air in his room fresh and clean-smelling by removing bedpans and emesis basins promptly after use and by providing adequate ventilation. Because he could easily aspirate vomitus when in a supine position, elevate his head or position him on his side.

Because pain can precipitate or intensify nausea, administer pain medications promptly as needed. If possible, give medications by injection or suppository to prevent exacerbating nausea. Be alert for abdominal distention and hypoactive bowel sounds when you administer an antiemetic: These signs may indicate gastric retention. If you detect these, immediately insert a nasogastric tube as required.

Prepare the patient for such procedures as computed tomography scan, ultrasound, endoscopy, and colonoscopy. Consult the nutritionist to determine the patient's metabolic demands such as total or partial parenteral nutrition.

PEDIATRIC POINTERS

Nausea, commonly described as stomachache, is one of the most common childhood complaints. Typically the result of overeating, nausea can also occur as part of diverse disorders ranging from acute infections to a conversion reaction caused by fear.

GERIATRIC POINTERS

Elderly patients have increased dental caries; tooth loss; decreased salivary gland function, which causes mouth dryness; reduced gastric acid output and motility; and decreased senses of taste and smell—any of which can contribute to nonpathologic nausea.

PATIENT COUNSELING

Advise the patient to avoid reading because eye movement can aggravate nausea. Also instruct him to avoid sudden position changes. Encourage him to practice good oral hygiene to remove unpleasant tastes and to moisten the mucous membranes. Tell the patient to avoid foods that may aggravate feelings of nausea such as spicy foods.

NECK PAIN

Neck pain may originate from any neck structure, ranging from the meninges and cervical vertebrae to its blood vessels, muscles, and lymphatic tissue. This symptom can also be referred from other areas of the body. Its location, onset, and pattern help determine its origin and underlying causes. Neck pain usually results from trauma and degenerative, congenital, inflammatory, metabolic, and neoplastic disorders.

 EMERGENCY ACTIONS If the patient's neck pain is due to trauma, first ensure proper cervical spine immobilization, preferably with a long backboard and a Philadelphia collar. (See *Applying a Philadelphia collar.*) Then take vital signs and perform a quick neurologic examination. If he shows signs of respiratory distress, give oxygen. Intubation or tracheostomy and mechanical ventilation may be necessary. Ask the patient (or a family member, if the

Applying a Philadelphia collar

A lightweight, molded polyethylene collar designed to hold the neck straight with the chin slightly elevated and tucked in, the Philadelphia cervical collar immobilizes the cervical spine, decreases muscle spasms, and relieves some pain. It also prevents further injury and promotes healing. When applying the collar, fit it snugly around the patient's neck and attach the Velcro fasteners or buckles at the back. Be sure to check the patient's airway and his neurovascular status to ensure that the collar isn't too tight. Also, make sure that the collar isn't placed too high in front, which can hyperextend the neck. In a patient with a neck sprain, hyperextension may cause the ligaments to heal in a shortened position; in a patient with a cervical spine fracture, it could cause serious neurologic damage.

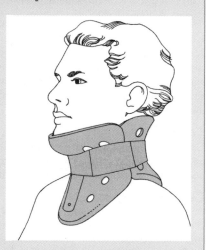

patient can't answer) how the injury occurred. Then examine the neck for abrasions, swelling, lacerations, erythema, and ecchymoses.

HISTORY

If the patient hasn't sustained trauma, find out the severity and onset of his neck pain. Where specifically in the neck does he feel pain? Does anything relieve or worsen the pain? Is there any particular event that precipitates the pain? Also ask about the development of other symptoms such as headaches. Next, focus on the patient's current and past illnesses and injuries, diet, drug history, and family health history.

PHYSICAL ASSESSMENT

Thoroughly inspect the patient's neck, shoulders, and cervical spine for swelling, masses, erythema, and ecchymoses. Assess active range of motion (ROM) in his neck by having him perform flexion, extension, rotation, and lateral side bending. Note the degree of pain produced by these movements. Examine his posture, and test and compare bilateral muscle strength. Check the sensation in his arms, and assess his hand grasp and arm reflexes. Attempt to elicit Brudzinski's and Kernig's signs if there's no history of neck trauma, and palpate the cervical lymph nodes for enlargement.

MEDICAL CAUSES

Cervical extension injury

Anterior or posterior neck pain may develop within hours or days following a whiplash injury. Anterior pain usually diminishes within several days, but posterior pain persists and may even intensify. Associated findings include tenderness, swelling and nuchal rigidity, arm or back pain, occipital headache, muscle spasms, visual blurring, and unilateral miosis on the affected side.

In an emergency
+ Ensure proper cervical spine immobilization.
+ Take vital signs and perform a quick neurologic examination.
+ Give oxygen as needed.
+ Ask how the injury occurred.
+ Examine the neck for abrasions, swelling, lacerations, erythema, and ecchymoses.

Key history points
+ Onset and description of pain
+ Alleviating, aggravating, or precipitating factors
+ Associated symptoms, such as headache
+ Medical and drug history

Critical assessment steps
+ Inspect the neck, shoulders, and cervical spine for swelling, masses, erythema, and ecchymoses.
+ Assess active ROM in the neck.
+ Examine posture.
+ Test and compare bilateral muscle strength.
+ Check sensation in the arms.
+ Assess hand grasp and arm reflexes.
+ If his condition permits, test for Brudzinski's and Kernig's signs.

Medical causes

Cervical extension injury
+ Anterior pain usually diminishes within several days after injury.
+ Posterior pain persists and may even intensify.

Medical causes
(continued)

Cervical spine fracture
✦ Survivors of such a fracture may experience severe neck pain.

Cervical spine tumor
✦ Metastatic tumors typically produce persistent neck pain.

Cervical spondylosis
✦ Posterior neck pain that's aggravated by and restricts movement.

Cervical stenosis
✦ Neck and arm pain, paresthesia, muscle weakness or paralysis, and decreased ROM may occur.

Herniated cervical disk
✦ Variable neck pain is aggravated by and restricts movement.

Hodgkin's lymphoma
✦ Generalized pain may eventually affect the neck.

Laryngeal cancer
✦ Neck pain radiates to the ear.

Lymphadenitis
✦ Enlarged and inflamed cervical lymph nodes cause acute pain.

Meningitis
✦ Neck pain may accompany nuchal rigidity.

Neck sprain
✦ Pain, slight swelling, stiffness, and restricted ROM result.

Paget's disease
✦ Cervical vertebrae deformity may produce severe neck pain, paresthesia, and arm weakness.

Cervical spine fracture
Fracture at C1 to C4 can cause sudden death; survivors may experience severe neck pain that restricts all movement, intense occipital headache, quadriplegia, deformity, and respiratory paralysis.

Cervical spine tumor
Metastatic tumors typically produce persistent neck pain that increases with movement and isn't relieved by rest; primary tumors cause mild to severe pain along a specific nerve root. Other findings depend on the lesions and may include paresthesia, arm and leg weakness that progresses to atrophy and paralysis, and bladder and bowel incontinence.

Cervical spondylosis
Cervical spondylosis, a degenerative process, produces posterior neck pain that's aggravated by and restricts movement. Pain may radiate down either arm and may accompany paresthesia, weakness, and stiffness.

Cervical stenosis
Cervical stenosis is a progressive disorder that commonly produces no symptoms. It may cause nonspecific neck and arm pain, paresthesia, muscle weakness or paralysis, and decreased ROM. The patient may report hand clumsiness and problems with gait and balance.

Herniated cervical disk
A herniated cervical disk characteristically causes variable neck pain that is aggravated by and restricts movement. It also causes referred pain along a specific dermatome, paresthesia and other sensory disturbances, and arm weakness.

Hodgkin's lymphoma
Hodgkin's lymphoma may eventually result in generalized pain that may affect the neck. Lymphadenopathy, the classic sign, may accompany paresthesia, muscle weakness, fever, fatigue, weight loss, malaise, and hepatomegaly.

Laryngeal cancer
Neck pain that radiates to the ear develops late in laryngeal cancer. The patient may also develop dysphagia, dyspnea, hemoptysis, stridor, hoarseness, and cervical lymphadenopathy.

Lymphadenitis
With lymphadenitis, enlarged and inflamed cervical lymph nodes cause acute pain and tenderness. Fever, chills, and malaise may also occur.

Meningitis
With meningitis, neck pain may accompany characteristic nuchal rigidity. Related findings include fever, headache, photophobia, positive Brudzinski's and Kernig's signs, and decreased level of consciousness (LOC).

Neck sprain
Minor sprains typically produce pain, slight swelling, stiffness, and restricted ROM. Ligament rupture causes pain, marked swelling, ecchymosis, muscle spasms, and nuchal rigidity with head tilt.

Paget's disease
Paget's disease commonly produces no symptoms in its early stages. As it progresses, cervical vertebrae deformity may produce severe, persistent neck pain along with paresthesia and arm weakness or paralysis.

Rheumatoid arthritis

Rheumatoid arthritis usually affects peripheral joints, but it can also involve the cervical vertebrae. Acute inflammation may cause moderate to severe pain that radiates along a specific nerve root; increased warmth, swelling, and tenderness in involved joints; stiffness, restricting ROM; paresthesia and muscle weakness; low-grade fever; anorexia; malaise; fatigue; and possible neck deformity. Some pain and stiffness remain after the acute phase.

Spinous process fracture

Fracture near the cervicothoracic junction produces acute pain radiating to the shoulders. Associated findings include swelling, exquisite tenderness, restricted ROM, muscle spasms, and deformity.

Subarachnoid hemorrhage

Subarachnoid hemorrhage is a life-threatening condition that may cause moderate to severe neck pain and rigidity, headache, and a decreased LOC. Kernig's and Brudzinski's signs are present. The patient may describe the headache as "the worst headache of my life."

Torticollis

With torticollis, severe neck pain accompanies recurrent unilateral stiffness and muscle spasms. Stiffness of the neck muscles is followed by a momentary twitching or contraction that pulls the head to the affected side.

Tracheal trauma

Fracture of the tracheal cartilage, a life-threatening condition, produces moderate to severe neck pain and respiratory difficulty. Torn tracheal mucosa produces mild to moderate pain and may result in airway occlusion, hemoptysis, hoarseness, and dysphagia.

SPECIAL CONSIDERATIONS

Promote patient comfort by giving an anti-inflammatory and an analgesic, as needed. Prepare him for diagnostic tests, such as X-rays, computed tomography scan, blood tests, and cerebrospinal fluid analysis.

PEDIATRIC POINTERS

The most common causes of neck pain in children are meningitis and trauma. A rare cause of neck pain is congenital torticollis.

PATIENT COUNSELING

Explain necessary activity limitations to the patient, such as avoiding flexion, extension, or rotation of the neck. If the patient needs to wear a cervical collar, make sure he knows how to apply it properly. Reinforce exercises that have been taught during physical therapy.

NIGHT BLINDNESS

Usually difficult to identify, night blindness (or nyctalopia) refers to impaired vision in the dark, especially after entering a darkened room or while driving at night. A symptom of choroidal and retinal degeneration, night blindness occurs in various ocular disorders and as an early indicator of vitamin A deficiency. In some patients, however, night blindness occurs without underlying pathology, simply re-

---

Medical causes
(continued)

Rheumatoid arthritis
+ Pain from inflammation may radiate along a specific nerve root.

Spinous process fracture
+ Fracture near the cervicothoracic junction produces acute pain that radiates to shoulders.

Subarachnoid hemorrhage
+ Moderate to severe neck pain and rigidity, headache, and decreased LOC may occur.

Torticollis
+ Severe neck pain accompanies recurrent unilateral stiffness and muscle spasms.

Tracheal trauma
+ Neck pain and respiratory difficulty occur.

Special considerations
+ Give an anti-inflammatory and an analgesic, as needed.

Peds points
+ The most common causes of neck pain in children are meningitis and trauma.

Teaching points
+ Activity limitations
+ Cervical collar application, if needed
+ Reinforcement of exercises

Key facts about night blindness
+ Impaired vision in the dark
+ Signals choroidal and retinal degeneration

Key history points

+ Onset and description
+ Associated ocular symptoms
+ History of glaucoma, cataracts, and familial vision degeneration

Critical assessment steps

+ Examine eyes for ptosis, abnormal tearing, discharge, and conjunctival injection.
+ Test visual acuity and visual fields in both eyes.
+ Check pupillary response.
+ Test six cardinal fields of gaze.

Medical causes

Cataracts

+ Night blindness and halo vision occur early.

Glaucoma

+ Night blindness occurs late.

Optic nerve atrophy

+ Night blindness, visual field and color vision defects, and decreased visual acuity may occur.

Retinitis pigmentosa

+ Night blindness and scattered black pigmentary bodies on the retina develop in adolescence.

Vitamin A deficiency

+ Night blindness, typically the first symptom, occurs with xerophthalmia and Bitot's spots.

Special considerations

+ Prepare patient for diagnostic tests.

flecting poor adaptation to the dark. In these patients, it's commonly accompanied by myopia.

HISTORY

If the patient complains of difficulty seeing at night, ask when he first noticed the problem. Is it intermittent or steadily worsening? Is it worse at certain times or in certain conditions? Also, ask about other ocular symptoms, such as eye pain, blurred or halo vision, floaters or spots, and photophobia.

Explore any history of glaucoma, cataracts, and familial degeneration of vision. If no ocular problems are apparent, briefly evaluate the patient's nutritional status for vitamin A deficiency.

PHYSICAL ASSESSMENT

Examine the eyes for ptosis, abnormal tearing, discharge, and conjunctival injection. Test visual acuity and visual fields in both eyes and, if trained and equipped, measure intraocular pressure. Check pupillary response, and evaluate extraocular muscle function by testing the six cardinal fields of gaze.

MEDICAL CAUSES

Cataracts

Night blindness and halo vision occur early in senile-type cataract formation. As the cataract matures, it causes gradual, painless visual blurring and vision loss, sometimes with visible lens opacity.

Glaucoma

Night blindness occurs late in chronic open-angle glaucoma, with halo vision, gradually impaired bilateral visual acuity, loss of peripheral vision and, possibly, slight eye pain.

Optic nerve atrophy

Optic nerve atrophy may cause night blindness, visual field and color vision defects, and decreased visual acuity. Pupillary reactions are sluggish, and optic disk pallor is evident.

Retinitis pigmentosa

Retinitis pigmentosa is usually a hereditary retinal degeneration in which night blindness is characteristically the first symptom, typically arising in adolescence. Scattered black pigmentary bodies form in a characteristic "bone-spicule" arrangement on the retina. As the disease progresses, the visual field gradually constricts, causing tunnel or "gun barrel" vision and, eventually, total blindness.

Vitamin A deficiency

Night blindness is typically the first symptom of vitamin A deficiency. Associated findings include xerophthalmia (conjunctival dryness) and Bitot's spots (gray-white conjunctival plaques). The patient may complain of visual blurring or vision loss. His skin may be dry and scaly. His mucous membranes may be shrunken and hardened.

SPECIAL CONSIDERATIONS

Prepare the patient for diagnostic testing, such as ophthalmoscopy, visual field testing, fluorescein angiography, and electroretinography. Genetic counseling is recommended for adults who risk transmitting hereditary disorders to their children.

Vitamin A supplementation and nutritional counseling may improve night vision in some patients.

PEDIATRIC POINTERS

Because children generally don't have adequate body reserves of vitamin A, they're especially prone to deficiency and resulting night blindness.

GERIATRIC POINTERS

Night blindness due to vitamin A deficiency usually occurs in elderly and disadvantaged patients. It's also a common effect of aging.

PATIENT COUNSELING

Because visual impairment is frightening to the patient, provide emotional support. Help decrease his anxiety and enhance cooperation by explaining scheduled diagnostic tests, such as electroretinography, in simple terms. Ensure patient safety, and explain that the patient shouldn't drive and should use assistive devices at night or in darkened or dim lighting as necessary.

NIPPLE DISCHARGE

Nipple discharge can occur spontaneously or can be elicited by nipple stimulation. It's characterized as intermittent or constant, as unilateral or bilateral, and by color, consistency, and composition. Its incidence increases with age and parity. This sign rarely occurs (but is more likely to be pathologic) in men and in nulligravid, regularly menstruating women. It's relatively common and usually normal in parous women. A thick, grayish discharge — benign epithelial debris from inactive ducts — can commonly be elicited in middle-age parous women. Colostrum, a thin, yellowish or milky discharge, typically occurs in the last weeks of pregnancy.

Nipple discharge can signal serious underlying disease, particularly when accompanied by other breast changes. Significant causes include endocrine disorders, cancer, certain drugs, and blocked lactiferous ducts.

HISTORY

Ask the patient when she first noticed the discharge, and determine its duration, extent, quantity, color, consistency, and smell, if any. Has she had other nipple and breast changes, such as pain, tenderness, itching, warmth, changes in contour, and lumps? If she reports a lump, question her about its onset, location, size, and consistency. Is the patient taking hormones (hormonal contraceptives or hormone replacement therapy)? Is the discharge spontaneous, or does it have to be expressed?

Obtain a complete gynecologic and obstetric history, and determine her normal menstrual cycle and the date of her last menses. Ask if she experiences breast swelling and tenderness, bloating, irritability, headaches, abdominal cramping, nausea, or diarrhea before or during menses. Note the number, date, and outcome of her pregnancies and, if she breast-fed, the approximate time of her last lactation. Also, check for any risk factors of breast cancer — family history, previous or current malignancies, nulliparity or first pregnancy after age 30, early menarche, or late menopause.

Peds points
- Children generally don't have adequate body reserves of vitamin A, which may cause night blindness.

Geri points
- Night blindness is a common effect of aging.

Teaching points
- Safety measures
- Use of assistive devices

Key facts about nipple discharge
- Characterized as intermittent or constant, as unilateral or bilateral, and by color, consistency, and composition
- Is relatively common in parous women

Key history points
- Onset, duration, and description of discharge
- Associated pain, tenderness, itching, warmth, changes in contour, and lumps
- Use of hormones
- Menstrual cycle history

Critical assessment steps

+ Characterize the discharge.
+ Check for nipple deviation, flattening, retraction, redness, asymmetry, thickening, excoriation, erosion, or cracking.
+ Inspect the breasts for asymmetry, irregular contours, dimpling, erythema, and peau d'orange.
+ With patient in supine position, palpate breasts and axillae for lumps.

Medical causes

Breast abscess
+ A thick, purulent discharge may be produced from a cracked nipple or an infected duct.

Breast cancer
+ Bloody, watery, or purulent discharge may emit from a normal-appearing nipple.

Choriocarcinoma
+ Galactorrhea may occur with persistent uterine bleeding and bogginess.

Herpes zoster
+ Bilateral, spontaneous, intermittent galactorrhea may occur.

Intraductal papilloma
+ Discharge is unilateral serous, serosanguineous, or bloody.

Mammary duct ectasia
+ A thick, sticky, grayish discharge from multiple ducts may be the first sign; discharge may be bilateral and is usually spontaneous.

PHYSICAL ASSESSMENT

Start your physical assessment by characterizing the discharge. If the discharge isn't frank, try to elicit it. (See *Eliciting nipple discharge.*) Then examine the nipples and breasts with the patient in four different positions: sitting with her arms at her sides; with her arms overhead; with her hands pressing on her hips; and leaning forward so her breasts are suspended. Check for nipple deviation, flattening, retraction, redness, asymmetry, thickening, excoriation, erosion, or cracking. Inspect her breasts for asymmetry, irregular contours, dimpling, erythema, and peau d'orange. With the patient in a supine position, palpate the breasts and axillae for lumps, giving special attention to the areolae. Note the size, location, delineation, consistency, and mobility of any lump you find.

MEDICAL CAUSES

Breast abscess

A breast abscess, most common in breast-feeding women, may produce a thick, purulent discharge from a cracked nipple or an infected duct. Associated findings include abrupt onset of high fever with chills; breast pain, tenderness, and erythema; a palpable soft nodule or generalized induration; and, possibly, nipple retraction.

Breast cancer

Breast cancer may cause bloody, watery, or purulent discharge from a normal-appearing nipple. Characteristic findings include a hard, irregular, fixed lump; erythema; dimpling; peau d'orange; changes in contour; nipple deviation, flattening, or retraction; axillary lymphadenopathy; and, possibly, breast pain.

Choriocarcinoma

Galactorrhea (a white or grayish milky discharge) may result from choriocarcinoma, a highly malignant neoplasm that can follow pregnancy. Other characteristics of choriocarcinoma include persistent uterine bleeding and bogginess after delivery or curettage, and vaginal masses.

Herpes zoster

Herpes zoster can stimulate the thoracic nerves, causing bilateral, spontaneous, intermittent galactorrhea. Other characteristics include shooting or burning pain, eruption of small red nodules or vesicles on the thorax and possibly the arms and legs, pruritus and paresthesia or hyperesthesia in affected areas, headache, and fever and malaise.

Intraductal papilloma

Intraductal papilloma is the primary cause of nipple discharge in the nonpregnant, non-breast-feeding woman. Unilateral serous, serosanguineous, or bloody nipple discharge—usually from only one duct—is its predominant sign. Discharge may be intermittent or profuse and constant, and can usually be stimulated by gentle pressure around the areola. Subareolar nodules, breast pain, and tenderness may occur.

Mammary duct ectasia

A thick, sticky, grayish discharge from multiple ducts may be the first sign of mammary duct ectasia. The discharge may be bilateral and is usually spontaneous. Other findings include a rubbery, poorly delineated lump beneath the areola, with a blue-green discoloration of the overlying skin; nipple retraction; and redness, swelling, tenderness, and burning pain in the areola and nipple.

Eliciting nipple discharge

If your patient has a history or evidence of nipple discharge, you can attempt to elicit it during your examination. Help the patient into a supine position, and gently squeeze her nipple between your thumb and index finger (as shown below left); note any discharge through the nipple. Then place your fingers on the areola, as shown below right, and palpate the entire areolar surface, watching for any discharge through areolar ducts.

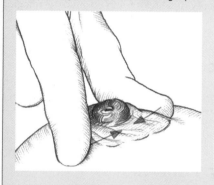

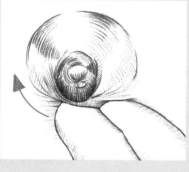

Paget's disease
With Paget's disease, serous or bloody discharge emits from denuded skin on the nipple, which is red, intensely itchy and, possibly, eroded or excoriated. The discharge is usually unilateral.

Prolactin-secreting pituitary tumor
Bilateral galactorrhea may occur with this tumor. Other findings include amenorrhea, infertility, decreased libido and vaginal secretions, headaches, and blindness.

Proliferative (fibrocystic) breast disease
Proliferative (fibrocystic) breast disease is a benign disorder that occasionally causes a bilateral clear, milky, or straw-colored discharge, which is rarely purulent or bloody. Multiple round, soft, tender nodules are usually palpable in both breasts, although they may occur singly. Usually, nodules are mobile and are located in the upper outer quadrant. Nodule size, tenderness, and discharge increase during the luteal phase of the menstrual cycle. Symptoms then regress after menses.

Trauma
Bilateral galactorrhea can result from trauma to the breasts. Depending on the cause and severity of the chest trauma, the patient may also have chest pain, dyspnea, bruising, flail chest, cardiac tamponade, pulmonary artery tears, ventricular rupture, shock, and bronchial, tracheal, or esophageal tears or rupture.

OTHER CAUSES

Drugs
Galactorrhea can be caused by psychotropic agents, particularly phenothiazines and tricyclic antidepressants; some antihypertensives (reserpine and methyldopa); hormonal contraceptives; cimetidine; metoclopramide; and verapamil.

Medical causes
(continued)

Paget's disease
+ Serous or bloody discharge emits from denuded skin on the nipple.

Prolactin-secreting pituitary tumor
+ Bilateral galactorrhea may occur.

Proliferative (fibrocystic) breast disease
+ Bilateral clear, milky, or straw-colored discharge occurs.

Trauma
+ Bilateral galactorrhea can result from trauma to the breasts.

Other causes
+ Antihypertensives, cimetidine, hormonal contraceptives, metoclopramide, psychotropic agents, or verapamil
+ Chest wall surgery

Special considerations

+ Clearly explain the nature and origin of the discharge.
+ Apply a breast binder.

Peds points

+ Nipple discharge in children and adolescents is rare.
+ Infants may experience a milky discharge between 3 days and 2 weeks after birth due to maternal hormonal influences.

Geri points

+ In postmenopausal women, breast changes are considered malignant until proven otherwise.

Teaching points

+ Importance of being aware of discharge characteristics
+ When to seek medical attention
+ Importance of breast self-examinations, medical appointments, and mammograms

Key facts about nipple retraction

+ Inward displacement of the nipple below the level of surrounding breast tissue
+ Results from scar tissue formation within a lesion or large mammary duct

Key history points

+ Onset of retraction
+ Other nipple changes
+ Associated breast pain, lumps, redness, swelling, or warmth
+ Risk factors for breast cancer

Surgery

Chest wall surgery may stimulate the thoracic nerves, causing intermittent bilateral galactorrhea.

SPECIAL CONSIDERATIONS

Although nipple discharge is usually insignificant, it can be frightening to the patient. Help relieve the patient's anxieties by clearly explaining the nature and origin of her discharge. Apply a breast binder, which may reduce discharge by eliminating nipple stimulation.

Diagnostic tests may include tissue biopsy (if a breast lump is found), cytologic study of the discharge, mammography, ultrasonography, transillumination, and serum prolactin.

PEDIATRIC POINTERS

Nipple discharge in children and adolescents is rare. When it does occur, it's almost always nonpathologic, as in the bloody discharge that sometimes accompanies onset of menarche. Infants of both sexes may experience a milky breast discharge beginning 3 days after birth and lasting up to 2 weeks due to maternal hormonal influences.

GERIATRIC POINTERS

In postmenopausal women, breast changes are considered malignant until proven otherwise.

PATIENT COUNSELING

Counsel your patient to be aware of discharge characteristics, including its consistency (thick or thinning), odor, origin (in single or multiple ducts), and relation to the menstrual cycle. If the discharge becomes bloody, instruct the patient to seek medical evaluation. Instruct the patient to perform breast self-examinations and to maintain appointments for breast examinations by a physician and for mammograms as recommended.

NIPPLE RETRACTION

Nipple retraction, the inward displacement of the nipple below the level of surrounding breast tissue, may indicate an inflammatory breast lesion or cancer. It results from scar tissue formation within a lesion or large mammary duct. As the scar tissue shortens, it pulls adjacent tissue inward, causing nipple deviation, flattening and, finally, retraction.

HISTORY

Ask the patient when she first noticed retraction of the nipple. Has she experienced other nipple changes, such as itching, discoloration, discharge, or excoriation? Has she noticed breast pain, lumps, redness, swelling, or warmth? Obtain a history, noting risk factors for breast cancer, such as a family history or previous malignancy.

PHYSICAL ASSESSMENT

Carefully examine both nipples and breasts with the patient sitting upright with her arms at her sides, with her hands pressing on her hips, and with her arms over-

ASSESSMENT TIP

Differentiating nipple retraction from inversion

Nipple retraction is sometimes confused with nipple inversion, a common abnormality that's congenital in many patients and doesn't usually signal underlying disease. A *retracted* nipple appears flat and broad, whereas an *inverted* nipple can be pulled out from the sulcus where it hides.

NIPPLE RETRACTION

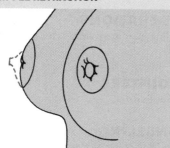

NIPPLE INVERSION

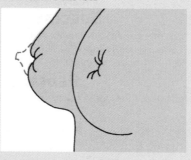

head; and with the patient leaning forward so her breasts hang. Look for redness, excoriation, and discharge; nipple flattening and deviation; and breast asymmetry, dimpling, or contour differences. (See *Differentiating nipple retraction from inversion.*)

Try to evert the nipple by gently squeezing the areola. With the patient in a supine position, palpate both breasts for lumps, especially beneath the areola. Mold breast skin over the lump or gently pull it up toward the clavicle, looking for accentuated nipple retraction. Also, palpate axillary lymph nodes.

MEDICAL CAUSES

Breast abscess
A breast abscess, most common in breast-feeding women, occasionally produces unilateral nipple retraction. More common findings include high fever with chills; breast pain, erythema, and tenderness; breast induration or soft mass; and cracked, sore nipples, possibly with purulent discharge.

Breast cancer
With breast cancer, unilateral nipple retraction is commonly accompanied by a hard, fixed, nontender nodule beneath the areola, as well as other breast nodules. Other nipple changes include itching, burning, erosion, and watery or bloody discharge. Breast changes commonly include dimpling, altered contour, peau d'orange, ulceration, tenderness (possibly pain), redness, and warmth. Axillary lymph nodes may be enlarged.

Mammary duct ectasia
Nipple retraction commonly occurs in mammary duct ectasia, along with a poorly defined, rubbery nodule beneath the areola, with a blue-green skin discoloration; areolar burning, itching, swelling, tenderness, and erythema; and nipple pain with a thick, sticky, grayish, multiductal discharge.

Critical assessment steps
+ Carefully examine both nipples and breasts with the patient sitting upright with her arms at her sides, with her hands pressing on her hips, and with her arms overhead and also with the patient leaning forward.
+ Look for redness, excoriation, and discharge; nipple flattening and deviation; and breast asymmetry, dimpling, or contour differences.
+ With patient in supine position, palpate both breasts for lumps.
+ Palpate axillary lymph nodes.

Medical causes

Breast abscess
+ Occasionally, unilateral nipple retraction occurs.

Breast cancer
+ Unilateral nipple retraction is commonly accompanied by a hard, fixed, nontender nodule beneath the areola.

Mammary duct ectasia
+ Nipple retraction commonly occurs with nipple pain, discharge, areolar abnormalities, and a poorly defined, rubbery nodule beneath the areola.

Medical causes
(continued)

Mastitis
+ Nipple retraction, deviation, cracking, or flattening may occur.

Other causes
+ Previous breast surgery

Special considerations
+ Prepare the patient for diagnostic tests.

Peds points
+ Nipple retraction doesn't occur in prepubescent females.

Teaching points
+ Breast self-examination

Key facts about nocturia
+ Excessive urination of 700 ml or more at night

Key history points
+ Onset, frequency, and pattern of nocturia
+ Precipitating factors
+ Volume voided
+ Associated color, odor, or consistency changes of urine
+ Pattern of fluid intake
+ Associated pain, burning, difficulty urinating, and CVA tenderness
+ Family history of renal or urinary tract disorders or endocrine and metabolic diseases
+ Drug history

Mastitis

Nipple retraction, deviation, cracking, or flattening may occur in mastitis, along with a firm and indurated or tender, flocculent, discrete breast nodule; warmth; erythema; tenderness; and edema. Fatigue, high fever, and chills may also be present.

OTHER CAUSES

Surgery
Previous breast surgery may cause underlying scarring and retraction.

SPECIAL CONSIDERATIONS

Prepare the patient for diagnostic tests, including mammography, cytology of nipple discharge, and biopsy.

PEDIATRIC POINTERS

Nipple retraction doesn't occur in prepubescent females.

PATIENT COUNSELING

Teach your patient breast self-examination, and advise her to always seek medical evaluation for breast changes.

NOCTURIA

Nocturia — excessive urination at night — may result from disruption of the normal diurnal pattern of urine concentration or from overstimulation of the nerves and muscles that control urination. Normally, more urine is concentrated during the night than during the day. As a result, most persons excrete three to four times more urine during the day and can sleep for 6 to 8 hours during the night without being awakened. The patient with nocturia may awaken one or more times during the night to empty his bladder and may excrete 700 ml or more of urine.

Although nocturia usually results from renal and lower urinary tract disorders, it may result from certain cardiovascular, endocrine, and metabolic disorders. This common sign may also result from drugs that induce diuresis, particularly when they're taken at night, and from the ingestion of large quantities of fluids — especially caffeinated beverages or alcohol — at bedtime.

HISTORY

Explore the history of the patient's nocturia. When did it begin? How often does it occur? Can the patient identify a specific pattern or precipitating factors? Also, note the volume of urine voided. Ask the patient about any change in the color, odor, or consistency of his urine. Has the patient changed his usual pattern or volume of fluid intake? Next, explore associated symptoms. Ask about pain or burning on urination, difficulty initiating a urine stream, costovertebral angle (CVA) tenderness, and flank, upper abdominal, or suprapubic pain.

Determine if the patient or his family has a history of renal or urinary tract disorders or endocrine and metabolic diseases, particularly diabetes. Is the patient taking a drug that increases urine output, such as a diuretic, a cardiac glycoside, or an antihypertensive?

Physical assessment

Focus your physical assessment on palpating and percussing the kidneys, the CVA, and the bladder. Carefully inspect the urinary meatus. Inspect a urine specimen for color, odor, and the presence of sediment.

Medical causes

Benign prostatic hyperplasia

Common in men older than age 50, benign prostatic hyperplasia (BPH) produces nocturia when significant urethral obstruction develops. Typically, it causes frequency, hesitancy, incontinence, reduced force and caliber of the urine stream and, possibly, hematuria. Oliguria may also occur. Palpation reveals a distended bladder and an enlarged prostate. The patient may also complain of lower abdominal fullness, perineal pain, and constipation.

Bladder neoplasm

A late sign of a bladder neoplasm, nocturia involves frequent voiding of small to moderate amounts of urine. Besides hematuria, the most common sign, associated characteristics include bladder distention, urinary frequency and urgency, dysuria, pyuria, vomiting, diarrhea, insomnia, and bladder, rectal, flank, back, or leg pain. Signs and symptoms of urinary tract infection (UTI), such as tenesmus, low-grade fever, and perineal pain, may also occur.

Cystitis

All three forms of cystitis may cause nocturia marked by frequent, small voidings and accompanied by dysuria and tenesmus.

Bacterial cystitis may also cause urinary urgency; hematuria; fatigue; suprapubic, perineal, flank, and lower back pain; and, occasionally, low-grade fever. Most common in women between ages 25 and 60, *chronic interstitial cystitis* is characterized by Hunner's ulcers (small, punctate, bleeding lesions in the bladder); it also causes gross hematuria. Because symptoms resemble bladder cancer, this must be ruled out.

Viral cystitis also causes urinary urgency, hematuria, and fever.

Diabetes insipidus

The result of antidiuretic hormone deficiency, diabetes insipidus usually produces nocturia early in its course. It's characterized by periodic voiding of moderate to large amounts of urine. Diabetes insipidus can also produce polydipsia and dehydration.

Diabetes mellitus

An early sign of diabetes mellitus, nocturia involves frequent, large voidings. Associated features include daytime polyuria, polydipsia, polyphagia, frequent UTIs, recurrent yeast infections, vaginitis, weakness, fatigue, weight loss and, possibly, signs of dehydration, such as dry mucous membranes and poor skin turgor.

Hypercalcemic nephropathy

With hypercalcemic nephropathy, nocturia involves the periodic voiding of moderate to large amounts of urine. Related findings include daytime polyuria, polydipsia and, occasionally, hematuria and pyuria.

Hypokalemic nephropathy

With hypokalemic nephropathy, nocturia involves the periodic voiding of moderate to large amounts of urine. Associated findings typically include polydipsia, day-

---

Medical causes
(continued)

Prostate cancer
+ Nocturia occurs late and is characterized by infrequent voiding of moderate amounts of urine.

Pyelonephritis (acute)
+ Nocturia is common and is usually characterized by infrequent voiding of moderate amounts of urine; urine may appear cloudy.

Renal failure (chronic)
+ Nocturia involving infrequent voiding of moderate amounts of urine occurs relatively early; oliguria or anuria may develop.

Other causes
+ Drugs that mobilize edematous fluid or produce diuresis

Special considerations
+ Maintain fluid balance.
+ Monitor vital signs, intake and output, and daily weight.
+ Document frequency of nocturia, amount, and specific gravity.
+ Plan administration of a diuretic for daytime hours, if possible.
+ Plan rest periods to compensate for sleep lost.

Peds points
+ With the exception of prostate disorders, causes of nocturia are generally the same for children and adults.

Geri points
+ Postmenopausal women have decreased bladder elasticity, but urine output remains constant, resulting in nocturia.

time polyuria, muscle weakness or paralysis, hypoactive bowel sounds, and increased susceptibility to pyelonephritis.

Prostate cancer
The second leading cause of cancer deaths in men, prostate cancer usually produces no symptoms in early stages. Later, it produces nocturia characterized by infrequent voiding of moderate amounts of urine. Other characteristic effects include dysuria (most common symptom), difficulty initiating a urine stream, interrupted urine stream, bladder distention, urinary frequency, weight loss, pallor, weakness, perineal pain, and constipation. Palpation reveals a hard, irregularly shaped, nodular prostate.

Pyelonephritis (acute)
Nocturia is common with acute pyelonephritis and is usually characterized by infrequent voiding of moderate amounts of urine. The urine may appear cloudy. Associated signs and symptoms include a high, sustained fever with chills, fatigue, unilateral or bilateral flank pain, CVA tenderness, weakness, dysuria, hematuria, urinary frequency and urgency, and tenesmus. Occasionally, anorexia, nausea, vomiting, diarrhea, and hypoactive bowel sounds may also occur.

Renal failure (chronic)
Nocturia occurs relatively early in chronic renal failure and is usually characterized by infrequent voiding of moderate amounts of urine. As the disorder progresses, oliguria or even anuria develops. Other widespread effects include fatigue, ammonia breath odor, Kussmaul's respirations, peripheral edema, elevated blood pressure, decreased level of consciousness, confusion, emotional lability, muscle twitching, anorexia, metallic taste in the mouth, constipation or diarrhea, petechiae, ecchymoses, pruritus, yellow- or bronze-tinged skin, nausea, and vomiting.

OTHER CAUSES

Drugs
Any drug that mobilizes edematous fluid or produces diuresis (for example, a diuretic or a cardiac glycoside) may cause nocturia; obviously, this effect depends on when the drug is administered.

SPECIAL CONSIDERATIONS
Patient care includes maintaining fluid balance, ensuring adequate rest, and providing patient education. Monitor vital signs, intake and output, and daily weight; continue to document the frequency of nocturia, amount, and specific gravity. Plan administration of a diuretic for daytime hours, if possible. Also plan rest periods to compensate for sleep lost because of nocturia.

Prepare the patient for diagnostic tests, which may include routine urinalysis; urine concentration and dilution studies; serum blood urea nitrogen, creatinine, and electrolyte levels; and cystoscopy.

PEDIATRIC POINTERS
In children, nocturia may be voluntary or involuntary. The latter is commonly known as enuresis, or bedwetting. With the exception of prostate disorders, causes of nocturia are generally the same for children and adults.

However, children with pyelonephritis are more susceptible to sepsis, which may display as fever, irritability, and poor skin perfusion. In addition, girls may experience vaginal discharge and vulvar soreness or pruritus.

GERIATRIC POINTERS

Postmenopausal women have decreased bladder elasticity, but urine output remains constant, resulting in nocturia.

PATIENT COUNSELING

Advise the patient to reduce fluid intake (especially of caffeinated and alcoholic beverages) before bedtime. Also advise him to void 15 to 20 minutes before retiring. Voiding once more just before retiring may be helpful.

NUCHAL RIGIDITY

Commonly an early sign of meningeal irritation, nuchal rigidity refers to stiffness of the neck that prevents flexion. To elicit this sign, attempt to passively flex the patient's neck and touch his chin to his chest. If nuchal rigidity is present, this maneuver triggers pain and muscle spasms. (Make sure that there's no cervical spinal misalignment, such as a fracture or dislocation, before testing for nuchal rigidity. Severe spinal cord damage could result.) The patient may also notice nuchal rigidity when he attempts to flex his neck during daily activities. This sign isn't reliable in children and infants.

Nuchal rigidity may herald life-threatening subarachnoid hemorrhage or meningitis. (See *Associated disorder: Meningitis*, page 458.) It may also be a late sign of cervical arthritis, in which joint mobility is gradually lost.

 EMERGENCY ACTIONS After eliciting nuchal rigidity, attempt to elicit **Kernig's and Brudzinski's signs. Quickly evaluate level of consciousness (LOC). Take vital signs. If you note signs of increased intracranial pressure (ICP), such as increased systolic pressure, bradycardia, and widened pulse pressure, start an I.V. line for drug administration and deliver oxygen as necessary, and keep the head of the bed at least as low as 30 degrees. Draw a sample for routine blood studies such as a complete blood count with a white blood cell count and electrolyte levels.**

HISTORY

Obtain a patient history, relying on family members if altered LOC prevents the patient from responding. Ask about the onset and duration of neck stiffness. Were there any precipitating factors? Also ask about associated signs and symptoms, such as headache, fever, nausea and vomiting, and motor and sensory changes. Check for a history of hypertension, head trauma, cerebral aneurysm or arteriovenous malformation, endocarditis, recent infection (such as sinusitis or pneumonia), or recent dental work. Then obtain a complete drug history.

If the patient has no other signs of meningeal irritation, ask about a history of arthritis or neck trauma. Can the patient recall pulling a muscle in his neck?

PHYSICAL ASSESSMENT

Perform a neurologic assessment followed by musculoskeletal and cardiopulmonary assessments. Inspect the patient's hands for swollen, tender joints, and palpate the neck for pain or tenderness.

Key facts about meningitis

+ Involves inflamed brain and spinal cord meninges
+ Usually results from bacterial infection

Causes

+ Bacteremia
+ Other infections, such as sinusitis, otitis media, encephalitis, myelitis, and brain abscess
+ Trauma or invasive procedures
+ Virus or other organism

Management

+ Appropriate I.V. antibiotics for at least 2 weeks, followed by oral antibiotics
+ Mannitol to decrease cerebral edema
+ Anticonvulsant (usually given I.V.) or sedative
+ Aspirin or acetaminophen

Supportive measures include:
+ Bed rest
+ Fever reduction
+ Fluid therapy (given cautiously if cerebral edema and increased ICP are present)
+ Appropriate therapy for any coexisting conditions
+ Possible prophylactic antibiotics after ventricular shunting procedures, skull fracture, or penetrating head wounds (use is controversial)

ASSOCIATED DISORDER

Meningitis

In meningitis, the brain and the spinal cord meninges become inflamed, usually as a result of bacterial infection. Such inflammation may involve all three meningeal membranes — the dura mater, arachnoid, and pia mater.

If the disease is recognized early and the infecting organism responds to treatment, the prognosis is good and complications are rare. However, mortality in untreated meningitis is 70% to 100%. The prognosis is poorer in infants and elderly patients.

CAUSES

Meningitis is almost always a complication of bacteremia, especially from:
+ pneumonia
+ empyema
+ osteomyelitis
+ endocarditis.

Other infections associated with the development of meningitis include:
+ sinusitis
+ otitis media
+ encephalitis
+ myelitis
+ brain abscess, usually caused by *Neisseria meningitidis, Haemophilus influenzae, Streptococcus pneumoniae,* or *Escherichia coli.*

In addition, meningitis may follow trauma or invasive procedures, including:
+ skull fracture
+ penetrating head wound
+ ventricular shunting.

Aseptic meningitis may result from a virus or other organism. Sometimes no causative organism can be found.

DIAGNOSIS

These diagnostic findings are common in patients with meningitis:
+ Lumbar puncture shows elevated cerebrospinal fluid (CSF) pressure (from obstructed CSF outflow at the arachnoid villi), cloudy or milky white CSF, high protein level, positive Gram stain and culture (unless a virus is responsible), and decreased glucose concentration.
+ Positive Brudzinski's and Kernig's signs indicate meningeal irritation.
+ Cultures of blood, urine, and nose and throat secretions reveal the offending organism.
+ Chest X-ray may reveal pneumonitis or lung abscess, tubercular lesions, or granulomas secondary to a fungal infection.
+ Sinus and skull X-rays may identify cranial osteomyelitis or paranasal sinusitis as the underlying infectious process, or skull fracture as the mechanism for entrance of microorganism.
+ White blood cell count reveals leukocytosis.
+ Computed tomography scan may reveal hydrocephalus or rule out cerebral hematoma, hemorrhage, or tumor as the underlying cause.

MEDICAL INTERVENTIONS

Treatment for meningitis may include:
+ appropriate I.V. antibiotics for at least 2 weeks, followed by oral antibiotics selected by culture and sensitivity testing (usual treatment)
+ digoxin to control arrhythmias
+ mannitol to decrease cerebral edema
+ anticonvulsant (usually given I.V.) or a sedative to reduce restlessness and prevent or control seizure activity
+ aspirin or acetaminophen to relieve headache and fever.

Supportive measures include:
+ bed rest to prevent increases in intracranial pressure (ICP)
+ fever reduction to prevent hyperthermia and increased metabolic demands that may increase ICP
+ fluid therapy (given cautiously if cerebral edema and increased ICP present) to prevent dehydration
+ appropriate therapy for any coexisting conditions, such as endocarditis or pneumonia
+ possible prophylactic antibiotics after ventricular shunting procedures, skull fracture, or penetrating head wounds to prevent infection (use is controversial).

Staff should take droplet precautions (in addition to standard precautions) for meningitis caused by *H. influenzae* and *N. meningitidis* until 24 hours after the start of effective therapy.

MEDICAL CAUSES

Cervical arthritis

With cervical arthritis, nuchal rigidity develops gradually. Initially, the patient may complain of neck stiffness in the early morning or after a period of inactivity. Stiffness then becomes increasingly severe and frequent. Pain on movement, especially with lateral motion or head turning, is common. Typically, arthritis also affects other joints, especially those in the hands.

Encephalitis

Encephalitis, a viral infection, may cause nuchal rigidity accompanied by other signs of meningeal irritation, such as positive Kernig's and Brudzinski's signs. Usually, nuchal rigidity appears abruptly and is preceded by headache, vomiting, and fever. The patient may display a rapidly decreasing LOC, progressing from lethargy to coma within 24 to 48 hours of onset. Associated features include seizures, ataxia, hemiparesis, nystagmus, and cranial nerve palsies, such as dysphagia and ptosis.

Meningitis

Nuchal rigidity is an early sign of meningitis and is accompanied by other signs of meningeal irritation — positive Kernig's and Brudzinski's signs, hyperreflexia and, possibly, opisthotonos. Other early features include fever with chills, headache, photophobia, and vomiting. Initially, the patient is confused and irritable; later, he may become stuporous and seizure-prone or may slip into coma. Cranial nerve involvement may cause ocular palsies, facial weakness, and hearing loss. An erythematous papular rash occurs in some forms of viral meningitis; a purpuric rash may occur in meningococcal meningitis.

Subarachnoid hemorrhage

Nuchal rigidity develops immediately after bleeding into the subarachnoid space. Examination may detect positive Kernig's and Brudzinski's signs. The patient may experience abrupt onset of severe headache, photophobia, fever, nausea and vomiting, dizziness, cranial nerve palsies, and focal neurologic signs, such as hemiparesis or hemiplegia. His LOC deteriorates rapidly, possibly progressing to coma. Signs of increased ICP, such as bradycardia and altered respirations, may also occur.

SPECIAL CONSIDERATIONS

Prepare the patient for diagnostic tests, such as computed tomography scans, magnetic resonance imaging, and cervical spinal X-rays.

Monitor vital signs, intake and output, and neurologic status closely. Avoid routine administration of opioid analgesics because these may mask signs of increasing ICP. Enforce strict bed rest; keep the head of the bed elevated at least 30 degrees to help minimize ICP.

Assist the patient in finding a comfortable position to obtain adequate rest.

PEDIATRIC POINTERS

Tests for nuchal rigidity are generally less reliable in children, especially infants. In younger children, move the head gently in all directions, observing for resistance. In older children, ask the child to sit upright and touch his chin to his chest. Resistance to this movement may indicate meningeal irritation.

PATIENT COUNSELING

Teach the patient with chronic sinusitis or other chronic infections the importance of seeking proper medical treatment. Explain signs and symptoms of meningitis to

---

Medical causes

Cervical arthritis
- Initially, nuchal rigidity may occur in the early morning or after a period of inactivity.
- Stiffness becomes increasingly severe and frequent.

Encephalitis
- Nuchal rigidity may occur with other signs of meningeal irritation.

Meningitis
- Nuchal rigidity is an early sign.
- Positive Kernig's and Brudzinski's signs, hyperreflexia and, possibly, opisthotonos occur.

Subarachnoid hemorrhage
- Nuchal rigidity develops immediately after bleeding into the subarachnoid space.

Special considerations
- Monitor vital signs, intake and output, and neurologic status.
- Avoid giving opioid analgesics.
- Enforce strict bed rest.
- Keep the head of the bed elevated at least 30 degrees.

Peds points
- Tests for nuchal rigidity are generally less reliable in children, especially infants.

Teaching points
- Importance of seeking proper medical treatment
- Signs and symptoms of meningitis to report

report to the health care provider. Provide reassurance and support to the patient and his family.

NYSTAGMUS

Nystagmus refers to the involuntary oscillations of one or, more commonly, both eyeballs. These oscillations are usually rhythmic and may be horizontal, vertical, rotary, or mixed. They may be transient or sustained and may occur spontaneously or on deviation or fixation of the eyes. Minor degrees of nystagmus at the extremes of gaze are normal. Nystagmus when the eyes are stationary and looking straight ahead is always abnormal. Although nystagmus is fairly easy to identify, the patient may be unaware of it unless it affects his vision.

Nystagmus may be classified as pendular or jerk. *Pendular nystagmus* consists of horizontal (pendular) or vertical (seesaw) oscillations that are equal in rate in both directions and resemble the movements of a clock's pendulum. *Jerk nystagmus* (convergence-retraction, downbeat, and vestibular), which is more common than pendular nystagmus, has a fast component and then a slow — perhaps unequal — corrective component in the opposite direction. (See *Classifying nystagmus*.)

Nystagmus is considered a *supranuclear* ocular palsy — that is, it results from pathology in the visual perceptual area, vestibular system, cerebellum, or brain stem rather than in the extraocular muscles or cranial nerves III, IV, and VI. Its causes are varied and include brain stem or cerebellar lesions, multiple sclerosis, encephalitis, labyrinthine disease, and drug toxicity. Occasionally, nystagmus is entirely normal; it's also considered a normal response in the unconscious patient during the doll's eye test (oculocephalic stimulation) or the cold caloric water test (oculovestibular stimulation).

HISTORY

Begin by asking the patient how long he's had nystagmus. Does it occur intermittently? Does it affect his vision? Ask about recent infection, especially of the ear or respiratory tract, and about head trauma and cancer. Does the patient or anyone in his family have a history of stroke? Then explore associated signs and symptoms. Ask about vertigo, dizziness, tinnitus, nausea or vomiting, numbness, weakness, bladder dysfunction, and fever.

PHYSICAL ASSESSMENT

Begin the physical assessment by evaluating the patient's level of consciousness (LOC) and vital signs. Be alert for signs of increased intracranial pressure (ICP), such as pupillary changes, drowsiness, elevated systolic pressure, and altered respiratory pattern. Next, assess nystagmus fully by testing extraocular muscle function: Ask the patient to focus straight ahead and then to follow your finger up, down, and in an "X" across his face. Note when nystagmus occurs as well as its velocity and direction. Finally, test reflexes, motor and sensory function, and the cranial nerves.

MEDICAL CAUSES

Encephalitis

With encephalitis, jerk nystagmus is typically accompanied by altered LOC ranging from lethargy to coma. Usually, it's preceded by sudden onset of fever, headache, and vomiting. Among other features are nuchal rigidity, seizures, aphasia, ataxia, photophobia, and cranial nerve palsies, such as dysphagia and ptosis.

Classifying nystagmus

The various types of jerk and pendular nystagmus are illustrated below.

JERK NYSTAGMUS

Convergence-retraction nystagmus refers to the irregular jerking of the eyes back into the orbit during upward gaze. It can indicate midbrain tegmental damage.

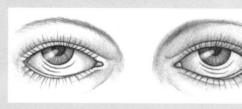

Downbeat nystagmus refers to the irregular downward jerking of the eyes during downward gaze. It can signal lower medullary damage.

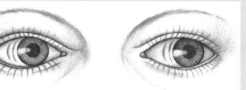

Vestibular nystagmus, the horizontal or rotary movement of the eyes, suggests vestibular disease or cochlear dysfunction.

PENDULAR NYSTAGMUS

Horizontal, or pendular, nystagmus refers to oscillations of equal velocity around a center point. It can indicate congenital loss of visual acuity or multiple sclerosis.

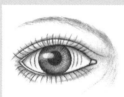
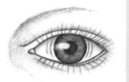

Vertical, or seesaw, nystagmus is the rapid, seesaw movement of the eyes: One eye appears to rise while the other appears to fall. It suggests an optic chiasm lesion.

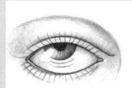
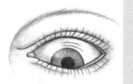

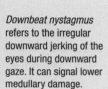
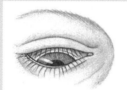
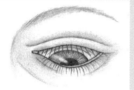

Head trauma

Brain stem injury may cause jerk nystagmus, which is usually horizontal. The patient may also display pupillary changes, altered respiratory pattern, coma, and decerebrate posture.

Medical causes
(continued)

Head trauma
✦ Brain stem injury may cause jerk nystagmus, which is usually horizontal.

Medical causes
(continued)

Labyrinthitis (acute)
✦ Sudden onset of jerk nystagmus is accompanied by dizziness, vertigo, tinnitus, and nausea.

Ménière's disease
✦ Acute attacks of jerk nystagmus, severe nausea, dizziness, vertigo, progressive hearing loss, and tinnitus occur.

Multiple sclerosis
✦ Jerk or pendular nystagmus may occur intermittently.

Stroke
✦ A stroke involving the posterior inferior cerebellar artery may cause sudden horizontal or vertical jerk nystagmus that may be gaze dependent.

Other causes
✦ Alcohol intoxication
✦ Barbiturate, phenytoin, or carbamazepine toxicity

Special considerations
✦ Prepare the patient for diagnostic tests.

Peds points
✦ In children, pendular nystagmus may be idiopathic, or it may result from early impaired vision associated with certain disorders.

Teaching points
✦ Safety measures
✦ Importance of avoiding sudden position changes

Labyrinthitis (acute)
Acute labyrinthitis is inner ear inflammation that causes sudden onset of jerk nystagmus, accompanied by dizziness, vertigo, tinnitus, nausea, and vomiting. The fast component of the nystagmus is toward the unaffected ear. Gradual sensorineural hearing loss may also occur.

Ménière's disease
Ménière's disease, an inner ear disorder, is characterized by acute attacks of jerk nystagmus, severe nausea and vomiting, dizziness, vertigo, progressive hearing loss, tinnitus, and diaphoresis. Typically, the direction of jerk nystagmus varies from one attack to the next. Attacks may last from 10 minutes to several hours.

Multiple sclerosis
With multiple sclerosis, jerk or pendular nystagmus may occur intermittently. Usually, it's preceded by diplopia, blurred vision, and paresthesia. Related signs and symptoms may include muscle weakness or paralysis, spasticity, hyperreflexia, intention tremor, gait ataxia, dysphagia, dysarthria, impotence, and emotional instability. The patient may also develop constipation, as well as urinary frequency, urgency, and incontinence.

Stroke
A stroke involving the posterior inferior cerebellar artery may cause sudden horizontal or vertical jerk nystagmus that may be gaze dependent. Other findings include dysphagia, dysarthria, loss of pain and temperature sensation on the ipsilateral face and contralateral trunk and limbs, ipsilateral Horner's syndrome (unilateral ptosis, pupillary constriction, and facial anhidrosis), and such cerebellar signs as ataxia and vertigo. Signs of increased ICP (such as altered LOC, bradycardia, widening pulse pressure, and elevated systolic pressure) may also occur.

OTHER CAUSES

Drugs and alcohol
Jerk nystagmus may result from barbiturate, phenytoin, or carbamazepine toxicity or from alcohol intoxication.

SPECIAL CONSIDERATIONS
Prepare the patient for diagnostic tests, such as electronystagmography and a cerebral computed tomography scan.

PEDIATRIC POINTERS
In children, pendular nystagmus may be idiopathic, or it may result from early impaired vision associated with such disorders as optic atrophy, albinism, congenital cataracts, or severe astigmatism.

PATIENT COUNSELING
Reinforce the need for safety measures to the patient and his family. Make sure the call bell is within reach and that the patient knows how and when to use it. Instruct the patient to avoid sudden position changes.

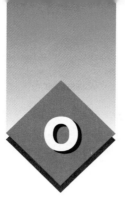

OCULAR DEVIATION

Ocular deviation refers to abnormal eye movement that may be conjugate (both eyes move together) or disconjugate (one eye moves separately from the other). This common sign may result from ocular, neurologic, endocrine, and systemic disorders that interfere with the muscles, nerves, or brain centers governing eye movement. Occasionally, it signals a life-threatening disorder such as a ruptured cerebral aneurysm.

Normally, eye movement is directly controlled by the extraocular muscles innervated by the oculomotor, trochlear, and abducens nerves (cranial nerves III, IV, and VI). Together, these muscles and nerves direct a visual stimulus to fall on corresponding parts of the retina. Disconjugate ocular deviation may result from unequal muscle tone (nonparalytic strabismus) or from muscle paralysis associated with cranial nerve damage (paralytic strabismus). Conjugate ocular deviation may result from disorders that affect the centers in the cerebral cortex and brain stem responsible for conjugate eye movement. Typically, such disorders cause gaze palsy — difficulty moving the eyes in one or more directions.

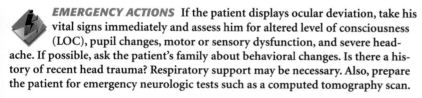

EMERGENCY ACTIONS If the patient displays ocular deviation, take his vital signs immediately and assess him for altered level of consciousness (LOC), pupil changes, motor or sensory dysfunction, and severe headache. If possible, ask the patient's family about behavioral changes. Is there a history of recent head trauma? Respiratory support may be necessary. Also, prepare the patient for emergency neurologic tests such as a computed tomography scan.

HISTORY

If the patient isn't in distress, find out how long he has had the ocular deviation. Is it accompanied by double vision, eye pain, or headache? Also, ask if he has noticed any associated motor or sensory changes, or fever.

Check for a history of hypertension, diabetes, allergies, and thyroid, neurologic, or muscular disorders. Then obtain a thorough ocular history. Has the patient ever had extraocular muscle imbalance, eye or head trauma, or eye surgery?

PHYSICAL ASSESSMENT

Perform a complete neurologic assessment, including a complete eye assessment. During the physical assessment, observe the patient for partial or complete ptosis. Does he spontaneously tilt his head or turn his face to compensate for ocular deviation? Check for eye redness or periorbital edema. Assess visual acuity; then evaluate

Key facts about ocular deviation
+ Abnormal eye movement
+ May be conjugate or disconjugate

In an emergency
+ Assess for altered LOC, pupil changes, motor or sensory dysfunction, and severe headache.
+ If possible, ask about behavioral changes or recent head trauma.

Key history points
+ Duration of ocular deviation
+ Associated double vision, eye pain, headache, motor or sensory changes, or fever
+ History of hypertension, diabetes, allergies, and thyroid, neurologic, or muscular disorders

Critical assessment steps
+ Perform a complete neurologic assessment, including a complete eye assessment.
+ Observe for partial or complete ptosis.
+ Observe for spontaneous head tilts or turns that compensate for ocular deviation.

ASSESSMENT TIP

Testing the six cardinal positions of gaze

To perform an assessment of extraocular function, sit directly in front of the patient and ask her to remain still while you hold a cylindrical object, such as a penlight, directly in front of and about 18″ (45.7 cm) away from her nose. Ask the patient to hold her head still and to watch the object as you move it clockwise through each of the six cardinal positions, returning the object to midpoint after each movement. (Three positions are shown here: left lateral, left superior, and left inferior.)

The ocular muscles must work with the muscle producing the opposite movement. Normally, when one muscle contracts, its opposite relaxes to produce a smooth motion.

Throughout the test, the patient's eyes should remain parallel as they move. Note any abnormal findings, such as nystagmus or the deviation of one eye away from the object.

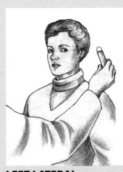

LEFT LATERAL

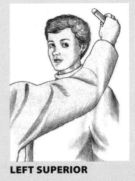

LEFT SUPERIOR

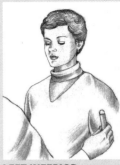

LEFT INFERIOR

extraocular muscle function by testing the six cardinal fields of gaze. (See *Testing the six cardinal positions of gaze*.)

MEDICAL CAUSES

Brain tumor

The nature of ocular deviation depends on the site and extent of the tumor. Associated signs and symptoms include headaches that are most severe in the morning, behavioral changes, memory loss, dizziness, confusion, vision loss, motor and sensory dysfunction, aphasia and, possibly, signs of hormonal imbalance. The patient's LOC may slowly deteriorate from lethargy to coma. Late signs include papilledema, vomiting, increased systolic blood pressure, widening pulse pressure, and decorticate posture.

Cerebral aneurysm

When an aneurysm near the internal carotid artery compresses the oculomotor nerve, it may produce features that resemble third cranial nerve palsy. Typically, ocular deviation and diplopia are the presenting signs. Other cardinal findings include ptosis, a dilated pupil on the affected side, and a severe, unilateral headache, usually in the frontal area. Rupture of the aneurysm abruptly intensifies the pain, which may be accompanied by nausea and vomiting. Bleeding from the site causes meningeal irritation, resulting in nuchal rigidity, back and leg pain, fever, irritability, occasional seizures, and blurred vision. Other signs and symptoms associated with intracranial bleeding include hemiparesis, dysphagia, and visual defects.

Medical causes

Brain tumor
✦ The nature of ocular deviation depends on the site and extent of the tumor.

Cerebral aneurysm
✦ Typically, ocular deviation and diplopia are the presenting signs.
✦ Ptosis, a dilated pupil on the affected side, and a severe, unilateral headache, (usually in the frontal area) may occur.

Diabetes mellitus

A leading cause of isolated third cranial nerve palsy, especially in the middle-age patient with long-standing mild diabetes, diabetes mellitus may cause ocular deviation and ptosis. Typically, the patient also complains of sudden onset of diplopia and pain.

Encephalitis

Encephalitis causes ocular deviation and diplopia in some patients. Typically, it begins abruptly with fever, headache, and vomiting, followed by signs of meningeal irritation (for example, nuchal rigidity) and of neuronal damage (for example, seizures, aphasia, ataxia, hemiparesis, cranial nerve palsies, and photophobia). The patient's LOC may rapidly deteriorate from lethargy to coma within 24 to 48 hours after onset.

Head trauma

The nature of ocular deviation depends on the site and extent of head trauma. The patient may have visible soft-tissue injury, bony deformity, facial edema, and clear or bloody otorrhea or rhinorrhea. Besides these obvious signs of trauma, he may also develop blurred vision, diplopia, nystagmus, behavioral changes, headache, motor and sensory dysfunction, and a decreased LOC that may progress to coma. Signs of increased intracranial pressure—such as bradycardia, increased systolic pressure, and widening pulse pressure—may also occur.

Multiple sclerosis

Ocular deviation may be an early sign of multiple sclerosis. Accompanying it are diplopia, blurred vision, and sensory dysfunction such as paresthesia. Other signs and symptoms include nystagmus, constipation, muscle weakness, paralysis, spasticity, hyperreflexia, intention tremor, gait ataxia, dysphagia, dysarthria, impotence, and emotional instability. In addition, the patient may experience urinary frequency, urgency, and incontinence.

Myasthenia gravis

With myasthenia gravis, ocular deviation may accompany the more common presenting signs of diplopia and ptosis. This disorder may affect only the eye muscles, or it may progress to other muscle groups, causing altered facial expression, difficulty chewing, dysphagia, weakened voice, and impaired fine hand movements. Signs of respiratory distress reflect weakness of the diaphragm and other respiratory muscles.

Ophthalmoplegic migraine

Most common in young adults, an ophthalmoplegic migraine produces ocular deviation and diplopia that persist for days after the pain subsides. Associated signs and symptoms include unilateral headache, possibly with ptosis on the same side; temporary hemiplegia; and sensory deficits. Irritability, depression, or slight confusion may also occur.

Orbital blowout fracture

In an orbital blowout fracture, the inferior rectus muscle may become entrapped, resulting in limited extraocular movement and ocular deviation. Typically, the patient's upward gaze is absent; other directions of gaze may be affected if edema is dramatic. The globe may also be displaced downward and inward. Associated signs and symptoms include pain, diplopia, nausea, periorbital edema, and ecchymosis.

Medical causes
(continued)

Diabetes mellitus
+ Ocular deviation and ptosis occur.

Encephalitis
+ Ocular deviation and diplopia occur in some patients.
+ Fever, headache, and vomiting are followed by signs of meningeal irritation and neuronal damage.

Head trauma
+ The nature of ocular deviation depends on the site and extent of head trauma.
+ The patient may have visible soft-tissue injury, bony deformity, facial edema, and clear or bloody otorrhea or rhinorrhea.

Multiple sclerosis
+ Ocular deviation may be an early sign.
+ Diplopia, blurred vision, and sensory dysfunction occur.

Myasthenia gravis
+ Ocular deviation may accompany the more common presenting signs of diplopia and ptosis.

Ophthalmoplegic migraine
+ Ocular deviation and diplopia persist for days after the pain subsides.

Orbital blowout fracture
+ The inferior rectus muscle may become entrapped, resulting in limited extraocular movement and ocular deviation.
+ Typically, upward gaze is absent.

Medical causes
(continued)

Orbital tumor
+ Ocular deviation occurs as the tumor gradually enlarges.

Stroke
+ The nature of ocular deviation depends on the site and extent of the stroke.

Thyrotoxicosis
+ Exophthalmos occurs, which causes limited extraocular movement and ocular deviation.
+ Usually, the upward gaze weakens first, followed by diplopia.

Special considerations
+ Monitor vital signs and neurologic status if you suspect an acute neurologic disorder.

Peds points
+ In children, the most common cause of ocular deviation is nonparalytic strabismus.

Teaching points
+ Explanation of disorder and its treatment
+ Changes in LOC to report
+ Ways to maintain a safe environment and reduce environmental stress

Key facts about oligomenorrhea
+ Abnormally infrequent menstrual bleeding (three to six menstrual cycles per year)
+ Is common in infertile, early postmenarchal, and perimenopausal women

---

Orbital tumor
Ocular deviation occurs as the tumor gradually enlarges. Associated findings include proptosis, diplopia and, possibly, blurred vision. The eyelid may also appear edematous.

Stroke
Stroke is a life-threatening disorder that may cause ocular deviation, depending on the site and extent of the stroke. Accompanying features of a stroke are also variable and include altered LOC, contralateral hemiplegia and sensory loss, dysarthria, dysphagia, homonymous hemianopsia, blurred vision, and diplopia. In addition, the patient may develop urine retention or incontinence or both, constipation, behavioral changes, headache, vomiting, and seizures.

Thyrotoxicosis
Thyrotoxicosis may produce exophthalmos — protruding eyes — which, in turn, causes limited extraocular movement and ocular deviation. Usually, the patient's upward gaze weakens first, followed by diplopia. Other features are lid retraction, a wide-eyed staring gaze, excessive tearing, edematous eyelids and, sometimes, inability to close the eyes. Cardinal features of thyrotoxicosis include tachycardia, palpitations, weight loss despite increased appetite, diarrhea, tremors, an enlarged thyroid, dyspnea, nervousness, diaphoresis, heat intolerance, and an atrial or ventricular gallop.

SPECIAL CONSIDERATIONS

Continue to monitor the patient's vital signs and neurologic status if you suspect an acute neurologic disorder. Take seizure precautions, if necessary. Also, prepare the patient for diagnostic tests, such as blood studies, orbital and skull X-rays, and computed tomography scan.

PEDIATRIC POINTERS

In children, the most common cause of ocular deviation is nonparalytic strabismus. Normally, children achieve binocular vision by age 3 to 4 months. Although severe strabismus is readily apparent, mild strabismus must be confirmed by tests for misalignment, such as the corneal light reflex test and the cover test. Testing is crucial — early corrective measures help preserve binocular vision and cosmetic appearance. Also, mild strabismus may indicate retinoblastoma, a tumor that may produce no symptoms before age 2 except for a characteristic whitish reflex in the pupil.

PATIENT COUNSELING

Explain the disorder and its treatment to the patient and his family. Teach them to recognize and report changes in LOC. Discuss ways to maintain a safe environment at home and to reduce environmental stress.

OLIGOMENORRHEA

In most women, menstrual bleeding occurs every 28 days plus or minus 4 days. Although some variation is normal, menstrual bleeding at intervals of greater than 36 days may indicate oligomenorrhea — abnormally infrequent menstrual bleeding characterized by three to six menstrual cycles per year. When menstrual bleeding does occur, it's usually profuse, prolonged (up to 10 days), and laden with clots and tissue. Occasionally, scant bleeding or spotting occurs between these heavy menses.

Oligomenorrhea may develop suddenly, or it may follow a period of gradually lengthening cycles. Although oligomenorrhea may alternate with normal menstrual bleeding, it can progress to secondary amenorrhea.

Because oligomenorrhea is commonly associated with anovulation, it's common in infertile, early postmenarchal, and perimenopausal women. This sign usually reflects abnormalities of the hormones that govern normal endometrial function. It may result from ovarian, hypothalamic, pituitary, and other metabolic disorders, and from the effects of certain drugs. It may also result from emotional or physical stress, such as sudden weight change, debilitating illness, or rigorous physical training.

HISTORY

After asking the patient's age, find out when menarche occurred. Has the patient ever experienced normal menstrual cycles? When did she begin having abnormal cycles? Ask her to describe the pattern of bleeding. How many days does the bleeding last, and how frequently does it occur? Are there clots and tissue fragments in her menstrual flow? Note when she last had menstrual bleeding.

Next, determine if she's having symptoms of ovulatory bleeding. Does she experience mild, cramping abdominal pain 14 days before she bleeds? Is the bleeding accompanied by premenstrual symptoms, such as breast tenderness, irritability, bloating, weight gain, nausea, and diarrhea? Does she have cramping or pain with bleeding? Also, check for a history of infertility. Does the patient have any children? Is she trying to conceive? Ask if she's currently using hormonal contraceptives or if she has ever used them in the past. If she has, find out when she stopped taking them.

 CULTURAL CUE *Be sensitive when you ask questions about sexual activity. In many cultures, women may be reluctant to discuss sexual matters with others.*

Then ask about previous gynecologic disorders such as ovarian cysts. If the patient is breast-feeding, has she experienced any problems with milk production? If she hasn't been breast-feeding recently, has she noticed milk leaking from her breasts? Ask about recent weight gain or loss. Is the patient less than 80% of her ideal weight? If so, does she claim that she's overweight? Ask if she's exercising more vigorously than usual.

Screen for metabolic disorders by asking about excessive thirst, frequent urination, or fatigue. Has the patient been jittery or had palpitations? Ask about headache, dizziness, and impaired peripheral vision. Complete the history by finding out what drugs the patient is taking.

PHYSICAL ASSESSMENT

Begin the physical assessment by taking the patient's vital signs and weighing her. Inspect for increased facial hair growth, sparse body hair, male distribution of fat and muscle, acne, and clitoral enlargement. Note if the skin is abnormally dry or moist, and check hair texture. Also, be alert for signs of psychological or physical stress. Rule out pregnancy by a blood or urine pregnancy test.

MEDICAL CAUSES

Adrenal hyperplasia

In adrenal hyperplasia, oligomenorrhea may occur with signs of androgen excess, such as clitoral enlargement, deepening voice, acne, and male distribution of hair, fat, and muscle mass.

Key history points
+ Current age
+ Menstrual history, including age of menarche and characteristics and duration of bleeding
+ Associated symptoms of ovulatory bleeding
+ Hormonal contraceptive use
+ Previous gynecologic disorders
+ Associated problems with breast-feeding
+ Weight gain or loss
+ Associated excessive thirst, frequent urination, fatigue, jitteriness, palpitations, headache, dizziness, and impaired peripheral vision
+ Drug history

Critical assessment steps
+ Take vital signs and weigh the patient.
+ Inspect for increased facial hair growth, sparse body hair, male distribution of fat and muscle, acne, and clitoral enlargement.
+ Note if the skin is abnormally dry or moist; check hair texture.
+ Be alert for signs of psychological or physical stress.
+ Rule out pregnancy.

Medical causes
Adrenal hyperplasia
+ Oligomenorrhea may occur with signs of androgen excess.

Medical causes
(continued)

Anorexia nervosa
✦ Sporadic oligomenorrhea or amenorrhea may occur along with a morbid fear of being fat and weight loss of more than 20% of ideal body weight.

Diabetes mellitus
✦ Oligomenorrhea may be an early sign.

Hypothyroidism
✦ Oligomenorrhea, fatigue, cold intolerance, constipation, bradycardia, and other signs and symptoms may occur.

Polycystic ovary disease
✦ About 25% of women with this disease have oligomenorrhea.

Prolactin-secreting pituitary tumor
✦ Oligomenorrhea or amenorrhea may be the first sign.

Thyrotoxicosis
✦ Oligomenorrhea may occur with reduced fertility.

Other causes
✦ Amphetamines, antihypertensives, and phenothiazine derivatives
✦ Drugs that increase androgen levels
✦ Hormonal contraceptives (when discontinued)

Special considerations
✦ Prepare the patient for diagnostic tests.

Anorexia nervosa
Anorexia nervosa may cause sporadic oligomenorrhea or amenorrhea. Its cardinal symptom, however, is a morbid fear of being fat associated with weight loss of more than 20% of ideal body weight. Typically, the patient displays dramatic skeletal muscle atrophy and loss of fatty tissue; dry or sparse scalp hair; lanugo on the face and body; and blotchy or sallow, dry skin. Other symptoms include constipation, decreased libido, and sleep disturbances.

Diabetes mellitus
Oligomenorrhea may be an early sign of diabetes mellitus. In juvenile-onset diabetes, the patient may have never had normal menses. Associated findings include excessive hunger, polydipsia, polyuria, weakness, fatigue, dry mucous membranes, poor skin turgor, irritability and emotional lability, and weight loss.

Hypothyroidism
Besides oligomenorrhea, hypothyroidism may result in fatigue; forgetfulness; cold intolerance; unexplained weight gain; constipation; bradycardia; decreased mental acuity; dry, flaky, inelastic skin; puffy face, hands, and feet; hoarseness; periorbital edema; ptosis; dry, sparse hair; and thick, brittle nails.

Polycystic ovary disease
About 25% of women with polycystic ovary disease have oligomenorrhea, but some may have amenorrhea, menometrorrhagia, or irregular menses. Infertility, anovulation, and enlarged, palpable ovaries are also common. Other features vary but may include signs of androgen excess — male distribution of body hair and muscle mass, facial hair growth, acne and, occasionally, obesity.

Prolactin-secreting pituitary tumor
Oligomenorrhea or amenorrhea may be the first sign of a prolactin-secreting pituitary tumor. Accompanying findings include unilateral or bilateral galactorrhea, infertility, loss of libido, and sparse pubic hair. Headache and visual field disturbances — such as diminished peripheral vision, blurred vision, diplopia, and hemianopia — signal tumor expansion.

Thyrotoxicosis
Thyrotoxicosis may produce oligomenorrhea along with reduced fertility. Cardinal findings include irritability, weight loss despite increased appetite, dyspnea, tachycardia, palpitations, diarrhea, tremors, diaphoresis, heat intolerance, an enlarged thyroid and, possibly, exophthalmos.

OTHER CAUSES

Drugs
Drugs that increase androgen levels — such as corticosteroids, corticotropin, anabolic steroids, danazol (Danocrine), and injectable and implanted contraceptives — may cause oligomenorrhea. Hormonal contraceptives may be associated with delayed resumption of normal menses when their use is discontinued; however, 95% of women resume normal menses within 3 months. Other drugs that may cause oligomenorrhea include phenothiazine derivatives and amphetamines, and antihypertensive drugs, which increase prolactin levels.

SPECIAL CONSIDERATIONS
Prepare the patient for diagnostic tests, such as blood hormone levels, thyroid studies, or pelvic imaging studies.

PEDIATRIC POINTERS

Teenage girls may experience oligomenorrhea associated with immature hormonal function. However, prolonged oligomenorrhea or the development of amenorrhea may signal congenital adrenal hyperplasia or Turner's syndrome.

GERIATRIC POINTERS

Oligomenorrhea in the perimenopausal woman usually indicates impending onset of menopause.

PATIENT COUNSELING

Ask the patient to record her basal body temperature to determine if she's having ovulatory cycles. Provide her with blank charts, and teach her how to keep them accurately. Have the patient use a home ovulation testing or urine luteinizing hormone kit to provide evidence of ovulation. Remind the patient that she may become pregnant because ovulation may still occur even though she isn't menstruating normally. Discuss contraceptive measures as appropriate.

OLIGURIA

A cardinal sign of renal and urinary tract disorders, oliguria is clinically defined as urine output of less than 400 ml/24 hours. Typically, this sign occurs abruptly and may herald serious — possibly life-threatening — hemodynamic instability. Its causes can be classified as prerenal (decreased renal blood flow), intrarenal (intrinsic renal damage), or postrenal (urinary tract obstruction); the pathophysiology differs for each classification. (See *How oliguria develops,* page 470.) Oliguria associated with a prerenal or postrenal cause is usually promptly reversible with treatment, although it may lead to intrarenal damage if untreated. However, oliguria associated with an intrarenal cause is usually more persistent and may be irreversible.

HISTORY

Begin by asking the patient about his usual daily voiding pattern, including frequency and amount. When did he first notice changes in this pattern and in the color, odor, or consistency of his urine? Ask about pain or burning on urination. Has the patient had a fever? Note his normal daily fluid intake. Has he recently been drinking more or less than usual? Has his intake of caffeine or alcohol changed drastically? Has he had recent episodes of diarrhea or vomiting that might cause fluid loss? Next, explore associated complaints, especially fatigue, loss of appetite, thirst, dyspnea, chest pain, or recent weight gain or loss (in dehydration).

Check for a history of renal, urinary tract, or cardiovascular disorders. Note recent traumatic injury or surgery associated with significant blood loss, as well as recent blood transfusions. Was the patient exposed to nephrotoxic agents, such as heavy metals, organic solvents, anesthetics, or radiographic contrast media? Next, obtain a drug history.

PHYSICAL ASSESSMENT

Begin the physical assessment by taking the patient's vital signs and weighing him. Assess his overall appearance for edema. Palpate both kidneys for tenderness and enlargement, and percuss for costovertebral angle (CVA) tenderness. Also, inspect the flank area for edema or erythema. Auscultate the heart and lungs for abnormal

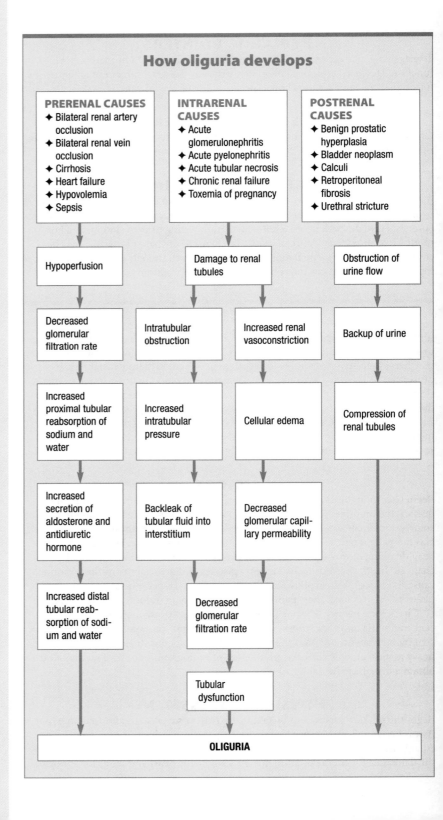

How oliguria develops

PRERENAL CAUSES
- Bilateral renal artery occlusion
- Bilateral renal vein occlusion
- Cirrhosis
- Heart failure
- Hypovolemia
- Sepsis

INTRARENAL CAUSES
- Acute glomerulonephritis
- Acute pyelonephritis
- Acute tubular necrosis
- Chronic renal failure
- Toxemia of pregnancy

POSTRENAL CAUSES
- Benign prostatic hyperplasia
- Bladder neoplasm
- Calculi
- Retroperitoneal fibrosis
- Urethral stricture

Hypoperfusion

Damage to renal tubules

Obstruction of urine flow

Decreased glomerular filtration rate

Intratubular obstruction

Increased renal vasoconstriction

Backup of urine

Increased proximal tubular reabsorption of sodium and water

Increased intratubular pressure

Cellular edema

Compression of renal tubules

Increased secretion of aldosterone and antidiuretic hormone

Backleak of tubular fluid into interstitium

Decreased glomerular capillary permeability

Increased distal tubular reabsorption of sodium and water

Decreased glomerular filtration rate

Tubular dysfunction

OLIGURIA

sounds, and the flank area for renal artery bruits. Assess the patient for edema or signs of dehydration such as dry mucous membranes.

Obtain a urine specimen, and inspect it for abnormal color, odor, or sediment. Use reagent strips to test for glucose, protein, and blood. Also, use a urinometer to measure specific gravity.

MEDICAL CAUSES

Acute tubular necrosis

An early sign of acute tubular necrosis, oliguria may occur abruptly (in shock) or gradually (in nephrotoxicity). Usually, it persists for about 2 weeks, followed by polyuria. Related features include signs of hyperkalemia (muscle weakness and cardiac arrhythmias), uremia (anorexia, confusion, lethargy, twitching, seizures, pruritus, and Kussmaul's respirations), and heart failure (edema, jugular vein distention, crackles, and dyspnea).

Calculi

Oliguria or anuria may result from calculi lodging in the kidneys, ureters, bladder outlet, or urethra. Associated signs and symptoms include urinary frequency and urgency, dysuria, and hematuria or pyuria. Usually, the patient experiences renal colic — excruciating pain that radiates from the CVA to the flank, the suprapubic region, and the external genitalia. This pain may be accompanied by nausea, vomiting, hypoactive bowel sounds, abdominal distention and, occasionally, fever and chills.

Glomerulonephritis (acute)

Acute glomerulonephritis produces oliguria or anuria. Other features are mild fever, fatigue, gross hematuria, proteinuria, generalized edema, elevated blood pressure, headache, nausea and vomiting, flank and abdominal pain, and signs of pulmonary congestion (dyspnea and productive cough).

Heart failure

Oliguria may occur in left-sided heart failure as a result of low cardiac output and decreased renal perfusion. Accompanying signs and symptoms include dyspnea, fatigue, weakness, peripheral edema, distended jugular veins, tachycardia, tachypnea, crackles, and a dry or productive cough. In advanced heart failure, the patient may also develop orthopnea, cyanosis, clubbing, ventricular gallop, diastolic hypertension, cardiomegaly, and hemoptysis.

Hypovolemia

Any disorder that decreases circulating fluid volume can produce oliguria. Associated findings in hypovolemia include orthostatic hypotension, apathy, lethargy, fatigue, gross muscle weakness, anorexia, nausea, profound thirst, dizziness, sunken eyeballs, poor skin turgor, and dry mucous membranes.

Pyelonephritis (acute)

Accompanying the sudden onset of oliguria in acute pyelonephritis are high fever with chills, fatigue, flank pain, CVA tenderness, weakness, nocturia, dysuria, hematuria, urinary frequency and urgency, and tenesmus. The urine may appear cloudy. Occasionally, the patient with acute pyelonephritis also experiences anorexia, nausea, diarrhea, and vomiting.

Renal artery occlusion (bilateral)

Renal artery occlusion may produce oliguria or, more commonly, anuria. Other features include severe, constant upper abdominal and flank pain, nausea and vom-

---

Medical causes

Acute tubular necrosis
✦ Oliguria may occur abruptly (in shock) or gradually (in nephrotoxicity) and persists for about 2 weeks, followed by polyuria.

Calculi
✦ Oliguria may result from calculi lodging in the kidneys, ureters, bladder outlet, or urethra.

Glomerulonephritis (acute)
✦ Oliguria or anuria occurs.

Heart failure
✦ Oliguria may occur in left-sided heart failure due to low cardiac output and decreased renal perfusion.

Hypovolemia
✦ Decreased circulating fluid volume can produce oliguria.

Pyelonephritis (acute)
✦ Oliguria, high fever with chills, fatigue, flank pain, CVA tenderness, weakness, nocturia, dysuria, hematuria, urinary frequency and urgency, and tenesmus occur.

Renal artery occlusion (bilateral)
✦ Oliguria or, more commonly, anuria may accompany severe, constant upper abdominal and flank pain, nausea and vomiting, and hypoactive bowel sounds.

Medical causes
(continued)

Renal failure (chronic)
✦ Oliguria is a major sign of end-stage chronic renal failure.

Renal vein occlusion (bilateral)
✦ Occasionally, oliguria occurs with acute low back and flank pain, CVA tenderness, fever, pallor, hematuria, enlarged and palpable kidneys, and edema.

Sepsis
✦ Oliguria, fever, chills, restlessness, confusion, diaphoresis, anorexia, vomiting, diarrhea, pallor, hypotension, and tachycardia occur.

Toxemia of pregnancy
✦ Oliguria may be accompanied by elevated blood pressure, dizziness, diplopia, blurred vision, nausea and vomiting, irritability, and frontal headache.

Urethral stricture
✦ Oliguria is accompanied by chronic urethral discharge, urinary frequency and urgency, dysuria, pyuria, and diminished urine stream.

Other causes
✦ Acyclovir, adrenergics, aminoglycosides, anticholinergics, chemotherapeutic drugs, diuretics, sulfonamides
✦ Contrast media

Special considerations
✦ Monitor vital signs, intake and output, and daily weight.
✦ Provide diet low in sodium, potassium, and protein.

iting, and hypoactive bowel sounds. The patient also develops a fever 1 to 2 days after the occlusion, as well as diastolic hypertension.

Renal failure (chronic)
Oliguria is a major sign of end-stage chronic renal failure. Associated findings reflect progressive uremia and include fatigue, weakness, irritability, uremic fetor, ecchymoses and petechiae, peripheral edema, elevated blood pressure, confusion, emotional lability, drowsiness, coarse muscle twitching, muscle cramps, peripheral neuropathies, anorexia, metallic taste in the mouth, nausea and vomiting, constipation or diarrhea, stomatitis, pruritus, pallor, and yellow- or bronze-tinged skin. Eventually, seizures, coma, and uremic frost may develop.

Renal vein occlusion (bilateral)
Renal vein occlusion occasionally causes oliguria accompanied by acute low back and flank pain, CVA tenderness, fever, pallor, hematuria, enlarged and palpable kidneys, edema and, possibly, signs of uremia.

Sepsis
Any condition that results in sepsis may produce oliguria, along with fever, chills, restlessness, confusion, diaphoresis, anorexia, vomiting, diarrhea, pallor, hypotension, and tachycardia. The patient may exhibit signs of local infection, such as dysuria and wound drainage. In severe infection, he may develop lactic acidosis marked by Kussmaul's respirations.

Toxemia of pregnancy
In severe preeclampsia, oliguria may be accompanied by elevated blood pressure, dizziness, diplopia, blurred vision, epigastric pain, nausea and vomiting, irritability, and severe frontal headache. Typically, the oliguria is preceded by generalized edema and sudden weight gain of more than 3 lb (1.4 kg) per week during the second trimester or more than 1 lb (0.5 kg) per week during the third trimester. If preeclampsia progresses to eclampsia, the patient develops seizures and may slip into coma.

Urethral stricture
Urethral stricture produces oliguria accompanied by chronic urethral discharge, urinary frequency and urgency, dysuria, pyuria, and diminished urine stream. As obstruction worsens, urine extravasation may lead to formation of urinomas and urosepsis.

OTHER CAUSES

Diagnostic studies
Radiographic studies that use contrast media may cause nephrotoxicity and oliguria.

Drugs
Oliguria may result from drugs that cause decreased renal perfusion (diuretics), nephrotoxicity (most notably, aminoglycosides and chemotherapeutic drugs), urine retention (adrenergics and anticholinergics), or urinary obstruction associated with precipitation of urinary crystals (sulfonamides and acyclovir).

SPECIAL CONSIDERATIONS

Monitor vital signs, intake and output, and daily weight. Depending on the cause of the oliguria, fluids are normally restricted to between 600 ml and 1 L more than the patient's urine output for the previous day. Provide a diet low in sodium, potassium, and protein.

Laboratory tests may be necessary to determine if the oliguria is reversible. Such tests include serum blood urea nitrogen and creatinine levels, urea and creatinine clearance, urine sodium levels, and urine osmolality. Abdominal X-rays, ultrasonography, computed tomography scan, cystography, and a renal scan may be required.

PEDIATRIC POINTERS

In the neonate, oliguria may result from edema or dehydration. Major causes include congenital heart disease, respiratory distress syndrome, sepsis, congenital hydronephrosis, acute tubular necrosis, and renal vein thrombosis. Common causes of oliguria in children between ages 1 and 5 are acute poststreptococcal glomerulonephritis and hemolytic-uremic syndrome. After age 5, causes of oliguria are similar to those in adults.

GERIATRIC POINTERS

In elderly patients, oliguria may result from gradual progression of an underlying disorder. It may also result from overall poor muscle tone secondary to inactivity, poor fluid intake, and infrequent voiding attempts.

PATIENT COUNSELING

Explain applicable fluid restrictions or increases to the patient. For example, the patient with renal calculi may require increased fluids, whereas the patient with renal failure may need to restrict fluid intake. Review the prescribed diet with the patient, and obtain a nutritional consult, if necessary.

ORTHOPNEA

Orthopnea—difficulty breathing in the supine position—is a common symptom of cardiopulmonary disorders that produce dyspnea. In many patients, it's a subtle symptom; the patient may complain that he can't catch his breath when lying down, or he may mention that he sleeps most comfortably in a reclining chair or propped up by pillows. Derived from this complaint is the common classification of two- or three-pillow orthopnea.

Orthopnea presumably results from increased hydrostatic pressure in the pulmonary vasculature related to gravitational effects in the supine position. It may be aggravated by obesity or pregnancy, which restricts diaphragmatic excursion. Assuming the upright position relieves orthopnea by placing much of the pulmonary vasculature above the left atrium, which reduces mean hydrostatic pressure, and by enhancing diaphragmatic excursion, which increases inspiratory volume.

HISTORY

Begin by asking about a history of cardiopulmonary disorders, such as myocardial infarction, rheumatic heart disease, valvular disease, asthma, emphysema, or chronic bronchitis. Does the patient smoke? If so, how much? Explore associated symptoms, noting especially complaints of cough, nocturnal or exertional dyspnea, fatigue, weakness, loss of appetite, or chest pain. Does the patient use alcohol or have a history of heavy alcohol use?

Peds points

✦ In a neonate, oliguria may result from edema or dehydration, congenital heart disease, respiratory distress syndrome, sepsis, congenital hydronephrosis, acute tubular necrosis, and renal vein thrombosis.

✦ Causes of oliguria in children ages 1 to 5 include hemolytic-uremic syndrome and acute poststreptococcal glomerulonephritis.

Geri points

✦ In elderly patients, oliguria may result from an underlying disorder, overall poor muscle tone secondary to inactivity, poor fluid intake, and infrequent voiding attempts.

Teaching points

✦ Fluid and dietary restrictions

Key facts about orthopnea

✦ Results from increased hydrostatic pressure in the pulmonary vasculature related to being in the supine position

Key history points

✦ History of cardiopulmonary disorders
✦ Smoking habits
✦ Associated cough, dyspnea, fatigue, loss of appetite, or chest pain

PHYSICAL ASSESSMENT

When examining the patient, check for other signs of increased respiratory effort, such as accessory muscle use, shallow respirations, and tachypnea. Also note barrel chest. Inspect the patient's skin for pallor or cyanosis, and the fingers for clubbing. Observe and palpate for edema, and check for jugular vein distention. Auscultate the lungs and heart. Monitor the patient's oxygen saturation.

MEDICAL CAUSES

Chronic obstructive pulmonary disease

Chronic obstructive pulmonary disease (COPD) typically produces orthopnea and other dyspneic complaints, accompanied by accessory muscle use, tachypnea, tachycardia, and paradoxical pulse. Auscultation may reveal diminished breath sounds, rhonchi, crackles, and wheezing. The patient may also exhibit a dry or productive cough with copious sputum. Other features include anorexia, weight loss, and edema. Barrel chest, cyanosis, and clubbing are usually late signs.

Left-sided heart failure

Orthopnea occurs late in left-sided heart failure. If heart failure is acute, orthopnea may begin suddenly; if chronic, it may become constant. The earliest symptom of left-sided heart failure is progressively severe dyspnea. Other common early symptoms include Cheyne-Stokes respirations, paroxysmal nocturnal dyspnea, fatigue, weakness, and a cough that may occasionally produce clear or blood-tinged sputum. Tachycardia, tachypnea, and crackles may also occur.

Other late findings include cyanosis, clubbing, ventricular gallop, and hemoptysis. Left-sided heart failure may also lead to such signs of shock as hypotension, thready pulse, and cold, clammy skin.

Mediastinal tumor

Orthopnea is an early sign of a mediastinal tumor, resulting from pressure of the tumor against the trachea, bronchus, or lung when the patient lies down. However, many patients are asymptomatic until the tumor enlarges. Then it produces retrosternal chest pain, dry cough, hoarseness, dysphagia, stertorous respirations, palpitations, and cyanosis. Examination reveals suprasternal retractions on inspiration, bulging of the chest wall, tracheal deviation, dilated jugular and superficial chest veins, and edema of the face, neck, and arms.

SPECIAL CONSIDERATIONS

To relieve orthopnea, place the patient in semi-Fowler's or high Fowler's position; if this doesn't help, have the patient lean over a bedside table with his chest forward. If necessary, administer oxygen via nasal cannula. A diuretic may be needed to reduce lung fluid. Monitor electrolyte levels closely after administering diuretics. Angiotensin-converting enzyme inhibitors should be used for patients with left-sided heart failure, unless contraindicated. Monitor intake and output closely.

An electrocardiogram, a chest X-ray, a pulmonary function test, and an arterial blood gas test may be necessary for further evaluation.

A central venous line or pulmonary artery catheter may be inserted to help measure central venous pressure and wedge and cardiac output, respectively.

PEDIATRIC POINTERS

Common causes of orthopnea in children include heart failure, croup syndrome, cystic fibrosis, and asthma. Sleeping in an infant seat may improve symptoms for a young child.

GERIATRIC POINTERS

If the elderly patient is using more than one pillow at night, consider noncardiogenic pulmonary reasons for this, such as gastroesophageal reflux disease, sleep apnea, arthritis, or simply the need for greater comfort.

PATIENT COUNSELING

Instruct the patient to notify the physician if he's using additional pillows regularly or if dyspnea worsens at night. Teach him to follow a low-sodium diet and to limit fluids. Tell him to weigh himself daily and to report a weight gain of 1⅛ to 2¼ lb (0.5 to 1 kg) in one day.

ORTHOSTATIC HYPOTENSION

In orthostatic hypotension, also called *postural hypertension,* the patient's blood pressure drops 15 to 20 mm Hg or more — with or without an increase in the heart rate of at least 20 beats/minute — when he rises from a supine to a sitting or standing position. (Blood pressure should be measured 5 minutes after the patient has changed his position.) This common sign indicates failure of compensatory vasomotor responses to adjust to position changes. It's typically associated with lightheadedness, syncope, or blurred vision and may occur in a hypotensive, normotensive, or hypertensive patient. Although commonly a nonpathologic sign in elderly patients, orthostatic hypotension may result from prolonged bed rest, fluid and electrolyte imbalance, endocrine or systemic disorders, and the effects of drugs.

To detect orthostatic hypotension, take and compare blood pressure readings with the patient supine, sitting, and then standing.

 EMERGENCY ACTIONS If you detect orthostatic hypotension, quickly check for tachycardia, altered level of consciousness (LOC), and pale, clammy skin. If these signs are present, suspect hypovolemic shock. Insert a large-bore I.V. line for fluid or blood replacement. Take the patient's vital signs every 15 minutes, and monitor his intake and output.

HISTORY

If the patient is in no danger, obtain a history. Ask the patient if he frequently experiences dizziness, weakness, or fainting when he stands. Also ask about associated symptoms, particularly fatigue, orthopnea, impotence, nausea, headache, abdominal or chest discomfort, and GI bleeding. Then obtain a complete drug history.

PHYSICAL ASSESSMENT

Begin the physical assessment by checking the patient's skin turgor. Palpate peripheral pulses, and auscultate the heart and lungs. Finally, test muscle strength and observe the patient's gait for unsteadiness.

MEDICAL CAUSES

Adrenal insufficiency

In adrenal insufficiency, orthostatic hypotension may be accompanied by fatigue, muscle weakness, poor coordination, anorexia, nausea and vomiting, fasting hypoglycemia, weight loss, abdominal pain, irritability, and a weak, irregular pulse. Another common feature is hyperpigmentation — bronze coloring of the skin — which is especially prominent on the face, lips, gums, tongue, buccal mucosa, el-

Geri points

✦ Consider noncardiogenic pulmonary reasons if patient is using more than one pillow in bed.

Teaching points

✦ Signs and symptoms to report
✦ Dietary and fluid restrictions
✦ Daily weight

Key facts about orthostatic hypotension

✦ Involves a blood pressure drop of 15 to 20 mm Hg or more upon rising from a supine to a sitting or standing position

In an emergency

✦ Check for tachycardia, altered LOC, and pale, clammy skin.
✦ Insert a large-bore I.V. line.
✦ Take vital signs frequently.

Key history points

✦ Dizziness, weakness, or fainting when standing
✦ Associated fatigue, orthopnea, nausea, headache, abdominal or chest discomfort, and GI bleeding
✦ Drug history

Critical assessment steps

✦ Check skin turgor.
✦ Palpate peripheral pulses.
✦ Auscultate the heart and lungs.

Medical causes

Adrenal insufficiency

✦ Orthostatic hypotension may be accompanied by such signs and symptoms as fatigue, muscle weakness, anorexia, abdominal pain, and hyperpigmentation.

Medical causes
(continued)

Amyloidosis
✦ Orthostatic hypotension is common.

Diabetic autonomic neuropathy
✦ Orthostatic hypotension, syncope, dysphagia, constipation or diarrhea, painless bladder distention with overflow incontinence, impotence, and retrograde ejaculation may occur.

Hyperaldosteronism
✦ Orthostatic hypotension with sustained elevated blood pressure occurs.

Hyponatremia
✦ Orthostatic hypotension is accompanied by headache, tachycardia, and abdominal cramps.

Hypovolemia
✦ Orthostatic hypotension is associated with apathy, fatigue, muscle weakness, anorexia, nausea, and profound thirst.

Other causes
✦ Antihypertensives, bretylium, levodopa, MAO inhibitors, morphine, nitrates, phenothiazines, spinal anesthesia, and tricyclic antidepressants
✦ Large doses of diuretics
✦ Prolonged bed rest
✦ Sympathectomy

bows, palms, knuckles, waist, and knees. Diarrhea, constipation, decreased libido, amenorrhea, and syncope may also occur along with enhanced taste, smell, and hearing, and cravings for salty food.

Amyloidosis
Orthostatic hypotension is commonly associated with amyloid infiltration of the autonomic nerves. Associated signs and symptoms vary widely and include angina, tachycardia, dyspnea, orthopnea, fatigue, and cough.

Diabetic autonomic neuropathy
Orthostatic hypotension may be accompanied by syncope, dysphagia, constipation or diarrhea, painless bladder distention with overflow incontinence, impotence, and retrograde ejaculation.

Hyperaldosteronism
Hyperaldosteronism typically produces orthostatic hypotension with sustained elevated blood pressure. Most other clinical effects of hyperaldosteronism result from hypokalemia, which increases neuromuscular irritability and produces muscle weakness, intermittent flaccid paralysis, fatigue, headache, paresthesia and, possibly, tetany with positive Trousseau's and Chvostek's signs. The patient may also exhibit vision disturbance, nocturia, polydipsia, and personality changes. Diabetes mellitus is a common finding.

Hyponatremia
In hyponatremia, orthostatic hypotension is typically accompanied by headache, profound thirst, tachycardia, nausea and vomiting, abdominal cramps, muscle twitching and weakness, fatigue, oliguria or anuria, cold clammy skin, poor skin turgor, irritability, seizures, and decreased LOC. Cyanosis, thready pulse, and eventually vasomotor collapse may occur in severe sodium deficit. Common causes include adrenal insufficiency, hypothyroidism, syndrome of inappropriate antidiuretic hormone secretion, and use of thiazide diuretics.

Hypovolemia
Mild to moderate hypovolemia may cause orthostatic hypotension associated with apathy, fatigue, muscle weakness, anorexia, nausea, and profound thirst. The patient may also develop dizziness, oliguria, sunken eyeballs, poor skin turgor, and dry mucous membranes.

OTHER CAUSES

Drugs
Certain drugs may cause orthostatic hypotension by reducing circulating blood volume, causing blood vessel dilation, or by depressing the sympathetic nervous system. These drugs include antihypertensives (especially guanethidine and the initial dosage of prazosin), tricyclic antidepressants, phenothiazines, levodopa, nitrates, monoamine oxidase inhibitors, morphine, bretylium, and spinal anesthesia. Large doses of diuretics can also cause orthostatic hypotension.

Treatments
Orthostatic hypotension is commonly associated with prolonged bed rest (24 hours or longer). It may also result from sympathectomy, which disrupts normal vasoconstrictive mechanisms.

SPECIAL CONSIDERATIONS

Monitor the patient's fluid balance by carefully recording his intake and output and weighing him daily. To help minimize orthostatic hypotension, advise the patient to change his position gradually. Elevate the head of the patient's bed, and help him to a sitting position with his feet dangling over the side of the bed. If he can tolerate this position, have him sit in a chair for brief periods. Immediately return him to bed if he becomes dizzy or pale or displays other signs of hypotension. Never leave the patient unattended while he's sitting or walking; evaluate his need for assistive devices, such as a cane or walker.

Prepare the patient for diagnostic tests, such as hematocrit, serum electrolyte and drug levels, urinalysis, 12-lead electrocardiogram, and chest X-ray.

PEDIATRIC POINTERS

Because normal blood pressure is lower in children than in adults, familiarize yourself with normal age-specific values to detect orthostatic hypotension. From birth to age 3 months, normal systolic pressure is 40 to 80 mm Hg; from age 3 months to 1 year, 80 to 100 mm Hg; and from ages 1 to 12, 100 mm Hg plus 2 mm Hg for every year over age 1. Diastolic blood pressure is first heard at about age 4; it's normally 60 mm Hg at this age and gradually increases to 70 mm Hg by age 12.

The causes of orthostatic hypotension in children may be the same as those in adults.

GERIATRIC POINTERS

Elderly patients commonly experience autonomic dysfunction, which can present as orthostatic hypotension. Postprandial hypotension occurs 45 to 60 minutes after a meal and has been documented in up to one-third of nursing home residents.

PATIENT COUNSELING

Patients with conditions that can lead to autonomic dysfunction should be made aware of the acute drop in blood pressure that can occur with positional changes. This is particularly important in patients with diabetes. When the problem appears, such patients need to avoid volume depletion and perform positional changes gradually instead of suddenly.

OTORRHEA

Otorrhea — drainage from the ear — may be bloody (otorrhagia), purulent, clear, or serosanguineous. Its onset, duration, and severity provide clues to the underlying cause. This sign may result from disorders that affect the external ear canal or the middle ear, including allergy, infection, neoplasms, trauma, and collagen diseases. Otorrhea may occur alone or with other symptoms such as ear pain.

HISTORY

Begin your evaluation by asking the patient when the otorrhea began, noting how he recognized it. Did he clean the drainage from deep within the ear canal, or did he wipe it from the auricle? Have him describe the color, consistency, and odor of the drainage. Is it clear, purulent, or bloody? Does it occur in one or both ears? Is it continuous or intermittent? If the patient wears cotton in his ear to absorb the drainage, ask how often he changes it.

Special considerations

+ Elevate the head of the bed, and help the patient to a sitting position with his feet dangling over the side of the bed; if tolerated, have him sit in a chair briefly.
+ Evaluate the need for assistive devices.

Peds points

+ The causes of orthostatic hypotension in children may be the same as those in adults.

Geri points

+ These patients commonly experience autonomic dysfunction, which can present as orthostatic hypotension.

Teaching points

+ Avoiding volume depletion
+ Performing positional changes gradually

Key facts about otorrhea

+ Drainage from the ear
+ May be bloody, purulent, clear, or serosanguineous

Key history points

+ Onset and description of drainage
+ Associated pain, tenderness, vertigo, or tinnitus
+ Medical history, including recent upper respiratory infection or head trauma

Critical assessment steps

+ Inspect the external ear, and apply pressure on the tragus and mastoid area to elicit tenderness; then insert an otoscope.
+ Observe for edema, erythema, crusts, or polyps.
+ Inspect the tympanic membrane.
+ Test hearing acuity.
+ Palpate the neck and preauricular, parotid, and postauricular areas for lymphadenopathy.
+ Test the function of cranial nerves VII, IX, X, and XI.

Medical causes

Allergy

+ Tympanic membrane perforation may cause clear or cloudy otorrhea, rhinorrhea, and itchy, watery eyes.

Aural polyps

+ Aural polyps may produce foul, purulent, and perhaps blood-streaked discharge.

Basilar skull fracture

+ Otorrhea may be clear, watery and positive for glucose, or bloody.

Dermatitis of the external ear canal

+ With contact dermatitis, vesicles produce clear, watery otorrhea.
+ Infectious eczematoid dermatitis causes purulent otorrhea.
+ With seborrheic dermatitis, otorrhea has greasy scales and flakes.

Then explore associated otologic symptoms, especially pain. Is there tenderness on movement of the pinna or tragus? Ask about vertigo, which is absent in disorders of the external ear canal. Also ask about tinnitus.

Next, check the patient's medical history for recent upper respiratory infection or head trauma. Also, ask how he cleans his ears and if he's an avid swimmer. Note a history of cancer, dermatitis, or immunosuppressant therapy.

PHYSICAL ASSESSMENT

Focus the physical assessment on the patient's external ear, middle ear, and tympanic membrane. (If his symptoms are unilateral, examine the uninvolved ear first to avoid cross-contamination.) Inspect the external ear, and apply pressure on the tragus and mastoid area to elicit tenderness. Then insert an otoscope, using the largest speculum that will comfortably fit into the ear canal. If necessary, clean cerumen, pus, or other debris from the canal. Observe for edema, erythema, crusts, or polyps. Inspect the tympanic membrane, which should look like a shiny, pearl gray cone. Note color changes, perforation, absence of the normal light reflex (a cone of light appearing toward the bottom of the drum), or a bulging membrane.

Next, test hearing acuity. Have the patient occlude one ear while you whisper some common two-syllable words toward the unoccluded ear. Stand behind him so he doesn't read your lips, and ask him to repeat what he heard. Perform the test on the other ear using different words. Then use a tuning fork to perform Weber's and Rinne tests.

Complete your assessment by palpating the patient's neck and his preauricular, parotid, and postauricular (mastoid) areas for lymphadenopathy. Also, test the function of cranial nerves VII, IX, X, and XI.

MEDICAL CAUSES

Allergy

An allergy associated with tympanic membrane perforation may cause clear or cloudy otorrhea, rhinorrhea, and itchy, watery eyes. The patient may also report nasal congestion and an itchy nose and throat.

Aural polyps

Aural polyps may produce foul, purulent, and perhaps blood-streaked discharge. If they occlude the external ear canal, the polyps may cause partial hearing loss.

Basilar skull fracture

With a basilar skull fracture, otorrhea may be clear and watery and positive for glucose, representing cerebrospinal fluid (CSF) leakage, or bloody, representing hemorrhage. Occasionally, inspection reveals blood behind the eardrum. The otorrhea may be accompanied by hearing loss, CSF or bloody rhinorrhea, periorbital ecchymosis (raccoon eyes), and mastoid ecchymosis (Battle's sign). Cranial nerve palsies, decreased level of consciousness, and headache are other common findings.

Dermatitis of the external ear canal

With contact dermatitis, vesicles produce clear, watery otorrhea with edema and erythema of the external ear canal.

Infectious eczematoid dermatitis causes purulent otorrhea with erythema and crusting of the external ear canal.

With seborrheic dermatitis, otorrhea consists of greasy scales and flakes. The scalp, forehead, and cheeks are also marked by pruritic, scaly lesions.

Mastoiditis

Mastoiditis causes thick, purulent, yellow otorrhea that becomes increasingly profuse. Its cardinal features include low-grade fever and dull aching and tenderness in the mastoid area. Postauricular erythema and edema may push the auricle out from the head; pressure within the edematous mastoid antrum may produce swelling and obstruction of the external ear canal, causing conductive hearing loss.

Myringitis (infectious)

With acute infectious myringitis, small, reddened, blood-filled blebs erupt in the external ear canal, the tympanic membrane and, occasionally, the middle ear. Spontaneous rupture of these blebs causes serosanguineous otorrhea. Other features include severe ear pain, tenderness over the mastoid process and, rarely, fever and hearing loss.

Chronic infectious myringitis causes purulent otorrhea, pruritus, and gradual hearing loss.

Otitis externa

Acute otitis externa, commonly known as *swimmer's ear,* usually causes purulent, yellow, sticky, foul-smelling otorrhea. Inspection may reveal white-green debris in the external ear canal. Associated findings include edema, erythema, pain, and itching of the auricle and external ear canal; severe tenderness with movement of the mastoid, tragus, mouth, or jaw; tenderness and swelling of surrounding nodes; and partial conductive hearing loss. The patient may also develop a low-grade fever and a headache ipsilateral to the affected ear.

Chronic otitis externa usually causes scanty, intermittent otorrhea that may be serous or purulent and possibly foul-smelling. Its primary symptom, however, is itching. Related findings include edema and slight erythema.

Otitis media

With acute otitis media, rupture of the tympanic membrane produces bloody, purulent otorrhea and relieves continuous or intermittent ear pain. Typically, a conductive hearing loss worsens over several hours.

With acute suppurative otitis media, the patient may also exhibit signs and symptoms of upper respiratory infection — sore throat, cough, nasal discharge, and headache. Other features include dizziness, fever, nausea, and vomiting.

Chronic otitis media causes intermittent, purulent, foul-smelling otorrhea commonly associated with perforation of the tympanic membrane. Conductive hearing loss occurs gradually and may be accompanied by pain, nausea, and vertigo.

Trauma

Bloody otorrhea may result from trauma, such as a blow to the external ear, a foreign body in the ear, or barotrauma. Usually, the bleeding is minimal or moderate; it may be accompanied by partial hearing loss.

Tumor

A benign tumor of the glomus jugulare (jugular bulb) may cause bloody otorrhea. Initially, the patient may complain of throbbing discomfort and tinnitus that resembles the sound of his heartbeat. Associated signs and symptoms include gradually progressive stuffiness in the affected ear, vertigo, conductive hearing loss and, possibly, a reddened mass behind the tympanic membrane.

Squamous cell carcinoma of the external ear (a malignant tumor) causes purulent otorrhea with itching; deep, boring ear pain; hearing loss; and, in late stages, facial paralysis.

Medical causes
(continued)

Mastoiditis
+ Thick, purulent, yellow otorrhea becomes increasingly profuse.

Myringitis (infectious)
+ Rupture of small, reddened, blood-filled blebs causes serosanguineous otorrhea.

Otitis externa
+ Acute form usually causes purulent, yellow, sticky, foul-smelling otorrhea.
+ Chronic form usually causes scanty, intermittent otorrhea that may be serous or purulent.

Otitis media
+ With acute otitis media, rupture of the tympanic membrane produces bloody, purulent otorrhea.
+ With acute suppurative otitis media, the patient may have otorrhea and exhibit signs and symptoms of upper respiratory infection.
+ Chronic otitis media causes intermittent, purulent, foul-smelling otorrhea commonly associated with perforation of the tympanic membrane.

Trauma
+ Bloody otorrhea may result.

Tumor
+ A benign tumor of the glomus jugulare may cause bloody otorrhea.
+ Squamous cell carcinoma of the external ear causes purulent otorrhea, whereas squamous cell carcinoma of the middle ear causes blood-tinged otorrhea.

Examining a child's ear

To examine a child's ear safely and accurately, restrain the child by having him sit on a parent's lap with the ear to be examined facing you. Have him put one arm around the parent's waist and the other down at his side, and then ask the parent to hold the child in place. Alternatively, if you are alone with the child, ask him to lie on his abdomen with his arms at his sides and his head turned so the affected ear faces the ceiling. Bend over him, restraining his upper body with your elbows and upper arms.

Special considerations
+ Apply warm, moist compresses; heating pads; or hot water bottles to the ears.
+ Use cotton wicks to clean the ear or to apply topical drugs.
+ Keep eardrops at room temperature; instillation of cold eardrops may cause vertigo.
+ If the patient has impaired hearing, ensure he understands what's explained to him.

Peds points
+ Perforation of the tympanic membrane secondary to otitis media is the most common cause of otorrhea in infants and young children.
+ Children may insert foreign bodies into their ears, resulting in infection, pain, and purulent discharge.

Teaching points
+ Safe ways to blow the nose and clean the ears
+ Use of earplugs while swimming
+ Signs and symptoms to report

In squamous cell carcinoma of the middle ear, blood-tinged otorrhea occurs early, typically accompanied by hearing loss on the affected side. Pain and facial paralysis are late features.

SPECIAL CONSIDERATIONS

Apply warm, moist compresses; heating pads; or hot water bottles to the patient's ears to relieve inflammation and pain. Use cotton wicks to gently clean the draining ear or to apply topical drugs. Keep eardrops at room temperature; instillation of cold eardrops may cause vertigo. If the patient has impaired hearing, ensure he understands everything that's explained to him, using written messages, if necessary.

PEDIATRIC POINTERS

When you examine or clean a child's ear, remember that the auditory canal lies horizontally and that the pinna must be pulled downward and backward. (See *Examining a child's ear*.) Perforation of the tympanic membrane secondary to otitis media is the most common cause of otorrhea in infants and young children. Children are also likely to insert foreign bodies into their ears, resulting in infection, pain, and purulent discharge.

PATIENT COUNSELING

Advise the patient with chronic ear problems to avoid forceful nose blowing when he has an upper respiratory infection so that infected secretions aren't channeled into the middle ear. Instruct him to blow his nose with his mouth open. Also, remind him to clean his ears with a washcloth only, and not to stick anything in his ear that might cause injury (such as a hairpin or a cotton-tipped applicator). If the patient is a swimmer, instruct him to wear earplugs and to wash and dry his ears thoroughly after swimming. Have him report recurring ear pain and drainage, especially in the absence of upper respiratory infection, because this may be a sign of cancer.

Tell the patient with a ruptured tympanic membrane that such a rupture usually heals spontaneously. However, warn him to avoid immersing his head in water while it heals; tell him to insert lubricated cotton balls into his ear canal before he showers or shampoos.

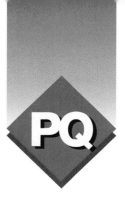

PALLOR

Pallor is abnormal paleness or loss of skin color, which may develop suddenly or gradually. Although generalized pallor affects the entire body, it's most apparent on the face, conjunctiva, oral mucosa, and nail beds. Localized pallor commonly affects a single limb.

How easily pallor is detected varies with skin color and the thickness and vascularity of underlying subcutaneous tissue. At times, it's merely a subtle lightening of skin color that may be difficult to detect in dark-skinned persons; sometimes it's evident only on the conjunctiva and oral mucosa.

Pallor may result from decreased peripheral oxyhemoglobin or decreased total oxyhemoglobin. The former reflects diminished peripheral blood flow associated with peripheral vasoconstriction, arterial occlusion, or low cardiac output. (Transient peripheral vasoconstriction may occur with exposure to cold, causing nonpathologic pallor.) The latter usually results from anemia, the chief cause of pallor. (See *How pallor develops,* page 482.)

 EMERGENCY ACTIONS If generalized pallor suddenly develops, quickly look for signs of shock, such as tachycardia, hypotension, oliguria, and decreased level of consciousness. Prepare to rapidly infuse fluids or blood. Keep emergency resuscitation equipment nearby.

HISTORY

If the patient's condition permits, take a complete history. Does the patient or anyone in his family have a history of anemia or of a chronic disorder that might lead to pallor, such as renal failure, heart failure, or diabetes? Ask about the patient's diet, particularly his intake of green vegetables.

Then explore the pallor more fully. Find out when the patient first noticed it. Is pallor constant or intermittent? Does it occur when he's exposed to the cold? Does it occur when he's under emotional stress? Explore associated signs and symptoms, such as dizziness, fainting, orthostasis, weakness and fatigue on exertion, dyspnea, chest pain, palpitations, menstrual irregularities, or loss of libido. If the pallor is confined to one or both legs, ask the patient if walking is painful. Do his legs feel cold or numb? If the pallor is confined to his fingers, ask about tingling and numbness.

PHYSICAL ASSESSMENT

Start the physical assessment by taking the patient's vital signs. Be sure to check for orthostatic hypotension. Auscultate the heart for gallops and murmurs and the

Key facts about pallor
+ Refers to abnormal paleness or loss of skin color
+ Develops suddenly or gradually
+ Can be difficult to detect in dark-skinned persons
+ Can be generalized or localized
+ Caused chiefly by anemia

In an emergency
+ Look for signs of shock with sudden generalized pallor.
+ Prepare to rapidly infuse fluids or blood.
+ Keep emergency resuscitation equipment nearby.

Key history points
+ Personal or family history of anemia, renal failure, heart failure, or diabetes
+ Diet
+ Date of onset

Critical assessment steps
+ Assess vital signs, checking for orthostatic hypotension, heart murmurs or gallops, and lung crackles.
+ Check skin temperature.
+ Note skin ulceration.
+ Palpate peripheral pulses.

How pallor develops

Pallor may result from decreased peripheral oxyhemoglobin or decreased total oxyhemoglobin. The flowchart below illustrates the progression to pallor.

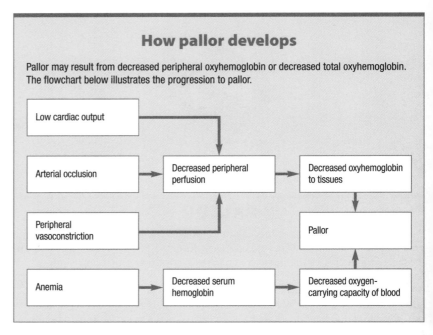

lungs for crackles. Check the patient's skin temperature — cold extremities commonly occur with vasoconstriction or arterial occlusion. Also, note skin ulceration. Examine the abdomen for splenomegaly. Finally, palpate peripheral pulses. An absent pulse in a pale extremity may indicate arterial occlusion, whereas a weak pulse may indicate low cardiac output.

 CULTURAL CUE Because skin color varies according to race and ethnic background, establish a baseline skin color so that changes can be more readily detected.

Medical causes

Anemia
+ Pallor begins gradually.
+ Skin is gray or sallow.

Arterial occlusion (acute)
+ Pallor begins abruptly in extremity with occlusion.
+ Line of demarcation separates cool, pale, cyanotic, and mottled skin from normal skin.

Arterial occlusive disease (chronic)
+ Pallor is specific to an extremity.
+ Pallor develops gradually and is aggravated by elevating the extremity.

MEDICAL CAUSES

Anemia
Typically, pallor develops gradually with anemia. The patient's skin may also appear sallow or grayish. Other effects include fatigue, dyspnea, tachycardia, bounding pulse, atrial gallop, systolic bruit over the carotid arteries and, possibly, crackles and bleeding tendencies.

Arterial occlusion (acute)
Pallor develops abruptly in the extremity with the occlusion, which usually results from an embolus. A line of demarcation develops, separating the cool, pale, cyanotic, and mottled skin below the occlusion from the normal skin above it. Accompanying the pallor may be severe pain, intense intermittent claudication, paresthesia, and paresis in the affected extremity. Absent pulses and increased capillary refill time below the occlusion are also characteristic.

Arterial occlusive disease (chronic)
With chronic arterial occlusive disease, pallor is specific to an extremity — usually one leg, but occasionally both legs or an arm. It develops gradually from obstructive arteriosclerosis or a thrombus and is aggravated by elevating the extremity. Associated findings include intermittent claudication, weakness, cool skin, diminished pulses in the extremity and, possibly, ulceration and gangrene.

Cardiac arrhythmias

Cardiac arrhythmias that seriously reduce cardiac output, such as complete heart block and attacks of tachyarrhythmia, may cause acute onset of pallor. Other features include irregular, rapid, or slow pulse; dizziness; weakness and fatigue; hypotension; confusion; palpitations; diaphoresis; oliguria; and, possibly, loss of consciousness.

Frostbite

Pallor is localized to the frostbitten area, such as the feet, hands, or ears. Typically, the area feels cold, waxy and, perhaps, hard if the frostbite is deep. The skin doesn't blanch and sensation may be absent. As the area thaws, the skin turns purplish blue. Blistering and gangrene may then follow if the frostbite is severe.

Orthostatic hypotension

With orthostatic hypotension, pallor occurs abruptly on rising from a recumbent position to a sitting or standing position. A precipitous drop in blood pressure, an increase in heart rate, and dizziness are also characteristic. At times, the patient loses consciousness for several minutes.

Raynaud's disease

Pallor of the fingers upon exposure to cold or stress is a hallmark of Raynaud's disease. Typically, the fingers abruptly turn pale, then cyanotic; with rewarming, they become red and paresthetic. With chronic disease, ulceration may occur.

Shock

Two forms of shock initially cause acute onset of pallor and cool, clammy skin. With hypovolemic shock, other early signs and symptoms include restlessness, thirst, slight tachycardia, and tachypnea. As shock progresses, the skin becomes increasingly clammy, pulse becomes more rapid and thready, and hypotension develops with narrowing pulse pressure. Other signs and symptoms include oliguria, subnormal body temperature, and decreased level of consciousness. With cardiogenic shock, the signs and symptoms are similar, but usually more profound.

Vasopressor syncope

Sudden onset of pallor immediately precedes or accompanies loss of consciousness during syncopal attacks. These common fainting spells may be triggered by emotional stress or pain and usually last only a few seconds or minutes. Before loss of consciousness, the patient may exhibit diaphoresis, nausea, yawning, hyperpnea, weakness, confusion, tachycardia, and dim vision. He then develops bradycardia, hypotension, a few clonic jerks, and dilated pupils with loss of consciousness.

SPECIAL CONSIDERATIONS

If the patient has chronic generalized pallor, prepare him for blood studies and, possibly, bone marrow biopsy. If the patient has localized pallor, he may require arteriography or other diagnostic studies to accurately determine the cause.

When pallor results from low cardiac output, administer blood and fluids as well as a diuretic, a cardiotonic, and an antiarrhythmic, as needed. Frequently monitor the patient's vital signs, intake and output, electrocardiogram results, and hemodynamic status.

PEDIATRIC POINTERS

In children, pallor stems from the same causes as it does in adults. It can also stem from a congenital heart defect or chronic lung disease.

Medical causes
(continued)
Cardiac arrhythmias
- Acute pallor may result from arrhythmias that seriously reduce cardiac output.

Frostbite
- Pallor is localized to the frostbitten area, which feels cold, waxy and, perhaps, hard.

Orthostatic hypotension
- Pallor occurs abruptly on rising from a recumbent position.

Raynaud's disease
- Upon exposure to cold or stress, the fingers abruptly turn pale, then cyanotic.

Shock
- With hypovolemic shock, acute pallor occurs early, along with restlessness, tachypnea, and cool, clammy skin.
- With cardiogenic shock, signs and symptoms are similar, but usually more profound.

Vasopressor syncope
- Sudden pallor immediately precedes or accompanies loss of consciousness.

Special considerations
- Administer blood and fluids, a diuretic, a cardiotonic, and an antiarrhythmic, as needed.
- Frequently monitor vital signs, ECG, and hemodynamic status.

Peds points
- Pallor in children can also stem from a congenital heart defect or chronic lung disease.

Teaching points
- ◆ Diet and rest (anemia)
- ◆ Cold-protection measures (frostbite and Raynaud's disease)
- ◆ Need to rise slowly (orthostatic hypotension)

Key facts about palpitations
- ◆ Usually felt over the precordium or in the throat or neck
- ◆ May be regular or irregular, fast or slow, paroxysmal or sustained

In an emergency
- ◆ Ask the patient about dizziness or shortness of breath.
- ◆ Take vital signs, noting hypotension and irregular or abnormal pulse.

Key history points
- ◆ History of cardiovascular or pulmonary disorder or hypoglycemia
- ◆ Recently prescribed cardiac glycosides
- ◆ Caffeine, tobacco, and alcohol use

Critical assessment steps
- ◆ Perform a complete cardiac and pulmonary assessment.
- ◆ Auscultate for gallops, murmurs, and abnormal breath sounds.

Medical causes
Anemia
- ◆ Palpitations occur on exertion, with pallor, fatigue, and dyspnea.

PATIENT COUNSELING

Teach the patient with anemia to eat foods rich in iron and to plan periods of rest throughout the day. Advise the patient with frostbite and Raynaud's disease to dress appropriately in cold weather and to limit time outdoors. Tell the patient with orthostatic hypotension or syncope to rise slowly from a recumbent to a standing position.

PALPITATIONS

Defined as a conscious awareness of one's own heartbeat, palpitations are usually felt over the precordium or in the throat or neck. The patient may describe them as pounding, jumping, turning, fluttering, or flopping, or as missing or skipping beats. Palpitations may be regular or irregular, fast or slow, paroxysmal or sustained.

Although usually insignificant, palpitations may result from a cardiac or metabolic disorder and from the effects of certain drugs. Nonpathologic palpitations may occur with a newly implanted prosthetic valve because the valve's clicking sound heightens the patient's awareness of his heartbeat. Transient palpitations may accompany emotional stress (such as fright, anger, or anxiety) or physical stress (such as exercise and fever). They can also accompany use of stimulants, such as tobacco and caffeine.

To help characterize the palpitations, ask the patient to simulate their rhythm by tapping his finger on a hard surface. An irregular "skipped beat" rhythm points to premature ventricular contractions, whereas an episodic racing rhythm that ends abruptly suggests paroxysmal atrial tachycardia.

 EMERGENCY ACTIONS If the patient complains of palpitations, ask him about dizziness and shortness of breath. Then inspect for pale, cool, clammy skin. Take the patient's vital signs, noting hypotension and irregular or abnormal pulse. If these signs are present, suspect cardiac arrhythmia. Prepare to begin cardiac monitoring and, if necessary, to deliver electroshock therapy. Start an I.V. line to administer an antiarrhythmic, if needed.

HISTORY

If the patient isn't in distress, take a complete cardiac history. Ask if he has a cardiovascular or pulmonary disorder, which may produce arrhythmias. Does the patient have a history of hypertension or hypoglycemia? Be sure to obtain a drug history. Has the patient recently started cardiac glycoside therapy? Also, ask about caffeine, tobacco, and alcohol consumption.

PHYSICAL ASSESSMENT

Perform a complete cardiac and pulmonary assessment. Then explore associated symptoms, such as weakness, fatigue, and angina. Be sure to auscultate for gallops, murmurs, and abnormal breath sounds.

MEDICAL CAUSES

Anemia
Palpitations may occur with anemia, especially on exertion. Pallor, fatigue, and dyspnea are also common. Associated signs include a systolic ejection murmur, bounding pulse, tachycardia, crackles, an atrial gallop, and a systolic bruit over the carotid arteries.

Anxiety attack (acute)

Anxiety is the most common cause of palpitations in children and adults. With this disorder, palpitations may be accompanied by diaphoresis, facial flushing, trembling, and an impending sense of doom. Almost invariably, the patient hyperventilates, which may lead to dizziness, weakness, and syncope. Other typical findings include tachycardia, precordial pain, shortness of breath, restlessness, and insomnia.

Cardiac arrhythmias

Paroxysmal or sustained palpitations may be accompanied by dizziness, weakness, and fatigue. The patient may also experience an irregular, rapid, or slow pulse rate; decreased blood pressure; confusion; pallor; chest pain; syncope; oliguria; and diaphoresis.

Hypertension

With hypertension, the patient may be asymptomatic or may complain of sustained palpitations alone or with headache, dizziness, tinnitus, and fatigue. His blood pressure typically exceeds 140/90 mm Hg. He may also experience nausea and vomiting, seizures, and decreased level of consciousness (LOC).

Hypocalcemia

Typically, hypocalcemia produces palpitations, weakness, and fatigue. It progresses from paresthesia to muscle tension and carpopedal spasms. The patient may also exhibit muscle twitching, hyperactive deep tendon reflexes, chorea, and positive Chvostek's and Trousseau's signs.

Hypoglycemia

Hypoglycemia occurs when blood glucose levels drop significantly and the sympathetic nervous system triggers adrenaline production. This may cause sustained palpitations, which may be accompanied by fatigue, irritability, hunger, cold sweats, tremors, tachycardia, anxiety, and headache. Eventually, the patient may develop central nervous system reactions, including blurred or double vision, muscle weakness, hemiplegia, and altered LOC.

Mitral prolapse

Mitral prolapse may cause paroxysmal palpitations accompanied by sharp, stabbing, or aching precordial pain. The hallmark of this disorder, however, is a midsystolic click followed by an apical systolic murmur. Associated signs and symptoms may include dyspnea, dizziness, severe fatigue, migraine headache, anxiety, paroxysmal tachycardia, crackles, and peripheral edema.

Mitral stenosis

Early features of mitral stenosis typically include sustained palpitations accompanied by exertional dyspnea and fatigue. Auscultation also reveals a loud S_1 or opening snap, and a rumbling diastolic murmur at the apex. Patients may also experience such related signs and symptoms as an atrial gallop and, with advanced mitral stenosis, orthopnea, dyspnea at rest, paroxysmal nocturnal dyspnea, peripheral edema, jugular vein distention, ascites, hepatomegaly, and atrial fibrillations.

Pheochromocytoma

This adrenal medulla tumor causes episodic hypermetabolism, commonly associated with paroxysmal palpitations. The cardinal sign of pheochromocytoma is dramatically elevated blood pressure, which may be sustained or paroxysmal. Associated signs and symptoms include tachycardia, headache, chest or abdominal pain, diaphoresis, warm and pale or flushed skin, paresthesia, tremors, insomnia, nausea and vomiting, and anxiety.

Medical causes
(continued)

Anxiety attack (acute)
✦ Palpitations may be accompanied by diaphoresis, facial flushing, and trembling.

Cardiac arrhythmias
✦ Paroxysmal or sustained palpitations may be accompanied by dizziness, weakness, and fatigue.

Hypertension
✦ Sustained palpitations may occur alone or with headache, dizziness, tinnitus, and fatigue.
✦ Blood pressure typically exceeds 140/90 mm Hg.

Hypocalcemia
✦ Palpitations occur with weakness and fatigue.

Hypoglycemia
✦ Sustained palpitations occur with fatigue, irritability, hunger, cold sweats, tremors, tachycardia, anxiety, and headache.

Mitral prolapse
✦ Paroxysmal palpitations accompany sharp, stabbing, or aching precordial pain and midsystolic click, followed by an apical systolic murmur.

Mitral stenosis
✦ Early on, sustained palpitations accompany exertional dyspnea and fatigue.

Pheochromocytoma
✦ Paroxysmal palpitations result from episodic hypermetabolism.
✦ The cardinal sign is dramatically elevated blood pressure.

Medical causes
(continued)

Thyrotoxicosis
◆ Sustained palpitations charac-teristically occur and may be ac-companied by tachycardia, dys-pnea, weight loss, tremors, di-aphoresis, and heat intolerance.

Other causes
◆ Drugs that precipitate cardiac arrhythmias or increase cardiac output
◆ Exercise

Special considerations
◆ Monitor for signs of reduced car-diac output.
◆ Provide supplemental oxygen.

Peds points
◆ Palpitations commonly result from fever and congenital heart defects.

Teaching points
◆ Diagnostic tests
◆ Anxiety-reduction techniques

Key facts about papular rash
◆ Consists of small, raised, cir-cumscribed papules
◆ May erupt anywhere on the body in various configurations
◆ May be acute or chronic

Key history points
◆ Time of onset
◆ Rash characteristics (itchy, burn-ing, or tender) and changes
◆ Medical and drug history
◆ Recent insect or rodent bite or exposure to infectious disease

Thyrotoxicosis
A characteristic symptom of thyrotoxicosis, sustained palpitations may be accom-panied by tachycardia, dyspnea, weight loss despite increased appetite, diarrhea, tremors, nervousness, diaphoresis, heat intolerance and, possibly, exophthalmos and an enlarged thyroid. The patient may also experience an atrial or ventricular gallop.

OTHER CAUSES

Drugs
Palpitations may result from drugs that precipitate cardiac arrhythmias or increase cardiac output, such as cardiac glycosides; sympathomimetics such as cocaine; gan-glionic blockers; beta blockers; calcium channel blockers; atropine; and minoxidil.

Exercise
Exercise can normally cause palpitations. In patients with coronary heart disease, exercise can also cause hypertension, mitral valve prolapse, and cardiomegaly.

SPECIAL CONSIDERATIONS
Monitor the patient for signs of reduced cardiac output, such as hypotension and reduced urinary output. Administer medications as needed, and prepare for proce-dures such as cardioversion. Provide supplemental oxygen, and take measures to reduce the workload of the heart, such as providing rest periods.

PEDIATRIC POINTERS
Palpitations in children commonly result from fever and congenital heart defects, such as patent ductus arteriosus and septal defects. Because many children can't de-scribe this complaint, focus your attention on objective measurements, such as car-diac monitoring, physical examination, and laboratory tests.

PATIENT COUNSELING
Prepare the patient for diagnostic tests, such as an electrocardiogram and Holter monitoring. Remember that even mild palpitations can cause the patient much concern. Maintain a quiet, comfortable environment to minimize anxiety and per-haps decrease palpitations.

PAPULAR RASH

A papular rash consists of small, raised, circumscribed — and perhaps discolored (red to purple) — lesions known as papules. It may erupt anywhere on the body in various configurations and may be acute or chronic. Papular rashes characterize many cutaneous disorders; they may also result from allergy and from infectious, neoplastic, and systemic disorders. (To compare papules with other skin lesions, see *Recognizing common skin lesions,* pages 488 and 489.)

HISTORY
Find out when the rash erupted. Has the patient noticed any changes in the rash since then? Is it itchy or burning, or painful or tender? Have the patient describe as-sociated signs and symptoms, such as fever, headache, and GI distress.

Obtain a medical history, including allergies, previous rashes or skin disorders, infections, childhood diseases, sexual history, sexually transmitted diseases (STDs), and cancers. Has the patient recently been bitten by an insect or a rodent or been exposed to anyone with an infectious disease? Finally, obtain a complete drug history.

Physical assessment

Fully evaluate the papular rash: Note its color, configuration, and location on the patient's body. Then complete a whole-body examination of the patient's skin, hair, and nails.

Medical causes

Acne vulgaris
With acne vulgaris, rupture of enlarged comedones produces inflamed—and possibly painful and pruritic—papules, pustules, nodules, or cysts on the face and sometimes the shoulders, chest, and back.

Anthrax (cutaneous)
Cutaneous anthrax begins as a small, painless, or pruritic macular or papular lesion resembling an insect bite. Within 2 days, it develops into a vesicle and then a painless ulcer with a characteristic black, necrotic center. Lymphadenopathy, malaise, headache, or fever may develop.

Dermatitis (perioral)
Perioral dermatitis is an inflammatory disorder that causes an erythematous eruption of discrete, tiny papules and pustules on the nasolabial fold, chin, and upper lip area. The lesions may be pruritic and painful.

Erythema migrans
Transmitted through a tick bite, erythema migrans is a systemic disorder characterized by a papular or macular rash starting from a single lesion (usually on the leg) that spreads at the margins while clearing centrally. The rash commonly appears on the thighs, trunk, or upper arms and is the classic early sign of Lyme disease, but about 25% of patients don't develop this skin manifestation. It may be accompanied by fever, chills, headache, malaise, nausea, vomiting, fatigue, backache, knee pain, and stiff neck.

Gonococcemia
In gonococcemia—a chronic STD—sporadic eruption of an erythematous macular rash is characteristic, although fistulas and petechiae may appear. The rash typically affects the distal extremities (palms and soles) and rapidly becomes maculopapular, vesiculopustular and, commonly, hemorrhagic. Bullae may form. The mature lesion is raised; has a gray, necrotic center; and is surrounded by erythema. Typically, it heals in 3 to 4 days. Eruptions are commonly accompanied by fever and joint pain.

Human immunodeficiency virus infection
Acute infection with human immunodeficiency virus (HIV) typically causes a generalized maculopapular rash. Other signs and symptoms include fever, malaise, sore throat, and headache. Lymphadenopathy and hepatosplenomegaly may also occur. Most patients don't recall these symptoms of acute infection.

Insect bites
Salivary secretions from insect bites—especially ticks, lice, flies, and mosquitoes—may produce an allergic reaction associated with a papular, macular, or petechial

Critical assessment steps
+ Note the color, configuration, and location of rash.

Medical causes
Acne vulgaris
+ Inflamed papules, pustules, nodules, or cysts appear on the face, shoulders, chest, and back.

Anthrax (cutaneous)
+ Intially appears as a small, painless, pruritic macular or papular lesion.
+ A vesicle develops and then evolves into a painless ulcer with a black, necrotic center.

Dermatitis (perioral)
+ Tiny, erythematous papules and pustules that may be pruritic and painful appear on the nasolabial fold, chin, and upper lip area.

Erythema migrans
+ Papular or macular rash starts as a single lesion and spreads at margins while clearing centrally.

Gonococcemia
+ Erythematous macular rash erupts sporadically on the palms and soles and rapidly becomes maculopapular, vesiculopustular, and hemorrhagic.

HIV
+ A generalized maculopapular rash occurs with acute infection.

Insect bites
+ A papular, macular, or petechial rash results from allergic reaction to salivary secretions from insect bites.

Guide to common skin lesions

◆ Macule — small flat blemish or discoloration with the same texture as the surrounding skin
◆ Vesicle — small, thin-walled, raised blister containing clear, serous, purulent, or bloody fluid
◆ Bulla — raised, thin-walled blister greater than 0.5 cm in diameter that contains clear or serous fluid
◆ Pustule — circumscribed, pus- or lymph-filled, elevated lesion that varies in diameter; may be firm or soft and white or yellow

Medical causes
(continued)

Kaposi's sarcoma
◆ Purple or blue papules or macules of vascular origin appear on the skin, mucous membrane, and viscera.
◆ Lesions decrease in size with firm pressure and then return to their original size within 10 to 15 seconds.

Lichen amyloidosis
◆ Discrete, firm, hemispherical, pruritic papules appear on the anterior tibiae, feet, and thighs.
◆ Papules may be brown or yellow and smooth or scaly.

Recognizing common skin lesions

Use the illustrations below to help you identify common skin lesions. Remember to keep a centimeter ruler handy to measure the size of the lesion accurately.

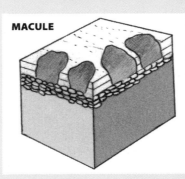

MACULE

A small (usually less than 1 cm in diameter), flat blemish or discoloration that can be brown, tan, red, or white and has the same texture as the surrounding skin

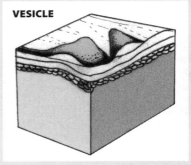

VESICLE

A small (less than 0.5 cm in diameter), thin-walled, raised blister containing clear, serous, purulent, or bloody fluid

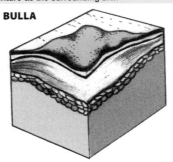

BULLA

A raised, thin-walled blister greater than 0.5 cm in diameter that contains clear or serous fluid

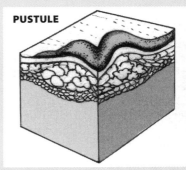

PUSTULE

A circumscribed, pus- or lymph-filled, elevated lesion that varies in diameter; may be firm or soft and white or yellow

rash. The rash is usually accompanied by such nonspecific signs and symptoms as fever, myalgia, headache, lymphadenopathy, nausea, and vomiting.

Kaposi's sarcoma
Kaposi's sarcoma is characterized by purple or blue papules or macules of vascular origin on the skin, mucous membranes, and viscera. These lesions decrease in size with firm pressure and then return to their original size within 10 to 15 seconds. They may become scaly and ulcerate with bleeding.

Lichen amyloidosis
Lichen amyloidosis, an idiopathic cutaneous disorder, produces discrete, firm, hemispherical, pruritic papules on the anterior tibiae, feet, and thighs. Papules may be brown or yellow and smooth or scaly.

**Guide to common
skin lesions**

+ Wheal — slightly raised, firm lesion of variable size and shape that's surrounded by edema
+ Papule — small, solid, raised lesion less than 1 cm in diameter with red to purple skin discoloration
+ Nodule — small, firm, circumscribed, elevated lesion 1 to 2 cm in diameter with possible skin discoloration
+ Tumor — solid, raised mass usually larger than 2 cm in diameter with possible skin discoloration

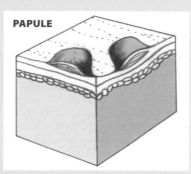

WHEAL

A slightly raised, firm lesion of variable size and shape that's surrounded by edema (skin may be red or pale)

PAPULE

A small, solid, raised lesion less than 1 cm in diameter with red to purple skin discoloration

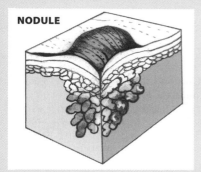

NODULE

A small, firm, circumscribed, elevated lesion 1 to 2 cm in diameter with possible skin discoloration

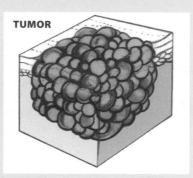

TUMOR

A solid, raised mass usually larger than 2 cm in diameter with possible skin discoloration

Lichen planus

Discrete, flat, angular or polygonal, violet papules, commonly marked with white lines or spots, are characteristic of lichen planus. The papules may be linear or may coalesce into plaques and usually appear on the lumbar region, genitalia, ankles, anterior tibiae, and wrists. Lesions usually develop first on the buccal mucosa as a lacy network of white or gray threadlike papules or plaques. Pruritus, distorted fingernails, and atrophic alopecia commonly occur.

Mononucleosis (infectious)

A maculopapular rash that resembles rubella is an early sign of infectious mononucleosis in 10% of patients. The rash is typically preceded by headache, malaise, and fatigue. It may be accompanied by sore throat, cervical lymphadenopathy, and fluc-

Medical causes
(continued)

Lichen planus
+ White lines or spots mark discrete, flat, angular or polygonal, violet papules.
+ Papules may be linear or may coalesce into plaques.

Mononucleosis (infectious)
+ A maculopapular rash that resembles rubella may be an early sign.
+ Headache, malaise, and fatigue typically precede the rash.

Medical causes
(continued)

Pityriasis rosea
+ Initially, an erythematous, slightly raised, oval lesion appears.
+ Later, yellow, erythematous patches with scaly edges appear on the trunk, arms, and legs.

Polymorphic light eruption
+ Papular, vesicular, or nodular rash appears on sun-exposed areas.

Psoriasis
+ Initially, small, erythematous papules appear.
+ Eventually, papules enlarge and coalesce, forming elevated, red, scaly plaques covered by characteristic silver scales.

Rosacea
+ Persistent erythema, telangiectasia, and recurrent eruption of papules and pustules on the forehead, malar areas, nose, and chin occur.

Sarcoidosis
+ Small, erythematous or yellow-brown papules appear on the face and upper back.

Seborrheic keratosis
+ Benign skin tumors begin as small, yellow-brown papules on the chest, back, or abdomen, eventually enlarging and becoming deeply pigmented.

Smallpox
+ Maculopapular rash develops on the mouth mucosa, pharynx, face, and forearms and then spreads to the trunk and legs.

tuating temperature with an evening peak of 101° to 102° F (38.3° to 38.9° C). Splenomegaly and hepatomegaly may also develop.

Pityriasis rosea
Pityriasis rosea begins with an erythematous "herald patch" — a slightly raised, oval lesion about 2 to 6 cm in diameter that may appear anywhere on the body. A few days to weeks later, yellow to tan or erythematous patches with scaly edges appear on the trunk, arms, and legs, commonly erupting along body cleavage lines in a characteristic "pine tree" pattern. These patches may be asymptomatic or slightly pruritic, are 0.5 to 1 cm in diameter, and typically improve with skin exposure.

Polymorphic light eruption
Abnormal reactions to light may produce papular, vesicular, or nodular rashes on sun-exposed areas. Other symptoms include pruritus, headache, and malaise.

Psoriasis
Psoriasis is a common chronic disorder that begins with small, erythematous papules on the scalp, chest, elbows, knees, back, buttocks, and genitalia. These papules are sometimes pruritic and painful. Eventually they enlarge and coalesce, forming elevated, red, scaly plaques covered by characteristic silver scales, except in moist areas such as the genitalia. These scales may flake off easily or thicken, covering the plaque. Associated features include pitted fingernails and arthralgia.

Rosacea
Rosacea, a hyperemic disorder, is characterized by persistent erythema, telangiectasia, and recurrent eruption of papules and pustules on the forehead, malar areas, nose, and chin. Eventually, eruptions occur more frequently and erythema deepens. Rhinophyma may occur in severe cases.

Sarcoidosis
Sarcoidosis, a multisystem granulomatous disorder, may produce crops of small, erythematous or yellow-brown papules around the eyes and mouth and on the nose, nasal mucosa, and upper back. Associated findings include dyspnea with a nonproductive cough, fatigue, arthralgia, weight loss, lymphadenopathy, vision loss, and dysphagia.

Seborrheic keratosis
With seborrheic keratosis, benign skin tumors begin as small, yellow-brown papules on the chest, back, or abdomen, eventually enlarging and becoming deeply pigmented. However, in blacks, these papules may remain small and affect only the malar part of the face (dermatosis papulosa nigra).

Smallpox
Initial signs and symptoms of smallpox (also known as variola major) include high fever, malaise, prostration, severe headache, backache, and abdominal pain. A maculopapular rash develops on the mucosa of the mouth, pharynx, face, and forearms and then spreads to the trunk and legs. Within 2 days, the rash becomes vesicular and, later, pustular. The lesions develop at the same time, appear identical, and are more prominent on the face and extremities. The pustules are round, firm, and deeply embedded in the skin. After 8 to 9 days, the pustules form a crust, and later the scab separates from the skin, leaving a pitted scar. In fatal cases, death results from encephalitis, extensive bleeding, or secondary infection.

Syphilis

A discrete, reddish brown, mucocutaneous rash and general lymphadenopathy herald the onset of secondary syphilis. The rash may be papular, macular, pustular, or nodular. It typically erupts between rolls of fat on the trunk and proximally on the arms, palms, soles, face, and scalp. Lesions in warm, moist areas enlarge and erode, producing highly contagious, pink or grayish white condylomata lata. The patient may also experience mild headache, malaise, anorexia, weight loss, nausea and vomiting, sore throat, low-grade fever, temporary alopecia, and brittle, pitted nails.

Systemic lupus erythematosus

Systemic lupus erythematosus (SLE) is characterized by a "butterfly rash" of erythematous maculopapules or discoid plaques that appears in a malar distribution across the nose and cheeks. Similar rashes may appear elsewhere, especially on exposed body areas. Other cardinal features of SLE include photosensitivity and nondeforming arthritis, especially in the hands, feet, and large joints. Common effects are patchy alopecia, mucous membrane ulceration, low-grade or spiking fever, chills, lymphadenopathy, anorexia, weight loss, abdominal pain, diarrhea or constipation, dyspnea, tachycardia, hematuria, headache, and irritability.

OTHER CAUSES

Drugs

Transient maculopapular rashes, usually on the trunk, may accompany reactions to many drugs, including antibiotics, such as tetracycline, ampicillin, cephalosporins, and sulfonamides; benzodiazepines such as diazepam; lithium; phenylbutazone; gold salts; allopurinol; isoniazid; and salicylates.

SPECIAL CONSIDERATIONS

Apply cool compresses or an antipruritic lotion. Administer an antihistamine for allergic reactions and an antibiotic for infection.

PEDIATRIC POINTERS

Common causes of papular rashes in children are infectious diseases, such as molluscum contagiosum and scarlet fever; scabies; insect bites; allergies and drug reactions; and miliaria, which occurs in three forms, depending on the depth of sweat gland involvement.

GERIATRIC POINTERS

In bedridden elderly patients, the first sign of pressure ulcers is commonly an erythematous area, sometimes with firm papules. If not properly managed, these lesions progress to deep ulcers and can lead to death.

PATIENT COUNSELING

Advise the patient to keep his skin clean and dry, to avoid scratching the rash, and to wear loose-fitting, nonirritating clothing. Instruct him to promptly report any change in the rash's color, size, or configuration as well as the onset of itching or bleeding. Also tell him to avoid excessive exposure to direct sunlight and to apply a protective sunscreen before going outdoors.

Warn patients with chronic conditions (such as SLE, psoriasis, or sarcoidosis) about the typical skin rashes that can develop. Tell them that these rashes can be an

Medical causes
(continued)

Syphilis
+ A discrete, reddish brown, mucocutaneous rash and general lymphadenopathy herald the onset of secondary syphilis.

SLE
+ A rash of erythematous maculopapules or discoid plaques appears in a malar distribution across the nose and cheeks.

Other causes
+ Antibiotics, benzodiazepines, lithium, phenylbutazone, gold salts, allopurinol, isoniazid, and salicylates

Special considerations
+ Apply cool compresses or an antipruritic lotion.
+ Administer an antihistamine for allergic reactions and an antibiotic for infection.

Peds points
+ Common causes of papular rashes in children are infectious diseases, scabies, insect bites, allergies, drug reactions, and miliaria.

Geri points
+ An erythematous area, sometimes with firm papules, may be the first sign of a pressure ulcer.

Teaching points
+ Skin care measures
+ Need to report change in rash color, size, or configuration and itching or bleeding

Key facts about paralysis

- Total loss of voluntary motor function from severe cortical or pyramidal tract damage
- Can be local or widespread, symmetrical or asymmetrical, transient or permanent, and spastic or flaccid
- Classified according to location and severity as paraplegia

In an emergency

- Immobilize the patient's spine, determine LOC, and take vital signs.
- Elevate the patient's head 30 degrees, if possible, in cases of increasing ICP.
- Evaluate respiratory status, and be prepared to maintain a patent airway.

Key history points

- Onset, duration, intensity, and progression of paralysis and events preceding development
- History of degenerative neurologic or neuromuscular disease, recent infectious illness, STD, cancer, or recent injury

Critical assessment steps

- Perform a complete neurologic examination.
- Assess strength in all major muscle groups.

Medical causes

ALS

- Spastic or flaccid paralysis occurs in the major muscle groups and progresses to total paralysis.

---

early sign of disease flare-up and that they should seek prompt treatment to prevent serious complications.

PARALYSIS

Paralysis, the total loss of voluntary motor function, results from severe cortical or pyramidal tract damage. It can occur with a cerebrovascular disorder, degenerative neuromuscular disease, trauma, tumor, or central nervous system infection. Acute paralysis may be an early indicator of a life-threatening disorder such as Guillain-Barré syndrome.

Paralysis can be local or widespread, symmetrical or asymmetrical, transient or permanent, and spastic or flaccid. It's commonly classified according to location and severity as paraplegia (sometimes transient paralysis of the legs), quadriplegia (permanent paralysis of the arms, legs, and body below the level of the spinal lesion), or hemiplegia (unilateral paralysis of varying severity and permanence). Incomplete paralysis with profound weakness (paresis) may precede total paralysis in some patients.

 EMERGENCY ACTIONS If paralysis has developed suddenly, suspect trauma or an acute vascular insult. After ensuring that the patient's spine is properly immobilized, quickly determine his level of consciousness (LOC) and take his vital signs. Elevated systolic blood pressure, widening pulse pressure, and bradycardia may signal increasing intracranial pressure (ICP). If possible, elevate the patient's head 30 degrees to decrease ICP.

Evaluate respiratory status, and be prepared to administer oxygen, insert an artificial airway, or provide intubation and mechanical ventilation, as needed. To help determine the nature of the patient's injury, ask him for an account of the precipitating events. If he's unable to respond, try to find an eyewitness.

HISTORY

If the patient is in no immediate danger, perform a complete neurologic assessment. Start with the history, relying on family members for information, if necessary. Ask about the onset, duration, intensity, and progression of paralysis and about the events preceding its development. Focus medical history questions on the incidence of degenerative neurologic or neuromuscular disease, recent infectious illness, sexually transmitted disease, cancer, or recent injury. Explore related signs and symptoms, noting fever, headache, vision disturbances, dysphagia, nausea and vomiting, bowel or bladder dysfunction, muscle pain or weakness, and fatigue.

PHYSICAL ASSESSMENT

Perform a complete neurologic examination, testing cranial nerve, motor, and sensory function and deep tendon reflexes. Assess strength in all major muscle groups, and note any muscle atrophy. Document all findings to serve as a baseline.

MEDICAL CAUSES

Amyotrophic lateral sclerosis

Amyotrophic lateral sclerosis (ALS) is an invariably fatal disorder that produces spastic or flaccid paralysis in the body's major muscle groups, eventually progressing to total paralysis. Earlier findings include progressive muscle weakness, fasciculations, and muscle atrophy, usually beginning in the arms and hands. Cramping and hyperreflexia are also common. Involvement of respiratory muscles and the brain stem produces dyspnea and, possibly, respiratory distress. Progressive cranial nerve paralysis causes dysarthria, dysphagial drooling, choking, and difficulty chewing.

Bell's palsy

Bell's palsy, a disease of cranial nerve VII, causes transient, unilateral facial muscle paralysis. The affected muscles sag, and eyelid closure is impossible. Other signs include increased tearing, drooling, and a diminished or absent corneal reflex.

Brain tumor

A tumor affecting the motor cortex of the frontal lobe may cause contralateral hemiparesis that progresses to hemiplegia. Onset is gradual, but paralysis is permanent without treatment. In early stages, frontal headache and behavioral changes may be the only indicators. Eventually, seizures, aphasia, and signs of increased ICP (decreased LOC and vomiting) develop.

Conversion disorder

Hysterical paralysis, a classic symptom of conversion disorder, is characterized by the loss of voluntary movement with no obvious physical cause. It can affect any muscle group, appears and disappears unpredictably, and may occur with histrionic behavior (manipulative, dramatic, vain, or irrational) or a strange indifference.

Encephalitis

Variable paralysis develops in the late stages of encephalitis. Earlier signs and symptoms include rapidly decreasing LOC (possibly coma), fever, headache, photophobia, vomiting, signs of meningeal irritation (nuchal rigidity, positive Kernig's and Brudzinski's signs), aphasia, ataxia, nystagmus, ocular palsies, myoclonus, and seizures.

Guillain-Barré syndrome

Guillain-Barré syndrome is characterized by a rapidly developing, but reversible, ascending paralysis. It commonly begins as leg muscle weakness and progresses symmetrically, sometimes affecting even the cranial nerves, producing dysphagia, nasal speech, and dysarthria. Respiratory muscle paralysis may be life-threatening. Other effects include transient paresthesia, orthostatic hypotension, tachycardia, diaphoresis, and bowel and bladder incontinence.

Head trauma

Cerebral injury can cause paralysis due to cerebral edema and increased intracranial pressure. Onset is usually sudden. Location and extent vary, depending on the injury. Associated findings also vary but include decreased LOC; sensory disturbances, such as paresthesia and loss of sensation; headache; blurred or double vision; nausea and vomiting; and focal neurologic disturbances.

Migraine headache

Hemiparesis, scotomas, paresthesia, confusion, dizziness, photophobia, or other transient symptoms may precede the onset of a throbbing unilateral headache and may persist after it subsides. The patient may also experience nausea and vomiting.

Multiple sclerosis

With multiple sclerosis, paralysis commonly waxes and wanes until the later stages, when it may become permanent. Its extent can range from monoplegia to quadriplegia. In most patients, vision and sensory disturbances (paresthesia) are the earliest symptoms. Later findings are widely variable and may include muscle weakness and spasticity, nystagmus, hyperreflexia, intention tremor, gait ataxia, dysphagia,

Medical causes
(continued)

Bell's palsy
✦ Transient paralysis affects muscles on one side of the face.

Brain tumor
✦ A contralateral hemiparesis that progresses to hemiplegia occurs with a tumor affecting the motor cortex of the frontal lobe.

Conversion disorder
✦ Loss of voluntary movement that can affect any muscle group and has no obvious physical cause.

Encephalitis
✦ Variable paralysis develops in the late stages.

Guillain-Barré syndrome
✦ A rapidly developing, reversible paralysis begins as leg muscle weakness and ascends symmetrically.

Head trauma
✦ Cerebral edema and increased ICP can produce sudden paralysis.

Migraine headache
✦ Hemiparesis and other transient symptoms may precede the onset of a throbbing unilateral headache and may persist after it subsides.

Multiple sclerosis
✦ Paralysis commonly waxes and wanes until the later stages, when it may become permanent.

Medical causes
(continued)

Myasthenia gravis
+ Muscle weakness and abnormal fatigability produce paralysis of certain muscle groups.
+ Paralysis is usually transient in early stages but becomes more persistent as the disease progresses.

Neurosyphilis
+ Irreversible hemiplegia may occur in the late stages.

Parkinson's disease
+ Extreme rigidity can progress to paralysis, particularly in the extremities.

Peripheral nerve trauma
+ Severe injury to a peripheral nerve or group of nerves results in the loss of motor and sensory function in the innervated area.

Peripheral neuropathy
+ Muscle weakness may lead to flaccid paralysis and atrophy.

Rabies
+ Progressive flaccid paralysis, vascular collapse, coma, and death occur within 2 weeks of contact with an infected animal.
+ Prodromal symptoms include fever; headache; hyperesthesia; paresthesia, coldness, and itching at the bite site; photophobia; tachycardia; shallow respirations; and excessive salivation, lacrimation, and perspiration.

Seizure disorders
+ Transient local paralysis can result from focal seizures.

dysarthria, impotence, and constipation. Urinary frequency, urgency, and incontinence may also occur.

Myasthenia gravis
Myasthenia gravis is a neuromuscular disease that causes profound muscle weakness and abnormal fatigability that may produce paralysis of certain muscle groups. Paralysis is usually transient in early stages but becomes more persistent as the disease progresses. Associated findings in myasthenia gravis depend on the areas of neuromuscular involvement; they include weak eye closure, ptosis, diplopia, lack of facial mobility, dysphagia, nasal speech, and frequent nasal regurgitation of fluids. Neck muscle weakness may cause the patient's jaw to drop and his head to bob. Respiratory muscle involvement can lead to respiratory distress — dyspnea, shallow respirations, and cyanosis.

Neurosyphilis
Irreversible hemiplegia may occur in the late stages of neurosyphilis. Dementia, cranial nerve palsies, meningitis, personality changes, tremors, and abnormal reflexes are other late findings.

Parkinson's disease
Tremors, bradykinesia, and lead-pipe or cogwheel rigidity are the classic signs of Parkinson's disease. Extreme rigidity can progress to paralysis, particularly in the extremities. In most cases, paralysis resolves with prompt treatment of the disease.

Peripheral nerve trauma
Severe injury to a peripheral nerve or group of nerves results in the loss of motor and sensory function in the innervated area. Muscles become flaccid and atrophied, and reflexes are lost. If transection isn't complete, paralysis may be temporary.

Peripheral neuropathy
Typically, peripheral neuropathy produces muscle weakness that may lead to flaccid paralysis and atrophy. Related effects include paresthesia, loss of vibration sensation, hypoactive or absent deep tendon reflexes, neuralgia, and skin changes such as anhidrosis.

Rabies
Rabies produces progressive flaccid paralysis, vascular collapse, coma, and death within 2 weeks of contact with an infected animal. Prodromal signs and symptoms — fever; headache; hyperesthesia; paresthesia, coldness, and itching at the bite site; photophobia; tachycardia; shallow respirations; and excessive salivation, lacrimation, and perspiration — develop almost immediately. Within 2 to 10 days, a phase of excitement begins, marked by agitation, cranial nerve dysfunction (pupil changes, hoarseness, facial weakness, ocular palsies), tachycardia or bradycardia, cyclic respirations, high fever, urine retention, drooling, and hydrophobia.

Seizure disorders
Seizures, particularly focal seizures, can cause transient local paralysis (Todd's paralysis). Any part of the body may be affected, although paralysis tends to occur contralateral to ae side of the irritable focus. Seizures may be preceded by an aura.

Spinal cord injury
Complete spinal cord transection results in permanent spastic paralysis below the level of injury. Reflexes may return after spinal shock resolves. Partial transection causes variable paralysis and paresthesia, depending on the location and extent of injury. (See *Understanding spinal cord syndromes.*)

Understanding spinal cord syndromes

When a patient's spinal cord is completely severed, he experiences partial motor and sensory loss. Most incomplete cord lesions fit into one of the syndromes described below.

Anterior cord syndrome, usually resulting from a flexion injury, causes motor paralysis and loss of pain and temperature sensation below the level of injury. Touch, proprioception, and vibration sensation are usually preserved.

Central cord syndrome is caused by hyperextension or flexion injury. Motor loss is variable and greater in the arms than in the legs; sensory loss is usually slight.

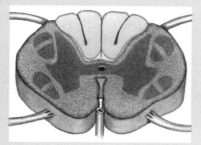

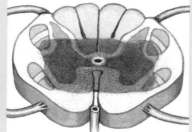

Brown-Séquard syndrome can result from flexion, rotation, or penetration injury. It's characterized by unilateral motor paralysis ipsilateral to the injury and by loss of pain and temperature sensation contralateral to the injury.

Posterior cord syndrome, produced by a cervical hyperextension injury, causes only a loss of proprioception and loss of light touch sensation. Motor function remains intact.

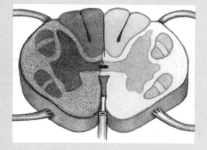

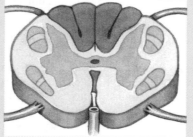

Spinal cord tumor

With a spinal cord tumor, paresis, pain, paresthesia, and variable sensory loss may occur along the nerve distribution pathway served by the affected cord segment. Eventually, these symptoms may progress to spastic paralysis with hyperactive deep tendon reflexes (unless the tumor is in the cauda equina, which produces hyporeflexia) and, perhaps, bladder and bowel incontinence. Paralysis is permanent without treatment.

Stroke

A stroke involving the motor cortex can produce contralateral paresis or paralysis. Onset may be sudden or gradual, and paralysis may be transient or permanent. Associated signs and symptoms vary widely and may include headache, vomiting,

Medical causes
(continued)

Spinal cord injury
+ Complete spinal cord transection results in permanent spastic paralysis below the level of the injury.
+ Partial transection causes variable paralysis and paresthesia, depending on the location and extent of injury.

Spinal cord tumor
+ Paresis, pain, paresthesia, and variable sensory loss may occur.

Stroke
+ Contralateral paresis or paralysis can result from a stroke involving the motor cortex.

Medical causes
(continued)
Subarachnoid hemorrhage
✦ Sudden paralysis (temporary or permanent) may occur.

Syringomyelia
✦ Segmental paresis leads to flaccid paralysis of hands and arms.

Thoracic aortic aneurysm
✦ Sudden transient bilateral paralysis may result from occlusion of spinal arteries by a ruptured thoracic aortic aneurysm.

TIA
✦ Transient unilateral paresis or paralysis may accompany paresthesia, blurred or double vision, dizziness, aphasia, dysarthria, decreased LOC, and other site-dependent effects.

West Nile encephalitis
✦ Paralysis may occur in more severe infections, accompanied by fever, headache, body aches, skin rash, and swollen lymph glands.

Other causes
✦ Neuromuscular blockers
✦ Electroconvulsive therapy

Special considerations
✦ Provide frequent position changes, meticulous skin care, and frequent chest physiotherapy to prevent complications from prolonged immobility.
✦ Perform passive ROM exercises, apply splints, and use footboards or other devices.
✦ Provide a liquid or soft diet, and keep suction equipment on hand as appropriate.

seizures, decreased LOC and mental acuity, dysarthria, dysphagia, ataxia, contralateral paresthesia or sensory loss, apraxia, agnosia, aphasia, vision disturbances, emotional lability, and bowel and bladder dysfunction.

Subarachnoid hemorrhage
A subarachnoid hemorrhage is a potentially life-threatening disorder that can produce sudden paralysis. The condition may be temporary, resolving with decreasing edema, or permanent, if tissue destruction has occurred. Other acute effects are severe headache, mydriasis, photophobia, aphasia, sharply decreased LOC, nuchal rigidity, vomiting, and seizures.

Syringomyelia
Syringomyelia, a degenerative spinal cord disease, produces segmental paresis, leading to flaccid paralysis of the hands and arms. Reflexes are absent, and loss of pain and temperature sensation is distributed over the neck, shoulders, and arms in a capelike pattern.

Thoracic aortic aneurysm
Occlusion of spinal arteries by a ruptured thoracic aortic aneurysm may cause sudden onset of transient bilateral paralysis. Severe chest pain radiating to the neck, shoulders, back, and abdomen and a sensation of tearing in the thorax are prominent symptoms. Related findings include syncope, pallor, diaphoresis, dyspnea, tachycardia, cyanosis, diastolic heart murmur, and abrupt loss of radial and femoral pulses or wide variations in pulses and blood pressure between arms and legs. Paradoxically, however, the patient appears to be in shock, and his systolic blood pressure is either normal or elevated.

Transient ischemic attack
Episodic transient ischemic attacks (TIA) may cause transient unilateral paresis or paralysis accompanied by paresthesia, blurred or double vision, dizziness, aphasia, dysarthria, decreased LOC, and other site-dependent effects.

West Nile encephalitis
Mild infections of West Nile encephalitis, a mosquito-borne flavivirus, are common and include fever, headache, and body aches, which are sometimes accompanied by skin rash and swollen lymph glands. More severe infections are marked by headache, high fever, neck stiffness, stupor, disorientation, coma, tremors, occasional convulsions, paralysis and, rarely, death.

OTHER CAUSES
Drugs
Therapeutic use of neuromuscular blockers, such as pancuronium or curare, produces paralysis.

Electroconvulsive therapy
Electroconvulsive therapy can produce acute, but transient, paralysis.

SPECIAL CONSIDERATIONS
Because a paralyzed patient is particularly susceptible to complications of prolonged immobility, provide frequent position changes, meticulous skin care, and frequent chest physiotherapy. He may benefit from passive range-of-motion exercises to maintain muscle tone, application of splints to prevent contractures, and the use of footboards or other devices to prevent footdrop. If his cranial nerves are affected, the patient will have difficulty chewing and swallowing. Provide a liquid

or soft diet, and keep suction equipment on hand in case aspiration occurs. Feeding tubes or total parenteral nutrition may be necessary with severe paralysis. Paralysis and accompanying vision disturbances may make ambulation hazardous; provide a call light, and show the patient how to call for help. As appropriate, arrange for physical, speech, or occupational therapy.

PEDIATRIC POINTERS

Although children may develop paralysis from an obvious cause—such as trauma, infection, or tumor—they may also develop it from a hereditary or congenital disorder, such as Tay-Sachs disease, Werdnig-Hoffmann disease, spina bifida, or cerebral palsy.

PATIENT COUNSELING

Because paralysis is a frightening experience, provide emotional support to the patient and his family. Allow the patient time to verbalize fears and concerns. Make referrals to social and psychological services as needed. Promote independence as much as possible.

PARESTHESIA

Paresthesia is an abnormal sensation or combination of sensations—commonly described as numbness, prickling, or tingling—felt along peripheral nerve pathways; these sensations generally aren't painful. Unpleasant or painful sensations, on the other hand, are termed *dysesthesia*. Paresthesia may develop suddenly or gradually and may be transient or permanent.

A common symptom of many neurologic disorders, paresthesia may also result from a systemic disorder or from a particular drug. It may reflect damage or irritation of the parietal lobe, thalamus, spinothalamic tract, or spinal or peripheral nerves—the neural circuit that transmits and interprets sensory stimuli.

HISTORY

First, explore the paresthesia. When did the abnormal sensations begin? Have the patient describe their character and distribution. Also, ask about associated signs and symptoms, such as sensory loss and paresis or paralysis. Next, take a medical history, including neurologic, cardiovascular, metabolic, renal, and chronic inflammatory disorders, such as arthritis or lupus. Has the patient recently sustained a traumatic injury or had surgery or an invasive procedure that may have damaged peripheral nerves?

PHYSICAL ASSESSMENT

Focus the physical examination on the patient's neurologic status. Assess his level of consciousness (LOC) and cranial nerve function. Test muscle strength and deep tendon reflexes (DTRs) in limbs affected by paresthesia. Systematically evaluate light touch, pain, temperature, vibration, and position sensation. Also, note skin color and temperature, and palpate pulses.

MEDICAL CAUSES

Arterial occlusion (acute)
With acute arterial occlusion, sudden paresthesia and coldness may develop in one or both legs with a saddle embolus. Paresis, intermittent claudication, and aching

Peds points
+ Children may develop paralysis from obvious causes or from hereditary or congenital disorders.

Teaching points
+ Referrals to social and psychological services

Key facts about paresthesia
+ Abnormal sensation or combination of sensations—commonly described as numbness, prickling, or tingling—along peripheral nerve pathways
+ May develop suddenly or gradually and may be transient or permanent

Key history points
+ Onset and nature of abnormal sensations
+ Associated signs and symptoms, such as sensory loss and paresis
+ Recent head injury, surgery, or invasive procedure
+ Medical history

Critical assessment steps
+ Assess LOC and cranial nerve function.
+ Test muscle strength and DTRs in limbs affected by paresthesia.
+ Systematically evaluate light touch, pain, temperature, vibration, and position sensation.
+ Note skin color and temperature, and palpate pulses.

Medical causes
Arterial occlusion (acute)
+ Sudden paresthesia and coldness may develop.

Medical causes
(continued)

Arterial occlusion (acute)
✦ Sudden paresthesia and coldness may develop.

Arteriosclerosis obliterans
✦ Paresthesia may occur in the affected leg, along with intermittent claudication.

Arthritis
✦ Paresthesia varies with location and type of arthritis.

Brain tumor
✦ Progressive contralateral paresthesia may occur with tumors affecting the sensory cortex.

Buerger's disease
✦ Feet become cold, cyanotic, and numb after exposure to cold.

Diabetes mellitus
✦ Paresthesia and a burning sensation in the hands and legs occur with diabetic neuropathy.

Guillain-Barré syndrome
✦ Transient paresthesia may precede muscle weakness.

Head trauma
✦ Paresthesia may accompany a concussion or contusion.

Heavy metal or solvent poisoning
✦ Acute or gradual paresthesia may occur with exposure products containing lead, mercury, thallium, or organophosphates.

Herniated disk
✦ Onset of paresthesia may occur along the distribution pathways of affected spinal nerves.

pain at rest are also characteristic. The extremity becomes mottled with a line of temperature and color demarcation at the level of occlusion. Pulses are absent below the occlusion, and capillary refill time is increased.

Arteriosclerosis obliterans
Arteriosclerosis obliterans produces paresthesia, intermittent claudication (most common symptom), diminished or absent popliteal and pedal pulses, pallor, paresis, and coldness in the affected leg.

Arthritis
Rheumatoid or osteoarthritic changes in the cervical spine may cause paresthesia in the neck, shoulders, and arms. The lumbar spine occasionally is affected, causing paresthesia in one or both legs and feet.

Brain tumor
Tumors affecting the sensory cortex in the parietal lobe may cause progressive contralateral paresthesia accompanied by agnosia, apraxia, agraphia, homonymous hemianopsia, and loss of proprioception.

Buerger's disease
With Buerger's disease, exposure to cold makes the feet cold, cyanotic, and numb; later, they redden, become hot, and tingle. Intermittent claudication, which is aggravated by exercise and relieved by rest, is also common. Other findings include weak peripheral pulses, migratory superficial thrombophlebitis and, later, ulceration, muscle atrophy, and gangrene.

Diabetes mellitus
Diabetic neuropathy can cause paresthesia with a burning sensation in the hands and legs. Other findings include insidious, permanent anosmia; fatigue; polyuria; polydipsia; weight loss; and polyphagia.

Guillain-Barré syndrome
With Guillain-Barré syndrome, transient paresthesia may precede muscle weakness, which usually begins in the legs and ascends to the arms and facial nerves. Weakness may progress to total paralysis. Other findings include dysarthria, dysphagia, nasal speech, orthostatic hypotension, bladder and bowel incontinence, diaphoresis, tachycardia and, possibly, signs of life-threatening respiratory muscle paralysis.

Head trauma
Unilateral or bilateral paresthesia may occur when head trauma causes a concussion or contusion; however, sensory loss is more common. Other findings include variable paresis or paralysis, decreased LOC, headache, blurred or double vision, nausea and vomiting, dizziness, and seizures.

Heavy metal or solvent poisoning
Exposure to industrial or household products containing lead, mercury, thallium, or organophosphates may cause paresthesia of acute or gradual onset. Mental status changes, tremors, weakness, seizures, and GI distress are also common.

Herniated disk
Herniation of a lumbar or cervical disk may cause acute or gradual onset of paresthesia along the distribution pathways of affected spinal nerves. Other neuromuscular effects include severe pain, muscle spasms, and weakness that may progress to atrophy unless herniation is relieved.

Herpes zoster

An early symptom of herpes zoster, paresthesia occurs in the dermatome supplied by the affected spinal nerve. Within several days, this dermatome is marked by a pruritic, erythematous, vesicular rash associated with sharp, shooting, or burning pain.

Hyperventilation syndrome

Usually triggered by acute anxiety, hyperventilation syndrome may produce transient paresthesia in the hands, feet, and perioral area, accompanied by agitation, vertigo, syncope, pallor, muscle twitching and weakness, carpopedal spasm, and cardiac arrhythmias.

Hypocalcemia

Asymmetrical paresthesia usually occurs in the fingers, toes, and circumoral area early in hypocalcemia. Other signs and symptoms are muscle weakness, twitching, or cramps; palpitations; hyperactive DTRs; carpopedal spasm; and positive Chvostek's and Trousseau's signs.

Migraine headache

Paresthesia in the hands, face, and perioral area may herald an impending migraine headache. Other prodromal symptoms include scotomas, hemiparesis, confusion, dizziness, and photophobia. These effects may persist during the characteristic throbbing headache and continue after it subsides.

Multiple sclerosis

With multiple sclerosis, demyelination of the sensory cortex or spinothalamic tract may produce paresthesia — typically one of the earliest symptoms. Like other effects of multiple sclerosis, paresthesia commonly waxes and wanes until the later stages, when it may become permanent. Associated findings include muscle weakness, spasticity, and hyperreflexia.

Peripheral nerve trauma

Injury to any major peripheral nerve can cause paresthesia — often dysesthesia — in the area supplied by that nerve. Paresthesia begins shortly after trauma and may be permanent. Other findings are flaccid paralysis or paresis, hyporeflexia, and variable sensory loss.

Peripheral neuropathy

Peripheral neuropathy can cause progressive paresthesia in all extremities. The patient also commonly displays muscle weakness, which may lead to flaccid paralysis and atrophy; loss of vibration sensation; diminished or absent DTRs; euralgia; and cutaneous changes, such as glossy, red skin and anhidrosis.

Rabies

Paresthesia, coldness, and itching at the site of an animal bite herald the prodromal stage of rabies. Other prodromal signs and symptoms are fever, headache, photophobia, hyperesthesia, tachycardia, shallow respirations, and excessive salivation, lacrimation, and perspiration.

Raynaud's disease

With Raynaud's disease, exposure to cold or stress makes the fingers turn pale, cold, and cyanotic; with rewarming, they become red, throbbing, aching, swollen, and paresthetic. Ulceration may occur in chronic cases.

Medical causes
(continued)

Herpes zoster
- ✦ Paresthesia occurs in dermatome supplied by affected spinal nerve.

Hyperventilation syndrome
- ✦ Transient paresthesia may occur in hands, feet, and perioral area.

Hypocalcemia
- ✦ Asymmetrical paresthesia usually occurs in fingers, toes, and circumoral area.

Migraine headache
- ✦ Paresthesia in hands, face, and perioral area may herald an impending migraine headache.

Multiple sclerosis
- ✦ An early symptom, paresthesia commonly waxes and wanes until the later stages.

Peripheral nerve trauma
- ✦ Injury to any major peripheral nerve can cause paresthesia in the area supplied by that nerve.

Peripheral neuropathy
- ✦ Progressive paresthesia can occur in all extremities.

Rabies
- ✦ Paresthesia, coldness, and itching at site of an animal bite herald prodromal stage of rabies.

Raynaud's disease
- ✦ Exposure to cold or stress turns fingers pale, cold, and cyanotic; with rewarming, they become red, throbbing, aching, swollen, and paresthetic.

Medical causes
(continued)

Seizure disorders
+ Paresthesia of the lips, fingers, and toes results from seizures originating in the parietal lobe.

Spinal cord injury
+ Paresthesia may occur in partial spinal cord transection.

Spinal cord tumors
+ Paresthesia, paresis, pain, and sensory loss occur.

Stroke
+ Although contralateral paresthesia may occur with stroke, sensory loss is more common.

SLE
+ SLE may cause paresthesia, but it is not a primary sign.

Thoracic outlet syndrome
+ Paresthesia occurs suddenly when the affected arm is raised and abducted.

TIA
+ Paresthesia typically occurs abruptly and is limited to an isolated part of the body.

Vitamin B deficiency
+ Paresthesia and weakness occur in the arms and legs.

Other causes
+ Phenytoin, chemotherapeutic agents, D-penicillamine, isoniazid, nitrofurantoin, chloroquine, and parenteral gold therapy
+ Radiation therapy

Seizure disorders

Seizures originating in the parietal lobe usually cause paresthesia of the lips, fingers, and toes. The paresthesia may act as auras that precede tonic-clonic seizures. After the seizure, the patient may complain of headache, fatigue, muscle soreness, and arm and leg weakness.

Spinal cord injury

Paresthesia may occur in partial spinal cord transection, after spinal shock resolves. It may be unilateral or bilateral, occurring at or below the level of the lesion. Associated sensory and motor loss is variable. (See *Understanding spinal cord syndromes*, page 495.) Spinal cord disorders may be associated with paresthesia on head flexion (Lhermitte's sign).

Spinal cord tumors

Paresthesia, paresis, pain, and sensory loss along nerve pathways served by the affected cord segment result from spinal cord tumors. Eventually, paresis may cause spastic paralysis with hyperactive DTRs (unless the tumor is in the cauda equina, which produces hyporeflexia) and, possibly, bladder and bowel incontinence.

Stroke

Although contralateral paresthesia may occur with stroke, sensory loss is more common. Associated features vary with the artery affected and may include contralateral hemiplegia, decreased LOC, and homonymous hemianopsia.

Systemic lupus erythematosus

Systemic lupus erythematosus (SLE) may cause paresthesia, but its primary signs and symptoms include nondeforming arthritis (usually of hands, feet, and large joints), photosensitivity, and a "butterfly rash" that appears across the nose and cheeks.

Thoracic outlet syndrome

Paresthesia occurs suddenly in this syndrome when the affected arm is raised and abducted. The arm also becomes pale and cool with diminished pulses. Unequal blood pressure between arms may be noted.

Transient ischemic attack

Paresthesia typically occurs abruptly with a transient ischemic attack (TIA) and is limited to one arm or another isolated part of the body. It usually lasts about 10 minutes and is accompanied by paralysis or paresis. Associated findings include decreased LOC, dizziness, unilateral vision loss, nystagmus, aphasia, dysarthria, tinnitus, facial weakness, dysphagia, and ataxic gait.

Vitamin B deficiency

Chronic thiamine or vitamin B_{12} deficiency may cause paresthesia and weakness in the arms and legs. Burning leg pain, hypoactive DTRs, and variable sensory loss are common in thiamine deficiency; vitamin B_{12} deficiency also produces mental status changes and impaired vision.

OTHER CAUSES

Drugs

Phenytoin, chemotherapeutic agents (such as vincristine, vinblastine, and procarbazine), D-penicillamine, isoniazid, nitrofurantoin, chloroquine, and parenteral gold therapy may produce transient paresthesia that disappears when the drug is discontinued.

Radiation therapy

Long-term radiation therapy eventually may cause peripheral nerve damage, resulting in paresthesia.

SPECIAL CONSIDERATIONS

Continue to monitor the patient's neurologic status. Help the patient perform daily activities as necessary. If he has sensory deficits, protect him from injury, heat, or pressure.

PEDIATRIC POINTERS

Although children may experience paresthesia associated with the same causes as adults, many are unable to describe this symptom. Nevertheless, hereditary polyneuropathies are usually first recognized in childhood.

PATIENT COUNSELING

Because paresthesia is commonly accompanied by patchy sensory loss, teach the patient safety measures. For example, have him test bathwater with a thermometer.

PEAU D'ORANGE

Usually a late sign of breast cancer, peau d'orange (orange peel skin) is the edematous thickening and pitting of breast skin. This slowly developing sign can also occur with breast or axillary lymph node infection, erysipelas, or Graves' disease. Its striking orange peel appearance stems from lymphatic edema around deepened hair follicles. (See *Recognizing peau d'orange,* page 502.)

HISTORY

Ask the patient when she first detected peau d'orange. Has she noticed any lumps, pain, or other breast changes? Does she have related signs and symptoms, such as malaise, achiness, and weight loss? Is she lactating, or has she recently weaned her infant? Has she had previous axillary surgery that might have impaired lymphatic drainage of a breast?

PHYSICAL ASSESSMENT

In a well-lit examining room, observe the patient's breasts. Estimate the extent of the peau d'orange, and check for erythema. Assess the nipples for discharge, deviation, retraction, dimpling, and cracking. Gently palpate the area of peau d'orange, noting warmth or induration. Then palpate the entire breast, noting any fixed or mobile lumps, and the axillary lymph nodes, noting enlargement. Finally, take the patient's temperature.

MEDICAL CAUSES

Breast abscess

Usually affecting lactating women with milk stasis, breast abscess is an infectious disorder that causes peau d'orange, malaise, breast tenderness and erythema, and a sudden fever that may be accompanied by shaking chills. A cracked nipple may produce a purulent discharge, and an indurated or palpable soft mass may be present.

Special considerations
+ Monitor neurologic status.
+ Help patient perform daily activities as necessary.
+ If sensory deficits are present, protect patient from injury.

Peds points
+ Children usually can't describe this symptom.
+ Hereditary polyneuropathies are first recognized in childhood.

Teaching points
+ Safety measures

Key facts about peau d'orange
+ Edematous thickening and pitting of breast skin that's usually a late sign of breast cancer

Key history points
+ Date of onset
+ Lumps, pain, or other changes
+ Lactation history
+ History of axillary surgery

Critical assessment steps
+ Estimate extent of peau d'orange; check for erythema and induration.
+ Assess nipples for discharge, deviation, retraction, dimpling, and cracking.
+ Palpate breast for lumps.
+ Palpate axillary lymph nodes, noting enlargement.

Medical causes
Breast abscess
+ Peau d'orange is accomanied by malaise, breast tenderness and erythema, and a sudden fever.

Recognizing peau d'orange

In peau d'orange, the skin appears to be pitted (as shown at right). This condition usually indicates late-stage breast cancer.

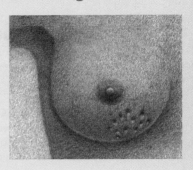

Medical causes
(continued)

Breast cancer
✦ Peau d'orange usually begins in the dependent part of the breast or the areola.
✦ Palpation typically reveals a firm, immobile mass that adheres to the skin above the area of peau d'orange.

Erysipelas
✦ A well-demarcated, erythematous, elevated area, typically with a peau d'orange texture, occurs.

Graves' disease
✦ Raised, thickened, hyperpigmented, peau d'orange–like areas that coalesce may occur.

Special considerations
✦ Once cancer is ruled out, treat the underlying disorder.

Teaching points
✦ Diagnostic tests

Breast cancer

Advanced breast cancer is the most likely cause of peau d'orange, which usually begins in the dependent part of the breast or the areola. Palpation typically reveals a firm, immobile mass that adheres to the skin above the area of peau d'orange. Inspection of the breasts may reveal changes in contour, size, or symmetry. Inspection of the nipples may reveal deviation, erosion, retraction, and a thin and watery, bloody, or purulent discharge. The patient may report a burning and itching sensation in the nipples as well as a sensation of warmth or heat in the breast. Breast pain may occur, but it isn't a reliable indicator of cancer.

Erysipelas

Erysipelas, a streptococcal infection, causes a well-demarcated, erythematous, elevated area, typically with a peau d'orange texture. Pain, warmth, and generalized signs and symptoms, such as fever and fatigue, also occur.

Graves' disease

Patients with Graves' disease (a thyroid disorder) may exhibit raised, thickened, hyperpigmented, peau d'orange–like areas that tend to coalesce. Other common signs and symptoms of hyperthyroidism include weight loss, palpitations, anxiety, heat intolerance, tremor, and amenorrhea.

SPECIAL CONSIDERATIONS

Prepare the patient for diagnostic tests, such as mammography, thermography, cytology of nipple discharge, and needle or open biopsy. If cancer is ruled out, treat the underlying disorder. For example, administer antibiotics to treat infectious causes.

PATIENT COUNSELING

Because peau d'orange usually signals advanced breast cancer, provide emotional support for the patient. Encourage her to express her fears and concerns. Clearly explain expected diagnostic tests, such as mammography and breast biopsy.

PERICARDIAL FRICTION RUB

Commonly transient, a pericardial friction rub is a scratching, grating, or crunching sound that occurs when two inflamed layers of the pericardium slide over each other. Ranging from faint to loud, this abnormal sound is best heard along the lower left sternal border during deep inspiration. (See *Comparing auscultation findings.*) It indicates pericarditis, which can result from acute infection, a cardiac or renal disorder, postpericardiotomy syndrome, or the use of certain drugs.

Occasionally, a pericardial friction rub can resemble a murmur (see *Pericardial friction rub or murmur?* page 504) or a pleural friction rub. However, the classic pericardial friction rub has three components. (See *Understanding pericardial friction rubs,* page 505.)

HISTORY

Obtain a complete medical history, noting especially cardiac dysfunction. Has the patient recently had a myocardial infarction or cardiac surgery? Has he ever had pericarditis or rheumatic disorder, such as rheumatoid arthritis or systemic lupus erythematosus? Does he have chronic renal failure or an infection? If the patient

ASSESSMENT TIP

Comparing auscultation findings

During auscultation, you may detect a pleural friction rub, crackles, or a pericardial friction rub — three abnormal sounds that are commonly confused. Use this chart to help clarify auscultation findings.

FINDING	CAUSE	QUALITY	LOCATION	TIMING
Pleural friction rub	Inflamed visceral and parietal pleural surfaces rub against each other.	Loud and grating, creaking, or squeaking	Best heard over the low axilla or the anterior, lateral, or posterior base of the lung	Occurs in late inspiration and early expiration but ceases when the patient holds his breath; persists during coughing
Crackles	Air suddenly enters fluid-filled airways.	Nonmusical clicking or rattling	Best heard at less distended and more dependent areas of the lungs, usually at the bases	Occurs chiefly during inspiration
Pericardial friction rub	Inflamed layers of the pericardium rub against each other.	Hard and grating, scratching, or crunching	Best heard along the lower left sternal border	Occurs in relation to heartbeat; most noticeable during deep inspiration and continues even when the patient holds his breath

Key facts about pericardial friction rub

✦ Occurs when two inflamed layers of the pericardium slide over each other, making a scratching, grating, or crunching sound
✦ Ranges from faint to loud
✦ Best heard along the lower left sternal border during deep inspiration

Key history points

✦ Complete medical history, noting cardiac dysfunction
✦ Recent MI or cardiac surgery
✦ History of pericarditis, rheumatoid arthritis, or SLE
✦ Chronic renal failure or an infection
✦ Description of chest pain

Guide to auscultation findings

✦ Pleural friction rub — loud and grating, creaking, or squeaking
✦ Crackles — nonmusical clicking or rattling
✦ Pericardial friction rub — hard and grating, scratching, or crunching

Pericardial friction rub or murmur?

Is the sound you hear a pericardial friction rub or a murmur? Here's how to tell. The classic pericardial friction rub has three sound components, which are related to the phases of the cardiac cycle. In some patients, however, the rub's presystolic and early diastolic sounds may be inaudible, causing the rub to resemble the murmur of mitral insufficiency or aortic stenosis and regurgitation.

If you don't detect the classic three-component sound, you can distinguish a pericardial friction rub from a murmur by auscultating again and asking yourself these questions:

HOW DEEP IS THE SOUND?
A pericardial friction rub usually sounds superficial; a murmur sounds deeper in the chest.

DOES THE SOUND RADIATE?
A pericardial friction rub usually doesn't radiate; a murmur may radiate widely.

DOES THE SOUND VARY WITH INSPIRATION OR CHANGES IN PATIENT POSITION?
A pericardial friction rub is usually loudest during inspiration and is best heard when the patient leans forward. A murmur varies in timing and duration with both factors.

Critical assessment steps

✦ Take the patient's vital signs, noting hypotension, tachycardia, irregular pulse, tachypnea, and fever.
✦ Inspect for jugular vein distention, edema, ascites, and hepatomegaly.
✦ Auscultate the lungs for crackles.

Medical causes

Pericarditis
✦ Pericardial friction rub is accompanied by sharp precordial or retrosternal pain that usually radiates to the left shoulder, neck, and back.
✦ Pain worsens with deep breathing, coughing, and lying flat.
✦ Pain lessens when patient sits up and leans forward.

Other causes

✦ Procainamide
✦ Chemotherapeutic drugs

Special considerations

✦ Monitor the patient's cardiovascular status.
✦ If the pericardial friction rub disappears, be alert for signs of cardiac tamponade.
✦ Ensure that the patient gets adequate rest.

complains of chest pain, ask him to describe its character and location. What relieves the pain? What worsens it?

PHYSICAL ASSESSMENT

Take the patient's vital signs, noting especially hypotension, tachycardia, irregular pulse, tachypnea, and fever. Inspect for jugular vein distention, edema, ascites, and hepatomegaly. Auscultate the lungs for crackles.

MEDICAL CAUSES

Pericarditis
A pericardial friction rub is the hallmark of acute pericarditis. This disorder also causes sharp precordial or retrosternal pain that usually radiates to the left shoulder, neck, and back. The pain worsens when the patient breathes deeply, coughs, or lies flat and, possibly, when he swallows. It abates when he sits up and leans forward. The patient may also develop fever, dyspnea, tachycardia, and arrhythmias.

With chronic constrictive pericarditis, a pericardial friction rub develops gradually and is accompanied by signs of decreased cardiac filling and output, such as peripheral edema, ascites, jugular vein distention on inspiration (Kussmaul's sign), and hepatomegaly. Dyspnea, orthopnea, paradoxical pulse, and chest pain may also occur.

OTHER CAUSES

Drugs
Procainamide and chemotherapeutic drugs can cause pericarditis.

SPECIAL CONSIDERATIONS

Continue to monitor the patient's cardiovascular status. If the pericardial friction rub disappears, be alert for signs of cardiac tamponade: pallor, hypotension, tachycardia, tachypnea, paradoxical pulse, increased jugular vein distention, and cool,

ASSESSMENT TIP

Understanding pericardial friction rubs

The complete, or classic, pericardial friction rub is triphasic. Its three sound components are linked to phases of the cardiac cycle. The *presystolic* component (A) reflects atrial systole and precedes the first heart sound (S_1). The *systolic* component (B) — usually the loudest — reflects ventricular systole and occurs between the S_1 and the second heart sound (S_2). The early diastolic component (C) reflects ventricular diastole and follows the S_2.

Sometimes, the early diastolic component merges with the presystolic component, producing a diphasic to-and-fro sound on auscultation. In other patients, auscultation may detect only one component — a monophasic rub, typically during ventricular systole.

TRIPHASIC RUB

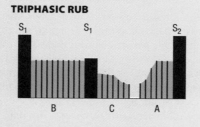

DIPHASIC RUB

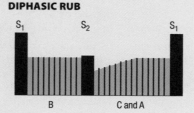

MONOPHASIC RUB

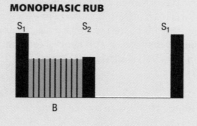

clammy skin. If these signs occur, prepare the patient for pericardiocentesis to prevent cardiovascular collapse.

Ensure that the patient gets adequate rest. Give an anti-inflammatory, antiarrhythmic, diuretic, or antimicrobial to treat the underlying cause. If necessary, prepare him for a pericardiectomy to promote adequate cardiac filling and contraction.

PEDIATRIC POINTERS

Bacterial pericarditis may develop during the first 2 decades of life, usually before age 6. Although a pericardial friction rub may occur, other signs and symptoms — such as fever, tachycardia, dyspnea, chest pain, jugular vein distention, and hepatomegaly — more reliably indicate this life-threatening disorder. A pericardial friction rub may also occur after surgery to correct congenital cardiac anomalies. However, it usually vanishes without development of pericarditis.

PATIENT COUNSELING

Explain the underlying disorder and its treatments to the patient. Encourage the patient to sit upright to relieve dyspnea and chest pain. To promote comfort and

Peds points

✦ A pericardial friction rub may develop with bacterial pericarditis, a life-threatening condition that usually occurs before age 6.
✦ A pericardial friction rub may occur after surgery to correct congenital cardiac anomalies.

Teaching points

✦ The underlying disorder and its treatments
✦ Pain-relief measures

ease anxiety, reassure the patient with acute pericarditis that his condition is temporary.

PERISTALTIC WAVES, VISIBLE

With intestinal obstruction, peristalsis temporarily increases in strength and frequency as the intestine contracts to force its contents past the obstruction. As a result, visible peristaltic waves may roll across the abdomen. Typically, these waves appear suddenly and vanish quickly, because increased peristalsis overcomes the obstruction or the GI tract becomes atonic. Peristaltic waves are best detected by stooping at the patient's side and inspecting his abdominal contour while he's in a supine position.

Visible peristaltic waves may also reflect normal stomach and intestinal contractions in thin patients or in malnourished patients with abdominal muscle atrophy.

HISTORY

After observing peristaltic waves, collect pertinent history data. For example, ask about a history of pyloric ulcer, stomach cancer, or chronic gastritis, which can lead to pyloric obstruction. Also ask about conditions leading to intestinal obstruction, such as intestinal tumors or polyps, gallstones, chronic constipation, and a hernia. Has the patient had recent abdominal surgery? Be sure to obtain a drug history.

Determine if the patient has related symptoms. Spasmodic abdominal pain, for example, accompanies small-bowel obstruction, whereas colicky pain accompanies pyloric obstruction. Is the patient experiencing nausea and vomiting? If he has vomited, ask about the consistency, amount, and color of the vomitus. Lumpy vomitus may contain undigested food particles; green or brown vomitus may contain bile or fecal matter.

PHYSICAL ASSESSMENT

With the patient in a supine position, inspect the abdomen for distention, surgical scars and adhesions, or visible loops of bowel. Auscultate for bowel sounds, noting high-pitched, tinkling sounds. Then jar the patient's bed (or roll the patient from side to side) and auscultate for a succussion splash—a splashing sound in the stomach from retained secretions caused by pyloric obstruction. Palpate the abdomen for rigidity and tenderness, and percuss for tympany. Check the skin and mucous membranes for dryness and poor skin turgor, indicating dehydration. Take the patient's vital signs, noting especially tachycardia and hypotension, which indicate hypovolemia.

MEDICAL CAUSES

Large-bowel obstruction

Visible peristaltic waves in the upper abdomen are an early sign of large-bowel obstruction. Obstipation, however, may be the earliest finding. Other characteristic signs and symptoms develop more slowly than in small-bowel obstruction. These include nausea, colicky abdominal pain (milder than in small-bowel obstruction), gradual and eventually marked abdominal distention, and hyperactive bowel sounds.

Pyloric obstruction

Peristaltic waves may be detected in a swollen epigastrium or in the left upper quadrant, usually beginning near the left rib margin and rolling from left to right.

Key facts about visible peristaltic waves

+ Occur when peristalsis increases in strength and frequency as the intestine contracts to force its contents past an obstruction
+ Consist of waves that appear suddenly and vanish quickly

Key history points

+ History of pyloric ulcer, stomach cancer, chronic gastritis, or intestinal obstruction
+ Recent abdominal surgery
+ Drug history

Critical assessment steps

+ Inspect the abdomen for distention, surgical scars, adhesions, or visible bowel loops.
+ Auscultate for bowel sounds and a succussion splash.
+ Palpate abdomen for rigidity and tenderness, and percuss for tympany.
+ Check skin and mucous membranes for dryness and poor skin turgor.

Medical causes

Large-bowel obstruction
+ Visible peristaltic waves in the upper abdomen are an early sign.

Pyloric obstruction
+ Peristaltic waves may be detected in a swollen epigastrium or in the left upper quadrant, usually beginning near the left rib margin and rolling from left to right.
+ Auscultation reveals a loud succussion splash.

Related findings include vague epigastric discomfort or colicky pain after eating, nausea, vomiting, anorexia, and weight loss. Auscultation reveals a loud succussion splash.

Small-bowel obstruction

Early signs of mechanical obstruction of the small bowel include peristaltic waves rolling across the upper abdomen and intermittent, cramping periumbilical pain. Associated signs and symptoms include nausea, vomiting of bilious or, later, fecal material, and constipation; in partial obstruction, diarrhea may occur. Hyperactive bowel sounds and slight abdominal distention also occur early.

SPECIAL CONSIDERATIONS

Because visible peristaltic waves are an early sign of intestinal obstruction, monitor the patient's status and prepare him for diagnostic evaluation and treatment. Withhold food and fluids, and explain the purpose and procedure of abdominal X-rays and barium studies, which can confirm obstruction.

If tests confirm obstruction, nasogastric suctioning may be performed to decompress the stomach and small bowel. Provide frequent oral hygiene, and watch for a thick, swollen tongue and dry mucous membranes, indicating dehydration. Frequently monitor vital signs and intake and output.

PEDIATRIC POINTERS

In infants, visible peristaltic waves may indicate pyloric stenosis. In small children, peristaltic waves may be visible normally because of the protuberant abdomen, or visible waves may indicate bowel obstruction stemming from congenital anomalies, volvulus, or the swallowing of a foreign body.

GERIATRIC POINTERS

In elderly patients who present with visible peristaltic waves, always check for fecal impaction, which is a common problem among those of this age-group. Also, obtain a detailed drug history; antidepressants and antipsychotics can predispose patients to constipation and bowel obstruction.

PATIENT COUNSELING

Advise patients suffering from chronic constipation and those taking an antidepressant or antipsychotic to increase their fluid intake and eat foods high in fiber, such as cereals, fruits, and vegetables. If no improvement occurs, administer a stool softener to prevent further complications such as bowel obstruction.

PHOTOPHOBIA

A common symptom, photophobia is an abnormal sensitivity to light. In many patients, photophobia simply indicates increased eye sensitivity without any underlying pathology. For example, it can stem from excessive wearing of contact lenses or use of poorly fitted lenses. However, in others, this symptom can result from a systemic disorder, an ocular disorder or trauma, or the use of certain drugs.

HISTORY

If your patient reports photophobia, find out when it began and how severe it is. Did it follow eye trauma, a chemical splash, or exposure to the rays of a sun lamp?

Medical causes

Small-bowel obstruction
- Peristaltic waves rolling across the upper abdomen and intermittent, cramping, periumbilical pain are early signs.

Special considerations
- Withhold food and fluids.
- Provide frequent oral hygiene.
- Frequently monitor vital signs and intake and output.

Peds points
- In infants, visible peristaltic waves may indicate pyloric stenosis.
- In small children, peristaltic waves may be visible normally or may indicate bowel obstruction.

Geri points
- Check for fecal impaction.
- Obtain detailed drug history.

Teaching points
- Diet and fluid requirements
- Stool softener

Key facts about photophobia
- Abnormal sensitivity to light
- Commonly indicates increased eye sensitivity without any underlying pathology
- May indicate a systemic disorder, an ocular disorder or trauma, or the use of certain drugs

Key history points
- Onset and severity
- Recent eye trauma, chemical splash, or exposure to rays of sun lamp
- Description of pain or discomfort

**Critical
assessment steps**

- Assess neurologic status.
- Assess visual activity, unless the cause is a chemical burn.
- Inspect the eyes' external structures and examine the conjunctivae.
- Characterize the amount and consistency of any discharge.
- Check pupillary reaction to light.

Medical causes

Burns
- Photophobia and eye pain may be accompanied by erythema and blistering on the face and lids, miosis, diffuse conjunctival injection, and corneal changes.

Conjunctivitis
- Photophobia occurs when conjunctivitis affects the cornea.

Corneal abrasion
- Photophobia is usually accompanied by excessive tearing, conjunctival injection, visible corneal damage, and foreign-body sensation in the eye.

Corneal foreign body
- Photophobia may occur with miosis, intense eye pain, foreign-body sensation, slightly impaired vision, conjunctival injection, and profuse tearing.

Corneal ulcer
- Severe photophobia and eye pain are aggravated by blinking.
- Impaired visual acuity, blurring, eye discharge, and sticky eyelids may also occur.

If photophobia results from trauma, avoid manipulating the eyes. Ask the patient about eye pain, and have him describe its location, duration, and intensity. Does he have a sensation of a foreign body in his eye? Does he have any other signs and symptoms, such as increased tearing and vision changes?

PHYSICAL ASSESSMENT

Take the patient's vital signs and assess neurologic status. Assess visual activity, unless the cause is a chemical burn. Follow this with a careful eye examination, inspecting the eyes' external structures for abnormalities. Examine the conjunctiva and sclera, noting their color. Characterize the amount and consistency of any discharge. Then check pupillary reaction to light. Evaluate extraocular muscle function by testing the six cardinal positions of gaze, and test visual acuity in both eyes. (See *Testing the six cardinal positions of gaze,* page 464.)

During your assessment, keep in mind that although photophobia can accompany life-threatening meningitis, it isn't a cardinal sign of meningeal irritation.

MEDICAL CAUSES

Burns
With a chemical burn, photophobia and eye pain may be accompanied by erythema and blistering on the face and lids, miosis, diffuse conjunctival injection, and corneal changes. The patient experiences blurred vision and may be unable to keep his eyes open. With an ultraviolet radiation burn, photophobia occurs with moderate to severe eye pain. These symptoms develop about 12 hours after exposure to the rays of a welding arc or sun lamp.

Conjunctivitis
When conjunctivitis affects the cornea, it causes photophobia. Other common findings include conjunctival injection, increased tearing, a foreign-body sensation, a feeling of fullness around the eyes, and eye pain, burning, and itching. Allergic conjunctivitis is distinguished by a stringy eye discharge and milky red injection. Bacterial conjunctivitis tends to cause brilliant red conjunctiva as well as a copious, mucopurulent, flaky eye discharge that may make the eyelids stick together. Fungal conjunctivitis produces a thick, purulent discharge; extreme redness; and crusting, sticky eyelids. Viral conjunctivitis causes copious tearing with little discharge as well as enlargement of the preauricular lymph nodes.

Corneal abrasion
A common finding with corneal abrasion, photophobia is usually accompanied by excessive tearing, conjunctival injection, visible corneal damage, and a foreign-body sensation in the eye. Blurred vision and eye pain may also occur.

Corneal foreign body
Photophobia may occur with miosis, intense eye pain, a foreign-body sensation, slightly impaired vision, conjunctival injection, and profuse tearing. A dark speck may be visible on the cornea.

Corneal ulcer
A corneal ulcer, a vision-threatening disorder, causes severe photophobia and eye pain that's aggravated by blinking. Impaired visual acuity may accompany blurring, eye discharge, and sticky eyelids. Conjunctival injection may occur even though the cornea appears white and opaque. A bacterial ulcer may also cause an irregularly shaped corneal ulcer and unilateral pupillary constriction. A fungal ulcer may be surrounded by progressively clearer rings.

Dry eye syndrome

Although dry eye syndrome may produce photophobia, it more characteristically causes eye pain, conjunctival injection, a foreign-body sensation, itching, excessive mucus secretion and, possibly, decreased tearing and difficulty moving the eyelids.

Iritis (acute)

Severe photophobia may result from acute iritis, along with marked conjunctival injection, moderate to severe eye pain, and blurred vision. The pupil may be constricted and may respond poorly to light.

Keratitis (interstitial)

Interstitial keratitis is a corneal inflammation that causes photophobia, eye pain, blurred vision, dramatic conjunctival injection, and grayish pink corneas.

Meningitis (acute bacterial)

A common symptom of acute bacterial meningitis, photophobia may occur with such other signs of meningeal irritation as nuchal rigidity, hyperreflexia, and opisthotonos. Brudzinski's and Kernig's signs can be elicited. Fever, an early finding, may be accompanied by chills. Related signs and symptoms may include headache, vomiting, ocular palsies, facial weakness, pupillary abnormalities, and hearing loss. With severe meningitis, seizures may occur along with stupor progressing to coma.

Migraine headache

Photophobia and noise sensitivity are prominent features of a common migraine headache. Typically severe, this aching or throbbing headache may also cause fatigue, blurred vision, nausea, and vomiting.

Uveitis

Both anterior and posterior uveitis can cause photophobia. Typically, anterior uveitis also produces moderate to severe eye pain, severe conjunctival injection, and a small, nonreactive pupil. Posterior uveitis develops slowly, causing visual floaters, eye pain, pupil distortion, conjunctival injection, and blurred vision.

OTHER CAUSES

Drugs

Mydriatics—such as phenylephrine, atropine, scopolamine, cyclopentolate, and tropicamide—can cause photophobia due to ocular dilation. Amphetamines, cocaine, and ophthalmic antifungals—such as trifluridine, vidarabine, and idoxuridine—can also cause photophobia.

SPECIAL CONSIDERATIONS

Promote the patient's comfort by darkening the room and telling him to close both eyes. Administer corticosteroids and antibiotic drops or ointment, as indicated. Take measures to treat the underlying disorder, if it can be identified. Saline eyedrops or other lubricating ointment can soothe dry eyes and may improve photophobia.

PEDIATRIC POINTERS

Suspect photophobia in any child who squints, rubs his eyes frequently, or wears sunglasses indoors and outside. Congenital disorders, such as albinism, and childhood diseases, such as measles and rubella, can cause photophobia.

Medical causes
(continued)

Dry eye syndrome
+ Photophobia may occur, but eye pain, conjunctival injection, a foreign-body sensation, itching, and excessive mucus secretion are more common symptoms.

Iritis (acute)
+ Severe photophobia occurs, along with conjunctival injection, eye pain, and blurred vision.

Keratitis (interstitial)
+ Photophobia occurs along with eye pain, blurred vision, dramatic conjunctival injection, and grayish pink corneas.

Meningitis (acute bacterial)
+ Photophobia occurs with such signs as nuchal rigidity, hyperreflexia, and opisthotonos.

Migraine headache
+ Photophobia and noise sensitivity are prominent features.

Uveitis
+ Photophobia results from both anterior and posterior uveitis.

Other causes
+ Mydriatics, amphetamines, cocaine, and ophthalmic antifungals

Special considerations
+ Darken the room and tell the patient to close his eyes.

Peds points
+ Suspect photophobia in a child who squints, rubs eyes frequently, or wears sunglasses indoors and outside.

Teaching points
+ Protection from light
+ Diagnostic tests

Key facts about pleural friction rub
+ Loud, coarse, grating, creaking, or squeaking sound that may be auscultated during late inspiration or early expiration
+ Indicates inflammation of the visceral and parietal pleural lining

In an emergency
+ Quickly look for signs of respiratory distress.
+ Check for hypotension, tachycardia, and decreased LOC.

If you detect signs of distress:
+ Open and maintain an airway.
+ Insert a large-bore I.V. line.
+ Elevate the patient's head 30 degrees.
+ Monitor cardiac status constantly, and check vital signs frequently.

Key history points
+ Description of chest pain
+ Activities that worsen or alleviate pain
+ Medical and smoking history

Critical assessment steps
+ Auscultate the lungs with the patient sitting upright.
+ Determine whether the friction rub is unilateral or bilateral.
+ Listen for absent or diminished breath sounds.
+ Palpate for decreased chest motion and percuss for flatness or dullness.

PATIENT COUNSELING
If photophobia persists at home, suggest that the patient wear dark glasses. Prepare the patient for diagnostic tests, such as corneal scraping and slit-lamp examination.

PLEURAL FRICTION RUB

Commonly resulting from a pulmonary disorder or trauma, this loud, coarse, grating, creaking, or squeaking sound may be auscultated over one or both lungs during late inspiration or early expiration. It's heard best over the low axilla or the anterior, lateral, or posterior bases of the lung fields with the patient upright. Sometimes intermittent, it may resemble crackles or a pericardial friction rub. (See *Comparing auscultation findings*, page 503.)

A pleural friction rub indicates inflammation of the visceral and parietal pleural lining, which causes congestion and edema. The resultant fibrinous exudate covers both pleural surfaces, displacing the fluid that's normally between them and causing the surfaces to rub together.

 EMERGENCY ACTIONS When you detect a pleural friction rub, quickly look for signs of respiratory distress: shallow or decreased respirations; crowing, wheezing, or stridor; dyspnea; increased accessory muscle use; intercostal or suprasternal retractions; cyanosis; and nasal flaring. Check for hypotension, tachycardia, and a decreased level of consciousness (LOC).

If you detect signs of distress, open and maintain an airway. Endotracheal intubation and supplemental oxygen may be necessary. Insert a large-bore I.V. line to deliver drugs and fluids. Elevate the patient's head 30 degrees. Monitor cardiac status constantly, and check vital signs frequently.

HISTORY
If the patient isn't in severe distress, explore related symptoms. Find out if he has had chest pain. If so, ask him to describe its location and severity. How long does his chest pain last? Does the pain radiate to his shoulder, neck, or upper abdomen? Does the pain worsen with breathing, movement, coughing, or sneezing? Does the pain abate if he splints his chest, holds his breath, or exerts pressure or lies on the affected side?

 CULTURAL CUE *Because pain is subjective and is exacerbated by anxiety, patients who are highly emotional may complain more readily of pleuritic pain than those who are habitually stoic about symptoms of illness.*

Ask the patient about a history of rheumatoid arthritis, a respiratory or cardiovascular disorder, recent trauma, asbestos exposure, or radiation therapy. If he smokes, obtain a history in pack-years.

PHYSICAL ASSESSMENT
Characterize the pleural friction rub by auscultating the lungs with the patient sitting upright and breathing deeply and slowly through his mouth. Is the friction rub unilateral or bilateral? Also, listen for absent or diminished breath sounds, noting their location and timing in the respiratory cycle. Do abnormal breath sounds clear with coughing? Observe the patient for clubbing and pedal edema, which may indicate a chronic disorder. Then palpate for decreased chest motion and percuss for flatness or dullness.

MEDICAL CAUSES

Asbestosis
Besides a pleural friction rub, asbestosis may cause exertional dyspnea, cough, chest pain, and crackles. Clubbing is a late sign. As the disease advances, dyspnea eventually occurs — even at rest.

Lung cancer
A pleural friction rub may be heard in the area of the lung that's affected by the cancer. Other effects include a cough (with possible hemoptysis), dyspnea, chest pain, weight loss, anorexia, fatigue, clubbing, fever, and wheezing.

Pleurisy
A pleural friction rub occurs early in pleurisy. However, the cardinal symptom is sudden, intense chest pain that's usually unilateral and located in the lower and lateral parts of the chest. Deep breathing, coughing, or thoracic movement aggravates the pain. Decreased breath sounds and inspiratory crackles may be heard over the painful area. Other findings include dyspnea, tachypnea, tachycardia, cyanosis, fever, and fatigue.

Pneumonia (bacterial)
A pleural friction rub occurs with bacterial pneumonia, which usually starts with a dry, painful, hacking cough that rapidly becomes productive. Related effects develop suddenly; these include shaking chills, high fever, headache, dyspnea, pleuritic chest pain, tachypnea, tachycardia, grunting respirations, nasal flaring, dullness to percussion, and cyanosis. Auscultation reveals decreased breath sounds and fine crackles.

Pulmonary embolism
A pulmonary embolism can cause a pleural friction rub over the affected area of the lung. Usually, the first symptom is sudden dyspnea, which may be accompanied by angina or unilateral pleuritic chest pain. Other clinical features include a nonproductive cough or a cough that produces blood-tinged sputum, tachycardia, tachypnea, low-grade fever, restlessness, and diaphoresis. Less common findings include massive hemoptysis, chest splinting, leg edema and — with a large embolus — cyanosis, syncope, and jugular vein distention. Crackles, diffuse wheezing, decreased breath sounds, and signs of circulatory collapse may also occur.

Rheumatoid arthritis
Rheumatoid arthritis occasionally causes a unilateral pleural friction rub, but more typical early findings include fatigue, persistent low-grade fever, weight loss, and vague arthralgia and myalgia. Later findings include warm, swollen, painful joints; joint stiffness after inactivity; subcutaneous nodules on the elbows; joint deformity; and muscle weakness and atrophy.

Systemic lupus erythematosus
Pulmonary involvement in systemic lupus erythematosus (SLE) can cause a pleural friction rub, hemoptysis, dyspnea, pleuritic chest pain, and crackles. More characteristic effects include a "butterfly rash," nondeforming joint pain and stiffness, and photosensitivity. Fever, anorexia, weight loss, and lymphadenopathy may also occur.

Medical causes

Asbestosis
+ Pleural friction rub may develop along with exertional dyspnea, cough, chest pain, and crackles.

Lung cancer
+ A pleural friction rub may be heard in the area of the lung that's affected by the cancer.

Pleurisy
+ A pleural friction rub occurs early in pleurisy.
+ The cardinal symptom is sudden, intense, unilateral chest pain located in the lower and lateral parts of the chest.

Pneumonia (bacterial)
+ A pleural friction rub occurs following a dry, painful, hacking, productive cough.

Pulmonary embolism
+ A pleural friction rub may occur over the affected area of the lung.
+ The first symptom is usually sudden dyspnea, which may be accompanied by angina or unilateral pleuritic chest pain.

Rheumatoid arthritis
+ A unilateral pleural friction rub may occur.
+ More typical early findings include fatigue, persistent low-grade fever, weight loss, and vague arthralgia and myalgia.

SLE
+ A pleural friction rub, accompanied by hemoptysis, dyspnea, pleuritic chest pain, and crackles, may occur with pulmonary involvement.

Medical causes
(continued)

Tuberculosis (pulmonary)
+ A pleural friction rub may occur over the affected part of the lung.

Other causes
+ Thoracic surgery
+ Radiation therapy

Special considerations
+ Monitor the patient's respiratory status and vital signs.
+ Administer an antitussive.
+ Administer oxygen and an antibiotic.

Peds points
+ Auscultate for a pleural friction rub in a child who has grunting respirations, reports chest pain, or protects his chest.

Geri points
+ Pleuritic chest pain may mimic cardiac chest pain.

Teaching points
+ Splinting maneuvers
+ Other pain relief measure

Key facts about polydipsia
+ May reflect decreased fluid intake, increased urine output, or excessive loss of water and salt

Key history points
+ Average fluid intake and output
+ Personal or family history of diabetes or kidney disease
+ Drug history

Tuberculosis (pulmonary)

With pulmonary tuberculosis, a pleural friction rub may occur over the affected part of the lung. Early signs and symptoms include weight loss, night sweats, low-grade fever in the afternoon, malaise, dyspnea, anorexia, and easy fatigability. Progression of the disorder usually produces pleuritic pain, fine crackles over the upper lobes, and a productive cough with blood-streaked sputum. Advanced tuberculosis can cause chest retraction, tracheal deviation, and dullness to percussion.

OTHER CAUSES

Treatments

Thoracic surgery and radiation therapy can cause pleural friction rub.

SPECIAL CONSIDERATIONS

Continue to monitor the patient's respiratory status and vital signs. If the patient's persistent dry, hacking cough tires him, administer an antitussive. (Avoid giving an opioid, which can further depress respirations.) Administer oxygen and an antibiotic. Prepare the patient for diagnostic tests such as chest X-rays.

PEDIATRIC POINTERS

Auscultate for a pleural friction rub in a child who has grunting respirations, reports chest pain, or protects his chest by holding it or lying on one side. A pleural friction rub in a child is usually an early sign of pleurisy.

GERIATRIC POINTERS

In elderly patients, the intensity of pleuritic chest pain may mimic that of cardiac chest pain.

PATIENT COUNSELING

Because pleuritic pain commonly accompanies a pleural friction rub, teach the patient splinting maneuvers to increase his comfort. Also, apply a heating pad over the affected area, and administer an analgesic for pain relief. Although coughing may be painful, instruct the patient not to suppress it because coughing and deep breathing help prevent respiratory complications. Inform the patient that the pain associated with a pleural friction rub may persist even after the cause of the rub has been resolved.

POLYDIPSIA

Polydipsia refers to excessive thirst, a common symptom associated with endocrine disorders and certain drugs. It may reflect decreased fluid intake, increased urine output, or excessive loss of water and salt.

HISTORY

Obtain a history. Find out how much fluid the patient drinks each day. How often and how much does he typically urinate? Does the need to urinate awaken him at night? Determine if he or anyone in his family has diabetes or kidney disease. What medications does he use? Has his lifestyle changed recently? If so, have these changes upset him?

PHYSICAL ASSESSMENT

If the patient has polydipsia, take his blood pressure and pulse when he's in supine and standing positions. A decrease of 10 mm Hg in systolic pressure and a pulse rate increase of 10 beats/minute from the supine to the sitting or standing position may indicate hypovolemia. If you detect these changes, ask the patient about recent weight loss. Check for signs of dehydration, such as dry mucous membranes and decreased skin turgor. Infuse I.V. replacement fluids as needed.

MEDICAL CAUSES

Diabetes insipidus

Diabetes insipidus characteristically produces polydipsia and may also cause excessive voiding of dilute urine and mild to moderate nocturia. Fatigue and signs of dehydration occur in severe cases.

Diabetes mellitus

Polydipsia is a classic finding with diabetes mellitus — a consequence of the hyperosmolar state. Other characteristic findings include polyuria, polyphagia, nocturia, weakness, fatigue, and weight loss. Signs of dehydration may occur. (See *Associated disorder: Diabetes mellitus,* page 514.)

 CULTURAL CUE *Diabetes is the fourth leading cause of death in Black, Native American, Hawaiian, and Filipino women. Also, Blacks are at greater risk for developing diabetes than Whites.*

Hypercalcemia

As hypercalcemia progresses, the patient develops polydipsia, polyuria, nocturia, constipation, paresthesia and, occasionally, hematuria and pyuria. Severe hypercalcemia can progress quickly to vomiting, decreased level of consciousness, and renal failure. Depression, mental lassitude, and increased sleep requirements are common.

Hypokalemia

An electrolyte imbalance — hypokalemia — can cause nephropathy, resulting in polydipsia, polyuria, and nocturia. Related hypokalemic signs and symptoms include muscle weakness or paralysis, fatigue, decreased bowel sounds, hypoactive deep tendon reflexes, and arrhythmias.

Renal disorders (chronic)

Chronic renal disorders, such as glomerulonephritis and pyelonephritis, damage the kidneys, causing polydipsia and polyuria. Associated signs and symptoms include nocturia, weakness, elevated blood pressure, pallor and, in later stages, oliguria.

Sickle cell anemia

As nephropathy develops in patients with sickle cell anemia, polydipsia and polyuria occur. They may be accompanied by abdominal pain and cramps, arthralgia and, occasionally, lower extremity skin ulcers and such bone deformities as kyphosis and scoliosis.

OTHER CAUSES

Drugs

Diuretics and demeclocycline may produce polydipsia. Phenothiazines and anticholinergics can cause dry mouth, making the patient so thirsty that he drinks compulsively.

Critical assessment steps

+ Obtain the patient's blood pressure and pulse when he's in supine and standing positions.
+ Check for signs of dehydration.

Medical causes

Diabetes insipidus
+ Polydipsia, excessive voiding, dilute urine, and nocturia are signs of diabetes insipidus.

Diabetes mellitus
+ Polydipsia is a classic finding with diabetes mellitus.
+ Polyuria, polyphagia, and nocturia may also occur.

Hypercalcemia
+ In later stages, polydipsia occurs with polyuria, nocturia, constipation, paresthesia and, occasionally, hematuria and pyuria.

Hypokalemia
+ Neuropathy from electrolyte imbalance can cause polydipsia, polyuria, and nocturia.

Renal disorders (chronic)
+ Polydipsia and polyuria signal kidney damage from chronic renal disorders.

Sickle cell anemia
+ Polydipsia and polyuria occur as nephropathy develops.

Other causes

+ Diuretics, demeclocycline, phenothiazines, and anticholinergics

Key facts about diabetes mellitus

- Characterized by hyperglycemia
- Caused by lack of insulin, insulin effect, or both
- Contributes to MI, stroke, renal failure, peripheral vascular disease, and new blindness
- Classified as type 1 (insulin insufficiency), type 2 (insulin resistance), or gestational (pregnancy related)

Causes

- Heredity
- Environment
- Lifestyle
- Pregnancy

Management

Type 1
- Insulin replacement and exercise
- Pancreas transplantation

Type 2
- Oral antidiabetic drugs

Type 1 and type 2
- Blood glucose monitoring
- Individualized meal planning

Gestational diabetes
- Nutrition therapy
- Injectable insulin if necessary
- Postpartum counseling
- Regular exercise and prevention of weight gain

ASSOCIATED DISORDER

Diabetes mellitus

Diabetes mellitus is a metabolic disorder characterized by hyperglycemia resulting from lack of insulin, lack of insulin effect, or both. A leading cause of death in the United States, diabetes mellitus is a contributing factor in about 50% of myocardial infarctions and about 75% of strokes as well as in renal failure and peripheral vascular disease. It's also the leading cause of new blindness.

There are three general classifications of diabetes mellitus:
- type 1, absolute insulin insufficiency
- type 2, insulin resistance with varying degrees of insulin secretory defects
- gestational diabetes, which emerges during pregnancy.

Onset of type 1 (insulin-dependent) usually occurs before age 30 (although it may occur at any age). The patient is usually thin and requires exogenous insulin and dietary management to achieve control. Conversely, type 2 (non-insulin-dependent) usually occurs in obese adults after age 40 and is treated with diet and exercise in combination with various oral antidiabetic drugs, although treatment may include insulin therapy.

CAUSES

Evidence indicates that diabetes mellitus has diverse causes, including heredity, environment (infection, diet, toxins, stress), lifestyle changes in genetically susceptible persons, and pregnancy.

DIAGNOSIS

In adult men and nonpregnant women, diabetes mellitus is diagnosed if two of the following criteria are obtained more than 24 hours apart by using the same test twice or any combination:
- fasting plasma glucose level of 126 mg/dl or more on at least two occasions
- typical symptoms of uncontrolled diabetes and random blood glucose level of 200 mg/dl or more
- blood glucose level of 200 mg/dl or more 2 hours after ingesting 75 g of oral dextrose. Diagnosis may also be based on:
- diabetic retinopathy on ophthalmologic examination

- other diagnostic and monitoring tests, including urinalysis for acetone and glycosylated hemoglobin (reflects glycemic control over the past 2 to 3 months).

MEDICAL INTERVENTION

Effective treatment of all types of diabetes mellitus optimizes blood glucose control and decreases complications. Treatment of type 1 diabetes mellitus includes:
- insulin replacement and exercise (current forms of insulin replacement include mixed-dose, split mixed-dose, and multiple daily injection regimens and continuous subcutaneous insulin infusions)
- pancreas transplantation (currently requires chronic immunosuppression).
  Treatment of type 2 diabetes mellitus includes:
- oral antidiabetic drugs to stimulate endogenous insulin production, increase insulin sensitivity at the cellular level, suppress hepatic gluconeogenesis, and delay GI absorption of carbohydrates.
  Treatment of both types of diabetes mellitus includes:
- careful monitoring of blood glucose levels
- individualized meal plan designed to meet nutritional needs, control blood glucose and lipid levels, and reach and maintain appropriate body weight (plan to be followed consistently with meals eaten at regular times)
- weight reduction (for obese patients with type 2 diabetes mellitus) or high calorie allotment, depending on growth stage and activity level (for those with type 1 diabetes mellitus).
  Treatment of gestational diabetes involves:
- medical nutrition therapy
- injectable insulin if blood glucose level isn't achieved with diet alone (oral antidiabetic agents are teratogenic and, therefore, are contraindicated during pregnancy)
- postpartum counseling to address the high risk of gestational diabetes in subsequent pregnancies and type 2 diabetes later in life
- regular exercise and prevention of weight gain to help prevent type 2 diabetes mellitus.

Special considerations

Carefully monitor the patient's fluid balance by recording his total intake and output. Weigh the patient at the same time each day, in the same clothing and using the same scale. Regularly check blood pressure and pulse in the supine and standing positions to detect orthostatic hypotension, which may indicate hypovolemia. Because thirst is usually the body's way of compensating for water loss, give the patient ample liquids.

Pediatric pointers

In children, polydipsia usually stems from diabetes insipidus or diabetes mellitus. Rare causes include pheochromocytoma, neuroblastoma, and Prader-Willi syndrome. However, some children develop habitual polydipsia that's unrelated to any disease.

Patient counseling

Teach the patient about his underlying disorder and its treatment. Discuss such self-care measures as diet, exercise, and home blood glucose monitoring. Explain the importance of reporting any significant weight gain or loss to his health care provider.

POLYPHAGIA

Polyphagia, also called *hyperphagia,* refers to voracious or excessive eating. This common symptom can be persistent or intermittent, resulting primarily from endocrine and psychological disorders as well as the use of certain drugs. Depending on the underlying cause, polyphagia may cause weight gain.

History

Begin your evaluation by asking the patient what he has eaten and drunk within the last 24 hours. (If he easily recalls this information, ask about his intake for the 2 previous days, for a broader view of his dietary habits.) Note the frequency of meals and the amount and types of food eaten. Find out if the patient's eating habits have changed recently. Has he always had a large appetite? Does his overeating alternate with periods of anorexia? Ask about conditions that may trigger overeating, such as stress, depression, or menstruation. Does the patient actually feel hungry, or does he eat simply because food is available? Does he ever vomit or have a headache after overeating?

Explore related signs and symptoms. Has the patient recently gained or lost weight? Does he feel tired, nervous, or excitable? Has he experienced heat intolerance, dizziness, palpitations, diarrhea, or increased thirst or urination? Obtain a complete drug history, including the use of laxatives or enemas.

Physical assessment

During the physical examination, weigh the patient. Tell him his current weight, and watch for any expression of disbelief or anger. Inspect the skin to detect dryness or poor turgor. Palpate the thyroid for enlargement.

Medical causes

Anxiety
+ Polyphagia may result from mild to moderate anxiety or emotional stress.

Bulimia
+ Polyphagia alternates with self-induced vomiting, fasting, or diarrhea.
+ Most commonly occurs in women ages 18 to 29.

Diabetes mellitus
+ Polyphagia occurs with weight loss, polydipsia, and polyuria.

Migraine headache
+ Polyphagia sometimes precedes a migraine headache.

Premenstrual syndrome
+ Appetite changes are common with premenstrual syndrome.

Thyrotoxicosis
+ Despite constant polyphagia, thyrotoxicosis can produce weight loss.

Other causes
+ Corticosteroids and cyproheptadine

Special considerations
+ Monitor the patient's eating habits and weight.

MEDICAL CAUSES

Anxiety
Polyphagia may result from mild to moderate anxiety or emotional stress. Mild anxiety typically produces restlessness, sleeplessness, irritability, repetitive questioning, and constant seeking of attention and reassurance. With moderate anxiety, selective inattention and difficulty concentrating may also occur. Other effects of anxiety may include muscle tension, diaphoresis, GI distress, palpitations, tachycardia, and urinary and sexual dysfunction.

Bulimia
Most common in women ages 18 to 29, bulimia causes polyphagia that alternates with self-induced vomiting, fasting, or diarrhea. The patient typically weighs less than normal but has a morbid fear of obesity. She appears depressed, has low self-esteem, and conceals her overeating.

Diabetes mellitus
With diabetes mellitus, polyphagia occurs with weight loss, polydipsia, and polyuria. It's accompanied by nocturia, weakness, fatigue, and such signs of dehydration as dry mucous membranes and poor skin turgor.

Migraine headache
Polyphagia sometimes precedes a migraine headache. The individual may experience changes in appetite or food cravings. Other prodromal signs and symptoms include fatigue, nausea, vomiting, and a visual aura. Light and noise sensitivity may also occur.

Premenstrual syndrome
Appetite changes, typified by food cravings and binges, are common with premenstrual syndrome. Abdominal bloating, the most common associated finding, may occur with behavioral changes, such as depression and insomnia. Headache, paresthesia, and other neurologic symptoms may also occur. Related findings include diarrhea or constipation, edema and temporary weight gain, palpitations, back pain, breast swelling and tenderness, oliguria, and easy bruising.

Thyrotoxicosis
Thyrotoxicosis can produce weight loss despite constant polyphagia. Other characteristics include weakness, nervousness, diarrhea, tremors, diaphoresis, and dyspnea. The patient's hair and nails are thin and brittle, and his thyroid is enlarged. He may also exhibit palpitations, tachycardia, heat intolerance, exophthalmos, and an atrial or ventricular gallop.

OTHER CAUSES

Drugs
Corticosteroids and cyproheptadine may increase appetite, causing weight gain.

SPECIAL CONSIDERATIONS

Monitor the patient's eating habits. Weigh him once or twice a week to monitor weight. Refer the patient to a registered dietitian for nutritional counseling, if indicated.

PEDIATRIC POINTERS

In children, polyphagia commonly results from juvenile diabetes. In infants ages 6 to 18 months, it can result from a malabsorptive disorder such as celiac disease. However, polyphagia may occur normally in a child who is experiencing a sudden growth spurt.

PATIENT COUNSELING

Offer the patient with polyphagia emotional support, and help him understand its underlying cause. As needed, refer the patient and his family for psychological counseling.

POLYURIA

A relatively common sign, polyuria is the daily production and excretion of more than 3 L of urine. It's usually reported by the patient as increased urination, especially when it occurs at night. Polyuria is aggravated by overhydration, consumption of caffeine or alcohol, and excessive ingestion of salt, glucose, or other hyperosmolar substances.

Polyuria usually results from the use of certain drugs, such as a diuretic, or from a psychological, neurologic, or renal disorder. It can reflect central nervous system dysfunction that diminishes or suppresses secretion of antidiuretic hormone (ADH), which regulates fluid balance. Alternatively, when ADH levels are normal, it can reflect renal impairment. In both of these pathophysiologic mechanisms, the renal tubules fail to reabsorb sufficient water, causing polyuria.

HISTORY

Explore the frequency and pattern of the polyuria. When did it begin? How long has it lasted? Was it precipitated by a certain event? Ask the patient to describe the pattern and amount of his daily fluid intake. Is the patient unusually tired or thirsty? Has he recently lost more than 5% of his body weight? Check for a history of visual deficits, headaches, or head trauma, which may precede diabetes insipidus. Also check for a history of urinary tract obstruction, diabetes mellitus, renal disorder, chronic hypokalemia or hypercalcemia, or psychiatric disorder (both past and present). Find out the schedule and dosage of any drugs the patient is taking.

PHYSICAL ASSESSMENT

Take vital signs, noting increased body temperature, tachycardia, and orthostatic hypotension (a 10 mm Hg or greater decrease in systolic blood pressure upon standing and a 10 beats per minute or greater increase in heart rate upon standing). Inspect for dry skin and mucous membranes, decreased skin turgor and elasticity, and reduced perspiration.

Perform a neurologic assessment, noting especially any change in the patient's level of consciousness. Then palpate the bladder and inspect the urethral meatus. Obtain a urine specimen and check its specific gravity.

Peds points

+ In children, polyphagia commonly results from juvenile diabetes.
+ In infants ages 6 to 18 months, polyphagia can result from a malabsorptive disorder.

Teaching points

+ Nutritional referral
+ Referral for personal or family counseling

Key facts about polyuria

+ Daily production and excretion of more than 3 L of urine

Key history points

+ Urinary frequency and pattern
+ Complaints of fatigue, increased thirst, or weight loss
+ History of visual deficits, headaches, head trauma, urinary tract obstruction, diabetes mellitus, renal disorder, chronic hypokalemia or hypercalcemia, or psychiatric disorder
+ Drug history

Critical assessment steps

+ Take vital signs, noting increased body temperature, tachycardia, and orthostatic hypotension.
+ Inspect for signs of dehydration.
+ Perform a neurologic assessment.
+ Obtain a urine specimen and check specific gravity.

Medical causes

Acute tubular necrosis
✦ Urine output is < 8 L/day.

Diabetes insipidus
✦ Polyuria of about 5 L/day occurs with a specific gravity of 1.005 or less.

Diabetes mellitus
✦ Polyuria is seldom > 5 L/day, and urine specific gravity is typically > 1.020.

Glomerulonephritis (chronic)
✦ Polyuria gradually progresses to oliguria.
✦ Urine output is usually < 4 L/day; specific gravity is about 1.010.

Hypercalcemia
✦ Nephropathy from elevated plasma calcium levels causes polyuria of < 5 L/day with a specific gravity of about 1.010.

Hypokalemia
✦ Nephropathy from prolonged potassium depletion causes polyuria of < 5 L/day with a specific gravity of about 1.010.

Postobstructive uropathy
✦ After resolution of a urinary tract obstruction, polyuria — usually > 5 L/day with a specific gravity of < 1.010 — occurs for up to several days before gradually subsiding.

Pyelonephritis
✦ Polyuria of < 5 L/day with a low but variable specific gravity occurs in acute disease.
✦ Chronic pyelonephritis produces polyuria of < 5 L/day that declines as renal function worsens.

MEDICAL CAUSES

Acute tubular necrosis
During the diuretic phase of acute tubular necrosis, polyuria of less than 8 L/day gradually subsides after 8 to 10 days. Urine specific gravity (1.010 or less) increases as polyuria subsides. Related findings include weight loss, decreasing edema, and nocturia.

Diabetes insipidus
With diabetes insipidus, polyuria of about 5 L/day with a specific gravity of 1.005 or less is common, although extreme polyuria — up to 30 L/day — occasionally occurs. Polyuria is commonly accompanied by polydipsia, nocturia, fatigue, and signs of dehydration, such as poor skin turgor and dry mucous membranes.

Diabetes mellitus
With diabetes mellitus, polyuria seldom exceeds 5 L/day, and urine specific gravity typically exceeds 1.020. The patient usually reports polydipsia, polyphagia, weight loss, weakness, frequent urinary tract infections and yeast vaginitis, fatigue, and nocturia. The patient may also display signs of dehydration and anorexia.

Glomerulonephritis (chronic)
Polyuria gradually progresses to oliguria with chronic glomerulonephritis. Urine output is usually less than 4 L/day; specific gravity is about 1.010. Related GI findings include anorexia, nausea, and vomiting. The patient may experience drowsiness, fatigue, edema, headache, elevated blood pressure, and dyspnea. Nocturia, hematuria, frothy or malodorous urine, and mild to severe proteinuria may also occur.

Hypercalcemia
Elevated plasma calcium levels may lead to nephropathy, usually producing polyuria of less than 5 L/day with a specific gravity of about 1.010. Accompanying signs and symptoms include polydipsia, nocturia, constipation, paresthesia and, occasionally, hematuria, and pyuria. With severe hypercalcemia, the patient's condition worsens rapidly and he experiences anorexia, vomiting, stupor progressing to coma, and renal failure.

Hypokalemia
Prolonged potassium depletion may lead to nephropathy, which results in polyuria — usually less than 5 L/day with a specific gravity of about 1.010. Associated findings include polydipsia, circumoral and foot paresthesia, hypoactive deep tendon reflexes, fatigue, hypoactive bowel sounds, nocturia, arrhythmias, and muscle cramping, weakness, or paralysis.

Postobstructive uropathy
After resolution of a urinary tract obstruction, polyuria — usually more than 5 L/day with a specific gravity of less than 1.010 — occurs for up to several days before gradually subsiding. Bladder distention and edema may occur with nocturia and weight loss. Occasionally, signs of dehydration appear.

Pyelonephritis
Acute pyelonephritis usually results in polyuria of less than 5 L/day with a low but variable specific gravity. Other findings include persistent high fever, flank pain (usually unilateral), hematuria, costovertebral angle tenderness, chills, weakness, dysuria, urinary frequency and urgency, tenesmus, and nocturia. Occasionally, nausea, anorexia, vomiting, and hypoactive bowel sounds occur.

Chronic pyelonephritis produces polyuria of less than 5 L/day that declines as renal function worsens. Urine specific gravity is usually about 1.010 but may be higher if proteinuria is present. Other effects include irritability, paresthesia, fatigue, nausea, vomiting, diarrhea, drowsiness, anorexia, pyuria and, in late stages, elevated blood pressure.

Sickle cell anemia

Sickle cell anemia may cause nephropathy, typically producing polyuria of less than 5 L/day with a specific gravity of about 1.020. Additional findings include polydipsia, fatigue, abdominal cramps, arthralgia, priapism and, occasionally, leg ulcers and bony deformities.

OTHER CAUSES

Diagnostic tests

Transient polyuria can result from radiographic tests that use contrast media.

Drugs

Diuretics characteristically produce polyuria. Cardiotonics, vitamin D, demeclocycline, phenytoin, lithium, methoxyflurane, and propoxyphene can also produce polyuria.

SPECIAL CONSIDERATIONS

Maintain adequate fluid balance when the patient has polyuria. Record intake and output accurately, and weigh the patient daily. Closely monitor the patient's vital signs to detect fluid imbalance, and encourage him to drink adequate fluids. Review his medications, and recommend modification where possible to help control symptoms.

Prepare the patient for serum electrolyte, osmolality, blood urea nitrogen, and creatinine studies to monitor fluid and electrolyte status, and for a fluid deprivation test to determine the cause of polyuria.

PEDIATRIC POINTERS

The major causes of polyuria in children are congenital nephrogenic diabetes insipidus, medullary cystic disease, polycystic renal disease, and distal renal tubular acidosis.

Because a child's fluid balance is more delicate than an adult's, check his urine specific gravity at each voiding, and be alert for signs of dehydration. These include a decrease in body weight, decreased skin turgor, dry mucous membranes, decreased urine output, absence of tears when crying, and pale, mottled, or gray skin.

GERIATRIC POINTERS

In elderly patients, chronic pyelonephritis is commonly associated with an underlying disorder. The possibility of associated malignant disease must be investigated.

PATIENT COUNSELING

Teach your patient about his underlying disorder and the need to replace fluids. Have him weigh himself daily and report any weight loss to his health care provider. Explain the signs and symptoms of dehydration and the importance of increasing fluid intake, especially in hot weather.

Medical causes
(continued)

Sickle cell anemia
✦ Nephropathy from the disease produces polyuria of < 5 L/day with a specific gravity of about 1.020.

Other causes
✦ Radiographic tests that use contrast media
✦ Diuretics
✦ Cardiotonics, vitamin D, demeclocycline, phenytoin, lithium, methoxyflurane, and propoxyphene

Special considerations
✦ Record intake and output, and weigh the patient daily.
✦ Encourage fluid intake to maintain adequate fluid balance.

Peds points
✦ The major causes of polyuria in children are congenital nephrogenic diabetes insipidus, medullary cystic disease, polycystic renal disease, and distal renal tubular acidosis.
✦ Because a child's fluid balance is more delicate than an adult's, check urine specific gravity at each voiding and be alert for signs of dehydration.

Geri points
✦ Chronic pyelonephritis is commonly associated with an underlying disorder.

Teaching points
✦ Facts about underlying disorder
✦ Fluid replacement
✦ Weight monitoring

PRURITUS

Commonly provoking scratching to gain relief, this unpleasant itching sensation affects the skin, certain mucous membranes, and the eyes. Most severe at night, pruritus may be exacerbated by increased skin temperature, poor skin turgor, local vasodilation, dermatoses, and stress.

The most common symptom of dermatologic disorders, pruritus may also result from a local or systemic disorder or from drug use. Physiologic pruritus, such as pruritic urticarial papules and plaques of pregnancy, may occur in primigravidas late in the third trimester. Pruritus can also stem from emotional upset or contact with skin irritants.

HISTORY

If the patient reports pruritus, have him describe its onset, frequency, and intensity. If pruritus occurs at night, ask whether it prevents him from falling asleep or awakens him after he falls asleep. (Generally, pruritus related to dermatoses prevents — but doesn't disturb — sleep.) Is the itching localized or generalized? When is it most severe? How long does it last? Is there a relationship to activities (exercising, bathing, applying makeup, or using perfumes)?

Ask the patient how he cleans his skin. In particular, look for excessive bathing, harsh soaps, contact allergy, and excessively hot water. Does he have occupational exposure to known skin irritants, such as glass fiber insulation or chemicals? Ask about the patient's general health and the medications he takes (new medications are suspect). Has he recently traveled abroad? Does he have any pets? Does anyone else in the house report itching? Does exercise, stress, fear, depression, or illness seem to aggravate the itching? Ask about contact with skin irritants, previous skin disorders, and related symptoms. Then obtain a complete drug history.

PHYSICAL ASSESSMENT

Observe the patient for signs of scratching, such as excoriation, purpura, scabs, scars, or lichenification. Look for primary lesions to help confirm dermatoses.

MEDICAL CAUSES

Anemia (iron deficiency)

Anemia occasionally produces pruritus. Initially asymptomatic, anemia can later cause exertional dyspnea, fatigue, listlessness, pallor, irritability, headache, tachycardia, poor muscle tone and, possibly, murmurs. Chronic anemia causes spoon-shaped (koilonychia) and brittle nails (cheilosis), cracked mouth corners, a smooth tongue (glossitis), and dysphagia.

Anthrax (cutaneous)

A cutaneous anthrax infection begins as a small, painless or pruritic, macular or papular lesion resembling an insect bite. Within 1 to 2 days, it develops into a vesicle and then a painless ulcer with a characteristic black, necrotic center. Lymphadenopathy, malaise, headache, or fever may develop.

Conjunctivitis

All forms of conjunctivitis cause eye itching, burning, and pain along with photophobia, conjunctival injection, a foreign-body sensation, excessive tearing, and a feeling of fullness around the eye. Allergic conjunctivitis may also cause milky redness and a stringy eye discharge. Bacterial conjunctivitis typically causes brilliant redness and a mucopurulent discharge that may make the eyelids stick together. Fungal conjunctivitis produces a thick, purulent discharge and crusting and sticking of the eyelid. Viral conjunctivitis may cause copious tearing—but little discharge—and preauricular lymph node enlargement.

Dermatitis

Several types of dermatitis can cause pruritus accompanied by a skin lesion. Atopic dermatitis begins with intense, severe pruritus and an erythematous rash on dry skin at flexion points (antecubital fossa, popliteal area, and neck). During a flare-up, scratching may produce edema, scaling, and pustules. With chronic atopic dermatitis, lesions may progress to dry, scaly skin with white dermatographism, blanching, and lichenification.

Mild irritants and allergies can cause contact dermatitis, with itchy, small vesicles that may ooze and scale and are surrounded by redness. A severe reaction can produce marked localized edema.

Dermatitis herpetiformis, most common in men between ages 20 and 50, initially causes intense pruritus and stinging. Between 8 and 12 hours later, symmetrically distributed lesions form on the buttocks, shoulders, elbows, and knees. Sometimes, they also form on the neck, face, and scalp. These lesions are erythematous and papular, bullous, or pustular.

Enterobiasis

Also known as pinworm or seatworm, this helminthic infection produces intense perianal pruritus, especially at night, when the female worm leaves the anus to deposit ova. Pruritus causes irritability, scratching, skin irritation and, sometimes, vaginitis.

Hemorrhoids

Anal pruritus may occur in patients with hemorrhoids along with rectal pain and constipation. External hemorrhoids may be seen outside the external anal sphincter; internal hemorrhoids are less obvious and less painful but more likely to cause rectal bleeding.

Hepatobiliary disease

An important diagnostic clue to liver and gallbladder disease, pruritus is commonly accompanied by jaundice and may be generalized or localized to the palms and soles. Other characteristics include right-upper-quadrant pain, clay-colored stools, chills and fever, flatus, belching and a bloated feeling, epigastric burning, and bitter fluid regurgitation. Later, liver disease may produce mental changes, ascites, bleeding tendencies, spider angiomas, palmar erythema, dry skin, fetor hepaticus, enlarged superficial abdominal veins, bilateral gynecomastia, testicular atrophy or menstrual irregularities, and hepatomegaly.

Herpes zoster

In herpes zoster, within 4 days of fever and malaise, pruritus, paresthesia or hyperesthesia, and severe, deep pain from cutaneous nerve involvement develop on the trunk or the arms and legs in a dermatome distribution. Up to 2 weeks after initial symptoms, red, nodular skin eruptions appear on the painful areas and become vesicular. About 10 days later, the vesicles rupture and form scabs.

Medical causes
(continued)

Dermatitis
✦ Pruritus may be accompanied by a skin lesion.
✦ Presentation varies by type of dermatitis.

Enterobiasis
✦ Intense perianal pruritus occurs, especially at night, when the female worm leaves the anus to deposit ova.

Hemorrhoids
✦ Anal pruritus, rectal pain, and constipation may occur.

Hepatobiliary disease
✦ Pruritus, often accompanied by jaundice, may be generalized or localized to the palms and soles.

Herpes zoster
✦ Within 4 days of fever and malaise, pruritus, paresthesia or hyperesthesia, and severe, deep pain from cutaneous nerve involvement develop on the trunk or arms and legs.

Medical causes
(continued)

Hodgkin's disease
✦ Severe, unexplained itching occasionally occurs.
✦ As the disease progresses, pruritus may become severe and unresponsive to treatment.

Lichen simplex chronicus
✦ Localized pruritus and a circumscribed scaling patch with sharp margins results from persistent rubbing and scratching of the skin.

Pediculosis
✦ Pruritus in the area of infestation is a prominent symptom of infestation.

Pityriasis rosea
✦ Pruritus that's aggravated by a hot bath or shower occasionally occurs.
✦ It begins as an erythematous herald patch and progresses to scaly, yellow, erythematous patches that erupt on the trunk or extremities and persist for 2 to 6 weeks.

Polycythemia vera
✦ Pruritus that's generalized or localized to the head, neck, face, and extremities may occur.
✦ Hot baths and showers typically aggravate it.
✦ The patient's oral mucosa may be deep purplish red, especially on the gingivae and tongue. The engorged gingivae ooze blood with slight trauma.

Psoriasis
✦ Pruritus and pain commonly occur.

Hodgkin's disease
Hodgkin's disease occasionally causes severe and unexplained itching. As the disease progresses, pruritus may become severe and unresponsive to treatment. Early nonspecific findings include persistent fever (occasionally, cyclic fever and chills), night sweats, fatigue, weight loss, malaise, and painless swelling of a cervical lymph node. Other lymph nodes may enlarge rapidly and cause pain, or they may enlarge slowly and be painless. Later findings include retroperitoneal node enlargement, hepatomegaly, splenomegaly, dyspnea, dysphagia, dry cough, hyperpigmentation, jaundice, and pallor.

Lichen simplex chronicus
Lichen simplex chronicus is due to persistent rubbing and scratching of the skin, causing localized pruritus and a circumscribed scaling patch with sharp margins. Later, the skin thickens and papules form. This condition usually affects areas easily reached, such as ankles, lower legs, anogenital area, back of neck, and ears.

Pediculosis
A prominent symptom of pediculosis, pruritus occurs in the area of infestation. Pediculosis capitis (head lice) may also cause scalp excoriation from scratching, along with matted, foul-smelling, lusterless hair; occipital and cervical lymphadenopathy; and oval, gray-white nits on hair shafts.

Pediculosis corporis (body lice) initially causes small red papules (usually on the shoulders, trunk, or buttocks), which become urticarial from scratching. Later, rashes or wheals may develop. Left untreated, pediculosis corporis produces dry, discolored, thickly encrusted, scaly skin with bacterial infection and scarring. In severe cases, it produces headache, fever, and malaise.

With pediculosis pubis (pubic lice), scratching commonly produces skin irritation. Nits or adult lice and erythematous, itching papules may appear in pubic hair or hair around the anus, abdomen, or thighs.

Pityriasis rosea
Pityriasis rosea occasionally produces mild pruritus that's aggravated by a hot bath or shower. It usually begins with an erythematous herald patch — a slightly raised, oval lesion about 2 to 6 cm in diameter. After a few days or weeks, scaly yellow-tan or erythematous patches erupt on the trunk and extremities and persist for 2 to 6 weeks. Occasionally, these patches are macular, vesicular, or urticarial.

Polycythemia vera
Polycythemia vera, a hematologic disorder, can produce pruritus that's generalized or localized to the head, neck, face, and extremities. The itching is typically aggravated by a hot bath or shower and can last from a few minutes to an hour. The patient's oral mucosa may be deep purplish red, especially on the gingivae and tongue. His engorged gingivae ooze blood with even slight trauma.

Related findings include headache, dizziness, fatigue, dyspnea, paresthesia, impaired mentation, tinnitus, double or blurred vision, scotoma, hypotension, intermittent claudication, urticaria, ruddy cyanosis, and ecchymosis. GI effects include gastric distress, weight loss, and hepatosplenomegaly.

Psoriasis
Pruritus and pain are common in psoriasis. This skin disorder typically begins with small erythematous papules that enlarge or coalesce to form red, elevated plaques with silver scales on the scalp, chest, elbows, knees, back, buttocks, and genitals. Nail pitting may occur.

Renal failure (chronic)

Pruritus may develop gradually or suddenly with chronic renal failure. It may be accompanied by ammonia breath odor, oliguria or anuria, lassitude, fatigue, irritability, decreased mental acuity, convulsions, coarse muscular twitching, muscle cramps, peripheral neuropathies, and coma. Renal failure also causes diverse GI signs and symptoms, such as anorexia, constipation or diarrhea, nausea, and vomiting.

Scabies

Typically, scabies causes localized pruritus that awakens the patient. It may become generalized and persist up to 2 weeks after treatment. Threadlike lesions several millimeters long appear with a swollen nodule or red papule.

Thyrotoxicosis

Generalized pruritus may precede or accompany the characteristic signs and symptoms of thyrotoxicosis: tachycardia, palpitations, weight loss despite increased appetite, diarrhea, tremors, an enlarged thyroid, dyspnea, nervousness, diaphoresis, heat intolerance and, possibly, exophthalmos.

Tinea pedis

Tinea pedis, also called athlete's foot, is a fungal infection that causes severe foot pruritus, pain with walking, scales and blisters between the toes, and a dry, scaly squamous inflammation on the entire sole. The affected skin may appear red and inflamed.

Urticaria

With urticaria, extreme pruritus and stinging occur as transient erythematous or whitish wheals form on the skin or mucous membranes. Prickly sensations typically precede the wheals, which may affect any part of the body and may range from pinpoint to palm-sized or larger.

Vaginitis

Vaginitis commonly causes localized pruritus and foul-smelling vaginal discharge that may be purulent, white or gray, and curdlike. Perineal pain and urinary symptoms, such as burning and frequency, may also occur.

OTHER CAUSES

Bedbug bites

Typically, bedbug bites produce itching and burning over the ankles and lower legs, along with clusters of purpuric spots.

Drug hypersensitivity

When mild and localized, an allergic reaction to such drugs as penicillin and sulfonamides can cause pruritus, erythema, an urticarial rash, and edema. However, with a severe drug reaction, anaphylaxis may occur.

SPECIAL CONSIDERATIONS

Administer a topical or oral corticosteroid, an antihistamine, or a tranquilizer, as ordered. If the patient doesn't have a localized infection or skin lesions, suspect a systemic disease and prepare him for a complete blood count and differential, erythrocyte sedimentation rate, protein electrophoresis, and radiologic studies.

Medical causes
(continued)

Renal failure (chronic)
+ Pruritus may develop gradually or suddenly.

Scabies
+ Localized pruritus that awakens the patient typically occurs.

Thyrotoxicosis
+ Generalized pruritus may precede or accompany the characteristic signs and symptoms of thyrotoxicosis.

Tinea pedis
+ Severe foot pruritus typically occurs.

Urticaria
+ Extreme pruritus and stinging occur as transient erythematous or whitish wheals form on the skin or mucous membranes.

Vaginitis
+ Localized pruritus commonly occurs with foul-smelling vaginal discharge that may be purulent, white or gray, and curdlike.

Other causes
+ Bedbug bites
+ Drug hypersensitivity

Special considerations
+ Administer a topical or oral corticosteroid, an antihistamine, or a tranquilizer, as ordered.

Peds points

◆ Many adult disorders also cause pruritus in children, but they may affect different parts of the body.
◆ Such childhood diseases as measles and chickenpox can also cause pruritus.

Teaching points

◆ Ways to control pruritus

Key facts about psychotic behavior

◆ Inability or unwillingness to recognize and acknowledge reality and to relate with others
◆ May begin suddenly or insidiously

Key history points

◆ Description of problem and any precipitating circumstances
◆ Drug history
◆ Alcohol or drug use
◆ Family's description of the patient's relationships, communication patterns, and role
◆ Family history of psychiatric or emotional illness

Critical assessment steps

◆ Assess the patient's appearance, behavior, mood, thought, coping mechanisms, and potential for self-destructive behavior.
◆ Watch for cognitive, linguistic, or perceptual abnormalities.
◆ Look for unusual gestures, posture, gait, tone of voice, and mannerisms.

PEDIATRIC POINTERS

Many adult disorders also cause pruritus in children, but they may affect different parts of the body. For instance, scabies may affect the head in infants but not in adults. Pityriasis rosea may affect the face, hands, and feet of adolescents.

Some childhood diseases, such as measles and chickenpox, can cause pruritus.

PATIENT COUNSELING

Suggest ways to control pruritus. For example, tell your patient to avoid scratching or rubbing the itchy areas. Advise him to keep fingernails short to avoid skin damage from any unconscious scratching. Recommend taking tepid baths, using little soap and rinsing thoroughly. Tell him to apply an emollient lotion after bathing to soften and cool the skin. Show the patient how to use topical ointments after bathing to soften and cool the skin.

PSYCHOTIC BEHAVIOR

Psychotic behavior reflects an inability or unwillingness to recognize and acknowledge reality and to relate with others. It may begin suddenly or insidiously, progressing from vague complaints of fatigue, insomnia, or headache to withdrawal, social isolation, and preoccupation with certain issues resulting in gross impairment in functioning.

Various behaviors together or separately can constitute psychotic behavior. These include delusions, illusions, hallucinations, bizarre language, and perseveration. *Delusions* are persistent beliefs that have no basis in reality or in the patient's knowledge or experience, such as delusions of grandeur. *Illusions* are misinterpretations of external sensory stimuli, such as a mirage in the desert. In contrast, *hallucinations* are sensory perceptions that don't result from external stimuli. *Bizarre language* reflects a communication disruption. It can range from echolalia (purposeless repetition of a word or phrase) and clang association (repetition of words or phrases that sound similar) to neologisms (creation and use of words whose meaning only the patient knows). *Perseveration,* a persistent verbal or motor response, may indicate organic brain disease. Motor changes include inactivity, excessive activity, and repetitive movements.

HISTORY

Because the patient's behavior can make it difficult — or potentially dangerous — to obtain pertinent information, conduct the interview in a calm, safe, and well-lit room. Provide enough personal space to avoid threatening or agitating the patient. Ask him to describe his problem and any circumstances that may have precipitated it. Obtain a drug history, noting especially use of an antipsychotic, and explore his use of alcohol and other drugs such as cocaine, indicating duration of use and amount. Ask about recent illnesses or accidents.

Interview the patient's family. Which family member does he seem closest to? How does the family describe the patient's relationships, communication patterns, and role? Has any family member ever been hospitalized for psychiatric or emotional illness? Ask about the patient's compliance with his drug regimen.

Finally, evaluate the patient's environment, educational and employment history, and socioeconomic status. Are community services available? How does the patient spend his leisure time? Does he have friends? Has he ever had a close emotional relationship?

PHYSICAL ASSESSMENT

Assess the patient's appearance, behavior, mood, thought, coping mechanisms, and potential for self-destructive behavior. As the patient talks, watch for cognitive, linguistic, or perceptual abnormalities such as delusions. Do thoughts and actions seem to match? Look for unusual gestures, posture, gait, tone of voice, and mannerisms. Does the patient appear to be responding to stimuli? For example, is he looking around the room?

MEDICAL CAUSES

Organic disorders

Various disorders, such as alcohol withdrawal syndrome, cocaine or amphetamine intoxication, cerebral hypoxia, and nutritional disorders, can produce psychotic behavior. Endocrine disorders, such as adrenal dysfunction, and severe infections, such as encephalitis, can also cause psychotic behavior. Neurologic causes include Alzheimer's disease and other dementias.

Psychiatric disorders

Psychotic behavior usually occurs with bipolar disorder, personality disorder, schizophrenia, and some pervasive developmental disorders.

OTHER CAUSES

Drugs

Certain drugs can cause psychotic behavior. (See *Psychotic behavior: An adverse drug effect,* page 526.) However, almost any drug can provoke psychotic behavior as a rare, severe adverse or idiosyncratic reaction.

Surgery

Postoperative delirium and depression may produce psychotic behavior.

SPECIAL CONSIDERATIONS

Continuously evaluate the patient's orientation to reality. Help him develop a conception of reality by calling him by his preferred name, telling him your name, describing where he is, and using clocks and calendars. (See *Controlling psychotic behavior,* page 527.)

Refer the patient for psychiatric evaluation. Administer an antipsychotic or other drugs, as needed, and prepare him for transfer to a mental health center, if necessary.

Don't overlook the patient's physiologic needs. Check his eating habits to avoid dehydration and malnutrition, and monitor his elimination patterns, especially if he's receiving an antipsychotic, which can cause constipation.

PEDIATRIC POINTERS

In children, psychotic behavior may result from early infantile autism, symbiotic infantile psychosis, or childhood schizophrenia — any of which can retard development of language, abstract thinking, and socialization. An adolescent patient who exhibits psychotic behavior may have a history of several days' drug use or lack of sleep or food, which must be evaluated and corrected before therapy can begin.

Medical causes

Organic disorders
✦ Psychotic behavior can result from alcohol withdrawal syndrome, cocaine or amphetamine intoxication, cerebral hypoxia, and nutritional disorders.
✦ Endocrine disorders, such as adrenal dysfunction, and severe infections, such as encephalitis, can also cause psychotic behavior.

Psychiatric disorders
✦ Psychotic behavior usually occurs with bipolar disorder, personality disorder, schizophrenia, and some pervasive developmental disorders.

Special considerations
✦ Continuously evaluate the patient's orientation to reality.
✦ Call the patient by his preferred name, tell him your name, describe where he is, and use clocks and calendars to help develop a conception of reality.
✦ Administer antipsychotic or other drugs, as needed.
✦ Monitor patient's eating and elimination habits.

Peds points
✦ In children, psychotic behavior may result from early infantile autism, symbiotic infantile psychosis, or childhood schizophrenia.
✦ An adolescent patient who exhibits psychotic behavior may have a history of several days' drug use or lack of sleep or food.

Other causes

Drugs

+ Albuterol
+ Alprazolam
+ Amantadine
+ Asparaginase
+ Atropine and anticholinergics
+ Bromocriptine
+ Cardiac glycosides
+ Cimetidine
+ Clonidine
+ Corticosteroids (prednisone, corticotropin, cortisone)
+ Cycloserine
+ Dapsone
+ Diazepam
+ Disopyramide
+ Disulfiram
+ Indomethacin
+ Lidocaine
+ Methyldopa
+ Propranolol
+ Thyroid hormones
+ Vincristine

Psychotic behavior: An adverse drug effect

Certain drugs can cause psychotic behavior and other psychiatric signs and symptoms, ranging from depression to violent behavior. Usually, these effects occur during therapy and resolve when the drug is discontinued. If your patient is receiving one of these common drugs and exhibits the behavior described below, the dosage may have to be changed or another drug may have to be substituted.

DRUG	PSYCHIATRIC SIGNS AND SYMPTOMS
albuterol	Hallucinations, paranoia
alprazolam	Anger, hostility
amantadine	Visual hallucinations, nightmares
asparaginase	Confusion, depression, paranoia
atropine and anticholinergics	Auditory, visual, and tactile hallucinations; memory loss; delirium; fear; paranoia
bromocriptine	Mania, delusions, sudden relapse of schizophrenia, paranoia, aggressive behavior
cardiac glycosides	Paranoia, euphoria, amnesia, visual hallucinations
cimetidine	Hallucinations, paranoia, confusion, depression, delirium
clonidine	Delirium, hallucinations, depression
corticosteroids (prednisone, corticotropin, cortisone)	Mania, catatonia, depression, confusion, paranoia, hallucinations
cycloserine	Anxiety, depression, confusion, paranoia, hallucinations
dapsone	Insomnia, agitation, hallucinations
diazepam	Suicidal thoughts, rage, hallucinations, depression
disopyramide	Agitation, paranoia, auditory and visual hallucinations, panic
disulfiram	Delirium, auditory hallucinations, paranoia, depression
indomethacin	Hostility, depression, paranoia, hallucinations
lidocaine	Disorientation, hallucinations, paranoia
methyldopa	Severe depression, amnesia, paranoia, hallucinations
propranolol	Severe depression, hallucinations, paranoia, confusion
thyroid hormones	Mania, hallucinations, paranoia
vincristine	Hallucinations

Teaching points

+ Importance of structured activities

PATIENT COUNSELING

Encourage the patient to become involved in structured activities. However, if he's nonverbal or incoherent, make sure to spend time with him. For example, sit or walk with him, or talk about the day, the season, the weather, or other concrete topics. Avoid making time commitments that you can't keep: This will only upset the patient and cause him to withdraw more.

Controlling psychotic behavior

A patient who displays psychotic behavior may be terrified and unable to differentiate between himself and his environment. To control his behavior and to prevent injury to the patient, staff, and others, follow these guidelines:

+ Remove potentially dangerous objects, such as belts or metal utensils, from the patient's environment.
+ Help the patient discern what's real and unreal in an honest and genuine way.
+ Be straightforward, concise, and nonthreatening when speaking to the patient. Discuss simple, concrete subjects, and avoid theories or philosophical issues.

+ Positively reinforce the patient's perceptions of reality, and correct his misperceptions in a matter-of-fact way.
+ *Never* argue with the patient but also don't support his misperceptions.
+ If the patient is frightened, stay with him.
+ Touch the patient to provide reassurance *only* if you've done this before and know that it's safe.
+ Move the patient to a safer, less-stimulating environment.
+ Provide one-on-one care if the patient's behavior is extremely bizarre, disturbing to other patients, or dangerous to himself.
+ Medicate the patient appropriately.

PTOSIS

Ptosis is the excessive drooping of one or both upper eyelids. This sign can be constant, progressive, or intermittent, and unilateral or bilateral. When it's unilateral, it's easy to detect by comparing the eyelids' relative positions. When it's bilateral or mild, it's difficult to detect — the eyelids may be abnormally low, covering the upper part of the iris or even part of the pupil instead of overlapping the iris slightly. Other clues include a furrowed forehead or a tipped-back head — both of these help the patient see under his drooping lids. With severe ptosis, the patient may not be able to raise his eyelids voluntarily. Because ptosis can resemble enophthalmos, exophthalmometry may be required.

Ptosis can be classified as congenital or acquired. Classification is important for proper treatment. *Congenital ptosis* results from levator muscle underdevelopment or disorders of the third cranial (oculomotor) nerve. *Acquired ptosis* may result from trauma to or inflammation of these muscles and nerves, or from certain drugs, a systemic disease, an intracranial lesion, or a life-threatening aneurysm. However, the most common cause is advanced age, which reduces muscle elasticity and produces senile ptosis. Ptosis occasionally indicates a life-threatening condition. For example, sudden unilateral ptosis can herald a cerebral aneurysm.

HISTORY

Ask the patient when he first noticed his drooping eyelid and whether it has worsened or improved. Find out if he has recently suffered a traumatic eye injury. (If he has, avoid manipulating the eye to prevent further damage.) Ask about eye pain or headache, and determine its location and severity. Has the patient experienced any vision changes? If so, have him describe them. Obtain a drug history, noting especially use of a chemotherapeutic drug.

Key facts about ptosis
+ Excessive drooping of one or both upper eyelids
+ Can be constant, progressive, or intermittent
+ Can be unilateral or bilateral
+ Can be congenital or acquired

Key history points
+ Date of onset and whether condition has worsened or improved
+ Recent traumatic eye injury
+ Eye pain or headache
+ Presence of vision changes
+ Drug history

Critical assessment steps

+ Assess degree of ptosis; check for eyelid edema, exophthalmos, and conjunctival injection.
+ Evaluate extraocular muscle function.
+ Examine pupil size, color, shape, and reaction to light.

Medical causes

Alcoholism

+ Ptosis can result from long-term alcohol abuse or from alcohol withdrawal.

Botulism

+ Cranial nerve dysfunction causes ptosis, dysarthria, dysphagia, and diplopia.

Cerebral aneurysm

+ Sudden ptosis, diplopia, dilated pupil, and inability to rotate the eye can occur.

Hemangioma

+ Ptosis may occur along with exophthalmos, limited extraocular movement, and blurred vision.

Levator muscle maldevelopment

+ Ptosis results from isolated dystrophy of the levator muscle.
+ Lid lag on downgaze is an important clue to diagnosis.

Myasthenia gravis

+ Gradual bilateral ptosis is commonly the first sign of disease.
+ Ptosis is accompanied by weak eye closure and diplopia.

Myotonic dystrophy

+ Mild to severe bilateral ptosis may occur.

PHYSICAL ASSESSMENT

Assess the degree of ptosis, and check for eyelid edema, exophthalmos, deviation, and conjunctival injection. Evaluate extraocular muscle function by testing the six cardinal fields of gaze. Carefully examine the pupils' size, color, shape, and reaction to light, and test visual acuity.

 CULTURAL CUE *Be aware that eyelid structure and size varies with racial background. For example, Asians tend to have larger eyelids, which makes the eyes appear less open.*

MEDICAL CAUSES

Alcoholism

Long-term alcohol abuse can cause ptosis and such complications as severe weight loss, jaundice, ascites, and mental disturbances. It may also result in signs and symptoms of withdrawal when drinking is stopped.

Botulism

With botulism, acute cranial nerve dysfunction causes the hallmark signs of ptosis, dysarthria, dysphagia, and diplopia. Other findings include dry mouth, sore throat, weakness, vomiting, diarrhea, hyporeflexia, and dyspnea.

Cerebral aneurysm

A cerebral aneurysm that compresses the oculomotor nerve can cause sudden ptosis, along with diplopia, a dilated pupil, and inability to rotate the eye. These may be the first signs of this life-threatening disorder. A ruptured aneurysm typically produces sudden severe headache, nausea, vomiting, and decreased level of consciousness (LOC). Other findings include nuchal rigidity, back and leg pain, fever, restlessness, irritability, occasional seizures, blurred vision, hemiparesis, sensory deficits, dysphagia, and visual defects.

Hemangioma

Hemangioma is an orbital tumor that can produce ptosis, exophthalmos, limited extraocular movement, and blurred vision. Periorbital tissues may become swollen.

Levator muscle maldevelopment

Ptosis from maldevelopment of the levator muscle of the upper eyelid — formerly classified as true congenital ptosis — is the result of an isolated dystrophy of the levator muscle affecting its contraction and relaxation. Lid lag on downgaze is an important clue to diagnosis.

Myasthenia gravis

Commonly the first sign of myasthenia gravis, gradual bilateral ptosis may be mild to severe and is accompanied by weak eye closure and diplopia. Other characteristics include muscle weakness and fatigue, which eventually may lead to paralysis. Depending on the muscles affected, other findings may include masklike facies, difficulty chewing or swallowing, dyspnea, cyanosis, and others.

Myotonic dystrophy

Myotonic dystrophy may cause mild to severe bilateral ptosis. Distinctive cataracts with iridescent dots in the cortex, miosis, diplopia, decreased tearing, and muscular and testicular atrophy may also occur.

Ocular muscle dystrophy

With ocular muscle dystrophy, bilateral ptosis progresses slowly to complete eyelid closure. Related signs and symptoms include progressive external ophthalmoplegia and muscle weakness and atrophy of the upper face, neck, trunk, and limbs.

Ocular trauma

Trauma to the nerve or muscles that control the eyelids can cause mild to severe ptosis. Depending on the damage, eye pain, lid swelling, ecchymosis, and decreased visual acuity may also occur.

Parinaud's syndrome

Parinaud's syndrome, a form of ophthalmoplegia, can cause ptosis, enophthalmos, nystagmus, lid retraction, dilated pupils with absent or poor light response, and papilledema. The patient's ocular muscles fail to move voluntarily.

Subdural hematoma (chronic)

Ptosis may be a late sign of a chronic subdural hematoma, along with unilateral pupillary dilation and sluggishness. Headache, behavioral changes, and decreased LOC commonly occur. Specific neurologic signs depend on the hematoma's location and size.

OTHER CAUSES

Drugs

Vinca alkaloids can produce ptosis.

Lead poisoning

With lead poisoning, ptosis usually develops over 3 to 6 months. Other findings include anorexia, nausea, vomiting, diarrhea, colicky abdominal pain, a lead line in the gums, decreased LOC, tachycardia, hypotension and, possibly, irritability and peripheral nerve weakness.

SPECIAL CONSIDERATIONS

If the patient has decreased visual acuity, orient him to his surroundings. Provide special spectacle frames that suspend the eyelid by traction with a wire crutch. These frames are usually used to help patients with temporary paresis or those who aren't good candidates for surgery.

PEDIATRIC POINTERS

Astigmatism and myopia may be associated with childhood ptosis. Parents typically discover congenital ptosis when their child is an infant. Usually, the ptosis is unilateral, constant, and accompanied by lagophthalmos, which causes the infant to sleep with his eyes open. If this occurs, teach proper eye care to prevent drying.

PATIENT COUNSELING

Because ptosis can affect body image and feelings of self-esteem, encourage the patient to verbalize his concerns about these issues. Prepare the patient for diagnostic studies, such as the Tensilon test and slit-lamp examination. If he needs surgery to correct levator muscle dysfunction, explain the procedure to him.

Key facts about absent or weak pulse

+ When generalized, indicates a life-threatening condition such as shock or arrhythmia
+ When localized, may indicate acute arterial occlusion

Key history points

+ History of heart disease
+ Medical and drug history

Critical assessment steps

+ Palpate the remaining arterial pulses for comparison.
+ Check other vital signs and evaluate cardiopulmonary status.

Medical causes

Aortic aneurysm (dissecting)

+ Weak or absent arterial pulses occur distal to the affected area when circulation to the innominate, left common carotid, subclavian, or femoral artery is affected.
+ Absent or diminished pulses occur in 50% of patients with proximal dissection.

Aortic stenosis

+ The carotid pulse is weak.
+ Paroxysmal or exertional dyspnea, chest pain, and syncope dominate the clinical picture.

Arterial occlusion

+ With acute occlusion, arterial pulses distal to the obstruction are unilaterally weak and then absent.
+ With chronic occlusion, pulses in the affected limb weaken gradually.

PULSE, ABSENT OR WEAK

An absent or weak pulse may be generalized or may affect only one extremity. When generalized, this sign is an important indicator of such life-threatening conditions as shock and arrhythmia. Localized loss or weakness of a pulse that's normally present and strong may indicate acute arterial occlusion, which could require emergency surgery. However, the pressure of palpation may temporarily diminish or obliterate superficial pulses, such as the posterior tibial or the dorsal pedal. Thus, bilateral weakness or absence of these pulses doesn't necessarily indicate underlying pathology. (See *Evaluating peripheral pulses.*)

HISTORY

After you detect an absent or weak pulse, review the patient's history of heart disease. Ask him what medications he's taking and whether he has any other illnesses. Also, question him about associated signs and symptoms, such as chest pain or dyspnea.

PHYSICAL ASSESSMENT

If you detect an absent or weak pulse, palpate the remaining arterial pulses to distinguish between localized or generalized loss or weakness. (See *Managing an absent or weak pulse,* pages 532 and 533.) Then check other vital signs and evaluate cardiopulmonary status.

MEDICAL CAUSES

Aortic aneurysm (dissecting)

When a dissecting aneurysm affects circulation to the innominate, left common carotid, subclavian, or femoral artery, it causes weak or absent arterial pulses distal to the affected area. Absent or diminished pulses occur in 50% of patients with proximal dissection and usually involve the brachiocephalic vessels. Pulse deficits are much less common in patients with distal dissection and tend to involve the left subclavian and femoral arteries. Tearing pain usually develops suddenly in the chest and neck and may radiate to the upper and lower back and abdomen. Other findings include syncope, loss of consciousness, weakness or transient paralysis of the legs or arms, the diastolic murmur of aortic insufficiency, systemic hypotension, and mottled skin below the waist.

Aortic stenosis

With aortic stenosis, the carotid pulse is sustained but weak. Dyspnea (especially paroxysmal dyspnea or dyspnea on exertion), chest pain, and syncope dominate the clinical picture. The patient commonly has an atrial gallop. Other findings include a harsh systolic ejection murmur, crackles, palpitations, fatigue, and narrowed pulse pressure.

Arterial occlusion

With acute occlusion, arterial pulses distal to the obstruction are unilaterally weak and then absent. The affected limb is cool, pale, and cyanotic, with increased capillary refill time, and the patient complains of moderate to severe pain and paresthesia. A line of color and temperature demarcation develops at the level of obstruction. Varying degrees of limb paralysis may also occur, along with intense intermit-

Evaluating peripheral pulses

The rate, amplitude, and symmetry of peripheral pulses provide important clues to cardiac function and the quality of peripheral perfusion. To gather these clues, palpate peripheral pulses lightly with the pads of your index, middle, and ring fingers, as space permits.

4+ = bounding
3+ = normal
2+ = difficult to palpate
1+ = weak, thready
0 = absent.
Use a stick figure to easily document the location and amplitude of all pulses.

RATE

Count all pulses for at least 30 seconds (60 seconds when recording vital signs). The normal rate is between 60 and 100 beats/minute.

SYMMETRY

Simultaneously palpate pulses (except for the carotid pulse) on both sides of the patient's body, and note any inequality. Always assess peripheral pulses methodically, moving from the arms to the legs.

AMPLITUDE

Palpate the blood vessel during ventricular systole. Describe pulse amplitude by using a scale such as the one here:

---

tent claudication. With chronic occlusion, occurring with such disorders as arteriosclerosis and Buerger's disease, pulses in the affected limb weaken gradually.

Cardiac arrhythmias

Cardiac arrhythmias may produce generalized weak pulses accompanied by cool, clammy skin. Other findings reflect the arrhythmia's severity and may include hypotension, chest pain, dyspnea, dizziness, and decreased level of consciousness (LOC).

Cardiac tamponade

Life-threatening cardiac tamponade causes a weak, rapid pulse accompanied by these classic findings: paradoxical pulse, jugular vein distention, hypotension, and muffled heart sounds. Narrowed pulse pressure, pericardial friction rub, and hepatomegaly may also occur. The patient may appear anxious, restless, and cyanotic and may have chest pain, clammy skin, dyspnea, and tachypnea.

Coarctation of the aorta

Findings of this disorder include bounding pulses in the arms and neck, with decreased pulsations and systolic pulse pressure in the lower extremities. Auscultation may reveal a systolic ejection click at the base and apex of the heart and, occasionally, over the carotid arteries that's often accompanied by a systolic ejection murmur at the base.

Peripheral vascular disease

Peripheral vascular disease causes a weakening and loss of peripheral pulses. The patient complains of aching pain distal to the occlusion that worsens with exercise and abates with rest. The skin feels cool and shows decreased hair growth. Impotence may occur in male patients with occlusion in the descending aorta or femoral areas.

(Text continues on page 534.)

Medical causes
(continued)

Cardiac arrhythmias
✦ Generalized weak pulses may accompany cool, clammy skin.

Cardiac tamponade
✦ A weak, rapid pulse accompanies these classic findings: paradoxical pulse, jugular vein distention, hypotension, and muffled heart sounds.
✦ Condition is life-threatening.

Coarctation of the aorta
✦ Bounding pulses occur in the arms and neck, with decreased pulsations and systolic pulse pressure in the lower extremities.

Peripheral vascular disease
✦ A weakening and loss of peripheral pulses occurs.

Managing an absent or weak pulse

An absent or weak pulse can result from any one of several life-threatening disorders. Your evaluation and interventions will vary, depending on whether the weak or absent pulse is generalized or localized to one extremity. They'll also depend on associated signs and symptoms. Use the flowchart below to help you establish priorities for successfully managing this emergency.

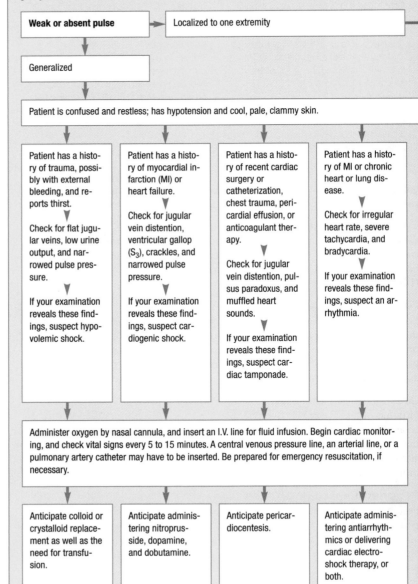

Weak or absent pulse → Localized to one extremity

Generalized

Patient is confused and restless; has hypotension and cool, pale, clammy skin.

Patient has a history of trauma, possibly with external bleeding, and reports thirst.	Patient has a history of myocardial infarction (MI) or heart failure.	Patient has a history of recent cardiac surgery or catheterization, chest trauma, pericardial effusion, or anticoagulant therapy.	Patient has a history of MI or chronic heart or lung disease.
Check for flat jugular veins, low urine output, and narrowed pulse pressure.	Check for jugular vein distention, ventricular gallop (S₃), crackles, and narrowed pulse pressure.	Check for jugular vein distention, pulsus paradoxus, and muffled heart sounds.	Check for irregular heart rate, severe tachycardia, and bradycardia.
If your examination reveals these findings, suspect hypovolemic shock.	If your examination reveals these findings, suspect cardiogenic shock.	If your examination reveals these findings, suspect cardiac tamponade.	If your examination reveals these findings, suspect an arrhythmia.

Administer oxygen by nasal cannula, and insert an I.V. line for fluid infusion. Begin cardiac monitoring, and check vital signs every 5 to 15 minutes. A central venous pressure line, an arterial line, or a pulmonary artery catheter may have to be inserted. Be prepared for emergency resuscitation, if necessary.

Anticipate colloid or crystalloid replacement as well as the need for transfusion.	Anticipate administering nitroprusside, dopamine, and dobutamine.	Anticipate pericardiocentesis.	Anticipate administering antiarrhythmics or delivering cardiac electroshock therapy, or both.

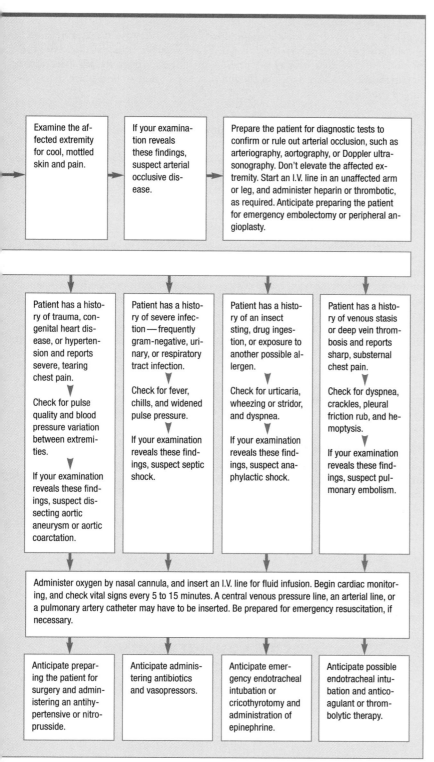

Examine the affected extremity for cool, mottled skin and pain.

If your examination reveals these findings, suspect arterial occlusive disease.

Prepare the patient for diagnostic tests to confirm or rule out arterial occlusion, such as arteriography, aortography, or Doppler ultrasonography. Don't elevate the affected extremity. Start an I.V. line in an unaffected arm or leg, and administer heparin or thrombotic, as required. Anticipate preparing the patient for emergency embolectomy or peripheral angioplasty.

Patient has a history of trauma, congenital heart disease, or hypertension and reports severe, tearing chest pain.

Check for pulse quality and blood pressure variation between extremities.

If your examination reveals these findings, suspect dissecting aortic aneurysm or aortic coarctation.

Patient has a history of severe infection — frequently gram-negative, urinary, or respiratory tract infection.

Check for fever, chills, and widened pulse pressure.

If your examination reveals these findings, suspect septic shock.

Patient has a history of an insect sting, drug ingestion, or exposure to another possible allergen.

Check for urticaria, wheezing or stridor, and dyspnea.

If your examination reveals these findings, suspect anaphylactic shock.

Patient has a history of venous stasis or deep vein thrombosis and reports sharp, substernal chest pain.

Check for dyspnea, crackles, pleural friction rub, and hemoptysis.

If your examination reveals these findings, suspect pulmonary embolism.

Administer oxygen by nasal cannula, and insert an I.V. line for fluid infusion. Begin cardiac monitoring, and check vital signs every 5 to 15 minutes. A central venous pressure line, an arterial line, or a pulmonary artery catheter may have to be inserted. Be prepared for emergency resuscitation, if necessary.

Anticipate preparing the patient for surgery and administering an antihypertensive or nitroprusside.

Anticipate administering antibiotics and vasopressors.

Anticipate emergency endotracheal intubation or cricothyrotomy and administration of epinephrine.

Anticipate possible endotracheal intubation and anticoagulant or thrombolytic therapy.

Medical causes
(continued)

Pulmonary embolism
✦ A generalized weak, rapid pulse occurs.

Shock
✦ With *anaphylactic shock,* pulses become rapid and weak and then uniformly absent within seconds or minutes after exposure to an allergen.
✦ With *cardiogenic shock,* peripheral pulses are absent and central pulses are weak, depending on the degree of vascular collapse.
✦ With *hypovolemic shock,* all peripheral pulses become weak and then uniformly absent, depending on the severity of hypovolemia.
✦ With *septic shock,* all pulses in the extremities first become weak and then become absent.

Thoracic outlet syndrome
✦ Gradual or abrupt weakness or loss of pulses in arms occurs, depending on how quickly vessels in neck compress.
✦ The pulse changes commonly occur after the patient works with his hands above his shoulders, lifts a weight, or abducts his arm.

Other causes
✦ Arteriovenous shunts for dialysis

Special considerations
✦ Monitor vital signs.
✦ Monitor hemodynamic status.

Pulmonary embolism
A pulmonary embolism causes a generalized weak, rapid pulse. It may also cause abrupt onset of chest pain, tachycardia, dyspnea, apprehension, syncope, diaphoresis, and cyanosis. Acute respiratory findings include tachypnea, dyspnea, decreased breath sounds, crackles, a pleural friction rub, and a cough — possibly with blood-tinged sputum.

Shock
With *anaphylactic shock,* pulses become rapid and weak and then uniformly absent within seconds or minutes after exposure to an allergen. This is preceded by hypotension, anxiety, restlessness, feelings of doom, intense itching, a pounding headache and, possibly, urticaria.

With *cardiogenic shock,* peripheral pulses are absent and central pulses are weak, depending on the degree of vascular collapse. Pulse pressure is narrow. Other signs include cold, pale, clammy skin; hypotension; tachycardia; rapid, shallow respirations; oliguria; restlessness; confusion; and obtundation.

With *hypovolemic shock,* all peripheral pulses become weak and then uniformly absent, depending on the severity of hypovolemia. As shock progresses, remaining pulses become thready and more rapid. Early signs of hypovolemic shock include restlessness, thirst, tachypnea, and cool, pale skin. Late signs include hypotension with narrowing pulse pressure, clammy skin, a drop in urine output to less than 25 ml/hour, confusion, decreased LOC and, possibly, hypothermia.

With *septic shock,* all pulses in the extremities first become weak. Depending on the degree of vascular collapse, pulses may then become uniformly absent. Shock is heralded by chills, sudden fever and, possibly, nausea, vomiting, and diarrhea. Typically, the patient experiences tachycardia, tachypnea, and flushed, warm, and dry skin. As shock progresses, he develops thirst, hypotension, anxiety, restlessness, and confusion. Then pulse pressure narrows, and the skin becomes cold, clammy, and cyanotic. The patient experiences severe hypotension, oliguria or anuria, respiratory failure, and coma.

Thoracic outlet syndrome
In thoracic outlet syndrome, the patient may develop gradual or abrupt weakness or loss of the pulses in the arms, depending on how quickly vessels in the neck compress. These pulse changes commonly occur after the patient works with his hands above his shoulders, lifts a weight, or abducts his arm. Paresthesia and pain occur along the ulnar distribution of the arm and disappear as soon as the patient returns his arm to a neutral position. The patient may also have asymmetrical blood pressure and cool, pale skin.

OTHER CAUSES

Treatments
Localized absent pulse may occur distal to arteriovenous shunts for dialysis.

SPECIAL CONSIDERATIONS
Continue to monitor the patient's vital signs to detect untoward changes in his condition. Monitor hemodynamic status by measuring daily weight and hourly or daily intake and output and by assessing central venous pressure.

PEDIATRIC POINTERS

Radial, dorsal pedal, and posterior tibial pulses aren't easily palpable in infants and small children, so be careful not to mistake these normally hard-to-find pulses for weak or absent pulses. Instead, palpate the brachial, popliteal, or femoral pulses to evaluate arterial circulation to the extremities. In children and young adults, weak or absent femoral and more distal pulses may indicate coarctation of the aorta.

PATIENT COUNSELING

Teach the patient how to check his pulse. Advise him to call his health care provider if he has difficulty palpating or is unable to palpate a pulse. Explain the importance of following a low-sodium diet and maintaining fluid restrictions, if necessary. Discuss signs and symptoms of fluid overload to report to the health care provider. Teach the patient to avoid activities that reduce circulation, such as prolonged sitting and crossing the legs.

PULSE, BOUNDING

Produced by large waves of pressure as blood ejects from the left ventricle with each contraction, a bounding pulse is strong and easily palpable and may be visible over superficial peripheral arteries. It's characterized by regular, recurrent expansion and contraction of the arterial walls and isn't obliterated by the pressure of palpation. A healthy person develops a bounding pulse during exercise, pregnancy, and periods of anxiety. However, this sign also results from fever and certain endocrine, hematologic, and cardiovascular disorders that increase the basal metabolic rate.

HISTORY

Ask the patient if he has noticed any weakness, fatigue, shortness of breath, or other health changes. Review his medical history for hyperthyroidism, anemia, or a cardiovascular disorder, and ask about his use of alcohol.

PHYSICAL ASSESSMENT

If you detect a bounding pulse, check other vital signs and then auscultate the heart and lungs for any abnormal sounds, rates, or rhythms. Then complete your cardiovascular assessment.

MEDICAL CAUSES

Alcoholism (acute)

With acute alcoholism, vasodilation produces a rapid, bounding pulse and flushed face. An odor of alcohol on the breath and an ataxic gait are common. Other findings include hypothermia, bradypnea, labored and loud respirations, nausea, vomiting, diuresis, decreased level of consciousness, and seizures.

Anemia

With anemia, a bounding pulse may be accompanied by capillary pulsations, a systolic ejection murmur, tachycardia, an atrial gallop (S_4), a ventricular gallop (S_3), and a systolic bruit over the carotid artery. Other findings include fatigue, pallor, dyspnea and, possibly, bleeding tendencies.

Peds points
+ Radial, dorsal pedal, and posterior tibial pulses aren't easily palpable in infants and small children.
+ In children and young adults, weak or absent femoral and more distal pulses may indicate coarctation of the aorta.

Teaching points
+ Techniques for checking pulse
+ Reporting of pulse changes

Key facts about bounding pulse
+ Produced by large waves of pressure as blood ejects with each left ventricle contraction
+ Easily palpable and may be visible over peripheral arteries

Key history points
+ Weakness, fatigue, shortness of breath, or other health changes
+ History of hyperthyroidism, anemia, or a cardiovascular disorder
+ Alcohol use

Critical assessment steps
+ Check vital signs; then auscultate heart and lungs for abnormal sounds, rates, or rhythms.

Medical causes
Alcoholism (acute)
+ A rapid, bounding pulse and flushed face result from vasodilation.

Anemia
+ Bounding pulse may be accompanied by systolic ejection murmur, tachycardia, and S_4 or S_3 gallop.

Medical causes
(continued)

Aortic insufficiency
+ Bounding pulse is characterized by rapid, forceful expansion of the arterial pulse followed by rapid contraction.
+ Widened pulse pressure also occurs.

Febrile disorder
+ Bounding pulse may occur with fever.

Thyrotoxicosis
+ A rapid, full, bounding pulse occurs along with tachycardia, palpitations, an S_3 or S_4 gallop, weight loss despite increased appetite, and heat intolerance.

Special considerations
+ If bounding pulse is accompanied by rapid or irregular heartbeat, connect the patient to a cardiac monitor for further evaluation.

Peds points
+ A bounding pulse can be normal in infants or children.
+ It can also result from patent ductus arteriosus if the left-to-right shunt is large.

Teaching points
+ Diet
+ Need for rest periods

Aortic insufficiency
Sometimes called a water-hammer pulse, bounding pulse associated with aortic insufficiency is characterized by rapid, forceful expansion of the arterial pulse followed by rapid contraction. Widened pulse pressure also occurs. Acute aortic insufficiency may produce findings associated with left-sided heart failure and cardiovascular collapse, such as weakness, severe dyspnea, hypotension, an S_3, and tachycardia. Additional findings include pallor, chest pain, palpitations, or strong, abrupt carotid pulsations. The patient may also experience pulsus bisferiens, an early systolic murmur, a murmur heard over the femoral artery during systole and diastole, and a high-pitched diastolic murmur that starts with the second heart sound. An apical diastolic rumble (Austin Flint murmur) may also occur, especially with heart failure. Most patients with chronic aortic insufficiency remain asymptomatic until their 40s or 50s, when exertional dyspnea, increased fatigue, orthopnea and, eventually, paroxysmal nocturnal dyspnea, angina, and syncope may develop.

Febrile disorder
Fever can cause a bounding pulse. Accompanying findings reflect the specific disorder but may include fatigue, chills, malaise, anorexia, tachycardia, tachypnea, and diaphoresis.

Thyrotoxicosis
Thyrotoxicosis produces a rapid, full, bounding pulse. Associated findings include tachycardia, palpitations, an S_3 or S_4 gallop, weight loss despite increased appetite, and heat intolerance. The patient may also develop diarrhea, an enlarged thyroid, dyspnea, tremors, nervousness, chest pain, exophthalmos, and signs of cardiovascular collapse. His skin will be warm, moist, and diaphoretic, and he may be hypersensitive to heat.

SPECIAL CONSIDERATIONS
Prepare the patient for diagnostic laboratory and radiographic studies. If a bounding pulse is accompanied by rapid or irregular heartbeat, you may need to connect the patient to a cardiac monitor for further evaluation.

PEDIATRIC POINTERS
A bounding pulse can be normal in infants or children because arteries lie close to the skin surface. It can also result from patent ductus arteriosus if the left-to-right shunt is large.

PATIENT COUNSELING
Counsel the patient about dietary modifications, such as increasing consumption of iron-rich foods for the patient with anemia and reducing sodium intake for the patient with aortic insufficiency. Refer the patient who abuses alcohol to Alcoholics Anonymous (AA), and offer to arrange a visit from an AA member. Encourage frequent rest periods to reduce metabolic demands.

PULSE PRESSURE, NARROWED

Pulse pressure, the difference between systolic and diastolic blood pressures, is measured by sphygmomanometry or intra-arterial monitoring. Normally, systolic pressure exceeds diastolic by about 40 mm Hg. Narrowed pressure—a difference of less than 30 mm Hg—occurs when peripheral vascular resistance increases, cardiac output declines, or intravascular volume markedly decreases. (See *Understanding pulse pressure changes,* page 538.)

With conditions that cause mechanical obstruction, such as aortic stenosis, pulse pressure is directly related to the severity of the underlying condition. Usually a late sign, narrowed pulse pressure alone doesn't signal an emergency, even though it commonly occurs with shock and other life-threatening disorders.

HISTORY

Ask the patient about specific cardiac symptoms, such as chest pain, dizziness, or syncope. Obtain his past medical history, and assess his risk factors for heart disease.

PHYSICAL ASSESSMENT

After you detect a narrowed pulse pressure, check for other signs of heart failure, such as hypotension, tachycardia, dyspnea, jugular vein distention, pulmonary crackles, and decreased urine output. Also check for changes in skin temperature or color, strength of peripheral pulses, and level of consciousness (LOC). Auscultate the heart for murmurs.

MEDICAL CAUSES

Aortic stenosis
Narrowed pulse pressure occurs late in significant stenosis. Aortic stenosis also produces an atrial or ventricular gallop; chest pain; a harsh, systolic ejection murmur; angina; dyspnea; paroxysmal nocturnal dyspnea; and syncope. Crackles, palpitations, fatigue, and diminished carotid pulses may also occur.

Cardiac tamponade
With cardiac tamponade, a life-threatening disorder, pulse pressure narrows by 10 to 20 mm Hg. Paradoxical pulse, jugular vein distention, hypotension, and muffled heart sounds are classic. The patient may be anxious, restless, and cyanotic, with clammy skin and chest pain. He may exhibit dyspnea, tachypnea, decreased LOC, and a weak, rapid pulse. Pericardial friction rub and hepatomegaly may also occur.

Heart failure
Narrowed pulse pressure occurs relatively late in heart failure and may accompany tachypnea, palpitations, dependent edema, steady weight gain despite nausea and anorexia, chest tightness, slowed mental response, hypotension, diaphoresis, pallor, and oliguria. Assessment reveals a ventricular gallop, inspiratory crackles and, possibly, a tender, palpable liver. Later, dullness develops over the lung bases, and hemoptysis, cyanosis, marked hepatomegaly, and marked pitting edema may occur.

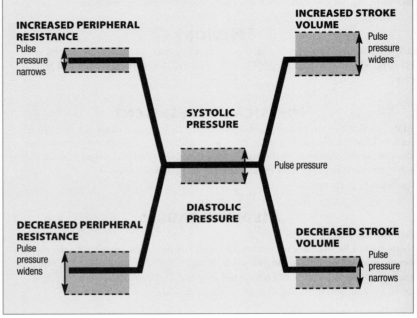

Understanding pulse pressure changes

Two major factors affect pulse pressure: the amount of blood that the ventricles eject into the arteries with each beat—known as *stroke volume*—and the arteries' *peripheral resistance* to blood flow. These two factors affect systolic and diastolic blood pressures and, as a result, pulse pressure. For example, pulse pressure narrows when systolic pressure falls (lower right), diastolic pressure rises (upper left), or both. These changes reflect decreased stroke volume, increased peripheral resistance, or both.

Pulse pressure widens when systolic pressure rises (upper right), diastolic pressure falls (lower left), or both. These changes reflect increased stroke volume, decreased peripheral resistance, or both.

INCREASED PERIPHERAL RESISTANCE
Pulse pressure narrows

INCREASED STROKE VOLUME
Pulse pressure widens

SYSTOLIC PRESSURE

Pulse pressure

DIASTOLIC PRESSURE

DECREASED PERIPHERAL RESISTANCE
Pulse pressure widens

DECREASED STROKE VOLUME
Pulse pressure narrows

Medical causes
(continued)

Shock
+ Narrowed pulse pressure occurs late.
+ Peripheral pulses first become weak and then uniformly absent in anaphylactic, hypovolemic, and septic shock.
+ In cardiogenic shock, peripheral pulses are absent and central pulses are weak.

Shock
With anaphylactic shock, narrowed pulse pressure occurs late, preceded by a rapid, weak pulse that soon becomes uniformly absent. Within seconds or minutes after exposure to an allergen, the patient experiences hypotension, anxiety, restlessness, and feelings of doom, along with intense itching, a pounding headache and, possibly, urticaria. Other findings include dyspnea, stridor, and hoarseness; chest or throat tightness; skin flushing; nausea, abdominal cramps, and urinary incontinence; and seizures.

With cardiogenic shock, narrowed pulse pressure occurs relatively late. Typically, peripheral pulses are absent and central pulses are weak. A drop in systolic pressure to 30 mm Hg below baseline, or a sustained reading below 80 mm Hg not attributable to medication, produces poor tissue perfusion. Poor perfusion produces tachycardia, tachypnea, cyanosis, oliguria, restlessness, confusion, obtundation, and cold, pale, clammy skin.

With hypovolemic shock, narrowed pulse pressure occurs as a late sign. All peripheral pulses become first weak and then uniformly absent. Deepening shock leads to hypotension, urine output of less than 25 ml/hour, confusion, decreased LOC and, possibly, hypothermia.

With septic shock, narrowed pulse pressure is a relatively late sign. All peripheral pulses become first weak and then uniformly absent. As shock progresses, the patient exhibits oliguria, thirst, anxiety, restlessness, confusion, and hypotension. Extremities become cool and cyanotic; the skin becomes cold and clammy. In time, he develops severe hypotension, persistent oliguria or anuria, respiratory failure, and coma.

SPECIAL CONSIDERATIONS

Monitor closely for changes in pulse rate or quality and for hypotension or diminished LOC. Prepare the patient for diagnostic studies, such as echocardiography, to detect valvular heart disease or cardiac tamponade secondary to a pericardial effusion.

PEDIATRIC POINTERS

In children, narrowed pulse pressure can result from congenital aortic stenosis as well as from disorders that affect adults.

PATIENT COUNSELING

Teach the patient about his disorder and its treatments. Explain any dietary and fluid restrictions. If fatigue is a problem, recommend rest periods throughout the day.

PULSE PRESSURE, WIDENED

Pulse pressure is the difference between systolic and diastolic blood pressures. Normally, systolic pressure is about 40 mm Hg higher than diastolic pressure. Widened pulse pressure — a difference of more than 50 mm Hg — commonly occurs as a physiologic response to fever, hot weather, exercise, anxiety, anemia, or pregnancy. However, it can also result from certain neurologic disorders — especially life-threatening increased intracranial pressure (ICP) — or from cardiovascular disorders that cause backflow of blood into the heart with each contraction, such as aortic insufficiency. Widened pulse pressure can easily be identified by monitoring of arterial blood pressure and is commonly detected during routine sphygmomanometric recordings.

EMERGENCY ACTIONS If the patient's level of consciousness (LOC) is decreased, and you suspect that his widened pulse pressure results from increased ICP, check his vital signs. Maintain a patent airway, and prepare to hyperventilate the patient with a handheld resuscitation bag to help reduce partial pressure of carbon dioxide levels and, thus, ICP. Perform a thorough neurologic examination to serve as a baseline for assessing subsequent changes. Use the Glasgow Coma Scale to evaluate the patient's LOC. (See *Glasgow Coma Scale*, page 396.) Also, check cranial nerve function — especially in cranial nerves III, IV, and VI — and assess pupillary reactions, reflexes, and muscle tone. Insertion of an ICP monitor may be necessary. Check for edema and auscultate for murmurs.

Special considerations
+ Monitor closely for changes in pulse rate or quality and for hypotension or diminished LOC.

Peds points
+ In children, narrowed pulse pressure can result from congenital aortic stenosis as well as from disorders that affect adults.

Teaching points
+ The disorder and its treatments
+ Diet and fluid restrictions
+ Rest periods

Key facts about widened pulse pressure
+ Systolic pressure is more than 50 mm Hg higher than diastolic pressure
+ Commonly occurs as a physiologic response to fever, hot weather, exercise, anxiety, anemia, or pregnancy

In an emergency
+ Suspect increased ICP if the patient's LOC is decreased.
+ Check vital signs.
+ Maintain a patent airway, and prepare to hyperventilate the patient with a handheld resuscitation bag.
+ Perform a neurologic examination.
+ Use the Glasgow Coma Scale to evaluate LOC.

Key history points
+ Medical, family, and drug histories
+ Associated symptoms

Critical assessment steps
+ Assess for signs and symptoms of heart failure.
+ Check for changes in skin temperature and color, strength of peripheral pulses, and LOC.
+ Auscultate the heart for murmurs.

Medical causes

Aortic insufficiency
+ Pulse pressure widens progressively as the valve deteriorates.

Arteriosclerosis
+ Pulse pressure widens following moderate hypertension.

Febrile disorders
+ Fever can cause widened pulse pressure.

Increased ICP
+ Widening pulse pressure is an intermediate to late sign of increased ICP.
+ Decreased LOC is the earliest and most sensitive indicator of this life-threatening condition.

Special considerations
+ If the patient displays increased ICP, continually reevaluate his neurologic status.
+ Watch for subtle changes in condition.

HISTORY

Obtain the patient's medical, family, and drug histories. If you don't suspect increased ICP, ask about such associated symptoms as chest pain, shortness of breath, weakness, fatigue, or syncope.

PHYSICAL ASSESSMENT

After you detect a widened pulse pressure, assess for signs and symptoms of heart failure, such as crackles, dyspnea, and jugular vein distention. Also check for changes in skin temperature and color, strength of peripheral pulses, and LOC. Auscultate the heart for murmurs. Check for peripheral edema.

MEDICAL CAUSES

Aortic insufficiency

With acute aortic insufficiency, pulse pressure widens progressively as the valve deteriorates, and a bounding pulse and an atrial gallop or ventricular gallop develop. These signs may be accompanied by chest pain; palpitations; pallor; strong, abrupt carotid pulsations; pulsus bisferiens; and signs of heart failure, such as crackles, dyspnea, and jugular vein distention. Auscultation may reveal several murmurs, such as an early diastolic murmur (common) and an apical diastolic rumble (Austin Flint murmur).

Arteriosclerosis

With arteriosclerosis, pulse pressure progressively widens. This sign is preceded by moderate hypertension and is accompanied by signs of vascular insufficiency, such as claudication, angina, and speech and vision disturbances.

Febrile disorders

Fever can cause widened pulse pressure. Accompanying symptoms vary depending on the specific disorder but may include fatigue, chills, malaise, anorexia, tachycardia, tachypnea, and diaphoresis.

Increased intracranial pressure

Widening pulse pressure is an intermediate to late sign of increased ICP. Although decreased LOC is the earliest and most sensitive indicator of this life-threatening condition, the onset and progression of widening pulse pressure also parallel rising ICP. (Even a gap of only 50 mm Hg can signal a rapid deterioration in the patient's condition.) Assessment reveals Cushing's triad: bradycardia, hypertension, and respiratory pattern changes. Other findings include headache, vomiting, and impaired or unequal motor movement. The patient may also exhibit vision disturbances, such as blurring or photophobia, and pupillary changes.

SPECIAL CONSIDERATIONS

If the patient displays increased ICP, continually reevaluate his neurologic status and compare your findings carefully with those of previous evaluations. Be alert for restlessness, confusion, unresponsiveness, or decreased LOC. Keep in mind, however, that increasing ICP is commonly signaled by subtle changes in the patient's condition, rather than the abrupt development of any one sign or symptom.

PEDIATRIC POINTERS

Increased ICP causes widened pulse pressure in children. Patent ductus arteriosus (PDA) can also cause it, but this sign may not be evident at birth. The older child with PDA experiences exertional dyspnea, with pulse pressure that widens even further on exertion.

GERIATRIC POINTERS

Recently, widened pulse pressure has been found to be a more powerful predictor of cardiovascular events in elderly patients than increased systolic or diastolic blood pressure.

PATIENT COUNSELING

Teach the patient about dietary modifications, such as restricting sodium and saturated fat. Encourage frequent rest periods to reduce metabolic demands. If the patient has a reduced LOC, explain safety measures to him and his family.

PULSE RHYTHM ABNORMALITY

An abnormal pulse rhythm is an irregular expansion and contraction of the peripheral arterial walls. It may be persistent or sporadic, and rhythmic or arrhythmic. Detected by palpating the radial or carotid pulse, an abnormal rhythm is typically reported first by the patient, who complains of feeling palpitations. This important finding reflects an underlying cardiac arrhythmia, which may range from benign to life-threatening. Arrhythmias are commonly associated with cardiovascular, renal, respiratory, metabolic, and neurologic disorders as well as the effects of drugs, diagnostic tests, and treatments. (See *Abnormal pulse rhythm: A clue to cardiac arrhythmias*, pages 542 to 545.)

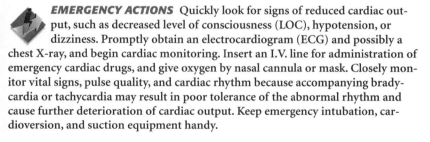 **EMERGENCY ACTIONS** Quickly look for signs of reduced cardiac output, such as decreased level of consciousness (LOC), hypotension, or dizziness. Promptly obtain an electrocardiogram (ECG) and possibly a chest X-ray, and begin cardiac monitoring. Insert an I.V. line for administration of emergency cardiac drugs, and give oxygen by nasal cannula or mask. Closely monitor vital signs, pulse quality, and cardiac rhythm because accompanying bradycardia or tachycardia may result in poor tolerance of the abnormal rhythm and cause further deterioration of cardiac output. Keep emergency intubation, cardioversion, and suction equipment handy.

HISTORY

If the patient's condition permits, ask if he's experiencing pain. If so, find out about onset and location. Does the pain radiate? Ask about a history of heart disease and treatments for arrhythmias. Obtain a drug history and check compliance. Also, ask about any caffeine or alcohol intake. Digoxin toxicity, cessation of an antiarrhythmic, and use of quinidine, a sympathomimetic (such as epinephrine), caffeine, or alcohol may cause arrhythmias.

PHYSICAL ASSESSMENT

Check the patient's apical and peripheral arterial pulses. An apical rate exceeding a peripheral arterial rate indicates a pulse deficit, which may also cause associated signs and symptoms of low cardiac output. Evaluate heart sounds: A long pause between S_1 *(lub)* and S_2 *(dub)* may indicate a conduction defect. A faint or absent S_1 and an easily audible S_2 may indicate atrial fibrillation or flutter. You may hear the two heart sounds close together on certain beats — possibly indicating premature

(Text continues on page 544.)

Abnormal pulse rhythm:
A clue to cardiac arrhythmias

An abnormal pulse rhythm may be your only clue that the patient has a cardiac arrhythmia, but this sign doesn't help you pinpoint the specific type of arrhythmia. For that, you need a cardiac monitor or an electrocardiogram (ECG) machine. These devices record the electrical current generated by the heart's conduction system and display this information on an oscilloscope screen or a strip-chart recorder. Besides rhythm disturbances, they can identify conduction defects and electrolyte imbalances.

The ECG strips below show some common cardiac arrhythmias that can cause abnormal pulse rhythms.

ARRHYTHMIA

Sinus arrhythmia

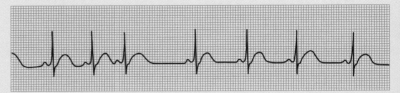

Premature atrial contractions (PACs)

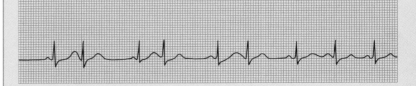

Paroxysmal atrial tachycardia

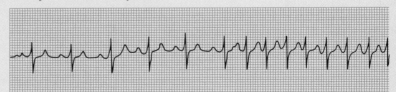

Atrial fibrillation

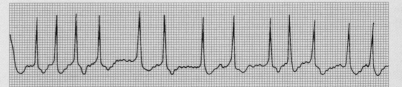

PULSE RHYTHM AND RATE	CLINICAL IMPLICATIONS
Irregular rhythm; fast, slow, or normal rate	✦ Reflex vagal tone inhibition (heart rate increases with inspiration and decreases with expiration) related to normal respiratory cycle ✦ May result from drugs, as in digitalis toxicity ✦ Occurs most often in children and young adults
Irregular rhythm during PACs; fast, slow, or normal rate	✦ Occasional PAC may be normal ✦ Isolated PACs indicate atrial irritation — for example, from anxiety or excessive caffeine intake; increasing PACs may herald other atrial arrhythmias ✦ May result from heart failure, chronic obstructive pulmonary disease (COPD), or use of cardiac glycosides, aminophylline, or an adrenergic
Regular rhythm with abrupt onset and termination of arrhythmia; heart rate exceeding 140 beats/minute	✦ May occur in otherwise normal, healthy persons who are suffering from physical or psychological stress, hypoxia, or digitalis toxicity; who use marijuana; or who consume excessive amounts of caffeine or other stimulants ✦ May precipitate angina or heart failure
Irregular rhythm; atrial rate exceeding 400 beats/minute; ventricular rate varies	✦ May result from heart failure, COPD, hypertension, sepsis, pulmonary embolus, mitral valve disease, atrial irritation, postcoronary bypass, or valve replacement surgery ✦ Preload inconsistent because atria don't contract; cardiac output changes with each beat; emboli may also result

(continued)

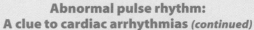

Abnormal pulse rhythm:
A clue to cardiac arrhythmias *(continued)*

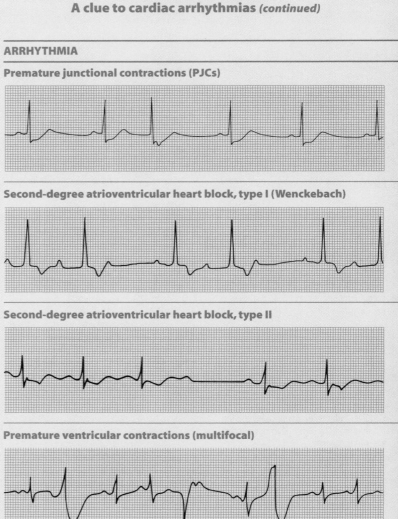

ARRHYTHMIA

Premature junctional contractions (PJCs)

Second-degree atrioventricular heart block, type I (Wenckebach)

Second-degree atrioventricular heart block, type II

Premature ventricular contractions (multifocal)

atrial contractions—or other variations in heart rate or rhythm. Take the patient's apical and radial pulses while you listen for heart sounds. With some arrhythmias, such as premature ventricular contractions, you may hear the beat with your stethoscope but not feel it over the radial artery. This indicates an ineffective contraction that failed to produce a peripheral pulse. Next, count the apical pulse for 60 seconds, noting the frequency of skipped peripheral beats.

PULSE RHYTHM AND RATE	CLINICAL IMPLICATIONS
Irregular rhythm during PJCs; fast, slow, or normal rate	✦ May result from myocardial infarction (MI) or ischemia, excessive caffeine intake or, most commonly, digitalis toxicity (from enhanced automaticity)
Irregular ventricular rhythm; fast, slow, or normal rate	✦ Often transient; may progress to complete heart block ✦ May result from inferior wall MI, digitalis or quinidine toxicity, vagal stimulation, electrolyte imbalance, or arteriosclerotic heart disease
Irregular ventricular rhythm; slow or normal rate	✦ May progress to complete heart block ✦ May result from degenerative disease of conduction system, ischemia of the atrioventricular node in an anterior MI, anteroseptal infarction, electrolyte imbalance, or digitalis or quinidine toxicity
Usually irregular rhythm with a long pause after the premature beat; fast, slow, or normal rate	✦ Arise from different ventricular sites or from the same site with changing patterns of conduction ✦ May result from caffeine or stress, alcohol ingestion, myocardial ischemia or infarction, myocardial irritation by pacemaker electrodes, hypocalcemia, hypercalcemia, digitalis toxicity, or exercise

MEDICAL CAUSES

Cardiac arrhythmias

An abnormal pulse rhythm may be the only sign of a cardiac arrhythmia. The patient may complain of palpitations, a fluttering heartbeat, or weak and skipped beats. Pulses may be weak and rapid or slow. Depending on the specific arrhythmia, dull chest pain or discomfort and hypotension may occur. Associated findings, if any, reflect decreased cardiac output. Neurologic findings, for example, include confusion, dizziness, light-headedness, decreased LOC and, sometimes, seizures. Other findings include decreased urine output, dyspnea, tachypnea, pallor, and diaphoresis.

Medical causes

Cardiac arrhythmias
✦ An abnormal pulse rhythm may be the only sign.
✦ The patient may complain of palpitations, a fluttering heartbeat, or weak and skipped beats.
✦ Dull chest pain or discomfort and hypotension may occur.

Special considerations

+ Sedate patient for cardioversion therapy if indicated.
+ Check vital signs frequently.
+ Collect blood samples for serum electrolyte, cardiac enzyme, and drug level studies.

Peds points

+ Arrhythmias also produce pulse rhythm abnormalities in children.

Teaching points

+ Diary of activities and symptoms
+ Medication compliance

Key facts about pulsus bisferiens

+ Hyperdynamic, double-beating pulse characterized by two systolic peaks separated by midsystolic dip
+ Typically has a taller or more forceful first peak
+ Occurs when a large volume of blood is rapidly ejected from the left ventricle

Key history points

+ History of cardiac disorders
+ Current medications
+ Date of onset of symptoms
+ Factors precipitating symptoms

Critical assessment steps

+ Take vital signs, and auscultate for abnormal heart or breath sounds.
+ Complete the cardiopulmonary assessment.

SPECIAL CONSIDERATIONS

The patient may require cardioversion therapy, before which he may need to be sedated. Prepare the patient for transfer to a cardiac or intensive care unit. To prevent falls and injury, don't leave him unattended while he's sitting or walking. Check vital signs frequently to detect bradycardia, tachycardia, hypertension or hypotension, tachypnea, and dyspnea. Also, monitor intake, output, and daily weight.

Collect blood samples for serum electrolyte, cardiac enzyme, and drug level studies. Prepare the patient for a chest X-ray and a 12-lead ECG. If possible, obtain a previous ECG with which to compare current findings. Prepare the patient for 24-hour Holter monitoring.

PEDIATRIC POINTERS

Arrhythmias also produce pulse rhythm abnormalities in children.

PATIENT COUNSELING

Explain to the patient the importance of keeping a diary of his activities and any symptoms that develop to correlate with the incidence of arrhythmias. Instruct the patient to avoid tobacco and caffeine, which increase arrhythmias. If he has a history of failing to comply with prescribed antiarrhythmic therapy, help him develop strategies to improve compliance.

PULSUS BISFERIENS

A bisferiens pulse is a hyperdynamic, double-beating pulse characterized by two systolic peaks separated by a midsystolic dip. Both peaks may be equal or either may be larger; usually, however, the first peak is taller or more forceful than the second. The first peak (percussion wave) is believed to be the pulse pressure; the second (tidal wave), reverberation from the periphery. Pulsus bisferiens occurs in conditions, such as aortic insufficiency, in which a large volume of blood is rapidly ejected from the left ventricle. The pulse can be palpated in peripheral arteries or observed on an arterial pressure wave recording. (See *Detecting pulsus bisferiens* and *Comparing arterial pressure waves,* page 548.)

HISTORY

After you detect a bisferiens pulse, review the patient's history for cardiac disorders. Next, find out what medication he's taking, if any, and ask if he has any other illnesses. Also ask about the development of any associated signs and symptoms, such as dyspnea, chest pain, or fatigue. Find out how long he has had these symptoms and if they change with activity or rest.

PHYSICAL ASSESSMENT

Take the patient's vital signs, and auscultate for abnormal heart or breath sounds. Then complete the cardiopulmonary assessment.

MEDICAL CAUSES

Aortic insufficiency

Aortic insufficiency is the most common organic cause of bisferiens pulse. Most patients with chronic aortic insufficiency are asymptomatic until ages 40 to 50.

ASSESSMENT TIP

Detecting pulsus bisferiens

To detect pulsus bisferiens, lightly palpate the carotid, brachial, radial, or femoral artery. (The pulse is easiest to palpate in the carotid artery.) At the same time, listen to the patient's heart sounds to determine if the two palpable peaks occur during systole. If they do, you'll feel the double pulse between the first and second heart sounds.

However, exertional dyspnea, worsening fatigue, orthopnea and, eventually, paroxysmal nocturnal dyspnea may develop.

Acute aortic insufficiency may produce signs and symptoms of left-sided heart failure and cardiovascular collapse, such as weakness, severe dyspnea, hypotension, ventricular gallop, and tachycardia. Additional findings include chest pain, palpitations, pallor, and strong, abrupt carotid pulsations. The patient may also exhibit widened pulse pressure and one or more murmurs, especially an apical diastolic rumble (Austin Flint murmur).

Aortic stenosis with aortic insufficiency

A bisferiens pulse is commonly seen in aortic stenosis that's accompanied by moderately severe aortic insufficiency. In aortic stenosis, the pulse rises slowly and the second wave of the double beat is the more forceful one. This disorder is commonly accompanied by dyspnea and fatigue. Chest pain and syncope aren't specific in the combined lesion, but they do suggest predominant aortic stenosis.

High cardiac output states

Pulsus bisferiens commonly occurs with high cardiac output states, such as anemia, thyrotoxicosis, fever, and exercise. Associated findings vary with the underlying cause and may include moderate tachycardia, a cervical venous hum, and widened pulse pressure.

Hypertrophic obstructive cardiomyopathy

About 40% of patients with hypertrophic obstructive cardiomyopathy have pulsus bisferiens because of a pressure gradient in the left ventricular outflow tract. Recorded more often than it's palpated, the pulse rises rapidly, and the first wave is the more forceful one. Associated findings include a systolic murmur, dyspnea, angina, fatigue, and syncope.

SPECIAL CONSIDERATIONS

Prepare the patient for diagnostic tests, such as an electrocardiogram, chest X-ray, cardiac catheterization, or angiography, to help determine the underlying cause of the abnormal pulse.

PEDIATRIC POINTERS

Pulsus bisferiens may be palpated in children with a large patent ductus arteriosus as well as those with congenital aortic stenosis and insufficiency.

PATIENT COUNSELING

Teach the patient about the treatment of the underlying disorder. If the patient complains of fatigue, encourage him to take frequent rest periods throughout the

Medical causes

Aortic insufficiency
✦ Aortic insufficiency is the most common organic cause of bisferiens pulse.

Aortic stenosis with aortic insufficiency
✦ The pulse rises slowly and the second wave of the double beat is the more forceful one.

High cardiac output states
✦ Pulsus bisferiens commonly occurs with high cardiac output states, such as anemia, thyrotoxicosis, fever, and exercise.

Hypertrophic obstructive cardiomyopathy
✦ Pulsus bisferiens occurs in about 40% of patients because of a pressure gradient in the left ventricular outflow tract.

Special considerations
✦ Prepare patient for diagnostic tests.

Peds points
✦ Pulsus bisferiens may be palpated in children with a large patent ductus arteriosus as well as those with congenital aortic stenosis and insufficiency.

Teaching points
✦ Facts about the disorder
✦ Signs and symptoms of heart failure

Comparing arterial pressure waves

The waveforms shown here help differentiate a normal arterial pulse from pulsus alternans, pulsus bisferiens, and pulsus paradoxus.

NORMAL ARTERIAL PULSE

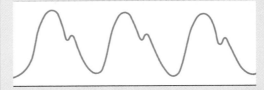

The percussion wave in a *normal arterial pulse* reflects ejection of blood into the aorta (early systole). The tidal wave is the peak of the pulse wave (later systole), and the dicrotic notch marks the beginning of diastole.

PULSUS ALTERNANS

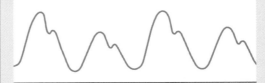

Pulsus alternans is a beat-to-beat alternation in pulse size and intensity. Although the rhythm of pulsus alternans is regular, the volume varies. If you take the blood pressure of a patient with this abnormality, you'll first hear a loud Korotkoff sound and then a soft sound, continually alternating. Pulsus alternans commonly accompanies states of poor contractility that occur with left-sided heart failure.

PULSUS BISFERIENS

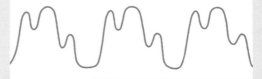

Pulsus bisferiens is a double-beating pulse with two systolic peaks. The first beat reflects pulse pressure; the second, reverberation from the periphery. Pulsus bisferiens commonly occurs with aortic insufficiency (aortic stenosis, aortic regurgitation), hypertrophic cardiomyopathy, or high cardiac output states.

PULSUS PARADOXUS

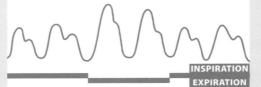

INSPIRATION
EXPIRATION

Pulsus paradoxus is an exaggerated decline in blood pressure during inspiration, resulting from an increase in negative intrathoracic pressure. A pulsus paradoxus that exceeds 10 mm Hg is considered abnormal and may result from cardiac tamponade, constrictive pericarditis, or severe lung disease.

day. Tell the patient to weigh himself daily and to report an increase of more than 3 lb (1.4 kg). Discuss signs and symptoms of heart failure to report to the health care provider.

PULSUS PARADOXUS

Pulsus paradoxus, or paradoxical pulse, is an exaggerated decline in blood pressure during inspiration. Normally, systolic pressure falls less than 10 mm Hg during inspiration. In pulsus paradoxus, it falls more than 10 mm Hg. (See *Comparing arterial pressure waves.*) When systolic pressure falls more than 20 mm Hg, the peripheral pulses may be barely palpable or may disappear during inspiration.

Pulsus paradoxus is thought to result from an exaggerated inspirational increase in negative intrathoracic pressure. Normally, systolic pressure drops during inspiration because of blood pooling in the pulmonary system. This, in turn, reduces left ventricular filling and stroke volume and transmits negative intrathoracic pressure to the aorta. Conditions associated with large intrapleural pressure swings, such as asthma, or those that reduce left-sided heart filling, such as pericardial tamponade, produce pulsus paradoxus. (See *Detecting and measuring pulsus paradoxus,* page 550.)

When you check for pulsus paradoxus, remember that irregular heart rhythms and tachycardia cause variations in pulse amplitude and must be ruled out before a true pulsus paradoxus can be identified.

 EMERGENCY ACTIONS A pulsus paradoxus may signal cardiac tamponade — a life-threatening complication of pericardial effusion that occurs when sufficient blood or fluid accumulates to compress the heart. When you detect pulsus paradoxus, quickly take the patient's other vital signs. Check for additional signs and symptoms of cardiac tamponade, such as dyspnea, tachypnea, diaphoresis, jugular vein distention, tachycardia, narrowed pulse pressure, and hypotension. Emergency pericardiocentesis to aspirate blood or fluid from the pericardial sac may be necessary. Then evaluate the effectiveness of pericardiocentesis by measuring the degree of pulsus paradoxus; it should decrease after aspiration.

HISTORY

If the patient doesn't have cardiac tamponade, find out if he has a history of chronic cardiac or pulmonary disease. Ask about the development of associated signs and symptoms, such as a cough or chest pain.

PHYSICAL ASSESSMENT

Auscultate for abnormal breath sounds. Next, complete your cardiac and pulmonary assessments.

MEDICAL CAUSES

Cardiac tamponade
Pulsus paradoxus commonly occurs with cardiac tamponade, but it may be difficult to detect if intrapericardial pressure rises abruptly and profound hypotension occurs. With severe tamponade, assessment also reveals these classic findings: hypotension, diminished or muffled heart sounds, and jugular vein distention. Related findings include chest pain, pericardial friction rub, narrowed pulse pressure, anxiety, restlessness, clammy skin, and hepatomegaly. Characteristic respiratory

Medical causes
(continued)

COPD
✦ Pulsus paradoxus results from the wide fluctuations in intrathoracic pressure that characterize COPD.
✦ Other findings include dyspnea, tachypnea, wheezing, cough, accessory muscle use, barrel chest, and clubbing.

Pericarditis (chronic constrictive)
✦ Pulsus paradoxus can occur in up to 50% of patients.
✦ Other findings include pericardial friction rub, chest pain, exertional dyspnea, orthopnea, hepatomegaly, and ascites.

Pulmonary embolism (massive)
✦ Pulsus paradoxus results from decreased left ventricular filling and stroke volume.
✦ Severe apprehension, dyspnea, tachypnea, and pleuritic chest pain also occur.

Right ventricular infarction
✦ Pulsus paradoxus may occur with elevated jugular venous or central venous pressure.

ASSESSMENT TIP

Detecting and measuring pulsus paradoxus

To accurately detect and measure pulsus paradoxus, use a sphygmomanometer or an intra-arterial monitoring device. Inflate the blood pressure cuff 10 to 20 mm Hg beyond the peak systolic pressure. Then deflate the cuff at a rate of 2 mm Hg/second until you hear the first Korotkoff sound during expiration. Note the systolic pressure. As you continue to slowly deflate the cuff, observe the patient's respiratory pattern. If a pulsus paradoxus is present, the Korotkoff sounds will disappear with inspiration and return with expiration. Continue to deflate the cuff until you hear Korotkoff sounds during both inspiration and expiration, and again note the systolic pressure. Subtract this reading from the first one to determine the degree of pulsus paradoxus. A difference of more than 10 mm Hg is abnormal.

You can also detect pulsus paradoxus by palpating the radial pulse over several cycles of slow inspiration and expiration. Marked pulse diminution during inspiration indicates pulsus paradoxus.

signs and symptoms include dyspnea, tachypnea, and cyanosis; the patient typically sits up and leans forward to facilitate breathing.

If cardiac tamponade develops gradually, pulsus paradoxus may be accompanied by weakness, anorexia, and weight loss. The patient may also report chest pain, but he won't have muffled heart sounds or severe hypotension.

Chronic obstructive pulmonary disease
The wide fluctuations in intrathoracic pressure that characterize chronic obstructive pulmonary disease (COPD) produce pulsus paradoxus and possibly tachycardia. Other findings vary but may include dyspnea, tachypnea, wheezing, productive or nonproductive cough, accessory muscle use, barrel chest, and clubbing. The patient may show labored, pursed-lip breathing after exertion or even at rest. Auscultation reveals decreased breath sounds, rhonchi, and crackles. Weight loss, cyanosis, and edema may occur.

Pericarditis (chronic constrictive)
Pulsus paradoxus can occur in up to 50% of patients with chronic constrictive pericarditis. Other findings include pericardial friction rub, chest pain, exertional dyspnea, orthopnea, hepatomegaly, and ascites. The patient also exhibits peripheral edema and Kussmaul's sign — jugular vein distention that becomes more prominent on inspiration.

Pulmonary embolism (massive)
Decreased left ventricular filling and stroke volume in massive pulmonary embolism produce pulsus paradoxus as well as syncope and severe apprehension, dyspnea, tachypnea, and pleuritic chest pain. The patient appears cyanotic, with jugular vein distention. He may succumb to circulatory collapse, with hypotension and a weak, rapid pulse. Pulmonary infarction may produce hemoptysis along with decreased breath sounds and a pleural friction rub over the affected area.

Right ventricular infarction
Right ventricular infarction may produce pulsus paradoxus and elevated jugular venous or central venous pressure. Other findings are similar to those of myocardial infarction. Signs of right-sided heart failure may occur, such as distended neck veins, hepatomegaly, and peripheral edema.

SPECIAL CONSIDERATIONS

Prepare the patient for an echocardiogram to visualize cardiac motion and to help determine the causative disorder. Also, monitor his vital signs and frequently check the degree of paradox. An increase in the degree of paradox may indicate recurring or worsening cardiac tamponade or impending respiratory arrest in severe COPD. Vigorous respiratory treatment, such as chest physiotherapy, may avert the need for endotracheal intubation.

PEDIATRIC POINTERS

Pulsus paradoxus commonly occurs in children with chronic pulmonary disease, especially during an acute asthma attack. Children with pericarditis may also develop pulsus paradoxus because of cardiac tamponade, although this disorder more commonly affects adults. A pulsus paradoxus above 20 mm Hg is a reliable indicator of cardiac tamponade in children; a change of 10 to 20 mm Hg is equivocal.

PATIENT COUNSELING

Review self-care techniques with the patient with COPD, such as pursed-lip, diaphragmatic breathing; coughing and deep-breathing exercises; and proper use of home oxygen equipment. If the patient requires pericardiocentesis, explain the procedure to him and help ease his anxiety.

PUPILS, NONREACTIVE

Nonreactive (fixed) pupils fail to constrict in response to light or to dilate when the light is removed. The development of a unilateral or bilateral nonreactive response indicates an important change in the patient's condition and may signal a life-threatening emergency and possibly brain death. It also occurs with use of certain optic drugs. (See *Assessing pupillary reaction*, page 552.)

A unilateral or bilateral nonreactive response indicates dysfunction of cranial nerves II and III, which mediate the pupillary light reflex. (See *Innervation of direct and consensual light reflexes*, page 553.)

 EMERGENCY ACTIONS If the patient is unconscious and develops unilateral or bilateral nonreactive pupils, quickly take his vital signs. Be alert for decerebrate or decorticate posture, bradycardia, elevated systolic blood pressure, widened pulse pressure, and the development of other untoward changes in the patient's condition. Remember, a unilateral dilated, nonreactive pupil may be an early sign of uncal brain herniation. Emergency surgery to decrease intracranial pressure (ICP) may be necessary. If the patient isn't already being treated for increased ICP, insert an I.V. line to administer a diuretic, an osmotic, or a corticosteroid. You may also need to start the patient on controlled hyperventilation.

HISTORY

If the patient is conscious, obtain a brief history. Ask him what type of eyedrops he's using, if any, and when they were last instilled. Also ask if he's experiencing any pain and, if so, try to determine its location, intensity, and duration.

Critical assessment steps

+ Check visual acuity in both eyes.
+ Test the pupillary reaction to accommodation.
+ Examine the cornea and iris for abnormalities.
+ Measure IOP.
+ Cover the affected eye with a protective metal shield.

Medical causes

Botulism

+ Nonreactive pupils and bilateral mydriasis usually appear 12 to 36 hours after ingestion of tainted food.
+ Other findings include blurred vision, diplopia, ptosis, strabismus, and extraocular muscle palsies.

Encephalitis

+ Initially sluggish pupils become dilated and nonreactive.
+ Decreased accommodation and other symptoms of cranial nerve palsies develop.
+ A decreased LOC, high fever, headache, vomiting, and nuchal rigidity occur within 48 hours.

Glaucoma (acute angle–closure)

+ Moderately dilated, nonreactive pupil occurs in the affected eye.
+ Sudden blurred vision, followed by excruciating pain in and around the affected eye occurs.
+ Patients commonly report seeing halos around white lights at night.

Assessing pupillary reaction

To evaluate pupillary reaction to light, first test the patient's direct light reflex. Darken the room, and cover one of the patient's eyes while you hold open the opposite eyelid. Using a bright penlight, bring the light toward the patient from the side and shine it directly into his opened eye. If normal, the pupil will promptly constrict. Next, test the consensual light reflex. Hold the patient's eyelids open, and shine the light into one eye while watching the pupil of the opposite eye. If normal, both pupils will promptly constrict. Repeat both procedures in the opposite eye.

PHYSICAL ASSESSMENT

Check the patient's visual acuity in both eyes. Then test the pupillary reaction to accommodation: Normally, both pupils constrict equally as the patient shifts his glance from a distant to a near object.

Next, hold a penlight at the side of each eye and examine the cornea and iris for any abnormalities. Measure intraocular pressure (IOP) with a tonometer, or estimate IOP by placing your second and third fingers over the patient's closed eyelid. If the eyeball feels rock hard, suspect elevated IOP. Ophthalmoscopic and slit-lamp examinations of the eye will need to be performed. If the patient has experienced ocular trauma, don't manipulate the affected eye. After the examination, be sure to cover the affected eye with a protective metal shield, but don't let the shield rest on the globe.

MEDICAL CAUSES

Botulism

Bilateral mydriasis and nonreactive pupils usually appear 12 to 36 hours after ingestion of tainted food. Other early findings of botulism include blurred vision, diplopia, ptosis, strabismus, and extraocular muscle palsies, along with anorexia, nausea, vomiting, diarrhea, and dry mouth. Vertigo, deafness, hoarseness, nasal voice, dysarthria, and dysphagia follow. Progressive muscle weakness and absent deep tendon reflexes usually evolve over 2 to 4 days, resulting in severe constipation and paralysis of respiratory muscles with respiratory distress.

Encephalitis

As encephalitis progresses, initially sluggish pupils become dilated and nonreactive. Decreased accommodation and other symptoms of cranial nerve palsies, such as dysphagia, develop. Within 48 hours after onset, encephalitis causes a decreased level of consciousness, high fever, headache, vomiting, and nuchal rigidity. Aphasia, ataxia, nystagmus, hemiparesis, and photophobia may occur with seizures.

Glaucoma (acute angle-closure)

Acute angle-closure glaucoma is an ophthalmic emergency that upon examination reveals a moderately dilated, nonreactive pupil in the affected eye. Conjunctival injection, corneal clouding, and decreased visual acuity also occur. The patient with acute angle-closure glaucoma experiences sudden onset of blurred vision, followed by excruciating pain in and around the affected eye. He commonly reports seeing halos around white lights at night. Severely elevated IOP commonly induces nausea and vomiting.

Innervation of direct and consensual light reflexes

Two reactions — direct and consensual — constitute the pupillary light reflex. Normally, when a light is shined directly onto the retina of one eye, the parasympathetic nerves are stimulated to cause brisk constriction of that pupil — the *direct light reflex*. The pupil of the opposite eye also constricts — the *consensual light reflex*.

The optic nerve (CN II) mediates the afferent arc of this reflex from each eye, whereas the oculomotor nerve (CN III) mediates the efferent arc to both eyes. A nonreactive or sluggish response in one or both pupils indicates dysfunction of these cranial nerves, usually due to degenerative disease of the central nervous system.

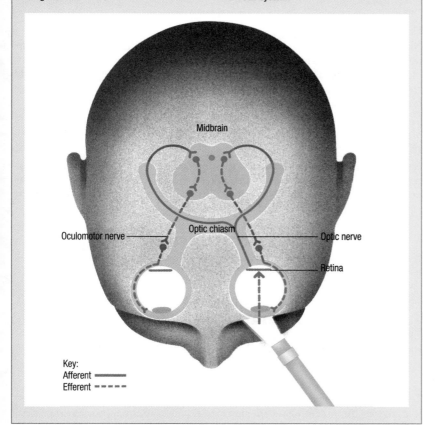

Midbrain

Oculomotor nerve

Optic chiasm

Optic nerve

Retina

Key:
Afferent ——————
Efferent – – – – –

Ocular trauma

Severe damage to the iris or optic nerve may produce a nonreactive, dilated pupil in the affected eye (traumatic iridoplegia). This sign is usually transitory but can be permanent. Slit-lamp examination commonly reveals a V-shaped notch in the pupillary rim, indicating a tear in the iris sphincter muscle. The patient usually experiences eye pain and may also develop eye edema and ecchymoses.

Oculomotor nerve palsy

Commonly, the first signs of this oculomotor ophthalmoplegia are a dilated, nonreactive pupil and loss of the accommodation reaction. These findings may occur in one eye or both, depending on whether the palsy is unilateral or bilateral.

Medical causes
(continued)

Ocular trauma
+ A nonreactive, dilated pupil may result from severe damage to the iris or optic nerve.
+ This sign is usually transitory but can be permanent.

Oculomotor nerve palsy
+ A dilated, nonreactive pupil and loss of the accommodation reaction is the first sign.
+ Findings may occur in one eye or both.
+ Symptom may signal life-threatening brain herniation.

Medical causes
(continued)

Uveitis
+ In anterior uveitis, a small, non-reactive pupil appears suddenly and is accompanied by severe eye pain, conjunctival injection, and photophobia.
+ With posterior uveitis, similar features develop insidiously.

Wernicke's disease
+ Nonreactive pupils occur late in disease.
+ Initial symptoms include an intention tremor accompanied by a sluggish pupillary reaction.

Other causes
+ Topical mydriatic or cycloplegic
+ Opiates
+ Atropine poisoning

Special considerations
+ If the patient is conscious, monitor his pupillary light reflex.

Peds points
+ The most common cause of nonreactive pupils in children is oculomotor nerve palsy from increased ICP.

Teaching points
+ Methods for instilling eye drops
+ Follow-up care

Key facts about sluggish pupils
+ Abnormally slow pupillary response to light
+ Can occur in one pupil or both
+ Indicates dysfunction of CNs II and III

Among the causes of total third cranial nerve palsy is life-threatening brain herniation. Central herniation causes bilateral midposition nonreactive pupils, whereas uncal herniation initially causes a unilateral dilated, nonreactive pupil. Other common findings include diplopia, ptosis, outward deviation of the eye, and inability to elevate or adduct the eye. Additional findings depend on the underlying cause of the palsy.

Uveitis
In anterior uveitis, a small, nonreactive pupil appears suddenly and is accompanied by severe eye pain, conjunctival injection, and photophobia. With posterior uveitis, similar features develop insidiously, along with blurred vision and distorted pupil shape.

Wernicke's disease
Nonreactive pupils are a late sign in Wernicke's disease, which initially produces an intention tremor accompanied by a sluggish pupillary reaction. Other ocular findings include diplopia, gaze paralysis, nystagmus, ptosis, decreased visual acuity, and conjunctival injection. The patient may also exhibit orthostatic hypotension, tachycardia, ataxia, apathy, and confusion.

OTHER CAUSES

Drugs
Instillation of a topical mydriatic and a cycloplegic may induce a temporarily nonreactive pupil in the affected eye. Opiates, such as heroin and morphine, cause pinpoint pupils with a minimal light response that can be seen only with a magnifying glass. Atropine poisoning produces widely dilated, nonreactive pupils.

SPECIAL CONSIDERATIONS
If the patient is conscious, monitor his pupillary light reflex to detect changes. If he's unconscious, close his eyes to prevent corneal exposure. (Use tape to secure the eyelids, if needed.)

PEDIATRIC POINTERS
Children have nonreactive pupils for the same reasons as adults. The most common cause is oculomotor nerve palsy from increased ICP.

PATIENT COUNSELING
Teach the patient the proper method for instilling eyedrops. If photophobia is present, suggest the patient wear dark glasses to ease discomfort. Stress the importance of follow-up care to check IOP.

PUPILS, SLUGGISH

A sluggish pupillary reaction is an abnormally slow pupillary response to light. It can occur in one pupil or both, unlike the normal reaction, which is always bilateral. A sluggish reaction accompanies degenerative disease of the central nervous system and diabetic neuropathy. It can occur normally in elderly people, whose pupils become smaller and less responsive with age.

A sluggish reaction in one or both pupils indicates dysfunction of cranial nerves (CNs) II and III, which mediate the pupillary light reflex. (See *Innervation of direct and consensual light reflexes,* page 553.)

HISTORY

If the patient is conscious, obtain a brief history. Ask him what type of eyedrops he's using, if any, and when they were last instilled. Also ask if he's experiencing pain or other ocular symptoms.

PHYSICAL ASSESSMENT

If you detect a sluggish pupillary reaction, determine the patient's visual function. Start by testing visual acuity in both eyes. Then test the pupillary reaction to accommodation; the pupils should constrict equally as the patient shifts his glance from a distant to a near object.

Next, hold a penlight at the side of each eye and examine the cornea and iris for irregularities, scars, and foreign bodies. Measure intraocular pressure (IOP) with a tonometer, or estimate IOP by placing your fingers over the patient's closed eyelid. If the eyeball feels rock hard, suspect elevated IOP. Also, ophthalmoscopic and slit-lamp examinations of the eye will need to be performed.

MEDICAL CAUSES

Diabetic neuropathy

A patient with long-standing diabetes mellitus may have a sluggish pupillary response. Additional findings include orthostatic hypotension, syncope, dysphagia, episodic constipation or diarrhea, painless bladder distention with overflow incontinence, retrograde ejaculation, and impotence.

Encephalitis

Encephalitis initially produces a bilateral sluggish pupillary response. Later, pupils become dilated and nonreactive, and decreased accommodation may occur, along with other cranial nerve palsies, such as dysphagia and facial weakness. Within 24 to 48 hours after onset, encephalitis causes a decreased level of consciousness, headache, high fever, vomiting, and nuchal rigidity. Also, aphasia, ataxia, nystagmus, hemiparesis, and photophobia may occur. The patient may exhibit seizure activity and myoclonic jerks.

Herpes zoster

The patient with herpes zoster affecting the nasociliary nerve may have a sluggish pupillary response. Examination of the conjunctiva reveals follicles. Additional ocular findings include a serous discharge, absence of tears, ptosis, and extraocular muscle palsy.

Iritis (acute)

With acute iritis, the affected eye exhibits a sluggish pupillary response and conjunctival injection. The pupil may remain constricted; if posterior synechiae have formed, the pupil will also be irregularly shaped. The patient reports sudden onset of eye pain and photophobia and may also have blurred vision.

Multiple sclerosis

Multiple sclerosis may produce small, irregularly shaped pupils that react better to accommodation than to light. Additional ocular findings may include ptosis, nystagmus, diplopia, and blurred vision. In most patients, vision problems and sensory impairment, such as paresthesia, are the earliest indications. Later, various features may develop, including muscle weakness and paralysis; intention tremor, spasticity, hyperreflexia, and gait ataxia; dysphagia and dysarthria; constipation; urinary urgency, frequency, and incontinence; impotence; and emotional instability.

Key history points
+ Medical history
+ Eyedrop use
+ Pain

Critical assessment steps
+ Test visual acuity and the pupillary reaction to accommodation.
+ Examine the cornea and iris for irregularities, scars, and foreign bodies.
+ Measure IOP.

Medical causes

Diabetic neuropathy
+ Sluggish pupillary response may occur with long-standing disease.

Encephalitis
+ Bilateral sluggish pupillary response is an initial symptom.
+ Later, pupils become dilated and nonreactive, and decreased accommodation may occur.

Herpes zoster
+ A sluggish pupillary response may occur if herpes zoster affects the nasociliary nerve.

Iritis (acute)
+ A sluggish pupillary response and conjunctival injection occurs in the affected eye.
+ The pupil may remain constricted.

Multiple sclerosis
+ Small, irregularly shaped pupils that react better to accommodation than to light may occur.
+ Additional ocular findings may include ptosis, nystagmus, diplopia, and blurred vision.

Medical causes

Myotonic dystrophy

+ Sluggish pupillary reaction may be accompanied by lid lag, ptosis, miosis and, possibly, diplopia.

Wernicke's disease

+ An intention tremor accompanied by a sluggish pupillary reaction is an early sign.
+ Additional ocular findings include diplopia, gaze paralysis, nystagmus, ptosis, decreased visual acuity, and conjunctival injection.

Special considerations

+ A sluggish pupillary reaction isn't diagnostically significant.

Peds points

+ Children experience sluggish pupillary reactions for the same reasons as adults.

Teaching points

+ Regular ophthalmologic exams
+ Facts about disease

Key facts about purpura

+ Extravasation of RBCs from the blood vessels into the skin, subcutaneous tissue, or mucous membranes
+ Involves easily-visible purplish or brownish red discolorations
+ Fails to blanch with pressure

Key history points

+ Onset and location of lesions
+ Drug history
+ History of easy bleeding
+ Recent illnesses or trauma

Myotonic dystrophy

With myotonic dystrophy, sluggish pupillary reaction may be accompanied by lid lag, ptosis, miosis and, possibly, diplopia. The patient may develop decreased visual acuity from cataract formation. Muscular weakness and atrophy and testicular atrophy may occur.

Wernicke's disease

Initially, Wernicke's disease produces an intention tremor accompanied by a sluggish pupillary reaction. Later, pupils may become nonreactive. Additional ocular findings include diplopia, gaze paralysis, nystagmus, ptosis, decreased visual acuity, and conjunctival injection. The patient may also exhibit orthostatic hypotension, tachycardia, ataxia, apathy, and confusion.

SPECIAL CONSIDERATIONS

A sluggish pupillary reaction isn't diagnostically significant, although it occurs with various disorders.

PEDIATRIC POINTERS

Children experience sluggish pupillary reactions for the same reasons as adults.

PATIENT COUNSELING

Encourage the patient with chronic illness to have regular ophthalmologic examinations to detect complications. Teach him about the course of his disease and the importance of avoiding stress, infection, and fatigue.

PURPURA

Purpura is the extravasation of red blood cells from the blood vessels into the skin, subcutaneous tissue, or mucous membranes. It's characterized by discoloration that's easily visible through the epidermis, usually purplish or brownish red. Purpuric lesions include petechiae, ecchymoses, and hematomas. (See *Identifying purpuric lesions*.) Purpura differs from erythema in that it doesn't blanch with pressure, because it involves blood in the tissues, not just dilated vessels.

Purpura results from damage to the endothelium of small blood vessels, a coagulation defect, ineffective perivascular support, capillary fragility and permeability, or a combination of these factors. These faulty hemostatic factors, in turn, can result from thrombocytopenia or another hematologic disorder, an invasive procedure or, of course, the use of an anticoagulant.

Additional causes are nonpathologic. Prolonged coughing or vomiting can produce crops of petechiae in loose face and neck tissue. Violent muscle contraction, as occurs in seizures or weight lifting, sometimes results in localized ecchymoses from increased intraluminal pressure and rupture. High fever, which increases capillary fragility, can also produce purpura.

HISTORY

Ask the patient when he first noticed the lesion and whether he has noticed other lesions on his body. Does he or his family have a history of a bleeding disorder or easy bruising? Find out what medications he's taking, if any, and ask him to describe his diet. Ask about recent trauma or transfusions and the development of associated signs, such as epistaxis, bleeding gums, hematuria, and hematochezia. Also

ASSESSMENT TIP

Identifying purpuric lesions

Purpuric lesions fall into three categories: petechiae, ecchymoses, and hematomas. Use the illustrations and the figures below to help you accurately identify purpuric lesions in your patients.

PETECHIAE
Petechiae are painless, round, pinpoint lesions, 1 to 3 mm in diameter. Caused by extravasation of red blood cells into cutaneous tissue, these red or brown lesions usually arise on dependent portions of the body. They appear and fade in crops and can group to form ecchymoses.

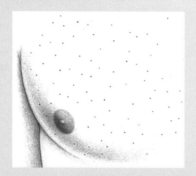

ECCHYMOSES
Ecchymoses, another form of blood extravasation, are larger than petechiae. These purple, blue, or yellow-green bruises vary in size and shape and can arise anywhere on the body as a result of trauma. Ecchymoses usually appear on the arms and legs of patients with bleeding disorders.

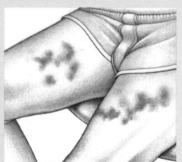

HEMATOMAS
Hematomas are palpable ecchymoses that are painful and swollen. Usually the result of trauma, superficial hematomas are red, whereas deep hematomas are blue. Hematomas commonly exceed 1 cm in diameter, but their size varies widely.

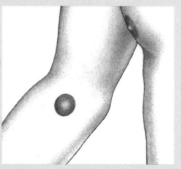

ask about systemic complaints that may suggest infection, such as fever. If the patient is female, ask about heavy menstrual flow.

CULTURAL CUE Make sure to ask your patient if he uses any type of folk medicine. Coin rubbing, practiced by cultures such as the Vietnamese, may produce ecchymoses on the back and abdomen; these marks may be misdiagnosed as abuse.

Critical assessment steps

+ Inspect the entire skin surface and mucous membranes.

Medical causes

Cholesterol emboli

+ Purpura typically occur in the lower extremities of patients with atherosclerotic vascular disease following anticoagulation therapy or an invasive arterial procedure.

DIC

+ Purpura occurs in varying degrees.
+ Cutaneous oozing, hematemesis, or bleeding from incision or needle insertion sites may occur.

Dysproteinemias

+ Petechiae and ecchymoses occur along with bleeding tendencies in multiple myeloma and cryoglobulinemia.

Easy bruising syndrome

+ Recurrent bruising on the legs, arms, and trunk, either spontaneously or following minor trauma, is a characteristic sign.

Fat emboli

+ Petechiae occur on the upper body a few days after a major injury.
+ Other findings include tachycardia, tachypnea, blood-tinged sputum, cyanosis, altered LOC, seizures, coma, or rash.

ITP

+ Scattered petechiae on the distal arms and legs is an early sign.
+ Deep-lying ecchymoses may also occur.

PHYSICAL ASSESSMENT

Inspect the patient's entire skin surface to determine the type, size, location, distribution, and severity of purpuric lesions. Also inspect the mucous membranes. Remember that the same mechanisms that cause purpura can also cause internal hemorrhage, although purpura isn't a cardinal indicator of this condition.

MEDICAL CAUSES

Cholesterol emboli

Purpura caused by cholesterol emboli are most commonly found in the lower extremities of patients with atherosclerotic vascular disease and usually occur after anticoagulation therapy or an invasive arterial procedure, such as angiogram or cardiac catheterization; however, they may occur spontaneously. Associated findings include livedo reticularis, cyanosis, gangrene, nodules, and ulceration of the skin.

Disseminated intravascular coagulation

Disseminated intravascular coagulation (DIC) can cause varying degrees of purpura, depending on its severity and underlying cause. The patient may have cutaneous oozing, hematemesis, or bleeding from incision or needle insertion sites. Other findings include acrocyanosis; nausea; dyspnea; seizures; severe muscle, back, and abdominal pain; and signs of acute tubular necrosis, such as oliguria.

Dysproteinemias

With multiple myeloma, petechiae and ecchymoses accompany other bleeding tendencies: hematemesis, epistaxis, gum bleeding, and excessive bleeding after surgery. Similar findings occur with cryoglobulinemia, which may also produce malignant maculopapular purpura. Hyperglobulinemia typically begins insidiously with occasional outbreaks of purpura over the lower legs and feet. These outbreaks eventually become more frequent and extensive, involving the entire lower leg and possibly the trunk. The purpura usually occurs after prolonged standing or exercise and may be heralded by skin burning or stinging. Leg edema, knee or ankle pain, and low-grade fever may precede or accompany the purpura, which gradually fades over 1 to 2 weeks. Persistent pigmentation develops after repeated outbreaks.

Easy bruising syndrome

Easy bruising syndrome is characterized by recurrent bruising on the legs, arms, and trunk, either spontaneously or following minor trauma. Bruising may be preceded by pain and is more common in women than in men, especially during menses.

Fat emboli

Petechiae that occur on the upper body a few days after a major injury are caused by fat emboli. The patient may experience fever, tachycardia, tachypnea, blood-tinged sputum, cyanosis, anxiety, restlessness, altered level of consciousness, seizures, coma, or rash.

Idiopathic thrombocytopenic purpura

Chronic idiopathic thrombocytopenic purpura (ITP) typically begins insidiously, with scattered petechiae that are usually found on the distal arms and legs. Deep-lying ecchymoses may also occur. Other findings include epistaxis, easy bruising, hematuria, hematemesis, and menorrhagia.

Leukemia

Leukemia produces widespread petechiae on the skin, mucous membranes, retina, and serosal surfaces that persist throughout the course of the disease. The patient may also exhibit swollen and bleeding gums, epistaxis, and other bleeding tendencies. Lymphadenopathy and splenomegaly are common.

Acute leukemias also produce severe prostration and high fever and may cause dyspnea, tachycardia, palpitations, and abdominal or bone pain. Confusion, headache, seizures, vomiting, papilledema, and nuchal rigidity may occur late in the disease. Chronic leukemias begin insidiously with minor bleeding tendencies, malaise, fatigue, pallor, low-grade fever, anorexia, and weight loss.

Liver disease

Hepatic disease may cause purpura, particularly ecchymoses, and other bleeding tendencies. Associated findings include hepatomegaly, ascites, right-upper-quadrant pain, jaundice, nausea, vomiting, and anorexia.

Meningococcemia

With meningococcemia, cutaneous and oropharyngeal petechia and purpura are initially discrete but become confluent, developing into hemorrhagic bullae and ulcerations. Fulminant infection results in extensive purpura and ecchymosis with irregular borders (purpura fulminans), most notably on the extremities. These lesions may develop necrotic centers. Associated symptoms include spiking fevers, chills, myalgia and arthralgia, and recent upper respiratory tract infection. Rapid progression of symptoms leads to headache, neck stiffness, and nuchal rigidity. Septic shock ensues within hours of onset of symptoms, accompanied by altered mental status and hypotension.

Myeloproliferative disorders

Myeloproliferative disorders, which include polycythemia vera, paradoxically can cause hemorrhage accompanied by ecchymoses and ruddy cyanosis. The oral mucosa takes on a deep purplish red hue, and slight trauma causes swollen gums to bleed. Other findings include pruritus, urticaria, and such nonspecific signs and symptoms as lethargy, weakness, fatigue, and weight loss. The patient typically complains of headache, a sensation of fullness in the head, and rushing in the ears; dizziness and vertigo; dyspnea; paresthesia of the fingers; double or blurred vision and scotoma; and epigastric distress. He may also experience intermittent claudication, hypertension, hepatosplenomegaly, and impaired mentation.

Nutritional deficiencies

With vitamin C deficiency (scurvy), the characteristic pattern of purpura is perifollicular petechiae, which coalesce to form ecchymoses, in the "saddle area" of the thighs and buttocks. Additional hemorrhaging occurs in arm and leg muscles (with phlebothrombosis), viscera, joints (with limb and joint pain), and nail beds. Related findings include scaly dermatitis; pallor; tender, swollen, bleeding gums and loosened teeth; dry mouth; and poor wound healing. Nonspecific symptoms include weakness, lethargy, and anorexia. Irritability, depression, insomnia, and hysteria may also develop.

Vitamin K deficiency produces abnormal bleeding tendencies, such as ecchymosis, gum bleeding, epistaxis, hematuria, and GI and intracranial bleeding.

Vitamin B_{12} deficiency can cause varying degrees of purpura. GI findings include anorexia, nausea, vomiting, weight loss, abdominal discomfort, and jaundice. Dyspnea, peripheral neuropathies, ataxia, glossitis and, occasionally, depression also occur.

Medical causes
(continued)

Leukemia
✦ Widespread, persistent petechiae appear on the skin, mucous membranes, retina, and serosal surfaces.

Liver disease
✦ Purpura, particularly ecchymoses, and other bleeding tendencies may occur.

Meningococcemia
✦ Cutaneous and oropharyngeal petechia and purpura are initially discrete but become confluent, developing into hemorrhagic bullae and ulcerations.
✦ Fulminant infection results in extensive purpura and ecchymosis with irregular borders, most notably on the extremities.

Myeloproliferative disorders
✦ Hemorrhage accompanied by ecchymoses and ruddy cyanosis can occur.
✦ The oral mucosa takes on a deep purplish red hue, and slight trauma causes swollen gums to bleed.

Nutritional deficiencies
✦ With vitamin C deficiency, purpura coalesces to form ecchymoses in the "saddle area" of the thighs and buttocks.
✦ Vitamin K deficiency produces abnormal bleeding tendencies, such as ecchymosis, gum bleeding, epistaxis, and hematuria.
✦ Vitamin B_{12} and folic acid deficiencies can cause varying degrees of purpura.

Medical causes
(continued)

Rocky Mountain spotted fever
✦ Initial skin lesions are small pink macules that evolve into blatant petechia and palpable purpura.
✦ The palms and soles are particularly affected.

Septicemia
✦ Purpura, especially in the form of petechiae, may result from thrombocytopenia or the effects of toxins.

SLE
✦ Purpura may occur with other cutaneous findings.
✦ Characteristic "butterfly rash" appears in the disorder's acute phase.

Trauma
✦ Local or widespread purpura may occur.

Other causes
✦ Invasive diagnostic procedures
✦ Anticoagulants
✦ Procedures that disrupt circulation

Folic acid deficiency also can cause varying degrees of purpura. The patient may be irritable and forgetful and may complain of fatigue, weakness, dyspnea, palpitations, nausea, anorexia, headaches, and fainting spells. Additional findings include pallor, slight jaundice, and glossitis.

Rocky Mountain spotted fever
The initial skin lesions of Rocky Mountain spotted fever are small pink macules that evolve into blatant petechia and palpable purpura. Hemorrhagic macules may develop. The palms and soles are particularly affected. Extensive cutaneous necrosis occurs in a small percentage of patients experiencing gangrene of the extremities, necessitating amputation. Associated signs and symptoms include fever, severe headache, generalized myalgia, photophobia, nausea, and vomiting. Late in the course of the illness, shock and death may occur.

Septicemia
Thrombocytopenia or the effects of toxins in acute infection can lead to purpura, especially in the form of petechiae. Associated findings include fever, chills, headache, tachycardia, lethargy, diaphoresis, and anorexia. Signs and symptoms specific to the area of infection — for example, cough, wound drainage, and urinary burning — also occur.

Systemic lupus erythematosus
Systemic lupus erythematosus (SLE) is a chronic inflammatory disorder that may produce purpura accompanied by other cutaneous findings, such as scaly patches on the scalp, face, neck, and arms; diffuse alopecia; telangiectasia; urticaria; and ulceration. The characteristic "butterfly rash" appears in the disorder's acute phase. Common associated signs and symptoms include nondeforming joint pain and stiffness, Raynaud's phenomenon, seizures, psychotic behavior, photosensitivity, fever, anorexia, weight loss, and lymphadenopathy.

Trauma
Traumatic injury can cause local or widespread purpura. Specific signs and symptoms depend on the type and location of the trauma.

OTHER CAUSES

Diagnostic tests
Invasive procedures, such as venipuncture and arterial catheterization, may produce local ecchymoses and hematomas caused by extravasated blood.

Drugs
The anticoagulants heparin and warfarin can produce purpura. Administration of warfarin can result in painful areas of erythema that become purpuric then necrotic with an adherent black eschar. The lesions develop between the 3rd and 10th day of drug administration.

Surgery and other procedures
Any procedure that disrupts circulation, coagulation, or platelet activity or production can cause purpura. Such procedures include pulmonary and cardiac surgery, radiation therapy, chemotherapy, hemodialysis, multiple blood transfusions with platelet-poor blood, and use of plasma expanders such as dextran.

SPECIAL CONSIDERATIONS

If the patient has a hematoma, apply pressure and cold compresses initially to help reduce bleeding and swelling. After the first 24 hours, apply hot compresses to help speed absorption of blood.

Prepare the patient for diagnostic tests. These may include a peripheral blood smear, bone marrow examination, and blood tests to determine platelet count, bleeding and coagulation times, capillary fragility, clot retraction, one-stage prothrombin time, partial thromboplastin time, and fibrinogen levels.

PEDIATRIC POINTERS

Neonates commonly exhibit petechiae, particularly on the head, neck, and shoulders, after vertex deliveries. Thought to result from the trauma of birth, these petechiae disappear within a few days. Other causes in infants include thrombocytopenia, vitamin K deficiency, and infantile scurvy.

The most common type of purpura in children is allergic purpura. Other causes in children include trauma, hemophilia, autoimmune hemolytic anemia, Gaucher's disease, thrombasthenia, congenital factor deficiencies, Wiskott-Aldrich syndrome, acute ITP, von Willebrand's disease, and the rare but life-threatening purpura fulminans, which usually follows bacterial or viral infection.

When you assess a child with purpura, be alert for signs of possible child abuse: bruises in different stages of resolution, from repeated beatings; bruise patterns resembling a familiar object, such as a belt, hand, or thumb and finger; and bruises on the face, buttocks, or genitalia, areas unlikely to be injured accidentally.

GERIATRIC POINTERS

Purpura can be a consequence of aging, when loss of collagen decreases connective tissue support of upper skin blood vessels. In an elderly or cachectic person, skin atrophy and inelasticity and loss of subcutaneous fat increase susceptibility to minor trauma, causing purpura to appear along the veins of the forearms, hands, legs, and feet. Chronic stasis usually affects elderly people, producing dusky reddish purpura on the legs after prolonged standing.

PATIENT COUNSELING

Reassure the patient that purpuric lesions aren't permanent and will fade if the underlying cause can be successfully treated. Warn him not to use cosmetic fade creams or other products in an attempt to reduce pigmentation

PUSTULAR RASH

A pustular rash is made up of crops of pustules — visible collections of pus within or beneath the epidermis, commonly in a hair follicle or sweat pore. These lesions vary greatly in size and shape and can be generalized or localized to the hair follicles or sweat glands. (See *Recognizing common skin lesions*, pages 488 and 489.) Pustules can result from a skin or systemic disorder, the use of certain drugs, or exposure to a skin irritant. Although many pustular lesions are sterile, a pustular rash usually indicates infection. Any vesicular eruption, or even acute contact dermatitis, can become pustular if secondary infection occurs.

Special considerations
+ Apply pressure and cold compresses to hematomas for the first 24 hours to reduce bleeding; then apply hot compresses to speed absorption of blood.

Peds points
+ Neonates commonly exhibit petechiae, particularly on the head, neck, and shoulders, after vertex deliveries.
+ The most common type of purpura in children is allergic purpura.
+ When assessing a child with purpura, be alert for signs of possible child abuse.

Geri points
+ Purpura can be a consequence of aging.
+ Skin atrophy and inelasticity and loss of subcutaneous fat increase susceptibility to minor trauma, causing purpura.
+ Chronic stasis produces dusky reddish purpura on the legs after prolonged standing.

Teaching points
+ Disease treatment as relates to purpura
+ Avoidance of fade creams

Key facts about pustular rash
+ Made up of crops of pustules — visible collections of pus within or beneath the epidermis, commonly in a hair follicle or sweat pore
+ Vary greatly in size and shape
+ Can be generalized or localized to the hair follicles or sweat glands

Key history points

+ Appearance, location, and onset of the first pustular lesion
+ Spread of lesions
+ Oral and topical medications
+ Family history of skin disorders

Critical assessment steps

+ Assess entire skin surface, noting if it's dry, oily, or moist.
+ Record the exact location and distribution of skin lesions, noting color, shape, and size.

Medical causes

Acne vulgaris
+ Pustules accompany papules, nodules, cysts, and open and closed comedones.
+ Lesions commonly appear on the face, shoulders, back, and chest.

Blastomycosis
+ Small, painless, nonpruritic macules or papules can enlarge to well-circumscribed, verrucous, crusted, or ulcerated lesions edged by pustules.

Folliculitis
+ Individual pustules, each pierced by a hair, occur.
+ Pruritus may also occur.

Furunculosis
+ Acute, deep-seated, red, hot, tender abscess evolves from a staphylococcus folliculitis.

Gonococcemia
+ A rash of scanty, pinpoint erythematous macules rapidly becomes vesiculopustular, maculopapular and, frequently, hemorrhagic.

HISTORY

Have the patient describe the appearance, location, and onset of the first pustular lesion. Did another type of skin lesion precede the pustule? Find out how the lesions spread. Ask what medications the patient takes and if he has applied any topical medication to his rash. If so, what type and when did he last apply it? Find out if he has a family history of a skin disorder.

PHYSICAL ASSESSMENT

Assess the entire skin surface, noting if it's dry, oily, moist, or greasy. Record the exact location and distribution of the skin lesions and their color, shape, and size.

MEDICAL CAUSES

Acne vulgaris
Pustules typify inflammatory lesions of acne vulgaris and are accompanied by papules, nodules, cysts, open comedones (blackheads) and closed comedones (whiteheads). Lesions commonly appear on the face, shoulders, back, and chest. Other findings include pain on pressure, pruritus, and burning. Chronic recurrent lesions produce scars.

Blastomycosis
Blastomycosis, a fungal infection, produces small, painless, nonpruritic macules or papules that can enlarge to well-circumscribed, verrucous, crusted, or ulcerated lesions edged by pustules. Localized infection may cause only one lesion; systemic infection may cause many lesions on the hands, feet, face, and wrists. Blastomycosis also produces signs of pulmonary infection, such as pleuritic chest pain and a dry, hacking or productive cough with occasional hemoptysis.

 CULTURAL CUE Blastomycosis is generally found in North America (where the fungus Blastomyces dermatitidis *inhabits the soil) and is endemic to the southeastern United States. Sporadic cases have also been reported in Africa.*

Folliculitis
This bacterial infection of hair follicles produces individual pustules, each pierced by a hair and possibly accompanied by pruritus. Folliculitis might progress to the hard painful nodules of furunculosis. "Hot tub" folliculitis produces pustules on areas covered by a bathing suit.

Furunculosis
A furuncle is an acute, deep-seated, red, hot, tender abscess that evolves from a staphylococcus folliculitis. Furuncles usually begin as small, tender red pustules at the base of hair follicles. They're likely to occur on the face, neck, forearm, groin, axillae, buttocks, and legs — areas that are prone to repeated friction. The pustules usually remain tense for 2 to 4 days and then become fluctuant. Rupture discharges pus and necrotic material. Then pain subsides, but erythema and edema may persist.

Gonococcemia
Gonococcemia produces a rash of scanty, pinpoint erythematous macules that rapidly become vesiculopustular, maculopapular and, frequently, hemorrhagic. Bullae may form. Mature lesions are elevated, with dirty gray necrotic centers and surrounding erythema. The rash appears on the distal part of the arms and legs, usually during the 1st day that other findings, such as fever and joint pain, occur. The rash disappears after 3 to 4 days but may recur with each episode of fever.

Impetigo contagiosa

Impetigo contagiosa is a vesiculopustular eruptive disorder, which occurs in non-bullous and bullous forms, that's usually caused by streptococci or staphylococci. Vesicles form and break, and a crust forms from the exudate: a thick, yellow crust in streptococcal impetigo and a thin, clear crust in staphylococcal impetigo. Both forms usually produce painless itching.

Nummular or annular dermatitis

With nummular or annular dermatitis, numerous coinlike (nummular) or ringed (annular) pustular lesions appear, usually on the extensor surfaces of the extremities, posterior trunk, buttocks, and lower legs; a few lesions may appear on the hands. The lesions commonly ooze a purulent exudate, itch severely, and rapidly become crusted and scaly. A few small, scaling patches may remain for some time.

Pustular miliaria

Pustular miliaria, an anhidrotic disorder, causes pustular lesions that begin as tiny erythematous papulovesicles located at sweat pores. Diffuse erythema may radiate from the lesion. The rash and associated burning and pruritus worsen with sweating.

Rosacea

Rosacea is a chronic hyperemic disorder that commonly produces telangiectasia with acute episodes of pustules, papules, and edema. Characterized by persistent erythema, rosacea may begin as a flush covering the forehead, malar region, nose, and chin. Intermittent episodes gradually become more persistent, and the skin—instead of returning to its normal color—develops varying degrees of erythema.

Scabies

Threadlike channels or burrows under the skin characterize scabies, which can also produce pustules, vesicles, and excoriations. The lesions are a few millimeters long with a swollen nodule or red papule that contains the itch mite.

Smallpox

Initial signs and symptoms of smallpox (variola major) include high fever, malaise, prostration, severe headache, backache, and abdominal pain. A maculopapular rash develops on the mucosa of the mouth, pharynx, face and forearms and then spreads to the trunk and legs. Within 2 days, the rash becomes vesicular and later pustular. The lesions develop at the same time, appear identical, and are more prominent on the face and extremities. The pustules are round, firm, and deeply embedded in the skin. After 8 to 9 days, the pustules form a crust, and later the scab separates from the skin, leaving a pitted scar.

Varicella zoster

When immunity to varicella declines, the virus reactivates along a dermatome, producing extremely painful and pruritic vesicles and pustules (herpes zoster, or shingles). Even with resolution of the rash, patients may experience chronic pain (postherpetic neuralgia) that may persist for months.

OTHER CAUSES

Drugs

Bromides and iodides commonly cause a pustular rash. Other drug causes include corticotropin, corticosteroids, dactinomycin, trimethadione, lithium, phenytoin, phenobarbital, isoniazid, hormonal contraceptives, androgens, and anabolic steroids.

Medical causes
(continued)

Impetigo contagiosa
- Vesicles form and break, and a crust forms from the exudate.

Nummular or annular dermatitis
- Numerous coinlike or ringed pustular lesions appear.

Pustular miliaria
- Pustular lesions begin as tiny erythematous papulovesicles at sweat pores.
- Diffuse erythema may radiate from the lesion.

Rosacea
- Acute episodes of pustules, papules, and edema occur with telangiectasia.
- Characterized by persistent erythema.

Scabies
- Threadlike channels or burrows under skin characterize scabies.

Smallpox
- A maculopapular rash develops on the mucosa of the mouth, pharynx, face, and forearms.

Varicella zoster
- Extremely painful and pruritic vesicles and pustules occur along a dermatome.

Other causes
- Bromides and iodides
- Corticotropin, corticosteroids, dactinomycin, trimethadione, lithium, phenytoin, phenobarbital, isoniazid, hormonal contraceptives, androgens, and anabolic steroids

Special considerations
+ Observe wound and skin isolation procedures until infection is ruled out.
+ If the organism is infectious, don't allow any drainage to touch unaffected skin.

Peds points
+ Varicella, erythema toxicum neonatorum, candidiasis, impetigo, infantile acropustulosis, and acrodermatitis enteropathica may produce a pustular rash in children.

Teaching points
+ Methods to prevent the spread of infection
+ Emotional support

Key facts about pyrosis
+ Substernal burning sensation that rises in the chest and may radiate to the neck or throat
+ Caused by reflux of gastric contents into the esophagus
+ Commonly accompanied by regurgitation

Key history points
+ History of heartburn
+ Factors triggering heartburn
+ Location of pain
+ Associated signs and symptoms, including regurgitation

Critical assessment steps
+ Perform an abdominal assessment.
+ Examine the mouth and throat.

SPECIAL CONSIDERATIONS

Observe wound and skin isolation procedures until infection is ruled out by a Gram stain or culture and sensitivity test of the pustule's contents. If the organism is infectious, don't allow any drainage to touch unaffected skin.

PEDIATRIC POINTERS

Among the various disorders that produce pustular rash in children are varicella, erythema toxicum neonatorum, candidiasis, impetigo, infantile acropustulosis, and acrodermatitis enteropathica.

PATIENT COUNSELING

Instruct the patient to keep his bathroom articles and linens separate from those of other family members. Associated pain and itching, altered body image, and the stress of isolation may result in anxiety, depression, and loss of sleep. Give medications to relieve pain and itching, and encourage the patient to express his feelings.

PYROSIS

Caused by reflux of gastric contents into the esophagus, pyrosis (heartburn) is a substernal burning sensation that rises in the chest and may radiate to the neck or throat. It's commonly accompanied by regurgitation, which also results from gastric reflux. Because increased intra-abdominal pressure contributes to reflux, pyrosis commonly occurs with pregnancy, ascites, or obesity. It also accompanies various GI disorders, connective tissue diseases, and the use of numerous drugs. Pyrosis usually develops after meals or when the patient lies down (especially on his right side), bends over, lifts heavy objects, or exercises vigorously. (See *How pyrosis occurs.*) It typically worsens with swallowing and improves when the patient sits upright or takes an antacid.

A patient experiencing a myocardial infarction (MI) may mistake chest pain for pyrosis. However, he'll probably develop other signs and symptoms — such as dyspnea, tachycardia, palpitations, nausea, and vomiting — that will help distinguish an MI from pyrosis. And, of course, his chest pain won't be relieved by an antacid.

HISTORY

Ask the patient if he has experienced heartburn before. Do certain foods or beverages trigger it? Does stress or fatigue aggravate his discomfort? Does movement, a certain body position, or ingestion of very hot or cold liquids worsen or help relieve the heartburn? Ask where the pain is located and whether it radiates to other areas. Also, find out if the patient regurgitates sour- or bitter-tasting fluids. (See *Regurgitation: Mechanism and causes,* page 566.) Does the patient have any associated signs and symptoms?

PHYSICAL ASSESSMENT

Perform an abdominal assessment. Because pyrosis can be a symptom of esophageal problems, be sure to include the mouth and throat in the examination.

How pyrosis occurs

Serving as a barrier to reflux, the lower esophageal sphincter (LES) normally relaxes only to allow food to pass from the esophagus into the stomach. However, hormonal fluctuations, mechanical stress, and the effects of certain foods and drugs can lower LES pressure. When LES pressure falls and intra-abdominal or intragastric pressure rises, the normally contracted LES relaxes inappropriately and allows reflux of gastric acid or bile secretions into the lower esophagus. There, the acids or secretions irritate and inflame the esophageal mucosa, producing pyrosis.

Persistent inflammation can cause LES pressure to decrease even more and may trigger a recurrent cycle of reflux and pyrosis.

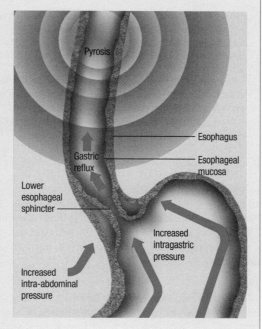

MEDICAL CAUSES

Esophageal cancer

Pyrosis may be a sign of esophageal cancer, depending on tumor size and location. The first and most common symptom is painless dysphagia that progressively worsens. Regurgitation and aspiration commonly occur at night. Eventually, partial obstruction and rapid weight loss occur, and the patient may complain of steady pain in the front and back of the chest. He may also experience hoarseness, sore throat, nausea, vomiting, and a feeling of substernal fullness.

Esophageal diverticula

Although usually asymptomatic, esophageal diverticula may cause pyrosis, regurgitation, and dysphagia. Other findings include chronic cough, halitosis, and a gurgling in the esophagus when liquids are swallowed. The patient may also complain of chest pain and a bad taste in the mouth.

Gastroesophageal reflux disease

Pyrosis, which is typically severe, is the most common symptom of gastroesophageal reflux disease (GERD). The pyrosis tends to be chronic, usually occurs 30 to 60 minutes after eating, and may be triggered by certain foods or beverages. It worsens when the patient lies down or bends and abates when he sits or stands upright or takes an antacid. Other findings include postural regurgitation, dysphagia, flatulent dyspepsia, and dull retrosternal pain that may radiate. (See *Associated disorder: Gastroesophageal reflux disease,* page 567.)

Medical causes

Esophageal cancer
✦ Painless dysphagia that progressively worsens is a common early symptom.
✦ Regurgitation and aspiration commonly occur at night.

Esophageal diverticula
✦ Pyrosis, regurgitation, and dysphagia may occur, although the disorder usually causes no symptoms.

GERD
✦ Pyrosis, which is typically severe, is the most common symptom.
✦ The pyrosis tends to be chronic, occurs 30 to 60 minutes after eating, and may be triggered by certain foods or beverages.

> ## Regurgitation: Mechanism and causes
>
> When gastric reflux moves up the esophagus and passes through the upper esophageal sphincter, regurgitation occurs. Unlike vomiting, regurgitation is effortless and unaccompanied by nausea. It usually happens when the patient is lying down or bending over and commonly accompanies pyrosis. Aspiration of regurgitated gastric contents can lead to recurrent pulmonary infections.
>
> In adults, regurgitation usually results from esophageal disorders such as achalasia. However, it can also occur when the gag reflex is absent, as in bulbar palsy, or when the patient has an overfilled stomach or esophagus.
>
> In infants, regurgitation can signal pyloric stenosis or dysphagia lusoria. Usually, however, infants "spit up" because their esophageal sphincters aren't fully developed during the first year of life.

Medical causes
(continued)

Hiatal hernia
+ Eructation occurs after eating, along with heartburn, regurgitation of sour-tasting fluid, and abdominal distention.

Obesity
+ Reflux and resulting pyrosis can result from increased intra-abdominal pressure.

Peptic ulcer disease
+ Pyrosis and indigestion usually signal the start of a peptic ulcer attack.

Scleroderma
+ Reflux with pyrosis may result from esophageal dysfunction.
+ Other symptoms include the sensation of food sticking behind the breastbone, odynophagia, bloating after meals, and weight loss.

Other causes
+ Acetohexamid
+ Tolbutamide
+ Lypressin
+ Aspirin
+ Anticholinergics and drugs that have anticholinergic effects
+ Large meals
+ Pregnancy

Hiatal hernia
With a hiatal hernia, eructation occurs after eating and is accompanied by heartburn, regurgitation of sour-tasting fluid, and abdominal distention. The patient complains of dull substernal or epigastric pain that may radiate to the shoulder. Other features include dysphagia, nausea, weight loss, dyspnea, tachypnea, a cough, and halitosis.

Obesity
With obesity, increased intra-abdominal pressure can contribute to reflux and resulting pyrosis. Other signs and symptoms may vary, depending on complications, but may include hypertension, cardiovascular disease, diabetes mellitus, renal disease, gallbladder disease, and psychosocial difficulties.

Peptic ulcer disease
Pyrosis and indigestion usually signal the start of a peptic ulcer attack. Most patients experience gnawing, burning pain in the left epigastrium, although some may report sharp pain. Typically, the pain arises 2 to 3 hours after eating or when the stomach is empty (usually at night), and is relieved by eating or taking an antacid or antisecretory drug. The pain may also occur after ingestion of coffee, aspirin, alcohol or, possibly, citrus juice.

Scleroderma
Scleroderma, a connective tissue disease, may cause esophageal dysfunction resulting in reflux with pyrosis, the sensation of food sticking behind the breastbone, odynophagia, bloating after meals, and weight loss. Other GI effects include abdominal distention, constipation or diarrhea, and malodorous floating stools. Early signs of scleroderma include blanching, pruritus, cyanosis, and stress- or cold-induced erythema of the fingers and toes. Later developments include finger and joint pain, stiffness, and swelling; skin thickening on the hands and forearms; masklike facies; and possibly flexion contractures. With advanced disease, cardiac and renal involvement may produce arrhythmias, dyspnea, cough, malignant hypertension, and signs of renal failure such as oliguria.

OTHER CAUSES

Drugs
Various drugs may cause or aggravate pyrosis, including acetohexamide, tolbutamide, lypressin, aspirin, anticholinergics, and drugs that have anticholinergic effects.

ASSOCIATED DISORDER

Gastroesophageal reflux disease

Gastroesophageal reflux disease (GERD) refers to backflow of gastric or duodenal contents or both into the esophagus and past the lower esophageal sphincter (LES) without associated belching or vomiting. The reflux of gastric contents causes acute epigastric pain, usually after a meal. The pain may radiate to the chest or arms. It commonly occurs in pregnant or obese persons. Lying down after a meal also contributes to reflux.

CAUSES
Causes of GERD include:
+ weakened esophageal sphincter
+ increased abdominal pressure, such as with obesity or pregnancy
+ hiatal hernia
+ medications, such as morphine, diazepam, calcium channel blockers, meperidine, and anticholinergic agents
+ food, alcohol, or cigarettes that lower LES pressure
+ nasogastric intubation for more than 4 days.

DIAGNOSIS
Diagnostic tests are aimed at determining the underlying cause of GERD:
+ Esophageal acidity test evaluates the competence of the LES and provides objective measure of reflux.
+ Acid perfusion test confirms esophagitis and distinguishes it from cardiac disorders.
+ Esophagoscopy allows visual examination of the lining of the esophagus to reveal the extent of the disease and confirm pathologic changes in mucosa.
+ Barium swallow identifies hiatal hernia as the cause.
+ Upper GI series detects hiatal hernia or motility problems.
+ Esophageal manometry evaluates resting pressure of the LES and determines sphincter competence.

MEDICAL INTERVENTIONS
Treatment may include:
+ diet therapy with frequent, small meals and avoidance of eating before going to bed to reduce abdominal pressure and the incidence of reflux
+ positioning, such as sitting up during and after meals and sleeping with the head of the bed elevated, to reduce abdominal pressure and prevent reflux
+ increased fluid intake to wash gastric contents out of the esophagus
+ antacids to neutralize acidic content of the stomach and minimize irritation
+ histamine-2 receptor antagonists to inhibit gastric acid secretion
+ proton pump inhibitors to reduce gastric acidity
+ cholinergic agents to increase LES pressure
+ smoking cessation to improve LES pressure (nicotine lowers LES pressure)
+ surgery (if hiatal hernia is the cause or the patient has refractory problems).

Lifestyle
Large meals or pregnancy may cause or aggravate pyrosis.

SPECIAL CONSIDERATIONS
Prepare the patient for diagnostic tests, such as barium swallow, upper GI series, esophagoscopy, and laboratory studies, to test esophageal motility and acidity.

PEDIATRIC POINTERS
A child may have difficulty distinguishing esophageal pain from pyrosis. To gain information, help him describe the sensation.

Key facts about GERD
+ Backflow of gastric or duodenal contents into esophagus and past LES without belching or vomiting
+ Causes acute epigastric pain that may radiate to the chest or arms
+ Commonly occurs in pregnant or obese persons

Causes
+ Weakened esophageal sphincter
+ Increased abdominal pressure
+ Hiatal hernia
+ Medications
+ Food, alcohol, or cigarettes that lower LES pressure
+ NG intubation for more than 4 days

Management
+ Diet therapy
+ Proper positioning
+ Increased fluid intake
+ Antacids, histamine-2 receptor antagonists, proton pump inhibitors, and cholinergic agents
+ Smoking cessation
+ Surgery

Special considerations
+ Prepare the patient for diagnostic tests.

Peds points
+ Help a child describe the sensation to aid differentiation between esophageal pain and pyrosis.

Geri points

+ Elderly patients with peptic ulcer disease commonly present with nonspecific abdominal discomfort or weight loss.
+ Elderly patients are at greater risk for complications from nonsteroidal anti-inflammatories.
+ Many develop pyrosis caused by intolerance to spicy foods.

Teaching points

+ Lifestyle changes, such as frequent, small meals and sitting upright for 2 hours after meals
+ Diet counseling
+ Measures to prevent increased intra-abdominal pressure
+ Smoking cessation and discontinuing use of drugs that reduce sphincter control

GERIATRIC POINTERS

Elderly patients with peptic ulcer disease commonly present with nonspecific abdominal discomfort or weight loss. Elderly patients are also at greater risk for complications from nonsteroidal anti-inflammatories, and many of them develop pyrosis caused by intolerance to spicy foods.

PATIENT COUNSELING

Advise the patient to eat frequent small meals, to sit upright (especially after a meal), and to avoid lying down for at least 2 hours after a meal. Instruct him to avoid highly seasoned foods, caffeine, acidic juices, carbonated beverages, alcohol, bedtime snacks, and foods high in fat or carbohydrates, which reduce lower esophageal sphincter (LES) pressure.

To prevent increased intra-abdominal pressure, instruct him to avoid bending, coughing, engaging in vigorous exercise, wearing tight clothing, or gaining weight. Also, advise him to refrain from smoking and using drugs that reduce sphincter control.

If the patient's pyrosis is severe, instruct him to sleep with extra pillows or wooden blocks under the head of the bed to reduce reflux by gravity. Tell him to take antacids (usually 1 hour after meals and at bedtime) or a histamine blocker as ordered. Medications that increase LES contraction, such as bethanechol, may be required.

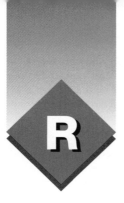

RECTAL PAIN

A common symptom of anorectal disorders, rectal pain is discomfort that arises in the anorectal area. Although the anal canal is separated from the rest of the rectum by the internal sphincter, the patient may refer to all local pain as rectal pain.

Because the mucocutaneous border of the anal canal and the perianal skin contains somatic nerve fibers, lesions in this area are especially painful. This pain may result from or be aggravated by diarrhea, constipation, or passage of hardened stools. It may also be aggravated by intense pruritus and continued scratching associated with drainage of mucus, blood, or fecal matter that irritates the skin and nerve endings.

HISTORY

Ask the patient to describe the pain. Is it sharp or dull, burning or knifelike? How often does it occur? Ask if the pain is worse during or immediately after defecation. Does the patient avoid having bowel movements because of anticipated pain? Find out what alleviates the pain.

Be sure to ask appropriate questions about the development of any associated signs and symptoms. For example, does the patient experience bleeding along with rectal pain? If so, find out how frequently this occurs and whether the blood appears on the toilet tissue, on the surface of the stool, or in the toilet bowl. Is the blood bright or dark red? Also, ask whether the patient has noticed other drainage, such as mucus or pus, and whether he's experiencing constipation or diarrhea. Ask when he last had a bowel movement. Obtain a dietary history.

PHYSICAL ASSESSMENT

Inspect the rectal area for bleeding; abnormal drainage such as pus; or protrusions, such as skin tags or thrombosed hemorrhoids. Also, check for inflammation and other lesions. A rectal examination may be necessary.

MEDICAL CAUSES

Abscess

A *perirectal abscess* can occur in various locations in the rectum and anus, causing pain in the perianal area. Typically, a superficial abscess produces constant, throbbing, local pain that's exacerbated by sitting or walking. The local pain associated with a deeper abscess may begin insidiously high in the rectum or even in the lower abdomen and is accompanied by an indurated anal mass. The patient may also de-

Key facts about rectal pain

+ Discomfort arising in the anorectal area
+ Common symptom of anorectal disorders

Key history points

+ Description of pain
+ Last bowel movement
+ Dietary history

Critical assessment steps

+ Inspect the rectal area for bleeding, drainage, or protrusions.
+ Check for inflammation and other lesions.

Medical causes

Abscess
+ A superficial abscess produces constant, throbbing, local pain that's exacerbated by sitting or walking.
+ The pain associated with a deeper abscess may begin insidiously high in the rectum or even in the lower abdomen and is accompanied by an indurated anal mass.
+ A prostatic abscess occasionally produces rectal pain.

Medical causes
(continued)

Anal fissure

✦ Sharp rectal pain occurs on defecation.

✦ A burning sensation and gnawing pain may continue up to 4 hours after defecation.

Anorectal fistula

✦ Pain develops when a tract formed between the anal canal and skin temporarily seals.

Cryptitis

✦ Dull anal pain or discomfort occurs with anal pruritus.

Hemorrhoids

✦ Rectal pain worsens during defecation and abates after it.

✦ Usually, rectal pain is accompanied by severe itching.

Proctalgia fugax

✦ Muscle spasms of rectum and pelvic floor produce sudden, severe episodes of rectal pain.

✦ The pain is sometimes associated with stress or anxiety and relieved by food and drink.

Other causes

✦ Anal intercourse

Special considerations

✦ Apply analgesic ointment or administer suppositories.

✦ Apply cold compresses to help shrink protruding hemorrhoids, prevent thrombosis, and reduce pain.

✦ If the patient's condition permits, place him in Trendelenburg's position with his buttocks elevated to further relieve pain.

velop such associated signs and symptoms as fever, malaise, anal swelling and inflammation, purulent drainage, and local tenderness.

A *prostatic abscess* occasionally produces rectal pain. Common associated findings include urine retention and frequency, dysuria, and fever. A rectal examination may reveal prostatic tenderness and gas.

Anal fissure

An anal fissure is a longitudinal crack in the anal lining that causes sharp rectal pain on defecation. The patient typically experiences a burning sensation and gnawing pain that can continue up to 4 hours after defecation. Fear of provoking this pain may lead to acute constipation. The patient may also develop anal pruritus and extreme tenderness and may report finding spots of blood on the toilet tissue after defecation.

Anorectal fistula

Pain develops when a tract formed between the anal canal and skin temporarily seals. It persists until drainage resumes. Other chief complaints of an anorectal fistula include pruritus and drainage of pus, blood, mucus and, occasionally, stool.

Cryptitis

Cryptitis results when particles of stool that are lodged in the anal folds decay and cause infection, which may produce dull anal pain or discomfort and anal pruritus. Intense pain may occur when the anal sphincter contracts.

Hemorrhoids

Thrombosed or prolapsed hemorrhoids cause rectal pain that may worsen during defecation and abate after it. The patient's fear of provoking the pain may lead to constipation. Usually, rectal pain is accompanied by severe itching. Internal hemorrhoids may also produce mild, intermittent bleeding that characteristically occurs as spotting on the toilet tissue or on the stool surface. External hemorrhoids are visible outside the anal sphincter.

Proctalgia fugax

With proctalgia fugax, muscle spasms of the rectum and pelvic floor produce sudden, severe episodes of rectal pain that last up to several minutes and then disappear. The patient may report being awakened by the pain, which is sometimes associated with stress or anxiety and relieved by food and drink.

OTHER CAUSES

Anal intercourse

Shearing forces may cause inflammation or tearing of the mucous membranes and discomfort.

SPECIAL CONSIDERATIONS

Apply analgesic ointment or administer suppositories. Administer a stool softener, if needed. If the rectal pain results from prolapsed hemorrhoids, apply cold compresses to help shrink protruding hemorrhoids, prevent thrombosis, and reduce pain. If the patient's condition permits, place him in Trendelenburg's position with his buttocks elevated to further relieve pain.

You may have to prepare the patient for an anoscopic examination and proctosigmoidoscopy to determine the cause of rectal pain. He may also need to provide a stool sample. Because the patient may feel embarrassed by treatments and diagnostic tests involving the rectum, provide emotional support and as much privacy as possible.

PEDIATRIC POINTERS

Observe any child with rectal pain for associated bleeding, drainage, and signs of infection (fever and irritability). Acute anal fissure is a common cause of rectal pain and bleeding in children, whose fear of provoking the pain may lead to constipation. Infants who seem to have pain on defecation should be evaluated for congenital anomalies of the rectum. Consider the possibility of sexual abuse in all children who complain of rectal pain.

GERIATRIC POINTERS

Because elderly people typically underreport their symptoms and have an increased risk of neoplastic disorders, they should always be thoroughly evaluated.

PATIENT COUNSELING

Teach the patient how to apply hot, moist compresses. Also teach him how to give himself a sitz bath; this will ease his discomfort by helping to relieve the sphincter spasm associated with most anorectal disorders. Stress the importance of following a proper diet and drinking plenty of fluids to maintain soft stools and thus avoid aggravating pain during defecation.

RESPIRATIONS, GRUNTING

Characterized by a deep, low-pitched grunting sound at the end of each breath, grunting respirations are a chief sign of respiratory distress in infants and children. They may be soft and heard only on auscultation, or loud and clearly audible without a stethoscope. Typically, the intensity of grunting respirations reflects the severity of respiratory distress. The grunting sound coincides with closure of the glottis, an effort to increase end-expiratory pressure in the lungs and prolong alveolar gas exchange, thereby enhancing ventilation and perfusion.

Grunting respirations indicate intrathoracic disease with lower respiratory involvement. Though most common in children, they sometimes occur in adults who are in severe respiratory distress. Whether they occur in children or adults, grunting respirations demand immediate medical attention.

 EMERGENCY ACTIONS If the patient exhibits grunting respirations, quickly place him in a comfortable position and check for signs of respiratory distress: wheezing; tachypnea (a minimum respiratory rate of 60 breaths/minute in infants, 40 breaths/minute in children ages 1 to 5, 30 breaths/minute in children older than age 5, or 20 breaths/minute in adults); accessory muscle use; substernal, subcostal, or intercostal retractions; nasal flaring; tachycardia (a minimum of 160 beats/minute in infants, 120 to 140 beats/minute in children ages 1 to 5, 120 beats/minute in children older than age 5, or 100 beats per minute in adults); cyanotic lips or nail beds; hypotension (less than 80/40 mm Hg in infants, less than 80/50 mm Hg in children ages 1 to 5, less than 90/55 mm Hg in children older than age 5, or less than 90/60 mm Hg in adults); and decreased level of consciousness. If you detect any of these signs, monitor oxygen saturation and administer oxygen and prescribed medications such as a bronchodilator. Also, have emergency equipment available, and prepare to intubate the

Peds points
✦ Observe any child with rectal pain for associated bleeding, drainage, and signs of infection.
✦ Acute anal fissure is a common cause of rectal pain and bleeding in children.
✦ Infants who seem to have pain on defecation should be evaluated for congenital anomalies of the rectum.
✦ Consider the possibility of sexual abuse in all children who complain of rectal pain.

Geri points
✦ Perform a thorough evaluation because elderly people typically underreport their symptoms and have an increased risk of neoplastic disorders.

Teaching points
✦ Methods to ease discomfort
✦ Proper diet and fluid intake

Key facts about grunting respirations
✦ Deep, low-pitched grunting sound at the end of each breath
✦ Coincides with closure of the glottis
✦ Indicates intrathoracic disease with lower respiratory involvement

In an emergency
✦ Quickly place patient in a comfortable position and check for signs of respiratory distress.
✦ Monitor oxygen saturation and administer oxygen and prescribed medications.
✦ Have emergency equipment available.
✦ Obtain ABG analysis.

Key history points

+ Onset of grunting respirations
+ Gestational age of infant
+ Personal history of frequent colds or upper respiratory tract infections
+ History of RSV
+ Change in activity level or feeding pattern

Critical assessment steps

+ Auscultate the lungs, noting diminished or abnormal sounds.
+ Characterize the color, amount, and consistency of any discharge or sputum.
+ Note the characteristics of the cough, if any.

Medical causes

Asthma

+ Grunting respirations may be apparent during severe attack.

Heart failure

+ Grunting respirations accompany increasing pulmonary edema as a late sign of heart failure.

Pneumonia

+ Grunting respirations accompany high fever, tachypnea, a productive cough, and lethargy.

Respiratory distress syndrome

+ Initially, audible expiratory grunting occurs with intercostal, subcostal, or substernal retractions; tachycardia; and tachypnea.
+ Cyanosis, frothy sputum, dramatic nasal flaring, lethargy, bradycardia, and hypotension characterizes severe distress.

patient if necessary. Obtain arterial blood gas analysis to determine oxygenation status.

HISTORY

After addressing the child's respiratory status, ask his parents when the grunting respirations began. If the patient is a premature infant, find out his gestational age. Ask the parents if anyone in the home has recently had an upper respiratory tract infection. Has the child had signs and symptoms of such an infection, such as a runny nose, cough, low-grade fever, or anorexia? Does he have a history of frequent colds or upper respiratory tract infections? Does he have a history of respiratory syncytial virus? Ask the parents to describe changes in the child's activity level or feeding pattern to determine if the child is lethargic or less alert than usual.

PHYSICAL ASSESSMENT

Begin the physical examination by auscultating the lungs, especially the lower lobes. Note diminished or abnormal sounds, such as crackles or sibilant rhonchi, which may indicate mucus or fluid buildup. Also, characterize the color, amount, and consistency of any discharge or sputum. Note the characteristics of the cough, if any.

MEDICAL CAUSES

Asthma

Grunting respirations may be apparent during a severe asthma attack, usually triggered by an upper respiratory tract infection or an allergic response. As the attack progresses, dyspnea, audible wheezing, chest tightness, and coughing occur. Patients may have a silent chest if air movement is poor.

Heart failure

A late sign of left-sided heart failure, grunting respirations accompany increasing pulmonary edema. Associated features include a productive cough, crackles, jugular vein distention, and chest wall retractions. Cyanosis may also be evident, depending on the underlying congenital cardiac defect.

Pneumonia

Life-threatening bacterial pneumonia is common after an upper respiratory tract infection or cold. *Pneumocystis carinii* pneumonia commonly affects children infected with human immunodeficiency virus. It causes grunting respirations accompanied by high fever, tachypnea, a productive cough, anorexia, and lethargy. Auscultation reveals diminished breath sounds, scattered crackles, and sibilant rhonchi over the affected lung. As the disorder progresses, the patient may also develop severe dyspnea, substernal and subcostal retractions, nasal flaring, cyanosis, and increasing lethargy. Some infants display GI signs, such as vomiting, diarrhea, and abdominal distention.

Respiratory distress syndrome

The result of lung immaturity in a premature infant (one who's less than 37 weeks' gestation) usually of low birth weight, respiratory distress syndrome initially causes audible expiratory grunting along with intercostal, subcostal, or substernal retractions; tachycardia; and tachypnea. Later, as respiratory distress tires the infant, apnea or irregular respirations replace the grunting. Severe respiratory distress is characterized by cyanosis, frothy sputum, dramatic nasal flaring, lethargy, bradycardia, and hypotension. Eventually, the infant becomes unresponsive. Auscultation reveals harsh, diminished breath sounds and crackles over the base of the lungs on deep inspiration. Oliguria and peripheral edema may also occur.

SPECIAL CONSIDERATIONS

Closely monitor the patient's condition. Keep emergency equipment nearby in case respiratory distress worsens. Prepare to administer oxygen using an oxygen hood or tent. Continually monitor arterial blood gas levels, and deliver the minimum amount of oxygen possible, to avoid causing retinopathy of prematurity from excessively high oxygen levels.

Begin inhalation therapy with a bronchodilator, and administer an I.V. antimicrobial if the patient has pneumonia (or, in some cases, status asthmaticus). Follow these measures with chest physical therapy as necessary.

Prepare the patient for chest X-rays. To prevent exposure to radiation, wear a lead apron and cover the child's genital area with a lead shield. If a blood culture is ordered, be sure to record on the laboratory slip any current antibiotic use.

PATIENT COUNSELING

Remember to explain all procedures to the patient's parents and to provide emotional support. Prepare the patient for the sights and sounds of the intensive care unit.

RESPIRATIONS, SHALLOW

Respirations are shallow when a diminished volume of air enters the lungs during inspiration. In an effort to obtain enough air, the patient with shallow respirations usually breathes at an accelerated rate. However, as he tires or as his muscles weaken, this compensatory increase in respirations diminishes, leading to inadequate gas exchange and such signs as dyspnea, cyanosis, confusion, agitation, loss of consciousness, and tachycardia.

Shallow respirations may develop suddenly or gradually and may last briefly or become chronic. They're a key sign of respiratory distress and neurologic deterioration. Causes include inadequate central respiratory control over breathing, neuromuscular disorders, increased resistance to airflow into the lungs, respiratory muscle fatigue or weakness, voluntary alterations in breathing, decreased activity from prolonged bed rest, and pain.

 EMERGENCY ACTIONS If you observe shallow respirations, be alert for impending respiratory failure or arrest. Is the patient severely dyspneic? Agitated or frightened? Look for signs of airway obstruction. If the patient is choking, perform four back blows and then four abdominal thrusts to try to expel the foreign object. Use suction if secretions occlude the patient's airway.

If the patient is also wheezing, check for stridor, nasal flaring, and use of accessory muscles. Administer oxygen with a face mask or a handheld resuscitation bag. Attempt to calm the patient. Administer epinephrine I.V.

If the patient loses consciousness, insert an artificial airway and prepare for endotracheal intubation and ventilatory support. Measure his tidal volume and minute volume with a Wright respirometer to determine the need for mechanical ventilation. (See *Measuring lung volumes,* page 574.) Check arterial blood gas (ABG) levels, heart rate, blood pressure, and oxygen saturation. Tachycardia, increased or decreased blood pressure, poor minute volume, and deteriorating ABG

Special considerations
+ Closely monitor the patient's condition and keep emergency equipment nearby.
+ Continually monitor ABG levels, and deliver the minimum amount of oxygen possible.
+ Begin inhalation therapy with a bronchodilator, and administer an I.V. antimicrobial if the patient has pneumonia.

Teaching points
+ Procedures

Key facts about shallow respirations
+ Diminished volume of air enters the lungs during inspiration
+ Triggers accelerated respiratory rate as patient attempts to obtain enough air
+ Leads to inadequate gas exchange as muscles tire and compensatory increase in respirations diminishes
+ May develop suddenly or gradually and may last briefly or become chronic

In an emergency
+ Be alert for impending respiratory failure or arrest.
+ Look for signs of airway obstruction.
+ Administer oxygen.
+ If the patient loses consciousness, insert an artificial airway and prepare for ET intubation and ventilatory support.

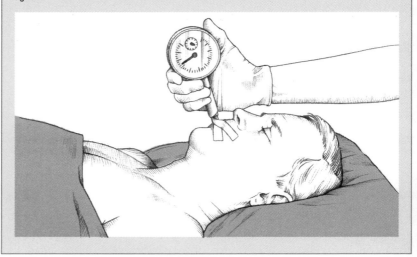

Measuring lung volumes

Use a Wright respirometer to measure tidal volume (the amount of air inspired with each breath) and minute volume (the volume of air inspired in a minute — or tidal volume multiplied by respiratory rate). You can connect the respirometer to an intubated patient's airway using an endotracheal tube (shown here) or a tracheostomy tube. If the patient isn't intubated, connect the respirometer to a face mask, making sure the seal over the patient's mouth and nose is airtight.

Key history points

+ Complete medical history (if not in severe respiratory distress)
+ Smoking and drug history
+ Onset and duration of shallow respirations
+ Factors that exacerbate or relieve shallow respirations

Critical assessment steps

+ Evaluate the patient's LOC and his orientation to time, person, and place.
+ Inspect the chest for deformities or abnormal movements.
+ Inspect the extremities for cyanosis and digital clubbing.
+ Auscultate for diminished, absent, or adventitious breath sounds and for abnormal or distant heart sounds.

levels or oxygen saturation signal the need for intubation and mechanical ventilation.

HISTORY

If the patient isn't in severe respiratory distress, begin with the history. Ask about chronic illness and any surgery or trauma. Has he had a tetanus booster in the past 10 years? Does he have asthma, allergies, or a history of heart failure or vascular disease? Does he have a chronic respiratory disorder or respiratory tract infection, tuberculosis, or a neurologic or neuromuscular disease? Does he smoke? Obtain a drug history, too, and explore the possibility of drug abuse.

Ask about the patient's shallow respirations: When did they begin? How long do they last? What makes them subside? What aggravates them? Ask about changes in appetite, weight, activity level, and behavior.

PHYSICAL ASSESSMENT

Begin the physical assessment by evaluating the patient's level of consciousness (LOC) and his orientation to time, person, and place. Observe spontaneous movements, and test muscle strength and deep tendon reflexes. Next, inspect the chest for deformities or abnormal movements such as intercostal retractions. Inspect the extremities for cyanosis and digital clubbing.

Palpate for expansion and diaphragmatic tactile fremitus, and percuss for hyperresonance or dullness. Auscultate for diminished, absent, or adventitious breath sounds and for abnormal or distant heart sounds. Do you note any peripheral edema? Finally, examine the abdomen for distention, tenderness, or masses.

MEDICAL CAUSES

Acute respiratory distress syndrome

Acute respiratory distress syndrome (ARDS) is a life-threatening syndrome that initially produces rapid, shallow respirations and dyspnea, at times after the patient appears stable. Hypoxemia leads to intercostal and suprasternal retractions, diaphoresis, and fluid accumulation, causing rhonchi and crackles. As hypoxemia worsens, the patient exhibits more difficulty breathing, restlessness, apprehension, decreased LOC, cyanosis and, possibly, tachycardia.

Amyotrophic lateral sclerosis

Respiratory muscle weakness in amyotrophic lateral sclerosis (ALS) causes progressive shallow respirations. Exertion may result in increased weakness and respiratory distress. ALS initially produces upper extremity muscle weakness and wasting, which in several years affect the trunk, neck, tongue, and muscles of the larynx, pharynx, and lower extremities. Associated signs and symptoms include muscle cramps and atrophy, hyperreflexia, slight spasticity of the legs, coarse fasciculations of the affected muscle, impaired speech, and difficulty chewing and swallowing.

Asthma

With asthma, bronchospasm and hyperinflation of the lungs cause rapid, shallow respirations. In adults, mild persistent signs and symptoms may worsen during severe attacks. Related respiratory effects include wheezing, rhonchi, a dry cough, dyspnea, prolonged expirations, intercostal and supraclavicular retractions on inspiration, nasal flaring, and use of accessory muscles. Chest tightness, tachycardia, diaphoresis, and flushing or cyanosis may occur.

Atelectasis

Decreased lung expansion or pleuritic pain causes sudden onset of rapid, shallow respirations. Other signs and symptoms of atelectasis include a dry cough, dyspnea, tachycardia, anxiety, cyanosis, and diaphoresis. Examination reveals dullness to percussion, decreased breath sounds and vocal fremitus, inspiratory lag, and substernal or intercostal retractions.

Bronchiectasis

With bronchiectasis, increased secretions obstruct airflow in the lungs, leading to shallow respirations and a productive cough with copious, foul-smelling, mucopurulent sputum (a classic finding). Other findings include hemoptysis, wheezing, rhonchi, coarse crackles during inspiration, and late-stage clubbing. The patient may complain of weight loss, fatigue, exertional weakness and dyspnea, fever, malaise, and halitosis.

Chronic bronchitis

Airway obstruction causes chronic shallow respirations in patients with chronic bronchitis. This disorder may begin with a nonproductive, hacking cough that later becomes productive. It may also cause prolonged expirations, wheezing, dyspnea, accessory muscle use, barrel chest, cyanosis, tachypnea, scattered rhonchi, coarse crackles, and clubbing (a late sign).

Coma

Rapid, shallow respirations result from neurologic dysfunction or restricted chest movement. Other manifestations depend on the underlying cause of the coma.

Emphysema

Increased breathing effort causes muscle fatigue, leading to chronic shallow respirations. The patient with emphysema may also display dyspnea, anorexia, malaise,

Medical causes

ARDS
- ✦ Rapid, shallow respirations and dyspnea appear initially, at times after the patient appears stable.

ALS
- ✦ Respiratory muscle weakness causes progressive shallow respirations.

Asthma
- ✦ Rapid, shallow respirations result from bronchospasm and hyperinflation of the lungs.

Atelectasis
- ✦ Decreased lung expansion or pleuritic pain causes sudden onset of rapid, shallow respirations.

Bronchiectasis
- ✦ Increased secretions obstruct airflow in the lungs, leading to shallow respirations and a productive cough with copious, foul-smelling, mucopurulent sputum (a classic finding).

Chronic bronchitis
- ✦ Chronic shallow respirations result from airway obstruction.

Coma
- ✦ Rapid, shallow respirations result from neurologic dysfunction or restricted chest movement.

Emphysema
- ✦ Increased breathing effort causes muscle fatigue, leading to chronic shallow respirations.

Medical causes
(continued)

Flail chest
+ Decreased air movement results in rapid, shallow respirations; paradoxical chest wall motion.

Fractured ribs
+ Pain on inspiration may cause shallow respirations.

Guillain-Barré syndrome
+ Progressive ascending paralysis causes rapid or progressive onset of shallow respirations.

Kyphoscoliosis
+ Skeletal cage distortion cause rapid, shallow respirations from reduced lung capacity.

Multiple sclerosis
+ Muscle weakness causes progressive shallow respirations.

Muscular dystrophy
+ Progressive thoracic deformity and muscle weakness cause shallow respirations to occur.

Myasthenia gravis
+ Progressive respiratory muscle weakness leads to shallow respirations, dyspnea, and cyanosis.

Obesity
+ The work of breathing may cause shallow respirations.

Parkinson's disease
+ Fatigue and weakness lead to progressive shallow respirations.

Pleural effusion
+ Restricted lung expansion causes shallow respirations.

tachypnea, diminished breath sounds, cyanosis, pursed-lip breathing, accessory muscle use, barrel chest, chronic productive cough, and clubbing (a late sign).

Flail chest
With flail chest, decreased air movement results in rapid, shallow respirations, paradoxical chest wall motion from rib instability, tachycardia, hypotension, ecchymoses, cyanosis, and pain over the affected area.

Fractured ribs
Pain on inspiration and possibly expiration may cause shallow respirations. The pain is usually described as sharp, severe chest pain. Other signs and symptoms include dyspnea, cough, and tenderness and edema at the fracture site.

Guillain-Barré syndrome
With Guillain-Barré syndrome, progressive ascending paralysis causes rapid or progressive onset of shallow respirations. Muscle weakness begins in the lower limbs and extends finally to the face. Associated findings include paresthesia, dysarthria, diminished or absent corneal reflex, nasal speech, dysphagia, ipsilateral loss of facial muscle control, and flaccid paralysis.

Kyphoscoliosis
Skeletal cage distortion can eventually cause rapid, shallow respirations from reduced lung capacity. Kyphoscoliosis also causes back pain, fatigue, tracheal deviation, ineffective coughing, and dyspnea.

Multiple sclerosis
Muscle weakness from multiple sclerosis causes progressive shallow respirations. Early features include diplopia, blurred vision, and paresthesia. Other possible findings include nystagmus, constipation, paralysis, spasticity, hyperreflexia, intention tremor, ataxic gait, dysphagia, dysarthria, urinary dysfunction, impotence, and emotional lability.

Muscular dystrophy
With muscular dystrophy, progressive thoracic deformity and muscle weakness cause shallow respirations to occur along with waddling gait, contractures, scoliosis, lordosis, and muscle atrophy or hypertrophy.

Myasthenia gravis
Progression of myasthenia gravis causes respiratory muscle weakness marked by shallow respirations, dyspnea, and cyanosis. Other effects include fatigue, weak eye closure, ptosis, diplopia, and difficulty chewing and swallowing.

Obesity
Morbid obesity may cause shallow respirations caused by the work of breathing associated with movement of the chest wall. Heart and breath sounds may be distant.

Parkinson's disease
Fatigue and weakness from Parkinson's disease lead to progressive shallow respirations. Typically, this disorder slowly progresses to increased rigidity (lead-pipe or cogwheel), masklike facies, stooped posture, shuffling gait, dysphagia, drooling, dysarthria, and pill-rolling tremor.

Pleural effusion
With pleural effusion, restricted lung expansion causes shallow respirations, beginning suddenly or gradually. Other findings include nonproductive cough, weight loss, dyspnea, and pleuritic chest pain. Examination reveals pleural friction rub,

tachycardia, tachypnea, decreased chest motion, flatness to percussion, egophony, decreased or absent breath sounds, and decreased tactile fremitus.

Pneumonia

Pulmonary consolidation results in rapid, shallow respirations. The patient may experience dyspnea, fever, shaking chills, chest pain, cough, tachycardia, decreased breath sounds, crackles, and rhonchi. He may also develop myalgias, fatigue, anorexia, headache, abdominal pain, cyanosis, and diaphoresis.

Pneumothorax

Pneumothorax causes sudden onset of shallow respirations and dyspnea. Related effects include tachycardia; tachypnea; sudden sharp, severe chest pain (commonly unilateral) worsening with movement; nonproductive cough; cyanosis; accessory muscle use; asymmetrical chest expansion; anxiety; restlessness; hyperresonance or tympany on the affected side; subcutaneous crepitation; decreased vocal fremitus; and diminished or absent breath sounds on the affected side.

Pulmonary edema

Pulmonary vascular congestion causes rapid, shallow respirations. Early signs and symptoms include exertional dyspnea, paroxysmal nocturnal dyspnea, nonproductive cough, tachycardia, tachypnea, dependent crackles, and a ventricular gallop. Severe pulmonary edema produces more rapid, labored respirations; widespread crackles; a productive cough with frothy, bloody sputum; worsening tachycardia; arrhythmias; cold, clammy skin; cyanosis; hypotension; and thready pulse.

Pulmonary embolism

A pulmonary embolism causes sudden, rapid, shallow respirations and severe dyspnea with angina or pleuritic chest pain. Other clinical features include tachycardia, tachypnea, a nonproductive cough or a productive cough with blood-tinged sputum, low-grade fever, restlessness, diaphoresis, pleural friction rub, crackles, diffuse wheezing, dullness to percussion, decreased breath sounds, and signs of circulatory collapse. Less common findings are massive hemoptysis, chest splinting, leg edema, and (with a large embolism) cyanosis, syncope, and jugular vein distention.

Spinal cord injury

Diaphragmatic breathing and shallow respirations may occur in injury to the C5 to C8 area. Other findings include quadriplegia with flaccidity followed by spastic paralysis, areflexia, hypotension, sensory loss below the level of injury, and bowel and bladder incontinence.

Upper airway obstruction

Partial airway obstruction causes acute shallow respirations with sudden gagging and dry, paroxysmal coughing; hoarseness; stridor; and tachycardia. Other findings include dyspnea, decreased breath sounds, wheezing, and cyanosis.

OTHER CAUSES

Drugs

Opioids, sedatives and hypnotics, tranquilizers, neuromuscular blockers, magnesium sulfate, and anesthetics can produce slow, shallow respirations.

Surgery

After abdominal or thoracic surgery, pain associated with chest splinting and decreased chest wall motion may cause shallow respirations.

Medical causes
(continued)

Pneumonia
+ Pulmonary consolidation results in rapid, shallow respirations.

Pneumothorax
+ Shallow respirations and dyspnea begin suddenly.

Pulmonary edema
+ Pulmonary vascular congestion causes rapid, shallow respirations.

Pulmonary embolism
+ Rapid, shallow respirations and severe dyspnea begin suddenly.

Spinal cord injury
+ Diaphragmatic breathing and shallow respirations may occur in injury to the C5 to C8 area.

Upper airway obstruction
+ Partial airway obstruction causes acute shallow respirations with sudden gagging and dry, paroxysmal coughing; hoarseness; stridor; and tachycardia.

Other causes
+ Opioids, sedatives and hypnotics, tranquilizers, neuromuscular blockers, magnesium sulfate, and anesthetics
+ Abdominal or chest surgery

Special considerations

+ Position the patient upright to ease his breathing.
+ Ensure adequate hydration, and use humidification as needed.
+ Administer oxygen, a broncho-dilator, a mucolytic, an expecto-rant, or an antibiotic, as ordered.
+ Turn the patient frequently.
+ Monitor the patient for increas-ing lethargy, which may indicate rising carbon dioxide levels.

Peds points

+ In children, shallow respirations commonly indicate a life-threatening condition.
+ Airway obstruction can occur rapidly because of the narrow passageways; if it does, admin-ister back blows or chest thrusts but not abdominal thrusts, which can damage internal organs.

Geri points

+ Stiffness or deformity of the chest wall associated with aging may cause shallow respirations.

Teaching points

+ Coughing and deep breathing
+ Emotional support

Key facts about stertorous respirations

+ Characterized by harsh, rattling, or snoring sound
+ Result from the vibration of re-laxed oropharyngeal structures during sleep or coma, causing partial airway obstruction
+ Occurs in about 10% of normal individuals, especially middle-age, obese men

SPECIAL CONSIDERATIONS

Prepare the patient for diagnostic tests: ABG analysis, pulmonary function tests, chest X-rays, or bronchoscopy.

Position the patient upright to ease his breathing. (Help a postoperative patient splint his incision while coughing.) If he's taking a drug that depresses respirations, follow all precautions and monitor him closely. Ensure adequate hydration, and use humidification as needed to thin secretions and to relieve inflamed, dry, or irritated airway mucosa. Administer oxygen, a bronchodilator, a mucolytic, an expectorant, or an antibiotic, as ordered.

Turn the patient frequently. He may require chest physiotherapy, incentive spirometry, or intermittent positive-pressure breathing. Monitor the patient for in-creasing lethargy, which may indicate rising carbon dioxide levels. Have emergency equipment at the patient's bedside.

PEDIATRIC POINTERS

In children, shallow respirations commonly indicate a life-threatening condition. Airway obstruction can occur rapidly because of the narrow passageways; if it does, administer back blows or chest thrusts but not abdominal thrusts, which can damage internal organs.

Causes of shallow respirations in infants and children include idiopathic (in-fant) respiratory distress syndrome, acute epiglottiditis, diphtheria, aspiration of a foreign body, croup, acute bronchiolitis, cystic fibrosis, and bacterial pneumonia.

Observe the child to detect apnea. As needed, use humidification and suction and administer supplemental oxygen. Give parenteral fluids to ensure adequate hy-dration. Chest physiotherapy may be required.

GERIATRIC POINTERS

Stiffness or deformity of the chest wall associated with aging may cause shallow respirations.

PATIENT COUNSELING

Have the patient cough and deep-breathe every hour to clear secretions and to counteract possible hypoventilation. Provide assistance with tracheal suctioning as needed. Because shallow respirations and respiratory distress can be frightening, provide your patient with emotional support and take measures to reduce anxiety.

RESPIRATIONS, STERTOROUS

Characterized by a harsh, rattling, or snoring sound, stertorous respirations usually result from the vibration of relaxed oropharyngeal structures during sleep or coma, causing partial airway obstruction. Less commonly, these respirations result from retained mucus in the upper airway.

This common sign occurs in about 10% of normal individuals, especially middle-age, obese men. It may be aggravated by use of alcohol or sedatives before bed, which increases oropharyngeal flaccidity, and by sleeping in the supine position, which allows the relaxed tongue to slip back into the airway. The major pathologic causes of stertorous respirations are obstructive sleep apnea and life-threatening upper airway obstruction associated with an oropharyngeal tumor or with uvular or palatal edema. This obstruction may also occur during the postictal phase of a generalized seizure when mucous secretions or a relaxed tongue blocks the airway.

Occasionally, stertorous respirations are mistaken for stridor, which is another sign of upper airway obstruction. However, stridor indicates laryngeal or tracheal obstruction, whereas stertorous respirations signal higher airway obstruction.

 EMERGENCY ACTIONS If you detect stertorous respirations, check the patient's mouth and throat for edema, redness, masses, or foreign objects. If edema is marked, quickly take vital signs, including oxygen saturation. Observe the patient for signs and symptoms of respiratory distress, such as dyspnea, tachypnea, use of accessory muscles, intercostal muscle retractions, and cyanosis. Elevate the head of the bed 30 degrees to help ease breathing and reduce the edema. Then administer supplemental oxygen by nasal cannula or face mask, and prepare to intubate the patient, perform a tracheostomy, or provide mechanical ventilation. Insert an I.V. line for fluid and drug access, and begin cardiac monitoring.

HISTORY

When possible, question the patient's partner about his snoring habits. Is the partner frequently awakened by the patient's snoring? Does the snoring improve if the patient sleeps with the window open? Has the partner also observed the patient talk in his sleep or sleepwalk? Ask about signs of sleep deprivation, such as personality changes, headaches, daytime somnolence, or decreased mental acuity.

PHYSICAL ASSESSMENT

When the patient is awake, perform a complete respiratory assessment, followed by an examination of his head, nose, and throat. If you detect stertorous respirations while the patient is sleeping, observe his breathing pattern for 3 to 4 minutes. Do noisy respirations cease when he turns on his side and recur when he assumes a supine position? Watch for periods of apnea and note their length.

MEDICAL CAUSES

Airway obstruction

Partial airway obstruction may lead to stertorous respirations accompanied by wheezing, dyspnea, tachypnea and, later, intercostal retractions and nasal flaring. If the obstruction becomes complete, the patient abruptly loses his ability to talk and displays diaphoresis, tachycardia, and inspiratory chest movement but absent breath sounds. Severe hypoxemia rapidly ensues, resulting in cyanosis, loss of consciousness, and cardiopulmonary collapse.

Obstructive sleep apnea

Loud and disruptive snoring is a major characteristic of obstructive sleep apnea, which commonly affects the obese. Typically, the snoring alternates with periods of sleep apnea, which usually end with loud gasping sounds. These episodes occur in a cyclic pattern throughout the night. Alternating tachycardia and bradycardia may occur as well as such sleep disturbances as somnambulism and talking during sleep. Some patients display hypertension and ankle edema. Most awaken in the morning with a generalized headache, feeling tired and unrefreshed. The most common complaint is excessive daytime sleepiness. Lack of sleep may cause depression, hostility, and decreased mental acuity.

Other causes

+ ET intubation or suction
+ Surgery

Special considerations

+ Administer a corticosteroid or an antibiotic and cool, humidified oxygen.

Peds points

+ In children, the most common cause of stertorous respirations is nasal or pharyngeal obstruction secondary to tonsillar or adenoid hypertrophy or the presence of a foreign body.

Geri points

+ Encourage the patient to seek treatment for sleep apnea or significant hypertrophy of tonsils or adenoids.

Teaching points

+ Weight loss
+ Set up and use of continuous or bilevel positive airway pressure

Key facts about costal and sternal retractions

+ Visible indentations of the soft tissue covering the chest wall
+ May be suprasternal, intercostal, subcostal, or substernal

In an emergency

+ Check quickly for other signs of respiratory distress.
+ Observe the depth and location of retractions.
+ Look for accessory muscle use, nasal flaring during inspiration, or grunting during expiration.
+ Auscultate the child's lungs to detect abnormal breath sounds.

OTHER CAUSES

Procedures

Endotracheal intubation, suction, or surgery may cause significant palatal or uvular edema, resulting in stertorous respirations.

SPECIAL CONSIDERATIONS

Monitor the patient's respiratory status carefully. Administer a corticosteroid or an antibiotic and cool, humidified oxygen to reduce palatal and uvular inflammation and edema.

Laryngoscopy and bronchoscopy (to rule out airway obstruction) or formal sleep studies may be necessary.

PEDIATRIC POINTERS

In children, the most common cause of stertorous respirations is nasal or pharyngeal obstruction secondary to tonsillar or adenoid hypertrophy or the presence of a foreign body.

GERIATRIC POINTERS

Encourage the patient to seek treatment for sleep apnea or significant hypertrophy of the tonsils or adenoids.

PATIENT COUNSELING

Encourage the obese patient to lose weight. Show the patient how to set up and use continuous or bilevel positive airway pressure, if indicated.

RETRACTIONS, COSTAL AND STERNAL

A cardinal sign of respiratory distress in infants and children, retractions are visible indentations of the soft tissue covering the chest wall. They may be suprasternal (directly above the sternum and clavicles), intercostal (between the ribs), subcostal (below the lower costal margin of the rib cage), or substernal (just below the xiphoid process). Retractions may be mild or severe, producing barely visible to deep indentations.

Normally, infants and young children use abdominal muscles for breathing, unlike older children and adults, who use the diaphragm. When breathing requires extra effort, accessory muscles assist respiration, especially inspiration. Retractions typically accompany accessory muscle use.

 EMERGENCY ACTIONS If you detect retractions in a child, check quickly for other signs of respiratory distress, such as cyanosis, tachypnea, tachycardia, and decreased oxygen saturation. Also, prepare the child for suctioning, insertion of an artificial airway, and administration of oxygen.

Observe the depth and location of retractions. Also, note the rate, depth, and quality of respirations. Look for accessory muscle use, nasal flaring during inspiration, or grunting during expiration. If the child has a cough, record the color, consistency, and odor of any sputum. Note whether the child appears restless or lethargic. Finally, auscultate the child's lungs to detect abnormal breath sounds. (See *Observing retractions*.)

ASSESSMENT TIP

Observing retractions

When you observe retractions in infants and children, note their exact location—an important clue to the cause and severity of respiratory distress. For example, subcostal and substernal retractions usually result from lower respiratory tract disorders; suprasternal retractions, from upper respiratory tract disorders.

Mild intercostal retractions alone may be normal. However, intercostal retractions accompanied by subcostal and substernal retractions may indicate moderate respiratory distress. Deep suprasternal retractions typically indicate severe distress.

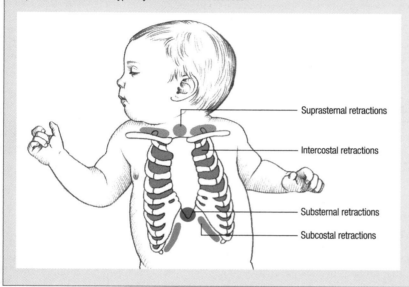

Suprasternal retractions

Intercostal retractions

Substernal retractions

Subcostal retractions

HISTORY

If the child's condition permits, ask his parents about his medical history. Was he born prematurely? Was he born with a low birth weight? Was the delivery complicated? Ask about recent signs of an upper respiratory tract infection, such as a runny nose, a cough, and a low-grade fever. How often has the child had respiratory problems during the past year? Has he been in contact with anyone who has had a cold, the flu, or other respiratory ailments? Did he ever have respiratory syncytial virus? Did he aspirate any food, liquid, or foreign body? Inquire about any personal or family history of allergies or asthma.

 CULTURAL CUE *When speaking to the parents of a child, determine who in the family makes the health care decisions. In the patriarchal family, a male, such as the father, makes health care decisions. In the matriarchal family, health care decisions are made by a female, such as the mother or grandmother.*

PHYSICAL ASSESSMENT

If the child isn't in severe distress, complete a cardiopulmonary assessment. If you haven't already done so, take the child's vital signs. Include the child's temperature in your assessment because a fever may signal a respiratory infection.

Key history points
+ Medical and birth history
+ Recent upper respiratory infection
+ Frequency of past respiratory problems
+ Recent exposure to cold, flu, or respiratory ailment
+ Aspiration of food, liquid, or foreign body
+ Personal or family history of allergies or asthma

Critical assessment steps
+ If the child isn't in severe distress, complete a cardiopulmonary assessment.
+ Take the child's vital signs, including his temperature.

Medical causes

Asthma attack
✦ Intercostal and suprasternal retractions may accompany attack.

Bronchiolitis
✦ Intercostal and subcostal retractions, nasal flaring, tachypnea, dyspnea, cough, restlessness, and a slight fever may occur.

Croup (spasmodic)
✦ Attacks of a barking cough, hoarseness, dyspnea, and restlessness occur.

Epiglottiditis
✦ This infection may precipitate severe respiratory distress with suprasternal, substernal, and intercostal retractions.

Heart failure
✦ Intercostal and substernal retractions occur along with nasal flaring, progressive tachypnea, grunting respirations, edema, and cyanosis.

Laryngotracheobronchitis (acute)
✦ Substernal and intercostal retractions follow low to moderate fever, runny nose, poor appetite, a barking cough, hoarseness, and inspiratory stridor.

Pneumonia (bacterial)
✦ Subcostal and intercostal retractions follow signs and symptoms of acute infection.

Respiratory distress syndrome
✦ Substernal and subcostal retractions are early signs of respiratory distress syndrome.

MEDICAL CAUSES

Asthma attack
Intercostal and suprasternal retractions may accompany an asthma attack. They're preceded by dyspnea, wheezing, a hacking cough, and pallor. Related features include cyanosis or flushing, crackles, rhonchi, diaphoresis, tachycardia, tachypnea, a frightened, anxious expression and, in patients with severe distress, nasal flaring.

Bronchiolitis
Most common in children younger than age 2, bronchiolitis—an acute lower respiratory tract infection—may cause intercostal and subcostal retractions, nasal flaring, tachypnea, dyspnea, cough, restlessness and a slight fever. Periodic apnea may occur in infants younger than age 6 months.

Croup (spasmodic)
Spasmodic croup causes attacks of a barking cough, hoarseness, dyspnea, and restlessness. As distress worsens, the child may display suprasternal, substernal, and intercostal retractions; nasal flaring; tachycardia; cyanosis; and an anxious, frantic expression. Croup attacks usually subside within a few hours but tend to recur.

Epiglottiditis
Epiglottiditis, a life-threatening bacterial infection, may precipitate severe respiratory distress with suprasternal, substernal, and intercostal retractions; stridor; nasal flaring; cyanosis; and tachycardia. Early features include sudden onset of a barking cough and high fever, sore throat, hoarseness, dysphagia, drooling, dyspnea, and restlessness. The child becomes panicky as edema makes breathing difficult. Total airway occlusion may occur in 2 to 5 hours.

Heart failure
Usually linked to a congenital heart defect in children, heart failure may cause intercostal and substernal retractions along with nasal flaring, progressive tachypnea, and—in severe respiratory distress—grunting respirations, edema, and cyanosis. Other findings include productive cough, crackles, jugular vein distention, tachycardia, right-upper-quadrant pain, anorexia, and fatigue.

Laryngotracheobronchitis (acute)
With acute laryngotracheobronchitis (a viral infection), substernal and intercostal retractions typically follow a low to moderate fever, runny nose, poor appetite, a barking cough, hoarseness, and inspiratory stridor. Associated signs and symptoms include tachycardia; shallow, rapid respirations; restlessness; irritability; and pale, cyanotic skin.

Pneumonia (bacterial)
Bacterial pneumonia begins with signs and symptoms of acute infection, such as high fever and lethargy, which are followed by subcostal and intercostal retractions, nasal flaring, dyspnea, tachypnea, grunting respirations, cyanosis, and a productive cough. Auscultation may reveal diminished breath sounds, scattered crackles, and sibilant rhonchi over the affected lung. GI effects may include vomiting, diarrhea, and abdominal distention.

Respiratory distress syndrome
Substernal and subcostal retractions are an early sign of respiratory distress syndrome, a life-threatening disorder that affects premature neonates shortly after birth. Associated early signs include tachypnea, tachycardia, and expiratory grunting. As respiratory distress worsens, intercostal and suprasternal retractions typically occur, and apnea or irregular respirations replace grunting. Other effects include

nasal flaring, cyanosis, lethargy, and eventual unresponsiveness as well as bradycardia and hypotension. Auscultation may detect crackles over the lung bases on deep inspiration and harsh, diminished breath sounds. Oliguria and peripheral edema may occur.

SPECIAL CONSIDERATIONS

Continue to monitor the child's vital signs. Keep suction equipment and an appropriate-sized airway at the bedside. If the infant weighs less than 15 lb (6.8 kg), place him in an oxygen hood. If he weighs more, place him in a cool mist tent. Perform chest physical therapy with postural drainage to help mobilize and drain excess lung secretions. A bronchodilator or, occasionally, a steroid may also be used.

Prepare the child for chest X-rays, cultures, pulmonary function tests, and arterial blood gas analysis.

PEDIATRIC POINTERS

When examining a child for retractions, know that crying may accentuate the contractions.

GERIATRIC POINTERS

Although retractions may occur at any age, they're more difficult to assess in an older patient who's obese or who has chronic chest wall stiffness or deformity.

PATIENT COUNSELING

Explain the procedures to the patient and his parents, and have the parents calm and comfort the child. Review all medications, dosages, and adverse reactions with the parents. Explain the importance of providing the child with a humidified environment and adequate hydration.

RHONCHI

Rhonchi are continuous adventitious breath sounds detected by auscultation. They're usually louder and lower pitched than crackles — more like a hoarse moan or a deep snore — though they may be described as rattling, sonorous, bubbling, rumbling, or musical. However, sibilant rhonchi, or wheezes, are high pitched.

Rhonchi are heard over large airways such as the trachea. They can occur in a patient with a pulmonary disorder when air flows through passages that have been narrowed by secretions, a tumor or foreign body, bronchospasm, or mucosal thickening. The resulting vibration of airway walls produces the rhonchi.

HISTORY

Begin with a history: Does the patient smoke? If so, obtain a history in pack-years. Has he recently lost weight or felt tired or weak? Does he have asthma or another pulmonary disorder? Is he taking any prescribed or over-the-counter drugs?

PHYSICAL ASSESSMENT

If you auscultate rhonchi, take the patient's vital signs, including oxygen saturation, and be alert for signs of respiratory distress. Characterize the patient's respirations as rapid or slow, shallow or deep, and regular or irregular. Inspect the chest, noting the use of accessory muscles. Is the patient audibly wheezing or gurgling? Auscul-

---

Special considerations
+ Keep suction equipment and an airway at the bedside.
+ If the infant weighs less than 15 lb, place him in an oxygen hood; if he weighs more, place him in a cool mist tent.
+ Perform chest physical therapy with postural drainage.

Peds points
+ When examining a child for retractions, know that crying may accentuate the contractions.

Geri points
+ Retractions are more difficult to assess in an older patient who is obese or who has chronic chest wall stiffness or deformity.

Teaching points
+ Medications
+ Humidified environment and adequate hydration

Key facts about rhonchi
+ Continuous adventitious breath sounds detected by auscultation
+ Sound louder and lower pitched than crackles
+ Heard over large airways such as the trachea
+ Can occur when air flows through passages that have been narrowed by secretions, a tumor or foreign body, bronchospasm, or mucosal thickening

Key history points
+ Smoking history
+ History of asthma or other pulmonary disorder
+ Current medications

Critical assessment steps

+ Characterize the patient's respirations as rapid or slow, shallow or deep, and regular or irregular.
+ Inspect the chest, noting the use of accessory muscles.
+ Auscultate for other abnormal breath sounds and note location.
+ Percuss the chest, and note frequency and productivity of cough.

Medical causes

ARDS
+ Initial features include dyspnea, rhonchi, crackles, and rapid, shallow respirations.

Aspiration of foreign body
+ Inspiratory and expiratory rhonchi and wheezing occur due to increased secretions.

Asthma
+ An asthma attack can cause rhonchi, crackles and, commonly, wheezing.

Bronchiectasis
+ Lower-lobe rhonchi and crackles occur.
+ Classic sign is a cough that produces mucopurulent, foul-smelling sputum.

Bronchitis
+ Sonorous rhonchi and wheezing occur due to bronchospasm or increased mucus in the airways.

Emphysema
+ Sonorous rhonchi may occur, but faint, high-pitched wheezing is more typical.

tate for other abnormal breath sounds, such as crackles and a pleural friction rub. If you detect these sounds, note their location. Are breath sounds diminished or absent? Next, percuss the chest. If the patient has a cough, note its frequency and characterize its sound. If it's productive, examine the sputum for color, odor, consistency, and blood.

During the examination, keep in mind that thick or excessive secretions, bronchospasm, or inflammation of mucous membranes may lead to airway obstruction. If necessary, suction the patient and keep equipment available for inserting an artificial airway. Keep a bronchodilator available to treat bronchospasm.

MEDICAL CAUSES

Acute respiratory distress syndrome
Fluid accumulation with acute respiratory distress syndrome (ARDS) — a life-threatening disorder — produces rhonchi and crackles. Initial features include rapid, shallow respirations and dyspnea, sometimes after the patient's condition appears stable. Developing hypoxemia leads to intercostal and suprasternal retractions, diaphoresis, and fluid accumulation. As hypoxemia worsens, the patient displays increased difficulty breathing, restlessness, apprehension, decreased level of consciousness, cyanosis, motor dysfunction and, possibly, tachycardia.

Aspiration of a foreign body
A retained foreign body in the bronchi can cause inspiratory and expiratory rhonchi and wheezing due to increased secretions. Diminished breath sounds may be auscultated over the obstructed area. Fever, pain, and cough may also occur.

Asthma
An asthma attack can cause rhonchi, crackles and, commonly, wheezing. Other features include apprehension, a dry cough that later becomes productive, prolonged expirations, and intercostal and supraclavicular retractions on inspiration. The patient may also exhibit increased accessory muscle use, nasal flaring, tachypnea, tachycardia, diaphoresis, and flushing or cyanosis.

Bronchiectasis
Bronchiectasis causes lower-lobe rhonchi and crackles, which coughing may help relieve. Its classic sign is a cough that produces mucopurulent, foul-smelling and, possibly, bloody sputum. Other findings include fever, weight loss, exertional dyspnea, fatigue, malaise, halitosis, weakness, and late-stage clubbing.

Bronchitis
Acute tracheobronchitis produces sonorous rhonchi and wheezing due to bronchospasm or increased mucus in the airways. Related findings include chills, sore throat, a low-grade fever (rising up to 102° F [38.9° C] in those with severe illness), muscle and back pain, and substernal tightness. A cough becomes productive as secretions increase.

With chronic bronchitis, auscultation may reveal scattered rhonchi, coarse crackles, wheezing, high-pitched piping sounds, and prolonged expirations. An early hacking cough later becomes productive. The patient also displays exertional dyspnea, increased accessory muscle use, barrel chest, cyanosis, tachypnea, and clubbing (a late sign).

Emphysema
Emphysema may cause sonorous rhonchi, but faint, high-pitched wheezing is more typical, together with weight loss, exertional dyspnea, accessory muscle use on inspiration, tachypnea, grunting expirations, and a mild, chronic, productive cough

with scant sputum. Other features include anorexia, malaise, barrel chest, peripheral cyanosis, and late-stage clubbing.

Pneumonia

Bacterial pneumonias can cause rhonchi and a dry cough that later becomes productive. Related signs and symptoms — shaking chills, high fever, myalgias, headache, pleuritic chest pain, tachypnea, tachycardia, dyspnea, cyanosis, diaphoresis, decreased breath sounds, and fine crackles — develop suddenly.

OTHER CAUSES

Diagnostic tests

Pulmonary function tests or bronchoscopy can loosen secretions and mucus, causing rhonchi.

Respiratory therapy

Respiratory therapy may produce rhonchi from loosened secretions and mucus.

SPECIAL CONSIDERATIONS

To ease the patient's breathing, place him in semi-Fowler's position and reposition him every 2 hours. Administer an antibiotic, a bronchodilator, and an expectorant. Also, provide humidification to thin secretions, to relieve inflammation, and to prevent drying. Pulmonary physiotherapy with postural drainage and percussion can also help loosen secretions. Use tracheal suctioning, if necessary, to help the patient clear secretions and to promote oxygenation and comfort. Promote coughing, deep breathing, and incentive spirometry.

Prepare the patient for diagnostic tests, such as arterial blood gas analysis, pulmonary function studies, sputum analysis, and chest X-rays.

PEDIATRIC POINTERS

Rhonchi in children can result from bacterial pneumonia, cystic fibrosis, and croup syndrome.

Because a respiratory tract disorder may begin abruptly and progress rapidly in an infant or a child, observe closely for signs of airway obstruction.

PATIENT COUNSELING

If appropriate, encourage increased activity to promote drainage of secretions. Teach deep-breathing and coughing techniques and splinting, if necessary. Encourage the patient to drink plenty of fluids to help liquefy secretions and prevent dehydration. Advise him not to suppress a moist cough.

ROMBERG'S SIGN

A positive Romberg's sign refers to a patient's inability to maintain balance when standing erect with his feet together and his eyes closed. Normally, the patient should be able to stand with his feet together and his eyes closed with minimal swaying for about 20 seconds (a negative Romberg's sign). (See *Assessing Romberg's sign,* page 586.)

If positive, Romberg's sign indicates a vestibular or proprioceptive disorder or a disorder of the spinal tracts (the posterior columns) that carry proprioceptive information — the perception of one's position in space, of joint movements, and of pressure sensations — to the brain. Insufficient vestibular or proprioceptive infor-

---

Medical causes
(continued)

Pneumonia
+ Bacterial pneumonias can cause rhonchi and a dry cough that later becomes productive.

Other causes
+ PFTs or bronchoscopy
+ Respiratory therapy

Special considerations
+ To ease breathing, place the patient in semi-Fowler's position.
+ Administer an antibiotic, a bronchodilator, and an expectorant.
+ Provide humidification.
+ Promote coughing, deep breathing, and incentive spirometry.

Peds points
+ Rhonchi in children can result from bacterial pneumonia, cystic fibrosis, and croup syndrome.
+ Because a respiratory tract disorder may begin abruptly and progress rapidly in an infant or a child, observe closely for signs of airway obstruction.

Teaching points
+ Deep-breathing and coughing techniques
+ Fluid intake

Key facts about Romberg's sign
+ Inability to maintain balance when standing erect with feet together and eyes closed
+ Indicates a vestibular or proprioceptive disorder or a disorder of the spinal tracts
+ May indicate cerebellar disorder

Assessing Romberg's sign

Observe the patient's balance as he stands with his eyes open, feet together, and arms at his sides. Then ask him to close his eyes. Hold your arms out on either side of him to protect him if he sways. If he falls to one side, the result of the Romberg's test is positive.

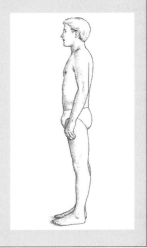

Key history points

+ Medical history including previous neurologic symptoms and disorders
+ Sensory changes and their onset

Critical assessment steps

+ Perform other neurologic screening tests, including proprioception.
+ Test the patient's awareness of body part position.
+ Test the patient's direction of movement.
+ Test sensation and two-point discrimination in all dermatomes.
+ Test and characterize the patient's DTRs.
+ Test the patient's vibratory sense.

Medical causes

Multiple sclerosis

+ Early features may include vision changes, diplopia, and paresthesia.

Peripheral nerve disease

+ Positive Romberg's sign may be accompanied by impotence, fatigue, and paresthesia, hyperesthesia, or anesthesia.

mation causes an inability to execute precise movements and maintain balance without visual cues. Difficulty performing this maneuver with eyes open or closed may indicate a cerebellar disorder.

HISTORY

Obtain the patient's medical history. Ask him about previous neurologic symptoms and disorders. Once you've detected a positive Romberg's sign, perform other neurologic screening tests. Also, ask the patient if he has noticed sensory changes, such as numbness and tingling in his limbs. If so, when did these changes begin?

PHYSICAL ASSESSMENT

First, test proprioception. If the patient can't maintain his balance with his eyes open, ask him to hop on one foot and then on the other. Next, ask him to do a knee bend and to walk a straight line, placing heel to toe. Lastly, ask him to walk a short distance so you can evaluate his gait.

Test the patient's awareness of body part position by changing the position of one of his fingers, or any other joint, while his eyes are closed. Ask him to describe the change you've made. Next, test the patient's direction of movement. Ask him to close his eyes and to touch his nose with the index finger of one hand and then with the other. Ask him to repeat this movement several times, gradually increasing his speed. Then test the accuracy of his movement by having him rapidly touch each finger of one hand to the thumb. Next, test sensation in all dermatomes, using a pin to assess sharp/dull differentiation. Also test two-point discrimination by touching two pins (one in each hand) to his skin simultaneously. Does he feel one or two pinpricks? Finally, test and characterize the patient's deep tendon reflexes (DTRs).

To test the patient's vibratory sense, ask him to close his eyes; then apply a mildly vibrating tuning fork to a bony prominence such as the medial malleolus. If the patient doesn't feel the stimulus initially, increase the vibration and then test the knee or hip. This procedure can also be done to test the fingers, elbow, and shoulder.

MEDICAL CAUSES

Multiple sclerosis

Early features of multiple sclerosis may include vision changes, diplopia, and paresthesia. Other findings include a positive Romberg's sign, nystagmus, constipation, muscle weakness and spasticity, and hyperreflexia. The patient may also have dysphagia, dysarthria, incontinence, urinary frequency and urgency, impotence, and emotional instability.

Peripheral nerve disease

Besides a positive Romberg's sign, advanced peripheral nerve disease may produce impotence, fatigue, and paresthesia, hyperesthesia, or anesthesia in the hands and feet. Related findings include incoordination, ataxia, burning pain in the affected area, progressive muscle weakness and atrophy, and loss of vibration sense. DTRs may be hypoactive.

Pernicious anemia

Pernicious anemia impairs myelin formation, which causes neurologic damage. A positive Romberg's sign and loss of proprioception in the lower limbs reflect peripheral nerve and spinal cord damage. Gait changes (usually ataxia), muscle weakness, impaired coordination, paresthesia, and sensory loss may be present. DTRs may be hypoactive or hyperactive. Other findings include a sore tongue, a positive Babinski's reflex, fatigue, blurred vision, diplopia, and light-headedness.

Spinal cerebellar degeneration

With spinal cerebellar degeneration, a positive Romberg's sign accompanies decreased visual acuity, fatigue, paresthesia, loss of vibration sense, incoordination, ataxic gait, and muscle weakness and atrophy. DTRs may be hypoactive.

Spinal cord disease

With spinal cord disease, a positive Romberg's sign may accompany pain, fasciculations, muscle weakness and atrophy, loss of sphincter tone, and loss of proprioception, vibration, and other senses. DTRs may be hypoactive at the level of the lesion and hyperactive above it.

Vestibular disorders

Besides a positive Romberg's sign, vestibular disorders commonly cause vertigo. Nystagmus, nausea, tinnitus, hearing loss, and vomiting may also occur.

SPECIAL CONSIDERATIONS

Help the patient with ambulation, especially in poorly lit areas. Also, keep a night-light on in his room, and raise the side rails of the bed.

PEDIATRIC POINTERS

Romberg's sign can't be tested in children until they can stand without support and follow commands. However, a positive sign in children commonly results from spinal cord disease.

PATIENT COUNSELING

Encourage the patient to ask for assistance and to use visual cues to maintain his balance. Instruct him in the use of assistive devices if necessary.

Medical causes
(continued)

Pernicious anemia
✦ A positive Romberg's sign and loss of proprioception in the lower limbs reflect peripheral nerve and spinal cord damage.

Spinal cerebellar degeneration
✦ Positive Romberg's sign accompanies decreased visual acuity, fatigue, paresthesia, loss of vibration sense, incoordination, ataxic gait, and muscle weakness and atrophy.

Spinal cord disease
✦ Positive Romberg's sign may accompany pain, fasciculations, muscle weakness and atrophy, and loss of sphincter tone, proprioception, and vibration.

Vestibular disorders
✦ Positive Romberg's sign may accompany vertigo.

Special considerations
✦ Help the patient with ambulation.
✦ Keep a night-light on and raise side rails of bed.

Peds points
✦ Romberg's sign can't be tested until a child can stand without support and follow commands.
✦ A positive sign in children commonly results from spinal cord disease.

Teaching points
✦ Safety measures
✦ Assistive devices

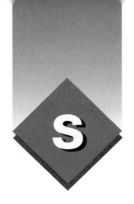

SALIVATION, DECREASED

Typically a common but minor complaint, diminished production or excretion of saliva (dry mouth) usually results from mouth breathing. However, this symptom can also result from salivary duct obstruction, Sjögren's syndrome, the use of an anticholinergic or other drug, and the effects of radiation. Also known as *xerostomia*, dry mouth can even result from vigorous exercise or autonomic stimulation — for example, as the result of fear.

HISTORY

Evaluate the patient's complaint of dry mouth by asking pertinent history questions: When did he first notice the symptom? Was he exercising at the time? Is he currently taking any medications? Is his sensation of dry mouth intermittent or continuous? Is it related to or relieved by a particular activity? Ask about related symptoms, such as burning or itching eyes, or changes in sense of smell or taste.

PHYSICAL ASSESSMENT

Inspect the patient's mouth, including the mucous membranes, for any abnormalities. Observe his eyes for conjunctival irritation, matted lids, and corneal epithelial thickening. Perform simple tests of smell and taste to detect impairment of these senses. Check for enlarged parotid and submaxillary glands. (See *Examining salivary glands and ductal openings*.) Palpate for tender or enlarged areas along the neck, too.

MEDICAL CAUSES

Dehydration
Decreased saliva production causes dry oral mucous membranes. Skin turgor is also decreased, and urine output may be low. Vital signs may reveal hypotension, tachycardia, and a low-grade fever.

Facial nerve paralysis
With facial nerve paralysis, a diminished saliva production occurs along with decreased sense of taste and facial muscle movement. The affected side of the face may sag and appear masklike.

Salivary duct obstruction
Usually associated with a salivary stone, salivary duct obstruction causes reduced salivation and local pain and swelling of the face or neck. The symptoms are most noticeable when eating or drinking.

Examining salivary glands and ductal openings

When a patient reports decreased salivation, assess the parotid and submaxillary glands for enlargement and the ductal openings for salivary flow.

To detect an enlarged parotid gland, ask the patient to clench his teeth, thereby tensing the masseter muscle. Then palpate the parotid duct (about 2″ [5 cm] long); you should be able to feel it against the tensed muscle, on the cheek just below the zygomatic arch. Next, check the ductal orifice, opposite the second molar. Using a gloved finger, palpate the orifice for enlargement, and observe for drainage.

Palpate the submaxillary gland. About the size of a walnut, this gland is located under the mandible, anterior to the angle of the jaw. Using a gloved finger, palpate the floor of the mouth for enlargement of the submaxillary ductal orifice.

Finally, test both ductal openings for salivary flow. Place cotton under the patient's tongue, have him sip pure lemon juice, and then remove the cotton and observe salivary flow from each opening. Document your findings.

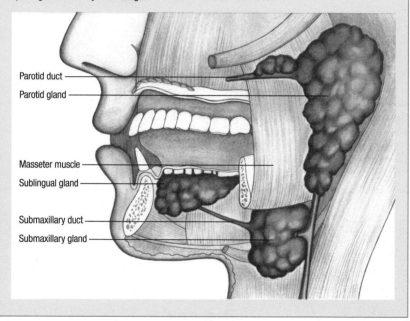

Sjögren's syndrome

Diminished secretions from the lacrimal, parotid, and submaxillary glands produce the hallmarks of Sjögren's syndrome: decreased or absent salivation and dry eyes with a persistent burning, gritty sensation. The patient may also experience dryness that involves the nose, respiratory tract, vagina, and skin.

Related oral signs and symptoms include difficulty chewing, talking, and swallowing as well as ulcers and soreness of the lips and mucosa. The parotid and submaxillary glands may be enlarged. Nasal crusting, epistaxis, fatigue, lethargy, nonproductive cough, abdominal discomfort, and polyuria may be present. These signs and symptoms may occur alone or with rheumatoid arthritis or another connective tissue disorder.

Medical causes
(continued)

Salivary duct obstruction
✦ Reduced salivation occurs with local pain and swelling of the face or neck.
✦ Symptoms are most noticeable when eating or drinking.

Sjögren's syndrome
✦ Diminished secretions from the lacrimal, parotid, and submaxillary glands produce decreased or absent salivation and dry eyes with a persistent burning, gritty sensation.

Other causes

+ Anticholinergics, antihistamines, TCAs, phenothiazines, clonidine and opioid analgesics
+ Irradiation of mouth or face

Special considerations

+ Allow extra time for speaking, eating, and swallowing.

Peds points

+ Mouth breathing and anticholinergic therapy are causes of decreased salivation in children.

Teaching points

+ Increasing fluid intake during meals and chewing gum or tart sugarless mints between meals
+ Proper oral hygiene

Key facts about increased salivation

+ Also known as *polysialia* or *ptyalism*
+ Results from GI disorders, systemic disorders, or use of certain drugs

Key history points

+ Associated fatigue, fever, headache, or sore throat
+ Recent exposure to toxins
+ Drug history

Critical assessment steps

+ Observe ability to swallow and chew.
+ Inspect the mouth for lesions; note their appearance.
+ Palpate lymph nodes, and determine if parotid glands are swollen or sore.

OTHER CAUSES

Drugs

Anticholinergics, antihistamines, tricyclic antidepressants, phenothiazines, clonidine, and opioid analgesics can cause decreased salivation, which disappears after discontinuation of therapy.

Radiation

Excessive irradiation of the mouth or face from chemotherapeutic treatments or dental X-rays may cause transient decreased salivation due to salivary gland atrophy, which can lead to difficulty swallowing, discomfort, and gum disease.

SPECIAL CONSIDERATIONS

If markedly reduced salivation interferes with speaking, eating, or swallowing, allow the patient extra time for these activities.

PEDIATRIC POINTERS

Mouth breathing and anticholinergic therapy are the primary causes of decreased salivation in children.

PATIENT COUNSELING

To relieve dry mouth, encourage the patient to increase his fluid intake during meals and to chew gum or tart sugarless mints between meals. To reduce the risk of cavities, advise him to brush his teeth, floss, use mouthwash, and avoid sugary desserts, candies, and drinks. Routine dental visits and fluoride treatments may also be beneficial.

Pilocarpine (5 to 10 mg orally three times daily) can relieve symptoms of dry mouth, but it must be used regularly.

SALIVATION, INCREASED

Increased salivation (also known as *polysialia* or *ptyalism*) is an uncommon symptom that can result from a GI disorder, especially of the mouth. It also accompanies certain systemic disorders and may result from the use of certain drugs or from exposure to toxins. Saliva may also accumulate because of difficulty swallowing. (See "Dysphagia," page 225.)

HISTORY

Ask the patient about related signs and symptoms, such as fatigue, fever, headache, or a sore throat. Also ask about exposure to industrial toxins such as mercury. Is the patient taking any medications? Note especially use of iodides, cholinergics, and miotics.

PHYSICAL ASSESSMENT

A patient who complains of increased salivation may have overproductive salivary glands or difficulty swallowing. To distinguish these, first test for a gag reflex and observe the patient's ability to swallow and chew. Is he drooling? Is his chewing uncoordinated? An impaired gag reflex, drooling, and chewing incoordination suggest difficulty swallowing.

Inspect the mouth and mucous membranes for lesions. If present, are they painful? Put on gloves and palpate the lesions, which may be suppurative or infectious. Describe them in your notes. Next, inspect the uvula, gingivae, and pharynx. Palpate the lymph nodes, and determine if the parotid glands are swollen or sore.

MEDICAL CAUSES

Bell's palsy

With Bell's palsy, paralysis of the facial nerve causes an inability to control salivation or close the eye on the affected side. The affected side of the face sags and is expressionless, the nasolabial fold flattens, and the palpebral fissure (the distance between the upper and lower eyelids) widens. The corneal reflex may be diminished or absent and the patient may have partial loss of taste or abnormal taste sensation.

Mercury poisoning

Stomatitis, characterized by increased salivation and a metallic taste, commonly occurs in those with mercury poisoning. The patient's teeth may be loose and his gums are painful, swollen, and prone to bleeding. A blue line appears on the gingivae. The patient may also experience personality changes, memory loss, abdominal cramps, diarrhea, paresthesia, and tremors of the eyelids, lips, tongue, and fingers.

Pregnancy

In the early months of pregnancy, many women experience increased salivation, nausea, gum swelling, and breast tenderness.

Stomatitis

Mucosal ulcers may be accompanied by moderately increased salivation, mouth pain, fever, and erythema. Spontaneous healing usually occurs in 7 to 10 days, but scarring and recurrence are possible.

Syphilis

With secondary syphilis, mucosal ulcers cause increased salivation that may persist up to 1 year. Related findings include fever, malaise, headache, anorexia, weight loss, nausea, vomiting, sore throat, and generalized lymphadenopathy. A bilaterally symmetrical rash appears on the arms, trunk, palms, soles, face, and scalp. Condylomata develop in the genital and perianal areas.

Tuberculosis

Certain forms of tuberculosis may produce solitary, irregularly-shaped mouth or tongue ulcers, covered with exudate, that cause increased salivation. Other findings include weight loss, anorexia, fever, fatigue, malaise, dyspnea, cough, night sweats (a common sign), and hemoptysis.

OTHER CAUSES

Drugs

Increased salivation may occur with iodide toxicity, but the earliest symptoms are a brassy taste and a burning sensation in the mouth and throat. Associated findings include sneezing, irritated eyelids, and (commonly) pain in the frontal sinus.

Pilocarpine and other miotics used to treat glaucoma may be absorbed systemically, increasing salivation. Cholinergics, such as bethanechol and neostigmine, may also cause this symptom.

SPECIAL CONSIDERATIONS

Though annoying to the patient, increased salivation doesn't require treatments beyond those needed to correct the underlying disorder.

Medical causes

Bell's palsy
+ Facial nerve paralysis causes an inability to control salivation.

Mercury poisoning
+ Stomatitis, characterized by increased salivation and a metallic taste, commonly occurs.

Pregnancy
+ In early months, many women experience increased salivation, nausea, gum swelling, and breast tenderness.

Stomatitis
+ Mucosal ulcers may be accompanied by moderately increased salivation, mouth pain, fever, and erythema.

Syphilis
+ With secondary syphilis, mucosal ulcers cause increased salivation that may persist up to 1 year.

Tuberculosis
+ Certain forms may produce mouth or tongue ulcers that cause increased salivation.

Other causes
+ Iodide toxicity
+ Pilocarpine and other miotics used to treat glaucoma
+ Cholinergics

Special considerations
+ Increased salivation doesn't require treatments beyond those needed to correct the underlying disorder.

Peds points

✦ Increased salivation in children may stem from the same conditions that affect adults or from congenital esophageal atresia.

Geri points

✦ Drooling is common in elderly people with Parkinson's disease.

Teaching points

✦ Proper oral hygiene

Key facts about scotoma

✦ Area of partial or complete blindness within an otherwise normal or slightly impaired visual field
✦ Usually located within the central 30-degree area
✦ Classified as absolute, relative, or scintillating

Key history points

✦ Medical history, including eye disorders, vision problems, or chronic systemic disorders
✦ Drug history

Critical assessment steps

✦ Test visual acuity.
✦ Inspect pupils for size, equality, and reaction to light.
✦ Make sure an ophthalmoscopic examination is performed and IOP is measured.
✦ Identify and characterize the scotoma using visual field tests.

PEDIATRIC POINTERS

Besides stemming from conditions that affect adults, increased salivation in children may also stem from congenital esophageal atresia. With this disorder, the infant is unable to swallow seemingly excessive saliva and frothy mucus.

GERIATRIC POINTERS

Drooling is common in elderly people with Parkinson's disease. It's caused by a reduction in automatic or conscious swallowing rather than by excessive salivation.

PATIENT COUNSELING

Teach the patient the importance of proper oral hygiene to prevent odor and dental problems. Remind him to seek regular dental care.

SCOTOMA

A scotoma is an area of partial or complete blindness within an otherwise normal or slightly impaired visual field. Usually located within the central 30-degree area, the defect ranges from absolute blindness to a barely detectable loss of visual acuity. Typically, the patient can pinpoint the scotoma's location in the visual field. (See *Locating scotomas.*)

A scotoma can result from a retinal, choroid, or optic nerve disorder. It can be classified as absolute, relative, or scintillating. An *absolute scotoma* refers to the total inability to see all sizes of test objects used in mapping the visual field. A *relative scotoma,* in contrast, refers to the ability to see only large test objects. A *scintillating scotoma* refers to the flashes or bursts of light commonly seen during a migraine headache.

HISTORY

Explore the patient's medical history, noting especially any eye disorders, vision problems, or chronic systemic disorders. Find out if he takes medications or uses eyedrops.

PHYSICAL ASSESSMENT

Test the patient's visual acuity and inspect his pupils for size, equality, and reaction to light. An ophthalmoscopic examination and measurement of intraocular pressure (IOP) are necessary. Then identify and characterize the scotoma using such visual field tests as the tangent screen examination, the Goldmann perimeter test, and the automated perimetry test. Two other visual field tests — confrontation testing and the Amsler grid — may also help in identifying a scotoma.

MEDICAL CAUSES

Chorioretinitis

Chorioretinitis, inflammation of the choroid and retina, produces a paracentral scotoma. Ophthalmoscopic examination reveals clouding and cells in the vitreous, subretinal hemorrhage, and neovascularization. The patient may have photophobia along with blurred vision.

Locating scotomas

Scotomas, or "blind spots," are classified according to the affected area of the visual field. The normal scotoma — shown in the temporal region of the right eye — appears in black in all the illustrations.

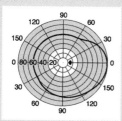

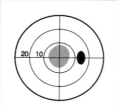

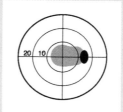

The *normally present scotoma* represents the position of the optic nerve head in the visual field. It appears between 10 and 20 degrees on this chart of the normal visual field.

A *central scotoma* involves the point of central fixation. It's always associated with decreased visual acuity.

A *centrocecal scotoma* involves the point of central fixation and the area between the blind spot and the fixation point.

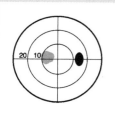

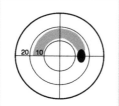

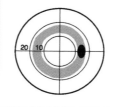

A *paracentral scotoma* affects an area of the visual field that is nasal or temporal to the point of central fixation.

An *arcuate scotoma* arches around the fixation point, usually ending on the nasal side of the visual field.

An *annular scotoma* forms a circular defect around the fixation point. It's common with retinal pigmentary degeneration.

Glaucoma

With glaucoma, prolonged elevation of IOP can cause an arcuate scotoma. Poorly controlled glaucoma can also cause cupping of the optic disk, loss of peripheral vision, and reduced visual acuity. The patient may also see rainbow-colored halos around lights.

Macular degeneration

Macular degeneration results in a central scotoma. Ophthalmoscopic examination reveals changes in the macular area. The patient may notice subtle changes in visual acuity, in color perception, and in the size and shape of objects.

Medical causes

Chorioretinitis

✦ A paracentral scotoma develops.
✦ Examination reveals clouding and cells in the vitreous, subretinal hemorrhage, and neovascularization.

Glaucoma

✦ Prolonged elevation of IOP can cause an arcuate scotoma.

Macular degeneration

✦ A central scotoma develops.
✦ Examination reveals changes in the macular area.

Medical causes
(continued)

Migraine headache
+ Transient scintillating scotomas can occur during the aura.

Optic neuritis
+ A central, circular, or centrocecal scotoma may develop along with vision loss or blurring and pain.
+ The scotoma may be unilateral or bilateral.

Retinitis pigmentosa
+ Annular scotoma progresses concentrically until only tunnel vision remains.

Special considerations
+ For the patient with an arcuate scotoma associated with glaucoma, emphasize regular testing of IOP and visual fields.
+ For the patient with a disorder involving the fovea centralis, teach him to use the Amsler grid.

Peds points
+ Use confrontation visual field testing in children.

Teaching points
+ Importance of compliance with drug therapy
+ Signs and symptoms to report
+ Available assistive devices

Key facts about scrotal swelling
+ Occurs when a condition affecting the testicles, epididymis, or scrotal skin produces edema or a mass
+ Can be unilateral or bilateral and painful or painless

Migraine headache

Transient scintillating scotomas, usually bilateral and typically homonymous, can occur during a classic migraine aura. Besides pain, characteristic associated symptoms include paresthesia of the lips, face, or hands; slight confusion; dizziness; and photophobia.

Optic neuritis

Inflammation, degeneration, or demyelination of the optic nerve produces a central, circular, or centrocecal scotoma. The scotoma may be unilateral with involvement of one nerve, or bilateral with involvement of both nerves. It can vary in size, density, and symmetry. The patient may report severe vision loss or blurring, lasting up to 3 weeks, and pain — especially with eye movement. Common ophthalmoscopic findings include hyperemia of the optic disk, retinal vein distention, blurred disk margins, and filling of the physiologic cup.

Retinitis pigmentosa

Retinitis pigmentosa initially involves loss of peripheral rods; the resulting annular scotoma progresses concentrically until only a central field of vision (tunnel vision) remains. The earliest symptom — impaired night vision — appears during adolescence. Associated signs include narrowing of the retinal blood vessels and pallor of the optic disk. Eventually, with invasion of the macula, blindness may occur.

SPECIAL CONSIDERATIONS

For the patient with an arcuate scotoma associated with glaucoma, emphasize regular testing of IOP and visual fields. For the patient with a disorder involving the fovea centralis (or the area surrounding it), teach him to periodically use the Amsler grid to detect progression of macular degeneration.

PEDIATRIC POINTERS

In young children, visual field testing is difficult and requires patience. Confrontation testing is the method of choice.

PATIENT COUNSELING

Explain to the patient the importance of complying with prescribed drug therapy to prevent progression and complications of the disease. Tell the patient to report any eye discharge, blurred or cloudy vision, halos, flashes of light, floaters, or changes in size and location of scotomas.

Inform the patient with bilateral central vision loss of the visual rehabilitation services available to him. Special devices, such as low-vision optical aids, are available to improve the quality of life in the patient with good peripheral vision.

SCROTAL SWELLING

Scrotal swelling occurs when a condition affecting the testicles, epididymis, or scrotal skin produces edema or a mass; the penis may be involved. Scrotal swelling can affect males of any age. It can be unilateral or bilateral and painful or painless.

The sudden onset of painful scrotal swelling suggests torsion of a testicle or testicular appendages, especially in a prepubescent male. This emergency requires immediate surgery to untwist and stabilize the spermatic cord or to remove the appendage.

EMERGENCY ACTIONS If severe pain accompanies scrotal swelling, ask when the swelling began. Using a Doppler stethoscope, evaluate blood flow to the testicle. If it's decreased or absent, suspect testicular torsion and prepare the patient for surgery. Withhold food and fluids, insert an I.V. line, and apply an ice pack to the scrotum to reduce pain and swelling. An attempt may be made to untwist the cord manually, but even if this is successful, the patient may still require surgery for stabilization.

HISTORY

If the patient isn't in distress, proceed with the medical history. Ask about injury to the scrotum, urethral discharge, cloudy urine, increased urinary frequency, and dysuria. Is the patient sexually active? When was his last sexual contact? Does he have a history of sexually transmitted disease? Find out about recent illnesses, particularly mumps. Does he have a history of prostate surgery or prolonged catheterization? Does changing his body position or level of activity affect the swelling?

 CULTURAL CUE *Patients of certain cultural backgrounds, such as Mexican-Americans, may need to establish a trusting relationship before discussing matters of a personal nature.*

PHYSICAL ASSESSMENT

Take the patient's vital signs, especially noting fever, and palpate his abdomen for tenderness. Then examine the entire genital area. Assess the scrotum with the patient in supine and standing positions. Note its size and color. Is the swelling unilateral or bilateral? Do you see signs of trauma or bruising? Are there rashes or lesions present? Gently palpate the scrotum for a cyst or a lump. Note especially tenderness or increased firmness. Check the testicles' position in the scrotum. Finally, transilluminate the scrotum to distinguish a fluid-filled cyst from a solid mass. (A solid mass can't be transilluminated.)

MEDICAL CAUSES

Epididymal cysts
Located in the head of the epididymis, epididymal cysts produce painless scrotal swelling. Most men, however, are asymptomatic and discover the cyst on self-examination.

Epididymitis
Key features of epididymitis are inflammation, pain, extreme tenderness, and swelling in the groin and scrotum. The patient waddles to avoid pressure on the groin and scrotum during walking. He may have high fever, malaise, urethral discharge and cloudy urine, and lower abdominal pain on the affected side. His scrotal skin may be hot, red, dry, flaky, and thin.

Hernia
Herniation of bowel into the scrotum can cause swelling and a soft or unusually firm scrotum. Occasionally, bowel sounds can be auscultated in the scrotum. If bowel obstruction occurs, anorexia, nausea, vomiting, and reduced bowel sounds may occur.

Hydrocele
With hydrocele, fluid accumulation produces gradual scrotal swelling that's usually painless. The scrotum may be soft and cystic or firm and tense. Palpation reveals a round, nontender scrotal mass.

In an emergency
If testicular torsion is suspected:
- ✦ Prepare patient for surgery.
- ✦ Withhold food and fluids.
- ✦ Insert I.V. line.
- ✦ Apply ice pack to the scrotum.

Key history points
- ✦ History of injury to scrotum, urethral discharge, cloudy urine, increased urinary frequency, dysuria, STD, prostate surgery, or prolonged catheterization
- ✦ Sexual activity
- ✦ Alleviating or aggravating body positions

Critical assessment steps
- ✦ Palpate abdomen for tenderness.
- ✦ Examine genital area.
- ✦ Assess scrotum with patient supine and standing.
- ✦ Check testicles' position in scrotum.

Medical causes
Epididymal cysts
- ✦ Painless scrotal swelling occurs.

Epididymitis
- ✦ Inflammation, pain, extreme tenderness, and swelling develop in the groin and scrotum.

Hernia
- ✦ Swelling and a soft or unusually firm scrotum are produced.

Hydrocele
- ✦ Fluid accumulation produces gradual scrotal swelling that's usually painless.

Medical causes
(continued)

Orchitis (acute)
✦ Sudden painful swelling of testicles occurs with hot, reddened scrotum; fever; chills; lower abdominal pain; nausea; vomiting; and extreme weakness.

Scrotal trauma
✦ Scrotal swelling, bruising, and severe pain result.

Spermatocele
✦ Moveable cystic mass develops; it may be transilluminated.

Testicular torsion
✦ Scrotal swelling; sudden, severe pain; and, possibly, elevation of the affected testicle within the scrotum occur.

Testicular tumor
✦ Scrotum swells and produces a sensation of excessive weight.

Other causes
✦ Blood effusion from surgery

Special considerations
✦ Place a rolled towel under the scrotum to help reduce swelling.
✦ For moderate swelling, suggest a loose-fitting athletic supporter.
✦ Apply heat or ice packs.

Peds points
✦ In children up to age 1, a hernia or hydrocele may cause scrotal swelling.
✦ In infants, scrotal swelling may stem from dermatitis.
✦ In prepubescent males, scrotal swelling usually results from torsion of spermatic cord.

Orchitis (acute)
Mumps, syphilis, or tuberculosis may precipitate acute orchitis, which causes sudden painful swelling of one or, at times, both testicles. Related findings include a hot, reddened scrotum; fever of up to 104° F (40° C); chills; lower abdominal pain; nausea; vomiting; and extreme weakness. Urinary signs are usually absent.

Scrotal trauma
Blunt trauma causes scrotal swelling with bruising and severe pain. The scrotum may appear dark or bluish. Nausea, vomiting, and difficulty urinating might also occur.

Spermatocele
A spermatocele, a usually painless cystic mass, lies above and behind the testicle and contains opaque fluid and sperm. Its onset may be acute or gradual. Less than 1 cm in diameter, it's movable and may be transilluminated.

Testicular torsion
Most common before puberty, testicular torsion is a urologic emergency that causes scrotal swelling; sudden, severe pain; and, possibly, elevation of the affected testicle within the scrotum. Testicular torsion may also cause nausea and vomiting.

Testicular tumor
Typically painless, smooth, and firm, a testicular tumor produces swelling and a sensation of excessive weight in the scrotum. With ureteral obstruction, the patient may have urinary complaints.

OTHER CAUSES

Surgery
An effusion of blood from surgery can produce a hematocele, leading to scrotal swelling.

SPECIAL CONSIDERATIONS

Keep the patient on bed rest and administer an antibiotic. Provide adequate fluids, fiber, and stool softeners. Place a rolled towel between the patient's legs and under the scrotum to help reduce severe swelling. Alternatively, if the patient has mild or moderate swelling, advise him to wear a loose-fitting athletic supporter lined with a soft cotton dressing. For several days, administer an analgesic to relieve his pain. Encourage sitz baths. Apply heat or ice packs to decrease inflammation.

Prepare the patient for needle aspiration of fluid-filled cysts and other diagnostic tests, such as lung tomography and computed tomography scan of the abdomen, to rule out malignant tumors.

PEDIATRIC POINTERS

A thorough physical assessment is especially important for children with scrotal swelling, who may be unable to provide history data. In children up to age 1, a hernia or hydrocele of the spermatic cord may stem from abnormal fetal development. In infants, scrotal swelling may stem from ammonia-related dermatitis if diapers aren't changed often enough. In prepubescent males, it usually results from torsion of the spermatic cord.

Other disorders that can produce scrotal swelling in children include epididymitis (rare before age 10), traumatic orchitis from contact sports, and mumps, which usually occurs after puberty.

PATIENT COUNSELING

Encourage the patient to perform testicular self-examinations at home. Encourage him to verbalize concerns and anxieties that he may have, such as reduced self-esteem, disturbed body image, and fertility issues.

SEIZURES, COMPLEX PARTIAL

A complex partial seizure occurs when a focal seizure begins in the temporal lobe and causes a partial alteration of consciousness—usually confusion. Psychomotor seizures can occur at any age, but incidence usually increases during adolescence and adulthood. Two-thirds of patients also have generalized seizures.

An aura—usually a complex hallucination, illusion, or sensation—typically precedes a psychomotor seizure. The hallucination may be audiovisual (images with sounds), auditory (abnormal or normal sounds or voices from the patient's past), or olfactory (unpleasant smells, such as rotten eggs or burning materials). Other types of auras include sensations of déjà vu, unfamiliarity with surroundings, or depersonalization. Some patients become fearful or anxious, experience lip smacking, or have an unpleasant feeling in the epigastric region that rises toward the chest and throat. The patient usually recognizes the aura and lies down before losing consciousness.

A period of unresponsiveness follows the aura. The patient may experience automatisms, appear dazed and wander aimlessly, perform inappropriate acts (such as undressing in public), be unresponsive, or utter incoherent phrases. After the seizure, the patient is confused, drowsy, and doesn't remember the seizure. Behavioral automatisms rarely last longer than 5 minutes, but postseizure confusion, agitation, and amnesia may persist.

Between attacks, the patient may exhibit slow and rigid thinking, outbursts of anger and aggressiveness, tedious conversation, a preoccupation with naive philosophical ideas, diminished libido, mood swings, and paranoid tendencies.

HISTORY

If you witness a complex partial seizure, never attempt to restrain the patient. Instead, lead him gently to a safe area. (*Exception:* Don't approach him if he's angry or violent.) Calmly encourage him to sit down, and remain with him until he's fully alert. After the seizure, ask him if he experienced an aura. Record all observations and findings.

PHYSICAL ASSESSMENT

If the patient has had a seizure, examine him for injury. Make sure he has a patent airway, and then perform a complete neurologic assessment.

MEDICAL CAUSES

Brain abscess

If the brain abscess is in the temporal lobe, complex partial seizures commonly occur after the abscess disappears. Related problems may include headache, nausea, vomiting, generalized seizures, and a decreased level of consciousness (LOC). The patient may also develop central facial weakness, auditory receptive aphasia, hemiparesis, and ocular disturbances.

Teaching points
+ Testicular self-examination

Key facts about complex partial seizures
+ Occur when focal seizures begin in the temporal lobe and cause partial alterations of consciousness
+ Typically preceded by auras

Key history points
+ Occurrence of aura

Critical assessment steps
+ Examine for injury after the seizure.
+ Ensure a patent airway.
+ Perform a complete neurologic assessment.

Medical causes
Brain abscess
+ If the temporal lobe is affected, complex partial seizures commonly occur after the abscess disappears.

Medical causes
(continued)

Head trauma

+ Trauma to the temporal lobe can produce complex partial seizures months or years later.
+ Seizures may decrease in frequency and eventually stop.

Temporal lobe tumor

+ Complex partial seizures may be the first sign.

Special considerations

+ After seizure, reorient patient to surroundings and protect him from injury.
+ Keep patient in bed until he's fully alert.
+ Remove harmful objects from the area.

Peds points

+ Complex partial seizures in children can result from birth injury, abuse, infection, or cancer.

Teaching points

+ Methods for coping with seizures
+ Safety measures

Key facts about generalized tonic-clonic seizures

+ Caused by paroxysmal, uncontrolled discharge of CNS neurons, leading to neurologic dysfunction
+ Extend to the entire brain

Head trauma

Severe trauma to the temporal lobe (especially from a penetrating injury) can produce complex partial seizures months or years later. The seizures may decrease in frequency and eventually stop. Head trauma also causes generalized seizures and behavior and personality changes.

Temporal lobe tumor

Complex partial seizures may be the first sign of a tumor in the temporal lobe. Other signs and symptoms include headache, pupillary changes, and mental dullness. Increased intracranial pressure may cause a decreased LOC, vomiting and, possibly, papilledema.

SPECIAL CONSIDERATIONS

After the seizure, remain with the patient to reorient him to his surroundings and to protect him from injury. Keep him in bed until he's fully alert, and remove harmful objects from the area.

Prepare the patient for diagnostic tests, such as EEG, computed tomography scans, or magnetic resonance imaging.

PEDIATRIC POINTERS

Complex partial seizures in children may resemble absence seizures (benign generalized seizures thought to originate subcortically). Complex partial seizures can result from birth injury, abuse, infection, or cancer. In about one-third of patients, their cause is unknown.

Repeated complex partial seizures commonly lead to generalized seizures. The child may experience a slight aura, which is rarely as clearly defined as that seen with generalized tonic-clonic seizures.

PATIENT COUNSELING

Offer emotional support to the patient and his family. Teach them how to cope with seizures. Discuss safety measures to take during a seizure.

SEIZURES, GENERALIZED TONIC-CLONIC

Like other types of seizures, generalized tonic-clonic seizures are caused by the paroxysmal, uncontrolled discharge of central nervous system (CNS) neurons, leading to neurologic dysfunction. Unlike most other types of seizures, however, this cerebral hyperactivity isn't confined to the original focus or to a localized area but extends to the entire brain.

Generalized tonic-clonic seizures usually occur singly. The patient may be asleep or awake and active. (See *What happens during a generalized tonic-clonic seizure.*) Possible complications include respiratory arrest due to airway obstruction from secretions, status epilepticus (occurring in 5% to 8% of patients), head or spinal injuries and bruises, Todd's paralysis and, rarely, cardiac arrest. Life-threatening status epilepticus is marked by prolonged seizure activity or by rapidly recurring seizures with no intervening periods of recovery. It's most commonly triggered by abrupt discontinuation of anticonvulsant therapy.

Generalized seizures may be caused by a brain tumor, vascular disorder, head trauma, infection, metabolic defect, drug or alcohol withdrawal syndrome, exposure to toxins, or a genetic defect. Generalized seizures may also result from a focal

What happens during a generalized tonic-clonic seizure

BEFORE THE SEIZURE

Prodromal signs and symptoms, such as myoclonic jerks, throbbing headache, and mood changes, may occur over several hours or days. The patient may have premonitions of the seizure. For example, he may report an aura, such as seeing a flashing light or smelling a characteristic odor.

DURING THE SEIZURE

If a generalized seizure begins with an aura, this indicates that irritability in a specific area of the brain quickly became widespread. Common auras include palpitations, epigastric distress rapidly rising to the throat, head or eye turning, and sensory hallucinations.

Next, *loss of consciousness* occurs as a sudden discharge of intense electrical activity overwhelms the brain's subcortical center. The patient falls and experiences brief, bilateral myoclonic contractures. Air forced through spasmodic vocal cords may produce a birdlike, piercing cry.

During the *tonic phase,* skeletal muscles contract for 10 to 20 seconds. The patient's eyelids are drawn up, his arms are flexed, and his legs are extended. His mouth opens wide, then snaps shut; he may bite his tongue. His respirations cease because of respiratory muscle spasm, and initial pallor of the skin and mucous membranes (the result of impaired venous return) changes to cyanosis secondary to apnea. The patient arches his back and slowly lowers his arms (as shown below). Other effects include dilated, nonreactive pupils; greatly increased heart rate and blood pressure; increased salivation and tracheobronchial secretions; and profuse diaphoresis.

During the *clonic phase,* lasting about 60 seconds, mild trembling progresses to violent contractures or jerks. Other motor activity includes facial grimaces (with possible tongue biting) and violent expiration of bloody, foamy saliva from clonic contractures of thoracic cage muscles. Clonic jerks slowly decrease in intensity and frequency. The patient is still apneic.

AFTER THE SEIZURE

The patient's movements gradually cease, and he becomes unresponsive to external stimuli. Other postseizure features include stertorous respirations from increased tracheobronchial secretions, equal or unequal pupils (but becoming reactive), and urinary incontinence due to brief muscle relaxation. After about 5 minutes, the patient's level of consciousness increases, and he appears confused and disoriented. His muscle tone, heart rate, and blood pressure return to normal.

After several hours' sleep, the patient awakens exhausted and may have a headache, sore muscles, and amnesia about the seizure.

Signs and symptoms of a generalized tonic-clonic seizure

Before seizure
+ Myoclonic jerks
+ Headache
+ Mood changes
+ Premonition of seizure

During seizure
+ Aura
+ Loss of consciousness
+ Myoclonic contractures
+ Birdlike, piercing cry
+ Skeletal muscle contraction
+ Drawn up eyelids
+ Flexed arms
+ Extended legs
+ Pallor or cyanosis
+ Arched back with lowered arms
+ Dilated, nonreactive pupils
+ Increased heart rate and blood pressure
+ Increased salivation and tracheobronchial secretions
+ Diaphoresis
+ Violent contractures or jerks
+ Facial grimacing

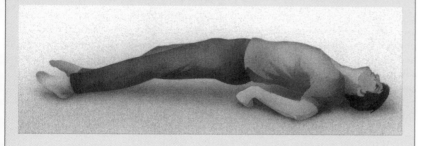

seizure. With recurring seizures, or epilepsy, the cause may be unknown. (See *How to respond to a seizure,* page 600.)

In an emergency

+ First check the patient's airway, breathing, and circulation (ensure that the cause isn't asystole or a blocked airway).
+ Stay with the patient and ensure a patent airway.
+ If possible, turn the patient to one side during the seizure.
+ If the seizure lasts longer than 4 minutes or if a second seizure occurs before full recovery from the first, suspect status epilepticus.
+ Administer diazepam or lorazepam by slow I.V. push.

Key history points

+ Description of seizure
+ Unusual sensations before the seizure
+ Seizure history
+ Drug history
+ Sleep deprivation or emotional or physical stress at time of seizure

Critical assessment steps

+ If the patient may have sustained a head injury, observe him closely for loss of consciousness, unequal or nonreactive pupils, and focal neurologic signs.
+ Examine the arms, legs, and face (including tongue) for injury, residual paralysis, or limb weakness.
+ Take vital signs.
+ Complete a neurologic assessment.

EMERGENCY ACTIONS

How to respond to a seizure

If you witness the beginning of the seizure, first check the patient's airway, breathing, and circulation, and ensure that the cause isn't asystole or a blocked airway. Stay with the patient and ensure a patent airway. Focus your care on observing the seizure and protecting the patient. Place a towel under his head to prevent injury, loosen his clothing, and move any sharp or hard objects out of his way. Never try to restrain the patient or force a hard object into his mouth; you might chip his teeth or fracture his jaw. Only at the start of the ictal phase can you safely insert a soft object into his mouth.

If possible, turn the patient to one side *during* the seizure to allow secretions to drain and to prevent aspiration. Otherwise, do this at the end of the clonic phase when respirations return. (If they fail to return, check for airway obstruction and suction the patient if necessary. Cardiopulmonary resuscitation, intubation, and mechanical ventilation may be needed.)

Protect the patient after the seizure by providing a safe area in which he can rest. As he awakens, reassure and reorient him. Check his vital signs and neurologic status. Carefully record these data as well as your observations during the seizure.

If the seizure lasts longer than 4 minutes or if a second seizure occurs before full recovery from the first, suspect status epilepticus. Establish an airway, start an I.V. line, give supplemental oxygen, and begin cardiac monitoring. Draw blood for appropriate studies. Turn the patient on his side, with his head in a semi-dependent position, to drain secretions and prevent aspiration. Periodically turn him to the opposite side, check his arterial blood gas levels for hypoxemia, and administer oxygen by mask, increasing the flow rate if necessary. If appropriate, administer diazepam or lorazepam by slow I.V. push, repeated two or three times at 10- to 20-minute intervals, to stop the seizures. If the patient isn't known to have epilepsy, an I.V. bolus of dextrose 50% (50 ml) with thiamine (100 mg) may be ordered. Dextrose may stop the seizures if the patient has hypoglycemia. If his thiamine level is low, also give thiamine to guard against further damage.

If the patient is intubated, expect to insert a nasogastric (NG) tube to prevent vomiting and aspiration. Be aware that if the patient hasn't been intubated, the NG tube itself can trigger the gag reflex and cause vomiting. Be sure to record your observations and the intervals between seizures.

HISTORY

If you didn't witness the seizure, obtain a description from the patient's companion. Ask when the seizure started and how long it lasted. Did the patient report any unusual sensations before the seizure began? Did the seizure start in one area of the body and spread, or did it affect the entire body right away? Did the patient fall on a hard surface? Did his eyes or head turn? Did he turn blue? Did he lose bladder control? Did he have any other seizures before recovering? Does he complain of headache and muscle soreness? Is he increasingly difficult to arouse when you check on him at 20-minute intervals?

Next, obtain a history. Has the patient ever had generalized or focal seizures before? If so, do they occur frequently? Do other family members also have them? Is the patient receiving drug therapy? Is he compliant? Also, ask about sleep deprivation and emotional or physical stress at the time the seizure occurred.

PHYSICAL ASSESSMENT

If the patient may have sustained a head injury, observe him closely for loss of consciousness, unequal or nonreactive pupils, and focal neurologic signs. Examine his arms, legs, and face (including tongue) for injury, residual paralysis, or limb weakness. If you haven't already done so, take the patient's vital signs. Then complete your neurologic assessment.

MEDICAL CAUSES

Alcohol withdrawal syndrome

Sudden withdrawal from alcohol dependence may cause seizures 7 to 48 hours later as well as status epilepticus. The patient may also be restless and exhibit hallucinations, profuse diaphoresis, and tachycardia.

Arsenic poisoning

Besides generalized seizures, arsenic poisoning may cause a garlicky breath odor, increased salivation, and generalized pruritus. GI effects include diarrhea, nausea, vomiting, and severe abdominal pain. Related effects include diffuse hyperpigmentation; sharply defined edema of the eyelids, face, and ankles; paresthesia of the extremities; alopecia; irritated mucous membranes; weakness; muscle aches; and peripheral neuropathy.

Brain abscess

Generalized seizures may occur in the acute stage of abscess formation or after the abscess disappears. Depending on the size and location of the abscess, decreased level of consciousness (LOC) varies from drowsiness to deep stupor. Early signs and symptoms reflect increased intracranial pressure (ICP) and include constant headache, nausea, vomiting, and focal seizures. Typical later features include ocular disturbances, such as nystagmus, impaired vision, and unequal pupils. Other findings vary with the abscess site but may include aphasia, hemiparesis, abnormal behavior, and personality changes.

Brain tumor

Generalized seizures may occur, depending on the tumor's location and type. Other findings include a slowly decreasing LOC, morning headache, dizziness, confusion, focal seizures, vision loss, motor and sensory disturbances, aphasia, and ataxia. Later findings include papilledema, vomiting, increased systolic blood pressure, widening pulse pressure, and (eventually) decorticate posture.

Cerebral aneurysm

Occasionally, generalized seizures may occur with an aneurysmal rupture. Premonitory signs and symptoms may last several days, but onset is typically abrupt with severe headache, nausea, vomiting, and decreased LOC. Depending on the site and amount of bleeding, related signs and symptoms vary but may include nuchal rigidity, irritability, hemiparesis, hemisensory defects, dysphagia, photophobia, diplopia, ptosis, and unilateral pupil dilation.

Eclampsia

Generalized seizures are a hallmark of eclampsia. Related findings include severe frontal headache, nausea and vomiting, vision disturbances, increased blood pressure, fever of up to 104° F (40° C), peripheral edema, and sudden weight gain. The patient may also exhibit oliguria, irritability, hyperactive deep tendon reflexes (DTRs), and decreased LOC.

Encephalitis

Seizures are an early sign of encephalitis, indicating a poor prognosis; they may also occur after recovery as a result of residual damage. Other findings include fever, headache, photophobia, nuchal rigidity, neck pain, vomiting, aphasia, ataxia,

Medical causes

Alcohol withdrawal syndrome
✦ Seizures as well as status epilepticus may occur 7 to 48 hours after sudden withdrawal.

Arsenic poisoning
✦ Generalized seizures may occur with a garlicky breath odor, increased salivation, generalized pruritus, diarrhea, nausea, vomiting, and abdominal pain.

Brain abscess
✦ Generalized seizures may occur in the acute stage of abscess formation or after the abscess disappears.
✦ Constant headache, nausea, vomiting, and focal seizures are early signs and symptoms.

Brain tumor
✦ Generalized seizures may occur, depending on the tumor's location and type.

Cerebral aneurysm
✦ Generalized seizures may occur.
✦ Onset is typically abrupt with severe headache, nausea, vomiting, and decreased LOC.

Eclampsia
✦ Generalized seizures are a hallmark.

Encephalitis
✦ Seizures are an early sign, indicating a poor prognosis.
✦ Seizures may also occur after recovery as a result of residual damage.

Medical causes
(continued)

Head trauma
✦ Generalized seizures may occur at the time of injury.
✦ Focal seizures may occur months later.

Hepatic encephalopathy
✦ Generalized seizures may occur late.

Hypertensive encephalopathy
✦ Seizures occur with increased blood pressure, decreased LOC, intense headache, vomiting, transient blindness, paralysis, and Cheyne-Stokes respirations.

Hypoglycemia
✦ Generalized seizures usually occur in severe cases.

Hyponatremia
✦ Seizures develop when sodium levels fall below 125 mEq/L, especially if the decrease is rapid.

Hypoparathyroidism
✦ Generalized seizures occur due to worsening tetany.

Hypoxic encephalopathy
✦ Generalized seizures, myoclonic jerks, and coma result.

Neurofibromatosis
✦ Multiple brain lesions cause focal and generalized seizures.

Renal failure (chronic)
✦ Onset of twitching, trembling, myoclonic jerks, and generalized seizures is rapid.

hemiparesis, nystagmus, irritability, cranial nerve palsies (causing facial weakness, ptosis, dysphagia), and myoclonic jerks.

Head trauma
In severe cases, generalized seizures may occur at the time of injury. (Months later, focal seizures may occur.) Severe head trauma may also cause a decreased LOC, leading to coma; soft-tissue injury of the face, head, or neck; clear or bloody drainage from the mouth, nose, or ears; facial edema; bony deformity of the face, head, or neck; Battle's sign; and lack of response to oculocephalic and oculovestibular stimulation. Motor and sensory deficits may occur along with altered respirations. Examination may reveal signs of increasing ICP, such as decreased response to painful stimuli, nonreactive pupils, bradycardia, increased systolic pressure, and widening pulse pressure. If the patient is conscious, he may exhibit vision deficits, behavioral changes, and headache.

Hepatic encephalopathy
Generalized seizures may occur late in hepatic encephalopathy. Associated late-stage findings in the comatose patient include fetor hepaticus, asterixis, hyperactive DTRs, and a positive Babinski's sign.

Hypertensive encephalopathy
Hypertensive encephalopathy, a life-threatening disorder, may cause seizures along with severely increased blood pressure, decreased LOC, intense headache, vomiting, transient blindness, paralysis, and (eventually) Cheyne-Stokes respirations.

Hypoglycemia
Generalized seizures usually occur with severe hypoglycemia, accompanied by blurred or double vision, motor weakness, hemiplegia, trembling, excessive diaphoresis, tachycardia, myoclonic twitching, and decreased LOC.

Hyponatremia
Seizures develop when serum sodium levels fall below 125 mEq/L, especially if the decrease is rapid. Hyponatremia also causes orthostatic hypotension, headache, muscle twitching and weakness, fatigue, oliguria or anuria, cold and clammy skin, decreased skin turgor, irritability, lethargy, confusion, and stupor or coma. Excessive thirst, tachycardia, nausea, vomiting, and abdominal cramps may also occur. Severe hyponatremia may cause cyanosis and vasomotor collapse, with a thready pulse.

Hypoparathyroidism
Worsening tetany causes generalized seizures. Chronic hypoparathyroidism produces neuromuscular irritability, Chvostek's sign, dysphagia, tetany, and hyperactive DTRs.

Hypoxic encephalopathy
Besides generalized seizures, hypoxic encephalopathy may produce myoclonic jerks and coma. Later, if the patient has recovered, dementia, visual agnosia, choreoathetosis, and ataxia may occur.

Neurofibromatosis
Multiple brain lesions from neurofibromatosis cause focal and generalized seizures. Inspection reveals café-au-lait spots, multiple skin tumors, scoliosis, and kyphoscoliosis. Related findings include dizziness, ataxia, monocular blindness, and nystagmus.

Renal failure (chronic)

End-stage renal failure produces rapid onset of twitching, trembling, myoclonic jerks, and generalized seizures. Related signs and symptoms include anuria or oliguria, fatigue, malaise, irritability, decreased mental acuity, muscle cramps, peripheral neuropathies, anorexia, and constipation or diarrhea. Integumentary effects include skin color changes (yellow, brown, or bronze), pruritus, and uremic frost. Other effects include ammonia breath odor, nausea and vomiting, ecchymoses, petechiae, GI bleeding, mouth and gum ulcers, hypertension, and Kussmaul's respirations.

Stroke

Seizures (focal more often than generalized) may occur within 6 months of an ischemic stroke. Associated signs and symptoms vary with the location and extent of brain damage. They include decreased LOC, contralateral hemiplegia, dysarthria, dysphagia, ataxia, unilateral sensory loss, apraxia, agnosia, and aphasia. The patient may also develop visual deficits, memory loss, poor judgment, personality changes, emotional lability, urine retention or urinary incontinence, constipation, headache, and vomiting.

OTHER CAUSES

Barbiturate withdrawal

In chronically intoxicated patients, barbiturate withdrawal may produce generalized seizures 2 to 4 days after the last dose. Status epilepticus is possible.

Diagnostic tests

Contrast agents used in radiologic tests may cause generalized seizures.

Drugs

Toxic blood levels of some drugs, such as theophylline, lidocaine, meperidine, penicillins, and cimetidine, may cause generalized seizures. Phenothiazines, tricyclic antidepressants, amphetamines, isoniazid, and vincristine may cause seizures in patients with preexisting epilepsy.

SPECIAL CONSIDERATIONS

Closely monitor the patient after the seizure for recurring seizure activity. Prepare him for a computed tomography scan or magnetic resonance imaging and EEG.

PEDIATRIC POINTERS

Generalized seizures are common in children. In fact, between 75% and 90% of epileptic patients experience their first seizure before age 20. Many children between ages 3 months and 3 years experience generalized seizures associated with fever; some of these children later develop seizures without fever. Generalized seizures may also stem from inborn errors of metabolism, perinatal injury, brain infection, Reye's syndrome, Sturge-Weber syndrome, arteriovenous malformation, lead poisoning, hypoglycemia, and idiopathic causes.

PATIENT COUNSELING

Advise the patient's family to observe and record his seizure activity to ensure proper treatment. Emphasize the importance of strict compliance with the drug regimen, and warn the patient about adverse reactions. Also, stress the importance of regular follow-up appointments for blood studies.

Medical causes
(continued)

Stroke
+ Seizures (focal more often than generalized) may occur within 6 months of an ischemic stroke.

Other causes
+ Barbiturate withdrawal
+ Contrast agents used in radiologic tests
+ Phenothiazines, TCAs, amphetamines, isoniazid, and vincristine (in patients with preexisting epilepsy)
+ Toxic blood levels of some drugs, such as theophylline, lidocaine, meperidine, penicillins, and cimetidine

Special considerations
+ Monitor the patient after the seizure for recurring seizure activity.

Peds points
+ Common in children, generalized seizures may stem from fever, epilepsy, inborn errors of metabolism, perinatal injury, brain infection, Reye's syndrome, Sturge-Weber syndrome, arteriovenous malformation, lead poisoning, hypoglycemia, and idiopathic causes.

Teaching points
+ Observing and recording seizure activity
+ Importance of compliance with drug regimen and follow-up appointments
+ Adverse reactions of prescribed drugs

SEIZURES, SIMPLE PARTIAL

Resulting from an irritable focus in the cerebral cortex, simple partial seizures typically last about 30 seconds and don't alter the patient's level of consciousness (LOC). The type and pattern reflect the location of the irritable focus. Simple partial seizures may be classified as motor (including both jacksonian seizures and epilepsia partialis continua) or somatosensory (including visual, olfactory, and auditory seizures).

A *focal motor seizure* is a series of unilateral clonic (muscle jerking) and tonic (muscle stiffening) movements of one part of the body. The patient's head and eyes characteristically turn away from the hemispheric focus — usually the frontal lobe near the motor strip. A tonic-clonic contraction of the trunk or extremities may follow.

A *jacksonian motor* seizure typically begins with a tonic contraction of a finger, the corner of the mouth, or one foot. Clonic movements follow, spreading to other muscles on the same side of the body, moving up the arm or leg, and eventually involving the whole side. Alternatively, clonic movements may spread to the opposite side, becoming generalized and leading to loss of consciousness. In the postictal phase, the patient may experience paralysis (Todd's paralysis) in the affected limbs, usually resolving within 24 hours.

Epilepsia partialis continua causes clonic twitching of one muscle group, usually in the face, arm, or leg. Twitching occurs every few seconds and persists for hours, days, or months without spreading. Spasms usually affect the distal arm and leg muscles more than the proximal ones; in the face, they affect the corner of the mouth, one or both eyelids and, occasionally, the neck or trunk muscles unilaterally.

A *focal somatosensory seizure* affects a localized body area on one side. Usually, this type of seizure initially causes numbness, tingling, or crawling or "electric" sensations; occasionally, it causes pain or burning sensations in the lips, fingers, or toes.

A *visual seizure* involves sensations of darkness or of stationary or moving lights or spots, usually red at first, then blue, green, and yellow. It can affect both visual fields or the visual field on the side opposite the lesion. The irritable focus is in the occipital lobe. In contrast, the irritable focus in an *auditory* or *olfactory seizure* is in the temporal lobe. (See *Body functions affected by focal seizures*.)

HISTORY

Record the patient's seizure activity in detail; your data may be critical in locating the lesion in the brain. Does the patient turn his head and eyes? If so, to what side? Where does movement first start? Does it spread? Because a partial seizure may become generalized, you'll need to watch closely for loss of consciousness, bilateral tonicity and clonicity, cyanosis, tongue biting, and urinary incontinence. (See "Seizures, generalized tonic-clonic," page 598.)

After the seizure, ask the patient to describe exactly what he remembers, if anything, about the seizure. Then obtain a history. Ask the patient what happened before the seizure. Can he describe an aura or did he recognize its onset? If so, how — by a smell, a visual disturbance, or a sound or visceral phenomenon, such as an unusual sensation in his stomach? How does this seizure compare with others he has had?

Also, explore fully any history, recent or remote, of head trauma. Check for a history of stroke or recent infection, especially with fever, headache, or a stiff neck.

Body functions affected by focal seizures

The site of the irritable focus determines which body functions are affected by a focal seizure, as shown in this illustration.

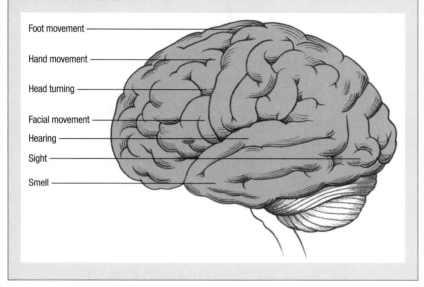

Foot movement
Hand movement
Head turning
Facial movement
Hearing
Sight
Smell

PHYSICAL ASSESSMENT

Take your patient's vital signs. Perform a complete physical assessment, focusing on the neurologic assessment. Check the patient's LOC, and test for residual deficits (such as weakness in the involved extremity) and sensory disturbances.

MEDICAL CAUSES

Brain abscess

Seizures can occur in the acute stage of abscess formation or after resolution of the abscess. Decreased LOC varies from drowsiness to deep stupor. Early signs and symptoms reflect increased intracranial pressure and include a constant, intractable headache, nausea, and vomiting. Later signs and symptoms include ocular disturbances, such as nystagmus, decreased visual acuity, and unequal pupils. Other findings vary according to the abscess site and may include aphasia, hemiparesis, and personality changes.

Brain tumor

Focal seizures are commonly the earliest indicators of a brain tumor. The patient may report morning headache, dizziness, confusion, vision loss, and motor and sensory disturbances. He may also develop aphasia, generalized seizures, ataxia, decreased LOC, papilledema, vomiting, increased systolic blood pressure, and widening pulse pressure. Eventually, he may assume a decorticate posture.

Head trauma

Any head injury can cause seizures, but penetrating wounds are characteristically associated with focal seizures. The seizures usually begin 3 to 15 months after in-

Critical assessment steps

- ◆ Take vital signs.
- ◆ Perform a complete physical assessment, focusing on the neurologic assessment.
- ◆ Check LOC.
- ◆ Test for residual deficits and sensory disturbances.

Medical causes

Brain abscess

- ◆ Seizures can occur in the acute stage of abscess formation or after resolution of the abscess.

Brain tumor

- ◆ Focal seizures are commonly the earliest indicators.
- ◆ Morning headache, dizziness, confusion, vision loss, and motor and sensory disturbances may occur.

Head trauma

- ◆ Penetrating wounds are associated with focal seizures.
- ◆ Seizures usually begin 3 to 15 months after injury, decrease in frequency after several years, and eventually stop.

Medical causes
(continued)
Multiple sclerosis
+ Focal or generalized seizures may occur in the late stages.

Neurofibromatosis
+ Multiple brain lesions cause focal seizures and, at times, generalized seizures.

Stroke
+ Focal seizures may occur up to 6 months after a stroke's onset.

Special considerations
+ Remain with the patient during the seizure, and reassure him.

Peds points
+ Focal seizures affect more children than adults.
+ Focal seizures in children can result from hemiplegic cerebral palsy, head trauma, child abuse, arteriovenous malformation, or Sturge-Weber syndrome.

Teaching points
+ Recording seizures
+ Importance of complying with drug regimen
+ Maintaining a safe environment

Key facts about bronze skin
+ Results from excessive circulating melanin
+ Tends to appear at pressure points and in creases on the palms and soles
+ May extend to the buccal mucosa and gums before covering the entire body

jury, decrease in frequency after several years, and eventually stop. The patient may develop generalized seizures and a decreased LOC that may progress to coma.

Multiple sclerosis
Focal or generalized seizures may occur with multiple sclerosis, usually during the late stages. Other findings include visual deficits, paresthesia, constipation, muscle weakness, spasticity, paralysis, hyperreflexia, intention tremor, gait ataxia, dysphagia, dysarthria, emotional lability, impotence, and urinary frequency, urgency, and incontinence.

Neurofibromatosis
With neurofibromatosis, multiple brain lesions cause focal seizures and, at times, generalized seizures. Inspection reveals café-au-lait spots, multiple skin tumors, scoliosis, and kyphoscoliosis. Related findings include dizziness, ataxia, progressive monocular blindness, nystagmus, and endocrine abnormalities.

Stroke
A major cause of seizures in patients older than age 50, a stroke may induce focal seizures up to 6 months after its onset. Related effects depend on the type and extent of the stroke but may include decreased LOC, contralateral hemiplegia, dysarthria, dysphagia, ataxia, unilateral sensory loss, apraxia, agnosia, and aphasia. A stroke may also cause vision deficits, memory loss, poor judgment, personality changes, emotional lability, headache, urinary incontinence or retention, and vomiting. It may result in generalized seizures.

SPECIAL CONSIDERATIONS
No emergency care is necessary during a focal seizure, unless it progresses to a generalized seizure. (See "Seizures, generalized tonic-clonic," page 598.) However, to ensure patient safety remain with the patient during the seizure, and reassure him.

Prepare the patient for such diagnostic tests as a computed tomography scan and EEG.

PEDIATRIC POINTERS
Affecting more children than adults, focal seizures are likely to spread and become generalized. They typically cause the child's eyes, or his head and eyes, to turn to the side; in neonates, they cause mouth twitching, staring, or both.

Focal seizures in children can result from hemiplegic cerebral palsy, head trauma, child abuse, arteriovenous malformation, or Sturge-Weber syndrome. About 25% of febrile seizures present as focal seizures.

PATIENT COUNSELING
After the seizure, instruct the patient to record his seizures. Also, emphasize the importance of complying with the prescribed drug regimen and maintaining a safe environment.

SKIN, BRONZE
The result of excessive circulating melanin, a bronze skin tone tends to appear at pressure points — such as the knuckles, elbows, toes, and knees — and in creases on the palms and soles. Eventually, this hyperpigmentation may extend to the buccal mucosa and gums before covering the entire body. Because bronzing develops

gradually, it's sometimes mistaken for a suntan. However, the hyperpigmentation can affect the entire body, not just sun-exposed areas. Sun exposure deepens the bronze color of exposed areas, but this effect fades. In fair-skinned patients, the bronze tone can range from light to dark. The tone also varies with the disorder.

HISTORY

Begin by asking the patient when the hyperpigmentation first appeared. Has its hue changed? When was he last exposed to the sun or artificial tanning source? Also, ask about a history of infection, illness, surgery, or trauma. Does he have abdominal pain, weakness, fatigue, diarrhea, or constipation? Has he recently lost weight? If the patient is receiving maintenance therapy for adrenal insufficiency, has his dosage been increased?

PHYSICAL ASSESSMENT

Examine the mucosa, gums, and scars for hyperpigmentation. Check for signs of dehydration and for abdominal distention, loss of body hair, and tissue and muscle wasting. Palpate for hepatosplenomegaly.

MEDICAL CAUSES

Adrenal hyperplasia

With adrenal hyperplasia, the skin assumes a dark bronze tone within a few months. Other findings include visual field deficits and headache (from an expanding pituitary lesion), and signs of masculinization in females such as clitoral enlargement, and male distribution of hair, fat, and muscle mass.

Biliary cirrhosis

Biliary cirrhosis causes bronze skin from melanosis of exposed areas of jaundiced skin: eyelids, palms, neck, and chest or back. The patient may also experience generalized pruritus, weakness, fatigue, jaundice, dark urine, pale stools with steatorrhea, decreased appetite with weight loss, and hepatomegaly.

Hemochromatosis

An early sign of hemochromatosis is progressive, generalized bronzing accentuated by metallic gray-bronze skin on sun-exposed areas, genitalia, and scars. Mucous membranes are affected less often. Early associated effects include weakness, lethargy, weight loss, abdominal pain, loss of libido, polydipsia, and polyuria.

 CULTURAL CUE *Hereditary hemochromatosis is the most common genetic disorder in whites, affecting 1 in 200 to 300 people of Northern European descent.*

Malnutrition

As weight loss, which occurs from malnutrition, depletes body nutrients, bronzing develops along with apathy, lethargy, anorexia, weakness, and slow pulse and respiratory rates. Patients may develop paresthesia in the extremities; dull, sparse, dry hair; brittle nails; dark, swollen cheeks; dry, flaky skin; red, swollen lips; muscle wasting; and gonadal atrophy in males.

Primary adrenal insufficiency

Bronze skin is a classic sign of primary adrenal insufficiency. Other findings include axillary and pubic hair loss, vitiligo, progressive fatigue, weakness, anorexia, nausea and vomiting, weight loss, orthostatic hypotension, weak and irregular pulse, abdominal pain, irritability, diarrhea or constipation, amenorrhea, and syncope.

Key history points

+ Onset of bronze skin
+ Last exposure to sun or tanning source
+ History of infection, illness, surgery, or trauma
+ Associated abdominal pain, weakness, fatigue, diarrhea, constipation, or weight loss
+ Current maintenance therapy for adrenal insufficiency

Critical assessment steps

+ Examine mucosa, gums, and scars for hyperpigmentation.
+ Check for dehydration, abdominal distention, loss of body hair, and tissue and muscle wasting.
+ Palpate for hepatosplenomegaly.

Medical causes

Adrenal hyperplasia
+ The skin assumes a dark bronze tone within a few months.

Biliary cirrhosis
+ Bronze skin results from melanosis of exposed areas of jaundiced skin.

Hemochromatosis
+ Progressive, generalized bronzing is accentuated by metallic gray-bronze skin.

Malnutrition
+ Bronzing, apathy, lethargy, anorexia, weakness, and slow pulse and respiratory rates occur.

Primary adrenal insufficiency
+ Bronze skin is a classic sign.

Medical causes
(continued)
Renal failure (chronic)
+ The skin becomes pallid, yellowish bronze, dry, and scaly.

Other causes
+ Prolonged therapy with high doses of a phenothiazine

Special considerations
+ Prepare the patient for diagnostic tests.

Peds points
+ Bronzing in children can result from celiac disease, the introduction of cereals, and, rarely, adrenoleukodystrophy.

Teaching points
+ Importance of rest periods
+ Referral to nutritional counseling, if appropriate

Key facts about clammy skin
+ Is moist, cool, and usually pale
+ Involves the release of epinephrine and norepinephrine, which causes cutaneous vasoconstriction and secretion of cold sweat from eccrine glands
+ Tends to occur on the palms, forehead, and soles

Key history points
+ History of type 1 diabetes or cardiac disorder
+ Drug history
+ Associated pain, chest pressure, nausea, epigastric distress, weakness, diarrhea, increased urination, or dry mouth

Renal failure (chronic)

With chronic renal failure, the skin becomes pallid, yellowish bronze, dry, and scaly. Other findings include ammonia breath odor, oliguria, fatigue, decreased mental acuity, seizures, muscle cramps, peripheral neuropathy, bleeding tendencies, pruritus and, occasionally, uremic frost and hypertension.

OTHER CAUSES

Drugs

Prolonged therapy with high doses of a phenothiazine may cause gradual bronzing of the skin.

SPECIAL CONSIDERATIONS

Prepare the patient for the adrenocorticotropic stimulation test, thyroid function studies, complete blood count, electrolyte analysis, electrocardiography, and a computed tomography scan of the pituitary gland.

PEDIATRIC POINTERS

Celiac disease can cause bronze skin in young children. Bronzing begins with the introduction of cereals and usually subsides later in childhood or adolescence. It also stems from adrenoleukodystrophy, a rare but life-threatening X-linked recessive disorder that affects boys and young men.

PATIENT COUNSELING

Encourage the patient to discuss his concerns about changes in body image. Encourage frequent rest periods if fatigue is a problem. A referral for nutritional counseling may be needed if the patient experiences weight loss, nausea, or vomiting.

SKIN, CLAMMY

Clammy skin — moist, cool, and usually pale — is a sympathetic response to stress, which triggers release of the hormones epinephrine and norepinephrine. These hormones cause cutaneous vasoconstriction and secretion of cold sweat from eccrine glands, particularly on the palms, forehead, and soles.

Clammy skin typically accompanies shock, acute hypoglycemia, anxiety reactions, arrhythmias, and heat exhaustion. It also occurs as a vasovagal reaction to severe pain associated with nausea, anorexia, epigastric distress, hyperpnea, tachypnea, weakness, confusion, tachycardia, pupillary dilation, or a combination of these findings. Marked bradycardia and syncope may follow.

HISTORY

Ask the patient if he has a history of type 1 diabetes mellitus or a cardiac disorder. Is the patient taking any medications, especially an antiarrhythmic? Is he experiencing pain, chest pressure, nausea, or epigastric distress? Does he feel weak? Does he have a dry mouth? Does he have diarrhea or increased urination?

PHYSICAL ASSESSMENT

Take vital signs and perform a cardiovascular assessment. Then proceed with the remainder of a complete physical assessment. Be sure to examine the pupils for dilation. Also, check for abdominal distention and increased muscle tension.

MEDICAL CAUSES

Anxiety

An acute anxiety attack commonly produces cold, clammy skin on the forehead, palms, and soles. Other features include pallor, dry mouth, tachycardia or bradycardia, palpitations, and hypertension or hypotension. The patient may also develop tremors, breathlessness, headache, muscle tension, nausea, vomiting, abdominal distention, diarrhea, increased urination, and sharp chest pain.

Cardiac arrhythmias

Cardiac arrhythmias may produce generalized cool, clammy skin along with mental status changes, dizziness, and hypotension. The pulse rate may be rapid, slow, or irregular. The patient may report palpitations, chest pain, diaphoresis, lightheadedness, and weakness.

Cardiogenic shock

With cardiogenic shock, generalized cool, moist, pale skin accompanies confusion, restlessness, hypotension, tachycardia, tachypnea, narrowing pulse pressure, cyanosis, and oliguria. Associated signs and symptoms include anginal pain, dyspnea, jugular vein distention, ventricular gallop, and a weak, rapid pulse.

Heat exhaustion

In the acute stage of heat exhaustion, generalized cold, clammy skin accompanies an ashen appearance, headache, confusion, syncope, giddiness and, possibly, a subnormal temperature, with mild heat exhaustion. The patient may exhibit a rapid and thready pulse, nausea, vomiting, tachypnea, oliguria, thirst, muscle cramps, and hypotension.

Hypoglycemia (acute)

With acute hypoglycemia, generalized cool, clammy skin or diaphoresis may accompany irritability, tremors, palpitations, hunger, headache, tachycardia, and anxiety. Central nervous system disturbances include blurred vision, diplopia, confusion, motor weakness, hemiplegia, and coma. These signs and symptoms typically resolve after the patient is given glucose.

Hypovolemic shock

With hypovolemic shock, generalized pale, cold, clammy skin accompanies subnormal body temperature, hypotension with narrowing pulse pressure, tachycardia, tachypnea, and rapid, thready pulse. Other findings are flat neck veins, increased capillary refill time, decreased urine output, confusion, and decreased level of consciousness.

Septic shock

The cold shock stage of septic shock causes generalized cold, clammy skin. Associated findings include rapid and thready pulse, severe hypotension, persistent oliguria or anuria, and respiratory failure.

Critical assessment steps

+ Take vital signs.
+ Perform cardiovascular and physical assessments.
+ Examine the pupils for dilation.
+ Check for abdominal distention and increased muscle tension.

Medical causes

Anxiety
+ Clammy skin occurs on the forehead, palms, and soles.

Cardiac arrhythmias
+ Generalized clammy skin occurs with mental status changes, dizziness, and hypotension.

Cardiogenic shock
+ Generalized clammy skin accompanies confusion, restlessness, hypotension, tachycardia, tachypnea, narrowing pulse pressure, cyanosis, and oliguria.

Heat exhaustion
+ Generalized clammy skin, an ashen appearance, headache, confusion, syncope, and giddiness develop.

Hypoglycemia (acute)
+ Generalized clammy skin or diaphoresis may occur.

Hypovolemic shock
+ Generalized clammy skin accompanies subnormal body temperature, hypotension, tachycardia, tachypnea, and rapid, thready pulse.

Septic shock
+ The cold shock stage causes generalized clammy skin.

Special considerations
+ Take vital signs frequently.
+ Monitor urine output.

Peds points
+ Infants in shock don't have clammy skin because of immature sweat glands.

Geri points
+ Elderly patients develop clammy skin easily because of decreased tissue perfusion.
+ Consider bowel ischemia in the differential diagnosis of older patients with cool, clammy skin.

Teaching points
+ Explanation of illness
+ Orientation to ICU, if applicable

Key facts about mottled skin
+ Patchy discoloration of the skin
+ Indicates changes of deep, middle, or superficial dermal blood vessels

Key history points
+ Onset of mottled skin (sudden or gradual)
+ Precipitating or alleviating factors
+ Associated pain, numbness, or tingling in extremity

Critical assessment steps
+ Observe the patient's skin color.
+ Palpate arms and legs for skin texture, swelling, and temperature differences.
+ Palpate for pulses.
+ Assess motor and sensory function.

SPECIAL CONSIDERATIONS

Take the patient's vital signs frequently, and monitor urine output. If clammy skin occurs with an anxiety reaction or pain, offer the patient emotional support, administer pain medication, and provide a quiet environment.

PEDIATRIC POINTERS

Infants in shock don't have clammy skin because of their immature sweat glands.

GERIATRIC POINTERS

Elderly patients develop clammy skin easily because of decreased tissue perfusion. Always consider bowel ischemia in the differential diagnosis of older patients who present with cool, clammy skin — especially if abdominal pain or bloody stools occur.

PATIENT COUNSELING

Because the patient with cool, clammy skin may be acutely ill, provide emotional support to him and his family. Explain what's happening using short, simple sentences. Orient them to the intensive care unit, if applicable, explaining the equipment and the unit's routines.

SKIN, MOTTLED

Mottled skin is patchy discoloration indicating primary or secondary changes of the deep, middle, or superficial dermal blood vessels. It can result from a hematologic, immune, or connective tissue disorder; chronic occlusive arterial disease; dysproteinemia; immobility; exposure to heat or cold; or shock. Mottled skin can be a normal reaction, such as the diffuse mottling that occurs when exposure to cold causes venous stasis in cutaneous blood vessels (cutis marmorata).

Mottling that occurs with other signs and symptoms usually affects the extremities, typically indicating restricted blood flow. For example, livedo reticularis, a characteristic network pattern of reddish blue discoloration, occurs when vasospasm of the middermal blood vessels slows local blood flow in dilated superficial capillaries and small veins. Shock causes mottling from systemic vasoconstriction.

HISTORY

Mottled skin may indicate an emergency condition requiring rapid evaluation and intervention. (See *Mottled skin: Knowing what to do.*) However, if the patient isn't in distress, obtain a history. Ask if the mottling began suddenly or gradually. What precipitated it? How long has he had it? Does anything make it go away? Does the patient have other symptoms, such as pain, numbness, or tingling in an extremity? If so, do they disappear with temperature changes?

PHYSICAL ASSESSMENT

Observe the patient's skin color, and palpate his arms and legs for skin texture, swelling, and temperature differences between extremities. Check capillary refill. Also, palpate for the presence (or absence) of pulses and for their quality. Note breaks in the skin, muscle appearance, and hair distribution. Also, assess motor and sensory function.

Mottled skin: Knowing what to do

If your patient's skin is pale, cool, clammy, and mottled at the elbows and knees or all over, he may be developing *hypovolemic shock*. Quickly take his vital signs, and be sure to note tachycardia or a weak, thready pulse. Observe the neck for flattened veins. Does the patient appear anxious? If you detect these signs and symptoms, place the patient in a supine position in bed with his legs elevated 20 to 30 degrees. Administer oxygen by nasal cannula or face mask, and begin cardiac monitoring. Insert a large-bore I.V. line for rapid fluid or blood product administration,

and prepare to insert a central line or a pulmonary artery catheter. Also prepare to catheterize the patient to monitor urine output.

Localized mottling in a pale, cool extremity that the patient says feels painful, numb, and tingling may signal acute arterial occlusion. Immediately check the patient's distal pulses: If they're absent or diminished, you'll need to insert an I.V. line in an unaffected extremity, and prepare the patient for arteriography or immediate surgery.

MEDICAL CAUSES

Arterial occlusion (acute)

Initial signs of acute arterial occlusion include temperature and color changes. Pallor may change to blotchy cyanosis and livedo reticularis. Color and temperature demarcation develop at the level of obstruction. Other effects include sudden onset of pain in the extremity and possibly paresthesia, paresis, and a sensation of cold in the affected area. Examination reveals diminished or absent pulses, cool extremities, increased capillary refill time, pallor, and diminished reflexes.

Arteriosclerosis obliterans

Atherosclerotic buildup narrows intra-arterial lumina, resulting in reduced blood flow through the affected artery. Obstructed blood flow to the extremities (most commonly the lower) produces such peripheral signs and symptoms as leg pallor, cyanosis, blotchy erythema, and livedo reticularis. Related findings include intermittent claudication (most common symptom), diminished or absent pedal pulses, and leg coolness. Other symptoms include coldness and paresthesia.

Buerger's disease

Buerger's disease is a form of vasculitis that produces unilateral or asymmetrical color changes and mottling, particularly livedo networking in the lower extremities. It also typically causes intermittent claudication and erythema along extremity blood vessels. During exposure to cold, the feet are cold, cyanotic, and numb; later they're hot, red, and tingling. Other findings include impaired peripheral pulses and peripheral neuropathy. Buerger's disease is typically exacerbated by smoking.

Hypovolemic shock

Vasoconstriction from hypovolemic shock commonly produces skin mottling, initially in the knees and elbows. As shock worsens, mottling becomes generalized. Early signs include sudden onset of pallor, cool skin, restlessness, thirst, tachypnea, and slight tachycardia. As shock progresses, associated findings include cool, clammy skin; rapid, thready pulse; hypotension; narrowed pulse pressure; decreased urine output; subnormal temperature; confusion; and decreased level of consciousness.

In an emergency

✦ If patient's skin is pale, cool, clammy, and mottled at elbows, knees, or all over, he may be developing hypovolemic shock. Quickly take vital signs, and note tachycardia or weak, thready pulse.
✦ Place patient in supine position in bed with legs elevated 20 to 30 degrees.
✦ Insert large-bore I.V. line for rapid fluid administration.

Medical causes

Arterial occlusion (acute)

✦ Temperature and color changes that develop at the level of obstruction are initial signs.

Arteriosclerosis obliterans

✦ Obstructed blood flow to the extremities produces leg pallor, cyanosis, blotchy erythema, and livedo reticularis.

Buerger's disease

✦ Color changes and mottling, particularly livedo networking in the lower extremities, occur.

Hypovolemic shock

✦ Vasoconstriction commonly produces skin mottling, initially in the knees and elbows.

Medical causes
(continued)

Livedo reticularis (idiopathic or primary)
+ Symmetrical, diffuse mottling can involve the hands, feet, arms, legs, buttocks, and trunk.

Polycythemia vera
+ Livedo reticularis (mottling) occurs.

Rheumatoid arthritis
+ Skin mottling may accompany joint pain and stiffness.

SLE
+ Livedo reticularis (mottling) occurs most commonly on outer arms.

Other causes
+ Prolonged immobility
+ Prolonged thermal exposure

Special considerations
+ Mottled skin typically results from a chronic condition.

Peds points
+ A common cause of mottled skin in children is systemic vasoconstriction from shock.

Geri points
+ Decreased tissue perfusion can easily cause mottled skin.
+ Conditions producing mottled skin in older patients include arterial occlusion, polycythemia vera, and bowel ischemia.

Teaching points
+ Avoidance of tight clothing and overexposure to cold or heating devices

Livedo reticularis (idiopathic or primary)

With livedo reticularis, symmetrical, diffuse mottling can involve the hands, feet, arms, legs, buttocks, and trunk. Initially, networking is intermittent and most pronounced on exposure to cold or stress; eventually, mottling persists even with warming.

Polycythemia vera

Polycythemia vera, a hematologic disorder, produces livedo reticularis, hemangiomas, purpura, rubor, ulcerative nodules, and scleroderma-like lesions. Other symptoms include headache, a vague feeling of fullness in the head, dizziness, vertigo, vision disturbances, dyspnea, and aquagenic pruritus.

Rheumatoid arthritis

Rheumatoid arthritis may cause skin mottling. Early nonspecific signs and symptoms progress to joint pain and stiffness with subcutaneous nodules, usually on the elbows. The patient may report morning stiffness.

Systemic lupus erythematosus

Systemic lupus erythematosus (SLE) is a connective tissue disorder that can cause livedo reticularis, most commonly on the outer arms. Other signs and symptoms include a butterfly rash, nondeforming joint pain and stiffness, photosensitivity, Raynaud's phenomenon, patchy alopecia, seizures, fever, anorexia, weight loss, lymphadenopathy, and emotional lability.

OTHER CAUSES

Immobility

Prolonged immobility may cause bluish mottling, most noticeably in dependent extremities.

Thermal exposure

Prolonged thermal exposure, such as from a heating pad or hot water bottle, may cause erythema Ab Igne — a localized, reticulated, brown-to-red mottling.

SPECIAL CONSIDERATIONS

Mottled skin typically results from a chronic condition.

PEDIATRIC POINTERS

A common cause of mottled skin in children is systemic vasoconstriction from shock. Other causes are the same as those for adults.

GERIATRIC POINTERS

In elderly patients, decreased tissue perfusion can easily cause mottled skin. Besides arterial occlusion and polycythemia vera, conditions that commonly affect patients in this age-group, bowel ischemia is common in elderly patients who present with livedo reticularis, especially if they also have abdominal pain or bloody stools.

PATIENT COUNSELING

Teach patients to avoid tight clothing and overexposure to cold or to heating devices, such as hot water bottles and heating pads. If the patient has a chronic condition, such as SLE or periarteritis nodosa, advise him to watch for mottled skin because it may indicate a flare-up of his disorder.

SKIN, SCALY

Scaly skin results when cells of the uppermost skin layer (stratum corneum) desiccate and shed, causing excessive accumulation of loosely adherent flakes of normal or abnormal keratin. Normally, skin cell loss is imperceptible; the appearance of scale indicates increased cell proliferation secondary to altered keratinization.

Scaly skin varies in texture from fine and delicate to branlike, coarse, or stratified. Scales are typically dry, brittle, and shiny, but they can be greasy and dull. Their color ranges from whitish gray, yellow, or brown to a silvery sheen.

Usually benign, scaly skin occurs with fungal, bacterial, and viral infections (cutaneous or systemic), lymphomas, and lupus erythematosus; it's also common in those with inflammatory skin disease. A form of scaly skin—generalized fine desquamation—commonly follows prolonged febrile illness, sunburn, and thermal burns. Red patches of scaly skin that appear or worsen in winter may result from dry skin (or from actinic keratosis, common in elderly patients). Certain drugs also cause scaly skin. Aggravating factors include cold, heat, immobility, and frequent bathing.

HISTORY

Begin the history by asking how long the patient has had scaly skin and whether he has had it before. Where did it first appear? Did a lesion or skin eruption, such as erythema, precede it? Has the patient used a new or different topical skin product recently? How often does he bathe? Has he had recent joint pain, illness, or malaise? Ask the patient about work exposure to chemicals, use of prescribed drugs, and a family history of skin disorders. Find out what kinds of soap, cosmetics, skin lotion, and hair preparations he uses.

PHYSICAL ASSESSMENT

Examine the entire skin surface. Is it dry, oily, moist, or greasy? Observe the general pattern of skin lesions, and record their location. Note their color, shape, and size. Are they thick or fine? Do they itch? Does the patient have other lesions besides scaly skin? Examine the mucous membranes of his mouth, lips, and nose, and inspect his ears, hair, and nails.

MEDICAL CAUSES

Bowen's disease

Bowen's disease, a common form of intraepidermal carcinoma, causes painless, erythematous plaques that are raised and indurated with a thick, hyperkeratotic scale and, possibly, ulcerated centers. The head and neck are the most commonly affected sites.

Dermatitis

Exfoliative dermatitis begins with rapidly developing generalized erythema. Desquamation with fine scales or thick sheets of all or most of the skin surface may cause life-threatening hypothermia. Other possible complications include cardiac output failure and septicemia. Systemic signs and symptoms include low-grade fever, chills, malaise, lymphadenopathy, and gynecomastia.

With nummular dermatitis, round, pustular lesions commonly ooze purulent exudate, itch severely, and rapidly become encrusted and scaly. Lesions appear on the extensor surfaces of the limbs, posterior trunk, and buttocks.

Key facts about scaly skin

+ Results when cells of the uppermost skin layer desiccate and shed
+ Causes accumulation of loosely adherent flakes of keratin

Key history points

+ Onset, duration, and location of scaly skin
+ Preceding lesion or skin eruption
+ Use of topical skin products or prescribed drugs and types of soap, cosmetics, skin lotion, and hair preparations used
+ Frequency of bathing
+ Recent joint pain, illness, or malaise
+ Exposure to chemicals
+ Family history of skin disorders

Critical assessment steps

+ Examine the entire skin surface.
+ Observe and record the pattern, location, and characteristics of skin lesions.
+ Inspect the mucous membranes of the mouth, lips, and nose.
+ Inspect the ears, hair, and nails.

Medical causes

Bowen's disease

+ Painless, erythematous plaques are raised and indurated with a thick, hyperkeratotic scale and, possibly, ulcerated centers.

Dermatitis

+ Scaling ranges from fine scales or thick sheets (exfoliative dermatitis) to scaly papules that progress to larger dry or moist, greasy scales with yellowish crusts (seborrheic dermatitis).

Medical causes
(continued)

Dermatophytosis

✦ Tinea capitis produces lesions with reddened, slightly elevated borders and a central area of dense scaling.
✦ Tinea pedis causes scaling and blisters between the toes.
✦ Tinea corporis produces crusty lesions.

Discoid lupus erythematosus

✦ Separate or coalescing lesions, ranging from pink to purple, are covered with a yellow or brown crust.
✦ Enlarged hair follicles are filled with scales.

Lymphoma

✦ Hodgkin's disease may cause pruritic scaling dermatitis that begins in the legs and spreads to the entire body.
✦ Non-Hodgkin's lymphoma produces erythematous patches with some scaling that become interspersed with nodules.

Pityriasis rosea

✦ Yellow-tan or erythematous patches with scaly edges erupt on the trunk and limbs a few days or weeks after onset.

Psoriasis

✦ Silvery white, micaceous scales cover erythematous plaques that have sharply defined borders.

Syphilis (secondary)

✦ Papulosquamous, slightly scaly eruptions are characteristic.

Seborrheic dermatitis begins with erythematous, scaly papules that progress to larger, dry or moist, greasy scales with yellowish crusts. This disorder primarily involves the center of the face, the chest and scalp and, possibly, the genitalia, axillae, and perianal regions. Pruritus occurs with scaling.

Dermatophytosis

Tinea capitis produces lesions with reddened, slightly elevated borders and a central area of dense scaling; these lesions may become inflamed and pus-filled (kerions). Patchy alopecia and itching may also occur. Tinea pedis causes scaling and blisters between the toes. The squamous type produces diffuse, fine, branlike scales. Adherent and silvery white, they're most prominent in skin creases and may affect the entire dorsum of the foot. Tinea corporis produces crusty lesions. As they enlarge, their centers heal, causing the classic ringworm shape.

Discoid lupus erythematosus

Discoid lupus erythematosus is a cutaneous form of lupus that may occur without systemic signs and symptoms. Separate or coalescing lesions (macules, papules, or plaques), ranging from pink to purple, are covered with a yellow or brown crust. Enlarged hair follicles are filled with scales, and telangiectasia may be present. After this inflammatory stage, the lesions heal and hypopigmentation or hyperpigmentation and noncontractile scarring and atrophy may occur. Discoid lupus commonly involves the face or sun-exposed areas of the neck, ears, scalp, lips, and oral mucosa. Alopecia may also occur.

Lymphoma

Hodgkin's disease and non-Hodgkin's lymphoma commonly cause scaly rashes. Hodgkin's disease may cause pruritic scaling dermatitis that begins in the legs and spreads to the entire body. Remissions and recurrences are common. Small nodules and diffuse pigmentation are related signs. This disease typically produces painless enlargement of the peripheral lymph nodes. Other signs and symptoms include fever, fatigue, weight loss, malaise, and hepatosplenomegaly.

Non-Hodgkin's lymphoma initially produces erythematous patches with some scaling that later become interspersed with nodules. Pruritus and discomfort are common; later, tumors and ulcers form. Progression produces nontender lymphadenopathy.

Pityriasis rosea

Pityriasis rosea, an acute, benign, and self-limiting disorder, produces widespread scales. It begins with an erythematous, raised, oval herald patch anywhere on the body. A few days or weeks later, yellow-tan or erythematous patches with scaly edges erupt on the trunk and limbs and sometimes on the face, hands, and feet. Pruritus also occurs.

Psoriasis

Silvery white, micaceous scales cover erythematous plaques that have sharply defined borders. Psoriasis usually appears on the scalp, chest, elbows, knees, back, buttocks, and genitalia. Associated signs and symptoms include nail pitting, pruritus, arthritis, and sometimes pain from dry, cracked, encrusted lesions.

Syphilis (secondary)

Papulosquamous, slightly scaly eruptions characterize secondary syphilis. A ring-shaped pattern of copper-red papules usually forms on the face, arms, palms, soles, chest, back, and abdomen. Annular papules may occur. Systemic findings include lymphadenopathy, malaise, weight loss, anorexia, nausea, vomiting, headache, sore throat, and low-grade fever.

Systemic lupus erythematosus

Systemic lupus erythematosus (SLE) produces a bright-red maculopapular eruption, sometimes with scaling. Patches are sharply defined and involve the nose and malar regions of the face in a butterfly pattern — a primary sign. Similar characteristic rashes appear on other body surfaces; scaling occurs along the lower lip or anterior hair line. Other primary signs and symptoms include photosensitivity and joint pain and stiffness. Vasculitis (leading to infarctive lesions, necrotic leg ulcers, or digital gangrene), Raynaud's phenomenon, patchy alopecia, and mucous membrane ulcers also can occur.

Tinea versicolor

Tinea versicolor, a benign fungal skin infection, typically produces macular hypopigmented, fawn-colored, or brown patches of varying sizes and shapes. All are slightly scaly. Lesions commonly affect the upper trunk, arms, and lower abdomen, sometimes the neck and, rarely, the face.

OTHER CAUSES

Drugs

Many drugs — including penicillins, sulfonamides, barbiturates, quinidine, diazepam, phenytoin, and isoniazid — can produce scaling patches.

SPECIAL CONSIDERATIONS

If scaling results from corticosteroid therapy, withhold the drug. Prepare the patient for such diagnostic tests as a Wood's light examination, skin scraping, and skin biopsy.

PEDIATRIC POINTERS

In children, scaly skin may stem from infantile eczema, pityriasis rosea, epidermolytic hyperkeratosis, psoriasis, various forms of ichthyosis, atopic dermatitis, a viral infection (especially hepatitis B virus, which can cause Gianotti-Crosti syndrome), seborrhea capitis (cradle cap), or an acute transient dermatitis. Desquamation may follow a febrile illness.

PATIENT COUNSELING

Teach the patient proper skin care, and suggest lubricating baths and emollients. Instruct him not to use hot water to bathe or shower.

SPLENOMEGALY

Because it occurs with various disorders and in up to 5% of normal adults, splenomegaly — an enlarged spleen — isn't a diagnostic sign by itself. Usually, however, it points to infection, trauma, or a hepatic, autoimmune, neoplastic, or hematologic disorder.

    Because the spleen functions as the body's largest lymph node, splenomegaly can result from any process that triggers lymphadenopathy. For example, it may reflect reactive hyperplasia (a response to infection or inflammation), proliferation or infiltration of neoplastic cells, extramedullary hemopoiesis, phagocytic cell proliferation, increased blood cell destruction, or vascular congestion associated with portal hypertension.

Medical causes
(continued)

SLE
✦ A bright-red maculopapular eruption that sometimes has scaling develops.

Tinea versicolor
✦ Slightly scaly, hypopigmented, fawn-colored, or brown patches commonly affect the upper trunk, arms, and lower abdomen.

Other causes
✦ Drugs such as penicillins, sulfonamides, barbiturates, quinidine, diazepam, phenytoin, and isoniazid

Special considerations
✦ If scaling results from corticosteroid therapy, withhold the drug.

Peds points
✦ Scaly skin may stem from infantile eczema, pityriasis rosea, epidermolytic hyperkeratosis, psoriasis, various forms of ichthyosis, atopic dermatitis, a viral infection, seborrhea capitis, or an acute transient dermatitis.

Teaching points
✦ Proper skin care

Key facts about splenomegaly
✦ Enlargement of the spleen
✦ May be detected by light palpation under the left costal margin

In an emergency

If the patient has a history of abdominal or thoracic trauma:
+ Don't palpate the abdomen because this may aggravate internal bleeding.
+ Examine for left-upper-quadrant pain and signs of shock, which may indicate splenic rupture.

If you suspect splenic rupture:
+ Insert an I.V. line for emergency fluid and blood replacement.
+ Administer oxygen.
+ Catheterize the patient.
+ Prepare the patient for possible surgery.

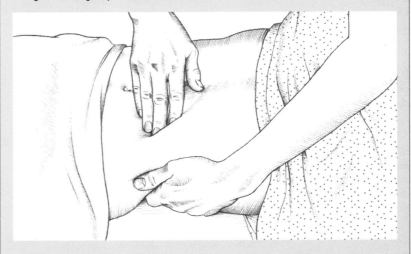

How to palpate for splenomegaly

Detecting splenomegaly requires skillful and gentle palpation to avoid rupturing the enlarged spleen. Follow these steps carefully:
+ Place the patient in the supine position and stand at his right side. Place your left hand under the left costovertebral angle and push lightly to move the spleen forward. Then press your right hand gently under the left front costal margin.
+ Have the patient take a deep breath and then exhale. As he exhales, move your right hand along the tissue contours under the border of the ribs, feeling for the spleen's edge. The enlarged spleen should feel like a firm mass that bumps against your fingers. Remember to begin palpation low enough in the abdomen to catch the edge of a massive spleen.
+ Grade the splenomegaly as slight (½" to 1½" [1 to 4 cm] below the costal margin), moderate (1½" to 3" [4 to 8 cm] below the costal margin), or great (greater than or equal to 3" below the costal margin).
+ Reposition the patient on his right side with his hips and knees flexed slightly to move the spleen forward. Then repeat the palpation procedure.

Splenomegaly may be detected by light palpation under the left costal margin. (See *How to palpate for splenomegaly*.) However, because this technique isn't always advisable or effective, splenomegaly may need to be confirmed by a computed tomography or radionuclide scan.

 EMERGENCY ACTIONS If the patient has a history of abdominal or thoracic trauma, don't palpate the abdomen because this may aggravate internal bleeding. Instead, examine the patient for left-upper-quadrant pain and signs of shock, such as tachycardia and tachypnea. If you detect these signs, suspect splenic rupture. Insert an I.V. line for emergency fluid and blood replacement, and administer oxygen. Also, catheterize the patient to evaluate urine output, and begin cardiac monitoring. Prepare the patient for possible surgery.

HISTORY

Begin by exploring associated signs and symptoms. Ask the patient if he has been unusually tired lately. Does he frequently have colds, sore throats, or other infections? Does he bruise easily? Ask about left-upper-quadrant pain, abdominal fullness, and early satiety.

PHYSICAL ASSESSMENT

Complete an abdominal assessment. Examine the patient's skin for pallor and ecchymoses. Palpate his axillae, groin, and neck for lymphadenopathy.

MEDICAL CAUSES

Cirrhosis

About one-third of patients with advanced cirrhosis develop moderate to marked splenomegaly. Among other late findings are jaundice, hepatomegaly, leg edema, hematemesis, and ascites. Signs of hepatic encephalopathy — such as asterixis, fetor hepaticus, slurred speech, and decreased level of consciousness that may progress to coma — are also common. Besides jaundice, skin effects may include severe pruritus, poor tissue turgor, spider angiomas, palmar erythema, pallor, and signs of bleeding tendencies. Endocrine effects may include menstrual irregularities or testicular atrophy, gynecomastia, and loss of chest and axillary hair. The patient may also develop fever and right-upper-abdominal pain that's aggravated by sitting up or leaning forward.

Endocarditis (subacute infective)

Endocarditis usually causes an enlarged, but nontender, spleen. Its classic sign, however, is a suddenly changing murmur or the discovery of a new murmur in the presence of fever. Other features include anorexia, pallor, weakness, fever, night sweats, fatigue, tachycardia, weight loss, arthralgia, petechiae, hematuria and, in chronic cases, clubbing. If embolization occurs, the patient may develop chest, abdominal, or limb pain; paralysis; hematuria; and blindness. Endocarditis may produce Osler's nodes (tender, raised, subcutaneous lesions on the fingers or toes), Roth's spots (hemorrhagic areas with white centers on the retina), and Janeway lesions (purplish macules on the palms or soles).

Hepatitis

Splenomegaly may occur with hepatitis. More characteristic findings include dark urine, clay-colored stools, anorexia, malaise, pruritus, hepatomegaly, vomiting, jaundice, and fatigue.

Histoplasmosis

Acute disseminated histoplasmosis commonly produces splenomegaly and hepatomegaly. It may also cause lymphadenopathy, jaundice, fever, anorexia, emaciation, and signs and symptoms of anemia, such as weakness, fatigue, pallor, and malaise. Occasionally, the patient's tongue, palate, epiglottis, and larynx become ulcerated, resulting in pain, hoarseness, and dysphagia.

CULTURAL CUE Histoplasmosis occurs worldwide, especially in the temperate areas of Asia, Africa, Europe, and North and South America. In the United States, it's most prevalent in the central and eastern states, especially in the Mississippi and Ohio River Valleys.

Hypersplenism (primary)

With hypersplenism, splenomegaly accompanies signs of pancytopenia — anemia, neutropenia, or thrombocytopenia. If the patient has anemia, findings may include

Key history points

+ Associated fatigue; frequent colds, sore throats, or other infections; bruising; left-upper-quadrant pain; abdominal fullness; and early satiety

Critical assessment steps

+ Complete an abdominal assessment.
+ Examine the skin for pallor and ecchymoses.
+ Palpate the axillae, groin, and neck for lymphadenopathy.

Medical causes

Cirrhosis
+ About one-third of patients with advanced cirrhosis develop splenomegaly.

Endocarditis (subacute infective)
+ The spleen is enlarged but nontender.

Hepatitis
+ Splenomegaly may occur.

Histoplasmosis
+ Splenomegaly and hepatomegaly occur.

Hypersplenism (primary)
+ Splenomegaly accompanies anemia, neutropenia, or thrombocytopenia.

Medical causes
(continued)

Leukemia
+ Moderate to severe splenomegaly is early sign.
+ Other signs include hepatomegaly, lymphadenopathy, fatigue, malaise, pallor, fever, gum swelling, bleeding tendencies, weight loss, anorexia, and abdominal, bone, and joint pain.

Lymphoma
+ Moderate to massive splenomegaly is late sign.

Mononucleosis (infectious)
+ Splenomegaly is most pronounced during second and third weeks of illness.

Pancreatic cancer
+ Moderate to severe splenomegaly may occur if a tumor compresses the splenic vein.

Polycythemia vera
+ Spleen may become enlarged, resulting in easy satiety, abdominal fullness, and left-upper-quadrant or pleuritic chest pain.

Splenic rupture
+ Splenomegaly may result from massive hemorrhage.

Special considerations
+ Prepare patient for diagnostic tests.

---

weakness, fatigue, malaise, and pallor. If he has severe neutropenia, frequent bacterial infections are likely. If he has severe thrombocytopenia, easy bruising or spontaneous, widespread hemorrhage may occur. The patient also experiences left-sided abdominal pain, and a feeling of fullness after eating a small amount of food.

Leukemia
Moderate to severe splenomegaly is an early sign of acute and chronic leukemia. With chronic granulocytic leukemia, splenomegaly is sometimes painful. Accompanying it may be hepatomegaly, lymphadenopathy, fatigue, malaise, pallor, fever, gum swelling, bleeding tendencies, weight loss, anorexia, and abdominal, bone, and joint pain. At times, acute leukemia also causes dyspnea, tachycardia, and palpitations. With advanced disease, the patient may display confusion, headache, vomiting, seizures, papilledema, and nuchal rigidity.

Lymphoma
Moderate to massive splenomegaly is a late sign of lymphoma and may be accompanied by hepatomegaly, painless lymphadenopathy, scaly dermatitis with pruritus, night sweats, fever, fatigue, weight loss, and malaise. Scaly rashes and pruritus may develop.

Mononucleosis (infectious)
A common sign of mononucleosis, splenomegaly is most pronounced during the second and third weeks of illness. Typically, it's accompanied by a triad of signs and symptoms: sore throat, cervical lymphadenopathy, and fluctuating temperature with an evening peak of 101° to 102° F (38.3° to 38.9° C). Occasionally, hepatomegaly, jaundice, and a maculopapular rash may also occur.

Pancreatic cancer
Pancreatic cancer may cause moderate to severe splenomegaly if tumor growth compresses the splenic vein. Other characteristic findings include abdominal or back pain, anorexia, nausea and vomiting, weight loss, GI bleeding, jaundice, pruritus, skin lesions, emotional lability, weakness, and fatigue. Palpation may reveal a tender abdominal mass and hepatomegaly; auscultation reveals a bruit in the periumbilical area and left upper quadrant.

Polycythemia vera
Late in polycythemia vera, the spleen may become markedly enlarged, resulting in easy satiety, abdominal fullness, and left-upper-quadrant or pleuritic chest pain. Signs and symptoms accompanying splenomegaly are widespread and numerous. The patient may exhibit deep, purplish red oral mucous membranes, headache, dyspnea, dizziness, vertigo, weakness, and fatigue. He may also develop finger and toe paresthesia, impaired mentation, tinnitus, blurred or double vision, scotoma, increased blood pressure, and intermittent claudication. Other signs and symptoms include pruritus, urticaria, ruddy cyanosis, epigastric distress, weight loss, hepatomegaly, and bleeding tendencies.

Splenic rupture
Splenomegaly may result from massive hemorrhage with splenic rupture. The patient may also experience left-upper-quadrant pain, abdominal rigidity, and Kehr's sign. Signs and symptoms of shock may also occur.

SPECIAL CONSIDERATIONS
Prepare the patient for diagnostic studies, such as a complete blood count, blood cultures, and radionuclide and computed tomography scans of the spleen.

PEDIATRIC POINTERS

In addition to the causes of splenomegaly previously described, children may develop splenomegaly in histiocytic disorders, congenital hemolytic anemia, Gaucher's disease, Niemann-Pick disease, hereditary spherocytosis, sickle cell disease, or beta-thalassemia (Cooley's anemia). Splenic abscess is the most common cause of splenomegaly in immunocompromised children.

PATIENT COUNSELING

Teach the patient about the disease process and his treatment options. Explain the importance of avoiding infection. Discuss the need for compliance with prescribed therapy and regular follow-up appointments.

STOOLS, CLAY-COLORED

Pale, putty-colored stools usually result from hepatic, gallbladder, or pancreatic disorders. Normally, bile pigments give the stool its characteristic brown color. However, hepatocellular degeneration or biliary obstruction may interfere with the formation or release of these pigments into the intestine, resulting in clay-colored stools. These stools are commonly associated with jaundice and dark "cola-colored" urine.

HISTORY

After documenting when the patient first noticed clay-colored stools, explore associated signs and symptoms, such as abdominal pain, nausea and vomiting, fatigue, anorexia, weight loss, and dark urine. Does the patient have trouble digesting fatty foods or heavy meals? Does he bruise easily?

Next, review the patient's medical history for gallbladder, hepatic, or pancreatic disorders. Has he ever had biliary surgery? Has he recently undergone barium studies? (Barium lightens stool color for several days.) Also, ask about antacid use because large amounts may lighten stool color. Note a history of alcoholism or exposure to other hepatotoxic substances.

PHYSICAL ASSESSMENT

After assessing the patient's general appearance, take his vital signs and check his skin and eyes for jaundice. Then examine the abdomen; inspect for distention and ascites, and auscultate for hypoactive bowel sounds. Percuss and palpate for masses and rebound tenderness. Finally, obtain urine and stool specimens for laboratory analysis.

MEDICAL CAUSES

Bile duct cancer

Commonly a presenting sign of bile duct cancer, clay-colored stools may be accompanied by progressive, profound jaundice; pruritus; anorexia and weight loss; bleeding tendencies; and a palpable mass. The patient may experience pain in the epigastrium or right upper quadrant that radiates to the back.

Biliary cirrhosis

With biliary cirrhosis, clay-colored stools typically follow unexplained pruritus that worsens at bedtime, weakness, fatigue, weight loss, and vague abdominal pain; these features may be present for years. Associated findings include jaundice, hy-

Medical causes
(continued)

Cholangitis (sclerosing)
✦ Fibrosis of the bile ducts, clay-colored stools, chronic or intermittent jaundice, pruritus, right-upper-quadrant pain, chills, and fever occur.

Cholelithiasis
✦ Obstruction of the common bile duct may result in clay-colored stools.
✦ Associated symptoms include dyspepsia and biliary colic.

Hepatic cancer
✦ Weight loss, weakness, and anorexia precede clay-colored stools.
✦ Later, nodular, firm hepatomegaly; jaundice; right-upper-quadrant pain; ascites; dependent edema; and fever develop.

Hepatitis
✦ Clay-colored stools signal the start of the icteric phase.
✦ Associated signs include mild weight loss, dark urine, anorexia, and tender hepatomegaly.

Pancreatic cancer
✦ Common bile duct obstruction may cause clay-colored stools.
✦ Classic associated features include abdominal or back pain, jaundice, pruritus, nausea and vomiting, anorexia, weight loss, fatigue, weakness, and fever.

Pancreatitis (acute)
✦ Clay-colored stools, dark urine, jaundice, and severe epigastric pain that's aggravated by lying down occur.

perpigmentation, and signs of malabsorption, such as nocturnal diarrhea, steatorrhea, purpura, and bone and back pain due to osteomalacia. The patient may also develop firm, nontender hepatomegaly, hematemesis, ascites, edema, and xanthomas on his palms, soles, and elbows.

Cholangitis (sclerosing)
Characterized by fibrosis of the bile ducts, cholangitis is a chronic inflammatory disorder that may cause clay-colored stools, chronic or intermittent jaundice, pruritus, right-upper-quadrant pain, chills, and fever. The patient may also experience weakness and fatigue.

Cholelithiasis
Stones in the biliary tract may cause clay-colored stools when they obstruct the common bile duct (choledocholithiasis). However, if the obstruction is intermittent, the stools may alternate between normal and clay color. Associated symptoms include dyspepsia and — in sudden, severe obstruction — characteristic biliary colic. This right-upper-quadrant pain intensifies over several hours, may radiate to the epigastrium or shoulder blades, and is unrelieved by antacids. The pain is accompanied by tachycardia, restlessness, nausea, intolerance to certain foods, vomiting, upper abdominal tenderness, fever, chills, and jaundice.

Hepatic cancer
Before clay-colored stools develop, the patient with hepatic cancer usually experiences weight loss, weakness, and anorexia. Later, he may develop nodular, firm hepatomegaly; jaundice; right-upper-quadrant pain; ascites; dependent edema; and fever. A bruit, hum, or rubbing sound may be heard on auscultation if the cancer involves a large part of the liver.

Hepatitis
With viral hepatitis, clay-colored stools signal the start of the icteric phase and are typically followed by jaundice within 1 to 5 days. Associated signs include mild weight loss and dark urine as well as continuation of some preicteric findings, such as anorexia and tender hepatomegaly. During the icteric phase, the patient may become irritable and develop right-upper-quadrant pain, splenomegaly, enlarged cervical lymph nodes, and severe pruritus. After jaundice disappears, the patient continues to experience fatigue, flatulence, abdominal pain or tenderness, and dyspepsia, although his appetite usually returns and hepatomegaly subsides. The posticteric phase generally lasts from 2 to 6 weeks, with full recovery in 6 months. (See *Associated disorder: Hepatitis.*)
    With cholestatic nonviral hepatitis, clay-colored stools occur with other signs of viral hepatitis.

Pancreatic cancer
Common bile duct obstruction associated with pancreatic cancer may cause clay-colored stools. Classic associated features include abdominal or back pain, jaundice, pruritus, nausea and vomiting, anorexia, weight loss, fatigue, weakness, and fever. Other possible effects include diarrhea, skin lesions (especially on the legs), emotional lability, splenomegaly, and signs of GI bleeding. Auscultation may reveal a bruit in the periumbilical area and left upper quadrant.

Pancreatitis (acute)
Acute pancreatitis may cause clay-colored stools, dark urine, and jaundice. Typically, it also causes severe epigastric pain that radiates to the back and is aggravated by lying down. Associated findings include nausea and vomiting, fever, abdominal rigidity and tenderness, hypoactive bowel sounds, and crackles at the lung bases.

ASSOCIATED DISORDER

Hepatitis

Viral hepatitis is a common infection of the liver that results in hepatic cell destruction, necrosis, and autolysis. In most patients, hepatic cells eventually regenerate with little or no residual damage. However, old age and serious underlying disorders make complications more likely. The prognosis is poor if edema and hepatic encephalopathy develop.

Five major forms of hepatitis are currently recognized:

+ Type A (infectious or short-incubation hepatitis) is most common among male homosexuals and in people with human immunodeficiency virus (HIV) infection. It's commonly spread via the fecal-oral route by the ingestion of fecal contaminants.
+ Type B (serum or long-incubation hepatitis) is most common among HIV-positive individuals. Routine screening of donor blood for the hepatitis B surface antigen has reduced the incidence of posttransfusion cases, but transmission by needles shared by drug abusers remains a major problem.
+ Type C accounts for about 20% of all viral hepatitis cases and most posttransfusion cases.
+ Type D (delta hepatitis) is responsible for about 50% of all cases of fulminant hepatitis, which has a high mortality. Developing in 1% of patients with viral hepatitis, fulminant hepatitis causes unremitting liver failure with encephalopathy. It progresses to coma and commonly leads to death within 2 weeks. In the United States, type D hepatitis occurs only in people who are frequently exposed to blood and blood products, such as I.V. drug users and hemophilia patients. Type D hepatitis is found only in patients with an acute or chronic episode of hepatitis B and requires the presence of hepatitis B surface antigen. The type D virus depends on the double-shelled type B virus to replicate. (For this reason, type D infection can't outlast a type B infection.)
+ Type E (formerly grouped with types C and D under the name non-A, non-B hepatitis) occurs primarily in patients who have recently returned from an endemic area (such as India, Africa, Asia, or Central America). It's more common in young adults and more severe in pregnant women.
+ Other types continue to be identified with growing patient populations and sophisticated laboratory identification techniques.

CAUSES

The five major forms of viral hepatitis result from infection with the causative viruses: A, B, C, D, or E.

DIAGNOSIS

These test results help confirm diagnosis of viral hepatitis:

+ Hepatitis profile study identifies antibodies specific to the causative virus, establishing the type of hepatitis.
+ Serum aspartate aminotransferase and serum alanine aminotransferase levels are increased in the prodromal stage.
+ Serum alkaline phosphatase level is slightly increased.
+ Serum bilirubin level may remain high into late disease, especially in severe cases.
+ Prothrombin time is prolonged (greater than 3 seconds longer than normal indicates severe liver damage).
+ White blood cell counts reveal transient neutropenia and lymphopenia followed by lymphocytosis.
+ Liver biopsy confirms suspicion of chronic hepatitis.

MEDICAL INTERVENTIONS

Treatment may include:

+ rest to minimize energy demands
+ avoidance of alcohol or other drugs to prevent further hepatic damage
+ diet therapy with small, high-calorie meals to combat anorexia
+ parenteral nutrition if patient can't eat because of persistent vomiting
+ vaccination against hepatitis A and B to provide immunity before transmission occurs
+ interferon alfa-2b and lamivudine for chronic hepatitis B; interferon and ribavirin for hepatitis C.

Key facts about hepatitis

+ An infection of the liver
+ Results in hepatic cell destruction, necrosis, and autolysis
+ Has five forms: types A, B, C, D, and E

Causes

+ Infection with causative viruses A, B, C, D, or E

Management

+ Rest
+ Avoidance of alcohol or drugs
+ Diet therapy
+ Parenteral nutrition (if patient can't eat)
+ Vaccination against hepatitis A and B
+ Interferon alfa-2b and lamivudine for chronic hepatitis B; interferon and ribavirin for hepatitis C

Other causes
+ Biliary surgery

Special considerations
+ Prepare patient for diagnostic tests.

Peds points
+ Clay-colored stools may occur in infants with biliary atresia.

Geri points
+ Because elderly patients with cholelithiasis have a greater risk of developing complications, surgery should be considered.

Teaching points
+ Ways to reduce abdominal pain
+ Dietary modifications
+ Need for restful environment

Key facts about stridor
+ Loud, harsh, musical respiratory sound
+ Results from an obstruction in the trachea or larynx

In an emergency
If you detect airway obstruction:
+ Try to clear the airway with back blows or abdominal thrusts.
+ Give oxygen or prepare for emergency endotracheal intubation.
+ Have equipment ready to suction any aspirated vomitus or blood.
+ Connect the patient to a cardiac monitor.
+ Position the patient upright.

With severe pancreatitis, findings include marked restlessness, tachycardia, mottled skin, and cold, sweaty extremities.

OTHER CAUSES

Biliary surgery
Biliary surgery may cause bile duct stricture, resulting in clay-colored stools.

SPECIAL CONSIDERATIONS

Prepare the patient for diagnostic tests, such as liver enzyme and serum bilirubin levels, hepatitis panels, sonograms, computed tomography, endoscope, retrograde cholangiopancreatography, and stool analysis.

PEDIATRIC POINTERS

Clay-colored stools may occur in infants with biliary atresia.

GERIATRIC POINTERS

Because elderly patients with cholelithiasis have a greater risk of developing complications if the condition isn't treated, surgery should be considered early on for treatment of persistent symptoms.

PATIENT COUNSELING

Discuss with the patient ways to reduce abdominal pain, such as assuming semi-Fowler's position or using analgesics. Explain any dietary restrictions or modifications and the importance of avoiding alcohol. Reinforce the need for a quiet, restful environment to conserve energy and decrease metabolic demands.

STRIDOR

A loud, harsh, musical respiratory sound, stridor results from an obstruction in the trachea or larynx. Usually heard during inspiration, this sign may also occur during expiration in severe upper airway obstruction. It may begin as low-pitched "croaking" and progress to high-pitched "crowing" as respirations become more vigorous.

Life-threatening upper airway obstruction can stem from foreign-body aspiration, increased secretions, intraluminal tumor, localized edema or muscle spasms, and external compression by a tumor or aneurysm.

EMERGENCY ACTIONS If you hear stridor, quickly check the patient's vital signs including oxygen saturation and examine him for other signs of partial airway obstruction — choking or gagging, tachypnea, dyspnea, shallow respirations, intercostal retractions, nasal flaring, tachycardia, cyanosis, and diaphoresis. (Be aware that abrupt cessation of stridor signals complete obstruction in which the patient has inspiratory chest movement but absent breath sounds. Unable to talk, he quickly becomes lethargic and loses consciousness.)

If you detect any signs of airway obstruction, try to clear the airway with back blows or abdominal thrusts (Heimlich maneuver). Next, administer oxygen by nasal cannula or face mask, or prepare for emergency endotracheal intubation or tracheostomy and mechanical ventilation. Have equipment ready to suction any aspirated vomitus or blood through the endotracheal or tracheostomy tube. Connect the patient to a cardiac monitor, and position him upright to ease breathing.

HISTORY

When the patient's condition permits, obtain a patient history from him or a family member. First, find out when the stridor began. Has he had it before? Does he have an upper respiratory tract infection? If so, how long has he had it?

Ask about a history of allergies, tumors, and respiratory and vascular disorders. Note recent exposure to smoke or noxious fumes or gases. Next, explore associated signs and symptoms. Does stridor occur with pain or a cough?

PHYSICAL ASSESSMENT

Examine the patient's mouth for excessive secretions, foreign matter, inflammation, and swelling. Assess his neck for swelling, masses, subcutaneous crepitation, and scars. Observe the patient's chest for delayed, decreased, or asymmetrical chest expansion. Auscultate for wheezes, rhonchi, crackles, rubs, and other abnormal breath sounds. Percuss for dullness, tympany, or flatness. Finally, note any burns or signs of trauma, such as ecchymoses and lacerations.

MEDICAL CAUSES

Airway trauma

Local trauma to the upper airway commonly causes acute obstruction, resulting in the sudden onset of stridor. Accompanying this sign are dysphonia, dysphagia, hemoptysis, cyanosis, accessory muscle use, intercostal retractions, nasal flaring, tachypnea, progressive dyspnea, and shallow respirations. Palpation may reveal subcutaneous crepitation in the neck or upper chest.

Anaphylaxis

With a severe allergic reaction (anaphylaxis), upper airway edema and laryngospasm cause stridor and other signs and symptoms of respiratory distress: nasal flaring, wheezing, accessory muscle use, intercostal retractions, and dyspnea. The patient may also develop nasal congestion and profuse, watery rhinorrhea. Typically, these respiratory effects are preceded by a feeling of impending doom or fear, weakness, diaphoresis, sneezing, nasal pruritus, urticaria, erythema, and angioedema. Common associated findings of anaphylaxis include chest or throat tightness, dysphagia and, possibly, signs of shock, such as hypotension, tachycardia, and cool, clammy skin.

Anthrax (inhalation)

Initial signs and symptoms of inhalation anthrax are flulike and include fever, chills, weakness, cough, and chest pain. The disease generally occurs in two stages with a period of recovery after the initial symptoms. The second stage develops abruptly with rapid deterioration marked by stridor, fever, dyspnea, and hypotension generally leading to death within 24 hours.

Aspiration of a foreign body

Sudden stridor is characteristic in this life-threatening situation. Related findings include abrupt onset of dry, paroxysmal coughing, gagging or choking, hoarseness, tachycardia, wheezing, dyspnea, tachypnea, intercostal muscle retractions, diminished breath sounds, cyanosis, and shallow respirations. The patient typically appears anxious and distressed.

Epiglottiditis

With epiglottiditis, a life-threatening inflammatory condition, stridor is caused by an erythematous, edematous epiglottis that obstructs the upper airway. Stridor occurs along with fever, sore throat, and a croupy cough. The cough may progress to

Key history points

+ Onset of stridor
+ Any previous instances of stridor
+ Current respiratory tract infection
+ History of allergies, tumors, or respiratory and vascular disorders
+ Recent exposure to smoke or noxious fumes or gases

Critical assessment steps

+ Examine the mouth.
+ Assess neck for swelling, masses, subcutaneous crepitation, and scars.
+ Observe chest for decreased or asymmetrical expansion.
+ Auscultate breath sounds.
+ Note burns or signs of trauma.

Medical causes

Airway trauma
+ Acute obstruction is common and results in the sudden onset of stridor.

Anaphylaxis
+ Upper airway edema and laryngospasm cause stridor.

Anthrax (inhalation)
+ The second stage involves stridor, fever, dyspnea, and hypotension generally leading to death within 24 hours.

Aspiration of foreign body
+ Sudden stridor is characteristic.

Epiglottiditis
+ Stridor, caused by erythematous, edematous epiglottis that obstructs the upper airway, occurs along with fever, sore throat, and a croupy cough.

Medical causes
(continued)

Hypocalcemia
✦ Laryngospasm can cause stridor.

Inhalation injury
✦ Laryngeal edema and bronchospasms, resulting in stridor, may develop within 48 hours after inhalation of smoke or noxious fumes.

Laryngeal tumor
✦ Stridor, a late sign, may be accompanied by dysphagia, dyspnea, enlarged cervical nodes, and pain that radiates to the ear.

Laryngitis (acute)
✦ Severe laryngeal edema, resulting in stridor and dyspnea, may occur.

Mediastinal tumor
✦ Compression of the trachea and bronchi results in stridor.

Thoracic aortic aneurysm
✦ If the trachea is compressed, stridor, dyspnea, wheezing, and a brassy cough may result.

Other causes
✦ Bronchoscopy or laryngoscopy
✦ Neck surgery, such as thyroidectomy
✦ Prolonged intubation

severe respiratory distress with sternal and intercostal retractions, nasal flaring, cyanosis, and tachycardia.

Hypocalcemia
With hypocalcemia, laryngospasm can cause stridor. Other findings include paresthesia, carpopedal spasm, hyperactive deep tendon reflexes, muscle twitching and cramping, and positive Chvostek's and Trousseau's signs.

Inhalation injury
Within 48 hours after inhalation of smoke or noxious fumes, the patient may develop laryngeal edema and bronchospasms, resulting in stridor. Associated signs and symptoms include singed nasal hairs, orofacial burns, coughing, hoarseness, sooty sputum, crackles, rhonchi, wheezes, and other signs and symptoms of respiratory distress, such as dyspnea, accessory muscle use, intercostal retractions, and nasal flaring.

Laryngeal tumor
Stridor is a late sign of laryngeal tumor and may be accompanied by dysphagia, dyspnea, enlarged cervical nodes, and pain that radiates to the ear. Typically, stridor is preceded by hoarseness, minor throat pain, and a mild, dry cough.

Laryngitis (acute)
Acute laryngitis may cause severe laryngeal edema, resulting in stridor and dyspnea. Its chief sign, however, is mild to severe hoarseness, perhaps with transient voice loss. Other findings include sore throat, dysphagia, dry cough, malaise, and fever.

Mediastinal tumor
Commonly producing no symptoms at first, a mediastinal tumor may eventually compress the trachea and bronchi, resulting in stridor. Its other effects include hoarseness, brassy cough, tracheal shift or tug, dilated neck veins, swelling of the face and neck, stertorous respirations, and suprasternal retractions on inspiration. The patient may also report dyspnea, dysphagia, and pain in the chest, shoulder, or arm.

Thoracic aortic aneurysm
If a thoracic aortic aneurysm compresses the trachea, it may cause stridor accompanied by dyspnea, wheezing, and a brassy cough. Other findings include hoarseness or complete voice loss, dysphagia, jugular vein distention, prominent chest veins, tracheal tug, paresthesia or neuralgia, and edema of the face, neck, and arms. The patient may also complain of substernal, lower back, abdominal, or shoulder pain.

OTHER CAUSES

Diagnostic tests
Bronchoscopy or laryngoscopy may precipitate laryngospasm and stridor.

Treatments
After prolonged intubation, the patient may exhibit laryngeal edema and stridor when the tube is removed. Aerosol therapy with epinephrine may reduce stridor. Reintubation may be necessary in some cases. Neck surgery, such as thyroidectomy, may cause laryngeal paralysis and stridor.

SPECIAL CONSIDERATIONS

Continue to monitor the patient's vital signs closely. Prepare him for diagnostic tests, such as arterial blood gas analysis and chest X-rays.

PEDIATRIC POINTERS

Stridor is a major sign of airway obstruction in children. When you hear this sign, you must intervene quickly to prevent total airway obstruction. This emergency can happen more rapidly in a child because his airway is narrower than an adult's.

Causes of stridor include foreign-body aspiration, croup syndrome, laryngeal diphtheria, pertussis, retropharyngeal abscess, and congenital abnormalities of the larynx.

Therapy for partial airway obstruction typically involves hot or cold steam in a mist tent or hood, parenteral fluids and electrolytes, and plenty of rest.

PATIENT COUNSELING

Having stridor can be frightening to the patient. Remain with him and talk to him using a calm voice. Explain all procedures and treatments to ease his anxiety.

SYNCOPE

A common neurologic sign, syncope (or fainting) refers to transient loss of consciousness associated with impaired cerebral blood supply or cerebral hypoxia. It usually occurs abruptly and lasts for seconds to minutes. An episode of syncope usually starts as a feeling of light-headedness. A patient can usually prevent an episode of syncope by lying down or sitting with his head between his knees. Typically, the patient lies motionless with his skeletal muscles relaxed but sphincter muscles controlled. However, the depth of unconsciousness varies — some patients can hear voices or see blurred outlines; others are unaware of their surroundings.

During a syncopal episode, the patient is strikingly pale with a slow, weak pulse, hypotension, and almost imperceptible breathing. If severe hypotension lasts for 20 seconds or longer, the patient may also develop convulsive, tonic-clonic movements.

Syncope may result from cardiac and cerebrovascular disorders, hypoxemia, and postural changes in the presence of autonomic dysfunction. It may also follow vigorous coughing (tussive syncope) and emotional stress, injury, shock, or pain (vasovagal syncope, or common fainting). Hysterical syncope may also follow emotional stress but isn't accompanied by other vasodepressor effects.

EMERGENCY ACTIONS If you see a patient faint, ensure a patent airway, patient safety, and take vital signs. Then place the patient in a supine position, elevate his legs, and loosen any tight clothing. Be alert for tachycardia, bradycardia, or an irregular pulse. Meanwhile, place him on a cardiac monitor to detect arrhythmias. If an arrhythmia appears, give oxygen and insert an I.V. line for drugs or fluids. Be ready to begin cardiopulmonary resuscitation. Cardioversion, defibrillation, or insertion of a temporary pacemaker may be required.

HISTORY

If the patient reports a fainting episode, gather information about the episode from him and his family. Did he feel weak, light-headed, nauseous, or sweaty just before he fainted? Did he get up quickly from a chair or from lying down? During the fainting episode, did he have muscle spasms or incontinence? How long was he un-

Special considerations
✦ Continue to monitor vital signs.
✦ Prepare the patient for diagnostic tests.

Peds points
✦ Causes of stridor in children include foreign-body aspiration, croup syndrome, laryngeal diphtheria, pertussis, retropharyngeal abscess, and congenital abnormalities of the larynx.

Teaching points
✦ Explanation of all procedures and treatments

Key facts about syncope
✦ Transient loss of consciousness associated with impaired cerebral blood supply or cerebral hypoxia
✦ Occurs abruptly and lasts for seconds to minutes

In an emergency
✦ Ensure a patent airway and patient safety.
✦ Take vital signs.
✦ Place patient in supine position.
✦ Place patient on cardiac monitor to detect arrhythmias.
If an arrhythmia appears:
✦ Be ready to begin CPR.
✦ Cardioversion, defibrillation, or insertion of a temporary pacemaker may be required.

Key history points
✦ Description and duration of fainting episode
✦ Precipitating factors
✦ Any associated headache
✦ History of fainting

Critical assessment steps

+ Take vital signs.
+ Examine for any injuries that may have occurred during his fall.
+ Perform a complete cardiac and neurologic assessment.

Medical causes

Aortic arch syndrome

+ Patient experiences syncope.
+ Weak or abruptly absent carotid pulses and unequal or absent radial pulses may be present.

Aortic stenosis

+ Syncope is a late sign.
+ Fatigue, orthopnea, paroxysmal nocturnal dyspnea, palpitations, and diminished carotid pulses occur.

Cardiac arrhythmias

+ Decreased cardiac output and impaired cerebral circulation may cause syncope.

Carotid sinus hypersensitivity

+ Syncope is triggered by compression of the carotid sinus.

Hypoxemia

+ Syncope, confusion, tachycardia, restlessness, and incoordination may occur.

Orthostatic hypotension

+ Syncope occurs when the patient rises quickly from a recumbent position.

TIAs

+ Syncope and decreased LOC may result.

---

conscious? When he regained consciousness, was he alert or confused? Did he have a headache? Has he fainted before? If so, how often does it occur?

PHYSICAL ASSESSMENT

Take the patient's vital signs and examine him for any injuries that may have occurred during his fall. Then perform a complete cardiac and neurologic assessment.

MEDICAL CAUSES

Aortic arch syndrome

With aortic arch syndrome, the patient experiences syncope and may exhibit weak or abruptly absent carotid pulses and unequal or absent radial pulses. Early signs and symptoms include night sweats, pallor, nausea, anorexia, weight loss, arthralgia, and Raynaud's phenomenon. He may also develop hypotension in the arms; neck, shoulder, and chest pain; paresthesia; intermittent claudication; bruits; vision disturbances; and dizziness.

Aortic stenosis

A cardinal late sign of aortic stenosis, syncope is accompanied by exertional dyspnea and angina. Related findings include marked fatigue, orthopnea, paroxysmal nocturnal dyspnea, palpitations, and diminished carotid pulses. Typically, auscultation reveals atrial and ventricular gallops as well as a harsh, crescendo-decrescendo systolic ejection murmur that's loudest at the right sternal border of the second intercostal space.

Cardiac arrhythmias

Any arrhythmia that decreases cardiac output and impairs cerebral circulation may cause syncope. Other effects — such as palpitations, pallor, confusion, diaphoresis, dyspnea, and hypotension — usually develop first. However, with Adams-Stokes syndrome, syncope may occur without warning. During syncope, the patient develops asystole, which may precipitate spasm and myoclonic jerks if prolonged. He also displays an ashen pallor that progresses to cyanosis, incontinence, bilateral Babinski's reflex, and fixed pupils.

Carotid sinus hypersensitivity

With carotid sinus hypersensitivity, syncope is triggered by compression of the carotid sinus, which may be caused by turning the head to one side or by wearing a tight collar. The fainting episode is usually of short duration.

Hypoxemia

Regardless of its cause, severe hypoxemia may produce syncope. Common related effects include confusion, tachycardia, restlessness, and incoordination. The patient may also have tachypnea, dyspnea, and cyanosis.

Orthostatic hypotension

With orthostatic hypotension, syncope occurs when the patient rises quickly from a recumbent position. Look for a drop of 10 to 20 mm Hg or more in systolic or diastolic blood pressure as well as tachycardia, pallor, dizziness, blurred vision, nausea, and diaphoresis.

Transient ischemic attacks

Marked by transient neurologic deficits, transient ischemic attacks (TIAs) may produce syncope and decreased level of consciousness. Other findings vary with the affected artery but may include vision loss, nystagmus, aphasia, dysarthria, unilateral numbness, hemiparesis or hemiplegia, tinnitus, facial weakness, dysphagia, and staggering or uncoordinated gait.

Vagal glossopharyngeal neuralgia

With vagal glossopharyngeal neuralgia, localized pressure may trigger pain in the base of the tongue, pharynx, larynx, tonsils, and ear, resulting in syncope that lasts for several minutes.

OTHER CAUSES

Drugs

Quinidine may cause syncope—and possibly sudden death—associated with ventricular fibrillation. Prazosin may cause severe orthostatic hypotension and syncope, usually after the first dose. Occasionally, griseofulvin, levodopa, and indomethacin can produce syncope.

SPECIAL CONSIDERATIONS

Continue to monitor the patient's vital signs closely. Prepare the patient for an electrocardiogram, Holter monitor, carotid duplex, carotid Doppler, and electrophysiology studies.

PEDIATRIC POINTERS

Syncope is much less common in children than in adults. It may result from a cardiac or neurologic disorder, allergies, or emotional stress.

PATIENT COUNSELING

Advise the patient to pace his activities, to rise slowly from a recumbent position, to avoid standing still for a prolonged time, and to sit or lie down as soon as he feels faint.

Medical causes
(continued)

Vagal glossopharyngeal neuralgia
+ Localized pressure may trigger pain in the base of the tongue, pharynx, larynx, tonsils, and ear, resulting in syncope.

Other causes
+ Griseofulvin
+ Indomethacin
+ Levodopa
+ Prazosin
+ Quinidine

Special considerations
+ Continue to monitor vital signs.
+ Prepare the patient for diagnostic studies.

Peds points
+ Syncope in children may result from a cardiac or neurologic disorder, allergies, or emotional stress.

Teaching points
+ Ways to prevent syncope, such as rising slowly from a recumbent position

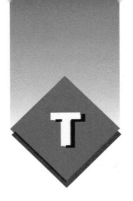

TACHYCARDIA

Easily detected by counting the apical, carotid, or radial pulse, tachycardia is a heart rate greater than 100 beats/minute. The patient with tachycardia usually complains of palpitations or of a "racing" heart. This common sign normally occurs in response to emotional or physical stress, such as excitement, exercise, pain, anxiety, and fever. It may also result from the use of stimulants, such as caffeine and tobacco. However, tachycardia may be an early sign of a life-threatening disorder, such as cardiogenic, hypovolemic, or septic shock. It may also result from a cardiovascular, respiratory, or metabolic disorder or from the effects of certain drugs, tests, or treatments. (See *What happens in tachycardia.*)

EMERGENCY ACTIONS After detecting tachycardia, first perform electrocardiography (ECG) to examine for reduced cardiac output, which may initiate or result from tachycardia. Take the patient's other vital signs and determine his level of consciousness (LOC). If the patient has increased or decreased blood pressure and is drowsy or confused, administer oxygen and begin cardiac monitoring. Insert an I.V. line for fluid, blood product, and drug administration, and gather emergency resuscitation equipment.

HISTORY

If the patient's condition permits, take a focused history. Find out if he has had palpitations before. If so, how were they treated? Explore associated symptoms. Is the patient dizzy or short of breath? Is he weak or fatigued? Is he experiencing episodes of syncope or chest pain? Next, ask about a history of trauma, diabetes, or cardiac, pulmonary, or thyroid disorders. Also, obtain an alcohol and drug history, including prescription, over-the-counter, and illicit drugs.

PHYSICAL ASSESSMENT

Inspect the patient's skin for pallor or cyanosis. Assess pulses, noting peripheral edema. Finally, auscultate the heart and lungs for abnormal sounds or rhythms.

MEDICAL CAUSES

Acute respiratory distress syndrome

Besides tachycardia, acute respiratory distress syndrome (ARDS) causes crackles, rhonchi, dyspnea, tachypnea, nasal flaring, and grunting respirations. Other findings include cyanosis, anxiety, decreased LOC, and abnormal chest X-ray findings.

Key facts about tachycardia

- Refers to a heart rate greater than 100 beats/minute
- Detected by counting the apical, carotid, or radial pulse

In an emergency

If patient has tachycardia, increased or decreased blood pressure, and is drowsy or confused:
- Give oxygen and begin cardiac monitoring.
- Insert an I.V. line.
- Gather resuscitation equipment.

Key history points

- Previous palpitations
- Associated symptoms, such as dizziness, shortness of breath, weakness, fatigue, episodes of syncope, or chest pain
- History of trauma, diabetes, or cardiac, pulmonary, or thyroid disorders
- Drug and alcohol use

Critical assessment steps

- Inspect for pallor or cyanosis.
- Assess pulses.
- Auscultate the heart and lungs.

What happens in tachycardia

Tachycardia represents the heart's effort to deliver more oxygen to body tissues by increasing the rate at which blood passes through the vessels. This sign can reflect overstimulation within the sinoatrial node, the atrium, the atrioventricular node, or the ventricles.

Because heart rate affects cardiac output (cardiac output = heart rate × stroke volume), tachycardia can lower cardiac output by reducing ventricular filling time and stroke volume (the output of each ventricle at every contraction). As cardiac output plummets, arterial pressure and peripheral perfusion decrease. Tachycardia further aggravates myocardial ischemia by increasing the heart's demand for oxygen while reducing the duration of diastole — the period of greatest coronary flow.

Adrenocortical insufficiency

With adrenocortical insufficiency, tachycardia commonly occurs with a weak pulse as well as progressive weakness and fatigue, which may become so severe that the patient requires bed rest. Other signs and symptoms include abdominal pain, nausea and vomiting, altered bowel habits, weight loss, orthostatic hypotension, irritability, bronze skin, decreased libido, and syncope. Some patients report an enhanced sense of taste, smell, and hearing.

Alcohol withdrawal syndrome

Tachycardia along with tachypnea, profuse diaphoresis, fever, insomnia, anorexia, and anxiety can occur in patients experiencing alcohol withdrawal. The patient is characteristically anxious, irritable, and prone to visual and tactile hallucinations.

Anaphylactic shock

With life-threatening anaphylactic shock, tachycardia and hypotension develop within minutes after exposure to an allergen, such as penicillin or an insect sting. Typically, the patient is visibly anxious and has severe pruritus, perhaps with urticaria and a pounding headache. Other findings may include flushed and clammy skin, a cough, dyspnea, nausea, abdominal cramps, seizures, stridor, change or loss of voice associated with laryngeal edema, and urinary urgency and incontinence.

Anemia

Tachycardia and bounding pulse are characteristic with anemia. Associated signs and symptoms include fatigue, pallor, dyspnea and, possibly, bleeding tendencies. Auscultation may reveal an atrial gallop, a systolic bruit over the carotid arteries, and crackles.

Anxiety

A "fight-or-flight" response produces tachycardia, tachypnea; chest pain; cold, clammy skin; dry mouth; nausea; and light-headedness. The symptoms dissipate as anxiety resolves.

Aortic insufficiency

With aortic insufficiency, tachycardia is accompanied by a "water-hammer" bounding pulse and a large, diffuse apical heave. With severe insufficiency, widened pulse pressure occurs. Auscultation reveals a hallmark diastolic murmur that starts with the second heart sound; is decrescendo, high-pitched, and blowing; and is heard best at the left sternal border of the second and third intercostal spaces. An atrial or ventricular gallop, an early systolic murmur, an Austin Flint murmur (apical diastolic rumble), or Duroziez's sign (a murmur over the femoral artery during systole and diastole) may also be heard. Other findings include angina, dyspnea, palpita-

Medical causes

ARDS
✦ Tachycardia, crackles, rhonchi, dyspnea, tachypnea, nasal flaring, and grunting respirations occur.

Adrenocortical insufficiency
✦ Tachycardia commonly occurs with a weak pulse and progressive weakness and fatigue.

Alcohol withdrawal syndrome
✦ Tachycardia, tachypnea, profuse diaphoresis, fever, insomnia, anorexia, and anxiety can occur.

Anaphylactic shock
✦ Tachycardia and hypotension develop within minutes after exposure to an allergen.

Anemia
✦ Tachycardia and bounding pulse are characteristic.

Anxiety
✦ Tachycardia, tachypnea; chest pain; cold, clammy skin; dry mouth; nausea; and light-headedness are produced.

Aortic insufficiency
✦ Tachycardia is accompanied by a bounding pulse and a large, diffuse apical heave.

Medical causes
(continued)

Aortic stenosis
✦ Tachycardia, a weak, thready pulse, and an atrial gallop occur.

Cardiac arrhythmias
✦ Tachycardia may occur along with hypotension, dizziness, palpitations, weakness, and fatigue.

Cardiac contusion
✦ Tachycardia, pain, dyspnea, hypotension, palpitations, sternal ecchymoses, and a pericardial friction rub may result.

Cardiac tamponade
✦ Tachycardia is commonly accompanied by paradoxical pulse, dyspnea, and tachypnea.

Cardiogenic shock
✦ Tachycardia; a weak, thready pulse; hypotension; tachypnea; clammy and cyanotic skin; and altered LOC are more profound than in other types of shock.

COPD
✦ Tachycardia occurs with cough, tachypnea, pursed-lip breathing, accessory muscle use, cyanosis, diminished breath sounds, rhonchi, crackles, and wheezing.

Diabetic ketoacidosis
✦ Tachycardia and a thready pulse are produced along with Kussmaul's respirations.

Febrile illness
✦ Fever can cause tachycardia, chills, and weakness.

tions, strong and abrupt carotid pulsations, pallor, and signs of heart failure, such as crackles and jugular vein distention.

Aortic stenosis
Typically, aortic stenosis causes tachycardia, a weak, thready pulse, and an atrial gallop. Its chief features, however, are exertional dyspnea, angina, dizziness, and syncope. Aortic stenosis also causes a harsh, crescendo-decrescendo systolic ejection murmur that's loudest at the right sternal border of the second intercostal space. Other findings include palpitations, crackles, and fatigue.

Cardiac arrhythmias
Tachycardia may occur with a cardiac arrhythmia. The patient may be hypotensive and report dizziness, palpitations, weakness, and fatigue. Depending on his heart rate, he may also exhibit tachypnea, decreased LOC, and pale, cool, clammy skin.

Cardiac contusion
The result of blunt chest trauma, cardiac contusion may cause tachycardia, substernal pain, dyspnea, hypotension, and palpitations. Assessment may detect sternal ecchymoses and a pericardial friction rub.

Cardiac tamponade
With life-threatening cardiac tamponade, tachycardia is commonly accompanied by paradoxical pulse, dyspnea, and tachypnea. The patient is visibly anxious and restless and has cyanotic, clammy skin and distended jugular veins. He may develop muffled heart sounds, pericardial friction rub, chest pain, hypotension, narrowed pulse pressure, and hepatomegaly.

Cardiogenic shock
Although many features of cardiogenic shock also appear in other types of shock, they're usually more profound in this type. Accompanying tachycardia are weak, thready pulse; narrowing pulse pressure; hypotension; tachypnea; cold, pale, clammy, and cyanotic skin; oliguria; restlessness; and altered LOC.

Chronic obstructive pulmonary disease
Although the clinical picture varies widely with chronic obstructive pulmonary disease (COPD), tachycardia is a common sign. Other characteristic findings include cough, tachypnea, dyspnea, pursed-lip breathing, accessory muscle use, cyanosis, diminished breath sounds, rhonchi, crackles, and wheezing. Clubbing and barrel chest are usually late findings.

Diabetic ketoacidosis
Diabetic ketoacidosis is a life-threatening disorder that commonly produces tachycardia and a thready pulse. Its cardinal sign, however, is Kussmaul's respirations — abnormally rapid, deep breathing. Other signs and symptoms of diabetic ketoacidosis include fruity breath odor, orthostatic hypotension, generalized weakness, anorexia, nausea, vomiting, and abdominal pain. The patient's LOC may vary from lethargy to coma.

Febrile illness
Fever can cause tachycardia, chills, diaphoresis, headache, and weakness. Related findings reflect the specific disorder.

Heart failure
Especially common with left-sided heart failure, tachycardia may be accompanied by a ventricular gallop, fatigue, dyspnea (exertional and paroxysmal nocturnal), orthopnea, and leg edema. Eventually, the patient develops widespread signs and

symptoms, such as palpitations, narrowed pulse pressure, hypotension, tachypnea, crackles, dependent edema, weight gain, slowed mental response, diaphoresis, pallor and, possibly, oliguria. Late signs include hemoptysis, cyanosis, and marked hepatomegaly and pitting edema.

Hyperosmolar hyperglycemic nonketotic syndrome

With hyperosmolar hyperglycemic nonketotic syndrome (HHNS), a rapidly deteriorating LOC is commonly accompanied by tachycardia, hypotension, tachypnea, seizures, oliguria, and severe dehydration with poor skin turgor and dry mucous membranes.

Hypertensive crisis

Life-threatening hypertensive crisis is characterized by tachycardia, tachypnea, diastolic blood pressure that exceeds 120 mm Hg, and systolic blood pressure that may exceed 200 mm Hg. Typically, the patient develops pulmonary edema with jugular vein distention, dyspnea, and pink, frothy sputum. Related findings include chest pain, severe headache, drowsiness, confusion, anxiety, tinnitus, epistaxis, muscle twitching, seizures, nausea, and vomiting. Focal neurologic signs, such as paresthesia, may also occur.

Hypoglycemia

A common sign of hypoglycemia, tachycardia is accompanied by hypothermia, nervousness, trembling, fatigue, malaise, weakness, headache, hunger, nausea, diaphoresis, and moist, clammy skin. Central nervous system effects include blurred or double vision, motor weakness, hemiplegia, seizures, and decreased LOC.

Hypovolemia

Tachycardia may occur with hypovolemia. Associated findings include hypotension, decreased urine output, fatigue, muscle weakness, decreased skin turgor, sunken eyeballs, thirst, syncope, and dry skin and tongue.

Hypovolemic shock

Mild tachycardia, an early sign of life-threatening hypovolemic shock, may be accompanied by tachypnea, restlessness, thirst, and pale, cool skin. As shock progresses, the patient's skin becomes clammy and his pulse, increasingly rapid and thready. He may also develop hypotension, narrowed pulse pressure, oliguria, subnormal body temperature, and decreased LOC.

Hypoxemia

With hypoxemia, tachycardia may accompany tachypnea, dyspnea, and cyanosis. Confusion, restlessness, and disorientation may progress to coma and syncope. Incoordination may also occur.

Myocardial infarction

Myocardial infarction may cause tachycardia or bradycardia. Its classic symptom, however, is crushing substernal chest pain that may radiate to the left arm, jaw, neck, or shoulder. Auscultation may reveal an atrial gallop, a new murmur, and crackles. Other signs and symptoms include pallor, clammy skin, dyspnea, diaphoresis, nausea and vomiting, anxiety, restlessness, and increased or decreased blood pressure.

Neurogenic shock

Tachycardia or bradycardia may accompany tachypnea, apprehension, oliguria, variable body temperature, decreased LOC, and warm, dry skin. Depending on the cause of shock, there also may be motor weakness of the limbs and diaphragm.

Medical causes
(continued)

Heart failure
✦ Tachycardia may occur with a ventricular gallop, fatigue, dyspnea, orthopnea, and leg edema.

HHNS
✦ A rapidly deteriorating LOC is accompanied by tachycardia, hypotension, tachypnea, seizures, oliguria, and severe dehydration.

Hypertensive crisis
✦ Tachycardia, diastolic blood pressure exceeding 120 mm Hg, systolic blood pressure that may exceed 200 mm Hg.

Hypoglycemia
✦ Tachycardia is accompanied by nervousness, weakness, headache, hunger, nausea, and diaphoresis.

Hypovolemia
✦ Tachycardia may occur.

Hypovolemic shock
✦ Mild tachycardia may be accompanied by tachypnea, restlessness, thirst, and pale, cool skin.

Hypoxemia
✦ Tachycardia may accompany dyspnea and cyanosis.

Myocardial infarction
✦ Tachycardia or bradycardia may occur along with crushing substernal chest pain.

Neurogenic shock
✦ Tachycardia or bradycardia may accompany tachypnea, apprehension, oliguria, variable body temperature, decreased LOC, and warm, dry skin.

Medical causes
(continued)

Orthostatic hypotension

✦ Tachycardia accompanies dizziness, syncope, pallor, blurred vision, diaphoresis, and nausea.

Pneumothorax

✦ Tachycardia and other signs and symptoms of distress, such as severe dyspnea and chest pain, tachypnea, and cyanosis, occur.

Pulmonary embolism

✦ Tachycardia is usually preceded by sudden dyspnea, angina, or pleuritic chest pain.

Septic shock

✦ Initially, chills, sudden fever, tachycardia, tachypnea and, possibly, nausea, vomiting, and diarrhea occur.

Thyrotoxicosis

✦ Tachycardia, an enlarged thyroid, nervousness, heat intolerance, weight loss despite increased appetite, tremors, and palpitations are classic features.

Other causes

✦ Cardiac catheterization and electrophysiologic studies
✦ Various drugs that affect the nervous system, circulatory system, or heart muscle, such as acetylcholinesterase inhibitors, alpha-adrenergic blockers, anticholinergics, beta-adrenergic bronchodilators, nitrates, phenothiazines, sympathomimetics, and vasodilators
✦ Excessive caffeine intake
✦ Alcohol intoxication
✦ Cardiac surgery
✦ Pacemaker malfunction or wire irritation

Orthostatic hypotension

Tachycardia accompanies the characteristic signs and symptoms of orthostatic hypotension, which include dizziness, syncope, pallor, blurred vision, diaphoresis, and nausea. Other signs and symptoms include dim vision, spots before the eyes and, possibly, signs of dehydration.

Pneumothorax

Life-threatening pneumothorax causes tachycardia and other signs and symptoms of distress, such as severe dyspnea and chest pain, tachypnea, and cyanosis. Related findings include dry cough, subcutaneous crepitation, absent or decreased breath sounds, cessation of normal chest movement on the affected side, and decreased vocal fremitus.

Pulmonary embolism

With pulmonary embolism, tachycardia is usually preceded by sudden dyspnea, angina, or pleuritic chest pain. Common associated signs and symptoms include weak peripheral pulses, cyanosis, tachypnea, low-grade fever, restlessness, diaphoresis, and a dry cough or a cough with blood-tinged sputum.

Septic shock

Initially, septic shock produces chills, sudden fever, tachycardia, tachypnea and, possibly, nausea, vomiting, and diarrhea. The patient's skin is flushed, warm, and dry; his blood pressure is normal or slightly decreased. Eventually, he may display anxiety; restlessness; thirst; oliguria or anuria; cool, clammy, cyanotic skin; rapid, thready pulse; and severe hypotension. His LOC may decrease progressively, perhaps culminating in a coma.

Thyrotoxicosis

Tachycardia is a classic feature of thyrotoxicosis. Others include an enlarged thyroid, nervousness, heat intolerance, weight loss despite increased appetite, diaphoresis, diarrhea, tremors, and palpitations. Although also considered characteristic, exophthalmos is sometimes absent.

OTHER CAUSES

Diagnostic tests

Cardiac catheterization and electrophysiologic studies may induce transient tachycardia.

Drugs and alcohol

Various drugs affect the nervous system, circulatory system, or heart muscle, resulting in tachycardia. Examples of these include sympathomimetics; phenothiazines; anticholinergics, such as atropine; thyroid drugs; vasodilators, such as hydralazine and nifedipine; acetylcholinesterase inhibitors, such as captopril; nitrates, such as nitroglycerin; alpha-adrenergic blockers, such as phentolamine; and beta-adrenergic bronchodilators, such as albuterol. Excessive caffeine intake and alcohol intoxication may also cause tachycardia.

Surgery and pacemakers

Cardiac surgery and pacemaker malfunction or wire irritation may cause tachycardia.

SPECIAL CONSIDERATIONS

Continue to monitor the patient closely. Explain ordered diagnostic tests, such as a thyroid panel, electrolyte and hemoglobin levels, hematocrit, pulmonary function studies, and 12-lead ECG. If appropriate, prepare him for an ambulatory ECG.

Normal pediatric heart rates

This chart lists the normal resting heart rate for girls and boys up to age 16.

AGE	HEART RATE (BEATS/MINUTE)	
	Girls	Boys
Neonate	130	130
2 years	110	110
4 years	100	100
6 years	100	100
8 years	90	90
10 years	90	90
12 years	90	85
14 years	85	80
16 years	80	75

PEDIATRIC POINTERS

When examining a child for tachycardia, recognize that normal heart rates for children are higher than those for adults. (See *Normal pediatric heart rates*.) In children, tachycardia may result from many of the adult causes previously described.

PATIENT COUNSELING

Educate the patient about the possibility of the tachyarrhythmia recurring. Explain that an antiarrhythmic and an internal defibrillator or ablation therapy may be indicated for symptomatic tachycardia.

TACHYPNEA

A common sign of cardiopulmonary disorders, tachypnea is an abnormally fast respiratory rate — 20 or more breaths/minute. Tachypnea may reflect the need to increase minute volume — the amount of air breathed each minute. Under these circumstances, it may be accompanied by an increase in tidal volume — the volume of air inhaled or exhaled per breath — resulting in hyperventilation. Tachypnea, however, may also reflect stiff lungs or overloaded ventilatory muscles, in which case tidal volume may actually be reduced.

Tachypnea may result from reduced arterial oxygen tension or arterial oxygen content, decreased perfusion, or increased oxygen demand. Heightened oxygen demand, for example, may result from fever, exertion, anxiety, and pain. It may also occur as a compensatory response to metabolic acidosis or may result from pulmonary irritation, stretch receptor stimulation, or a neurologic disorder that upsets medullary respiratory control. Generally, respirations increase by 4 breaths/minute for every 1° F (17.2° C) increase in body temperature.

Special considerations
+ Continue to monitor the patient.
+ Explain ordered diagnostic tests.
+ If appropriate, prepare patient for an ambulatory ECG.

Peds points
+ Normal heart rates for children are higher than those for adults.

Teaching points
+ Possibility of tachyarrhythmia recurring
+ Use of antiarrhythmics, internal defibrillator, or ablation therapy as possible treatments

Key facts about tachypnea
+ Refers to an abnormally fast respiratory rate (20 or more breaths/minute)

In an emergency

If the patient has paradoxical chest movement:

+ Suspect flail chest.
+ Immediately splint the chest with your hands or with sandbags.
+ Administer supplemental oxygen.
+ If possible, place the patient in semi-Fowler's position.
+ Insert an I.V. line.
+ Begin cardiac monitoring.

Key history points

+ Onset and description of tachypnea
+ History of pulmonary or cardiac conditions or anxiety attacks
+ Associated signs and symptoms, such as diaphoresis or chest pain
+ Drug history

Critical assessment steps

+ Take vital signs, including oxygen saturation.
+ Auscultate the chest for abnormal heart and breath sounds.
+ Record the color, amount, and consistency of any sputum.
+ Check for jugular vein distention.
+ Examine the skin for pallor, cyanosis, edema, and warmth or coolness.

Medical causes

ARDS

+ Tachypnea, an early feature, gradually worsens as fluid accumulates in the lungs.

Alcohol withdrawal syndrome

+ Tachypnea is a late sign.

Anaphylactic shock

+ Tachypnea develops within minutes after allergen exposure.

 EMERGENCY ACTIONS After detecting tachypnea, quickly evaluate cardiopulmonary status; obtain a set of vital signs with oxygen saturation; check for cyanosis, chest pain, dyspnea, tachycardia, and hypotension. If the patient has paradoxical chest movement, suspect flail chest and immediately splint his chest with your hands or with sandbags. Then administer supplemental oxygen by nasal cannula or face mask and, if possible, place the patient in semi-Fowler's position to help ease his breathing. Intubation and mechanical ventilation may be necessary if respiratory failure occurs. Also, insert an I.V. line for fluid and drug administration and begin cardiac monitoring.

HISTORY

If the patient's condition permits, obtain a medical history. Find out when the tachypnea began. Did it follow activity? Has he had it before? Does the patient have a history of asthma, chronic obstructive pulmonary disease (COPD), or any other pulmonary or cardiac conditions? Have him describe associated signs and symptoms, such as diaphoresis, chest pain, and recent weight loss. Is he anxious about anything or does he have a history of anxiety attacks? Note whether he takes any drugs for pain relief. If so, how effective are they?

PHYSICAL ASSESSMENT

Begin the physical assessment by taking the patient's vital signs, including oxygen saturation, if you haven't already done so. Observe the patient's overall behavior. Does he seem restless, confused, or fatigued? Then auscultate the chest for abnormal heart and breath sounds. If the patient has a productive cough, record the color, amount, and consistency of sputum. Finally, check for jugular vein distention, and examine the skin for pallor, cyanosis, edema, and warmth or coolness.

MEDICAL CAUSES

Acute respiratory distress syndrome

Tachypnea and apprehension may be the earliest features of acute respiratory distress syndrome (ARDS). Tachypnea gradually worsens as fluid accumulates in the patient's lungs, causing them to stiffen. It's accompanied by accessory muscle use, grunting expirations, suprasternal and intercostal retractions, crackles, and rhonchi. Eventually, ARDS produces hypoxemia, resulting in tachycardia, dyspnea, cyanosis, respiratory failure, and shock.

Alcohol withdrawal syndrome

A late sign in the acute phase of alcohol withdrawal syndrome, tachypnea typically accompanies anorexia, insomnia, tachycardia, fever, and diaphoresis. The patient may also experience anxiety, irritability, and bizarre visual or tactile hallucinations.

Anaphylactic shock

With life-threatening anaphylactic shock, tachypnea develops within minutes after exposure to an allergen, such as penicillin or insect venom. Accompanying signs and symptoms include anxiety, pounding headache, skin flushing, intense pruritus and, possibly, diffuse urticaria. The patient may exhibit widespread edema, affecting the eyelids, lips, tongue, hands, feet, and genitalia. Other findings include cool, clammy skin; rapid, thready pulse; cough; dyspnea; stridor; and change or loss of voice associated with laryngeal edema.

Anemia

Tachypnea may occur with anemia, depending on the duration and severity of the disorder. Associated signs and symptoms include fatigue, pallor, dyspnea, tachycardia, postural hypotension, bounding pulse, an atrial gallop, and a systolic bruit over the carotid arteries.

Anxiety
Tachypnea may occur during high-anxiety states because of the "fight-or-flight" response. Associated signs and symptoms include tachycardia, restlessness, chest pain, nausea, and light-headedness, all of which dissipate as the anxiety state resolves.

Aspiration of a foreign body
Life-threatening upper airway obstruction may result from aspiration of a foreign body. With a partial obstruction, the patient abruptly develops a dry, paroxysmal cough with rapid, shallow respirations. Other signs and symptoms include dyspnea, gagging or choking, intercostal retractions, nasal flaring, cyanosis, decreased or absent breath sounds, hoarseness, and stridor or coarse wheezing. Typically, the patient appears frightened and distressed. A complete obstruction may rapidly cause asphyxia and death.

Asthma
Tachypnea is common with life-threatening asthma attacks, which commonly occur at night. These attacks usually begin with mild wheezing and a dry cough that progresses to mucus expectoration. Eventually, the patient becomes apprehensive and develops prolonged expirations, intercostal and supraclavicular retractions on inspiration, accessory muscle use, severe audible wheezing, rhonchi, flaring nostrils, tachycardia, diaphoresis, and flushing or cyanosis.

Bronchiectasis
Although bronchiectasis may produce tachypnea, its classic sign is a chronic productive cough that produces copious amounts of mucopurulent, foul-smelling sputum and, occasionally, hemoptysis. Related findings include coarse crackles on inspiration, exertional dyspnea, rhonchi, and halitosis. The patient may also exhibit fever, malaise, weight loss, fatigue, and weakness. Clubbing is a common late sign.

Bronchitis (chronic)
Mild tachypnea may occur in chronic bronchitis (a form of COPD), but it isn't typically a predominant sign. Usually, chronic bronchitis begins with a dry, hacking cough, which later produces copious amounts of sputum. Other characteristics include dyspnea, prolonged expirations, wheezing, scattered rhonchi, accessory muscle use, and cyanosis. Clubbing and barrel chest are late signs.

Cardiac arrhythmias
Depending on the patient's heart rate, tachypnea may occur along with hypotension, dizziness, palpitations, weakness, and fatigue. The patient's level of consciousness (LOC) may be decreased.

Cardiac tamponade
With life-threatening cardiac tamponade, tachypnea may accompany tachycardia, dyspnea, and paradoxical pulse. Related findings include muffled heart sounds, pericardial friction rub, chest pain, hypotension, narrowed pulse pressure, and hepatomegaly. The patient is noticeably anxious and restless. His skin is clammy and cyanotic, and his jugular veins are distended.

Cardiogenic shock
Besides tachypnea, the patient in cardiogenic shock commonly displays cold, pale, clammy, cyanotic skin; hypotension; tachycardia; narrowed pulse pressure; a ventricular gallop; oliguria; decreased LOC; and jugular vein distention.

Medical causes
(continued)

Anemia
+ Tachypnea may occur, depending on the disorder.

Anxiety
+ Tachypnea may occur because of the "fight-or-flight" response.

Aspiration of a foreign body
+ A dry paroxysmal cough with rapid, shallow respirations develops abruptly.

Asthma
+ Tachypnea is common.
+ Attacks begin with mild wheezing and a dry cough that progresses to mucus expectoration.

Bronchiectasis
+ Tachypnea may occur with the classic chronic productive cough.

Bronchitis (chronic)
+ Mild tachypnea may occur but isn't typically a predominant sign.

Cardiac arrhythmias
+ Tachypnea may occur along with hypotension, dizziness, palpitations, weakness, and fatigue.

Cardiac tamponade
+ Tachypnea may accompany tachycardia, dyspnea, and paradoxical pulse.

Cardiogenic shock
+ Tachypnea, clammy skin, hypotension, tachycardia, narrowed pulse pressure, a ventricular gallop, oliguria, decreased LOC, and jugular vein distention result.

Medical causes
(continued)

Emphysema
✦ Tachypnea is accompanied by exertional dyspnea.

Febrile illness
✦ Fever can cause tachypnea, tachycardia, chills, diaphoresis, headache, and weakness.

Flail chest
✦ Tachypnea usually appears early in this life-threatening disorder.

Head trauma
✦ When trauma affects the brain stem, central neurogenic hyperventilation may occur with other signs of neurogenic dysfunction.

HHNS
✦ Rapidly deteriorating LOC occurs with tachypnea, tachycardia, hypotension, seizures, oliguria, and signs of dehydration.

Hypovolemic shock
✦ Tachypnea is an early sign that may be accompanied by cool, pale skin; restlessness; thirst; and mild tachycardia.

Hypoxia
✦ Lack of oxygen increases the rate and depth of breathing.

Interstitial fibrosis
✦ Tachypnea develops gradually and may become severe.

Lung abscess
✦ Tachypnea is usually paired with dyspnea and accentuated by fever.

Emphysema
Emphysema is a chronic pulmonary disorder that commonly produces tachypnea accompanied by exertional dyspnea. Emphysema may also cause anorexia, malaise, peripheral cyanosis, pursed-lip breathing, accessory muscle use, and chronic productive cough. Percussion yields a hyperresonant tone; auscultation reveals wheezing, crackles, and diminished breath sounds. Clubbing and barrel chest are late signs.

Febrile illness
Fever can cause tachypnea, tachycardia, chills, diaphoresis, headache, and weakness. Related findings depend on the specific disorder.

Flail chest
Tachypnea usually appears early in flail chest, a life-threatening disorder. Other findings include paradoxical chest wall movement, rib bruises and palpable fractures, localized chest pain, hypotension, and diminished breath sounds. The patient may also develop signs of respiratory distress, such as dyspnea and accessory muscle use.

Head trauma
When trauma affects the brain stem, the patient may display central neurogenic hyperventilation, a form of tachypnea marked by rapid, even, and deep respirations. The tachypnea may be accompanied by other signs of life-threatening neurogenic dysfunction, such as coma, unequal and nonreactive pupils, seizures, hemiplegia, flaccidity, and hypoactive or absent deep tendon reflexes.

Hyperosmolar hyperglycemic nonketotic syndrome
With hyperosmolar hyperglycemic nonketotic syndrome (HHNS), rapidly deteriorating LOC occurs with tachypnea, tachycardia, hypotension, seizures, oliguria, and signs of dehydration, such as dry mouth and poor skin turgor. Confusion progressing to coma may also occur.

Hypovolemic shock
An early sign of life-threatening hypovolemic shock, tachypnea is accompanied by cool, pale skin; restlessness; thirst; and mild tachycardia. As shock progresses, the patient's skin becomes clammy; his pulse is increasingly rapid and thready. Other findings include hypotension, narrowed pulse pressure, oliguria, subnormal body temperature, and decreased LOC.

Hypoxia
Hypoxia (lack of oxygen) from any cause increases the rate (and often the depth) of breathing. The patient may be restless. He may also have impaired judgment, tachycardia, dyspnea, and cyanosis. Associated symptoms are related to the cause of the hypoxia.

Interstitial fibrosis
With interstitial fibrosis, tachypnea develops gradually and may become severe. Associated features include exertional dyspnea, pleuritic chest pain, a paroxysmal dry cough, crackles, late inspiratory wheezing, cyanosis, fatigue, and weight loss. Clubbing is a late sign.

Lung abscess
With lung abscess, tachypnea is usually paired with dyspnea and accentuated by fever. However, the chief sign is a productive cough with copious amounts of purulent, foul-smelling, usually bloody sputum. Other findings include chest pain, halitosis, diaphoresis, chills, fatigue, weakness, anorexia, weight loss, and clubbing.

Neurogenic shock

Tachypnea is characteristic in this life-threatening type of shock. Tachypnea is commonly accompanied by apprehension, bradycardia or tachycardia, oliguria, fluctuating body temperature, and decreased LOC that may progress to coma. The patient's skin is warm, dry, and perhaps flushed. He may experience nausea and vomiting.

Plague

The onset of the pneumonic form of plague (*Yersinia pestis*) is usually sudden. The infection is characterized by chills, fever, headache, and myalgia. Pulmonary signs and symptoms include tachypnea, productive cough, chest pain, dyspnea, hemoptysis, and increasing respiratory distress and cardiopulmonary insufficiency.

Pneumonia (bacterial)

A common sign in bacterial pneumonia, tachypnea is usually preceded by a painful, hacking, dry cough that rapidly becomes productive. Other signs and symptoms quickly follow, including high fever, shaking chills, headache, dyspnea, pleuritic chest pain, tachycardia, grunting respirations, nasal flaring, and cyanosis. Auscultation reveals diminished breath sounds and fine crackles; percussion yields a dull tone.

Pneumothorax

Tachypnea, a common sign of life-threatening pneumothorax, is typically accompanied by severe, sharp, and commonly unilateral chest pain that's aggravated by chest movement. Associated signs and symptoms include dyspnea, tachycardia, accessory muscle use, asymmetrical chest expansion, dry cough, cyanosis, anxiety, and restlessness. Examination of the affected lung reveals hyperresonance or tympany, subcutaneous crepitation, decreased vocal fremitus, and diminished or absent breath sounds. The patient with tension pneumothorax also develops a deviated trachea.

Pulmonary edema

Pulmonary edema is a life-threatening disorder that produces early signs of tachypnea accompanied by exertional dyspnea, paroxysmal nocturnal dyspnea and, later, orthopnea. Other features of pulmonary edema include a dry cough, crackles, tachycardia, and a ventricular gallop. With severe pulmonary edema, respirations become increasingly rapid and labored, tachycardia worsens, and crackles become more diffuse. The patient's cough also produces frothy, bloody sputum. Signs of shock — such as hypotension, thready pulse, and cold, clammy skin — may also occur.

Pulmonary embolism (acute)

Tachypnea occurs suddenly with pulmonary embolism and is usually accompanied by dyspnea. The patient may complain of angina or pleuritic chest pain. Other common characteristics include tachycardia, a dry or productive cough with blood-tinged sputum, low-grade fever, restlessness, and diaphoresis. Less-common signs include massive hemoptysis, chest splinting, leg edema, and — with a large embolus — jugular vein distention and syncope. Other findings include pleural friction rub, crackles, diffuse wheezing, dullness on percussion, diminished breath sounds, and signs of shock, such as hypotension and a weak, rapid pulse.

Septic shock

Early in septic shock, the patient usually experiences tachypnea; sudden fever; chills; flushed, warm, yet dry skin; and possibly nausea, vomiting, and diarrhea. He may also develop tachycardia and normal or slightly decreased blood pressure. As

Medical causes
(continued)

Tumor
+ A lung, pleural, or mediastinal tumor may cause tachypnea.

Other causes
+ Overdose of salicylates

Special considerations
+ Continue to monitor vital signs.
+ Keep suction and emergency equipment nearby.
+ Prepare to intubate the patient and to provide mechanical ventilation if necessary.

Peds points
+ Pediatric causes include congenital heart defects, meningitis, metabolic acidosis, cystic fibrosis, hunger, and anxiety.

Geri points
+ Tachypnea may have various causes in elderly patients, such as pneumonia, heart failure, COPD, anxiety, or failure to take cardiac and respiratory medications appropriately.

Teaching points
+ Explanation that slight increases in respiratory rate may be normal

Key facts about taste abnormalities
+ Involves a loss of taste (ageusia), partial loss of taste (hypogeusia), a distorted sense of taste (dysgeusia), or an unpleasant sense of taste (cacogeusia)

---

this life-threatening type of shock progresses, the patient may display anxiety; restlessness; decreased LOC; hypotension; cool, clammy, and cyanotic skin; rapid, thready pulse; thirst; and oliguria that may progress to anuria.

Tumor
A lung, pleural, or mediastinal tumor may cause tachypnea along with exertional dyspnea, cough, hemoptysis, and pleuritic chest pain. Other effects include tracheal shift, jugular vein distention, weight loss, anorexia, and fatigue.

OTHER CAUSES

Drugs
Tachypnea may result from an overdose of salicylates.

SPECIAL CONSIDERATIONS

Continue to monitor the patient's vital signs closely. Be sure to keep suction and emergency equipment nearby. Prepare to intubate the patient and to provide mechanical ventilation if necessary. Prepare the patient for diagnostic studies, such as arterial blood gas analysis, blood cultures, chest X-rays, pulmonary function tests, and an electrocardiogram.

PEDIATRIC POINTERS

When assessing a child for tachypnea, be aware that the normal respiratory rate varies with the child's age. If you detect tachypnea, first rule out the causes listed above. Then consider these pediatric causes: congenital heart defects, meningitis, metabolic acidosis, and cystic fibrosis. Keep in mind, however, that hunger and anxiety may also cause tachypnea.

GERIATRIC POINTERS

Tachypnea may have a various causes in elderly patients, such as pneumonia, heart failure, COPD, anxiety, or failure to take cardiac and respiratory medications appropriately. Mild increases in respiratory rate may be unnoticed.

PATIENT COUNSELING

Reassure the patient that slight increases in respiratory rate may be normal. Provide emotional support because high levels of anxiety can worsen the patient's tachypnea.

TASTE ABNORMALITIES

There are several types of taste impairment. *Ageusia* is complete loss of taste; *hypogeusia,* partial loss of taste; and *dysgeusia,* a distorted sense of taste. In *cacogeusia,* food may taste unpleasant or even revolting.

The sensory receptors for taste are the taste buds, which are concentrated over the tongue's surface and scattered over the palate, pharynx, and larynx. These buds can differentiate among sweet, salty, sour, and bitter stimuli. More complex flavors are perceived by taste and olfactory receptors together. In fact, much of what the layman calls taste is actually smell; food odors typically stimulate the olfactory system more strongly than food tastes stimulate the taste buds.

Any factor that interrupts transmission of taste stimuli to the brain may cause taste abnormalities. (See *Tracing taste pathways to the brain.*) Such factors include trauma, infection, vitamin and mineral deficiencies, neurologic and oral disorders,

Tracing taste pathways to the brain

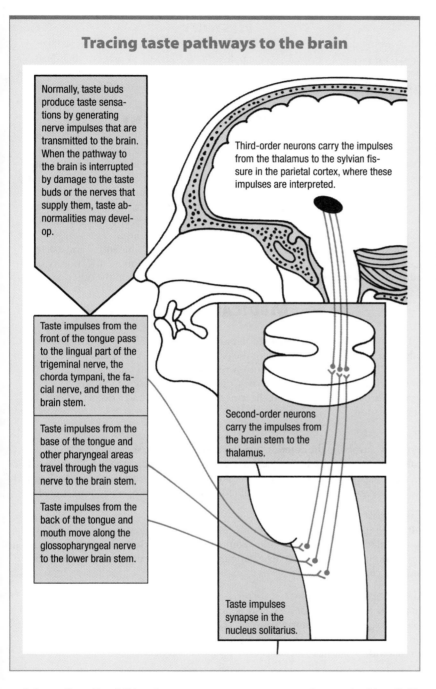

Normally, taste buds produce taste sensations by generating nerve impulses that are transmitted to the brain. When the pathway to the brain is interrupted by damage to the taste buds or the nerves that supply them, taste abnormalities may develop.

Third-order neurons carry the impulses from the thalamus to the sylvian fissure in the parietal cortex, where these impulses are interpreted.

Taste impulses from the front of the tongue pass to the lingual part of the trigeminal nerve, the chorda tympani, the facial nerve, and then the brain stem.

Taste impulses from the base of the tongue and other pharyngeal areas travel through the vagus nerve to the brain stem.

Taste impulses from the back of the tongue and mouth move along the glossopharyngeal nerve to the lower brain stem.

Second-order neurons carry the impulses from the brain stem to the thalamus.

Taste impulses synapse in the nucleus solitarius.

and drug effects. In addition, because tastes are most accurately perceived in a fluid medium, mouth dryness may interfere with taste.

Two major nonpathologic causes of impaired taste are aging, which normally reduces the number of taste buds, and heavy smoking (especially pipe smoking), which dries the tongue.

Key history points

+ Onset of taste abnormality
+ History of oral or other disorders
+ Recent flu, head trauma, or radiation treatments
+ Smoking habits
+ Drug history

Critical assessment steps

+ Evaluate taste: Withdraw the tongue with a gauze sponge, apply various flavors (such as salt or sugar) on the tongue, and ask patient to identify the tastes.
+ Inspect the oral cavity for lesions, sores, and mucosal or taste bud abnormalities.
+ Evaluate sense of smell: Pinch one nostril and ask the patient to close his eyes and sniff through the open nostril to identify nonirritating odors such as coffee. Repeat test on the other nostril.

Medical causes

Basilar skull fracture

+ If the first cranial nerve is involved, the patient usually can't detect aromatic flavors.

Bell's palsy

+ Taste loss in the anterior two-thirds of the tongue is common.

Common cold

+ Impaired taste is usually secondary to loss of smell.

Geographic tongue

+ Taste abnormalities occur with areas of loss and regrowth of filiform papillae.

Influenza

+ The patient may have hypogeusia, dysgeusia, or both.

HISTORY

After noting the patient's age, find out when his taste abnormality began. Then search for possible causes. Does the patient have a history of oral or other disorders? Has he recently had the flu or suffered head trauma? Does he smoke? Is he receiving radiation treatments? Is he currently taking any medications?

PHYSICAL ASSESSMENT

Thoroughly evaluate the patient's sense of taste. Gently withdraw his tongue slightly with a gauze sponge. Then use a moistened applicator to place a few crystals of salt or sugar on one side of the tongue. Ask the patient to identify the taste sensation while his tongue is protruded. Repeat the test on the other side of the tongue. To test bitter taste sensation, apply a tiny amount of quinine to the base of the tongue. To test sour taste sensation, apply a tiny amount of dilute vinegar on the base of the tongue. Inspect the oral cavity for lesions, sores, and mucosal abnormalities. Observe the taste buds for any obvious abnormalities.

Finally, evaluate the patient's sense of smell. Pinch off one nostril and ask the patient to close his eyes and sniff through the open nostril to identify nonirritating odors, such as coffee, lime, and wintergreen. Repeat the test on the other nostril.

MEDICAL CAUSES

Basilar skull fracture

If the first cranial nerve is involved in basilar skull fracture, the patient can't detect odors on the affected side. Usually, the patient can't detect aromatic flavors, although he can still correctly identify sweet, salty, sour, and bitter stimuli. Other findings include epistaxis, rhinorrhea, otorrhea, Battle's sign, raccoon eyes, headache, nausea and vomiting, hearing and vision loss, and a decreased level of consciousness.

Bell's palsy

Taste loss involving the anterior two-thirds of the tongue is common with Bell's palsy. Hemifacial muscle weakness or paralysis is also characteristic. The affected side of the patient's face sags and is masklike. Associated signs include drooling and tearing, diminished or absent corneal reflex, and difficulty blinking the affected eye.

Common cold

Although impaired taste is a common complaint with the common cold, it's usually secondary to loss of smell. Other common features include rhinorrhea with nasal congestion, sore throat, headache, fatigue, myalgia, arthralgia, malaise, and a dry, hacking cough.

Geographic tongue

In geographic tongue disorder, taste abnormalities occur along with many areas of loss and regrowth of filiform papillae. These areas are continually changing and produce a maplike appearance with denuded red patches surrounded by thick white borders.

Influenza

After influenza the patient may have hypogeusia, dysgeusia, or both. Typically, he also reports an impaired sense of smell. The patient with influenza commonly complains of sore throat, fever with chills, headache, weakness, malaise, muscle aches, cough and, occasionally, hoarseness and rhinorrhea.

Oral cancer

About one-half of all oral tumors involve the tongue, especially the posterior portion and the lateral borders. These tumors may destroy or damage taste buds, resulting in impaired taste. The patient also has difficulty chewing and speaking and may develop halitosis.

Sjögren's syndrome

With Sjögren's syndrome, an autosomal recessive disorder, impaired sense of taste results from extreme mouth dryness associated with inadequate production of saliva. Ocular dryness is also characteristic; initially, it causes burning and pain around the eyes and under the lids. Later, the patient develops photosensitivity, impaired vision, and eye fatigue and redness. Other signs and symptoms include mouth soreness; difficulty chewing, swallowing, and talking; a dry cough; hoarseness; epistaxis; dry, scaly skin; decreased sweating; abdominal distress; and polyuria. Physical examination may reveal corneal ulceration, nasal crusting, and enlarged lacrimal, parotid, and submaxillary glands.

Thalamic syndrome

Thalamic syndrome, which is caused by a lesion in the thalamus, may produce a distorted sense of taste. Typically, this symptom is preceded by contralateral sensory loss (both deep and cutaneous), transient hemiparesis, and homonymous hemianopia. Later, the patient gradually regains sensation and may then experience pain or hyperpathia.

Thrush

With thrush, cream-colored or bluish white patches of exudates on the tongue, mouth, or pharynx cause altered taste, pain, and a burning sensation. The condition may cause respiratory distress in infants.

Viral hepatitis (acute)

Hypogeusia commonly precedes jaundice by 1 to 2 weeks. Associated signs and symptoms in the preicteric phase of hepatitis include altered sense of smell, anorexia, nausea and vomiting, fatigue, malaise, headache, photophobia, sore throat, and a cough. The patient may also experience muscle and joint aches.

Vitamin B$_{12}$ deficiency

With a vitamin B$_{12}$ deficiency, hypogeusia is accompanied by an impaired sense of smell, anorexia, weight loss, abdominal discomfort, and glossitis. The patient may also exhibit yellow skin, peripheral neuropathy, dyspnea, ataxic gait, and dementia.

Zinc deficiency

A deficiency of zinc is common in patients with idiopathic hypogeusia, suggesting that zinc plays an important role in normal taste sensation. Common associated findings include cacogeusia, a distorted sense of smell, anorexia, soft and misshapen nails, and sparse hair growth. Palpation may reveal an enlarged liver and spleen.

OTHER CAUSES

Drugs

Drugs that may distort the sense of taste include penicillamine, captopril, griseofulvin, lithium, rifampin, antithyroid preparations, procarbazine, vincristine, and vinblastine.

Medical causes
(continued)

Oral cancer
+ Tumors involving the tongue may destroy or damage taste buds.

Sjögren's syndrome
+ Impaired sense of taste results from extreme mouth dryness associated with inadequate production of saliva.

Thalamic syndrome
+ A distorted sense of taste is preceded by contralateral sensory loss, transient hemiparesis, and homonymous hemianopia.

Thrush
+ Cream-colored or bluish white patches of exudates on the tongue, mouth, or pharynx cause altered taste, pain, burning.

Viral hepatitis (acute)
+ Hypogeusia commonly precedes jaundice by 1 to 2 weeks.

Vitamin B$_{12}$ deficiency
+ Hypogeusia is accompanied by impaired sense of smell, anorexia, weight loss, abdominal discomfort, and glossitis.

Zinc deficiency
+ Idiopathic hypogeusia may occur with cacogeusia.

Other causes
+ Antithyroid preparations, captopril, griseofulvin, lithium, penicillamine, procarbazine, rifampin, vincristine, and vinblastine
+ Irradiation of the head or neck

Special considerations
+ Modify patient's diet if necessary.

Peds points
+ Children may be unable to differentiate between abnormal taste sensation and taste dislike.

Teaching points
+ Good oral hygiene
+ Use of spices to enhance flavor
+ Referral to a dietitian as needed

Key facts about increased tearing
+ Also known as *epiphora*
+ Usually results from inadequate tear drainage due to obstruction of the lacrimal drainage system or malposition of the lower lid

Key history points
+ Onset and description of tearing
+ Accompanying pain, irritation, or discharge
+ History of eye trauma or ocular and systemic disorders
+ Drug history
+ Possible occupational hazards

Critical assessment steps
+ Examine both eyes.
+ Examine the eyelids for lesions and edema.
+ Check for ptosis.
+ Examine the conjunctiva for redness and abnormal drainage.
+ Note the color of the sclera.
+ Using a flashlight, examine the cornea and iris for scars, irregularities, and foreign bodies.

Radiation therapy

Irradiation of the head or neck may cause excessive dryness of the mouth, resulting in impaired taste sensation.

SPECIAL CONSIDERATIONS

Modify the patient's diet, if necessary, so that he can distinguish and enjoy as many tastes as possible.

PEDIATRIC POINTERS

Recognize that young children typically can't differentiate between an abnormal taste sensation and a simple taste dislike.

PATIENT COUNSELING

Encourage good oral hygiene before and after meals. Suggest to the patient that using spices may enhance flavor. Refer the patient to a dietitian if reduced or absent sense of taste is adversely affecting his nutritional status.

TEARING, INCREASED

Tears normally bathe the eyes, keeping the epithelium moist and flushing away foreign bodies. Excessive lacrimation (tear production), also known as *epiphora,* usually results from inadequate tear drainage due to obstruction of the lacrimal drainage system or malposition of the lower lid. Reflex tearing occurs with any disturbance of the corneal epithelium.

Lacrimation may be classified as psychic or neurogenic. *Psychic lacrimation* normally occurs in response to emotional or physical stress, such as pain, and is the most common cause of increased tearing. *Neurogenic lacrimation* is triggered by reflex stimulation associated with ocular trauma or inflammation or with exposure to environmental irritants, such as strong light, dry or hot wind, or airborne allergens. This type of lacrimation may also accompany eyestrain, yawning, vomiting, and laughing.

HISTORY

If the patient complains of increased tearing, begin by fully exploring this sign. When did it begin? Is it constant or intermittent? Minimal or extensive? Is increased tearing accompanied by pain or irritation? Is there any other drainage or discharge from the eye? Next, ask about recent eye trauma and about ocular and systemic disorders. Then record what drugs the patient is taking. Note his occupation and the nature of his work. For example, does he read extensively, look at a computer screen frequently, or work with small or fine objects? Is he exposed to any chemicals or dust in the workplace?

PHYSICAL ASSESSMENT

After taking vital signs, examine both eyes — unless the history suggests a perforating or penetrating injury. Carefully inspect the external structures. Do the eyelashes contain debris? Examine the eyelids for lesions and edema. Ask the patient to look straight ahead at a fixed object while you check for ptosis. Are the lid margins turned inward or outward? Examine the eyeballs. Do they appear sunken or bulging? Examine the conjunctiva for redness and abnormal drainage. Also, note the color of the sclera. Hold a flashlight at the side of either eye and examine the cornea and iris for scars, irregularities, and foreign bodies. Evaluate extraocular muscle function by testing the six cardinal fields of gaze. Finally, test the patient's visual acuity.

MEDICAL CAUSES

Conjunctival foreign bodies and abrasions

Increased tearing may accompany localized conjunctival injection, severe eye pain, and photophobia. A foreign-body sensation may be present. Typically, visual acuity isn't affected.

Conjunctivitis

Typically, increased tearing is accompanied by conjunctival injection and itching. Allergic conjunctivitis also causes a stringy discharge. With bacterial conjunctivitis, other features include copious, purulent discharge; burning; a foreign-body sensation; and possibly eye pain if the cornea is involved. Associated signs of fungal conjunctivitis include lid edema, burning, and a copious, thick, purulent discharge that may form sticky crusts on the lids. The patient complains of photophobia and pain if the cornea is involved. Highly contagious viral conjunctivitis also causes a foreign-body sensation, slight exudate, and lid edema.

Corneal abrasion

Marked by severe corneal pain that's aggravated by blinking, a corneal abrasion also causes increased tearing. Associated features are a foreign-body sensation, blurred vision, conjunctival injection, and photophobia, which makes opening the lids difficult.

Corneal foreign body

When a foreign body lodges in the cornea, the patient experiences increased tearing, blurred vision, a foreign-body sensation, photophobia, eye pain, miosis, and conjunctival injection. A dark speck may also be visible in the cornea.

Corneal ulcers

With corneal ulcers, a vision-threatening disorder, increased tearing is accompanied by severe photophobia and eye pain. Typically, an early symptom of a corneal ulcer is pain that's aggravated by blinking. Ulcers also cause blurred vision, conjunctival injection, and a white, opaque cornea. Bacterial ulcers also produce a copious, purulent discharge that may form sticky crusts on the lids.

Dacryocystitis

Increased tearing and a purulent discharge are the chief complaints with dacryocystitis, which is commonly unilateral. Associated signs and symptoms include pain and tenderness around the tear sac with marked eyelid edema and redness near the lacrimal punctum. Pressure on the tear sac expresses a thick, purulent discharge or, in chronic cases, a mucoid discharge.

Dry eye syndrome

Excessive dryness of the cornea and conjunctiva can cause reflex stimulation of the lacrimal gland and excess tearing. Other signs and symptoms include eye pain, conjunctival injection, and itching.

Episcleritis

Commonly unilateral, episcleritis causes increased tearing, photophobia, and — if the sclera is inflamed — eye pain and tenderness on palpation. Inspection reveals conjunctival injection and edema, a purplish pink sclera, and episcleral edema.

Medical causes

Conjunctival foreign bodies and abrasions

✦ Increased tearing may occur with localized conjunctival injection, eye pain, and photophobia.

Conjunctivitis

✦ Increased tearing, conjunctival injection, and itching occur.

Corneal abrasion

✦ Corneal pain is accompanied by increased tearing.

Corneal foreign body

✦ Increased tearing, blurred vision, a foreign-body sensation, photophobia, eye pain, miosis, and conjunctival injection occur.

Corneal ulcers

✦ Increased tearing, severe photophobia, and eye pain occur.

Dacryocystitis

✦ Increased tearing and a purulent discharge are the chief complaints.

Dry eye syndrome

✦ Excessive dryness of the cornea and conjunctiva can result in excess tearing.

Episcleritis

✦ Increased tearing and photophobia occur.

Medical causes
(continued)

Herpes zoster
+ Increased tearing may occur if the trigeminal nerve is affected.

Lid contractions
+ Increased tearing usually results from stricture of the canaliculi.

Psoriasis vulgaris
+ If lesions affect the eyelids and extend into the conjunctiva, they may cause irritation, increased tearing, and a foreign-body sensation.

Punctum misplacement
+ Increased tearing may be accompanied by keratitis.

Thyrotoxicosis
+ Increased tearing usually occurs in both eyes.

Other causes
+ Miotics

Special considerations
+ Obtain tear specimen for culture.
+ Prepare patient for Schirmer's test and irrigation of lacrimal drainage system.

Peds points
+ The most common pediatric causes of increased tearing include allergies, conjunctivitis, and the common cold.

Teaching points
+ Importance of not touching the unaffected eye and not sharing eye makeup or pillowcases
+ Good hand-washing techniques

Herpes zoster
Increased tearing usually occurs when herpes zoster affects the trigeminal nerve. It's accompanied by severe unilateral facial and eye pain that's followed by the eruption of vesicles within several days. The patient's eyelids are red and swollen with scanty serous discharge. Other common findings include a white, cloudy cornea and conjunctival injection.

Lid contractions
With lid contractions, increased tearing usually results from stricture of the canaliculi. Because lid contractions are caused by burns or chemical or mechanical trauma, lid scars are also commonly visible.

Psoriasis vulgaris
When psoriasis vulgaris lesions affect the eyelids and extend into the conjunctiva, they may cause irritation, increased tearing, and a foreign-body sensation. The lesions are typically preceded by signs of chronic conjunctivitis, such as copious mucoid discharge and conjunctival injection.

Punctum misplacement
Increased tearing is characteristic when ectropion involves the punctum, causing misplacement. It may be accompanied by exposure keratitis.

Thyrotoxicosis
Thyrotoxicosis may cause increased tearing, usually in both eyes. Other ocular effects include ptosis, lid edema, photophobia, a foreign-body sensation, conjunctival injection, chemosis, diplopia and, at times, exophthalmos. Common associated features are heat intolerance, weight loss despite increased appetite, nervousness, sweating, diarrhea, tremors, tachycardia, palpitations, and an enlarged thyroid.

OTHER CAUSES

Cholinergics
Miotics, such as pilocarpine, may increase tearing.

SPECIAL CONSIDERATIONS
Obtain a tear specimen for culture. Isolate the patient until a definite diagnosis is made. Also, prepare him for Schirmer's test to measure tear production and secretion, and for irrigation of the lacrimal drainage system.

PEDIATRIC POINTERS
The most common pediatric causes of increased tearing include allergies, conjunctivitis, and the common cold.

PATIENT COUNSELING
Instruct the patient not to touch the unaffected eye to avoid possible cross-contamination. Teach the patient not to share eye makeup or pillowcases and to practice good hand-washing techniques.

THROAT PAIN

Throat pain—also known as a *sore throat*—refers to discomfort in any part of the pharynx: the nasopharynx, the oropharynx, or the hypopharynx. This common symptom ranges from a sensation of scratchiness to severe pain. It's typically accompanied by ear pain because cranial nerves IX and X innervate the pharynx as well as the middle and external ear.

Throat pain may result from infection, trauma, allergy, cancer, or a systemic disorder. It may also follow surgery and endotracheal intubation. Nonpathologic causes include dry mucous membranes associated with mouth breathing and laryngeal irritation associated with alcohol consumption, inhaling smoke or chemicals like ammonia, and vocal strain.

HISTORY

Ask the patient when he first noticed the pain and have him describe it. Has he had throat pain before? Is it accompanied by fever, ear pain, or dysphagia? Review the patient's medical history for throat problems, allergies, and systemic disorders.

PHYSICAL ASSESSMENT

Carefully examine the pharynx, noting redness, exudate, or swelling. Examine the oropharynx, using a warmed metal spatula or tongue blade, and the nasopharynx, using a warmed laryngeal mirror or a fiber-optic nasopharyngoscope. Laryngoscopic examination of the hypopharynx may be required. (If necessary, spray the soft palate and pharyngeal wall with a local anesthetic to prevent gagging.) Observe the tonsils for redness, swelling, or exudate. Obtain an exudate specimen for culture. Then examine the nose, using a nasal speculum. Also, check the patient's ears, especially if he reports ear pain. Finally, palpate the neck and oropharynx for nodules or lymph node enlargement.

MEDICAL CAUSES

Agranulocytosis

With agranulocytosis, sore throat may accompany other signs and symptoms of infection, such as fever, chills, and headache. Typically, sore throat follows progressive fatigue and weakness. Other findings include nausea and vomiting, anorexia, and bleeding tendencies. Rough-edged ulcers with gray or black membranes may appear on the gums, palate, or perianal area.

Allergic rhinitis

Occurring seasonally or year-round, allergic rhinitis may produce sore throat as well as nasal congestion with a thin nasal discharge, postnasal drip, paroxysmal sneezing, decreased sense of smell, frontal or temporal headache, and itchy eyes, nose, and throat. Examination reveals pale and glistening nasal mucosa with edematous nasal turbinates, watery eyes, reddened conjunctiva and eyelids and, possibly, swollen lids.

Bronchitis (acute)

Acute bronchitis may produce lower throat pain associated with fever, chills, cough, and muscle and back pain. Auscultation reveals rhonchi, wheezing and, at times, crackles.

Chronic fatigue syndrome

Chronic fatigue syndrome is a nonspecific symptom complex that's characterized by incapacitating fatigue. Associated findings besides sore throat include myalgia, lymphadenopathy, and cognitive dysfunction.

Key facts about throat pain
+ Discomfort in pharynx
+ Ranges from sensation of scratchiness to severe pain

Key history points
+ Onset of throat pain
+ Accompanying fever, ear pain, or dysphagia
+ Medical history, including throat problems and allergies

Critical assessment steps
+ Examine the pharynx, oropharynx, and nasopharynx.
+ Obtain exudate specimen for culture.
+ Examine the nose.
+ Check the ears.
+ Palpate neck and oropharynx.

Medical causes
Agranulocytosis
+ Sore throat may follow progressive fatigue and weakness.

Allergic rhinitis
+ Sore throat occurs with other signs and symptoms, such as nasal congestion.

Bronchitis (acute)
+ Lower throat pain, fever, chills, cough, and muscle and back pain may occur.

Chronic fatigue syndrome
+ Incapacitating fatigue occurs with sore throat, myalgia, lymphadenopathy, and cognitive dysfunction.

Medical causes
(continued)

Common cold
✦ Sore throat may accompany other signs and symptoms, such as cough and nasal congestion.

Contact ulcers
✦ Ulcers appear symmetrically on the posterior vocal cords, resulting in sore throat.

Foreign body
✦ A foreign body lodged in the palatine or lingual tonsil and pyriform sinus may produce localized throat pain.

GERD
✦ Chronic sore throat and hoarseness may occur.

Glossopharyngeal neuralgia
✦ Unilateral, knifelike throat pain occurs in the tonsillar fossa.

Herpes simplex virus
✦ Sore throat may result from lesions on the oral mucosa.

Influenza
✦ Sore throat, fever, headache, weakness, malaise, and muscle aches are common complaints.

Laryngeal cancer
✦ With extrinsic laryngeal cancer, pain or burning in the throat occurs when drinking citrus juice or hot liquids, or the patient feels a lump in the throat.
✦ With intrinsic laryngeal cancer, hoarseness persists for longer than 3 weeks.

Common cold
With the common cold, sore throat may accompany cough, sneezing, nasal congestion, mouth breathing, rhinorrhea, fatigue, headache, myalgia, and arthralgia. The patient may also have a transient loss of taste and smell.

Contact ulcers
Common in men with stressful jobs, contact ulcers appear symmetrically on the posterior vocal cords, resulting in sore throat. The pain is aggravated by talking and may be accompanied by referred ear pain and, occasionally, hemoptysis. Typically, the patient also has a history of chronic throat clearing or acid reflux.

Foreign body
A foreign body lodged in the palatine or lingual tonsil and pyriform sinus may produce localized throat pain. The pain may persist after the foreign body is dislodged until mucosal irritation resolves.

Gastroesophageal reflux disease
Gastroesophageal reflux disease (GERD) may cause chronic sore throat and hoarseness. The arytenoids may also appear red and swollen, resulting in a sensation of a lump in the throat. Pyrosis, usually severe, is the most common symptom of this disorder.

Glossopharyngeal neuralgia
Triggered by a specific pharyngeal movement, such as yawning, chewing or swallowing, glossopharyngeal neuralgia causes unilateral, knifelike throat pain in the tonsillar fossa that may radiate to the ear. Eating spicy foods may also trigger this pain.

Herpes simplex virus
Sore throat in those infected with the herpes simplex virus may result from lesions on the oral mucosa, especially the tongue, gingivae, and cheeks. After causing brief prodromal discomfort, lesions erupt into erythematous vesicles that eventually rupture and leave a painful ulcer, followed by a yellowish crust. In generalized infection, the vesicles accompany submaxillary lymphadenopathy, halitosis, increased salivation, anorexia, and fever of up to 105° F (40.6° C).

Influenza
Patients with influenza commonly complain of sore throat, fever with chills, headache, weakness, malaise, muscle aches, cough and, occasionally, hoarseness and rhinorrhea. Chills generally subside after the first few days, but intermittent fever, weakness, and cough may persist for up to 1 week.

Laryngeal cancer
With extrinsic laryngeal cancer, the chief symptom is pain or burning in the throat when drinking citrus juice or hot liquids, or a lump in the throat; with intrinsic laryngeal cancer, it's hoarseness that persists for longer than 3 weeks. Later signs and symptoms of metastasis include dysphagia, dyspnea, a cough, enlarged cervical lymph nodes, and pain that radiates to the ear.

Laryngitis (acute)
Acute laryngitis produces sore throat. Its cardinal sign, however, is mild to severe hoarseness, perhaps with temporary loss of voice. Other findings are malaise, low-grade fever, dysphagia, dry cough, and tender, enlarged cervical lymph nodes.

Mononucleosis (infectious)
Sore throat is one of the three classic findings in mononucleosis. The other two classic signs are cervical lymphadenopathy and fluctuating temperature with an evening peak of 101° to 102° F (38.3° to 38.9° C). Splenomegaly and hepatomegaly may also develop.

Necrotizing ulcerative gingivitis (acute)
Also known as *trench mouth,* necrotizing ulcerative gingivitis usually begins abruptly with sore throat and tender gums that ulcerate and bleed. A gray exudate may cover the gums and pharyngeal tonsils. Related signs and symptoms include a foul taste in the mouth, halitosis, cervical lymphadenopathy, headache, malaise, and fever.

Peritonsillar abscess
A complication of bacterial tonsillitis, peritonsillar abscess typically causes severe throat pain that radiates to the ear. Accompanying the pain may be dysphagia, drooling, dysarthria, halitosis, fever with chills, malaise, and nausea. The patient usually tilts his head toward the side of the abscess. Examination may also reveal a deviated uvula, trismus, and tender cervical lymphadenopathy.

Pharyngeal burns
First- or second-degree burns of the posterior pharynx may cause throat pain and dysphagia. Laryngeal edema, bronchospasm, and stridor may occur if the larynx is involved in the burn.

Pharyngitis
Whether bacterial, fungal, or viral, pharyngitis may cause sore throat and localized erythema and edema. *Bacterial pharyngitis* begins abruptly with a unilateral sore throat. Associated signs and symptoms include dysphagia, fever, malaise, headache, abdominal pain, myalgia, and arthralgia. Inspection reveals an exudate on the tonsil or tonsillar fossae, uvular edema, soft palate erythema, and tender cervical lymph nodes.

Also known as thrush, *fungal pharyngitis* causes diffuse sore throat — commonly described as a burning sensation — accompanied by pharyngeal erythema and edema. White plaques mark the pharynx, tonsil, tonsillar pillars, base of the tongue, and oral mucosa; scraping these plaques uncovers a hemorrhagic base.

With *viral pharyngitis,* findings include diffuse sore throat, malaise, fever, and mild erythema and edema of the posterior oropharyngeal wall. Tonsillary enlargement may be present along with anterior cervical lymphadenopathy.

Pharyngomaxillary space abscess
A complication of untreated pharyngeal or tonsillar infection or tooth extraction, pharyngomaxillary space abscess causes mild throat pain. Inspection reveals a bulge in the medial wall of the pharynx accompanied by swelling of the neck and at the jaw angle on the affected side. Other signs and symptoms include fever, dysphagia, trismus and, possibly, signs of respiratory distress or toxemia.

Sinusitis (acute)
Acute sinusitis may cause sore throat with purulent nasal discharge and postnasal drip, resulting in halitosis. Other effects include headache, malaise, cough, fever, and facial pain and swelling associated with nasal congestion.

Medical causes
(continued)

Laryngitis (acute)
+ Sore throat occurs with mild to severe hoarseness.

Mononucleosis (infectious)
+ Sore throat, cervical lymphadenopathy, and fluctuating temperature are classic findings.

Necrotizing ulcerative gingivitis (acute)
+ Sore throat and gums that ulcerate and bleed develop abruptly.

Peritonsillar abscess
+ Severe throat pain radiates to the ear.

Pharyngeal burns
+ Throat pain and dysphagia may result.

Pharyngitis
+ Bacterial form begins abruptly with a unilateral sore throat.
+ Fungal form causes a diffuse, burning sore throat.
+ Viral form causes a diffuse sore throat, malaise, fever, and mild erythema and edema of the posterior oropharyngeal wall.

Pharyngomaxillary space abscess
+ Mild throat pain develops along with a bulge in the medial wall of the pharynx and swelling of the neck on the affected side.

Sinusitis (acute)
+ Sore throat occurs with purulent nasal discharge and postnasal drip.

Medical causes
(continued)

Tongue cancer
+ Localized throat pain may occur around a white lesion or ulcer.

Tonsillar cancer
+ Throat pain that may radiate to the ear is the presenting symptom.

Tonsillitis
+ Throat pain may range from mild to severe.

Uvulitis
+ Throat pain or a sensation of something in the throat may occur.

Other causes
+ Endotracheal intubation
+ Local surgery, such as tonsillectomy and adenoidectomy

Special considerations
+ Provide analgesic sprays or lozenges to relieve throat pain.
+ Prepare the patient for throat culture, CBC, and a Monospot test.

Peds points
+ Pediatric causes of sore throat include acute epiglottiditis, herpangina, scarlet fever, acute follicular tonsillitis, and retropharyngeal abscess.

Teaching points
+ Importance of completing full course of antibiotic treatment
+ Ways to soothe the throat

Tongue cancer
With tongue cancer, the patient experiences localized throat pain that may occur around a raised white lesion or ulcer. The pain may radiate to the ear and be accompanied by dysphagia.

Tonsillar cancer
Sore throat is the presenting symptom in tonsillar cancer. Unfortunately, the cancer is usually quite advanced before the appearance of this symptom. The pain may radiate to the ear and is accompanied by a superficial ulcer on the tonsil or one that extends to the base of the tongue.

Tonsillitis
With *acute tonsillitis,* mild to severe sore throat is usually the first symptom. The pain may radiate to the ears and be accompanied by dysphagia and headache. Related findings include malaise, fever with chills, halitosis, myalgia, arthralgia, and tender cervical lymphadenopathy. Examination reveals edematous, reddened tonsils with a purulent exudate.

Chronic tonsillitis causes mild sore throat, malaise, and tender cervical lymph nodes. The tonsils appear smooth, pink and, possibly, enlarged, with a purulent debris in the crypts. Halitosis and a foul taste in the mouth are other common findings.

Unilateral or bilateral throat pain just above the hyoid bone occurs with *lingual tonsillitis.* The lingual tonsils appear red and swollen and are covered with exudate. Other findings include a muffled voice, dysphagia, and tender cervical lymphadenopathy on the affected side.

Uvulitis
Uvulitis is an inflammation that can cause throat pain or a sensation of something in the throat. The uvula is usually swollen and red but, in allergic uvulitis, it's pale.

OTHER CAUSES

Treatments
Endotracheal intubation and local surgery, such as tonsillectomy and adenoidectomy, commonly cause sore throat.

SPECIAL CONSIDERATIONS
Provide analgesic sprays or lozenges to relieve throat pain. Also, prepare the patient for throat culture, complete blood count, and a Monospot test.

PEDIATRIC POINTERS
Sore throat is a common complaint in children and may result from many of the same disorders that affect adults. Other pediatric causes of sore throat include acute epiglottiditis, herpangina, scarlet fever, acute follicular tonsillitis, and retropharyngeal abscess.

PATIENT COUNSELING
If the patient is taking antibiotics, stress the importance of completing the full course of treatment, even if symptoms improve after only a few days. Tell the patient that he's presumed noninfectious after 24 hours of antibiotic coverage. Suggest gargling with salt water to soothe the throat.

THYROID ENLARGEMENT

An enlarged thyroid can result from inflammation, physiologic changes, iodine deficiency, and thyroid tumors. Depending on the medical cause, hyperfunction or hypofunction may occur with resulting excess or deficiency, respectively, of the hormone thyroxine. If no infection is present, enlargement is usually slow and progressive. An enlarged thyroid that causes visible swelling in the front of the neck is called a *goiter*.

History

The patient's history commonly reveals the cause of thyroid enlargement. Important data includes a family history of thyroid disease, when the thyroid enlargement began, any previous irradiation of the thyroid or the neck, recent infections, and the use of thyroid replacement drugs.

Physical assessment

Begin the physical assessment by inspecting the patient's trachea for midline deviation. Although you can usually see the enlarged gland, you should always palpate it. (See *Palpating the thyroid gland,* page 650.)

During palpation, be sure to note the size, shape, and consistency of the gland, and the presence or absence of nodules. Using the bell of a stethoscope, listen over the lateral lobes for a bruit. The bruit is usually continuous.

Medical causes

Hypothyroidism

Besides an enlarged thyroid, signs and symptoms of hypothyroidism include weight gain despite anorexia; fatigue; cold intolerance; constipation; menorrhagia; slowed intellectual and motor activity; dry, pale, cool skin; dry, sparse hair; and thick, brittle nails. Eventually, the face assumes a dull expression with periorbital edema.

 CULTURAL CUE *Goiters are common in areas of the world that are deficient in iodine, such as Asia, Latin America, Africa, and parts of Europe.*

Thyroiditis

Autoimmune thyroiditis usually produces no symptoms other than thyroid enlargement. In subacute granulomatous thyroiditis, moderate thyroid enlargement may follow an upper respiratory infection or a sore throat. The thyroid may be painful and tender. Dysphagia may also occur.

Thyrotoxicosis

One of the classic features of thyrotoxicosis is an enlarged thyroid gland. Associated signs and symptoms include nervousness; heat intolerance; fatigue; weight loss despite increased appetite; diarrhea; sweating; palpitations; tremors; smooth, warm, flushed skin; fine, soft hair; exophthalmos; nausea and vomiting due to increased GI motility and peristalsis; and, in females, oligomenorrhea or amenorrhea.

Tumors

An enlarged thyroid may result from a malignant tumor or a nonmalignant tumor (such as an adenoma). A malignant tumor usually appears as a single nodule in the neck; a nonmalignant tumor may appear as multiple nodules in the neck. Associated signs and symptoms include hoarseness, loss of voice, and dysphagia.

Key facts about thyroid enlargement
+ Can result from inflammation, physiologic changes, iodine deficiency, and thyroid tumors

Key history points
+ Onset of enlargement
+ Use of thyroid replacement drugs

Critical assessment steps
+ Palpate the enlarged gland; note size, shape, and consistency of gland.
+ Using bell of stethoscope, listen over lobes for a bruit.

Medical causes
Hypothyroidism
+ Enlarged thyroid; weight gain, fatigue; cold intolerance; dry, pale, cool skin; dry, sparse hair; and thick, brittle nails result.

Thyroiditis
+ Autoimmune thyroiditis usually produces no symptoms other than thyroid enlargement.
+ In subacute granulomatous thyroiditis, thyroid enlargement may follow an upper respiratory infection or a sore throat.

Thyrotoxicosis
+ An enlarged thyroid gland is a classic feature.

Tumors
+ An enlarged thyroid may be accompanied by hoarseness, loss of voice, and dysphagia.

Palpating the thyroid gland

To palpate the thyroid gland, you'll need to stand behind the patient. Give the patient a cup of water, and have him extend his neck slightly. Place the fingers of both hands on the patient's neck, just below the cricoid cartilage and just lateral to the trachea. Tell the patient to take a sip of water and swallow. The thyroid gland should rise as he swallows. Use your fingers to palpate laterally and downward to feel the whole thyroid gland. Palpate over the midline to feel the isthmus of the thyroid.

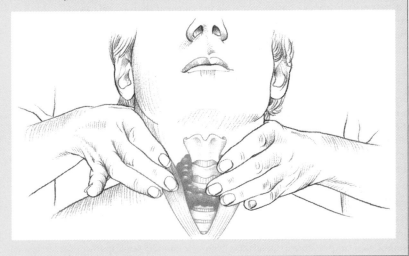

Other causes
+ Goitrogens in various drugs and foods

Special considerations
+ Prepare the patient for diagnostic tests and surgery or radiation therapy, if necessary.
+ Specific interventions depend on whether the patient is hypothyroid, has thyroiditis, or is recovering from a thyroidectomy.

OTHER CAUSES

Goitrogens

Goitrogens are drugs and substances in foods that decrease thyroxine production. Drugs include lithium, sulfonamides, phenylbutazone, and para-aminosalicylic acid. Foods containing goitrogens include peanuts, cabbage, soybeans, strawberries, spinach, rutabagas, and radishes.

SPECIAL CONSIDERATIONS

Prepare the patient with an enlarged thyroid for tests, such as needle aspiration, ultrasound, and radioactive thyroid scanning. Also prepare him for surgery or radiation therapy, if necessary.

The hypothyroid patient will need a warm room and moisturizing lotion for his skin. A gentle laxative and stool softener may help with constipation. Provide a high-bulk, low-calorie diet, and encourage activity to promote weight loss. Warn the patient to report any infection immediately; if he develops a fever, monitor his temperature until it's stable. After thyroid replacement begins, watch for signs and symptoms of hyperthyroidism, such as restlessness, sweating, and excessive weight loss. Avoid administering a sedative, if possible, or reduce the dosage because hypothyroidism delays metabolism of many drugs.

For patients with thyroiditis, give an antibiotic and watch for elevations in temperature, which may indicate developing resistance to the antibiotic. Examine the patient's neck for unusual swelling or redness. Provide a liquid diet if the patient has difficulty swallowing. Check for signs of hyperthyroidism, such as nervousness, tremor, and weakness, which are common with subacute thyroiditis. The patient with severe hyperthyroidism (thyroid storm) will need close monitoring of temperature, volume status, heart rate, and blood pressure.

After thyroidectomy, check vital signs every 15 to 30 minutes until the patient's condition stabilizes. Be alert for signs of tetany secondary to parathyroid injury during surgery. Monitor postoperative serum calcium levels, and keep 10% calcium gluconate available for I.V. use as needed. Evaluate dressings frequently for excessive bleeding, and watch for signs of airway obstruction, such as difficulty in talking, increased swallowing, or stridor. Keep tracheotomy equipment handy.

PEDIATRIC POINTERS

Congenital goiter, a syndrome of infantile myxedema or cretinism, is characterized by mental retardation, growth failure, and other signs and symptoms of hypothyroidism. Early treatment can prevent mental retardation. Genetic counseling is important because subsequent children are at risk.

PATIENT COUNSELING

Instruct the patient to watch for signs and symptoms of hypothyroidism, such as lethargy, restlessness, dry skin, and sensitivity to cold. If the patient has Graves' disease, proptosis may cause his eyes to become dry, so advise him to use artificial tears frequently. If the hyperthyroid patient is receiving therapy with radioactive iodine, tell him not to expectorate or cough freely after treatment because his saliva is radioactive for 24 hours. If the patient has a goiter, support him as he expresses his feelings related to his appearance.

After thyroidectomy or radioactive destruction of the thyroid gland, explain to the patient that lifelong thyroid hormone replacement therapy is necessary. Tell him to watch for signs of overdose, such as nervousness and palpitations.

TINNITUS

Tinnitus literally means ringing in the ears; although many other abnormal sounds fall under this term. For example, tinnitus may be described as the sound of escaping air, running water, or the inside of a seashell or as a sizzling, buzzing, or humming noise. Occasionally, it's described as a roaring or musical sound. This common symptom may be unilateral or bilateral and constant or intermittent. Although the brain may adjust to or suppress constant tinnitus, tinnitus may be so disturbing that some patients contemplate suicide as their only source of relief.

Tinnitus can be classified in several ways. *Subjective tinnitus* is heard only by the patient; *objective tinnitus* is also heard by the observer who places a stethoscope near the patient's affected ear. *Tinnitus aurium* refers to noise that the patient hears in his ears; *tinnitus cerebri,* to noise that he hears in his head.

Tinnitus is usually associated with neural injury within the auditory pathway, resulting in altered, spontaneous firing of sensory auditory neurons. Commonly resulting from an ear disorder, tinnitus may also stem from a cardiovascular or systemic disorder or from the effects of drugs. Nonpathologic causes of tinnitus include acute anxiety and presbycusis.

HISTORY

Ask the patient to describe the sound he hears, including its onset, pattern, pitch, location, and intensity. Ask whether the sound is accompanied by other symptoms,

Critical assessment steps

+ Inspect the ears and examine the tympanic membrane.
+ Perform Weber's and Rinne tests.
+ Auscultate for bruits in the neck.

Medical causes

Acoustic neuroma
+ Unilateral tinnitus precedes unilateral sensorineural hearing loss and vertigo.

Anemia
+ Mild tinnitus may occur.

Atherosclerosis of the carotid artery
+ Constant tinnitus can be stopped by applying pressure over the carotid artery.

Cervical spondylosis
+ Osteophytic growths may compress the vertebral arteries, resulting in tinnitus.

Ear canal obstruction
+ Tinnitus may occur with conductive hearing loss, itching, blockage, and a feeling of fullness or pain in the ear.

Eustachian tube patency
+ Tinnitus, audible breath sounds, loud and distorted voice sounds, and a sense of fullness in the ear can occur.

Hypertension
+ Bilateral, high-pitched tinnitus may occur.

Intracranial arteriovenous malformation
+ A large malformation may cause tinnitus accompanied by a bruit over the mastoid process.

such as vertigo, headache, or hearing loss. Next, take a health history, including a complete drug history.

PHYSICAL ASSESSMENT

Using an otoscope, inspect the patient's ears and examine the tympanic membrane. To check for hearing loss, perform Weber's and Rinne tuning fork tests. Also, auscultate for bruits in the neck. Then compress the jugular or carotid artery to see if this affects the tinnitus. Finally, examine the nasopharynx for masses that might cause eustachian tube dysfunction and tinnitus.

MEDICAL CAUSES

Acoustic neuroma
Acoustic neuroma, a tumor of the eighth cranial nerve, causes unilateral tinnitus that precedes early symptoms of unilateral sensorineural hearing loss and vertigo. Facial paralysis, headache, nausea, vomiting, and papilledema may also occur.

Anemia
Severe anemia may produce mild, reversible tinnitus. Other common effects include pallor, weakness, fatigue, exertional dyspnea, tachycardia, bounding pulse, atrial gallop, and a systolic bruit over the carotid arteries.

Atherosclerosis of the carotid artery
With atherosclerosis of the carotid artery, the patient has constant tinnitus that can be stopped by applying pressure over the carotid artery. Auscultation over the upper part of the neck, on the auricle, or near the ear on the affected side may detect a bruit. Palpation may reveal a weak carotid pulse.

Cervical spondylosis
With cervical spondylosis, a degenerative disorder, osteophytic growths may compress the vertebral arteries, resulting in tinnitus. Typically, a stiff neck and pain aggravated by activity accompany tinnitus. Other features include brief vertigo, nystagmus, hearing loss, paresthesia, weakness, and pain that radiates down the arms.

Ear canal obstruction
When cerumen or a foreign body blocks the ear canal, tinnitus may occur with conductive hearing loss, itching, blockage, and a feeling of fullness or pain in the ear.

Eustachian tube patency
Normally, the eustachian tube remains closed, except during swallowing. However, persistent patency of this tube can cause tinnitus, audible breath sounds, loud and distorted voice sounds, and a sense of fullness in the ear. Examination with a pneumatic otoscope reveals movement of the tympanic membrane with respirations. At times, breath sounds can be heard with a stethoscope placed over the auricle.

Hypertension
Bilateral, high-pitched tinnitus may occur with severe hypertension. Diastolic blood pressure exceeding 120 mm Hg may also cause severe, throbbing headache; restlessness; nausea; vomiting; blurred vision; seizures; and decreased level of consciousness.

Intracranial arteriovenous malformation
A large intracranial arteriovenous malformation may cause pulsating tinnitus accompanied by a bruit over the mastoid process. Other manifestations include severe headache, seizures, and progressive neurologic deficits.

Labyrinthitis (suppurative)

With suppurative labyrinthitis, tinnitus may accompany sudden, severe attacks of vertigo, unilateral or bilateral sensorineural hearing loss, nystagmus, dizziness, nausea, and vomiting.

Ménière's disease

Ménière's disease, a labyrinthine disease, is characterized by attacks of tinnitus, vertigo, a feeling of fullness or blockage in the ear, and fluctuating sensorineural hearing loss. These attacks last from 10 minutes to several hours; they occur over a few days or weeks and are followed by a remission. Severe nausea, vomiting, diaphoresis, and nystagmus may also occur during attacks.

Ossicle dislocation

Acoustic trauma, such as a slap on the ear, may dislocate the ossicle, resulting in tinnitus and sensorineural hearing loss. Bleeding from the middle ear may also occur.

Otitis externa (acute)

Although not a major complaint with otitis externa, tinnitus may result if debris in the external ear canal impinges on the tympanic membrane. More typical findings include pruritus, foul-smelling purulent discharge, and severe ear pain that's aggravated by manipulation of the tragus or auricle, teeth clenching, mouth opening, and chewing. The external ear canal typically appears red and edematous and may be occluded by debris, causing partial hearing loss.

Otitis media

Otitis media may cause tinnitus and conductive hearing loss. However, its more typical features include ear pain, a red and bulging tympanic membrane, high fever, chills, and dizziness.

Otosclerosis

With otosclerosis, the patient may describe ringing, roaring, or whistling tinnitus or a combination of these sounds. He may also report progressive hearing loss, which may lead to bilateral deafness, and vertigo.

Presbycusis

Presbycusis, an otologic effect of aging, produces tinnitus and a progressive, symmetrical, bilateral sensorineural hearing loss, usually of high-frequency tones.

Tympanic membrane perforation

With tympanic membrane perforation, tinnitus and hearing loss go hand-in-hand. Tinnitus is usually the chief complaint in a small perforation; hearing loss, in a larger perforation. These symptoms typically develop suddenly and may be accompanied by pain, vertigo, and a feeling of fullness in the ear.

OTHER CAUSES

Drugs and alcohol

An overdose of salicylates commonly causes reversible tinnitus. Quinine, alcohol, and indomethacin may also cause reversible tinnitus. Common drugs that may cause irreversible tinnitus include the aminoglycoside antibiotics (especially kanamycin, streptomycin, and gentamicin) and vancomycin.

Medical causes
(continued)

Labyrinthitis (suppurative)
✦ Tinnitus may accompany sudden, severe attacks of vertigo, unilateral or bilateral sensorineural hearing loss, nystagmus, dizziness, nausea, and vomiting.

Ménière's disease
✦ Attacks of tinnitus, vertigo, a feeling of fullness or blockage in the ear, and fluctuating sensorineural hearing loss may last from 10 minutes to several hours.

Ossicle dislocation
✦ Tinnitus and sensorineural hearing loss result.

Otitis externa (acute)
✦ Tinnitus may result if debris in the external ear canal impinges on the tympanic membrane.

Otitis media
✦ Tinnitus and conductive hearing loss may occur.

Otosclerosis
✦ Patient may describe ringing, roaring, or whistling tinnitus or a combination of these sounds.

Presbycusis
✦ Tinnitus and a progressive, symmetrical, bilateral sensorineural hearing loss occur.

Tympanic membrane perforation
✦ Tinnitus is usually the chief complaint in a small perforation; hearing loss, in a larger perforation.

Other causes

+ Alcohol
+ Aminoglycoside antibiotics, indomethacin, quinine, or vancomycin
+ Noise
+ Overdose of salicylates

Special considerations

+ Educate the patient about strategies for adapting to the tinnitus.
+ A hearing aid may be used to amplify environmental sounds, thereby obscuring tinnitus.

Peds points

+ Maternal use of ototoxic drugs during the third trimester of pregnancy can cause labyrinthine damage in the fetus, resulting in tinnitus.

Teaching points

+ Avoidance of excessive noise, ototoxic agents, and factors that may cause cochlear damage

Key facts about tracheal deviation

+ Signals an underlying condition that can compromise pulmonary function and possibly cause respiratory distress
+ Occurs with disorders that produce mediastinal shift due to asymmetrical thoracic volume or pressure

In an emergency

+ Be alert for signs and symptoms of respiratory distress.
+ If possible, place the patient in semi-Fowler's position to aid respiratory excursion and improve oxygenation.

Noise

Chronic exposure to noise, especially high-pitched sounds, can damage the ear's hair cells, causing tinnitus and a bilateral hearing loss. These symptoms may be temporary or permanent.

SPECIAL CONSIDERATIONS

Tinnitus is typically difficult to treat successfully. After ruling out any reversible causes, it's important to educate the patient about strategies for adapting to the tinnitus, including biofeedback and masking devices.

In addition, a hearing aid may be prescribed to amplify environmental sounds, thereby obscuring tinnitus. For some patients, a device that combines features of a masker and a hearing aid may be used to block out tinnitus.

PEDIATRIC POINTERS

A pregnant woman's use of ototoxic drugs during the third trimester of pregnancy can cause labyrinthine damage in the fetus, resulting in tinnitus. Many of the disorders described above can also cause tinnitus in children.

PATIENT COUNSELING

Advise the patient to avoid further exposure to excessive noise, ototoxic agents, and other factors that may cause cochlear damage. Inform him that even people with normal hearing may experience intermittent periods of mild, high-pitched tinnitus that can last for several minutes.

TRACHEAL DEVIATION

Normally, the trachea is located at the midline of the neck — except at the bifurcation, where it shifts slightly toward the right. Visible deviation from its normal position signals an underlying condition that can compromise pulmonary function and possibly cause respiratory distress. A hallmark of life-threatening tension pneumothorax, tracheal deviation occurs with disorders that produce mediastinal shift due to asymmetrical thoracic volume or pressure. A nonlesion pneumothorax can produce tracheal deviation to the ipsilateral side. (See *Detecting slight tracheal deviation.*)

 EMERGENCY ACTIONS Be alert for signs and symptoms of respiratory distress (tachypnea, dyspnea, decreased or absent breath sounds, stridor, nasal flaring, accessory muscle use, asymmetrical chest expansion, restlessness, and anxiety). If possible, place the patient in semi-Fowler's position to aid respiratory excursion and improve oxygenation. Give supplemental oxygen, and intubate the patient if necessary. Insert an I.V. line for fluid and drug administration. In addition, palpate for subcutaneous crepitation in the neck and chest, a sign of tension pneumothorax. Chest tube insertion may be necessary to release trapped air or fluid and to restore normal intrapleural and intrathoracic pressure gradients.

HISTORY

If the patient doesn't display signs of distress, ask about a history of pulmonary or cardiac disorders, surgery, trauma, or infection. If he smokes, determine how much. Ask about associated signs and symptoms, especially breathing difficulty, pain, and cough.

ASSESSMENT TIP

Detecting slight tracheal deviation

Although gross tracheal deviation is visible, detection of slight deviation requires palpation and perhaps even an X-ray. Try palpation first.

    With the tip of your index finger, locate the patient's trachea by palpating between the sternocleidomastoid muscles. Then compare the trachea's position to an imaginary line drawn vertically through the suprasternal notch. Any deviation from midline is usually considered abnormal.

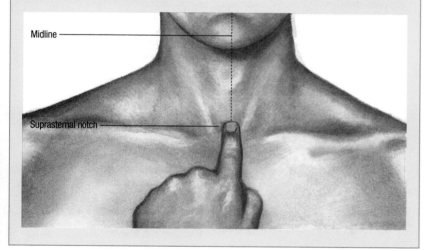

Midline

Suprasternal notch

PHYSICAL ASSESSMENT

Take the patient's vital signs and observe for respiratory distress. If the patient's condition allows, perform a complete cardiopulmonary assessment.

MEDICAL CAUSES

Atelectasis

Extensive lung collapse can produce tracheal deviation toward the affected side. Respiratory findings of atelectasis include dyspnea, tachypnea, pleuritic chest pain, dry cough, dullness on percussion, decreased vocal fremitus and breath sounds, inspiratory lag, and substernal or intercostal retraction.

Hiatal hernia

With hiatal hernia, intrusion of abdominal viscera into the pleural space causes tracheal deviation toward the unaffected side. The degree of attendant respiratory distress depends on the extent of herniation. Other effects include pyrosis, regurgitation or vomiting, and chest or abdominal pain.

Kyphoscoliosis

Kyphoscoliosis can cause rib cage distortion and mediastinal shift, producing tracheal deviation toward the compressed lung. Respiratory effects include dry cough, dyspnea, asymmetrical chest expansion and, possibly, asymmetrical breath sounds. Backache and fatigue are also common.

In an emergency
(continued)
+ Give supplemental oxygen, and intubate the patient if necessary.
+ Insert an I.V. line for fluid and drug administration.
+ Palpate for subcutaneous crepitation in the neck and chest, a sign of tension pneumothorax.
+ Chest tube insertion may be necessary.

Key history points
+ History of pulmonary or cardiac disorders, surgery, trauma, or infection
+ Smoking habits
+ Associated signs and symptoms, such as breathing difficulty, pain, and cough

Critical assessment steps
+ Observe for respiratory distress.
+ Perform a complete cardiopulmonary assessment.

Medical causes
Atelectasis
+ Extensive lung collapse can produce tracheal deviation toward the affected side.

Hiatal hernia
+ Intrusion of abdominal viscera into the pleural space causes tracheal deviation toward the unaffected side.

Kyphoscoliosis
+ Rib cage distortion and mediastinal shift produces tracheal deviation toward the compressed lung.

Tension pneumothorax

In tension pneumothorax, a life-threatening condition, a lacerated lung or hole in the chest wall causes air to enter the pleural space, thus creating positive pleural pressure. When air is unable to leave, each inspiration traps air in the pleural space. This causes collapse of the ipsilateral lung and marked impairment of venous return, which can severely compromise cardiac output and may cause a mediastinal shift. As the mediastinum shifts toward the unaffected lung, ventilation is further impaired. On expiration, the vena cava is distorted, decreasing venous return. As a result, cardiac output and blood pressure are reduced.

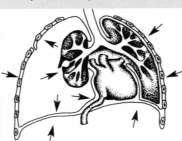

CAUSES
Tension pneumothorax may be caused by:
+ penetrating chest wound treated with an air-tight dressing
+ fractured ribs
+ mechanical ventilation

+ high-level positive end-expiratory pressure that causes alveolar blebs to rupture
+ chest tube occlusion or malfunction.

DIAGNOSIS
These test results help diagnosis tension pneumothorax:
+ Chest X-rays confirm the diagnosis by revealing air in the pleural space and, possibly, a mediastinal shift.
+ Arterial blood gas analysis may reveal hypoxemia, possibly with respiratory acidosis and hypercapnia. Partial pressure of arterial oxygen levels may decrease.

MEDICAL INTERVENTION
Correction of tension pneumothorax typically involves:
+ immediate treatment with large-bore needle insertion into the pleural space through the second intercostal space to reexpand the lung
+ insertion of a thoracostomy tube to promote lung reexpansion
+ analgesics to promote comfort and encourage deep breathing and coughing
+ monitoring of blood pressure and pulse for early detection of physiologic compromise
+ monitoring of respiratory rate and breath sounds to detect early signs of respiratory compromise
+ oxygen administration to enhance oxygenation and improve hypoxia.

Medical causes
(continued)

Mediastinal tumor
+ If large, a mediastinal tumor can press against the trachea and nearby structures, causing tracheal deviation and dysphagia.

Pleural effusion
+ If the effusion is large, the mediastinum can shift to the contralateral side, producing tracheal deviation.

Mediastinal tumor
Although it may produce no symptoms in its early stages, a mediastinal tumor, when large, can press against the trachea and nearby structures, causing tracheal deviation and dysphagia. Other late findings include stridor, dyspnea, brassy cough, hoarseness, and stertorous respirations with suprasternal retraction. The patient may experience shoulder, arm, or chest pain as well as edema of the neck, face, or arm. His neck and chest wall veins may be dilated.

Pleural effusion
A large pleural effusion can shift the mediastinum to the contralateral side, producing tracheal deviation. Related effects include dry cough, dyspnea, pleuritic pain, pleural friction rub, tachypnea, decreased chest motion, decreased or absent breath sounds, egophony, flatness on percussion, decreased tactile fremitus, fever, and weight loss.

Pulmonary fibrosis

Asymmetrical pulmonary fibrosis can cause tracheal deviation as the mediastinum shifts toward the affected side. Associated findings reflect the underlying condition and pattern of fibrosis. Dyspnea, cough, clubbing, malaise, and fever commonly occur.

Pulmonary tuberculosis

With a large cavitation, tracheal deviation toward the affected side accompanies asymmetrical chest excursion, dullness on percussion, increased tactile fremitus, amphoric breath sounds, and inspiratory crackles. Insidious early effects include fatigue, anorexia, weight loss, fever, chills, and night sweats. Productive cough, hemoptysis, pleuritic chest pain, and dyspnea develop as tuberculosis progresses.

Tension pneumothorax

Tension pneumothorax, an acute, life-threatening condition, produces tracheal deviation toward the unaffected side. It's marked by a sudden onset of respiratory distress accompanied by sharp chest pain, dry cough, severe dyspnea, tachycardia, wheezing, cyanosis, accessory muscle use, nasal flaring, air hunger, and asymmetrical chest movement. Restless and anxious, the patient may also develop subcutaneous crepitation in the neck and upper chest, decreased vocal fremitus, decreased or absent breath sounds on the affected side, jugular vein distention, and hypotension. (See *Associated disorder: Tension pneumothorax.*)

Thoracic aortic aneurysm

A thoracic aortic aneurysm usually causes the trachea to deviate to the right. Highly variable associated findings may include stridor, dyspnea, wheezing, brassy cough, hoarseness, and dysphagia. Edema of the face, neck, or arm may occur with distended chest wall and neck veins. The patient may also experience substernal, neck, shoulder, or lower back pain, possibly with paresthesia or neuralgia.

SPECIAL CONSIDERATIONS

Because tracheal deviation usually signals a severe underlying disorder that can cause respiratory distress at any time, monitor the patient's respiratory and cardiac status constantly, and make sure that emergency equipment is readily available. Prepare the patient for diagnostic tests, such as chest X-rays, bronchoscopy, an electrocardiogram, and arterial blood gas analysis.

PEDIATRIC POINTERS

Keep in mind that respiratory distress typically develops more rapidly in children than in adults.

GERIATRIC POINTERS

In elderly patients, tracheal deviation to the right commonly stems from an elongated, atherosclerotic aortic arch, but this deviation isn't considered abnormal.

PATIENT COUNSELING

Teach the patient to perform coughing and deep-breathing exercises properly. Discuss signs and symptoms of respiratory difficulty to report, such as shortness of breath and increased respiratory rate. Provide reassurance and emotional support because the patient may be frightened by his limited breathing capacity.

Medical causes
(continued)

Pulmonary fibrosis
+ Tracheal deviation occurs as the mediastinum shifts toward the affected side.

Pulmonary tuberculosis
+ Tracheal deviation toward the affected side accompanies asymmetrical chest excursion, amphoric breath sounds, and inspiratory crackles.

Tension pneumothorax
+ Tracheal deviation is toward the unaffected side.

Thoracic aortic aneurysm
+ The trachea usually deviates to the right.

Special considerations
+ Monitor respiratory and cardiac status constantly.
+ Make sure that emergency equipment is readily available.

Peds points
+ Respiratory distress typically develops more rapidly in children than in adults.

Geri points
+ Tracheal deviation to the right commonly stems from an elongated, atherosclerotic aortic arch, but this deviation isn't considered abnormal.

Teaching points
+ How to perform coughing and deep-breathing exercises
+ Signs and symptoms of respiratory difficulty to report

Key facts about tremors

+ Refer to rhythmic oscillations that result from alternating contraction of opposing muscle groups
+ Characterized by their location, amplitude, and frequency
+ Classified as resting, intention, or postural

Key history points

+ Onset, duration, and progression of tremor
+ Aggravating or alleviating factors
+ Other symptoms, such as behavioral changes or memory loss
+ History of neurologic, endocrine, or metabolic disorders
+ Drug and alcohol history

Critical assessment steps

+ Assess overall appearance and demeanor, noting mental status.
+ Test ROM and strength in all major muscle groups while observing for chorea, athetosis, dystonia, and other involuntary movements.
+ Check DTRs and, if possible, observe the patient's gait.

Medical causes

Alcohol withdrawal syndrome

+ Resting and intention tremors may appear as soon as 7 hours after the last drink and progressively worsen.

Alkalosis

+ A severe intention tremor may occur along with twitching, carpopedal spasms, agitation, diaphoresis, and hyperventilation.

TREMORS

The most common type of involuntary muscle movement, tremors are regular rhythmic oscillations that result from alternating contraction of opposing muscle groups. They're typical signs of extrapyramidal or cerebellar disorders and can also result from certain drugs.

Tremors can be characterized by their location, amplitude, and frequency. They're classified as resting, intention, or postural. *Resting tremors* occur when an extremity is at rest and subside with movement. They include the classic pill-rolling tremor of Parkinson's disease. Conversely, *intention tremors* occur only with movement and subside with rest. *Postural (or action) tremors* appear when an extremity or the trunk is actively held in a particular posture or position. A common type of postural tremor is called an essential tremor.

Stress or emotional upset tends to aggravate a tremor. Alcohol commonly diminishes postural tremors.

HISTORY

Begin the patient history by asking the patient about the tremor's onset. Was onset sudden or gradual? Also, ask about the tremor's duration, progression, and any aggravating or alleviating factors. Does the tremor interfere with the patient's normal activities? Does he have other symptoms? Has he noticed any behavioral changes or memory loss? (The patient's family or friends may provide more accurate information on this.)

Explore the patient's personal and family medical history for a neurologic (especially seizures), endocrine, or metabolic disorder. Obtain a complete drug history, noting especially the use of phenothiazines. Also, ask about alcohol use.

PHYSICAL ASSESSMENT

Assess the patient's overall appearance and demeanor, noting mental status. Test range of motion and strength in all major muscle groups while observing for chorea, athetosis, dystonia, and other involuntary movements. Check deep tendon reflexes and, if possible, observe the patient's gait.

MEDICAL CAUSES

Alcohol withdrawal syndrome

Acute alcohol withdrawal after long-term dependence may first be manifested by resting and intention tremors that appear as soon as 7 hours after the last drink and progressively worsen. Other early signs and symptoms include diaphoresis, tachycardia, elevated blood pressure, anxiety, restlessness, irritability, insomnia, headache, nausea, and vomiting. Severe withdrawal may produce profound tremors, agitation, confusion, hallucinations and, possibly, seizures.

Alkalosis

Severe alkalosis may produce a severe intention tremor along with twitching, carpopedal spasms, agitation, diaphoresis, and hyperventilation. The patient may complain of dizziness, tinnitus, palpitations, and peripheral and circumoral paresthesia.

Cerebellar tumor

An intention tremor is a cardinal sign of a cerebellar tumor; related findings may include ataxia, nystagmus, incoordination, muscle weakness and atrophy, and hypoactive or absent deep tendon reflexes.

Graves' disease

Fine tremors of the hand, nervousness, weight loss, fatigue, palpitations, dyspnea, and increased heat intolerance are some of the typical signs of Graves' disease. It's also characterized by an enlarged thyroid gland (goiter) and exophthalmos.

Hypercapnia

Hypercapnia (elevated partial pressure of carbon dioxide) may result in a rapid, fine intention tremor. Other common findings include headache, fatigue, blurred vision, weakness, lethargy, and decreased level of consciousness (LOC).

Hypoglycemia

Acute hypoglycemia may produce a rapid, fine intention tremor accompanied by confusion, weakness, tachycardia, diaphoresis, and cold, clammy skin. Early patient complaints typically include mild generalized headache, profound hunger, nervousness, and blurred or double vision. The tremor may disappear as hypoglycemia worsens and hypotonia and decreased LOC become evident.

Kwashiorkor

Coarse intention and resting tremors may occur in the advanced stages of kwashiorkor. Examination reveals myoclonus, rigidity of all extremities, hyperreflexia, hepatomegaly, and pitting edema in the hands, feet, and sacral area. Other signs include a flat affect, pronounced hair loss, and dry, peeling skin.

Multiple sclerosis

An intention tremor that waxes and wanes may be an early sign of multiple sclerosis. Commonly, visual and sensory impairments are the earliest findings. Associated effects vary greatly and may include nystagmus, muscle weakness, paralysis, spasticity, hyperreflexia, ataxic gait, dysphagia, and dysarthria. Constipation, urinary frequency and urgency, incontinence, impotence, and emotional lability may also occur.

Parkinson's disease

Tremors, a classic early sign of Parkinson's disease, usually begin in the fingers and may eventually affect the foot, eyelids, jaw, lips, and tongue. The slow, regular, rhythmic resting tremor takes the form of flexion-extension or abduction-adduction of the fingers or hand, or pronation-supination of the hand. Flexion-extension of the fingers combined with abduction-adduction of the thumb yields the characteristic pill-rolling tremor.

Leg involvement produces flexion-extension foot movement. Lightly closing the eyelids causes them to flutter. The jaw may move up and down, and the lips may purse. The tongue, when protruded, may move in and out of the mouth in tempo with tremors elsewhere in the body. The rate of the tremor holds constant over time, but its amplitude varies.

Other characteristic findings include cogwheel or lead-pipe rigidity, bradykinesia, propulsive gait with forward-leaning posture, monotone voice, masklike facies, drooling, dysphagia, dysarthria, and occasionally oculogyric crisis (eyes fix upward, with involuntary tonic movements) or blepharospasm (eyelids close completely).

Porphyria

Involvement of the basal ganglia in porphyria can produce a resting tremor with rigidity, accompanied by chorea and athetosis. As the disease progresses, generalized seizures may appear along with aphasia and hemiplegia.

Medical causes
(continued)

Cerebellar tumor
- An intention tremor is a cardinal sign.

Graves' disease
- Fine hand tremors, weight loss, fatigue, and an enlarged thyroid gland characterize Graves' disease.

Hypercapnia
- A rapid, fine intention tremor may occur.

Hypoglycemia
- A rapid, fine intention tremor is accompanied by confusion, weakness, tachycardia, diaphoresis, and cold, clammy skin; the tremor may disappear as hypoglycemia worsens.

Kwashiorkor
- Coarse intention and resting tremors may occur in the advanced stages.

Multiple sclerosis
- An intention tremor that waxes and wanes may be an early sign.

Parkinson's disease
- Tremors usually begin in the fingers and may eventually affect the foot, eyelids, jaw, lips, and tongue.

Porphyria
- Involvement of the basal ganglia can produce a resting tremor with rigidity, accompanied by chorea and athetosis.

Medical causes
(continued)

Thalamic syndrome

✦ Contralateral ataxic tremors and other abnormal movements occur along with Weber's syndrome, paralysis of vertical gaze, and stupor or coma.

Thyrotoxicosis

✦ A rapid, fine intention tremor of the hands and tongue occurs along with clonus, hyperreflexia, and Babinski's reflex.

Wernicke's disease

✦ An intention tremor is an early sign.

West Nile encephalitis

✦ Severe infections are marked by headache, high fever, neck stiffness, stupor, disorientation, coma, tremors, occasional seizures, and paralysis.

Other causes

✦ Amphetamines, lithium toxicity, metoclopramide, metyrosine, phenothiazines and other antipsychotics, phenytoin, and sympathomimetics
✦ Manganese toxicity
✦ Mercury poisoning

Special considerations

✦ Assist the patient with activities as necessary.
✦ Take precautions against possible injury during activities.

Peds points

✦ Pediatric-specific causes of pathologic tremors include cerebral palsy, fetal alcohol syndrome, and maternal drug addiction.

Thalamic syndrome

Central midbrain syndromes are heralded by contralateral ataxic tremors and other abnormal movements, along with Weber's syndrome (oculomotor palsy with contralateral hemiplegia), paralysis of vertical gaze, and stupor or coma.

Anteromedial-inferior thalamic syndrome produces varying combinations of tremor, deep sensory loss, and hemiataxia. However, the main effect of this syndrome may be an extrapyramidal dysfunction, such as hemiballismus or hemichoreoathetosis.

Thyrotoxicosis

Neuromuscular effects of thyrotoxicosis include a rapid, fine intention tremor of the hands and tongue, along with clonus, hyperreflexia, and Babinski's reflex. Other common signs and symptoms include tachycardia, cardiac arrhythmias, palpitations, anxiety, dyspnea, diaphoresis, heat intolerance, weight loss despite increased appetite, diarrhea, an enlarged thyroid and, possibly, exophthalmos.

Wernicke's disease

An intention tremor is an early sign of Wernicke's disease. Other features of Wernicke's disease include ocular abnormalities (such as gaze paralysis and nystagmus), ataxia, apathy, and confusion. Orthostatic hypotension and tachycardia may also develop.

West Nile encephalitis

In West Nile encephalitis, mild infections are common and include fever, headache, and body aches, commonly accompanied by rash and swollen lymph glands. More severe infections are marked by headache, high fever, neck stiffness, stupor, disorientation, coma, tremors, occasional seizures, paralysis and, rarely, death.

OTHER CAUSES

Drugs

Phenothiazines (particularly piperazine derivatives such as fluphenazine) and other antipsychotics may cause resting and pill-rolling tremors. Infrequently, metoclopramide and metyrosine also cause these tremors. Lithium toxicity, sympathomimetics (such as terbutaline and pseudoephedrine), amphetamines, and phenytoin can all cause tremors that disappear with dose reduction.

Manganese toxicity

Early signs of manganese poisoning include resting tremor, chorea, propulsive gait, cogwheel rigidity, personality changes, amnesia, and masklike facies.

Mercury poisoning

Mercury is a chronic form of poisoning that's characterized by irritability, copious amounts of saliva, loose teeth, gum disease, slurred speech and tremors.

SPECIAL CONSIDERATIONS

Severe intention tremors may interfere with the patient's ability to perform activities of daily living. Assist the patient with these activities as necessary, and take precautions against possible injury during such activities as walking or eating.

PEDIATRIC POINTERS

A normal neonate may display coarse tremors with stiffening — an exaggerated hypocalcemic startle reflex — in response to noises and chills. Pediatric-specific causes of pathologic tremors include cerebral palsy, fetal alcohol syndrome, and maternal drug addiction.

PATIENT COUNSELING

Encourage the patient to express his feelings about changes in his body image to reduce anxiety and depression. Because reinforcing independence may help maintain self-esteem, encourage the patient to do as much of his own personal care as possible. Provide assistive devices, if necessary, to help with activities of daily living.

TUNNEL VISION

Resulting from severe constriction of the visual field that leaves only a small central area of sight, tunnel vision (also known as *gun barrel vision* or *tubular vision*) is typically described as the sensation of looking through a tunnel or gun barrel. It may be unilateral or bilateral and usually develops gradually. (See *Comparing tunnel vision with normal vision,* page 662.) This abnormality results from chronic open-angle glaucoma and advanced retinal degeneration. Tunnel vision also can result from laser photocoagulation therapy, which aims to correct retinal detachment. Also a common complaint of malingerers, tunnel vision can be verified or discounted by visual field examination performed by an ophthalmologist.

HISTORY

Ask the patient when he first noticed a loss of peripheral vision, and have him describe the progression of vision loss. Ask him to describe in detail exactly what and how far he can see peripherally. Explore the patient's personal and family history for ocular problems, especially progressive blindness that began at an early age.

PHYSICAL ASSESSMENT

To rule out malingering, observe the patient as he walks. A patient with severely limited peripheral vision typically bumps into objects (and may even have bruises), whereas the malingerer manages to avoid them.

If your assessment findings suggest tunnel vision, refer the patient to an ophthalmologist for further evaluation.

MEDICAL CAUSES

Chronic open-angle glaucoma

With chronic open-angle glaucoma, bilateral tunnel vision occurs late and slowly progresses to complete blindness. Other late findings include mild eye pain, halo vision, and reduced visual acuity (especially at night) that isn't correctable with glasses.

Retinal pigmentary degeneration

This group of hereditary disorders, such as retinitis pigmentosa, produces an annular scotoma that progresses concentrically, causing tunnel vision and eventually resulting in complete blindness, usually by age 50. Impaired night vision, the earliest symptom, typically appears during the first or second decade of life. An ophthalmoscopic examination may reveal narrowed retinal blood vessels and a pale optic disk.

SPECIAL CONSIDERATIONS

To protect the patient from injury, be sure to remove all potentially dangerous objects and orient him to his surroundings. Because visual impairment is frightening, reassure the patient and clearly explain diagnostic procedures, such as tonometry, perimeter examination, and visual field testing.

Teaching points
+ Reinforcement of independence
+ Use of assistive devices as needed

Key facts about tunnel vision
+ Also known as *gun barrel vision* or *tubular vision*
+ Results from severe constriction of the visual field
+ Leaves only a small central area of sight

Key history points
+ Onset and description of loss of peripheral vision
+ Personal and family history of ocular problems.

Critical assessment steps
+ If your assessment findings suggest tunnel vision, refer the patient to an ophthalmologist for further evaluation.

Medical causes

Chronic open-angle glaucoma
+ Bilateral tunnel vision occurs late and slowly progresses to complete blindness.

Retinal pigmentary degeneration
+ An annular scotoma progresses concentrically, causing tunnel vision and eventually resulting in complete blindness, usually by age 50.
+ Impaired night vision, the earliest symptom, typically appears during the first or second decade of life.

Special considerations

✦ Remove all potentially dangerous objects and orient the patient to his surroundings.
✦ Clearly explain diagnostic procedures.

Peds points

✦ In children with retinitis pigmentosa, night blindness foreshadows tunnel vision, which usually doesn't develop until later in the disease process.

Teaching points

✦ Use of eye moments to avoid bumping into objects

Comparing tunnel vision with normal vision

The patient with tunnel vision experiences drastic constriction of his peripheral visual field. The illustrations here convey the extent of this constriction, comparing test findings for normal and tunnel vision.

Normal field of vision in the right eye, as shown on a perimetry chart

Normal field of vision in the right eye, as shown on a perimetry chart

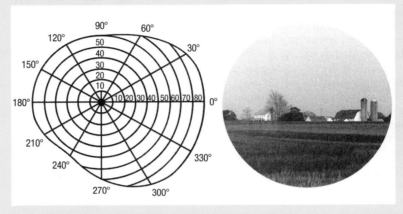

Tunnel vision in the right eye, as shown on a perimetry chart

Tunnel vision in the right eye, as seen in advanced glaucoma during perimeter examination

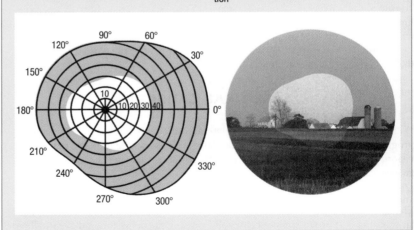

PEDIATRIC POINTERS

In children with retinitis pigmentosa, night blindness foreshadows tunnel vision, which usually doesn't develop until later in the disease process.

PATIENT COUNSELING

If tunnel vision is permanent, teach the patient to move his eyes from side to side when he walks to avoid bumping into objects.

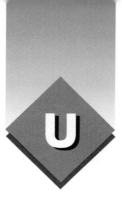

URETHRAL DISCHARGE

Urethral discharge from the urinary meatus may be purulent, mucoid, or thin; sanguineous or clear; and scant or profuse. It usually develops suddenly, most commonly in men with a prostate infection.

HISTORY

Ask the patient when he first noticed the discharge, and have him describe its color, consistency, and quantity. Does he experience pain or burning on urination? Does he have difficulty initiating a urine stream? Does he experience urinary frequency? Ask the patient about other associated signs and symptoms, such as fever, chills, and perineal fullness. Explore his history for prostate problems, sexually transmitted disease, or urinary tract infection. Ask the patient if he has had recent sexual contacts or a new sexual partner.

PHYSICAL ASSESSMENT

Inspect the patient's urethral meatus for inflammation and swelling. Using proper technique, obtain a culture specimen. (See *Collecting a urethral discharge specimen,* page 664.) Then obtain a urine specimen for urinalysis, culture, and possibly a three-glass urine test. (See *How to perform the three-glass urine test,* page 665.) In the male patient, the prostate gland may have to be palpated.

MEDICAL CAUSES

Prostatitis

Acute prostatitis is characterized by purulent urethral discharge. Initial signs and symptoms include sudden fever, chills, low back pain, myalgia, perineal fullness, and arthralgia. Urination becomes increasingly frequent and urgent, and the urine may appear cloudy. Dysuria, nocturia, and some degree of urinary obstruction may also occur. The prostate may be tense, boggy, tender, and warm.

Although chronic prostatitis commonly produces no symptoms, it may produce a persistent urethral discharge that's thin, milky, or clear and sometimes sticky. The discharge appears at the meatus after a long interval between voidings, as in the morning. Associated effects include a dull aching in the prostate or rectum, sexual dysfunction such as ejaculatory pain, and urinary disturbances such as frequency, urgency, and dysuria.

Key facts about urethral discharge
+ May be purulent, mucoid, or thin; sanguineous or clear

Key history points
+ Onset and description of discharge
+ Associated pain or burning on urination
+ History of prostate problems, STD, or UTI
+ Sexual habits and partners

Critical assessment steps
+ Inspect the urethral meatus for inflammation and swelling.
+ Obtain a culture specimen.
+ Obtain a urine specimen for urinalysis and culture

Medical causes
Prostatitis
+ Acute form involves purulent urethral discharge, sudden fever, chills, low back pain, myalgia, perineal fullness, and arthralgia.
+ Chronic form may produce a persistent urethral discharge that's thin, milky, or clear and appears at the meatus after a long interval between voidings.

Medical causes
(continued)

Reiter's syndrome
+ Urethral discharge occurs 1 to 2 weeks after sexual contact.

Urethritis
+ Scant or profuse urethral discharge that's either thin and clear, mucoid, or thick and purulent is produced.

Special considerations
+ Suggest that the patient take hot sitz baths several times daily, increase his fluid intake, void frequently, and avoid caffeine, tea, and alcohol.
+ Monitor for urine retention.

Peds points
+ Evaluate a child with urethral discharge for evidence of sexual and physical abuse.

Geri points
+ Urethral discharge in elderly males isn't usually related to an STD.

Teaching points
+ Importance of either stopping or engaging in sexual activity

Key facts about urinary frequency
+ Refers to increased incidence of the urge to void without an increase in the total volume of urine produced
+ Is a cardinal sign of UTI

Collecting a urethral discharge specimen

To obtain a urethral specimen from a male patient, follow these steps:
+ Instruct the patient not to void for 1 hour before specimen collection to prevent flushing of secretions from the urethra.
+ Provide privacy for the patient.
+ Help the patient onto an examination table and into a supine position, and expose his penis. Have him grasp and raise his penis to allow visualization of the urethra.
+ Wash your hands, and put on sterile gloves.
+ Insert a thin, sterile urogenital alginate swab no more than ¾″ (2 cm) into the urethra. Rotate the swab, and leave it in place for 10 to 30 seconds to absorb organisms.
+ Remove the swab, allow it to dry, and then send it to the laboratory.
+ Help the patient off the examination table, and tell him to dress.

Reiter's syndrome
Reiter's syndrome is a self-limiting syndrome that usually affects males. Urethral discharge and other signs of acute urethritis occur 1 to 2 weeks after sexual contact. Asymmetrical arthritis, conjunctivitis of one or both eyes, and ulcerations on the oral mucosa, glans penis, palms, and soles may also occur.

Urethritis
Urethritis, which is commonly sexually transmitted (as in gonorrhea), typically produces scant or profuse urethral discharge that's either thin and clear, mucoid, or thick and purulent. Other effects include urinary hesitancy, urgency, and frequency; dysuria; and itching and burning around the meatus.

SPECIAL CONSIDERATIONS
To help the patient relieve symptoms, suggest that he take hot sitz baths several times daily, increase his fluid intake, void frequently, and avoid caffeine, tea, and alcohol. Monitor him for urine retention.

PEDIATRIC POINTERS
Carefully evaluate a child with urethral discharge for evidence of sexual and physical abuse.

GERIATRIC POINTERS
Urethral discharge in elderly males isn't usually related to a sexually transmitted disease.

PATIENT COUNSELING
Advise the patient with acute prostatitis to discontinue sexual activity until acute symptoms subside. However, encourage the patient with chronic prostatitis to regularly engage in sexual activity because ejaculation may relieve pain.

URINARY FREQUENCY

Urinary frequency refers to increased incidence of the urge to void without an increase in the total volume of urine produced. Usually resulting from decreased bladder capacity, urinary frequency is a cardinal sign of urinary tract infection

How to perform the three-glass urine test

If your male patient complains of urinary frequency and urgency, dysuria, flank or lower back pain, or other signs or symptoms of urethritis, and if his urine specimen is cloudy, perform the three-glass urine test.

First ask him to void into three conical glasses labeled with numbers 1, 2, and 3. First-voided urine goes into glass #1, midstream urine into glass #2, and the remainder into glass #3. Tell the patient to avoid interrupting the stream of urine when shifting glasses, if possible.

Next, observe each glass for pus and mucus shreds. Also, note urine color and odor. Glass #1 will contain matter from the anterior urethra, glass #2 matter from the bladder, and glass #3 sediment from the prostate and seminal vesicles.

Some common findings are shown here. However, confirming diagnosis requires microscopic examination and a bacteriology report.

	SPECIMEN 1	SPECIMEN 2	SPECIMEN 3
Acute or subacute urethritis	Cloudy	Clear	Clear
Acute posterior urethritis	Cloudy	Clear or cloudy	Cloudy
Chronic anterior urethritis	Small shreds	Clear	Clear
Chronic posterior urethritis	Large shreds	Clear	Clear
Chronic urethritis - (anterior and posterior)	Small and large shreds	Clear	Clear
Prostatitis	Clear or large shreds	Clear	Cloudy or large shreds
Cystitis and pyelonephritis	Cloudy	Cloudy	Cloudy

(UTI). (See *Associated disorder: Urinary tract infection,* page 666.) However, it can also stem from another urologic disorder, neurologic dysfunction, or pressure on the bladder from a nearby tumor or from organ enlargement (as with pregnancy).

HISTORY

Ask the patient how many times per day he voids. How does this compare to his previous pattern of voiding? Ask about the onset and duration of the abnormal frequency and about any associated urinary signs or symptoms, such as dysuria, urgency, incontinence, hematuria, discharge, or lower abdominal pain with urination.

Ask also about neurologic symptoms, such as muscle weakness, numbness, or tingling. Explore his medical history for UTI, other urologic problems or recent urologic procedures, and neurologic disorders. With a male patient, ask about a history of prostatic enlargement. If the patient is a female of childbearing age, ask whether she is or could be pregnant.

Key history points
- Normal and current voiding patterns
- Onset and duration of urinary frequency
- Associated dysuria, urgency, incontinence, hematuria, discharge, or lower abdominal pain with urination
- History of UTI, other urologic problems or recent urologic procedures, and neurologic disorders
- History of prostatic enlargement if applicable
- Possibility of pregnancy if applicable

Key facts about UTI

+ Describes infections of the upper and lower urinary tract
+ Typically develop as an ascending infection from the urethra
+ Gram-negative bacteria cause most bacterial UTIs

Precipitating factors

+ Female gender
+ Increased sexual activity
+ Pregnancy
+ Urinary tract abnormalities
+ Obstructed urine flow
+ Impaired bladder innervation
+ Urinary stasis
+ Incomplete bladder emptying
+ Chronic health problems
+ Urinary tract instrumentation
+ Age

Management

+ Antibiotics
+ Fluids to dilute the urine
+ Frequent voiding
+ Proper perineal hygiene
+ Analgesics and warm sitz baths

Critical assessment steps

+ Obtain a clean-catch midstream specimen.
+ Palpate the suprapubic area, abdomen, and flanks, noting any tenderness.
+ Examine the urethral meatus for redness, discharge, or swelling.
+ In a male patient, the physician may palpate the prostate gland.

ASSOCIATED DISORDER

Urinary tract infection

Urinary tract infection (UTI) is a general term used to describe infections of the upper and lower urinary tract. Upper UTIs affect the kidneys, whereas lower UTIs affect the urinary bladder (cystitis) and urethra (urethritis). Lower UTIs are nearly 10 times more common in women than in men and affect approximately 10% to 20% of all women at least once. Lower UTI is also a prevalent bacterial disease in children, with girls most commonly affected.

UTIs typically develop as an ascending infection from the urethra. Infection of the kidney by bacteria usually occurs secondary to ascending infection from the bladder. Kidney infection commonly results from ureterovesical reflux in which an incompetent valve allows urine to flow back into the ureters during voiding.

Gram-negative bacteria cause most bacterial UTIs. Gram-negative and gram-positive bacteria may occasionally cause pyelonephritis (an infectious inflammation of the renal pelvis, tubules, and interstitial tissue). UTIs usually respond readily to treatment, but recurrence and resistant bacterial flare-up during therapy are possible.

CAUSES

Factors that increase the risk of developing a UTI include:
+ female gender
+ increased sexual activity
+ pregnancy

+ structural and functional urinary tract abnormalities (such as strictures)
+ obstructed urine flow
+ impaired bladder innervation
+ urinary stasis
+ incomplete bladder emptying
+ chronic health problems
+ urinary tract instrumentation (such as bladder catheterization and cystoscopy)
+ age.

DIAGNOSIS

The following tests help diagnose a UTI:
+ Urine culture reveals microorganism; a bacterial count above 100,000 confirms the diagnosis.
+ Urine microscopy is positive for pyuria, hematuria, or bacteriuria.
+ Voiding cystoureterography or excretory urography may detect congenital anomalies that predispose the patient to recurrent UTIs.

MEDICAL INTERVENTIONS

Treatment of a UTI may include:
+ antibiotics to eradicate the microorganism
+ fluids to dilute the urine
+ frequent voiding to reduce urinary stasis
+ proper perineal hygiene to reduce the risk of infection
+ analgesics and warm sitz baths to promote comfort.

PHYSICAL ASSESSMENT

Obtain a clean-catch midstream specimen for urinalysis and culture and sensitivity tests. Then palpate the patient's suprapubic area, abdomen, and flanks, noting any tenderness. Examine his urethral meatus for redness, discharge, or swelling. In a male patient, the physician may palpate the prostate gland.

If the patient's medical history reveals symptoms or a history of neurologic disorders, perform a neurologic assessment.

MEDICAL CAUSES

Benign prostatic hyperplasia

With benign prostatis hyperplasia (BPH), prostatic enlargement causes urinary frequency, along with nocturia and possibly incontinence and hematuria. Initial effects are reduced caliber and force of the urine stream, urinary hesitancy and tenesmus, inability to stop the urine stream, a feeling of incomplete voiding, and occasionally urine retention. Assessment reveals bladder distention.

Bladder calculus

Bladder irritation may lead to urinary frequency and urgency, dysuria, terminal hematuria, and suprapubic pain from bladder spasms. The patient may have overflow incontinence if the calculus lodges in the bladder neck. Greatest discomfort usually occurs at the end of micturition if the stone lodges in the bladder neck. This may also cause overflow incontinence and referred pain to the lower back or heel.

Bladder cancer

Urinary frequency, urgency, dribbling, and nocturia may develop from bladder irritation; however, the first sign of bladder cancer commonly is gross, painless, intermittent hematuria (usually with clots). Patients with invasive lesions commonly have suprapubic or pelvic pain from bladder spasms.

Multiple sclerosis

Urinary frequency, urgency, and incontinence are common urologic findings in patients with multiple sclerosis. Typically, visual problems (such as diplopia and blurred vision) and sensory impairment (such as paresthesia) are the earliest symptoms. Other findings may include constipation, muscle weakness, paralysis, spasticity, hyperreflexia, intention tremor, ataxic gait, dysarthria, impotence, and emotional lability.

Prostate cancer

In advanced stages of prostate cancer, urinary frequency may occur, along with hesitancy, dribbling, nocturia, dysuria, bladder distention, perineal pain, constipation, and a hard, irregularly shaped prostate.

Prostatitis

Acute prostatitis commonly produces urinary frequency, along with urgency, dysuria, nocturia, and purulent urethral discharge. Other findings include fever, chills, low back pain, myalgia, arthralgia, and perineal fullness. The prostate may be tense, boggy, tender, and warm. Signs and symptoms of chronic prostatitis are usually the same as those of the acute form, but to a lesser degree. The patient may also experience pain on ejaculation.

Rectal tumor

The pressure exerted by a rectal tumor on the bladder may cause urinary frequency. Early findings include changed bowel habits, commonly starting with an urgent need to defecate on arising or obstipation alternating with diarrhea; blood or mucus in the stool; and a sense of incomplete evacuation.

Reiter's syndrome

Reiter's syndrome is a self-limiting syndrome in which urinary frequency occurs with symptoms of acute urethritis 1 to 2 weeks after sexual contact. Other symptoms include asymmetrical arthritis of knees, ankles, and metatarsophalangeal joints; unilateral or bilateral conjunctivitis; and small painless ulcers on the mouth, tongue, glans penis, palms of the hands, and soles of the feet.

Reproductive tract tumor

A tumor in the female reproductive tract may compress the bladder, causing urinary frequency. Other findings vary but may include abdominal distention, menstrual disturbances, vaginal bleeding, weight loss, pelvic pain, and fatigue.

Medical causes

BPH
+ Prostatic enlargement causes urinary frequency, along with nocturia and possibly incontinence and hematuria.

Bladder calculus
+ Irritation may lead to urinary frequency and urgency, dysuria, terminal hematuria, and suprapubic pain from bladder spasms.

Bladder cancer
+ Urinary frequency, urgency, dribbling, and nocturia may develop.
+ The first sign commonly is gross, painless, intermittent hematuria.

Multiple sclerosis
+ Urinary frequency, urgency, and incontinence are common.

Prostate cancer
+ Urinary frequency may occur in advanced stages.

Prostatitis
+ Urinary frequency, urgency, dysuria, nocturia, and purulent urethral discharge are produced.

Rectal tumor
+ Pressure from the tumor on the bladder may cause urinary frequency.

Reiter's syndrome
+ Urinary frequency occurs 1 to 2 weeks after sexual contact.

Reproductive tract tumor
+ A tumor in the female reproductive tract may compress the bladder, causing urinary frequency.

Medical causes
(continued)

Spinal cord lesion
+ Urinary frequency, continuous overflow, dribbling, urgency, urinary hesitancy, and bladder distention result.

Urethral stricture
+ Bladder decompensation produces urinary frequency, along with urgency and nocturia.

UTI
+ Urinary frequency, urgency, dysuria, hematuria, and cloudy urine occur.

Other causes
+ Diuretics, including caffeine
+ Radiation therapy

Special considerations
+ If mobility is impaired, keep a bedpan or commode by the bed.
+ Document the patient's daily intake and output amounts.

Peds points
+ UTI is a common cause of urinary frequency in children.

Geri points
+ Men older than age 50 are prone to non–sex-related UTIs.
+ In postmenopausal women, decreased estrogen levels cause urinary frequency.

Teaching points
+ Safer sex practices
+ Proper way to clean genital area
+ Increasing fluid intake and frequency of voiding

Spinal cord lesion
Incomplete spinal cord transection results in urinary frequency, continuous overflow, dribbling, urgency when voluntary control of sphincter function weakens, urinary hesitancy, and bladder distention. Other effects occur below the level of the lesion and include weakness, paralysis, sensory disturbances, hyperreflexia, and impotence.

Urethral stricture
Bladder decompensation produces urinary frequency, along with urgency and nocturia. Early signs include hesitancy, tenesmus, and reduced caliber and force of the urine stream. Eventually, overflow incontinence may occur. Urinoma and urosepsis may develop.

Urinary tract infection
UTI is a common cause of urinary frequency. It may also produce urgency, dysuria, hematuria, cloudy urine and, in males, urethral discharge. The patient may report bladder spasms or a feeling of warmth during urination and a fever.

OTHER CAUSES

Diuretics
Diuretics, which include caffeine, reduce the body's total volume of water and salt by increasing urine excretion. Excessive intake of coffee, tea, and other caffeinated beverages leads to urinary frequency.

Treatments
Radiation therapy may cause bladder inflammation, leading to urinary frequency.

SPECIAL CONSIDERATIONS

Prepare the patient for diagnostic tests, such as urinalysis, culture and sensitivity tests, imaging tests, ultrasonography, cystoscopy, cystometry, postvoid residual tests, and a complete neurologic workup. If the patient's mobility is impaired, keep a bedpan or commode near his bed. Accurately document the patient's daily intake and output amounts.

PEDIATRIC POINTERS

UTI is a common cause of urinary frequency in children, especially girls. Congenital anomalies that can cause UTI include a duplicated ureter, congenital bladder diverticulum, and an ectopic ureteral orifice.

GERIATRIC POINTERS

Men older than age 50 are prone to frequent non–sex-related UTIs. In postmenopausal women, decreased estrogen levels cause urinary frequency, urgency, and nocturia.

PATIENT COUNSELING

Instruct sexually active patients in safer sex practices. Advise girls to clean the genital area from front to back to reduce contamination by *Escherichia coli*. Women should increase fluid intake, especially water, void frequently throughout the day, and clean themselves in the same manner as girls.

URINARY HESITANCY

Urinary hesitancy—difficulty starting a urine stream generally followed by a decrease in the force of the stream—can result from a urinary tract infection (UTI), a partial lower urinary tract obstruction, a neuromuscular disorder, or use of certain drugs. Occurring at all ages and in both sexes, it's most common in older men with prostatic enlargement. It also occurs in women with gravid uterus, tumors in the reproductive system, such as uterine fibroids, or ovarian, uterine, or vaginal cancer. Urinary hesitancy usually arises gradually, commonly going unnoticed until urine retention causes bladder distention and discomfort.

HISTORY

Ask the patient when he first noticed hesitancy and if he has ever had the problem before. Ask about other urinary problems, especially reduced force or interruption of the urine stream. Ask if he has ever been treated for a prostate problem or UTI or obstruction. Obtain a drug history.

PHYSICAL ASSESSMENT

Inspect the patient's urethral meatus for inflammation, discharge, and other abnormalities. Examine the anal sphincter and test sensation in the perineum. Obtain a clean-catch specimen for urinalysis and culture. In a male patient, the prostate gland requires palpation. A female patient requires a gynecologic examination.

MEDICAL CAUSES

Benign prostatic hyperplasia

Characteristic early findings of benign prostatic hyperplasia (BPH) include urinary hesitancy, reduced caliber and force of urine stream, perineal pain, a feeling of incomplete voiding, inability to stop the urine stream and, occasionally, urine retention. As obstruction increases, urination becomes more frequent, with nocturia, urinary overflow, incontinence, bladder distention, and possibly hematuria.

Prostate cancer

In patients with advanced prostate cancer, urinary hesitancy may occur, accompanied by frequency, dribbling, nocturia, dysuria, bladder distention, perineal pain, and constipation. Digital rectal examination commonly reveals a hard, nodular prostate.

Spinal cord lesion

A lesion below the micturition center that has destroyed the sacral nerve roots causes urinary hesitancy, tenesmus, and constant dribbling from retention and overflow incontinence. Associated findings are urinary frequency and urgency, dysuria, and nocturia.

Urethral stricture

Partial obstruction of the lower urinary tract produces urinary hesitancy, tenesmus, and decreased force and caliber of the urine stream. Urinary frequency and urgency, nocturia, and eventually overflow incontinence may develop. Pyuria usually indicates accompanying infection. Increased obstruction may lead to urine extravasation and formation of urinomas.

Key facts about urinary hesitancy

◆ Involves difficulty starting a urine stream followed by a decrease in the force of the stream
◆ Is most common in men with prostatic enlargement

Key history points

◆ Onset of hesitancy
◆ Other urinary problems
◆ Previous hesitancy, prostate problem, UTI, or obstruction
◆ Drug history

Critical assessment steps

◆ Inspect the urethral meatus.
◆ Examine the anal sphincter and test sensation in the perineum.
◆ Obtain a clean-catch specimen.
◆ Have the prostate gland palpated or a gynecologic examination performed as appropriate.

Medical causes

BPH

◆ Early findings include urinary hesitancy and reduced caliber and force of urine stream.

Prostate cancer

◆ Urinary hesitancy may occur in the advanced stages.

Spinal cord lesion

◆ A lesion below the micturition center that has destroyed the sacral nerve roots causes urinary hesitancy.

Urethral stricture

◆ Urinary frequency and urgency, nocturia, and eventually overflow incontinence may develop.

Medical causes
(continued)

UTI
+ Urinary hesitancy may occur along with frequency, possible hematuria, dysuria, nocturia, and cloudy urine.

Other causes
+ Anticholinergics and drugs with anticholinergic properties
+ General anesthesia

Special considerations
+ Monitor voiding pattern.
+ Palpate for bladder distention.
+ Apply local heat to the perineum or the abdomen.

Peds points
+ Posterior strictures in male infants may result in a less forceful urine stream.

Teaching points
+ Signs and symptoms of UTI to report
+ Self-catheterization

Key facts about urinary incontinence
+ Refers to the uncontrollable passage of urine
+ May be transient or permanent
+ Classified as stress, overflow, urge, or total

Key history points
+ Onset and description of incontinence
+ Description of normal urinary pattern and fluid intake

Urinary tract infection

Urinary hesitancy may be associated UTI. Characteristic urinary changes include frequency, possible hematuria, dysuria, nocturia, and cloudy urine. Associated findings include bladder spasms; costovertebral angle tenderness; suprapubic, low back, pelvic, or flank pain; urethral discharge in males; fever; chills; malaise; nausea; and vomiting.

OTHER CAUSES

Drugs

Anticholinergics and drugs with anticholinergic properties (such as tricyclic antidepressants and some nasal decongestants and cold remedies) may cause urinary hesitancy. Urinary hesitancy also may occur in those recovering from general anesthesia.

SPECIAL CONSIDERATIONS

Monitor the patient's voiding pattern. Frequently palpate for bladder distention. Apply local heat to the perineum or the abdomen to enhance muscle relaxation and aid urination. Prepare the patient for tests, such as cystometrography or cystourethrography.

PEDIATRIC POINTERS

The most common cause of urinary obstruction in male infants is posterior strictures. Infants with this problem may have a less forceful urine stream and may also present with fever due to UTI, failure to thrive, or a palpable bladder.

PATIENT COUNSELING

Teach the patient signs and symptoms of UTI to report. Also, teach him how to perform a clean, intermittent self-catheterization.

URINARY INCONTINENCE

Incontinence, the uncontrollable passage of urine, can result from a bladder abnormality, a neurologic disorder, or an alteration in pelvic muscle strength. A common urologic sign, incontinence may be transient or permanent and may involve large volumes of urine or scant dribbling. It can be classified as stress, overflow, urge, or total incontinence. *Stress incontinence* refers to intermittent leakage resulting from a sudden physical strain, such as a cough, sneeze, laugh, or quick movement. *Overflow incontinence* is a dribble resulting from urine retention, which fills the bladder and prevents it from contracting with sufficient force to expel a urine stream. *Urge incontinence* refers to the inability to suppress a sudden urge to urinate. *Total incontinence* is continuous leakage resulting from the bladder's inability to retain urine.

HISTORY

Ask the patient when he first noticed the incontinence and whether it began suddenly or gradually. Have him describe his typical urinary pattern: Does incontinence usually occur during the day or at night? Does he have any urinary control, or is he totally incontinent? If he is occasionally able to control urination, ask him the usual times and amounts voided. Determine his normal fluid intake. Ask about other urinary problems, such as hesitancy, frequency, urgency, nocturia, and decreased force or interruption of the urine stream. Also ask if he has ever sought treatment for incontinence or found a way to deal with it himself.

Obtain a medical history, especially noting urinary tract infection (UTI), prostate conditions, spinal injury or tumor, stroke, or surgery involving the bladder, prostate, or pelvic floor. Ask a woman how many pregnancies she has had and how many childbirths.

PHYSICAL ASSESSMENT

After completing the history, have the patient empty his bladder. Inspect the urethral meatus for obvious inflammation or anatomic defect. Have female patients bear down; note any urine leakage. Gently palpate the abdomen for bladder distention, which signals urine retention. Perform a complete neurologic assessment, noting motor and sensory function and obvious muscle atrophy.

MEDICAL CAUSES

Benign prostatic hyperplasia

Overflow incontinence is common with benign prostatic hyperplasia (BPH) as a result of urethral obstruction and urine retention. The disorder begins with a group of signs and symptoms known as prostatism: reduced caliber and force of urine stream, urinary hesitancy, and a feeling of incomplete voiding. As obstruction increases, urination becomes more frequent, with nocturia and, possibly, hematuria. Examination reveals bladder distention and an enlarged prostate.

Bladder calculus

Overflow incontinence may occur if the stone lodges in the bladder neck. Associated findings vary but may include those of an irritable bladder: urinary frequency and urgency, dysuria, hematuria, and suprapubic pain from bladder spasms. Pelvic pain and pain referred to the tip of the penis, vulva, low back, or heel may occur. Pain may be exacerbated by movement.

Bladder cancer

With bladder cancer, the patient commonly presents with urge incontinence and hematuria; obstruction by a tumor may produce overflow incontinence. Symptoms may be absent during the early stages. Other urinary signs and symptoms include frequency, dysuria, nocturia, dribbling, and suprapubic pain from bladder spasms after voiding. A mass may be palpable on bimanual examination.

Diabetic neuropathy

Diabetic neuropathy may cause painless bladder distention with overflow incontinence. Related findings include episodic constipation or diarrhea (which is commonly nocturnal), impotence and retrograde ejaculation, orthostatic hypotension, syncope, and dysphagia.

Guillain-Barré syndrome

Urinary incontinence may occur early in Guillain-Barré syndrome as a result of peripheral and autonomic nerve dysfunction. The most prominent sign is progressive, profound muscle weakness, which typically starts in the legs and extends to the arms and facial nerves within 24 to 72 hours. Associated findings include paresthesia; dysarthria; nasal speech; dysphagia; orthostatic hypotension; fecal incontinence; diaphoresis; drooling; pain in the shoulders, thighs, or lumbar region; and tachycardia.

Key history points
(continued)

✦ History of UTI, prostate conditions, spinal injury or tumor, stroke, or surgery involving the bladder, prostate, or pelvic floor

Critical assessment steps

✦ Have the patient empty his bladder.
✦ Inspect the urethral meatus for inflammation or defect.
✦ Have female patients bear down; note any urine leakage.
✦ Gently palpate the abdomen for bladder distention.

Medical causes

BPH

✦ Overflow incontinence results from urethral obstruction and urine retention.

Bladder calculus

✦ Overflow incontinence may occur if the stone lodges in the bladder neck.

Bladder cancer

✦ The patient commonly presents with urge incontinence and hematuria.
✦ Obstruction by a tumor may produce overflow incontinence.

Diabetic neuropathy

✦ Bladder distention with overflow incontinence may occur.

Guillain-Barré syndrome

✦ Urinary incontinence may occur early because of peripheral and autonomic nerve dysfunction.

Medical causes
(continued)

Multiple sclerosis
✦ Urinary incontinence, urgency, and frequency are common.

Prostate cancer
✦ Urinary incontinence usually appears only in advanced stages.

Prostatitis (chronic)
✦ Urinary incontinence may occur as a result of urethral obstruction from an enlarged prostate.

Spinal cord injury
✦ Overflow incontinence follows rapid bladder distention.

Stroke
✦ Urinary incontinence may be transient or permanent.

Urethral stricture
✦ Eventually, overflow incontinence may occur.

UTI
✦ Incontinence, urinary urgency, dysuria, hematuria, and cloudy urine occur.

Other causes
✦ Prostatectomy

Special considerations
✦ Obtain a urine specimen.
✦ Start bladder retraining.
✦ If incontinence has a neurologic basis, monitor for urine retention.

Multiple sclerosis
Urinary incontinence, urgency, and frequency are common urologic findings in multiple sclerosis. In most patients, vision problems and sensory impairment occur early. Other findings include constipation, muscle weakness, paralysis, spasticity, hyperreflexia, intention tremor, ataxic gait, dysarthria, impotence, and emotional lability.

Prostate cancer
Urinary incontinence usually appears only in the advanced stages of prostate cancer. Urinary frequency and hesitancy, nocturia, dysuria, bladder distention, perineal pain, constipation, and a hard, irregularly shaped, nodular prostate are other common late findings.

Prostatitis (chronic)
Urinary incontinence may occur as a result of urethral obstruction from an enlarged prostate. Other findings include urinary frequency and urgency, dysuria, hematuria, bladder distention, persistent urethral discharge, dull perineal pain that may radiate, ejaculatory pain, and decreased libido.

Spinal cord injury
Complete spinal cord transection above the sacral level causes flaccid paralysis of the bladder. Overflow incontinence follows rapid bladder distention. Other findings include paraplegia, sexual dysfunction, sensory loss, muscle atrophy, anhidrosis, and loss of reflexes distal to the injury.

Stroke
Urinary incontinence may be transient or permanent in stroke patients. Associated findings reflect the site and extent of the lesion and may include impaired mentation, emotional lability, behavioral changes, altered level of consciousness, and seizures. Headache, vomiting, visual deficits, and decreased visual acuity are possible. Sensorimotor effects include contralateral hemiplegia, dysarthria, dysphagia, ataxia, apraxia, agnosia, aphasia, and unilateral sensory loss.

Urethral stricture
Eventually, overflow incontinence may occur with urethral stricture. As obstruction increases, urine extravasation may lead to formation of urinomas and urosepsis.

Urinary tract infection
Besides incontinence, a UTI may produce urinary urgency, dysuria, hematuria, cloudy urine and, in males, urethral discharge. Bladder spasms or a feeling of warmth during urination may occur.

OTHER CAUSES

Surgery
Urinary incontinence may occur after prostatectomy as a result of urethral sphincter damage.

SPECIAL CONSIDERATIONS

Prepare the patient for diagnostic tests, such as cystoscopy, cystometry, and a complete neurologic workup. Obtain a urine specimen.

Begin management of incontinence by implementing a bladder retraining program. If the patient's incontinence has a neurologic basis, monitor him for urine retention, which may require periodic catheterizations. A patient with permanent urinary incontinence may require surgical creation of a urinary diversion.

PEDIATRIC POINTERS

Causes of incontinence in children include infrequent or incomplete voiding. These may also lead to UTI. Ectopic ureteral orifice is an uncommon congenital anomaly associated with incontinence. A complete diagnostic evaluation usually is necessary to rule out organic disease.

GERIATRIC POINTERS

Diagnosing a UTI in elderly patients can be problematic because many present only with urinary incontinence or changes in mental status, anorexia, or malaise. Also, many elderly patients without UTIs present with dysuria, frequency, urgency, or incontinence.

PATIENT COUNSELING

To prevent stress incontinence, teach the patient Kegel exercises to help strengthen the pelvic floor muscles. If appropriate, teach the patient self-catheterization techniques. Reassure your patient that episodes of incontinence don't signal a failure of the program. Encourage him to maintain a persistent, tolerant attitude.

URINARY URGENCY

A sudden compelling urge to urinate, accompanied by bladder pain, is a classic symptom of urinary tract infection (UTI). As inflammation decreases bladder capacity, discomfort results from the accumulation of even small amounts of urine. Repeated, frequent voiding in an effort to alleviate this discomfort produces urine output of only a few milliliters at each voiding.

Urgency without bladder pain may point to an upper-motor-neuron lesion that has disrupted bladder control.

HISTORY

Ask the patient about the onset of urinary urgency and whether he has ever experienced it before. Ask about other urologic symptoms, such as dysuria and cloudy urine. Also ask about neurologic symptoms such as paresthesia. Examine his medical history for recurrent or chronic UTIs or for surgery or procedures involving the urinary tract.

PHYSICAL ASSESSMENT

Obtain a clean-catch specimen for urinalysis and culture. Note urine character, color, and odor, and use a reagent strip to test for pH, glucose, and blood. Then palpate the suprapubic area and both flanks for distention and tenderness. If the patient's history or symptoms suggest neurologic dysfunction, perform a neurologic assessment.

MEDICAL CAUSES

Bladder calculus

Bladder irritation from a calculus can lead to urinary urgency and frequency, dysuria, terminal hematuria, and suprapubic pain from bladder spasms. Pain may be referred to the penis, vulva, lower back, or heel.

Peds points

+ Causes of incontinence in children include infrequent or incomplete voiding and an ectopic ureteral orifice.

Geri points

+ Elderly patients with UTIs may present only with urinary incontinence or changes in mental status, anorexia, or malaise.

Teaching points

+ How to perform Kegel exercises
+ Self-catheterization

Key facts about urinary urgency

+ Refers to a sudden compelling urge to urinate

Key history points

+ Onset and history of urgency
+ Other symptoms, such as dysuria, cloudy urine, and paresthesia
+ History of UTIs or surgery or procedures involving the urinary tract

Critical assessment steps

+ Obtain a clean-catch specimen for urinalysis and culture.
+ Note urine character, color, and odor, and use a reagent strip to test for pH, glucose, and blood.

Medical causes

Bladder calculus

+ Bladder irritation can lead to urinary urgency and frequency, dysuria, terminal hematuria, and suprapubic pain.

Medical causes
(continued)

Multiple sclerosis
- Urinary urgency can occur with or without the frequent UTIs.

Reiter's syndrome
- Urgency occurs with other symptoms of acute urethritis 1 to 2 weeks after sexual contact.

Spinal cord lesion
- Urinary urgency can result when voluntary control of sphincter function weakens.

Urethral stricture
- Bladder decompensation produces urinary urgency, frequency, and nocturia.

UTI
- Urinary urgency or frequency, hematuria, dysuria, nocturia, and cloudy urine develop.

Other causes
- Radiation therapy

Special considerations
- Increase the patient's fluid intake if not contraindicated.
- Administer an antibiotic and a urinary anesthetic.

Peds points
- In young children, urinary urgency may appear as a change in toilet habits.

Multiple sclerosis
Urinary urgency can occur with or without the frequent UTIs that can accompany multiple sclerosis. Commonly, visual and other sensory impairments are the earliest findings. Other findings include urinary frequency, incontinence, constipation, muscle weakness, paralysis, spasticity, intention tremor, hyperreflexia, ataxic gait, dysphagia, dysarthria, impotence, and emotional lability.

Reiter's syndrome
Reiter's syndrome is a self-limiting syndrome that primarily affects males. Urgency occurs with other symptoms of acute urethritis 1 to 2 weeks after sexual contact. Arthritic and ocular symptoms and skin lesions usually develop within several weeks after sexual contact. These symptoms include asymmetrical arthritis of knees, ankles, or metatarsal phalangeal joints; conjunctivitis; and ulcers on the penis, or skin, or in the mouth.

Spinal cord lesion
Urinary urgency can result from incomplete spinal cord transection when voluntary control of sphincter function weakens. Urinary frequency, difficulty initiating and inhibiting a urine stream, and bladder distention and discomfort may also occur. Neuromuscular effects distal to the lesion include weakness, paralysis, hyperreflexia, sensory disturbances, and impotence.

Urethral stricture
Bladder decompensation produces urinary urgency, frequency, and nocturia. Early signs and symptoms include hesitancy, tenesmus, and reduced caliber and force of the urine stream. Eventually, overflow incontinence may occur.

Urinary tract infection
Urinary urgency is commonly associated with a UTI. Other characteristic urinary changes include frequency, hematuria, dysuria, nocturia, and cloudy urine. Urinary hesitancy may also occur. Associated findings include bladder spasms; costovertebral angle tenderness; suprapubic, low back, or flank pain; urethral discharge in males; fever; chills; malaise; nausea; and vomiting.

OTHER CAUSES

Treatments
Radiation therapy may irritate and inflame the bladder, causing urinary urgency.

SPECIAL CONSIDERATIONS

Prepare the patient for the diagnostic workup, including a complete urinalysis, culture and sensitivity studies, and possibly neurologic tests.

Increase the patient's fluid intake, especially water, if not contraindicated, to dilute the urine and diminish the feeling of urgency. Administer an antibiotic and a urinary anesthetic, such as phenazopyridine.

PEDIATRIC POINTERS

In young children, urinary urgency may appear as a change in toilet habits, such as a sudden onset of bed-wetting or daytime accidents in a toilet-trained child. Urgency may also result from urethral irritation by bubble bath salts. Girls may experience vaginal discharge and vulvar soreness or pruritus.

PATIENT COUNSELING

Instruct sexually active patients in safer sex practices. Advise women and girls about proper genital hygiene — such as cleaning from front to back to reduce contamination from fecal bacteria. Instruct women to maintain adequate fluid intake, allowing frequent daily voiding.

URTICARIA

Urticaria, also known as *hives,* is a vascular skin reaction characterized by the eruption of transient pruritic wheals — smooth, slightly elevated patches with well-defined erythematous margins and pale centers of various shapes and sizes. It's produced by the local release of histamine or other vasoactive substances as part of a hypersensitivity reaction. (See *Recognizing common skin lesions,* pages 488 and 489.)

Acute urticaria evolves rapidly and usually has a detectable cause, commonly hypersensitivity to certain drugs, foods, insect bites, inhalants, or contactants; emotional stress; or environmental factors. Although individual lesions usually subside within 12 to 24 hours, new crops of lesions may erupt continuously, thus prolonging the attack.

Urticaria lasting longer than 6 weeks is classified as chronic. The lesions may recur for months or years, and the underlying cause is usually unknown. Occasionally, a diagnosis of psychogenic urticaria is made.

Angioedema, or giant urticaria, is characterized by the acute eruption of wheals involving the mucous membranes and, occasionally, the arms, legs, or genitals.

 EMERGENCY ACTIONS In an acute case of urticaria, quickly evaluate respiratory status and take vital signs. Ensure patent I.V. access if you note any respiratory difficulty or signs of impending anaphylactic shock. Also, as appropriate, give local epinephrine or apply ice to the affected site to decrease absorption through vasoconstriction. Maintain a patent airway, give oxygen as needed, and institute cardiac monitoring. Have resuscitation equipment at hand, and be prepared to begin cardiopulmonary resuscitation. Intubation or a tracheostomy may be required.

HISTORY

If the patient isn't in distress, obtain a complete history. Does he have any known allergies? Does the urticaria follow a seasonal pattern? Do certain foods or drugs seem to aggravate it? Is there a relationship to physical exertion? Is the patient routinely exposed to chemicals on the job or at home? Has the patient recently changed or used new skin products? Obtain a detailed drug history, including prescription and over-the-counter drugs. Note any history of chronic or parasitic infection, skin disease, or a GI disorder.

PHYSICAL ASSESSMENT

Obtain the patient's vital signs. Perform a complete cardiopulmonary assessment, noting signs and symptoms of shock or respiratory distress. Finish your examination by assessing for urticaria in other areas because new crops may continue to appear.

Teaching points
+ Safer sex practices
+ Proper genital hygiene for women and girls
+ Adequate fluid intake and frequent daily voiding

Key facts about urticaria
+ Is a vascular skin reaction
+ Characterized by the eruption of transient pruritic wheals in response to the local release of histamine or other vasoactive substances

In an emergency
+ Evaluate respiratory status and take vital signs.
+ Ensure patent I.V. access.
+ As appropriate, give local epinephrine or apply ice.
+ Maintain a patent airway.
+ Give oxygen as needed.
+ Institute cardiac monitoring.
+ Be prepared to begin CPR.

Key history points
+ Known allergies
+ Pattern of urticaria or aggravating factors
+ Exposure to chemicals
+ Drug history

Critical assessment steps
+ Obtain vital signs.
+ Perform a complete cardiopulmonary assessment, noting signs and symptoms of shock or respiratory distress.
+ Assess for urticaria in other areas because new crops may continue to appear.

Medical causes

Anaphylaxis
✦ Diffuse urticaria and angioedema develops; wheals range from pinpoint to palm-size or larger.

Hereditary angioedema
✦ Patches of nonpitting, nonpruritic edema develop on an extremity or the face.

Lyme disease
✦ Urticaria may result from erythema chronicum migrans.

Other causes
✦ Various drugs (most commonly aspirin, atropine, codeine, dextrans, immune serums, insulin, morphine, penicillin, quinine, sulfonamides, and vaccines)
✦ Radiographic contrast medium

Special considerations
✦ Apply a bland skin emollient or one containing menthol and phenol.
✦ Expect to give an antihistamine, a systemic corticosteroid, or a tranquilizer.
✦ Tepid baths and cool compresses may decrease pruritus.

Peds points
✦ Pediatric forms of urticaria include acute papular urticaria and urticaria pigmentosa (rare).

Teaching points
✦ Importance of wearing medical identification for allergies
✦ Risks of delayed symptoms
✦ Signs and symptoms to report
✦ Ways to prevent anaphylaxis
✦ Proper use of an anaphylaxis kit

MEDICAL CAUSES

Anaphylaxis
Anaphylaxis is marked by the rapid eruption of diffuse urticaria and angioedema, with wheals ranging from pinpoint to palm-size or larger. Lesions are usually pruritic and stinging; paresthesia commonly precedes their eruption. Other acute findings include profound anxiety; weakness; diaphoresis; sneezing; shortness of breath; profuse rhinorrhea; nasal congestion; dysphagia; and warm, moist skin.

Hereditary angioedema
Hereditary angioedema is an autosomal dominant disorder in which cutaneous involvement is manifested by nonpitting, nonpruritic edema of an extremity or the face. Respiratory mucosal involvement can produce life-threatening acute laryngeal edema.

Lyme disease
Although not diagnostic of this tick-borne disease, urticaria may result from the characteristic skin lesion (erythema chronicum migrans). Later effects of Lyme disease include constant malaise and fatigue, intermittent headache, fever, chills, lymphadenopathy, neurologic and cardiac abnormalities, and arthritis.

OTHER CAUSES

Drugs
Many drugs can produce urticaria. Among the most common are aspirin, atropine, codeine, dextrans, immune serums, insulin, morphine, penicillin, quinine, sulfonamides, and vaccines. In addition, radiographic contrast medium commonly produces urticaria, especially when administered I.V.

SPECIAL CONSIDERATIONS

To help relieve the patient's discomfort, apply a bland skin emollient or one containing menthol and phenol. Expect to give an antihistamine, a systemic corticosteroid or, if stress is a suspected contributing factor, a tranquilizer. Tepid baths and cool compresses may also enhance vasoconstriction and decrease pruritus.

PEDIATRIC POINTERS

Pediatric forms of urticaria include acute papular urticaria (usually after insect bites) and urticaria pigmentosa (rare). Hereditary angioedema may be causative.

PATIENT COUNSELING

Explain the importance of wearing medical identification for allergies. Discuss the risks of delayed symptoms and the need to report any recurrence of dyspnea, urticaria, chest tightness, angioedema, or other symptoms. Teach the patient ways to prevent anaphylaxis, such as avoiding the causative food or drug. Tell him to carry an anaphylaxis kit containing epinephrine and an antihistamine and make sure he knows how to use it.

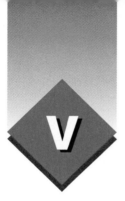

VAGINAL BLEEDING, POSTMENOPAUSAL

Postmenopausal vaginal bleeding — bleeding that occurs 6 or more months after menopause — is an important indicator of gynecologic cancer, but it can also result from infection, a local pelvic disorder, estrogenic stimulation, atrophy of the endometrium, and physiologic thinning and drying of the vaginal mucous membranes. Bleeding from the vagina may be indicative of bleeding from another gynecologic location, such as the ovaries, fallopian tubes, uterus, cervix, or vagina. Bleeding from these areas exits the body through the vagina. It usually occurs as slight, brown or red spotting developing either spontaneously or following coitus or douching, but it may also occur as oozing of fresh blood or as bright red hemorrhage. Many patients — especially those with a history of heavy menstrual flow — minimize the importance of this bleeding, delaying diagnosis.

HISTORY

Determine the patient's age and her age at menopause. Ask when she first noticed the abnormal bleeding. Then obtain a thorough obstetric and gynecologic history. When did she begin menstruating? Were her menses regular? If not, ask her to describe any menstrual irregularities. How old was she when she first had intercourse? How many sexual partners has she had? Has she had any children? Has she had fertility problems? If possible, obtain an obstetric and gynecologic history of the patient's mother, and ask about a family history of gynecologic cancer. Determine if the patient has any associated symptoms and if she's taking estrogen.

PHYSICAL ASSESSMENT

Observe the external genitalia, noting the character of any vaginal discharge and the appearance of the labia, vaginal rugae, and clitoris. Carefully palpate the patient's breasts and lymph nodes for nodules or enlargement. The patient will require pelvic and rectal examinations.

MEDICAL CAUSES

Atrophic vaginitis

When bloody staining occurs in atrophic vaginitis, it usually follows coitus or douching. Characteristic white, watery vaginal discharge may be accompanied by pruritus, dyspareunia, and a burning sensation in the vagina and labia. Sparse pubic hair, a pale vagina with decreased rugae and small hemorrhagic spots, clitoral atrophy, and shrinking of the labia minora may also occur.

Medical causes
(continued)

Cervical cancer
+ Spotting or heavier bleeding occurs early.
+ Pink-tinged, smelly discharge and postcoital pain occur.

Cervical or endometrial polyps
+ Spotting (possibly mucopurulent and pink) may occur after coitus, douching, or straining at stool.

Endometrial hyperplasia or cancer
+ Early bleeding is brownish and scant or red and profuse.
+ Bleeding becomes heavier and more frequent.

Ovarian tumor (feminizing)
+ Endometrial shedding may occur and cause heavy bleeding.

Vaginal cancer
+ Spotting or bleeding may be preceded by thin, watery discharge.

Other causes
+ Unopposed estrogen replacement therapy

Special considerations
+ Stop estrogen until a diagnosis is made.

Geri points
+ Endometrial atrophy is the predominant cause of postmenopausal bleeding.

Teaching points
+ Reassurance that most postmenopausal vaginal bleeding is benign

Cervical cancer
Early invasive cervical cancer causes vaginal spotting or heavier bleeding, usually after coitus or douching but occasionally spontaneously. Related findings include persistent, pink-tinged, and foul-smelling vaginal discharge and postcoital pain. As the cancer spreads, back and sciatic pain, leg swelling, anorexia, weight loss, hematuria, dysuria, rectal bleeding, and weakness may occur.

Cervical or endometrial polyps
Cervical or endometrial polyps are small, pedunculated growths that may cause spotting (possibly as a mucopurulent, pink discharge) after coitus, douching, or straining at stool. Many endometrial polyps produce no symptoms, however.

Endometrial hyperplasia or cancer
With endometrial hyperplasia or cancer, bleeding occurs early, can be brownish and scant or bright red and profuse, and usually follows coitus or douching. Bleeding later becomes heavier and more frequent, leading to clotting and anemia. Bleeding may be accompanied by pelvic, rectal, lower back, and leg pain. The uterus may be enlarged.

Ovarian tumor (feminizing)
Estrogen-producing ovarian tumors can stimulate endometrial shedding and cause heavy bleeding unassociated with coitus or douching. A palpable pelvic mass, increased cervical mucus, breast enlargement, and spider angiomas may be present.

Vaginal cancer
With vaginal cancer, characteristic spotting or bleeding may be preceded by a thin, watery vaginal discharge. Bleeding may be spontaneous but usually follows coitus or douching. A firm, ulcerated vaginal lesion may be present; dyspareunia, urinary frequency, bladder and pelvic pain, rectal bleeding, and vulvar lesions may develop later.

OTHER CAUSES

Drugs
Unopposed estrogen replacement therapy is a common cause of abnormal vaginal bleeding. This can usually be reduced by adding progesterone (in women who haven't had a hysterectomy) and by adjusting the patient's estrogen dosage.

SPECIAL CONSIDERATIONS
Prepare the patient for diagnostic tests, such as ultrasonography to outline a cervical or uterine tumor; endometrial biopsy, colposcopy, or dilatation and curettage with hysteroscopy to obtain tissue for histologic examination; testing for occult blood in the stool; and vaginal and cervical cultures to detect infection. Discontinue estrogen until a diagnosis is made.

GERIATRIC POINTERS
Some 80% of postmenopausal vaginal bleeding is benign; endometrial atrophy is the predominant cause. Malignancy should be ruled out.

PATIENT COUNSELING
Reassure the patient that most postmenopausal vaginal bleeding is benign and not cancer related.

VAGINAL DISCHARGE

Common in women of childbearing age, physiologic vaginal discharge is mucoid, clear or white, nonbloody, and odorless. Produced by the cervical mucosa and, to a lesser degree, by the vulvar glands, this discharge may occasionally be scant or profuse due to estrogenic stimulation and changes during the patient's menstrual cycle. However, a marked increase in discharge or a change in discharge color, odor, or consistency can signal disease. The discharge may result from infection, sexually transmitted disease, reproductive tract disease, fistulas, and certain drugs. In addition, the prolonged presence of a foreign body, such as a tampon or diaphragm, in the patient's vagina can cause irritation and an inflammatory exudate, as can frequent douching, feminine hygiene products, contraceptive products, bubble baths, and colored or perfumed toilet papers.

HISTORY

Ask the patient to describe the onset, color, consistency, odor, and texture of her vaginal discharge. How does the discharge differ from her usual vaginal secretions? Is the onset related to her menstrual cycle? Also, ask about associated symptoms, such as dysuria and perineal pruritus and burning. Does she have spotting after coitus or douching? Ask about recent changes in her sexual habits and hygiene practices. Is she or could she be pregnant? Next, ask if she has had vaginal discharge before or has ever been treated for a vaginal infection. What treatment did she receive? Did she complete the course of medication? Ask about her current use of medications, especially antibiotics, oral estrogens, and contraceptives.

PHYSICAL ASSESSMENT

Examine the external genitalia and note the character of the discharge. (See *Identifying causes of vaginal discharge,* page 680.) Observe vulvar and vaginal tissues for redness, edema, and excoriation. Palpate the inguinal lymph nodes to detect tenderness or enlargement. Palpate the abdomen for tenderness. A pelvic examination may be required. Obtain vaginal discharge specimens for testing.

MEDICAL CAUSES

Atrophic vaginitis

With atrophic vaginitis, a thin, scant, watery white vaginal discharge may be accompanied by pruritus, burning, tenderness, and bloody spotting after coitus or douching. Sparse pubic hair, a pale vagina with decreased rugae and small hemorrhagic spots, clitoral atrophy, and shrinking of the labia minora may also occur.

Bacterial vaginosis

Bacterial vaginosis results in a thin, foul-smelling, green or gray-white discharge that adheres to the vaginal walls and can be easily wiped away, leaving healthy-looking tissue. Pruritus, redness, and other signs of vaginal irritation may occur but are usually minimal.

Candidiasis

Infection with *Candida albicans* causes a profuse, white, curdlike discharge with a yeasty, sweet odor. Onset is abrupt, usually just before menses or during a course of antibiotics. Exudate may be lightly attached to the labia and vaginal walls and is commonly accompanied by vulvar redness and edema. The inner thighs may be covered with a fine, red dermatitis and weeping erosions. Intense labial itching and burning may also occur. Some patients experience external dysuria.

Key facts about vaginal discharge
+ May be mucoid, clear or white, nonbloody, and odorless

Key history points
+ Onset and description
+ Associated symptoms, such as dysuria and perineal pruritus
+ Recent changes in sexual habits or hygiene practices
+ Previous discharge or infection and treatment used
+ Current drug use

Critical assessment steps
+ Note the character of the discharge.
+ Observe vulvar and vaginal tissues for redness, edema, and excoriation.
+ A pelvic examination may be required.
+ Obtain vaginal discharge specimens for testing.

Medical causes
Atrophic vaginitis
+ A thin, scant, watery white vaginal discharge may be accompanied by pruritus, burning, tenderness, and bloody spotting after coitus or douching.

Bacterial vaginosis
+ Thin, foul-smelling, green or gray-white discharge adheres to the vaginal walls and can be easily wiped away.

Candidiasis
+ A profuse, white, curdlike discharge with a yeasty, sweet odor is produced abruptly.
+ Exudate may be lightly attached to the labia and vaginal walls.

Identifying causes of vaginal discharge

The color, consistency, amount, and odor of your patient's vaginal discharge provide important clues about the underlying disorder. For quick reference, use this chart to match common characteristics of vaginal discharge and their possible causes.

CHARACTERISTICS	POSSIBLE CAUSES
Thin, scant, watery white discharge	Atrophic vaginitis
Thin, green or gray-white, foul-smelling discharge	Bacterial vaginosis
White, curdlike, profuse discharge with yeasty, sweet odor	Candidiasis
Mucopurulent, foul-smelling discharge	Chancroid
Yellow, mucopurulent, odorless, or acrid discharge	Chlamydial infection
Scant, serosanguineous, or purulent discharge with foul odor	Endometritis
Copious mucoid discharge	Genital herpes
Profuse, mucopurulent discharge, possibly foul-smelling	Genital warts
Yellow or green, foul-smelling discharge from the cervix or occasionally from Bartholin's or Skene's ducts	Gonorrhea
Chronic, watery, bloody, or purulent discharge, possibly foul-smelling	Gynecologic cancer
Frothy, green-yellow, and profuse (or thin, white, and scant) foul-smelling discharge	Trichomoniasis

Medical causes
(continued)

Chlamydial infection
+ A yellow, mucopurulent, odorless, or acrid vaginal discharge is produced.

Endometritis
+ A scant, serosanguineous discharge with a foul odor can result.

Genital warts
+ A profuse, mucopurulent vaginal discharge, which may be foul-smelling if the warts are infected, may be produced.

Gonorrhea
+ Occasionally, yellow or green, foul-smelling discharge can be expressed from Bartholin's or Skene's ducts.

Chlamydial infection
A chlamydial infection causes a yellow, mucopurulent, odorless, or acrid vaginal discharge. Other findings include dysuria, dyspareunia, and vaginal bleeding after douching or coitus, especially following menses. Many women remain asymptomatic.

Endometritis
A scant, serosanguineous discharge with a foul odor can result from bacterial invasion of the endometrium. Associated findings include fever, lower back and abdominal pain, abdominal muscle spasm, malaise, dysmenorrhea, and an enlarged uterus.

Genital warts
Genital warts are mosaic, papular vulvar lesions that can cause a profuse, mucopurulent vaginal discharge, which may be foul-smelling if the warts are infected. Patients with genital warts frequently complain of burning or paresthesia in the vaginal introitus.

Gonorrhea
Although 80% of women with gonorrhea are asymptomatic, others have a yellow or green, foul-smelling discharge that can be expressed from Bartholin's or Skene's

ducts. Other findings include dysuria, urinary frequency and incontinence, bleeding, and vaginal redness and swelling. Severe pelvic and lower abdominal pain and fever may develop.

Gynecologic cancer
Endometrial or cervical cancer produces a chronic, watery, bloody or purulent vaginal discharge that may be foul-smelling. Other findings include abnormal vaginal bleeding and, later, weight loss; pelvic, back, and leg pain; fatigue; urinary frequency; and abdominal distention.

Herpes simplex (genital)
A copious mucoid discharge results from genital herpes, but the initial complaint is painful, indurated vesicles and ulcerations on the labia, vagina, cervix, anus, thighs, or mouth. Erythema, marked edema, and tender inguinal lymph nodes may occur with fever, malaise, and dysuria.

Trichomoniasis
Trichomoniasis can cause a foul-smelling discharge, which may be frothy, green-yellow, and profuse or thin, white, and scant. Other findings include pruritus; a red, inflamed vagina with tiny petechiae; dysuria and urinary frequency; and dyspareunia, postcoital spotting, menorrhagia, or dysmenorrhea. About 70% of patients are asymptomatic.

OTHER CAUSES
Contraceptive creams and jellies
These products can increase vaginal secretions.

Drugs
Drugs that contain estrogen, including hormonal contraceptives, can cause increased mucoid vaginal discharge. Antibiotics, such as tetracycline, may increase the risk of a candidal vaginal infection and discharge.

Radiation therapy
Irradiation of the reproductive tract can cause a watery, odorless vaginal discharge.

SPECIAL CONSIDERATIONS
Obtain swabs and cultures of the discharge to identify the causative organism. Administer antibiotics, antivirals, or other medications, as appropriate. Observe standard precautions to prevent the spread of infection.

PEDIATRIC POINTERS
Female neonates who have been exposed to maternal estrogens in utero may have a white mucous vaginal discharge for the first month after birth; a yellow mucous discharge indicates a pathologic condition. In the older child, a purulent, foul-smelling, and possibly bloody vaginal discharge commonly results from a foreign object placed in the vagina. The possibility of sexual abuse should also be considered.

GERIATRIC POINTERS
The postmenopausal vaginal mucosa becomes thin due to decreased estrogen levels. Together with a rise in vaginal pH, this reduces resistance to infectious agents, increasing the incidence of vaginitis.

Medical causes
(continued)
Gynecologic cancer
✦ Chronic, watery, bloody or purulent vaginal discharge may be foul-smelling.

Herpes simplex (genital)
✦ Copious mucoid discharge results.

Trichomoniasis
✦ A foul-smelling discharge, which may be frothy, green-yellow, and profuse or thin, white, and scant, may be produced.

Other causes
✦ Antibiotics
✦ Contraceptive creams and jellies
✦ Drugs that contain estrogen
✦ Irradiation of reproductive tract

Special considerations
✦ Obtain cultures of the discharge.
✦ Give antibiotics, antivirals, or other drugs, as appropriate.

Peds points
✦ Female neonates who have been exposed to maternal estrogens in utero may have a white mucous vaginal discharge for the first month after birth; a yellow mucous discharge indicates a pathologic condition.
✦ In an older child, purulent, foul-smelling, and possibly bloody vaginal discharge commonly results from a foreign object placed in the vagina. Consider the possibility of sexual abuse.

Geri points
✦ Incidence of vaginitis increases in older patients.

Teaching points

✦ Importance of keeping the perineum clean and dry, avoiding tight-fitting clothing
✦ Douching with vinegar and water to relieve discomfort
✦ Compliance with prescribed drugs
✦ Avoiding intercourse until symptoms of infection clear
✦ Safer sex methods

Key facts about venous hum

✦ Is a functional or innocent murmur heard above the clavicles throughout the cardiac cycle
✦ Is loudest during diastole
✦ May be low-pitched, rough, or noisy
✦ Commonly accompanies a thrill

Key history points

✦ History of anemia or thyroid disorders
✦ Associated palpitations, dyspnea, nervousness, tremors, heat intolerance, weight loss, fatigue, or malaise

Critical assessment steps

✦ Take vital signs, noting especially tachycardia, hypertension, a bounding pulse, and widened pulse pressure.
✦ Auscultate the heart for gallops or murmurs.
✦ Examine the skin and mucous membranes for pallor.

PATIENT COUNSELING

Teach the patient to keep her perineum clean and dry. Also, tell her to avoid wearing tight-fitting clothing and nylon underwear and to instead wear cotton-crotched underwear and pantyhose. If appropriate, suggest that the patient douche with a solution of 5 tbs of white vinegar to 2 qt (2 L) of warm water to help relieve her discomfort.

If the patient has a vaginal infection, tell her to continue taking the prescribed medication even if her symptoms clear or she menstruates. Also, advise her to avoid intercourse until her symptoms clear and then to have her partner use condoms until she completes her course of medication. If her condition is sexually transmitted, instruct her on safer sex methods.

VENOUS HUM

A venous hum is a functional or innocent murmur heard above the clavicles throughout the cardiac cycle. Loudest during diastole, it's low-pitched, rough, or noisy. The hum commonly accompanies a thrill or, possibly, a high-pitched whine. It's best heard by applying the bell of the stethoscope to the medial aspect of the right supraclavicular area while the patient sits upright or by placing the stethoscope bell in the second or third parasternal interspace while the patient stands upright. (See *Detecting a venous hum.*)

A venous hum is a common, normal finding in children and pregnant women. However, it also occurs in hyperdynamic states, such as anemia and thyrotoxicosis. The hum results from increased blood flow through the internal jugular veins, especially on the right side, which causes audible vibrations in the tissues.

Occasionally, a venous hum may be mistaken for an intracardiac murmur or a thyroid bruit. However, a venous hum disappears with jugular vein compression and waxes and wanes with head turning. In contrast, both an intracardiac murmur and a thyroid bruit persist despite jugular compression and head turning.

HISTORY

Determine if the patient has a history of anemia or thyroid disorders. If he does, ask what medication or other treatments he has received. If he doesn't, ask if he has had associated signs and symptoms, such as palpitations, dyspnea, nervousness, tremors, heat intolerance, weight loss, fatigue, or malaise.

PHYSICAL ASSESSMENT

Take the patient's vital signs, noting especially tachycardia, hypertension, a bounding pulse, and widened pulse pressure. Auscultate his heart for gallops or murmurs. Examine his skin and mucous membranes for pallor.

MEDICAL CAUSES

Anemia

A venous hum is common with severe anemia (hemoglobin level below 7 g/dl). Additional findings include pale skin and mucous membranes, dyspnea, crackles, tachycardia, bounding pulse, atrial gallop, systolic bruits over both carotid arteries, bleeding tendencies, weakness, fatigue, and malaise.

Detecting a venous hum

To detect a venous hum, have your patient sit upright and then place the bell of the stethoscope over his right supraclavicular area. Gently lift his chin and turn his head toward the left, which increases the loudness of the hum.

If you still can't hear the hum, press his jugular vein with your thumb. The hum will disappear with pressure but will suddenly return, temporarily louder than before, when you release your thumb — a result of the turbulence created by pressure changes.

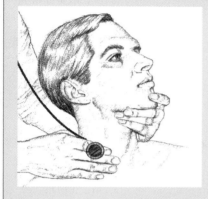
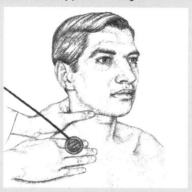

Thyrotoxicosis

Thyrotoxicosis may cause a loud venous hum, audible whether the patient is sitting or in a supine position. Auscultation may also reveal an atrial or ventricular gallop. Additional findings include tachycardia, palpitations, weight loss despite increased appetite, diarrhea, an enlarged thyroid, dyspnea, nervousness, difficulty concentrating, and tremors, diaphoresis, and heat intolerance. Exophthalmos may be present. Women may have oligomenorrhea or amenorrhea; men, gynecomastia. Both sexes may have decreased libido.

SPECIAL CONSIDERATIONS

Prepare the patient for diagnostic tests, which may include an electrocardiogram, complete blood count, and thyroid hormone (T_3 and T_4) assays.

PEDIATRIC POINTERS

A cervical venous hum occurs normally in more than two-thirds of children between ages 5 and 15.

PATIENT COUNSELING

Teach the patient ways to manage his underlying disorder, such as increasing dietary iron intake if anemic or taking antithyroid medication if hyperthyroid. Encourage rest periods to conserve energy and reduce metabolic demands.

Medical causes
Anemia
+ In severe cases, a venous hum occurs with pale skin and mucous membranes, dyspnea, crackles, tachycardia, bounding pulse, atrial gallop, systolic bruits over the carotid arteries, bleeding tendencies, weakness, fatigue, and malaise.

Thyrotoxicosis
+ A loud venous hum may be audible whether the patient is sitting or in a supine position.
+ An atrial or ventricular gallop may be present.

Special considerations
+ Prepare the patient for diagnostic tests.

Peds points
+ A cervical venous hum occurs normally in more than two-thirds of children between ages 5 and 15.

Teaching points
+ Ways to manage the disorder
+ Importance of rest periods

VERTIGO

Vertigo is an illusion of movement in which the patient feels that he's revolving in space (subjective vertigo) or that his surroundings are revolving around him (objective vertigo). He may complain of feeling as if he's being pulled sideways, as though drawn by a magnet.

A common symptom, vertigo usually begins abruptly and may be temporary or permanent, mild or severe. It may worsen when the patient moves and subside when he lies down. It's commonly confused with dizziness — a sensation of imbalance and light-headedness that's nonspecific. However, unlike dizziness, vertigo is commonly accompanied by nausea, vomiting, nystagmus, and tinnitus or hearing loss. Although the patient's limb coordination is unaffected, vertiginous gait may occur.

Vertigo may result from a neurologic or otologic disorder that affects the equilibratory apparatus (the vestibule, semicircular canals, eighth cranial nerve, vestibular nuclei in the brain stem and their temporal lobe connections, and eyes). However, this symptom may also result from alcohol intoxication, hyperventilation, postural changes (benign postural vertigo), the effects of certain drugs, tests, or procedures.

HISTORY

Ask your patient to describe the onset and duration of his vertigo, being careful to distinguish this symptom from dizziness. Does he feel that he's moving or that his surroundings are moving around him? How often do the attacks occur? Do they follow position changes, or are they unpredictable? Find out if the patient can walk during an attack, if he leans to one side, and if he has ever fallen. Ask if he experiences motion sickness and if he prefers one position during an attack. Obtain a recent drug history. Note any evidence of alcohol abuse.

PHYSICAL ASSESSMENT

Perform a neurologic assessment, focusing particularly on eighth cranial nerve function. Observe the patient's gait and posture for abnormalities.

MEDICAL CAUSES

Acoustic neuroma
Acoustic neuroma is a tumor of the eighth cranial nerve that causes mild, intermittent vertigo and unilateral sensorineural hearing loss. Other findings include tinnitus, postauricular or suboccipital pain, and — with cranial nerve compression — facial paralysis.

Benign positional vertigo
With benign positional vertigo, debris in a semicircular canal produces vertigo on head position change, which lasts a few minutes. It's usually temporary and can be effectively treated with positional maneuvers.

Brain stem ischemia
Brain stem ischemia produces sudden, severe vertigo that may become episodic and later persistent. Associated findings include ataxia, nausea, vomiting, increased blood pressure, tachycardia, nystagmus, and lateral deviation of the eyes toward the side of the lesion. Hemiparesis and paresthesia may also occur.

Head trauma

Persistent vertigo, occurring soon after injury, accompanies spontaneous or positional nystagmus and, if the temporal bone is fractured, hearing loss. Associated findings include headache, nausea, vomiting, and decreased level of consciousness (LOC). Behavioral changes, diplopia or visual blurring, seizures, motor or sensory deficits, and signs of increased intracranial pressure may also occur.

Herpes zoster

Infection of the eighth cranial nerve with herpes zoster produces sudden onset of vertigo accompanied by facial paralysis, hearing loss in the affected ear, and herpetic vesicular lesions in the auditory canal.

Labyrinthitis

Severe vertigo begins abruptly with this inner ear infection. Vertigo may occur in a single episode or may recur over months or years. Associated findings of labyrinthitis include nausea, vomiting, progressive sensorineural hearing loss, and nystagmus.

Ménière's disease

With Ménière's disease, labyrinthine dysfunction causes abrupt onset of vertigo, lasting minutes, hours, or days. Unpredictable episodes of severe vertigo and unsteady gait may cause the patient to fall. During an attack, any sudden motion of the head or eyes can precipitate nausea and vomiting.

Motion sickness

Motion sickness is characterized by vertigo, nausea, vomiting, and headache in response to rhythmic or erratic motions. Headache, dizziness, fatigue, diaphoresis, hypersalivation, and dyspnea may also occur.

Multiple sclerosis

Episodic vertigo may occur early in multiple sclerosis and become persistent. Other early findings include diplopia, visual blurring, and paresthesia. Multiple sclerosis may also produce nystagmus, constipation, muscle weakness, paralysis, spasticity, hyperreflexia, intention tremor, and ataxia.

Seizures

Temporal lobe seizures may produce vertigo, usually associated with other symptoms of partial complex seizures. The seizures may be heralded by an aura and followed by several minutes of mental confusion.

Vestibular neuritis

With vestibular neuritis, severe vertigo usually begins abruptly and lasts several days, without tinnitus or hearing loss. Other findings include nausea, vomiting, and nystagmus.

OTHER CAUSES

Diagnostic tests

Caloric testing (irrigating the ears with warm or cold water) can induce vertigo.

Drugs and alcohol

High or toxic doses of certain drugs or alcohol may produce vertigo. These drugs include salicylates, aminoglycosides, antibiotics, quinine, and hormonal contraceptives.

Medical causes
(continued)

Herpes zoster
+ Infection of the eighth cranial nerve produces sudden onset of vertigo, facial paralysis, hearing loss in the affected ear, and herpetic vesicular lesions in the auditory canal.

Labyrinthitis
+ Severe vertigo begins abruptly and may occur in a single episode or recur over months or years.

Ménière's disease
+ Labyrinthine dysfunction causes abrupt onset of vertigo, lasting minutes, hours, or days.

Motion sickness
+ Vertigo, nausea, vomiting, and headache occur in response to rhythmic or erratic motions.

Multiple sclerosis
+ Episodic vertigo may occur early and become persistent.

Seizures
+ Temporal lobe seizures may produce vertigo.

Vestibular neuritis
+ Severe vertigo usually begins abruptly and lasts several days.

Other causes
+ Use of overly warm or cold eardrops or irrigating solutions
+ Caloric testing
+ Ear surgery
+ High or toxic doses of certain drugs

Special considerations

+ Place the patient in a comfortable position.
+ Monitor vital signs and LOC.
+ Keep the bed's side rails up, or help the patient to a chair if he's standing when vertigo occurs.
+ Give drugs to control nausea and vomiting and decrease labyrinthine irritability.

Peds points

+ Ear infection and vestibular neuritis may cause vertigo.

Teaching points

+ Moving around with assistance
+ Avoiding sudden position changes and dangerous tasks

Key facts about vesicular rash

+ Appears as a scattered or linear distribution of blisterlike lesions that are usually less than 0.5 cm in diameter
+ May be filled with clear, cloudy, or bloody fluid

Key history points

+ Onset and characteristics of rash
+ Drug history
+ Associated signs and symptoms
+ Family history of skin disorders
+ History of allergies
+ Recent infections, insect bites, or exposure to allergens

Critical assessment steps

+ Note if skin is dry, oily, or moist.
+ Observe the distribution of the lesions; record their location.

Surgery and other procedures

Ear surgery may cause vertigo that lasts for several days. Also, administration of overly warm or cold eardrops or irrigating solutions can cause vertigo.

SPECIAL CONSIDERATIONS

Place the patient in a comfortable position, and monitor his vital signs and LOC. Keep the side rails up if he's in bed, or help him to a chair if he's standing when vertigo occurs. Darken the room and keep him calm. Administer drugs to control nausea and vomiting and meclizine or dimenhydrinate to decrease labyrinthine irritability.

Prepare the patient for diagnostic tests, such as electronystagmography, EEG, and X-rays of the middle and inner ears.

PEDIATRIC POINTERS

Ear infection is a common cause of vertigo in children. Vestibular neuritis may also cause this symptom.

PATIENT COUNSELING

If the patient is experiencing vertigo, tell him not to get out of bed or walk without assistance. Instruct the patient not to make sudden position changes and to avoid tasks that can be dangerous such as driving.

VESICULAR RASH

A vesicular rash is a scattered or linear distribution of blisterlike lesions — sharply circumscribed and filled with clear, cloudy, or bloody fluid. The lesions, which are usually less than 0.5 cm in diameter, may occur singly or in groups. (See *Recognizing common skin lesions,* pages 488 and 489.) They sometimes occur with bullae — fluid-filled lesions larger than 0.5 cm in diameter.

A vesicular rash may be mild or severe and temporary or permanent. It can result from infection, inflammation, or allergic reactions.

HISTORY

Ask your patient when the rash began, how it spread, and whether it has appeared before. Did other skin lesions precede eruption of the vesicles? Obtain a thorough drug history. If the patient has used a topical medication, what type did he use and when was it last applied? Also, ask about associated signs and symptoms. Find out if he has a family history of skin disorders, and ask about allergies, recent infections, insect bites, and exposure to allergens.

PHYSICAL ASSESSMENT

Examine the patient's skin, noting if it's dry, oily, or moist. Observe the general distribution of the lesions and record their exact location. Note the color, shape, and size of the lesions, and check for crusts, scales, scars, macules, papules, or wheals. Palpate the vesicles or bullae to determine if they're flaccid or tense. Slide your finger across the skin to see if the outer layer of epidermis separates easily from the basal layer (Nikolsky's sign).

MEDICAL CAUSES

Burns (second degree)

Second-degree burns include thermal burns that affect the epidermis and part of the dermis, which cause vesicles and bullae, erythema, swelling, pain, and moistness.

Dermatitis

With *contact dermatitis,* a hypersensitivity reaction produces an eruption of small vesicles surrounded by redness and marked edema. The vesicles may ooze, scale, and cause severe pruritus.

Dermatitis herpetiformis produces a chronic inflammatory eruption marked by vesicular, papular, bullous, pustular, or erythematous lesions. Usually, the rash is symmetrically distributed on the buttocks, shoulders, extensor surfaces of the elbows and knees, and sometimes the face, scalp, and neck. Other symptoms include severe pruritus, burning, and stinging.

 CULTURAL CUE *Dermatitis herpetiformis is more common in people of Northern European descent; it rarely occurs in Asians and Blacks.*

With *nummular dermatitis,* groups of pinpoint vesicles and papules appear on erythematous or pustular lesions that are nummular (coinlike) or annular (ringlike). Often, the pustular lesions ooze a purulent exudate, itch severely, and rapidly become crusted and scaly. Two or three lesions may develop on the hands, but the lesions typically develop on the extensor surfaces of the limbs and on the buttocks and posterior trunk.

Dermatophytid

Dermatophytid, also known as *ringworm,* is an allergic reaction to fungal infection. It produces vesicular lesions on the hands, usually in response to tinea pedis. The lesions are extremely pruritic and tender and may be accompanied by fever, anorexia, generalized adenopathy, and splenomegaly.

Herpes simplex

Herpes simplex is a common viral infection that produces groups of vesicles on an inflamed base, most commonly on the lips and lower face. In about 25% of cases of herpes simplex, the genital region is the site of involvement. Vesicles are preceded by itching, tingling, burning, or pain; develop singly or in groups; are 2 to 3 mm in size; and do not coalesce. Eventually, they rupture, forming a painful ulcer followed by a yellowish crust.

Herpes zoster

With herpes zoster, a vesicular rash is preceded by erythema and, occasionally, by a nodular skin eruption and unilateral, sharp, pain along a dermatome. About 5 days later, the lesions erupt and the pain becomes burning. Vesicles dry and scab about 10 days after eruption. Associated findings include fever, malaise, pruritus, and paresthesia or hyperesthesia of the involved area. Herpes zoster involving the cranial nerves produces facial palsy, hearing loss, dizziness, loss of taste, eye pain, and impaired vision.

Insect bites

With insect bites, vesicles appear on red hivelike papules and may become hemorrhagic. Nonspecific signs and symptoms may also occur, such as fever, myalgia, headache, lymphadenopathy, nausea, and vomiting.

Critical assessment steps *(continued)*

- ✦ Note characteristics of lesions; check for crusts, scales, scars, macules, papules, or wheals.
- ✦ Slide your finger across the skin to see if the outer layer of epidermis separates easily from the basal layer.

Medical causes

Burns (second degree)
- ✦ Vesicles and bullae, erythema, swelling, pain, and moistness are produced.

Dermatitis
- ✦ With contact dermatitis, small vesicles are surrounded by redness and marked edema.
- ✦ With dermatitis herpetiformis, vesicular, papular, bullous, pustular, or erythematous lesions form.
- ✦ With nummular dermatitis, groups of pinpoint vesicles and papules appear on erythematous or pustular lesions.

Dermatophytid
- ✦ Pruritic and tender vesicular lesions develop on the hands.

Herpes simplex
- ✦ Vesicles that are 2 to 3 mm in size and on an inflamed base, most commonly appear on the lips and lower face.

Herpes zoster
- ✦ A vesicular rash is preceded by erythema and, occasionally, by a nodular skin eruption and pain along a dermatome.

Insect bites
- ✦ Vesicles appear on red papules.

Medical causes
(continued)

Pompholyx (dyshidrosis or dyshidrosis eczema)
✦ Symmetrical vesicular lesions appear on the palms and soles.

Scabies
✦ Small vesicles erupt on an erythematous base and may be at the end of a threadlike burrow.

Smallpox
✦ A maculopapular rash on the mucosa of the mouth, pharynx, face and forearms spreads, then turns vesicular within 2 days.

Tinea pedis
✦ Vesicles and scaling develop between the toes.

Special considerations
✦ If necessary, start an I.V. line.
✦ Obtain cultures to determine the standard causative organism.
✦ Be alert for signs of secondary infection.
✦ Give the patient an antibiotic and apply corticosteroid or antimicrobial ointment to the lesions.

Peds points
✦ Pediatric causes include staphylococcal infections, varicella, hand-foot-and-mouth disease, contact dermatitis, and miliaria rubra.

Teaching points
✦ Importance of frequent handwashing
✦ Avoiding touching lesions
✦ Use of tepid baths or cold compresses to relieve itching

Pompholyx (dyshidrosis or dyshidrosis eczema)
Pompholyx is a common, recurrent disorder that produces symmetrical vesicular lesions that can become pustular. The pruritic lesions are more common on the palms than on the soles and may be accompanied by minimal erythema.

Scabies
With scabies, small vesicles erupt on an erythematous base and may be at the end of a threadlike burrow. Burrows are a few millimeters long, with a swollen nodule or red papule that contains the mite. Pustules and excoriations may also occur. Men may develop burrows on the glans, shaft, and scrotum; women may develop burrows on the nipples. Both sexes may develop burrows on the webs of the fingers, wrists, elbows, axillae, and waistline. Associated pruritus worsens with inactivity and warmth and at night.

Smallpox
Initial signs and symptoms of smallpox (variola major) include high fever, malaise, prostration, severe headache, backache, and abdominal pain. A maculopapular rash develops on the mucosa of the mouth, pharynx, face and forearms and then spreads to the trunk and legs. Within 2 days the rash becomes vesicular and later pustular. The lesions develop at the same time, appear identical, and are more prominent on the face and extremities. The pustules are round, firm, and deeply embedded in the skin. After 8 to 9 days, the pustules form a crust. Later, the scab separates from the skin, leaving a pitted scar. In fatal cases, death results from encephalitis, extensive bleeding, or secondary infection.

Tinea pedis
Tinea pedis, a fungal infection, causes vesicles and scaling between the toes and, possibly, scaling over the entire sole. Severe infection causes inflammation, pruritus, and difficulty walking.

SPECIAL CONSIDERATIONS
Any skin eruption that covers a large area may cause substantial fluid loss through the vesicles, bullae, or other weeping lesions. If necessary, start an I.V. line to replace fluids and electrolytes. Keep the patient's environment warm and free from drafts, cover him with sheets or blankets as necessary, and take his rectal temperature every 4 hours because increased fluid loss and increased blood flow to inflamed skin may lead to hyperthermia.

Obtain cultures to determine the standard causative organism. Use precautions until infection is ruled out. Be alert for signs of secondary infection. Give the patient an antibiotic and apply corticosteroid or antimicrobial ointment to the lesions.

PEDIATRIC POINTERS
Vesicular rashes in children are caused by staphylococcal infections (staphylococcal scalded skin syndrome is a life-threatening infection occurring in infants), varicella, hand-foot-and-mouth disease, contact dermatitis, and miliaria rubra.

PATIENT COUNSELING
Tell the patient to wash his hands often and not to touch the lesions. Tell the patient not to scratch the rash to avoid infection and scarring. Suggest a tepid bath using little soap and rinsing thoroughly to help relieve itching. Cold compresses may also relieve itching.

VISION LOSS

Vision loss—the inability to perceive visual stimuli—can be sudden or gradual and temporary or permanent. The deficit can range from a slight impairment of vision to total blindness. It can result from an ocular, a neurologic, or a systemic disorder or from trauma or the use of certain drugs. The ultimate visual outcome may depend on early, accurate diagnosis and treatment.

HISTORY

Sudden vision loss can signal an ocular emergency. (See *Managing sudden vision loss,* page 690.)

If the patient's vision loss occurred gradually, ask him if the vision loss affects one eye or both and all or only part of the visual field. Is the visual loss transient or persistent? Did the visual loss occur abruptly, or did it develop over hours, days, or weeks? What is the patient's age? Ask the patient if he has experienced photosensitivity, and ask him about the location, intensity, and duration of any eye pain. You should also obtain an ocular history and a family history of eye problems or systemic diseases that may lead to eye problems, such as hypertension; diabetes mellitus; thyroid, rheumatic, or vascular disease; infections; and cancer.

PHYSICAL ASSESSMENT

Don't touch the patient's eye if he has perforating or penetrating ocular trauma. The first step in performing the eye examination is to assess visual acuity, with best available correction in each eye. (See *Testing visual acuity,* page 691.)

Carefully inspect both eyes, noting edema, foreign bodies, drainage, or conjunctival or scleral redness. Observe whether lid closure is complete or incomplete, and check for ptosis. Using a flashlight, examine the cornea and iris for scars, irregularities, and foreign bodies. Observe the size, shape, and color of the pupils, and test the direct and consensual light reflex (see "Pupils, nonreactive," page 551) and the effect of accommodation. Evaluate extraocular muscle function by testing the six cardinal fields of gaze.

MEDICAL CAUSES

Amaurosis fugax
With amaurosis fugax, recurrent attacks of unilateral vision loss may last from a few seconds to a few minutes. Vision is normal at other times. Transient unilateral weakness, hypertension, and elevated intraocular pressure (IOP) in the affected eye may also occur.

Cataract
With a cataract, usually, painless and gradual visual blurring precedes vision loss. As the cataract progresses, the pupil turns milky white. Night blindness and halo vision may be early signs of this disorder.

Concussion
Immediately or shortly after blunt head trauma, which causes a concussion, vision may be blurred, double, or lost. Generally, vision loss is temporary. Other findings include headache, anterograde and retrograde amnesia, transient loss of consciousness, nausea, vomiting, dizziness, irritability, confusion, lethargy, and aphasia.

Key facts about vision loss
+ Ranges from slight impairment to total blindness

Key history points
+ Characteristics of vision loss
+ Associated photosensitivity or pain
+ Ocular history

Critical assessment steps
+ Don't touch the patient's eye if he has perforating or penetrating ocular trauma.
+ Assess visual acuity, with best available correction in each eye.
+ Inspect the eyes, noting edema, foreign bodies, drainage, or conjunctival or scleral redness.
+ Using a flashlight, examine the cornea and iris.
+ Observe the size, shape, and color of the pupils.
+ Test the direct and consensual light reflex and the effect of accommodation.

Medical causes
Amaurosis fugax
+ Recurrent attacks of unilateral vision loss may last from a few seconds to a few minutes.
+ Vision is normal at other times.

Cataract
+ Painless and gradual visual blurring precedes vision loss.

Concussion
+ Vision may be temporarily blurred, doubled, or lost.

Managing sudden vision loss

Sudden vision loss can signal central retinal artery occlusion or acute angle-closure glaucoma — ocular emergencies that require immediate intervention. If your patient reports sudden vision loss, immediately notify an ophthalmologist for an emergency examination, and perform these interventions:

For a patient with suspected central retinal artery occlusion, perform light massage over his closed eyelid. Increase his carbon dioxide level by administering a set flow of oxygen and carbon dioxide through a Venturi mask, or have the patient rebreathe in a paper bag to retain exhaled carbon dioxide. These steps will dilate the artery and, possibly, restore blood flow to the retina.

For a patient with suspected acute angle-closure glaucoma, measure intraocular pressure (IOP) with a tonometer. (You can also estimate IOP without a tonometer by placing your fingers over the patient's closed eyelid. A rock-hard eyeball usually indicates increased IOP.) Expect to instill timolol drops and administer I.V. acetazolamide to help decrease IOP.

Medical causes
(continued)

Diabetic retinopathy
◆ Retinal edema and hemorrhage lead to visual blurring, which may progress to blindness.

Endophthalmitis
◆ Permanent unilateral vision loss may result as well as headache, photophobia, and ocular discharge.

Glaucoma
◆ Gradual visual blurring may progress to total blindness.
◆ Acute angle-closure glaucoma may produce blindness within 3 to 5 days.
◆ Chronic open-angle glaucoma causes peripheral vision loss.

Herpes zoster
◆ When the nasociliary nerve is affected, bilateral vision loss is accompanied by eyelid lesions, conjunctivitis, skin lesions, and ocular muscle palsies.

Hyphema
◆ Blood in the anterior chamber can reduce vision to light perception only.

Keratitis
◆ Complete unilateral vision loss may occur with an opaque cornea, increased tearing, irritation, and photophobia.

Diabetic retinopathy
With diabetic retinopathy, retinal edema and hemorrhage lead to visual blurring, which may progress to blindness. The patient may also have a loss of central vision and color vision.

Endophthalmitis
Typically, endophthalmitis follows penetrating trauma, I.V. drug use, or intraocular surgery, causing possibly permanent unilateral vision loss; a sympathetic inflammation may affect the other eye. The patient with endophthalmitis may also experience headache, photophobia, and ocular discharge.

Glaucoma
Glaucoma produces gradual visual blurring that may progress to total blindness. Acute angle-closure glaucoma is an ocular emergency that may produce blindness within 3 to 5 days. Findings are rapid onset of unilateral inflammation and pain, pressure over the eye, moderate pupil dilation, nonreactive pupillary response, a cloudy cornea, reduced visual acuity, photophobia, and perception of blue or red halos around lights. Nausea and vomiting may also occur.

Chronic open-angle glaucoma is usually bilateral, with an insidious onset and a slowly progressive course. It causes peripheral vision loss, aching eyes, halo vision, and reduced visual acuity (especially at night).

Herpes zoster
When herpes zoster affects the nasociliary nerve, bilateral vision loss is accompanied by eyelid lesions, conjunctivitis, skin lesions that usually appear on the nose, and ocular muscle palsies.

Hyphema
With a hyphema, blood in the anterior chamber can reduce vision to light perception only. Other effects include moderate pain, conjunctival injection, and eyelid edema. Most hyphemas are the direct result of blunt trauma to the normal eye.

Keratitis
Keratitis (inflammation of the cornea) may lead to complete unilateral vision loss. Other findings include an opaque cornea, increased tearing, irritation, and photophobia.

Testing visual acuity

Use a Snellen letter chart to test visual acuity in the literate patient older than age 6. Have the patient sit or stand 20′ (6 m) from the chart. Then, tell him to cover his left eye and read aloud the smallest line of letters that he can see. Record the fraction assigned to that line on the chart (the numerator indicates distance from the chart; the denominator indicates the distance at which a normal eye can read the chart). Normal vision is 20/20. Repeat the test with the patient's right eye covered.

If your patient can't read the largest letter from a distance of 20′, have him approach the chart until he can read it. Then, record the distance between him and the chart as the numerator of the fraction. For example, if he can see the top line of the chart at a distance of 3′ (1 m), record the test result as 3/200.

Use a Snellen symbol chart to test children ages 3 to 6 and illiterate patients. Follow the same procedure as for the Snellen letter chart, but ask the patient to indicate the direction of the E's fingers as you point to each symbol.

SNELLEN LETTER CHART   **SNELLEN SYMBOL CHART**

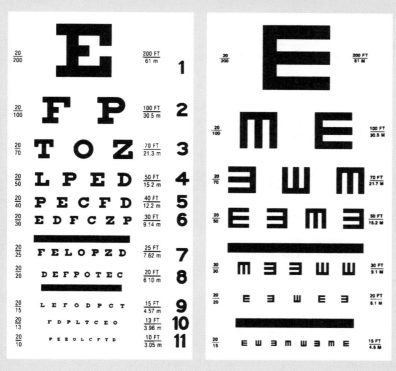

Ocular trauma

Following eye injury, sudden unilateral or bilateral vision loss may occur. Vision loss may be total or partial and permanent or temporary. The eyelids may be reddened, edematous, and lacerated; intraocular contents may be extruded.

Medical causes
(continued)

Ocular trauma
✦ Vision loss is sudden, total or partial, permanent or temporary

Medical causes
(continued)

Optic atrophy
+ Irreversible loss of the visual field and changes in color vision result.

Optic neuritis
+ Unilateral vision loss is temporary but severe.

Paget's disease
+ Bilateral vision loss may develop because of bony impingements on the cranial nerves.

Papilledema
+ Acute papilledema may lead to momentary blurring or transiently obscured vision; chimeric papilledema may cause vision loss.

Pituitary tumor
+ Blurred vision progresses to hemianopia and, possibly, unilateral blindness as tumor grows.

Retinal artery occlusion (central)
+ Unilateral vision loss is sudden.
+ Permanent blindness may occur within hours.

Retinal detachment
+ Painless vision loss may be gradual or sudden and total or partial.

Retinal vein occlusion (central)
+ Unilateral decrease in visual acuity may occur with variable vision loss.

Senile macular degeneration
+ Painless blurring or loss of central vision occurs.

Optic atrophy
Optic atrophy (degeneration of the optic nerve) can develop spontaneously or follow inflammation or edema of the nerve head, causing irreversible loss of the visual field with changes in color vision. Pupillary reactions are sluggish, and optic disk pallor is evident.

Optic neuritis
Optic neuritis usually produces temporary but severe unilateral vision loss. Pain around the eye occurs, especially with movement of the globe. This may occur with visual field defects and a sluggish pupillary response to light. Ophthalmoscopic examination commonly reveals hyperemia of the optic disk, blurred disk margins, and filling of the physiologic cup.

Paget's disease
With Paget's disease, bilateral vision loss may develop as a result of bony impingements on the cranial nerves. This occurs with hearing loss, tinnitus, vertigo, and severe, persistent bone pain. Cranial enlargement may be noticeable frontally and occipitally, and headaches may occur. Sites of bone involvement are warm and tender, and impaired mobility and pathologic fractures are common.

Papilledema
Papilledema is characterized by swelling of the optic disk from increased intracranial pressure; both optic disks are affected. Acute papilledema may lead to momentary blurring or transiently obscured vision, whereas chimeric papilledema may lead to vision loss.

Pituitary tumor
As a pituitary adenoma grows, blurred vision progresses to hemianopia and, possibly, unilateral blindness. Double vision, nystagmus, ptosis, limited eye movement, and headaches may also occur.

Retinal artery occlusion (central)
Retinal artery occlusion is a painless ocular emergency that causes sudden unilateral vision loss, which may be partial or complete. Pupil examination reveals a sluggish direct pupillary response and a normal consensual response. Permanent blindness may occur within hours.

Retinal detachment
Depending on the degree and location of retinal detachment, painless vision loss may be gradual or sudden and total or partial. Macular involvement causes total blindness.

With partial vision loss, the patient may describe visual field defects or a shadow or curtain over the visual field as well as visual floaters.

Retinal vein occlusion (central)
Most common in geriatric patients, retinal vein occlusion is a painless disorder that causes a unilateral decrease in visual acuity with variable vision loss. IOP may be elevated in both eyes.

Senile macular degeneration
Occurring in elderly patients, senile macular degeneration causes painless blurring or loss of central vision. Vision loss may proceed slowly or rapidly, eventually affecting both eyes. Visual acuity may be worse at night.

Temporal arteritis

Vision loss and visual blurring with a throbbing, unilateral headache characterize temporal arteritis. Other findings include malaise, anorexia, weight loss, weakness, low-grade fever, generalized muscle aches, and confusion.

Uveitis

Inflammation of the uveal tract may result in unilateral vision loss. Anterior uveitis produces moderate to severe eye pain, severe conjunctival injection, photophobia, and a small, nonreactive pupil. Posterior uveitis may produce insidious onset of blurred vision, conjunctival injection, visual floaters, pain, and photophobia. Associated posterior scar formation distorts the shape of the pupil.

Vitreous hemorrhage

With vitreous hemorrhage, sudden unilateral vision loss may result from intraocular trauma, ocular tumors, or systemic disease (especially diabetes, hypertension, sickle cell anemia, or leukemia). Visual floaters and partial vision with a reddish haze may occur. The patient's vision loss may be permanent.

OTHER CAUSES

Drugs

Chloroquine therapy may cause patchy retinal pigmentation that typically leads to blindness. Phenylbutazone may cause vision loss and increased susceptibility to retinal detachment. Cardiac glycoside derivatives, indomethacin, ethambutol, quinine sulfate, and methanol toxicity may also cause vision loss.

SPECIAL CONSIDERATIONS

If the patient reports photophobia, darken the room and suggest that he wear sunglasses during the day. Obtain cultures of any drainage, and instruct him not to touch the unaffected eye with anything that has come in contact with the affected eye.

PEDIATRIC POINTERS

Children who complain of slowly progressive vision loss may have an optic nerve glioma (a slow-growing, usually benign tumor) or retinoblastoma (a malignant tumor of the retina). Congenital rubella and syphilis may cause vision loss in infants. Retrolental fibroplasia may cause vision loss in premature infants. Other congenital causes of vision loss include Marfan syndrome, retinitis pigmentosa, and amblyopia.

GERIATRIC POINTERS

In elderly patients, reduced visual acuity may be caused by morphologic changes in the choroid, pigment epithelium, and retina or by decreased function of the rods, cones, and other neural elements. Elderly patients often have difficulty turning their eyes upward. IOP also increases with age.

PATIENT COUNSELING

Any degree of vision loss can be extremely frightening to your patient. To ease his fears, orient him to his environment and make sure it's safe, and announce your presence each time you approach him. Instruct him to wash his hands often and to avoid rubbing his eyes. If necessary, prepare him for surgery.

Medical causes
(continued)

Temporal arteritis
+ Vision loss and visual blurring with a headache occur.

Uveitis
+ Inflammation of the uveal tract may cause unilateral vision loss.

Vitreous hemorrhage
+ Unilateral vision loss is sudden.

Other causes
+ Cardiac glycoside derivatives
+ Chloroquine therapy
+ Ethambutol, indomethacin, phenylbutazone, and quinine sulfate
+ Methanol toxicity

Special considerations
+ For photophobia patients, darken the room and suggest wearing sunglasses during the day.

Peds points
+ Optic nerve gliomas and retinoblastomas may cause vision loss in children.
+ Congenital rubella and syphilis may cause vision loss in infants.

Geri points
+ Reduced visual acuity may be caused by morphologic changes in the choroid, pigment epithelium, and retina or by decreased function of the rods, cones, and other neural elements.

Teaching points
+ Orientation to environment
+ Importance of frequent handwashing and avoiding rubbing the eyes

Key facts about visual blurring

+ Refers to the loss of visual acuity with indistinct visual details

Key history points

+ Associated eye pain, trauma, sudden vision loss, or discharge
+ Onset of visual blurring
+ Medical and drug history

Critical assessment steps

+ Inspect the eye; note lid edema, drainage, conjunctival or scleral redness, an irregularly shaped iris, and excessive blinking.
+ Assess for pupillary changes.
+ Test visual acuity in both eyes.

Medical causes

Brain tumor
+ Visual blurring may occur along with decreased LOC, headache, memory loss, and other neuro-logic signs and symptoms.

Cataract
+ Gradual blurring may occur.

Concussion
+ Vision may be blurred, double, or temporarily lost.

Conjunctivitis
+ Visual blurring may be accompanied by photophobia, pain, burning, tearing, itching, and a feeling of fullness around the eyes.

VISUAL BLURRING

Visual blurring is a common symptom that refers to the loss of visual acuity with indistinct visual details. It may result from eye injury, a neurologic or eye disorder, or a disorder with vascular complications, such as diabetes mellitus. Visual blurring may also result from mucus passing over the cornea, a refractive error, improperly fitted contact lenses, or certain drugs.

HISTORY

If your patient has visual blurring accompanied by sudden, severe eye pain, a history of trauma, or sudden vision loss, order an ophthalmologic examination. If the patient has a penetrating or perforating eye injury, don't touch the eye.

If the patient isn't in distress, ask him how long he has had the visual blurring. Does it occur only at certain times? Ask about associated signs and symptoms, such as pain or discharge. If visual blurring followed injury, obtain details of the accident, and ask if vision was impaired immediately after the injury. Obtain a medical and drug history.

PHYSICAL ASSESSMENT

Inspect the patient's eye, noting lid edema, drainage, or conjunctival or scleral redness. Also note an irregularly shaped iris, which may indicate previous trauma, and excessive blinking, which may indicate corneal damage. Assess the patient for pupillary changes. Test visual acuity in both eyes. (See *Testing visual acuity*, page 691.)

MEDICAL CAUSES

Brain tumor

Visual blurring may occur with a brain tumor. Associated findings include decreased level of consciousness (LOC), headache, apathy, behavioral changes, memory loss, decreased attention span, dizziness, and confusion. A tumor can also cause aphasia, seizures, ataxia, and signs of hormonal imbalance. Its later effects are papilledema, vomiting, increased systolic blood pressure, widened pulse pressure, and decorticate posture.

Cataract

A cataract is a painless disorder that causes gradual visual blurring. Other effects of a cataract include halo vision (an early sign), visual glare in bright light, progressive vision loss, and a gray pupil that later turns milky white.

Concussion

Immediately or shortly after blunt head trauma, which causes a concussion, vision may be blurred, double, or temporarily lost. Other findings include changes in LOC and behavior.

Conjunctivitis

With conjunctivitis, visual blurring may be accompanied by photophobia, pain, burning, tearing, itching, and a feeling of fullness around the eyes. Other findings include redness near the fornices (brilliant red suggests a bacterial cause; milky red, an allergic cause) and drainage (copious, mucopurulent, and flaky in bacterial conjunctivitis; stringy in allergic conjunctivitis). Copious tearing, minimal exudate, and an enlarged preauricular lymph node occur with viral conjunctivitis.

Corneal abrasions

With corneal abrasions, visual blurring may occur with severe eye pain, especially when the eyelid moves over the abrasion. The patient may also have photophobia, redness, and excessive tearing.

Diabetic retinopathy

With diabetic retinopathy, retinal edema and hemorrhage produce gradual blurring, which may progress to blindness. The patient may also have a loss of central vision and color vision.

Eye tumor

If the eye tumor involves the macula, visual blurring may be the presenting symptom. Related findings include varying visual field losses.

Glaucoma

With acute angle-closure glaucoma, an ocular emergency, unilateral visual blurring and severe pain begin suddenly. Other findings include halo vision; a moderately dilated, nonreactive pupil; conjunctival injection; a cloudy cornea; and decreased visual acuity. Severely elevated intraocular pressure (IOP) may cause nausea and vomiting.

With chronic angle-closure glaucoma, transient visual blurring and halo vision may precede pain and blindness.

Hypertension

Hypertension may cause visual blurring and a constant morning headache that decreases in severity during the day. If diastolic blood pressure exceeds 120 mm Hg, the patient may report a severe, throbbing headache. Associated findings include restlessness, confusion, nausea, vomiting, seizures, and decreased LOC.

Hyphema

Blunt eye trauma with hemorrhage into the anterior chamber causes visual blurring. Other effects of hyphemas include moderate pain, diffuse conjunctival injection, visible blood in the anterior chamber, ecchymoses, eyelid edema, and a hard eye.

Iritis

Acute iritis causes sudden visual blurring, moderate to severe eye pain, photophobia, conjunctival injection, and a constricted pupil. Assessment reveals a poor pupillary response to light.

Migraine headache

A migraine may cause visual blurring and paroxysmal attacks of severe, throbbing, unilateral or bilateral headache. Other effects include nausea, vomiting, sensitivity to light and noise, and sensory or visual auras.

Multiple sclerosis

Blurred vision, diplopia, and paresthesia may occur in the early stages of multiple sclerosis. Later effects vary and may include nystagmus, muscle weakness, paralysis, spasticity, hyperreflexia, intention tremor, and ataxic gait. Urinary frequency, urgency, and incontinence may also occur.

Medical causes
(continued)

Corneal abrasions
✦ Visual blurring may occur with severe eye pain.

Diabetic retinopathy
✦ Retinal edema and hemorrhage produce gradual blurring.

Eye tumor
✦ If the macula is involved, blurring may be the presenting symptom.

Glaucoma
✦ With acute angle-closure glaucoma, unilateral visual blurring and severe pain begin suddenly.
✦ With chronic angle-closure glaucoma, transient visual blurring and halo vision may precede pain and blindness.

Hypertension
✦ Visual blurring and a constant morning headache occur.

Hyphema
✦ Blunt eye trauma with hemorrhage into the anterior chamber causes visual blurring.

Iritis
✦ Sudden blurring, eye pain, photophobia, conjunctival injection, and a constricted pupil develop.

Migraine headache
✦ Blurring and paroxysmal attacks of headache may occur.

Multiple sclerosis
✦ Blurred vision, diplopia, and paresthesia may occur early.

Medical causes
(continued)

Optic neuritis
◆ Inflammation, degeneration, or demyelinization of the optic nerve causes an acute attack of blurring and vision loss.

Retinal detachment
◆ Sudden blurring may be followed by visual floaters and recurring light flashes.

Retinal vein occlusion (central)
◆ Gradual unilateral visual blurring and varying degrees of vision loss occur.

Senile macular degeneration
◆ Initially, painless visual blurring worsens at night.

Serous retinopathy (central)
◆ Blurring may accompany darkened vision in the affected eye.

Stroke
◆ Brief attacks of bilateral visual blurring may precede or accompany a stroke.

Temporal arteritis
◆ Sudden blurred vision is accompanied by vision loss and a throbbing unilateral headache.

Uveitis (posterior)
◆ Blurred vision, conjunctival injection, visual floaters, pain, and photophobia may develop.

Vitreous hemorrhage
◆ Sudden unilateral visual blurring and varying vision loss occur.

Optic neuritis
Inflammation, degeneration, or demyelinization of the optic nerve usually causes an acute attack of visual blurring and vision loss. Related findings include scotomas and eye pain. Ophthalmoscopic examination reveals hyperemia of the optic disk, large vein distention, blurred disk margins, and filling of the physiologic cup.

Retinal detachment
Sudden visual blurring may be the initial symptom of retinal detachment. Blurring worsens, accompanied by visual floaters and recurring flashes of light. Progressive detachment increases vision loss.

Retinal vein occlusion (central)
Retinal vein occlusion is a painless disorder that causes gradual unilateral visual blurring and varying degrees of vision loss. IOP may be elevated in both eyes.

Senile macular degeneration
Senile macular degeneration may cause painless visual blurring (initially worse at night), loss of central vision and slowly or rapidly progressive vision loss. Vision loss may proceed, eventually affecting both eyes.

Serous retinopathy (central)
With serous retinopathy, visual blurring may accompany darkened vision in the affected eye. The patient may report a blind spot in his visual field and that straight lines appear distorted.

Stroke
Brief attacks of bilateral visual blurring may precede or accompany a stroke. Associated findings include decreased LOC, contralateral hemiplegia, dysarthria, dysphagia, ataxia, unilateral sensory loss, and apraxia. Stroke may also cause agnosia, aphasia, homonymous hemianopia, diplopia, disorientation, memory loss, and poor judgment. Other features include urine retention or urinary incontinence, constipation, personality changes, emotional lability, headache, vomiting, and seizures.

Temporal arteritis
Most common in women older than age 60, temporal arteritis causes sudden blurred vision accompanied by vision loss and a throbbing unilateral headache in the temporal or frontotemporal region. Prodromal signs and symptoms include malaise, anorexia, weight loss, weakness, low-grade fever, and generalized muscle aches. Other findings include confusion; disorientation; swollen, nodular, tender temporal arteries; and erythema of overlying skin.

Uveitis (posterior)
Uveitis may produce insidious onset of blurred vision, conjunctival injection, visual floaters, pain, and photophobia. Associated posterior scar formation distorts the shape of the pupil.

Vitreous hemorrhage
Sudden unilateral visual blurring and varying vision loss occur with vitreous hemorrhage. Visual floaters or dark streaks may also occur. The patient may have partial vision with a reddish haze.

OTHER CAUSES

Drugs

Visual blurring may stem from the effects of cycloplegics, guanethidine, reserpine, clomiphene, phenylbutazone, thiazide diuretics, antihistamines, anticholinergics, or phenothiazines.

SPECIAL CONSIDERATIONS

Prepare the patient for diagnostic tests, such as tonometry, slit-lamp examination, X-rays of the skull and orbit and, if a neurologic lesion is suspected, a computed tomography scan.

PEDIATRIC POINTERS

Visual blurring in children may stem from congenital syphilis, congenital cataracts, refractive errors, eye injuries or infections, and increased intracranial pressure. Refer the child to an ophthalmologist if appropriate.

Test vision in school-age children as you would in adults; test children ages 3 to 6 with the Snellen symbol chart. (See *Testing visual acuity*, page 691.) Test toddlers with Allen cards, each illustrated with a familiar object, such as an animal. Ask the child to cover one eye and identify the objects as you flash them. Then, ask him to identify them as you gradually back away. Record the maximum distance at which he can identify at least three pictures.

PATIENT COUNSELING

As necessary, teach the patient how to instill ophthalmic medication. If visual blurring leads to permanent vision loss, provide emotional support, orient the patient to his surroundings, and provide for his safety. If necessary, prepare him for surgery.

VISUAL FLOATERS

Visual floaters are particles of blood or cellular debris that move about in the vitreous. As these enter the visual field, they appear as spots or dots. Chronic floaters may occur normally in elderly or myopic patients. However, the sudden onset of visual floaters commonly signals retinal detachment, an ocular emergency.

 EMERGENCY ACTIONS Sudden onset of visual floaters may signal retinal detachment. Does the patient also see flashing lights or spots in the affected eye? Is he experiencing a curtainlike loss of vision? If so, notify an ophthalmologist immediately. Restrict his eye movements until the diagnosis is made.

HISTORY

If the patient's condition permits, obtain a drug and allergy history. Ask about any nearsightedness (a predisposing factor), use of corrective lenses, eye trauma, or other eye disorders. Also ask about a history of granulomatous disease, diabetes mellitus, or hypertension, which may have predisposed him to retinal detachment, vitreous hemorrhage, or uveitis.

Other causes

+ Cycloplegics, guanethidine, reserpine, clomiphene, phenylbutazone, thiazide diuretics, antihistamines, anticholinergics, or phenothiazines

Special considerations

+ Prepare the patient for diagnostic tests.

Peds points

+ Blurring may stem from congenital syphilis or cataracts, refractive errors, eye injuries or infections, and increased ICP.

Teaching points

+ How to instill drugs
+ Orientation to the environment

Key facts about visual floaters

+ Particles of blood or cellular debris that move about in vitreous
+ Appear as spots or dots on the visual field

In an emergency

+ Notify an ophthalmologist and restrict eye movemenet if you suspect retinal detachment.

Key history points

+ Drug and allergy history
+ Use of corrective lenses
+ History of nearsightedness

Critical assessment steps

+ Inspect the eyes for injury.
+ Determine visual acuity.

Medical causes

Retinal detachment
+ Floaters and light flashes appear suddenly in the visual field where the retina is detached.

Uveitis (posterior)
+ Visual floaters, gradual eye pain, photophobia, blurred vision, and conjunctival injection may occur.

Vitreous hemorrhage
+ A shower of red or black dots or a red haze occurs across the visual field.

Special considerations

+ Ensure the patient's safety as needed.

Peds points

+ Visual floaters in children usually follow trauma.

Geri points

+ Elderly patients may experience increased myopia caused by lens changes.

Teaching points

+ Importance of not touching or rubbing eyes
+ Avoiding straining or sudden movements

PHYSICAL ASSESSMENT

If appropriate, inspect the patient's eyes for signs of injury, such as bruising or edema, and determine his visual acuity. (See *Testing visual acuity,* page 691.)

MEDICAL CAUSES

Retinal detachment

Floaters and light flashes appear suddenly in the portion of the visual field where the retina is detached from the choroid. As the retina detaches further (a painless process), gradual vision loss occurs, likened to a cloud or curtain falling in front of the eyes. Ophthalmoscopic examination reveals a gray, opaque, detached retina with an indefinite margin. Retinal vessels appear almost black.

Uveitis (posterior)

Uveitis may cause visual floaters accompanied by gradual eye pain, photophobia, blurred vision, and conjunctival injection. Associated posterior scar formation distorts the shape of the pupil.

Vitreous hemorrhage

Rupture of retinal vessels produces a shower of red or black dots or a red haze across the visual field. Vision is suddenly blurred in the affected eye, and visual acuity may be greatly reduced.

SPECIAL CONSIDERATIONS

Encourage bed rest and provide a calm environment. Depending on the cause, the patient may require eye patches, surgery, a corticosteroid, or other drug therapy. If bilateral eye patches are necessary—as with retinal detachment—you will need to ensure the patient's safety. Place pillows or towels behind the patient's head to maintain the appropriate patient position.

PEDIATRIC POINTERS

Visual floaters in children usually follow trauma that causes retinal detachment or vitreous hemorrhage. However, they may also result from vitreous debris, a benign congenital condition that has no other signs or symptoms.

GERIATRIC POINTERS

Elderly patients may experience increased myopia caused by lens changes. Also, the closest distance at which one can see clearly slowly decreases with age.

PATIENT COUNSELING

If both of the patient's eyes are patched, you should identify yourself when you approach him and orient him to time frequently. Provide sensory stimulation, such as a radio or tape player. Be sure to warn him not to touch or rub his eyes and to avoid straining or sudden movements.

VOMITING

Vomiting is the forceful expulsion of gastric contents through the mouth. Characteristically preceded by nausea, vomiting results from a coordinated sequence of abdominal muscle contractions and reverse esophageal peristalsis.

A common sign of GI disorders, vomiting also occurs with fluid and electrolyte imbalances; infections; and metabolic, endocrine, labyrinthine, central nervous system (CNS), and cardiac disorders. It can also result from drug therapy, surgery, or radiation.

Vomiting occurs normally during the first trimester of pregnancy, but its subsequent development may signal complications. It can also result from stress, anxiety, pain, alcohol intoxication, overeating, or ingestion of distasteful foods or liquids.

HISTORY

Ask your patient to describe the onset, duration, and intensity of his vomiting. What started the vomiting? What makes it subside? If possible, collect, measure, and inspect the character of the vomitus. (See *Vomitus: Characteristics and causes,* page 700.) Explore any associated complaints, particularly nausea, abdominal pain, anorexia and weight loss, changes in bowel habits or stools, excessive belching or flatus, and bloating or fullness.

Obtain a medical history, noting GI, endocrine, and metabolic disorders; recent infections; and cancer, including chemotherapy or radiation therapy. Ask about current medication use and alcohol consumption. If the patient is a female of childbearing age, ask if she is or could be pregnant. Ask which contraceptive method she's using.

PHYSICAL ASSESSMENT

Inspect the abdomen for distention, and auscultate for bowel sounds and bruits. Palpate for rigidity and tenderness, and test for rebound tenderness. Next, palpate and percuss the liver for enlargement. Assess other body systems as appropriate.

During the assessment, keep in mind that projectile vomiting *unaccompanied* by nausea may indicate increased intracranial pressure (ICP), a life-threatening emergency. If this occurs in a patient with CNS injury, you should quickly check his vital signs. Be alert for widened pulse pressure or bradycardia.

MEDICAL CAUSES

Adrenal insufficiency
Common GI findings associated with adrenal insufficiency include vomiting, nausea, anorexia, and diarrhea. Other findings include weakness; fatigue; weight loss; bronze skin; orthostatic hypotension; and weak, irregular pulse.

Anthrax (GI)
With anthrax, initial signs and symptoms after eating contaminated meat from an infected animal include vomiting, loss of appetite, nausea, and fever. Signs and symptoms may progress to abdominal pain, severe bloody diarrhea, and hematemesis.

Appendicitis
With appendicitis, vomiting and nausea may follow or accompany abdominal pain. Pain typically begins as vague epigastric or periumbilical discomfort and rapidly progresses to severe, stabbing pain in the right lower quadrant. The patient general-

Vomitus: Characteristics and causes

When you collect a sample of the patient's vomitus, observe it carefully for clues to the underlying disorder. Here's what vomitus may indicate:

BILE-STAINED (GREENISH) VOMITUS
Obstruction below the pylorus, as from a duodenal lesion

BLOODY VOMITUS
Upper GI bleeding (if bright red may result from gastritis or a peptic ulcer; if dark red, from esophageal or gastric varices)

BROWN VOMITUS WITH A FECAL ODOR
Intestinal obstruction or infarction

BURNING, BITTER-TASTING VOMITUS
Excessive hydrochloric acid in gastric contents

COFFEE-GROUND VOMITUS
Digested blood from slowly bleeding gastric or duodenal lesion

UNDIGESTED FOOD
Gastric outlet obstruction, as from gastric tumor or ulcer

Medical causes
(continued)

Bulimia
✦ Characterized by polyphagia that alternates with self-induced vomiting, fasting, or diarrhea.

Cholecystitis (acute)
✦ Nausea and mild vomiting commonly follow severe right-upper-quadrant pain that may radiate to the back or shoulders.

Cholelithiasis
✦ Nausea and vomiting accompany severe unlocalized right-upper-quadrant or epigastric pain after ingestion of fatty foods.

Cirrhosis
✦ Nausea and vomiting, anorexia, aching abdominal pain, and constipation or diarrhea occur early.

E. coli 0157:H7
✦ Vomiting, watery or bloody diarrhea, nausea, fever, and abdominal cramps occur.

---

ly has a positive McBurney's sign — severe pain and tenderness on palpation about 2″ (5 cm) from the right anterior superior spine of the ilium, on a line between that spine and the umbilicus. Associated findings usually include abdominal rigidity and tenderness, anorexia, constipation or diarrhea, cutaneous hyperalgesia, fever, tachycardia, and malaise.

Bulimia
Most common in women ages 18 to 29, bulimia is characterized by polyphagia that alternates with self-induced vomiting, fasting, or diarrhea. It's commonly accompanied by anorexia. The patient typically weighs less than normal but has a morbid fear of obesity. Self-induced vomiting may be evidenced by calloused knuckles.

Cholecystitis (acute)
With acute cholecystitis, nausea and mild vomiting commonly follow severe right-upper-quadrant pain that may radiate to the back or shoulders. Associated findings include abdominal tenderness and, possibly, rigidity and distention, fever, and diaphoresis.

Cholelithiasis
Nausea and vomiting accompany severe unlocalized right-upper-quadrant or epigastric pain after ingestion of fatty foods. Other findings in cholelithiasis include abdominal tenderness and guarding, flatulence, belching, epigastric burning, pyrosis, tachycardia, and restlessness.

Cirrhosis
Insidious early signs and symptoms of cirrhosis typically include nausea and vomiting, anorexia, aching abdominal pain, and constipation or diarrhea. Later findings include jaundice, hepatomegaly, and abdominal distention.

Escherichia coli 0157:H7
The signs and symptoms of E. coli include vomiting, watery or bloody diarrhea, nausea, fever, and abdominal cramps. In children younger than age 5 and elderly

patients, hemolytic uremic syndrome may develop in which the red blood cells are destroyed, and this may ultimately lead to acute renal failure.

Ectopic pregnancy

Vomiting, nausea, vaginal bleeding, and lower abdominal pain occur in ectopic pregnancy, a potentially life-threatening disorder. The patient with an ectopic pregnancy may have a tender adrenal mass and a 1- to -2-month history of amenorrhea.

Electrolyte imbalances

Electrolyte imbalances such as hyponatremia, hypernatremia, hypokalemia, and hypercalcemia frequently cause nausea and vomiting. Other effects include arrhythmias, tremors, seizures, anorexia, malaise, and weakness.

Food poisoning

Vomiting is a common finding in food poisoning. Diarrhea, severe, cramping abdominal pain, prostration, and fever also usually occur.

Gastritis

Nausea and vomiting of mucus or blood are common with gastritis, especially after ingestion of alcohol, aspirin, spicy foods, or caffeine. Epigastric pain, belching, and fever may occur.

Gastroenteritis

Gastroenteritis causes nausea, vomiting (often of undigested food), diarrhea, and abdominal cramping. Fever, malaise, hyperactive bowel sounds, and abdominal pain and tenderness may also occur.

Heart failure

Nausea and vomiting may occur, especially with right-sided heart failure. Associated findings include tachycardia, ventricular gallop, fatigue, dyspnea, crackles, peripheral edema, and jugular vein distention.

Hepatitis

Vomiting commonly follows nausea as an early sign of viral hepatitis. Other early findings include fatigue, myalgia, arthralgia, headache, photophobia, anorexia, pharyngitis, cough, and fever.

Hyperemesis gravidarum

Unremitting nausea and vomiting that last beyond the first trimester characterize hyperemesis gravidarum, a disorder of pregnancy. Vomitus contains undigested food, mucus, and small amounts of bile early in the disorder; later, it has a coffee-ground appearance. Associated findings include weight loss, headache, and delirium.

Increased intracranial pressure

Projectile vomiting that isn't preceded by nausea is a sign of increased ICP. The patient may exhibit a decreased level of consciousness (LOC) and Cushing's triad (bradycardia, hypertension, and respiratory pattern changes). He may also have headache, widened pulse pressure, impaired motor movement, vision disturbances, pupillary changes, and papilledema.

Medical causes
(continued)

Ectopic pregnancy
✦ Vomiting, nausea, vaginal bleeding, and lower abdominal pain occur.

Electrolyte imbalances
✦ Nausea and vomiting frequently occur along with arrhythmias, tremors, seizures, anorexia, malaise, and weakness.

Food poisoning
✦ Vomiting, diarrhea, cramping abdominal pain, prostration, and fever are common.

Gastritis
✦ Nausea and vomiting of mucus or blood are common.

Gastroenteritis
✦ Nausea, vomiting (often of undigested food), diarrhea, and abdominal cramping occur.

Heart failure
✦ Nausea and vomiting may occur, especially with right-sided heart failure.

Hepatitis
✦ Nausea and vomiting, fatigue, myalgia, arthralgia, headache, photophobia, anorexia, pharyngitis, cough, and fever are early findings.

Hyperemesis gravidarum
✦ Nausea and vomiting is unremitting and lasts beyond the first trimester.

Increased ICP
✦ Projectile vomiting isn't preceded by nausea.

Medical causes
(continued)

Intestinal obstruction
+ Nausea and vomiting (bilious or fecal) are common.

Labyrinthitis
+ Nausea, vomiting, vertigo, hearing loss, and nystagmus occur.

Ménière's disease
+ Sudden, brief, recurrent attacks of nausea and vomiting, dizziness, vertigo, hearing loss, tinnitus, and nystagmus occur.

Mesenteric artery ischemia
+ Nausea and vomiting and cramping abdominal pain occur, especially after meals.

Mesenteric venous thrombosis
+ Nausea, vomiting, and abdominal pain occur along with diarrhea or constipation, hematemesis, and melena.

Metabolic acidosis
+ Nausea, vomiting, anorexia, diarrhea, Kussmaul's respirations, and decreased LOC may occur.

Migraine headache
+ Nausea and vomiting are prodromal signs and symptoms.

Motion sickness
+ Rhythmic or erratic motion causes nausea and vomiting.

Myocardial infarction
+ Nausea and vomiting may occur, but the cardinal symptom is severe substernal chest pain.

Pancreatitis (acute)
+ Vomiting is an early sign.

Intestinal obstruction
Nausea and vomiting (bilious or fecal) are common with intestinal obstruction, especially of the upper small intestine. Abdominal pain is usually episodic and colicky but can become severe and steady. Constipation occurs early in large intestinal obstruction and late in small intestinal obstruction. Obstipation, however, may signal complete obstruction. In partial obstruction bowel sounds are typically high pitched and hyperactive; in complete obstruction, hypoactive or absent. Abdominal distention and tenderness also occur, possibly with visible peristaltic waves and a palpable abdominal mass.

Labyrinthitis
Nausea and vomiting commonly occur with labyrinthitis, an acute inner ear inflammation. Other findings in labyrinthitis include severe vertigo, progressive hearing loss, nystagmus, and possibly otorrhea.

Ménière's disease
Ménière's disease causes sudden, brief, recurrent attacks of nausea and vomiting, dizziness, vertigo, hearing loss, tinnitus, diaphoresis, and nystagmus. Hearing loss may be progressive and tinnitus may persist between attacks.

Mesenteric artery ischemia
Mesenteric artery ischemia is a life-threatening disorder that may cause nausea and vomiting and severe, cramping abdominal pain, especially after meals. Other findings include diarrhea or constipation, abdominal tenderness and bloating, anorexia, weight loss, and abdominal bruits.

Mesenteric venous thrombosis
With mesenteric venous thrombosis, insidious or acute onset of nausea, vomiting, and abdominal pain occurs along with diarrhea or constipation, abdominal distention, hematemesis, and melena.

Metabolic acidosis
Metabolic acidosis may produce nausea, vomiting, anorexia, diarrhea, Kussmaul's respirations, and decreased LOC.

Migraine headache
Nausea and vomiting are prodromal signs and symptoms of a migraine headache. Fatigue, photophobia, light flashes, increased noise sensitivity, and possibly partial vision loss and paresthesia also occur.

Motion sickness
Rhythmic or erratic motion causes nausea and vomiting that may be accompanied by headache, vertigo, dizziness, fatigue, diaphoresis, and dyspnea.

Myocardial infarction
Nausea and vomiting may occur, but the cardinal symptom of myocardial infarction is severe substernal chest pain, which may radiate to the left arm, jaw, or neck. Dyspnea, pallor, clammy skin, diaphoresis, and restlessness also occur.

Pancreatitis (acute)
Vomiting, usually preceded by nausea, is an early sign of pancreatitis. Associated findings include steady, severe epigastric or left-upper-quadrant pain that may radiate to the back, abdominal tenderness and rigidity, hypoactive bowel sounds, anorexia, vomiting, and fever. Tachycardia, restlessness, hypotension, skin mottling, and cold, sweaty extremities may occur in severe cases.

Peptic ulcer

Nausea and vomiting may follow sharp, burning or gnawing epigastric pain, especially when the stomach is empty or after ingestion of alcohol, caffeine, or aspirin. Attacks are relieved by eating or taking antacids. Hematemesis or melena may also occur.

Peritonitis

With peritonitis, nausea and vomiting usually accompany acute abdominal pain in the area of inflammation. Other findings include high fever with chills; tachycardia; hypoactive or absent bowel sounds; abdominal distention, rigidity, and tenderness; weakness; pale, cold skin; diaphoresis; hypotension; signs of dehydration; and shallow respirations.

Preeclampsia

Nausea and vomiting are common with preeclampsia, a disorder of pregnancy. Rapid weight gain, epigastric pain, generalized edema, elevated blood pressure, oliguria, severe frontal headache, and blurred or double vision also occur.

Renal and urologic disorders

Cystitis, pyelonephritis, calculi, and other renal and urologic disorders can cause vomiting. Accompanying findings reflect the specific disorder. Persistent nausea and vomiting are typical findings in patients with acute or worsening chronic renal failure.

Thyrotoxicosis

With thyrotoxicosis, nausea and vomiting may accompany the classic findings of severe anxiety, heat intolerance, weight loss despite increased appetite, diaphoresis, diarrhea, tremors, tachycardia, and palpitations. Other findings include exophthalmos, ventricular or atrial gallop, and an enlarged thyroid gland.

Ulcerative colitis

Vomiting, nausea, and anorexia may occur, but the most common sign of ulcerative colitis is recurrent diarrhea with blood, pus, and mucus. Fever, chills, and weight loss are other common signs and symptoms.

OTHER CAUSES

Drugs

Drugs that commonly cause vomiting include antineoplastics, opiates, ferrous sulfate, levodopa, oral potassium, chloride replacements, estrogens, sulfasalazine, antibiotics, quinidine, anesthetics, and overdoses of cardiac glycosides and theophylline. Syrup of ipecac is used to treat overdoses by inducing vomiting.

Radiation and surgery

Radiation therapy may cause nausea and vomiting if it disrupts the gastric mucosa. Postoperative nausea and vomiting are common, especially after abdominal surgery.

SPECIAL CONSIDERATIONS

Draw blood to determine fluid, electrolyte, and acid-base balance. (Prolonged vomiting can cause dehydration, electrolyte imbalances, and metabolic alkalosis.) Keep the patient's room fresh and clean smelling by removing bedpans and emesis basins promptly after use. Elevate his head or position him on his side to prevent

---

Medical causes
(continued)
Peptic ulcer
✦ Nausea and vomiting may follow epigastric pain.

Peritonitis
✦ Nausea and vomiting usually accompany acute abdominal pain.

Preeclampsia
✦ Nausea and vomiting occur with rapid weight gain, epigastric pain, edema, elevated blood pressure, oliguria, headache, and blurred or double vision.

Renal and urologic disorders
✦ Vomiting may occur.

Thyrotoxicosis
✦ Nausea and vomiting may accompany the classic findings.

Ulcerative colitis
✦ Vomiting, nausea, and anorexia may occur with the common sign of recurrent diarrhea with blood, pus, and mucus.

Other causes
✦ Anesthetics, antibiotics, antineoplastics, chloride replacements, estrogens, ferrous sulfate, levodopa, opiates, oral potassium, quinidine, sulfasalazine
✦ Overdoses of cardiac glycosides and theophylline
✦ Radiation therapy
✦ Surgery

Special considerations
✦ Draw blood to determine electrolyte and acid-base balance.
✦ Position the patient to prevent aspiration of vomitus.

Special considerations
(continued)

✦ Monitor vital signs and intake and output.
✦ Maintain hydration.
✦ Give pain medications promptly. If possible, give these by injection or suppository.
✦ If an opioid is used to treat pain, monitor bowel sounds, flatus, and bowel movements.

Peds points

✦ In a neonate, pyloric obstruction may cause projectile vomiting; Hirschsprung's disease may cause fecal vomiting.
✦ Intussusception may lead to vomiting of bile and fecal matter.

Geri points

✦ Rule out intestinal ischemia first because it's especially common in patients of this age-group.

Teaching points

✦ Deep-breathing techniques
✦ Replacing fluid losses

Key facts about vulvar lesions

✦ Refer to cutaneous lumps, nodules, papules, vesicles, or ulcers that appear on the vulva

Key history points

✦ Onset of vulvar lesions
✦ Associated features, such as as swelling, pain, or discharge
✦ Potential for STD exposure

Critical assessment steps

✦ Examine the lesion.
✦ Obtain cultures.

---

aspiration of vomitus. Continuously monitor vital signs and intake and output (including vomitus and liquid stools). If necessary, administer I.V. fluids or have the patient sip clear liquids to maintain hydration.

Because pain can precipitate or intensify nausea and vomiting, administer pain medications promptly. If possible, give these by injection or suppository to prevent exacerbating associated nausea. If an opioid is used to treat pain, monitor bowel sounds, flatus, and bowel movements carefully because they may slow down GI motility and exacerbate vomiting. If you administer an antiemetic, be alert for abdominal distention and hypoactive bowel sounds, which may indicate gastric retention. If this occurs, insert a nasogastric tube.

PEDIATRIC POINTERS

In a neonate, pyloric obstruction may cause projectile vomiting, whereas Hirschsprung's disease may cause fecal vomiting. Intussusception may lead to vomiting of bile and fecal matter in an infant or toddler. Because an infant may aspirate vomitus as a result of his immature cough and gag reflexes, position him on his side or abdomen and clear any vomitus immediately.

GERIATRIC POINTERS

Although elderly patients can develop several of the disorders mentioned earlier, always rule out intestinal ischemia first — it's especially common in patients of this age-group, and it has a high mortality rate.

PATIENT COUNSELING

Have the patient breathe deeply to ease his nausea and help prevent further vomiting. Advise him to replace fluid losses to avoid dehydration. A patient suffering from migraine headaches should be advised that vomiting may be a prodromal symptom and antimigraine medication should be taken.

VULVAR LESIONS

Vulvar lesions are cutaneous lumps, nodules, papules, vesicles, or ulcers that result from benign or malignant tumors, dystrophies, dermatoses, or infection. They can appear anywhere on the vulva and may go undetected until a gynecologic examination. Usually, however, the patient notices lesions because of associated symptoms, such as pruritus, dysuria, or dyspareunia.

HISTORY

Ask the patient when she first noticed a vulvar lesion, and find out about associated features, such as swelling, pain, tenderness, itching, or discharge. Does she have lesions elsewhere on her body? Ask about signs and symptoms of systemic illness, such as malaise, fever, or rash on other body areas. Is the patient sexually active? Could she have been exposed to a sexually transmitted disease (STD)?

PHYSICAL ASSESSMENT

Examine the lesion, perform a pelvic examination, and obtain cultures. (See *Recognizing common vulvar lesions*.) Examine the rest of the skin for rashes and lesions.

Recognizing common vulvar lesions

Various disorders can cause vulvar lesions. For example, sexually transmitted diseases account for most vulvar lesions in premenopausal women, whereas vulvar tumors and cysts account for most lesions in women ages 50 to 70. The illustrations below will help you recognize some of the most common lesions.

Primary genital herpes produces multiple ulcerated lesions surrounded by red halos.

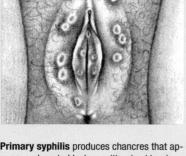

Basal cell carcinoma can produce an ulcerated lesion with raised, poorly rolled edges.

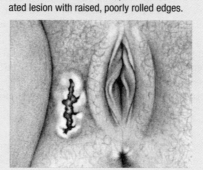

Primary syphilis produces chancres that appear as ulcerated lesions with raised borders.

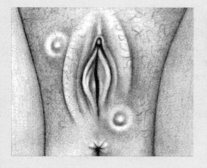

Epidermal inclusion cysts produce a round lump that usually appears on the labia majora.

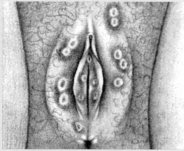

Squamous cell carcinoma can produce a large, granulomatous-appearing ulcer.

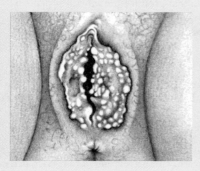

Bartholin's duct cysts produce a tense, nontender, palpable lump that usually appears on the labia minora.

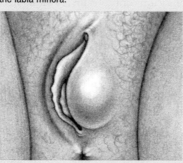

Medical causes

Basal cell carcinoma
+ The tumor is nodular and has a central ulcer and a raised, poorly rolled border.

Benign cysts
+ Epidermal inclusion cysts (usually round) appear on labia majora.
+ Bartholin's duct cysts are usually unilateral and appear on posterior labia minora.
+ Bartholin's abscess causes gradual pain and tenderness.

Genital warts
+ Painless red and pink swellings grow on vulva, vagina, and cervix.

Gonorrhea
+ Vulvar lesions, which usually are confined to Bartholin's glands, may develop along with pruritus, a burning sensation, pain, and a green-yellow vaginal discharge,

Herpes simplex (genital)
+ Fluid-filled vesicles appear on cervix and, possibly, on vulva, labia, perianal skin, or vagina.

Molluscum contagiosum
+ Raised vulvar papules are 1 to 2 mm in diameter and pearly or flesh colored with umbilicated centers and a white core.

Pediculosis pubis
+ Erythematous vulvar papules occur with pruritus and irritation.

Squamous cell carcinoma
+ Invasive carcinoma may produce vulvar pruritus, pain, and a lump.
+ Carcinoma in situ produces a vulvar lesion that may be white or red, raised, well defined, moist, crusted, and isolated.

MEDICAL CAUSES

Basal cell carcinoma

Most common in postmenopausal women, basal cell carcinoma is a nodular tumor that has a central ulcer and a raised, poorly rolled border. Although it typically doesn't produce symptoms, the tumor may occasionally cause pruritus, bleeding, discharge, and a burning sensation.

Benign cysts

Epidermal inclusion cysts, the most common benign vulvar cysts, appear primarily on the labia majora, are usually round, and typically produce no symptoms. Occasionally, they become erythematous and tender.

Bartholin's duct cysts are usually unilateral, tense, nontender, and palpable; they appear on the posterior labia minora and may cause minor discomfort during intercourse or, when large, difficulty with intercourse or even walking. Bartholin's abscess, infection of a Bartholin's duct cyst, causes gradual pain and tenderness and possibly vulvar swelling, redness, and deformity.

Genital warts

Genital warts is an STD that produces painless warts on the vulva, vagina, and cervix. Genital warts start as tiny red or pink swellings that grow and become pedunculated. Multiple swellings with a cauliflower appearance are common. Other findings include pruritus, erythema, and a profuse, mucopurulent vaginal discharge. Patients frequently complain of burning or paresthesia in the vaginal introitus.

Gonorrhea

With gonorrhea, vulvar lesions, which usually are confined to Bartholin's glands, may develop along with pruritus, a burning sensation, pain, and a green-yellow vaginal discharge, but most patients with gonorrhea are asymptomatic. Other findings include dysuria and urinary incontinence; vaginal redness, swelling, bleeding, and engorgement; and severe pelvic and lower abdominal pain.

Herpes simplex (genital)

With genital herpes simplex, fluid-filled vesicles appear on the cervix and, possibly, on the vulva, labia, perianal skin, vagina, or mouth. The vesicles, initially painless, may rupture and develop into extensive, shallow, painful ulcers, with redness, marked edema, and tender inguinal lymph nodes. Other findings include fever, malaise, and dysuria.

Molluscum contagiosum

Molluscum contagiosum is a viral infection that produces raised vulvar papules that are 1 to 2 mm in diameter and pearly or flesh colored with umbilicated centers, and that have a white core. Pruritic lesions may also appear on the face, eyelids, breasts, and inner thighs.

Pediculosis pubis

Infection with pediculosis pubis produces erythematous vulvar papules with pruritus and skin irritation. Adult pubic lice and nits are visible on pubic hair with magnification.

Squamous cell carcinoma

Invasive carcinoma occurs primarily in postmenopausal women and may produce vulvar pruritus, pain, and a vulvar lump. As the tumor enlarges, it may encroach on the vagina, anus, and urethra, causing bleeding, discharge, or dysuria. Carcinoma in situ is most common in premenopausal women, producing a vulvar lesion that may be white or red, raised, well defined, moist, crusted, and isolated.

Squamous cell hyperplasia

Squamous cell hyperplasia are vulvar lesions that may be well delineated or poorly defined; localized or extensive; and red, brown, white, or both red and white. However, intense pruritus, possibly with vulvar pain, intense burning, and dyspareunia, is the cardinal symptom of squamous cell hyperplasia. With lichen sclerosis, a type of vulvar dystrophy, vulvar skin has a parchmentlike appearance. Fissures may develop between the clitoris and urethra or other vulvar areas.

Syphilis

Chancres, the primary vulvar lesions of syphilis, may appear on the vulva, vagina, or cervix 10 to 90 days after initial contact. Usually painless, they start as papules that then erode, with indurated, raised edges and clear bases. Condylomata lata, highly contagious secondary vulvar lesions, are raised, gray, flat-topped, and commonly ulcerated. Other findings include a maculopapular, pustular, or nodular rash; headache; malaise; anorexia; weight loss; fever; nausea; vomiting; generalized lymphadenopathy; and a sore throat.

Viral disease (systemic)

Varicella, measles, and other systemic viral diseases may produce vulvar lesions. The characteristics of the lesions depend on the particular viral infection.

SPECIAL CONSIDERATIONS

Expect to administer a systemic antibiotic, an antiviral, a topical corticosteroid, a topical testosterone, or an antipruritic.

PEDIATRIC POINTERS

Vulvar lesions in children may result from congenital syphilis or gonorrhea. Evaluate for sexual abuse.

GERIATRIC POINTERS

Vulvar dystrophies and neoplasia increase in frequency with advancing age. All vulvar lesions must be suspected of being malignant until proven otherwise. Also, many women remain sexually active well into their older years and may come from a time when STDs weren't openly discussed. These patients should be questioned about sexual activities and educated about safer sex practices.

PATIENT COUNSELING

Show the patient how to give herself a sitz bath to promote healing and comfort. If she has an STD, encourage her to inform her sexual partners and persuade them to be treated. Advise her to avoid sexual contact until the lesions are no longer contagious. Provide information on safer sex practices.

Medical causes
(continued)

Squamous cell hyperplasia
+ Vulvar lesions may be well delineated or poorly defined; localized or extensive; and red, brown, white, or both red and white.

Syphilis
+ Papules with indurated, raised edges and clear bases may appear on the vulva, vagina, or cervix 10 to 90 days after initial contact.

Viral disease (systemic)
+ Varicella, measles, and other systemic viral diseases may produce vulvar lesions.

Special considerations
+ Expect to give a systemic antibiotic, an antiviral, a topical corticosteroid, a topical testosterone, or an antipruritic.

Peds points
+ Vulvar lesions in children may result from congenital syphilis or gonorrhea. Evaluate for sexual abuse.

Geri points
+ Vulvar dystrophies and neoplasia increase in frequency with advancing age.

Teaching points
+ Sitz baths
+ Safer sex practices

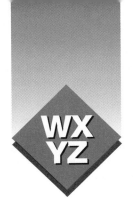

WEIGHT GAIN, EXCESSIVE

Weight gain occurs when ingested calories exceed body requirements for energy, causing increased adipose tissue storage. It can also occur when fluid retention causes edema. When weight gain results from overeating, emotional factors — most commonly anxiety, guilt, and depression — and social factors may be the primary causes.

Among elderly people, weight gain commonly reflects a sustained food intake in the presence of the normal, progressive fall in basal metabolic rate. Among women, a progressive weight gain occurs with pregnancy, whereas a periodic weight gain usually occurs with menstruation.

Weight gain, a primary sign of many endocrine disorders, also occurs with conditions that limit activity, especially cardiovascular and pulmonary disorders. It can also result from drug therapy that increases appetite or causes fluid retention or from cardiovascular, hepatic, and renal disorders that cause edema.

HISTORY

Determine your patient's previous patterns of weight gain and loss. Does he have a family history of obesity, thyroid disease, or diabetes mellitus? Assess his eating and activity patterns. Has his appetite increased? Does he exercise regularly or at all? Next, ask about associated symptoms. Has he experienced vision disturbances, hoarseness, paresthesia, or increased urination and thirst? Has he become impotent? If the patient is female, has she had menstrual irregularities or experienced weight gain during menstruation?

Form an impression of the patient's mental status. Is he anxious or depressed? Does he respond slowly? Is his memory poor? What medications is he using?

CULTURAL CUE *Body weight is influenced by gender and race. For example, Black men tend to weigh less than White men and Black women tend to weigh more than White women of the same age. Socioeconomic status also affects weight gain. Individuals of lower socioeconomic status tend to have more pronounced obesity than those of middle-class or upper middle-class status.*

PHYSICAL ASSESSMENT

During your physical assessment, measure skin-fold thickness to estimate fat reserves. (See *Evaluating nutritional status,* pages 710 and 711.) Note fat distribution and the presence of localized or generalized edema and overall nutritional status. Inspect for other abnormalities, such as abnormal body hair distribution or hair loss and dry skin. Take and record the patient's vital signs.

Key facts about excessive weight gain

+ Occurs when ingested calories exceed body requirements for energy, causing increased adipose tissue storage, or when fluid retention causes edema

Key history points

+ Previous pattern of weight gain and loss
+ Family history of obesity, thyroid disease, or diabetes mellitus
+ Eating and activity patterns
+ Exercise habits
+ Associated vision disturbances, hoarseness, paresthesia, or increased urination and thirst, impotence, or menstrual irregularities
+ Drug history

Critical assessment steps

+ Measure skin-fold thickness.
+ Note fat distribution and the presence of edema.
+ Note overall nutritional status.
+ Inspect for other abnormalities, such as abnormal body hair distribution or hair loss and dry skin.
+ Take vital signs.

Medical causes

Acromegaly

Acromegaly causes moderate weight gain. Other findings include coarsened facial features, prognathism, enlarged hands and feet, increased sweating, oily skin, deep voice, back and joint pain, lethargy, sleepiness, and heat intolerance. Occasionally, hirsutism may occur.

Diabetes mellitus

The increased appetite associated with diabetes mellitus may lead to weight gain, although weight loss sometimes occurs instead. Other findings include fatigue, polydipsia, polyuria, nocturia, weakness, polyphagia, and somnolence.

Heart failure

Despite anorexia, weight gain may result from edema. Other typical findings in heart failure include paroxysmal nocturnal dyspnea, tachypnea, tachycardia, nausea, orthopnea, and fatigue.

Hypercortisolism

Excessive weight gain, usually over the trunk and the back of the neck (buffalo hump), characteristically occurs in hypercortisolism. Other cushingoid features include slender extremities, moon face, weakness, purple striae, emotional lability, and increased susceptibility to infection. Gynecomastia may occur in men; hirsutism, acne, and menstrual irregularities may occur in women.

Hyperinsulinism

Hyperinsulinism increases appetite, leading to weight gain. Emotional lability, indigestion, weakness, diaphoresis, tachycardia, vision disturbances, and syncope also occur.

Hypogonadism

Weight gain is common in hypogonadism. Prepubertal hypogonadism causes eunuchoid body proportions with relatively sparse facial and body hair and a high-pitched voice. Postpubertal hypogonadism causes loss of libido, impotence, and infertility.

Hypothyroidism

With hypothyroidism, weight gain occurs despite anorexia. Related signs and symptoms include fatigue; cold intolerance; constipation; menorrhagia; slowed intellectual and motor activity; dry, pale, cool skin; dry, sparse hair; and thick, brittle nails. Myalgia, hoarseness, hypoactive deep tendon reflexes, bradycardia, and abdominal distention may occur. Eventually, the face assumes a dull expression with periorbital edema.

Nephrotic syndrome

With nephrotic syndrome, weight gain results from edema. In severe cases, anasarca develops—increasing body weight up to 50%. Related effects include abdominal distention, orthostatic hypotension, and lethargy.

Pancreatic islet cell tumor

Pancreatic islet cell tumor causes excessive hunger, which leads to weight gain. Other findings include emotional lability, weakness, malaise, fatigue, restlessness, diaphoresis, palpitations, tachycardia, vision disturbances, and syncope.

Medical causes

Acromegaly
✦ Moderate weight gain occurs with coarsened facial features, prognathism, enlarged hands and feet, increased sweating, oily skin, deep voice, back and joint pain, lethargy, sleepiness, and heat intolerance.

Diabetes mellitus
✦ The increased appetite associated with diabetes mellitus may lead to weight gain.

Heart failure
✦ Weight gain may result from edema.

Hypercortisolism
✦ Excessive weight gain, usually over the trunk and the back of the neck (buffalo hump), occurs.

Hyperinsulinism
✦ Increased appetite leads to weight gain.

Hypogonadism
✦ Weight gain is common.

Hypothyroidism
✦ Weight gain occurs despite anorexia.

Nephrotic syndrome
✦ Weight gain results from edema.
✦ In severe cases, anasarca develops—increasing body weight up to 50%.

Pancreatic islet cell tumor
✦ Excessive hunger leads to weight gain.

Evaluating nutritional status

If your patient has excessive weight loss or gain, you can help assess his nutritional status by measuring his skin-fold thickness and midarm circumference and by calculating his midarm muscle circumference. Skin-fold measurements reflect adipose tissue mass (subcutaneous fat accounts for about 50% of the body's adipose tissue). Midarm measurements reflect skeletal muscle and adipose tissue mass.

Use the steps described here to gather these measurements. Then express them as a percentage of standard by using this formula:

$$\frac{\text{Actual measurement}}{\text{Standard measurement}} \times 100 = \underline{\hspace{1cm}}\%$$

Standard anthropometric measurements vary according to the patient's age and sex and can be found in a chart of normal anthropometric values. The abridged chart at right lists standard arm measurements for adult men and women.

TEST	STANDARD	
Triceps skin fold	Men	12.5 mm
	Women	16.5 mm
Midarm circumference	Men	29.3 mm
	Women	28.5 mm
Midarm muscle circumference	Men	25.3 mm
	Women	23.2 mm

A triceps or subscapular skin-fold measurement below 60% of the standard value indicates severe depletion of fat reserves; measurement between 60% and 90% indicates moderate to mild depletion; and above 90% indicates significant fat reserves. A midarm circumference of less than 90% of the standard value indicates caloric deprivation; greater than 90% indicates adequate or ample muscle and fat. A midarm muscle circumference of less than 90% indicates protein depletion; greater than 90% indicates adequate or ample protein reserves.

Medical causes
(continued)

Preeclampsia
✦ Rapid weight gain may accompany nausea and vomiting, epigastric pain, elevated blood pressure, and visual blurring or double vision.

Other causes
✦ Corticosteroids, cyproheptadine, hormonal contraceptives, lithium, phenothiazines, and tricyclic antidepressants

Preeclampsia
With preeclampsia, rapid weight gain (exceeding the normal weight gain of pregnancy) may accompany nausea and vomiting, epigastric pain, elevated blood pressure, and visual blurring or double vision.

OTHER CAUSES

Drugs
Corticosteroids, phenothiazines, and tricyclic antidepressants cause weight gain from fluid retention and increased appetite. Other drugs that can lead to weight

To measure the triceps skin fold, locate the midpoint of the patient's upper arm, using a nonstretch tape measure. Mark the midpoint with a felt-tip pen. Then grasp the skin with your thumb and forefinger about 1 cm above the midpoint. Place the calipers at the midpoint and squeeze them for about 3 seconds. Record the measurement registered on the handle gauge to the nearest 0.5 mm. Take two more readings and average all three to compensate for any measurement error.

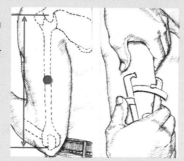

To measure the subscapular skin fold, use your thumb and forefinger to grasp the skin just below the angle of the scapula, in line with the natural cleavage of the skin. Apply the calipers and proceed as you would when measuring the triceps skin fold. Both subscapular and triceps skin-fold measurements are reliable measurements of fat loss or gain during hospitalization.

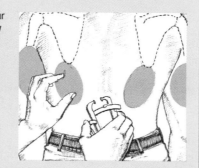

To measure midarm circumference, return to the midpoint you marked on the patient's upper arm. Then use a tape measure to determine the arm circumference at this point. This measurement reflects both skeletal muscle and adipose tissue mass and helps evaluate protein and calorie reserves. To calculate midarm muscle circumference, multiply the triceps skin-fold thickness (in centimeters) by 3.143, and subtract this figure from the midarm circumference. Midarm muscle circumference reflects muscle mass alone, providing a more sensitive index of protein reserves.

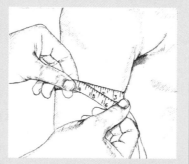

gain include hormonal contraceptives, which cause fluid retention; cyproheptadine, which increases appetite; and lithium, which can induce hypothyroidism.

SPECIAL CONSIDERATIONS

Psychological counseling may be necessary for patients with weight gain, particularly when it results from emotional problems or when uneven weight distribution alters body image. If the patient is obese or has a cardiopulmonary disorder, exercises should be monitored closely. Further studies to rule out possible secondary causes should include serum thyroid-stimulating hormone determination and dexamethasone suppression testing. Laboratory tests for serum cholesterol, triglyc-

Special considerations

- ✦ Psychological counseling may be necessary.
- ✦ If the patient is obese or has a cardiopulmonary disorder, exercises should be monitored closely.
- ✦ Studies to rule out possible secondary causes should include serum thyroid-stimulating hormone determination and dexamethasone suppression testing.
- ✦ Laboratory tests for serum cholesterol, triglyceride, and glucose levels should be performed.

Peds points

+ Weight gain can result from an endocrine disorder or from inactivity caused by Prader-Willi syndrome, Down syndrome, Werdnig-Hoffmann disease, muscular dystrophy, and cerebral palsy.
+ Nonpathologic causes include poor eating habits, sedentary recreation, and emotional problems.

Geri points

+ Desired weights increase with age.

Teaching points

+ Importance of weight control
+ Behavior modification and dietary compliance
+ Appropriate exercise

Key facts about excessive weight loss

+ Can reflect decreased food intake, decreased food absorption, increased metabolic requirements, or a combination of the three

Key history points

+ Diet, weight, and drug history
+ Sources of anxiety or depression
+ Changes in bowel habits, nausea, vomiting, abdominal pain, excessive thirst, excessive urination, or heat intolerance

Critical assessment steps

+ Check height and weight.
+ Take vital signs and note general appearance.
+ Examine the skin and mouth.

eride, and glucose levels should be performed because high levels of these substances are cardiac risk factors.

PEDIATRIC POINTERS

Weight gain in children can result from an endocrine disorder, such as hypercortisolism. Other causes include inactivity caused by Prader-Willi syndrome, Down syndrome, Werdnig-Hoffmann disease, late stages of muscular dystrophy, and severe cerebral palsy.

Nonpathologic causes include poor eating habits, sedentary recreation, and emotional problems, especially among adolescents. Regardless of the cause, discourage fad diets and provide a balanced weight loss program. The incidence of obesity is increasing among children.

GERIATRIC POINTERS

Desired weights (weights associated with lowest mortality rates) increase with age.

PATIENT COUNSELING

Educating the patient about weight control is extremely important. Stress the benefits of behavior modification and dietary compliance. Help the patient plan an appropriate exercise routine.

WEIGHT LOSS, EXCESSIVE

Weight loss can reflect decreased food intake, decreased food absorption, increased metabolic requirements, or a combination of the three. Its causes include endocrine, neoplastic, GI, and psychiatric disorders; nutritional deficiencies; infections; and neurologic lesions that cause paralysis and dysphagia. However, weight loss may accompany conditions that prevent sufficient food intake, such as painful oral lesions, ill-fitting dentures, and loss of teeth. It may be the metabolic effect of poverty, fad diets, excessive exercise, or certain drugs.

Weight loss may occur as a late sign in such chronic diseases as heart failure and renal disease. In these diseases, however, it's the result of anorexia. (See "Anorexia," page 42.)

HISTORY

Begin with a thorough diet history because weight loss almost always is caused by inadequate caloric intake. If the patient hasn't been eating properly, try to determine why. Ask him about previous weight and if the recent loss was intentional. Be alert to lifestyle or occupational changes that may be a source of anxiety or depression. For example, has he gotten separated or divorced? Has he recently changed jobs?

Inquire about recent changes in bowel habits, such as diarrhea or bulky, floating stools. Has the patient had nausea, vomiting, or abdominal pain, which may indicate a GI disorder? Has he had excessive thirst, excessive urination, or heat intolerance, which may signal an endocrine disorder? Take a careful drug history, noting especially use of diet pills and laxatives.

PHYSICAL ASSESSMENT

Carefully check the patient's height and weight. Ask about his previous weight. Take his vital signs and note his general appearance: Is he well nourished? Do his clothes fit? Is muscle wasting evident? Ask about exact weight changes (with approximate dates).

Next, examine the patient's skin for turgor and abnormal pigmentation, especially around the joints. Does he have pallor or jaundice? Examine his mouth, including the condition of his teeth or dentures. Look for signs of infection or irritation on the roof of the mouth, and note any hyperpigmentation of the buccal mucosa. Also check the patient's eyes for exophthalmos and his neck for swelling; evaluate his lungs for adventitious sounds. Inspect his abdomen for signs of wasting, and palpate for masses, tenderness, and an enlarged liver.

Conventional laboratory and radiologic investigations, such as complete blood count, serum albumin levels, urinalysis, chest X-ray, and upper GI series usually reveal the cause of weight loss.

MEDICAL CAUSES

Adrenal insufficiency
Weight loss occurs with adrenal insufficiency, along with anorexia, weakness, fatigue, irritability, syncope, nausea, vomiting, abdominal pain, and diarrhea or constipation. Hyperpigmentation may occur at the joints, belt line, palmar creases, lips, gums, tongue, and buccal mucosa.

Anorexia nervosa
Anorexia nervosa, a psychogenic disorder that's most common in young women, is characterized by a severe, self-imposed weight loss ranging from 10% to 50% of premorbid weight, which typically was normal or not more than 5 lb (2.3 kg) over ideal weight. Related findings include skeletal muscle atrophy, loss of fatty tissue, hypotension, constipation, dental caries, susceptibility to infection, blotchy or sallow skin, cold intolerance, hairiness on the face and body, dryness or loss of scalp hair, and amenorrhea. The patient usually demonstrates restless activity and vigor and may also have a morbid fear of becoming fat. Self-induced vomiting or use of laxatives or diuretics may lead to dehydration or to metabolic alkalosis or acidosis.

Cancer
Weight loss is often a sign of cancer. Other findings reflect the type, location, and stage of the tumor and can include fatigue, pain, nausea, vomiting, anorexia, abnormal bleeding, and a palpable mass.

Crohn's disease
With Crohn's disease, weight loss occurs with chronic cramping, abdominal pain, and anorexia. Other signs and symptoms include diarrhea, nausea, fever, tachycardia, abdominal tenderness and guarding, hyperactive bowel sounds, abdominal distention, and pain. Perianal lesions and a palpable mass in the right or left lower quadrant may also be present.

Cryptosporidiosis
Weight loss may occur with cryptosporidiosis, an opportunistic protozoan infection. Other findings include profuse watery diarrhea, abdominal cramping, flatulence, anorexia, malaise, fever, nausea, vomiting, and myalgia.

Depression
Weight loss or weight gain may occur with severe depression, along with insomnia or hypersomnia, anorexia, apathy, fatigue, and feelings of worthlessness. Indecisiveness, incoherence, and suicidal thoughts or behavior may also occur.

Critical assessment steps (continued)
+ Look for signs of infection or irritation on the roof of the mouth; note hyperpigmentation of the buccal mucosa.
+ Check the eyes for exophthalmos and the neck for swelling.
+ Evaluate breath sounds.
+ Inspect the abdomen for wasting; palpate for masses, tenderness, and an enlarged liver.

Medical causes

Adrenal insufficiency
+ Weight loss, anorexia, weakness, fatigue, irritability, syncope, nausea, vomiting, abdominal pain, and diarrhea or constipation occur.

Anorexia nervosa
+ Self-imposed weight loss ranges from 10% to 50% of premorbid weight.

Cancer
+ Weight loss occurs with findings specific to the tumor.

Crohn's disease
+ Weight loss, cramping, abdominal pain, and anorexia occur.

Cryptosporidiosis
+ Weight loss may occur with diarrhea, abdominal cramping, flatulence, anorexia, malaise, fever, nausea, vomiting, and myalgia.

Depression
+ Weight loss or gain may occur with insomnia or hypersomnia, anorexia, apathy, fatigue, and feelings of worthlessness.

Medical causes
(continued)

Diabetes mellitus
◆ Weight loss may occur despite increased appetite.

Esophagitis
◆ Painful inflammation of the esophagus leads to avoidance of eating and weight loss.

Gastroenteritis
◆ Malabsorption and dehydration cause sudden weight loss in acute viral infections or gradual weight loss in parasitic infections.

Herpes simplex 1
◆ Blisters in and around mouth make eating painful, causing decreased food intake and weight loss.

Leukemia
◆ Acute form causes progressive weight loss; severe prostration; high fever; swollen, bleeding gums; and bleeding tendencies.
◆ Chronic form causes progressive weight loss, malaise, fatigue, pallor, enlarged spleen, bleeding tendencies, anemia, skin eruptions, anorexia, and fever.

Lymphoma
◆ Gradual weight loss may occur.

Pulmonary tuberculosis
◆ Weight loss, fatigue, weakness, anorexia, night sweats, and low-grade fever occur.

Stomatitis
◆ Inflammation of the oral mucosa causes weight loss due to decreased eating.

Diabetes mellitus
Weight loss may occur with diabetes mellitus, despite increased appetite. Other findings include polydipsia, weakness, fatigue, blurred vision, and polyuria with nocturia.

Esophagitis
Painful inflammation of the esophagus leads to temporary avoidance of eating and subsequent weight loss. Intense pain in the mouth and anterior chest occurs, along with hypersalivation, dysphagia, tachypnea, and hematemesis. If a stricture develops, dysphagia and weight loss will recur.

Gastroenteritis
Malabsorption and dehydration cause weight loss in gastroenteritis. The loss may be sudden in acute viral infections or reactions or gradual in parasitic infection. Other findings include poor skin turgor, dry mucous membranes, tachycardia, hypotension, diarrhea, abdominal pain and tenderness, hyperactive bowel sounds, nausea, vomiting, fever, and malaise.

Herpes simplex 1
With herpes simplex 1, painful fluid-filled blisters in and around the mouth, especially the tongue, gums, and cheeks, make eating painful causing decreased food intake and weight loss. Fever and pharyngitis may also occur.

Leukemia
Acute leukemia causes progressive weight loss accompanied by severe prostration; high fever; swollen, bleeding gums; and bleeding tendencies. Dyspnea, tachycardia, palpitations, and abdominal or bone pain may occur. As the disease progresses, neurologic symptoms may eventually develop.

Chronic leukemia, which occurs insidiously in adults, causes progressive weight loss with malaise, fatigue, pallor, enlarged spleen, bleeding tendencies, anemia, skin eruptions, anorexia, and fever.

Lymphoma
Hodgkin's disease and non-Hodgkin's lymphoma cause gradual weight loss. Associated findings include fever, fatigue, night sweats, malaise, hepatosplenomegaly, and lymphadenopathy. Scaly rashes and pruritus may develop.

Pulmonary tuberculosis
Pulmonary tuberculosis causes gradual weight loss, along with fatigue, weakness, anorexia, night sweats, and low-grade fever. Other clinical effects include a cough with bloody or mucopurulent sputum, dyspnea, and pleuritic chest pain. Examination may reveal dullness on percussion, crackles after coughing, increased tactile fremitus, and amphoric breath sounds.

Stomatitis
Inflammation of the oral mucosa (usually red, swollen, and ulcerated) in stomatitis causes weight loss due to decreased eating. Associated findings include fever, increased salivation, malaise, mouth pain, anorexia, and swollen, bleeding gums.

Thyrotoxicosis
With thyrotoxicosis, increased metabolism causes weight loss. Other characteristic signs and symptoms include nervousness, heat intolerance, diarrhea, increased appetite, palpitations, tachycardia, diaphoresis, fine tremor, and possibly an enlarged thyroid and exophthalmos. A ventricular or atrial gallop may be heard.

Ulcerative colitis

Weight loss is a late sign of ulcerative colitis, which is initially characterized by bloody diarrhea with pus or mucus. Weakness, crampy lower abdominal pain, tenesmus, anorexia, low-grade fever, and occasional nausea and vomiting may also occur. Bowel sounds are hyperactive, and constipation may occur late. With fulminant colitis, severe and steady abdominal pain and diarrhea, high fever, and tachycardia occur.

OTHER CAUSES

Drugs

Amphetamines and inappropriate dosage of thyroid preparations commonly lead to weight loss. Laxative abuse may cause a malabsorptive state that leads to weight loss. Chemotherapeutic agents cause stomatitis, which, when severe, causes weight loss.

SPECIAL CONSIDERATIONS

If the patient has a chronic disease, administer hyperalimentation or tube feedings to maintain nutrition and to prevent edema, poor healing, and muscle wasting. Take daily calorie counts and weigh him weekly. Consult a nutritionist to determine an appropriate diet with adequate calories.

PEDIATRIC POINTERS

In infants, weight loss may be caused by failure-to-thrive syndrome. In children, severe weight loss may be the first indication of diabetes mellitus. Chronic, gradual weight loss occurs in children with marasmus—nonedematous protein-calorie malnutrition.

Weight loss may also occur as a result of child abuse or neglect; an infection causing high fevers; hand-foot-and-mouth disease, which causes painful oral sores; a GI disorder causing vomiting and diarrhea; or celiac disease.

GERIATRIC POINTERS

Some elderly patients experience mild, gradual weight loss due to changes in body composition, such as loss of height and lean body mass, and lower basal metabolic rate, leading to decreased energy requirements. Rapid, unintentional weight loss, however, is highly predictive of morbidity and mortality in the elderly. Other nondisease causes of weight loss in this group include tooth loss, difficulty chewing, and social isolation. Alcoholism may also cause weight loss.

PATIENT COUNSELING

Refer your patient for psychological counseling if weight loss negatively affects his body image. Teach the patient about his diet and recommend that he keep a food diary. Determine his food preferences and try to incorporate them into his diet. Encourage oral hygiene before meals to make the food more palatable.

Medical causes
(continued)

Thyrotoxicosis
+ Increased metabolism causes weight loss.

Ulcerative colitis
+ Weight loss is a late sign.

Other causes
+ Amphetamines
+ Chemotherapeutic agents
+ Inappropriate dosage of thyroid preparations
+ Laxative abuse

Special considerations
+ Take daily calorie counts and weigh the patient weekly.
+ Consult a nutritionist.

Peds points
+ In infants, weight loss may be due to failure-to-thrive syndrome.
+ In children, severe weight loss may be the first indication of diabetes mellitus.

Geri points
+ Some elderly patients experience mild, gradual weight loss due to changes in body composition.
+ Rapid, unintentional weight loss is highly predictive of morbidity and mortality in the elderly.
+ Other causes include tooth loss, difficulty chewing, social isolation, and alcoholism.

Teaching points
+ Proper diet
+ Good oral hygiene
+ Referral to psychological counseling, if appropriate

WHEEZING

Wheezes are adventitious breath sounds with a high-pitched, musical, squealing, creaking, or groaning quality. Also known as *sibilant rhonchi,* they're caused by air flowing at a high velocity through a narrowed airway. When they originate in the large airways, they can be heard by placing an unaided ear over the chest wall or at the mouth. When they originate in smaller airways, they can be heard by placing a stethoscope over the anterior or posterior chest. Unlike crackles and rhonchi, wheezes can't be cleared by coughing.

Usually, prolonged wheezing occurs during expiration when bronchi are shortened and narrowed. Causes of airway narrowing include bronchospasm; mucosal thickening or edema; partial obstruction from a tumor, a foreign body, or secretions; and extrinsic pressure, as in tension pneumothorax or goiter. With airway obstruction, wheezing occurs during inspiration. (See *Associated disorder: Asthma.*)

EMERGENCY ACTIONS Examine the degree of the patient's respiratory distress. Is he responsive? Is he restless, confused, anxious, or afraid? Are his respirations abnormally fast, slow, shallow, or deep? Are they irregular? Can you hear wheezing through his mouth? Does he exhibit increased use of accessory muscles; increased chest wall motion; intercostal, suprasternal, or supraclavicular retractions; stridor; or nasal flaring? Take his other vital signs, noting hypotension or hypertension, decreased oxygen saturation, and an irregular, weak, rapid, or slow pulse.

Help him relax, administer humidified oxygen by face mask, and encourage slow, deep breathing. Have endotracheal intubation and emergency resuscitation equipment readily available. Call the respiratory therapy department to supply intermittent positive-pressure breathing and nebulization treatments with bronchodilators. Insert an I.V. line for administration of drugs, such as diuretics, steroids, bronchodilators, and sedatives. Perform the abdominal thrust maneuver, as indicated, for airway obstruction.

HISTORY

If the patient isn't in respiratory distress, obtain a history. What provokes his wheezing? Does he have asthma or allergies? Does he smoke or have a history of a pulmonary, cardiac, or circulatory disorder? Does he have cancer? Ask about recent surgery, illness, or trauma or changes in appetite, weight, exercise tolerance, or sleep patterns. Obtain a drug history. Ask about exposure to toxic fumes or any respiratory irritants. If he has a cough, ask how it sounds, when it starts, and how often it occurs. Does he have paroxysms of coughing? Is his cough dry, sputum producing, or bloody?

Ask the patient about chest pain. If he reports pain, determine its quality, onset, duration, intensity, and radiation. Does it increase with breathing, coughing, or certain positions?

PHYSICAL ASSESSMENT

Examine the patient's nose and mouth for congestion, drainage, or signs of infection, such as halitosis. If he produces sputum, obtain a sample for examination. Check for cyanosis, pallor, clamminess, masses, tenderness, swelling, distended jugular veins, and enlarged lymph nodes. Inspect his chest for abnormal configuration and asymmetrical motion, and determine if the trachea is midline. (See *Detecting slight tracheal deviation,* page 655.) Percuss for dullness or hyperresonance, and auscultate for crackles, rhonchi, or pleural friction rubs. Note absent or hy-

Asthma

Asthma is a chronic inflammatory airway disorder characterized by airflow obstruction and airway hyperresponsiveness to various stimuli. It's a type of chronic obstructive pulmonary disease, a long-term pulmonary disease characterized by increased airflow resistance. Asthma's widespread but variable airflow obstruction is caused by bronchospasm, edema of the airway mucosa, and increased mucus production.

Asthma may result from sensitivity to extrinsic or intrinsic allergens. *Extrinsic,* or *atopic,* asthma begins in childhood; typically, patients are sensitive to specific external allergens. *Intrinsic,* or *nonatopic,* patients with asthma react to internal, nonallergenic factors. Most episodes occur after a severe respiratory tract infection, especially in adults. However, many patients with asthma, especially children, have intrinsic and extrinsic asthma. A significant number of adults acquire an allergic form of asthma or experience an exacerbation of existing asthma from being exposed to agents in the workplace.

CAUSES

Extrinsic causes of asthma include:
+ pollen
+ animal dander
+ house dust or mold
+ kapok or feather pillows
+ food additives containing sulfites
+ other sensitizing substances such as nonsteroidal anti-inflammatory drugs.
  Intrinsic causes of asthma include:
+ emotional stress
+ fatigue
+ endocrine changes
+ temperature variations
+ humidity variations
+ exposure to noxious fumes
+ anxiety
+ coughing or laughing
+ genetic factors.

DIAGNOSIS

These tests help diagnose asthma:
+ Pulmonary function studies reveal signs of airway obstructive disease, a decreased or low but still within normal range vital capacity, and increased total lung and residual capacities. Pulmonary function may be normal between attacks. Partial pressure of arterial oxygen (Pao_2) and partial pressure of arterial carbon dioxide ($Paco_2$) are usually decreased, except in severe asthma, when $Paco_2$ may be normal or increased, indicating severe bronchial obstruction.
+ Serum immunoglobulin E levels may increase from an allergic reaction.
+ Sputum analysis may indicate the presence of Curschmann's spirals (casts of airways), Charcot-Leyden crystals, and eosinophils.
+ Complete blood count with differential reveals an increased eosinophil count.
+ Chest X-rays can be used to diagnose or monitor the progress of asthma and may show hyperinflation with areas of atelectasis.
+ Arterial blood gas (ABG) analysis detects hypoxemia (decreased Pao_2; decreased, normal, or increasing $Paco_2$) and guides treatment.
+ Skin testing may identify specific allergens. Results read in 1 or 2 days detect an early reaction; after 4 or 5 days, a late reaction.
+ Bronchial challenge testing evaluates the clinical significance of allergens identified by skin testing.
+ Electrocardiography shows sinus tachycardia during an attack; a severe attack may show signs of cor pulmonale (such as right axis deviation and peaked P wave) that resolve after the attack.

MEDICAL INTERVENTION

These approaches are typically used to correct asthma:
+ Prevention by identifying and avoiding precipitating factors, such as environmental allergens or irritants, is considered the best treatment.
+ Desensitization to specific antigens, which decreases the severity of attacks upon future exposure, can be helpful if the stimuli can't be removed entirely.
+ Low-flow humidified oxygen may be needed to treat dyspnea, cyanosis, and hypoxemia. The amount delivered should maintain Pao_2 between 65 and 85 mm Hg, as determined by ABG analysis.

(continued)

Key facts about asthma
+ Characterized by airflow obstruction and airway hyperresponsiveness to various stimuli
+ May result from sensitivity to extrinsic or intrinsic allergens

Causes
+ Extrinsic causes include pollen, animal dander, dust or mold, kapok or feather pillows, food additives containing sulfites, and NSAIDs.
+ Intrinsic causes include emotional stress, fatigue, endocrine changes, temperature variations, humidity variations, exposure to noxious fumes, anxiety, coughing or laughing, and genetic factors.

Management
+ Prevention by identifying and avoiding precipitating factors
+ Desensitization to specific antigens
+ Low-flow humidified oxygen to treat dyspnea, cyanosis, and hypoxemia
+ Mechanical ventilation if the patient doesn't respond to initial ventilatory support and drugs or if the patient develops respiratory failure
+ Drug therapy with anticholinergic bronchodilators, bronchodilators, corticosteroids, mast cell stabilizers, or leukotriene modifiers

Asthma *(continued)*

♦ Mechanical ventilation is necessary if the patient doesn't respond to initial ventilatory support and drugs or if the patient develops respiratory failure.

Drug therapy for asthma is typically based on the severity of disease. Here are some common asthma medications and their effects:

♦ Anticholinergic bronchodilators, such as ipratropium, block acetylcholine, another chemical mediator.
♦ Bronchodilators — including the methylxanthines (theophylline and aminophylline) and the beta$_2$-adrenergic agonists (albuterol and terbutaline) decrease bronchoconstriction, reduce bronchial airway edema, and increase pulmonary ventilation.
♦ Corticosteroids, such as hydrocortisone sodium succinate, prednisone, methylprednisolone, and beclomethasone, are used for their anti-inflammatory and immunosuppressive effects, which decrease inflammation and edema of the airways.

♦ Mast cell stabilizers (cromolyn and nedocromil) are used for patients with atopic asthma who have seasonal disease. When given prophylactically, they block the acute obstructive effects of antigen exposure by inhibiting the degranulation of mast cells, thereby preventing the release of chemical mediators responsible for anaphylaxis.
♦ Leukotriene modifiers, including zileuton and leukotriene receptor antagonists (LTRAs), such as montelukast and zafirlukast, inhibit the potent bronchoconstriction and inflammatory effects of the cysteinyl leukotrienes. LTRAs can be used as adjunctive therapy to avoid high-dose inhaled corticosteroids. Although this class of medications doesn't replace inhaled corticosteroids as first-line anti-inflammatory treatment, it can be used successfully in cases where poor compliance with inhaled corticosteroid use is suspected.

Medical causes

Anaphylaxis
♦ Tracheal edema or bronchospasm can result in severe wheezing and stridor.

Aspiration of a foreign body
♦ Partial obstruction produces sudden onset of wheezing and possibly stridor; a dry, paroxysmal cough; gagging; and hoarseness.

Aspiration pneumonitis
♦ Wheezing may accompany tachypnea, marked dyspnea, cyanosis, tachycardia, fever, productive cough, and pink, frothy sputum.

Asthma
♦ Wheezing heard at the mouth during expiration is an initial and cardinal sign.

poactive breath sounds, abnormal heart sounds, gallops, or murmurs. Also note arrhythmias, bradycardia, or tachycardia. (See *Evaluating breath sounds,* pages 720 and 721.)

MEDICAL CAUSES

Anaphylaxis
Anaphylaxis is an allergic reaction that can cause tracheal edema or bronchospasm, resulting in severe wheezing and stridor. Initial signs and symptoms of anaphylaxis include fright, weakness, sneezing, dyspnea, nasal pruritus, urticaria, erythema, and angioedema. Respiratory distress occurs with nasal flaring, accessory muscle use, and intercostal retractions. Other findings include nasal edema and congestion; profuse, watery rhinorrhea; chest or throat tightness; and dysphagia. Cardiac effects include arrhythmias and hypotension.

Aspiration of a foreign body
Partial obstruction by a foreign body produces sudden onset of wheezing and possibly stridor; a dry, paroxysmal cough; gagging; and hoarseness. Other findings include tachycardia, dyspnea, decreased breath sounds, and possibly cyanosis. A retained foreign body may cause inflammation leading to fever, pain, and swelling.

Aspiration pneumonitis
With aspiration pneumonitis, wheezing may accompany tachypnea, marked dyspnea, cyanosis, tachycardia, fever, productive (eventually purulent) cough, and pink, frothy sputum.

Asthma

Wheezing is an initial and cardinal sign of asthma. It's heard at the mouth during expiration. An initially dry cough later becomes productive with thick mucus. Other findings include apprehension, prolonged expiration, intercostal and supraclavicular retractions, rhonchi, accessory muscle use, nasal flaring, and tachypnea. Asthma also produces tachycardia, diaphoresis, and flushing or cyanosis.

Bronchial adenoma

Bronchial adenoma is an insidious disorder that produces unilateral, possibly severe wheezing. Common features are chronic cough and recurring hemoptysis. Symptoms of airway obstruction may occur later.

Bronchiectasis

With bronchiectasis, excessive mucus commonly causes intermittent and localized or diffuse wheezing. A copious, foul-smelling, mucopurulent cough is classic. The cough is accompanied by hemoptysis, rhonchi, and coarse crackles. Weight loss, fatigue, weakness, exertional dyspnea, fever, malaise, halitosis, and late-stage clubbing may also occur.

Bronchitis (chronic)

Chronic bronchitis causes wheezing that varies in severity, location, and intensity. Associated findings include prolonged expiration, coarse crackles, scattered rhonchi, and a hacking cough that later becomes productive. Other effects include dyspnea, accessory muscle use, barrel chest, tachypnea, clubbing, edema, weight gain, and cyanosis.

Bronchogenic carcinoma

Obstruction from bronchogenic carcinoma may cause localized wheezing. Typical findings include a productive cough, dyspnea, hemoptysis (initially blood-tinged sputum, possibly leading to massive hemorrhage), anorexia, and weight loss. Upper extremity edema and chest pain may also occur.

Chemical pneumonitis (acute)

With acute chemical pneumonitis, mucosal injury causes increased secretions and edema, leading to wheezing, dyspnea, orthopnea, crackles, malaise, fever, and a productive cough with purulent sputum. The patient may also have signs of conjunctivitis, pharyngitis, laryngitis, and rhinitis.

Emphysema

Mild to moderate wheezing may occur with emphysema, a form of chronic obstructive pulmonary disease. Related findings include dyspnea, malaise, tachypnea, diminished breath sounds, peripheral cyanosis, pursed-lip breathing, anorexia, and malaise. Accessory muscle use, barrel chest, a chronic productive cough, and clubbing may also occur.

Inhalation injury

Wheezing may eventually occur with inhalation injury. Early findings include hoarseness and coughing, singed nasal hairs, orofacial burns, and soot-stained sputum. Later effects are crackles, rhonchi, and respiratory distress.

Pneumothorax (tension)

Tension pneumothorax, a life-threatening disorder, causes respiratory distress with possible wheezing, dyspnea, tachycardia, tachypnea, and sudden, severe, sharp chest pain (often unilateral). Other findings include a dry cough, cyanosis, accessory muscle use, asymmetrical chest wall movement, anxiety, and restlessness. Examina-

Medical causes
(continued)

Bronchial adenoma
+ Unilateral, possibly severe wheezing occurs with chronic cough and recurring hemoptysis.

Bronchiectasis
+ Excessive mucus causes intermittent and localized or diffuse wheezing.

Bronchitis (chronic)
+ Chronic bronchitis causes wheezing that varies in severity, location, and intensity.

Bronchogenic carcinoma
+ Obstruction may cause localized wheezing.

Chemical pneumonitis (acute)
+ Mucosal injury causes increased secretions and edema, leading to wheezing, dyspnea, orthopnea, crackles, malaise, fever, and a productive cough with purulent sputum.

Emphysema
+ Mild to moderate wheezing may occur.

Inhalation injury
+ Wheezing may eventually occur after hoarseness and coughing, singed nasal hairs, orofacial burns, and soot-stained sputum.

Pneumothorax (tension)
+ Wheezing, dyspnea, tachycardia, tachypnea, and sudden, severe, sharp chest pain (often unilateral) may occur.

ASSESSMENT TIP

Evaluating breath sounds

Diminished or absent breath sounds indicate some interference with airflow. If pus, fluid, or air fills the pleural space, breath sounds will be quieter than normal. If a foreign body or secretions obstruct a bronchus, breath sounds will be diminished or absent over distal lung tissue. Increased thickness of the chest wall, such as with a patient who's obese or extremely muscular, may cause breath sounds to be decreased, distant, or inaudible. Absent breath sounds typically indicate loss of ventilation power.

When air passes through narrowed airways or through moisture, or when the membranes lining the chest cavity become inflamed, adventitious breath sounds will be heard. These include crackles, rhonchi, wheezes, and pleural friction rubs. Usually, these sounds indicate pulmonary disease.

Follow the auscultation sequences shown to assess the patient's breath sounds. Have the patient take full, deep breaths, and compare sound variations from one side to the other. Note the location, timing, and character of any abnormal breath sounds.

POSTERIOR

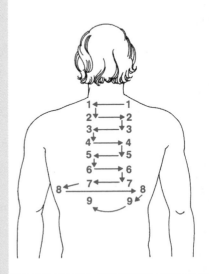

---

tion reveals hyperresonance or tympany and diminished or absent breath sounds on the affected side, subcutaneous crepitation, decreased vocal fremitus, and tracheal deviation.

Pulmonary coccidioidomycosis

Pulmonary coccidioidomycosis may cause wheezing and rhonchi along with cough, fever, chills, pleuritic chest pain, headache, weakness, fatigue, sore throat, backache, malaise, anorexia, and an itchy, macular rash.

Pulmonary edema

Wheezing may occur with pulmonary edema , a life-threatening disorder. Other signs and symptoms of pulmonary edema include coughing, exertional and paroxysmal nocturnal dyspnea and, later, orthopnea. Examination reveals tachycardia, tachypnea, dependent crackles, and a diastolic gallop. Severe pulmonary edema produces rapid, labored respirations; diffuse crackles; a productive cough with frothy, bloody sputum; arrhythmias; cold, clammy, cyanotic skin; hypotension; and thready pulse.

Pulmonary tuberculosis

In late stages, fibrosis causes wheezing. Common findings include a mild to severe productive cough with pleuritic chest pain and fine crackles, night sweats, anorexia, weight loss, fever, malaise, dyspnea, and fatigue. Other features are dullness to percussion, increased tactile fremitus, and amphoric breath sounds.

Medical causes
(continued)

Pulmonary coccidioidomycosis

◆ Wheezing and rhonchi may occur with cough, fever, chills, pleuritic chest pain, headache, weakness, fatigue, sore throat, backache, malaise, anorexia, and an itchy, macular rash.

Pulmonary edema

◆ Wheezing may occur with coughing, exertional and paroxysmal nocturnal dyspnea and, later, orthopnea.

Pulmonary tuberculosis

◆ Fibrosis causes wheezing in the late stages.

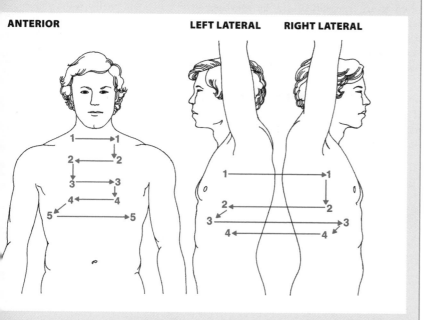

ANTERIOR   **LEFT LATERAL**   **RIGHT LATERAL**

CULTURAL CUE *Those living in Appalachian regions have a 50% higher mortality from tuberculosis than the national average. They also have a higher incidence of pneumonia, influenza, and black lung disease. The higher rate of respiratory tract diseases may be related to the high-risk occupations of the region, such as those in the mining, timber, and textile industries.*

Thyroid goiter

Thyroid goiter may not produce symptoms, or it may cause wheezing, dysphagia, and respiratory difficulty related to a compressed airway. The neck will appear swollen and distended.

Tracheobronchitis

Auscultation of the patient with tracheobronchitis may detect wheezing, rhonchi, and moist or coarse crackles. The patient also has a cough, slight fever, sudden chills, muscle and back pain, and substernal tightness.

SPECIAL CONSIDERATIONS

Prepare the patient for diagnostic tests, such as chest X-rays, arterial blood gas analysis, pulmonary function tests, and sputum culture.

Ease the patient's breathing by placing him in semi-Fowler's position and repositioning him frequently. Perform pulmonary physiotherapy as necessary.

Administer an antibiotic to treat infection, a bronchodilator to relieve bronchospasm and maintain patent airways, a steroid to reduce inflammation, and a

---

Medical causes
(continued)

Thyroid goiter
◆ Wheezing, dysphagia, and respiratory difficulty related to a compressed airway may develop.

Tracheobronchitis
◆ Wheezing, rhonchi, and moist or coarse crackles may be auscultated.

Special considerations
◆ Place the patient in semi-Fowler's position.
◆ Perform pulmonary physiotherapy as necessary.
◆ Administer an antibiotic to treat infection, a bronchodilator to relieve bronchospasm and maintain patent airways, a steroid to reduce inflammation, and a mucolytic or expectorant to increase the flow of secretions.
◆ Provide humidification.

mucolytic or expectorant to increase the flow of secretions. Provide humidification to thin secretions.

PEDIATRIC POINTERS

Children are especially susceptible to wheezing because their small airways allow rapid obstruction. Primary causes of wheezing include bronchospasm, mucosal edema, and accumulation of secretions. These may occur with such disorders as cystic fibrosis, aspiration of a foreign body, acute bronchiolitis, and pulmonary hemosiderosis.

PATIENT COUNSELING

If appropriate, encourage increased activity to promote drainage and prevent pooling of secretions. Encourage regular deep breathing and coughing. Also encourage the patient to drink fluids to liquefy secretions and prevent dehydration.

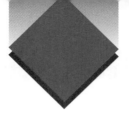

Appendices and index

Additional signs and symptoms

Amnesia

Amnesia is a disturbance in, or loss of, memory. *Anterograde amnesia* denotes memory loss for events that occurred after the onset of the causative trauma or disease. *Retrograde amnesia* involves memory loss for events that occurred before the onset.

Organic (true) amnesia results from temporal lobe dysfunction. It characteristically spares patches of memory. A common symptom in patients with seizures or head trauma, organic amnesia can also be an early indicator of Alzheimer's disease. *Hysterical amnesia* has a psychogenic origin and characteristically causes complete memory loss. *Treatment-induced amnesia* is usually transient.

Analgesia

A sign of central nervous system disease, analgesia is the absence of sensitivity to pain that commonly indicates a specific type and location of spinal cord lesion. It always occurs with loss of temperature sensation (thermanesthesia). Analgesia can also occur with such sensory deficits as paresthesia, loss of proprioception and vibratory sense, and tactile anesthesia in disorders involving the peripheral nerves, spinal cord, and brain. Analgesia is tested for by lightly touching different dermatomes with a pin.

Apnea

Apnea is the cessation of spontaneous respiration. Common causes include trauma, cardiac arrest, neurologic disease, aspiration of foreign objects, bronchospasm, and drug overdose — life-threatening emergencies that require immediate intervention.

Apneustic respirations

Apneustic respirations are characterized by prolonged, gasping inspirations, with a pause at full inspiration. This irregular breathing pattern is an important localizing sign of severe brain stem damage.

Asterixis

Also known as a *liver flap* or *flapping tremor,* asterixis is a bilateral, coarse movement, characterized by sudden relaxation of muscle groups holding a sustained posture. This elicited sign is most commonly observed in the wrists and fingers but may also appear during any sustained voluntary action. Typically, it signals hepatic, renal, or pulmonary disease. Asterixis may signal serious metabolic deterioration.

Athetosis

An extrapyramidal sign, athetosis is characterized by slow, continuous, and twisting involuntary movements that typically involve the face, neck, and distal extremities, such as the forearm, wrist, and hand. Facial grimaces, jaw and tongue movements, and occasional phonation are associated with neck movements. Athetosis worsens during stress and voluntary activity, may subside during relaxation, and disappears during sleep.

Usually beginning during childhood, athetosis resulting from hypoxia at birth, kernicterus, or a genetic disorder. In adults, athetosis usually results from vascular or neoplastic lesions, degenerative disease, drug toxicity, or hypoxia.

Barrel chest

A rounded configuration of the chest in which the anteroposterior diameter enlarges to approximate the transverse diameter is called *barrel chest.* The diaphragm is depressed and the sternum is pushed forward with the ribs attached in a horizontal — not angular — fashion. As a result, the chest appears continuously in the inspiratory position. Typically a late sign of chronic obstructive pulmonary disease, barrel chest results from augmented lung volumes due to chronic airflow obstruction.

Biot's respirations

Biot's respirations (also known as *ataxic respirations*) involve an irregular and unpredictable respiratory rate, rhythm, and depth. This rare sign is a late and ominous sign of neurologic deterioration; it may reflect increased pressure on the medulla coinciding with brain stem compression.

Breast dimpling

Puckering or retraction of skin on the breast, called *breast dimpling,* results from abnormal attachment of the skin to underlying tissue. It suggests an inflammatory or malignant mass beneath the skin surface and usually represents a late sign of breast cancer.

Dimpling usually affects women older than age 40 but also occasionally affects men.

Breast ulcer

A breast ulcer involves the destruction of the skin and subcutaneous tissue on the nipple, areola, or the breast itself. It's usually a late sign of cancer, appearing well after the confirming diagnosis. However, it may be the presenting sign of breast cancer in men, who are more apt to dismiss earlier breast changes. Breast ulcers can also result from trauma, infection, or radiation.

Breath with ammonia odor

The odor of ammonia on the breath — also called *uremic fetor* and commonly described as urinous or "fishy" breath — is a sign that typically occurs in end-stage chronic renal failure. Ammonia breath odor reflects the long-term metabolic disturbances and biochemical abnormalities associated with uremia and end-stage chronic renal failure. It's produced by metabolic end products blown off by the lungs and the breakdown of urea (to ammonia) in the saliva.

Buffalo hump

A buffalo hump is an accumulation of cervicodorsal fat. This sign may indicate hypercortisolism or Cushing's syndrome. Hypercortisolism itself may result from long-term glucocorticoid therapy, adrenal carcinoma, adrenal adenoma, ectopic corticotropin production, or Cushing's disease.

Café-au-lait spots

Café-au-lait spots appear as flat, light brown, uniformly hyperpigmented macules or patches on the skin surface. This sign is an important indicator of neurofibromatosis and other congenital melanotic disorders. Café-au-lait spots usually appear during the first 3 years of life but may develop at any age. They can be differentiated from freckles and other benign birthmarks by their larger size (a few millimeters to ⅝″ [1.6 cm] or larger) and irregular shape. They usually have no significance; however, six or more café-au-lait spots may be associated with an underlying neurologic disorder.

Cat's cry

This mewing, kittenlike sound occurs during infancy and is the primary indicator of cri du chat (also known as *cat's cry*) syndrome. The chromosomal defect responsible (deletion of the short arm of chromosome 5) usually appears spontaneously but may be inherited from a carrier parent. The characteristic cry is thought to result from abnormal laryngeal development.

This syndrome affects about 1 in 50,000 neonates and causes profound mental retardation and failure to thrive. Most of those affected can have a normal life span, although a small number have serious organ defects and other life-threatening medical conditions.

Cheyne-Stokes respirations

Cheyne-Stokes respirations are characterized by a waxing and waning period of hyperpnea that alternates with a shorter period of apnea. The most common pattern of periodic breathing, these respirations can occur normally in patients with heart or lung disease or those who live at high altitudes. This sign usually indicates increased intracranial pressure from a deep cerebral or brain stem lesion or a metabolic disturbance in the brain. Cheyne-Stokes respirations may indicate a major change in the patient's behavior — usually for the worse.

Clubbing

Clubbing is a painless, usually bilateral increase in soft tissue around the terminal phalanges of the fingers or toes. It's a nonspecific sign of pulmonary and cyanotic cardiovascular disorders. With early clubbing, the normal 160-degree angle between the nail and the nail base approximates 180 degrees. As clubbing progresses, this angle widens and the base of the nail becomes visibly swollen. With late clubbing, the angle where the nail meets the now-convex nail base extends more than halfway up the nail.

Cogwheel rigidity

Muscle rigidity that reacts with superimposed ratchetlike movements when the muscle is passively stretched is called *cogwheel rigidity*. A cardinal sign of Parkinson's disease, cogwheel rigidity an be elicited by stabilizing the patient's forearm and then moving his wrist through the range of motion while observing and feeling for these movements. Cogwheel rigidity usually appears in the arms but can sometimes be elicited in the ankle.

Cold intolerance

Cold intolerance — the increased sensitivity to cold temperatures — reflects damage to the body's temperature-regulating mechanism, based on interactions between the hypothalamus and the thyroid gland. Typically, the symptom results from tumors or a hormonal deficiency. In elderly patients, cold intolerance reflects normal age-related physiologic changes.

Corneal reflex, absent

The corneal reflex is tested by drawing a fine-pointed wisp of sterile cotton from a corner of each eye to the cornea. If bilateral eye blinking occurs, the reflex is present. When the reflex is absent, neither eyelid closes when the cornea of one is touched.

The site of the afferent fibers for this reflex is in the ophthalmic branch of the trigeminal nerve (cranial nerve [CN] V); the efferent fibers are located in the facial nerve (CN VII). Unilateral or bilateral absence of the corneal reflex may result from damage to these nerves.

Cry, high-pitched

A high-pitched cry (also called a *cerebral cry*) is characterized by a brief, sharp, piercing vocal sound produced by a neonate or infant. This cry is a late sign of increased intracranial pressure (ICP). The acute onset of a high-pitched cry demands emergency treatment to prevent permanent brain damage or death.

In neonates, increased ICP may result from intracranial bleeding associated with birth trauma or from congenital malformations, such as craniostenosis and Arnold-Chiari syndrome. In fact, a high-pitched cry may be an early sign of congenital malformation. In infants, increased ICP may result from meningitis, head trauma, or child abuse.

Depression

Depression is a mood disturbance that's characterized by feelings of sadness, despair, and loss of interest or pleasure in activities. These feelings may be accompanied by somatic complaints, such as changes in appetite, sleep disturbances, restlessness or lethargy, and decreased concentration. Thoughts of injuring one's self, death, or suicide may also occur.

The criterion for major depression is one or more episodes of depressed mood, or decreased interest or the ability to take pleasure in all or most activities, lasting at least 2 weeks. Depression has numerous causes, including genetic and family history, medical and psychiatric disorders, and the use of certain drugs. It can also occur in the postpartum period.

Doll's eye sign, absent

The absence of the doll's eye sign (a negative oculocephalic reflex) is detected by rapid, gentle turning of the patient's head from side to side. The eyes remain fixed in midposition, instead of the normal response of moving laterally toward the side opposite the direction the head is turned.

The absence of doll's eye sign indicates injury to the midbrain or pons, involving cranial nerves III and VI. It typically accompanies coma caused by lesions of the cerebellum and brain stem. Absent doll's eye sign is necessary for a diagnosis of brain death.

Drooling

Drooling is the flow of saliva from the mouth. This sign results from an excess in salivation or a failure to swallow or retain saliva. It may stem from facial muscle paralysis or weakness that prevents mouth closure, from neuromuscular disorders or local pain that causes dysphagia or, less commonly, from the effects of drugs or toxins that induce salivation. Because it signals an inability to handle secretions, drooling warns of potential aspiration.

Dysmenorrhea

Dysmenorrhea (painful menstruation) may involve sharp, intermittent pain or dull, aching pain. It's usually characterized by mild to severe cramping or colicky pain in the pelvis or lower abdomen that may radiate to the thighs and lower sacrum. This pain may precede menstruation by several days or may accompany it. The pain gradually subsides as bleeding tapers off.

Dysmenorrhea may be idiopathic, as in premenstrual syndrome and primary dysmenorrhea. It commonly results from endometriosis and other pelvic disorders. It may also result from structural abnormalities such as an imperforate hymen. Stress and poor health may aggravate dysmenorrhea; rest and mild exercise may relieve it.

Dyspareunia

Dyspareunia (painful or difficult coitus) may occur with attempted penetration or during or after coitus. It may stem from friction of the penis against perineal tissue or from jarring of deeper adnexal structures.

Dyspareunia commonly accompanies pelvic disorders. However, it may also result from diminished vaginal lubrication associated with aging, the effects of drugs, and psychological factors — most notably, fear of pain or injury. Other psychological factors include guilty feelings about sex, fear of pregnancy or of injury to the fetus during pregnancy, and anxiety caused by a disrupted sexual relationship or by a new sexual partner. Inadequate vaginal lubrication associated with insufficient foreplay and mental or physical fatigue may also cause dyspareunia.

Dystonia

Dystonia is characterized by slow, involuntary movements of large-muscle groups in the limbs, trunk, and neck. This extrapyramidal sign may involve flexion of the foot, hyperextension of the legs, extension and pronation of the arms, arching of the back, and extension and rotation of the neck (spasmodic torticollis). It's typically aggravated by walking and emotional stress and relieved by sleep. Dystonia may be intermittent — lasting just a few minutes — or continuous and painful. Occasionally, it causes permanent contractures, resulting in a grotesque posture. Although dystonia may be hereditary or idiopathic, it usually results from extrapyramidal disorders or drugs.

Enophthalmos

Enophthalmos is the backward displacement of the eye into the orbit. This sign usually results from trauma, but it may also be due to severe dehydration and eye disorders. In elderly people, senile atrophy of orbital fat may produce physiologic enophthalmos.

Because enophthalmos allows the upper lid to droop over the sunken eye, this sign is commonly mistaken for ptosis. However, exophthalmometry can differentiate these two signs.

Enuresis

Enuresis is nighttime urinary incontinence in girls age 5 and older and boys age 6 and older. This sign rarely continues into adulthood but may occur in some adults with sleep apnea. *Primary enuresis* describes a child who has never achieved bladder control; *secondary enuresis* describes a child who achieved bladder control for at least 3 months but has lost it.

Among factors that may contribute to enuresis are delayed development of detrusor muscle control, unusually deep or sound sleep, organic disorders (such as urinary tract infection or obstruction), and psychological stress. Psychological stress — probably the most important factor — commonly results from the birth of a sibling, the death of a parent or loved one, divorce, or premature, rigorous toilet training.

Erectile dysfunction

Erectile dysfunction is the inability to achieve and maintain penile erection sufficient to complete satisfactory sexual intercourse. Ejaculation may or may not be affected.

Erectile dysfunction can be classified as primary or secondary. A man with *primary erectile dysfunction* has never been potent with a sexual partner but may achieve normal erections in other situations. *Secondary erectile dysfunction* carries a more favorable prognosis because, despite his present erectile dysfunction, the patient has completed satisfactory intercourse in the past.

Organic causes of erectile dysfunction include vascular disease, diabetes mellitus, hypogonadism, a spinal cord lesion, alcohol and drug abuse, and surgical complications. Psychogenic causes range from performance anxiety and marital discord to moral or religious conflicts. Fatigue, poor health, age, and drugs can also disrupt normal sexual function.

Eructation

The characteristic sound that occurs when gas or acidic fluid rises from the stomach is called *eructation*. Occasionally, this sign results from a GI disorder. More commonly, however, eructation results from aerophagia — the unconscious swallowing of air — or from ingestion of gas-producing food. Eructation may relieve associated symptoms, most notably nausea, heartburn, dyspepsia, and bloating.

Fasciculations

Fasciculations are local muscle contractions. They represent the spontaneous discharge of a muscle fiber bundle innervated by a single motor nerve filament. These contractions cause visible dimpling or wavelike twitching of the skin, but they aren't strong enough to cause a joint to move. They occur irregularly at frequencies ranging from once every several seconds to two or three times per second; infrequently, myokymia — continuous, rapid fasciculations that cause a rippling effect — may occur.

Benign, nonpathologic fasciculations are common and normal. They commonly occur in tense, anxious, or overtired people and typically affect the eyelid, thumb, or calf. However, fasciculations may also indicate a severe neurologic disorder, most notably a diffuse motor neuron disorder that causes loss of control over muscle fiber discharge. They're also an early sign of pesticide poisoning.

Fecal incontinence

Fecal incontinence is the involuntary passage of feces. This sign follows the loss or impairment of external anal sphincter control. It can result from various GI, neurologic, and psychological disorders; the effects of drugs; or surgery. In some patients, it may even be a purposeful manipulative behavior. Although usually not a sign of severe illness, it can greatly affect the patient's physical and psychological well-being.

Fetor hepaticus

Fetor hepaticus, a distinctive musty, sweet breath odor characterizes hepatic encephalopathy, a life-threatening complication of severe liver disease.

Fontanel bulging

A bulging fontanel is widened, tense, and pulsating. Occurring in infants, it's a cardinal sign of meningitis associated with increased intracranial pressure — a medical emergency. It can also be an indication of encephalitis or fluid overload. Because prolonged coughing, crying, or lying down can cause transient, physiologic bulging, the infant's head should be observed and palpated while the infant is upright and relaxed to detect pathologic bulging.

Fontanel depression

Depression of the anterior fontanel below the surrounding bony ridges of the skull may be a sign of dehydration, possibly from insufficient fluid intake, but typically reflects excessive fluid loss from severe vomiting or diarrhea. Fontanel depression may also reflect insensible water loss, pyloric stenosis, or tracheoesophageal fistula. To detect fontanel depression, it's best to assess the fontanel when the infant is in an upright position and isn't crying.

Gag reflex abnormalities

The gag reflex, or pharyngeal reflex, is a protective mechanism that prevents aspiration of food, fluid, and vomitus. This sign is elicited by touching the posterior wall of the oropharynx with a tongue depressor or by suctioning the throat. Prompt elevation of the palate, constriction of the pharyngeal musculature, and a sensation of gagging indicate a normal gag reflex. An abnormal gag reflex — either decreased or absent — interferes with the ability to swallow and, more important, increases susceptibility to life-threatening aspiration.

An impaired gag reflex can result from any lesion that affects its mediators — cranial nerves IX (glossopharyngeal) and X (vagus) or the pons or medulla. It can also occur during a coma, in muscle diseases such as severe myasthenia gravis, or as a temporary result of anesthesia.

Gait, bizarre

A bizarre gait (also called a *hysterical gait*) has no consistent pattern and no obvious organic basis; rather, it's produced unconsciously by a person with a somatoform disorder (hysterical neurosis) or consciously by a malingerer. It may mimic an organic impairment but characteristically has a more theatrical or bizarre quality with key elements missing, such as a spastic gait without hip circumduction, or leg "paralysis" with normal reflexes and motor strength. Its manifestations may include wild gyrations, exaggerated stepping, leg dragging, or mimicking unusual walks, such as that of a tightrope walker.

Gait, propulsive

A gait characterized by a stooped, rigid posture is called a *propulsive* or *festinating gait*. The patient's head and neck are bent forward; his flexed, stiffened arms are held away from the body; his fingers are extended; and his knees and hips are stiffly bent. During ambulation, this posture results in a forward shifting of the body's center of gravity and consequent impairment of balance, causing increasingly rapid, short, shuffling steps with involuntary acceleration (festination) and lack of control over forward motion (propulsion) or backward motion (retropul-

sion). Propulsive gait is a cardinal sign of advanced Parkinson's disease.

Gait, scissors

A stiff, short gait in which the thighs overlap with each step is classified as a scissors gait. Resulting from bilateral spastic paresis (diplegia), the patient's legs flex slightly at the hips and knees, so he looks as if he's crouching. With each step, his thighs adduct and his knees hit or cross in a scissorslike movement. His steps are short, regular, and laborious, as if he were wading through waist-deep water. His feet may be plantarflexed and turned inward, with a shortened Achilles tendon; as a result, he walks on his toes or on the balls of his feet and may scrape his toes on the ground.

Gait, spastic

Spastic gait — sometimes referred to as *paretic, hemiplegic,* or *weak gait* — is a stiff, foot-dragging walk that's caused by unilateral leg muscle hypertonicity. This gait indicates focal damage to the corticospinal tract. The affected leg becomes rigid, with a marked decrease in flexion at the hip and knee and possibly plantar flexion and equinovarus deformity of the foot. Because the patient's leg doesn't swing normally at the hip or knee, his foot tends to drag or shuffle, scraping his toes on the ground. To compensate, the pelvis of the affected side tilts upward in an attempt to lift the toes, causing the patient's leg to abduct and circumduct. Also, arm swing is hindered on the same side as the affected leg. Spastic gait usually develops after a period of flaccidity (hypotonicity) in the affected leg.

Gait, steppage

Steppage gait is a gait in which the foot hangs with the toes pointing down. Other names for this gait include equine, paretic, prancing, or weak. Steppage gait typically results from footdrop caused by weakness or paralysis of pretibial and peroneal muscles, usually from lower motor neuron lesions. Footdrop causes the toes to scrape the ground during ambulation. To compensate, the hip rotates outward and the hip and knee flex in an exaggerated fashion to lift the advancing leg off the ground. The foot is thrown forward and the toes hit the ground first, producing an audible slap. The rhythm of the gait is usually regular, with even steps and normal upper body posture and arm swing.

Gait, waddling

Waddling gait (a ducklike walk) is an important sign of muscular dystrophy, spinal muscle atrophy or, rarely, congenital hip displacement. The gait results from deterioration of the pelvic girdle muscles — primarily the gluteus medius, hip flexors, and hip extensors. Weakness in these muscles hinders stabilization of the weight-bearing hip during walking, causing the opposite hip to drop and the trunk to lean toward that side in an attempt to maintain balance.

Typically, the legs assume a wide stance and the trunk is thrown back to further improve stability, exaggerating lordosis and abdominal protrusion. In severe cases, leg and foot muscle contractures may cause equinovarus deformity of the foot combined with circumduction or bowing of the legs.

Gum swelling

Gum swelling involves an increase in the size of existing gum cells (hypertrophy) or an increase in their number (hyperplasia). This common sign may involve one or many papillae — the triangular bits of gum between adjacent teeth.

Gum swelling usually results from the effects of phenytoin; less commonly, from nutritional deficiency and certain systemic disorders. Physiologic gum swelling and bleeding may occur during the first and second trimesters of pregnancy when hormonal changes make the gums highly vascular; even slight irritation causes swelling and gives the papillae a characteristic raspberry hue (pregnancy epulis). Irritating dentures may also cause swelling associated with red, soft, movable masses on the gums.

Heat intolerance

Heat intolerance is the inability to withstand high temperatures or to maintain a comfortable body temperature. This symptom produces a continuous feeling of being overheated and, at times, profuse diaphoresis. Most cases of heat intolerance result from thyrotoxicosis. Although rare, hypothalamic disease may also cause intolerance to heat and cold.

Heberden's nodes

Heberden's nodes, painless, irregular, cartilaginous or bony enlargements of the distal interphalangeal joints of the finger, reflect degeneration of articular cartilage. This degeneration irritates the bone and stimulates osteoblasts, causing bony enlargement. Approximately 2 to 3 mm in diameter, Heberden's nodes develop on one or both sides of the dorsal midline. The dominant hand usually has larger nodes, which affect one or more fingers but not the thumb. Osteoarthritis is the most common cause of Heberden's nodes. Less commonly, repeated fingertip trauma may lead to node formation in only one joint ("baseball finger").

Hiccups

Also called a *singultus,* a hiccup is an involuntary, spasmodic contraction of the diaphragm followed by sudden closure of the glottis. The characteristic sound of hiccups reflects the vibration of closed vocal cords as air suddenly rushes into the lungs.

Although hiccups are usually benign and transient, in a patient with a neurologic disorder they may indicate increasing intracranial pressure or extension of a brain stem lesion. They may also occur after ingestion of hot or cold liquids or other irritants, after exposure to cold, or with irritation from a drainage tube. Persistent hiccups cause considerable distress and may lead to vomiting. Increased serum levels of carbon dioxide may inhibit hiccups; decreased levels may accentuate them.

Hyperpigmentation

Hyperpigmentation (also called *hypermelanosis*) is excessive skin coloring. It usually reflects overproduction, abnormal location, or maldistribution of the pigment melanin. This sign can also reflect abnormalities of other skin pigments: carotenoids (yellow), oxyhemoglobin (red), and hemoglobin (blue).

Hyperpigmentation most commonly results from exposure to sunlight. However, it can also result from metabolic, endocrine, neoplastic, and inflammatory disorders; chemical poisoning; drugs; genetic defects; thermal burns; ionizing radiation; and localized activation by sunlight of certain photosensitizing chemicals on the skin.

Many types of benign hyperpigmented lesions occur normally. Some, such as acanthosis nigricans and carotenemia, may also accompany certain disorders. Chronic nutritional insufficiency may lead to dyspigmentation — increased pigmentation in some areas and decreased pigmentation in others.

Hypopigmentation

Hypopigmentation (also called *hypomelanosis*) is a decrease in normal skin, hair, mucous membrane, or nail color. This sign results from deficiency, absence, or abnormal degradation of the pigment melanin. Its causes include genetic disorders, nutritional deficiency, chemicals and drugs, inflammation, infection, and physical trauma.

Janeway lesions

Janeway lesions are small erythematous lesions on the palms and soles that disappear spontaneously. These lesions are slightly raised but usually flat, irregular, and nontender. They blanch with pressure or elevation of the affected extremity; occasionally, they form a diffuse rash over the trunk and extremities.

Janeway lesions were once a common finding in those with infective endocarditis, possibly reflecting an immunologic reaction to the infecting organisms (usually bacteria). These lesions are rarely seen today because the disease is now detected and managed at an earlier stage.

Kehr's sign

Kehr's sign, referred left shoulder pain due to diaphragmatic irritation by intraperitoneal blood, is a cardinal sign of hemorrhage within the peritoneal cavity. It usually arises when the patient assumes the supine position or lowers his head. Such positioning increases the contact of free blood or clots with the left diaphragm, involving the phrenic nerve. A classic symptom of a ruptured spleen, Kehr's sign also occurs in ruptured ectopic pregnancy.

Lid lag

Also called *Graefe's sign,* lid lag—the inability of the upper eyelid to follow the eye's downward movements—is a cardinal sign of thyrotoxicosis. Testing for lid lag involves holding a finger, penlight, or other target above the patient's eye level and then moving it downward and observing eyelid movement as his eyes follow the target. This sign is demonstrated when a rim of sclera appears between the upper lid margin and the iris when the patient lowers his eyes, when one lid closes more slowly than the other, or when both lids close slowly and incompletely with jerky movements.

Low birth weight

Neonates born weighing less than the normal minimum birth weight of 5½ lb (2,500 g) are classified as having a low birth weight. The premature neonate (born before the 37th week of gestation) weighs an appropriate amount for his gestational age and probably would have matured normally if carried to term. Conversely, the small-for-gestational age (SGA) neonate weighs less than the normal amount for his age; however, his organs are mature.

In the premature neonate, low birth weight usually results from a disorder that prevents the uterus from retaining the fetus, interferes with the normal course of pregnancy, causes premature separation of the placenta, or stimulates uterine contractions before term. In the SGA neonate, intrauterine growth may be retarded by a disorder that interferes with placental circulation, fetal development, or maternal health.

Regardless of the cause, low birth weight is associated with higher neonate morbidity and mortality. Low birth weight can also signal a life-threatening emergency.

Masklike facies

A total loss of facial expression, masklike facies results from bradykinesia usually due to extrapyramidal damage. The rate of eye blinking is reduced to 1 to 4 blinks per minute, producing a characteristic "reptilian" stare. Although a neurologic disorder is the most common cause, masklike facies can also result from certain systemic diseases and the effects of drugs and toxins. The sign often develops insidiously, at first mistaken by the observer for depression or apathy.

McBurney's sign

Characterized by tenderness elicited when the right lower abdominal quadrant over McBurney's point is palpated, McBurney's sign is a telltale indicator of localized peritoneal inflammation in acute appendicitis. Before McBurney's sign is elicited, the abdomen is inspected for distention, auscultated for hypoactive or absent bowel sounds, and tested for tympany.

McMurray's sign

A palpable, audible click or pop elicited by rotating the tibia on the femur, McMurray's sign is commonly an indicator of medial meniscal injury. It results when gentle manipulation of the leg traps torn cartilage and then lets it snap free. Because eliciting this sign forces the surface of the tibial plateau against the femoral condyles, such manipulation is contraindicated in patients with suspected fractures of the tibial plateau or femoral condyles and should only be performed by a person trained to elicit McMurray's sign.

A positive McMurray's sign augments other findings commonly associated with meniscal injury, such as severe joint line tenderness, locking or clicking of the joint, and decreased range of motion.

Menorrhagia

Menorrhagia is abnormally heavy or long menstrual bleeding. A form of dysfunctional uterine bleeding, menorrhagia can result from endocrine and hematologic disorders, stress, and certain drugs and procedures.

Metrorrhagia

Uterine bleeding that occurs irregularly between menstrual periods is called *metrorrhagia.* It's usually light bleeding, although it can range from staining to hemorrhage. Usually, metrorrhagia reflects slight physiologic bleeding from the endometrium during ovulation. However, metrorrhagia may be the only indication of an underlying gynecologic disorder. It can also result from stress, drugs, treatments, and intrauterine devices.

Miosis

Miosis (pupillary constriction) occurs normally as a response to fatigue, increased light, or administration of a miotic; as part of the eye's accommodation reflex; and as part of the aging process. However, it can also stem from an ocular or neurologic disorder, trauma, use of a systemic drug, or contact lens overuse. A rare form of miosis — Argyll Robertson pupils — can stem from tabes dorsalis and diverse neurologic disorders. Occurring bilaterally, these miotic (often pinpoint), unequal, and irregularly shaped pupils don't dilate properly with mydriatic use and fail to react to light, although they do constrict on accommodation.

Moon face

Moon face, a distinctive facial adiposity, usually indicates hypercortisolism resulting from ectopic or excessive pituitary production of corticotropin, adrenal adenoma or carcinoma, or long-term glucocorticoid therapy. Its typical characteristics include marked facial roundness and puffiness, a double chin, a prominent upper lip, and full supraclavicular fossae.

Muscle atrophy

Muscle atrophy, or wasting, is the loss of muscle size and contour. It results from denervation or prolonged muscle disuse. When deprived of regular exercise, muscle fibers lose bulk and length, producing a visible loss of muscle and apparent emaciation or deformity in the affected area. Even slight atrophy usually causes some loss of motion or power.

Atrophy usually results from neuromuscular disease or injury. However, it may also stem from certain metabolic and endocrine disorders and prolonged immobility. Some muscle atrophy also occurs with aging.

Muscle flaccidity

Flaccid, or hypotonic, muscles are profoundly weak and soft and have decreased resistance to movement, increased mobility, and greater than normal range of motion. The result of disrupted muscle innervation, flaccidity can be localized to a limb or muscle group or generalized over the entire body. Its onset may be acute, as in trauma, or chronic, as in neurologic disease.

Nasal flaring

Nasal flaring is the abnormal dilation of the nostrils. Usually occurring during inspiration, nasal flaring may occasionally occur during expiration or throughout the respiratory cycle. It indicates respiratory dysfunction, ranging from mild difficulty to potentially life-threatening respiratory distress.

Paroxysmal nocturnal dyspnea

An attack of dyspnea that abruptly awakens the patient is called *paroxysmal nocturnal dyspnea*. Common findings include diaphoresis, coughing, wheezing, and chest discomfort. The attack abates after the patient sits up or stands for several minutes, but may recur every 2 to 3 hours.

Paroxysmal nocturnal dyspnea is a sign of left-sided heart failure. It may result from decreased respiratory drive, impaired left ventricular function, enhanced reabsorption of interstitial fluid, or increased thoracic blood volume.

Pica

Pica is the craving and ingestion of normally inedible substances, such as plaster, charcoal, clay, wool, ashes, paint, or dirt. In children, the most commonly affected group, pica typically results from nutritional deficiencies. It's commonly seen in pregnant patients and may be associated with iron deficiency anemia. However, in adults, pica may reflect a psychological disturbance. Depending on the substance eaten, pica can lead to poisoning and GI disorders.

Postnasal drip

Nasal discharge, frequent throat clearing, and mucoid or mucopurulent secretions in the posterior pharynx suggest postnasal drip. This symptom typically results from infection or allergies — a thick, tenacious, and purulent discharge suggests infection, whereas a watery discharge usually suggests an allergy. Postnasal drip may also result from environmental irritants.

Priapism

A urologic emergency, priapism is characterized by a persistent, painful erection that's unrelated to sexual excitation. This relatively rare sign may begin during sleep and appear to be a normal erection, but it may last for several hours or days. It's usually accompanied by a severe, constant, dull aching in the penis. Despite the pain, the patient may be too embarrassed to seek medical help. He may try to achieve detumescence through continued sexual activity.

Without prompt treatment, penile ischemia and thrombosis occur. In about half of all cases, priapism is idiopathic and develops without apparent predisposing factors. Secondary priapism can result from a blood disorder, neoplasm, trauma, or use of certain drugs.

Psoas sign

Psoas sign is evident if the patient experiences increased abdominal pain when he moves his leg against resistance. A positive psoas sign indicates direct or reflexive irritation of the psoas muscles. This sign, which can be elicited on the right or left side, usually indicates appendicitis but may also occur with localized abscesses. It's elicited in a patient with abdominal or lower back pain *after* completion of an abdominal examination to prevent spurious assessment findings.

Pulsus alternans

Pulsus alternans (alternating pulse) is a beat-to-beat change in the size and intensity of a peripheral pulse. It's a sign of severe left-sided heart failure. Although pulse rhythm remains regular, strong and weak contractions alternate. An alternation in the intensity of heart sounds and of existing heart murmurs may accompany this sign.

Although most easily detected by sphygmomanometry, pulsus alternans can be detected by palpating the bra-chial, radial, or femoral artery when systolic pressure varies from beat to beat by more than 20 mm Hg. Because the small changes in arterial pressure that occur during normal respirations may obscure this abnormal pulse, you'll need to have the patient hold his breath during palpation. Apply *light* pressure to avoid obliterating the weaker pulse.

Purple striae

Purple striae — thin, purple streaks on the skin — characteristically occur in hypercortisolism along with other cushingoid signs, such as a buffalo hump and moon face. Although hypercortisolism can be caused by adrenocortical carcinoma, adrenal adenoma, and pituitary adenoma, it usually results from excessive use of glucocorticoids. Although purple striae are most common over the abdominal area, they may also occur over the breasts, hips, buttocks, thighs, and axillae.

Raccoon eyes

Raccoon eyes are bilateral periorbital ecchymoses that don't result from facial soft-tissue trauma. Usually an indicator of basilar skull fracture, this sign develops when damage at the time of fracture tears the meninges and causes the venous sinuses to bleed into the arachnoid villi and the cranial sinuses. Raccoon eyes may be the only indicator of a basilar skull fracture, which isn't always visible on skull X-rays. Their appearance signals the need for careful assessment to detect any underlying trauma because a basilar skull fracture can injure cranial nerves, blood vessels, and the brain stem. Raccoon eyes can also occur after a craniotomy if the surgery causes a meningeal tear.

Rebound tenderness

Rebound tenderness (also known as *Blumberg's sign*) is characterized by intense, elicited abdominal pain caused by rebound of palpated tissue. This sign is a reliable indicator of peritonitis. The tenderness may be localized, as in an abscess, or generalized, as in perforation of an intra-abdominal organ. Rebound tenderness usually occurs with abdominal pain, tenderness, and rigidity. When a patient has sudden, severe abdominal pain, this symptom is usually elicited to detect peritoneal inflammation.

Rhinorrhea

Rhinorrhea is the free discharge of thin nasal mucus. Common but rarely serious, rhinorrhea can be self-limiting or chronic, resulting from a nasal, sinus, or systemic disorder or from a basilar skull fracture. Rhinorrhea can also result from sinus or cranial surgery, excessive use of vasoconstricting nose drops or sprays, or inhalation of an irritant, such as tobacco smoke, dust, and fumes. Depending on the cause, the discharge may be clear, purulent, bloody, or serosanguineous.

Salt craving

A salt craving is a compensatory response to the body's failure to adequately conserve sodium. Causes include adrenal insufficiency (primary) and adrenal crisis, a potentially fatal condition.

Seizures, absence

Absence seizures are benign, generalized seizures thought to originate subcortically. These brief episodes of unconsciousness usually last 3 to 20 seconds and can occur 100 or more times a day. Absence seizures usually begin between ages 4 and 12. Their first sign may be deteriorating school work and behavior. The cause of these seizures is unknown.

Absence seizures occur without warning. The patient suddenly stops all purposeful activity and stares blankly ahead, as if he were daydreaming. They may produce automatisms, such as repetitive lip smacking, or mild clonic or myoclonic movements, including mild jerking of the eyelids. The patient may drop an object that he's holding, and muscle relaxation may cause him to drop his head or arms or to slump. After the attack, the patient resumes activity, typically unaware of the episode.

Setting-sun sign

Setting-sun sign (also known as *sunset eyes*) in an infant or young child is a late and ominous sign of increased intracranial pressure on cranial nerves III, IV, and VI. Both eyes are rotated downward, typically revealing an area of sclera above the irises; occasionally, the irises appear to be forced outward. Pupils are sluggish, responding to light unequally.

Skin turgor, decreased

Pinched skin that "holds" for up to 30 seconds, then slowly returns to its normal contour is considered to have decreased turgor. Skin turgor is commonly assessed over the hand, arm or sternum, areas normally free from wrinkles and wide variations in tissue thickness, by picking up a fold of skin and releasing it.

Decreased skin turgor results from dehydration or volume depletion, which moves interstitial fluid into the vascular bed to maintain circulating blood volume, leading to slackness in the skin's dermal layer. It's a normal finding in elderly patients and in people who have lost weight rapidly; it also occurs with disorders affecting the GI, renal, endocrine, and other systems.

Spider angioma

Also known as an *arterial spider,* a *spider nevus,* a *spider telangiectasia,* a *stellate angioma,* or a *vascular spider,* a spider angioma is a fiery red vascular lesion with an elevated central body, branching spiderlike legs, and a surrounding flush. A form of telangiectasia, this characteristic lesion ranges from a few millimeters to several centimeters in diameter and may occur singly or in multiples. Spider angiomas usually appear on the face and neck; less commonly, they occur on the shoulders, thorax, arms, backs of the hands and fingers, and mucous membranes of the lips and nose.

Spider angiomas are typically associated with cirrhosis but can also be found in hyperestrogenic states such as pregnancy or in those taking hormonal contraceptives. They may erupt in the second or third month of pregnancy, enlarge and multiply, then disappear about 6 weeks after delivery. These lesions may also appear in elderly patients.

Tics

A tic is an involuntary, repetitive movement of a specific group of muscles — usually those of the face, neck, shoulders, trunk, and hands. This sign typically occurs suddenly and intermittently. It may involve a single isolated movement, such as lip smacking, grimacing, blinking, sniffing, tongue thrusting, throat clearing, hitching up one shoulder, or protruding the chin or it may involve a complex set of movements. Mild tics, such as twitching of an eyelid, are especially common.

Tics are usually psychogenic and may be aggravated by stress or anxiety. Psychogenic tics commonly begin between ages 5 and 10 as voluntary, coordinated, and purposeful actions that the child feels compelled to perform to decrease anxiety. However, tics are also associated with Tourette syndrome, which typically begins during childhood.

Tracheal tugging

Tracheal tugging (also known as *Cardarelli's sign, Castellino's sign,* or *Oliver's sign*) is a visible recession of the larynx and trachea that occurs in synchrony with cardiac systole. Tracheal tugging commonly results from an aneurysm or a tumor near the aortic arch. It may signal dangerous compression or obstruction of major airways. The tugging movement, best observed with the patient's neck hyperextended, reflects abnormal transmission of aortic pulsations because of compression and distortion of the heart, esophagus, great vessels, airways, and nerves.

Trismus

Commonly known as *lockjaw,* trismus is the prolonged and painful tonic spasm of the masticatory jaw muscles. It's a characteristic early sign of tetanus produced by the neuromuscular effects of tetanospasmin, a potentially lethal exotoxin. It can also result from drug therapy; occasionally, a milder form may accompany neuromuscular involvement in other disorders or infection or disease of the jaw, teeth, parotid glands, or tonsils.

Uremic frost

Uremic frost is a fine white powder, believed to be urate crystals, that covers the skin. It's a characteristic sign of end-stage renal failure or uremia. The frost typically appears on the face, neck, axillae, groin, and genitalia.

Urine cloudiness

Cloudy, murky, or turbid urine reflecting the presence of bacteria, mucus, leukocytes or erythrocytes, epithelial cells, fat, or phosphates (in alkaline urine) is characteristic of urinary tract infection but can also result from prolonged storage of a urine specimen at room temperature.

Violent behavior

Violent behavior is defined as the use of physical force to violate, injure, or abuse an object or person. Marked by the sudden loss of self-control, this behavior may also be self-directed. It may result from an organic or psychiatric disorder or from the use of certain drugs.

Wristdrop

Wristdrop is the flexed position of the hand due to paresis of the extensor muscles of the hand, wrist, and fingers. This weakness may be slight or severe and temporary or permanent. Wristdrop may occur unilaterally and suddenly with a radial nerve injury or bilaterally and gradually with a neurologic disorder, such as myasthenia gravis, Guillain-Barré syndrome, or multiple sclerosis.

Selected references

Andrews, M., and Boyle, J. *Transcultural Concepts in Nursing Care,* 4th ed. Philadelphia: Lippincott Williams & Wilkins, 2003.

Berry, B., and Pinard, A. "Assessing Tissue Oxygenation," *Critical Care Nurse* 22(3):22-40, June 2002.

Better ElderCare: A Nurse's Guide to Caring for Older Adults. Springhouse, Pa.: Springhouse Corp., 2002.

Bickley, L.S., and Szilagyi, P.G. *Bates' Guide to Physical Examination and History Taking,* 8th ed. Philadelphia: Lippincott Williams & Wilkins, 2003.

Braunwald, E., et al., eds. *Harrison's Principles of Internal Medicine,* 15th ed. New York: McGraw-Hill Book Co., 2001.

Copel, L. *Nurse's Clinical Guide: Psychiatric and Mental Health Care,* 2nd ed. Springhouse, Pa.: Springhouse Corp., 2000.

Craven R., and Hirnle, C. *Fundamentals of Nursing Human Health and Function,* 4th ed. Philadelphia: Lippincott Williams & Wilkins, 2003.

Eliopoulos, C. *Gerontological Nursing,* 5th ed. Philadelphia: Lippincott Williams & Wilkins, 2001.

Fetrow, C.W., and Avila, J.R. *Professional's Handbook of Complementary and Alternative Medicines,* 3rd ed. Springhouse, Pa.: Lippincott Williams & Wilkins, 2004.

Green-Hernandez, C., et al. *Primary Care Pediatrics.* Philadelphia: Lippincott Williams & Wilkins, 2001.

Hickey, J. *The Clinical Practice of Neurological and Neurosurgical Nursing,* 5th ed. Philadelphia: Lippincott Williams & Wilkins, 2003.

Kemp, C. "Bioterrorism: Introduction and Major Agents," *Journal of the American Academy of Nurse Practitioners* 13(11):483-91, November 2001.

Kozier, B., et al. *Fundamentals of Nursing Concepts, Process, and Practice,* 7th ed. Upper Saddle River, N.J.: Prentice Hall Health, 2004.

Mastering ACLS. Springhouse, Pa.: Springhouse Corp., 2002.

Netlina, S.M. *The Lippincott Manual of Nursing Practice,* 7th ed. Philadelphia: Lippincott Williams & Wilkins, 2001.

Pillitteri, A. *Maternal and Child Health Nursing,* 4th ed. Philadelphia: Lippincott Williams & Wilkins, 2003.

Procedures for Nurse Practitioners. Springhouse, Pa.: Springhouse Corp., 2001.

Professional Guide to Pathophysiology. Philadelphia: Lippincott Williams & Wilkins, 2003.

Shives, L., and Isaacs, A. *Basic Concepts of Psychiatric-Mental Health Nursing,* 5th ed. Philadelphia: Lippincott Williams & Wilkins, 2002.

Simpson, K., and Creehan, P. *AWHONN's Perinatal Nursing,* 2nd ed. Philadelphia: Lippincott Williams & Wilkins, 2001.

SkillMasters: Expert ECG Interpretation. Springhouse, Pa.: Lippincott Williams & Wilkins, 2003.

Temte, S.L., et al. "Bioterrorism: A Primary Care Perspective" [Online]. Available: *www.patientcareonline.com* [2003, October 6].

Index

i refers to an illustration; t refers to a table.

i refers to an illustration; t refers to a table.

i refers to an illustration; t refers to a table.

i refers to an illustration; t refers to a table.

i refers to an illustration; t refers to a table.

i refers to an illustration; t refers to a table.

i refers to an illustration; t refers to a table.

i refers to an illustration; t refers to a table.

i refers to an illustration; t refers to a table.

i refers to an illustration; t refers to a table.

i refers to an illustration; t refers to a table.

i refers to an illustration; t refers to a table.

i refers to an illustration; t refers to a table.

i refers to an illustration; t refers to a table.